Public Health Science and Nursing Practice

Public Health Science and Nursing Practice

Caring for Populations

Christine L. Savage, PhD, RN, CARN, FAAN
*Professor and Chair, Department of Community
    Public Health*
Johns Hopkins University School of Nursing
    & Public Health
Baltimore, MD

Joan E. Kub, PhD, MA, PHCNS-BC, FAAN
*Coordinator of MSN/MPH and MSN in PHN tracks
Associate Professor*
Johns Hopkins University School of Nursing,
    Public Health, & Medicine
Baltimore, MD

Sara L. Groves, DrPH, MSN, PHCNS-BC
Assistant Professor
Johns Hopkins University School of Nursing
Baltimore, MD

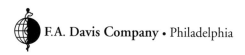 F.A. Davis Company • Philadelphia

F. A. Davis Company
1915 Arch Street
Philadelphia, PA 19103
www.fadavis.com

Printed in the United States of America

Last digit indicates print number: 10 9 8 7 6 5 4 3 2 1

Publisher, Nursing: Terri Wood Allen
Content Project Manager: Echo K. Gerhart
Electronic Project Manager: Kate Crowley
Design and Illustration Manager: Carolyn O'Brien

As new scientific information becomes available through basic and clinical research, recommended treatments and drug therapies undergo changes. The author(s) and publisher have done everything possible to make this book accurate, up to date, and in accord with accepted standards at the time of publication. The author(s), editors, and publisher are not responsible for errors or omissions or for consequences from application of the book, and make no warranty, expressed or implied, in regard to the contents of the book. Any practice described in this book should be applied by the reader in accordance with professional standards of care used in regard to the unique circumstances that may apply in each situation. The reader is advised always to check product information (package inserts) for changes and new information regarding dose and contraindications before administering any drug. Caution is especially urged when using new or infrequently ordered drugs.

Library of Congress Cataloging-in-Publication Data

Savage, Christine L., author.
 Public health science and nursing practice : caring for populations / Christine L. Savage, Joan E. Kub, Sara L. Groves.
  p. ; cm.
 Includes bibliographical references and index.
 ISBN 978-0-8036-2199-2 (alk. paper)
 I. Kub, Joan E., author. II. Groves, Sara L., author. III. Title.
 [DNLM: 1. Public Health Nursing. 2. Community Health Nursing. 3. Health Planning. 4. Population Characteristics. WY 108]

RT97
610.73'4—dc23

2014031458

Public health and nursing go hand in hand. In the *2010 Future of Nursing* report by the Institute of Medicine, the rationale for setting a goal that 80% of all nurses would hold a bachelor of science degree in nursing included the importance of demonstrated competencies in public health as key to the practice of nursing. As nurses, we apply public health science on a daily basis as we strive to prevent disease; reduce mortality and morbidity in those who are ill; and contribute to the health of the communities we serve. Our goal is to lead you on the journey of discovering how the public health sciences are an integral part of nursing practice and how nurses implement effective public health interventions.

About this Book

This book presents public health in a way that captures the adventure of tackling health from a community- and population-based perspective. Public health helps us to answer the question "Why is this happening?" and implement interventions that improve the health of populations. Public health issues are usually messy, real-world problems that do not always have obvious solutions. You will learn through the examples provided how to gather the needed information to understand important health issues, especially those included in *Healthy People 2020*. You will have an opportunity to explore population-level, evidence-based interventions and learn how to evaluate the effectiveness of the interventions. We aim to provide you with the knowledge needed to achieve the competencies in public health increasingly needed by professional nurses across multiple settings. You will be provided with numerous examples of how public health nurses integrate nursing and public health, with a focus on promoting the health of populations.

The application of public health knowledge in the provision of care and the prevention of disease is not new to the nursing profession. Florence Nightingale is often viewed as the first nurse epidemiologist because of her work in the Crimean War. She applied public health science to nursing practice in a way that saved lives and improved outcomes both in the context of war and back

in England with the development of professional nursing in hospital and home settings. As nurses practicing in the 21st century, we follow in her footsteps. Consider nurses working in primary care with mothers and children or those working in low-income countries facing epidemics of tuberculosis and HIV/AIDS. How does knowledge of public health science enhance our ability to address these complex health issues? Before we can improve health outcomes, we must understand the natural history of disease, the social context in which these health issues arise, and the resources critical to addressing all of the barriers to care. Knowledge of public health and how it applies to nursing practice has taken on increased importance as we move from a fee-for-service model of care to a health-care system that rewards prevention of disease.

Nurses providing direct clinical care must have knowledge of pharmacology, pathophysiology, and physical health assessment. Because nurses also provide care to communities and populations, they must also know how to apply the basics of the public health sciences such as epidemiology, social and behavioral sciences, and environmental health. They must also meet the Quad Council generalist core competencies such as community assessment, health planning, and health policy. To help you to do that, we have employed a problem-based learning approach to the presentation of the material in this book so that you can apply the principles of public health to real-life nursing settings.

Throughout the book, case studies demonstrate how the application of the public health sciences and public health practice to nursing practice is essential to the promotion of health and the prevention of disease. At times, the focus will be on solving health-related mysteries and how that leads to the implementation of interventions to address the health problems at the population level. At other times, the focus will be the application of the public health sciences to the development and implementation of evidence-based, population-level interventions aimed at addressing the health issue.

Although there have been significant improvements in health during the past 100 years, achieving our stated health goals, whether it be *Healthy People* goals and objectives or the global goals, continues to be a challenge. The ability for each individual, family, and community to lead a healthy and productive life involves an interaction between ourselves, our environment, and the communities in which we live. Understanding the multiple determinants of health, including social determinants that significantly influence health disparities and health inequities, is an essential skill for nurses. The public health sciences help us understand the complexity of the interaction of external and internal forces that shape our health. The premise of this book is that all nurses require adequate knowledge of the public health sciences and how to apply it to nursing practice across all settings and populations. With this knowledge, we can truly contribute to the building of a healthy world.

Organization of the Text

The philosophical approach to this text is that all professional nurses incorporate population-level interventions no matter what the setting. We include not only chapters on the traditional public health settings such as the public health department and school health, but also chapters on acute and primary care settings. The book uses a constructivist learning approach by which the learner constructs her or his own knowledge. Thus, the content is delivered by applying the information within the context of the real world.

This text uses a problem-based learning approach so that the student can apply the content to nursing practice. It is organized into four units. Unit I, Basis for Public Health Nursing Knowledge and Skills, covers the essential knowledge based in the public health sciences and core public health nursing competencies needed to solve health problems and implement evidenced-based interventions at the population level. This unit provides the basic public health knowledge needed by all generalist nurses. The content covered in these chapters is applied across the next three units of the book. Unit II, Community Health Across Populations: Public Health Issues, covers health issues that span populations and settings including communicable and noncommunicable disease, health disparity, behavioral health, and global health. Unit III, Public Health Planning, covers the settings in which nurses practice. Finally, Unit IV, Public Health Nursing—Special Populations, covers public health policy, culture, vulnerability, and disaster management.

Key Features

▲ CASE STUDIES

Throughout the book, the student will find case studies embedded in the chapters that provide essential content within the context of actual nursing practice. This approach begins with the issue and walks the reader through the process of deciding how best to address the problem presented. In some of the cases presented, the object is to solve the mystery (**Solving the Mystery**), such as the case in Chapter 8 that walks through solving the mystery of why people are presenting at the emergency department with severe gastrointestinal symptoms. Other cases (**Applying Public Health Science**) describe how nurses apply the public health sciences such as epidemiology to help develop and implement evidence-based interventions at the population level. There is a standard case study at the end of selected chapters. For instructors, there is online access on the Davis*Plus* website for the book to a problem-based learning exercise that can be used to further apply the content presented in the chapter.

■ HEALTHY PEOPLE 2020

Healthy People 2020 is referenced throughout, and boxes are presented that demonstrate how nursing can contribute to meeting *Healthy People 2020* objectives.

■ EVIDENCE-BASED PRACTICE BOXES

Evidence-Based Practice (EBP) boxes illustrate how research and its resulting evidence can support and inform public health nursing practice. Cutting-edge EBP is a strong underpinning of the book as a whole.

LEARNING OUTCOMES AND KEY TERMS

Each chapter begins with Learning Outcomes and a list of Key Terms that appear in boldface and color at first mention in a chapter.

Teaching/Learning Package

Instructor Resources

Instructor Resources on Davis*Plus* include the following:

- NCLEX-Style Test Bank
- PowerPoint Presentations

- Instructor's Guide
- QSEN Crosswalk
- Quad Council Competencies
- Faculty Guide to Problem-Based Learning
- Problem-Based Learning PowerPoint Presentation

Student Resources

Student Resources on Davis*Plus* include the following:

- QSEN Crosswalk
- Quad Council Competencies

- Student Guide to Problem-Based Learning
- Student NCLEX-Style Test Bank
- List of Web Resources

We hope you will enjoy this book and, most of all, we hope as nurses you will always care for the health of populations no matter the setting, thus increasing the contribution of nursing to the goal of optimal health for all.

Contributors

Jacqueline Agnew, MPH, PhD, RN, FAAN
*Professor, Department of Environmental Health
  Sciences*
The Johns Hopkins Bloomberg School of Public Health
Baltimore, Maryland
Chapter 6

Kathleen Ballman, DNP, ACNP-BC, CEN, EMT-P
*Associate Professor of Clinical Nursing, Coordinator,
  Adult-Gerontology Acute Care Nurse Practitioner
  Program*
University of Cincinnati, College of Nursing
Cincinnati, Ohio
Chapter 15

Derryl E. Block, PhD, MPH, MSN, RN
Dean, College of Health and Human Sciences
Northern Illinois University
DeKalb, Illinois
Chapter 22

Jenny Bradley, MSN, RN
Nurse Manager, Emergency Department
MultiCare Auburn Medical Center
Auburn, Washington
Chapter 25

Susan Bulecza, DNP, RN, PHCNS-BC
State Public Health Nursing Director
Florida Department of Health
Tallahassee, Florida
Chapter 14

Maureen Farrell Cadorette, PhD, RN, BSN, MPH,
  COHN-S
Assistant Scientist
Johns Hopkins Bloomberg School of Public Health
Baltimore, Maryland
Chapter 6

Julie Anne Cook, RN, MSN/MPH, APHN-BC
Occupational Health Specialist
Suburban Hospital Johns Hopkins Medicine
Bethesda, Maryland
Chapter 10

Christine Colella, DNP, CS, CNP
*Associate Professor of Clinical Nursing, Director, NP
  programs*
University of Cincinnati, College of Nursing
Cincinnati, Ohio
Chapter 16

Mary K. Donnelly, DNP, MPH, CRNP
Instructor
Johns Hopkins University School of Nursing
Baltimore, Maryland
Chapter 19

Elaine R. Feeney, PhD, RN
Adjunct Faculty
Towson University
Baltimore, Maryland
Chapter 11

Sheila T. Fitzgerald, PhD, ANP, MSN, BS
*Associate Professor, Director, Occupational
  and Environmental Health Nursing Program*
Johns Hopkins Bloomberg School of Public Health
Baltimore, Maryland
Chapter 21

Gordon Gillespie, PhD, RN, PHCNS-BC, CEN,
  CPEN, FAEN
*Associate Professor & Robert Wood Johnson Foundation
  Nurse Faculty Scholar*
University of Cincinnati
Cincinnati, Ohio
Chapters 21 & 25

Emily Johnson, MSN, RN, CPNP-PC
Part-time Clinical Faculty, Pediatric Nurse Practitioner
Johns Hopkins University School of Nursing
Baltimore, Maryland
Chapter 19

Elizabeth S. Kasameyer, RN, BSN, MSN/MPH, DrPH
 Risk Assessment Certificate
Johns Hopkins Bloomberg School of Public Health
Baltimore, Maryland
Chapter 6

Rebecca C. Lee, PhD, RN, PHCNS-BC, CTN-A
Associate Professor
University of Cincinnati College of Nursing
Cincinnati, Ohio
Chapter 24

Jeanne Leffers, PhD, RN
Professor Emeritus
University of Massachusetts Dartmouth College
 of Nursing
North Dartmouth, Massachusetts
Chapter 18

Barbara B. Little, DNP, MPH, RN, APHN-BC, CNE
Senior Teaching Faculty
Florida State University
Tallahassee, Florida
Chapter 14

William A. Mase, Dr.PH, MPH, MA
Assistant Professor
Georgia Southern University
Statesboro, Georgia
Chapter 3

Donna Mazyck, MS, RN, NCSN
Executive Director
National Association of School Nurse
Silver Spring, Maryland
Chapter 19

Kathleen Michael, PhD, RN, CRRN
Associate Professor
University of Maryland School of Nursing
Baltimore, Maryland
Chapter 20

Rose Chalo Nabirye, PhD, MPH, BNS
Senior Lecturer and Chair, Department of Nursing
School of Health Sciences, College of Health Sciences
Makerere University
Kampala, Uganda
Chapter 13

Mary R. Nicholson, RN, BSN, MSN CIC
Infection Control Practitioner, Manager
The Christ Hospital
Cincinnati, Ohio
Chapter 15

Krysten North, MPH
Chapter 24

Donna Shambley-Ebron, PhD, RN, CTN-A
Associate Professor
University of Cincinnati, College of Nursing
Cincinnati, Ohio
Chapter 23

Sarah Szanton, PhD, ANP, FAAN
Associate Professor and PhD Program Director
Associate Director for Policy, Center on Innovative Care
 in Aging
Joint Appointment with the Department of Health
 Policy and Management,
Johns Hopkins Bloomberg School of Public Health
Johns Hopkins School of Nursing
Baltimore, Maryland
Chapter 24

Christine Vandenhouten, PhD, RN, APHN-BC
Assistant Professor
University of Wisconsin, Green Bay Professional
 Program in Nursing
Green Bay, Wisconsin
Chapter 3

Tenner Goodwin Veenema, PhD, MPH, RN, FAAN
Associate Professor
Johns Hopkins University School of Nursing
Baltimore, Maryland
Chapter 25

Jo Ann C. Abegglen, DNP, APRN, PNP
Associate Professor of Nursing
Brigham Young University College of Nursing
Provo, Utah

Evelyn L. Acheson, PhD, RN
Director, WHO Collaborating Center (Affiliate), Graduate Faculty
University of Oklahoma
Tulsa, Oklahoma

Kathleen Anderson, MS, RNP-C
Assistant Clinical Professor
Binghamton University
Binghamton, New York

Lori Barber, RN, MN, LNC
Professor of Nursing
Utah Valley University
Orem, Utah

Margaret K. Bassett, MPH, MS, BSN
Associate Professor
Radford University
Radford, Virginia

Susan Benson, MPH, RN
Clinical Faculty
University of Texas at El Paso
El Paso, Texas

Lisa Marie Bernardo, PhD, MPH, RN, HFS
Associate Professor
University of Pittsburgh School of Nursing
Pittsburgh, Pennsylvania

Joan T. Bickes, MSN, APRN, BC
Assistant Professor (Clinical)
Wayne State University
Detroit, Michigan

Anne Bongiorno, PhD, APRN, BC, CNE
Associate Professor
SUNY Plattsburgh
Plattsburgh, New York

Judith D. Brock, BA, BSN, MPH
Assistant Professor of Nursing
Mesa State College
Grand Junction, Colorado

Voncelia Brown, PhD, RN
Assistant Professor
Salisbury University
Salisbury, Maryland

Marta A. Browning, MSN, RN
Clinical Associate Professor of Nursing
University of Alabama in Huntsville
Huntsville, Alabama

Annie Collins, RN, MSN
Assistant Professor
Washburn University
Topeka, Kansas

Elizabeth B. Daniels, MN, RN
Assistant Professor
Medical College of Georgia
Athens, Georgia

Karen J. Egenes, EdD, RN, CNE
Associate Professor and Chair, Dept. of Health Promotion
Loyola University Chicago, Marcella Niehoff School of Nursing
Chicago, Illinois

Aida L. Egues, DNP, RN, PHCNS-BC, CNE
Assistant Professor
New York College of Technology of the City University of New York
Brooklyn, New York

Priscilla Faulkner, MS, MA, CNS, CDE
Assistant Professor
University of Northern Colorado School of Nursing
Greeley, Colorado

Sue Gabriel, EdD, MSN, MFS, RN, SANE-A, CFN, FABFN, FABFE
Associate Professor
BryanLGH College of Health Sciences, College of Nursing
Lincoln, Nebraska

Candace Graber, RN, MSN, AOCNS
Faculty
Platt College
Aurora, Colorado

Linda P. Grimsley, DSN, RN
Chair & Associate Professor, Department of Nursing
Albany State College
Albany, Georgia

Mary Alice Hodge, PhD, RN
Director, BSN Programs
Gardner-Webb University
Boiling Springs, North Carolina

Beverley E. Holland, PhD, ARNP
BSN Department Chair, Associate Professor
Bellarmine University
Louisville, Kentucky

Debbie Hooser, DNSc, RN
Associate Professor of Nursing
Baptist College of Health Sciences
Memphis, Tennessee

Faye Hummel, PhD, RN, CTN
Professor
University of Northern Colorado School of Nursing
Greeley, Colorado

Mary Agnes Kendra, PhD, RN
Associate Professor of Nursing
The University of Akron
Akron, Ohio

Judith L. Keswick, RN, PHN, MSN
Associate Professor of Nursing, Stanislaus
California State University
Turlock, California

Malena King-Jones, PhD, RN, MS
Assistant Professor
D'Youville College School of Nursing
Buffalo, New York

Sandra Kundrik Leh, PhD, RN
Assistant Professor of Nursing
Cedar Crest College
Allentown, Pennsylvania

Ginny Langham, MSN, RN
Instructor
Auburn Montgomery School of Nursing
Montgomery, Alabama

Cheryl Leiningen, MA, RN, APN-BC
Assistant Professor, Program Coordinator
New Jersey City University
Jersey City, New Jersey

Alice L. March, PhD, RN, FNP-C, CNE
Assistant Professor
The University of Alabama
Tuscaloosa, Alabama

Karen May, MSN, RN
Assistant Professor
Neumann University
Aston, Pennsylvania

Elizabeth Henderson McIntosh, CRNP, FNP, MSN
Nurse Practitioner, Clinical Faculty
Auburn University
Montgomery, Alabama

Jeanne Pfeiffer, DNP, MPH, RN, CIC
Clinical Assistant Professor
University of Minnesota School of Nursing
Minneapolis, Minnesota

Rebecca Presswood, MS, RN
Instructor, Associate Degree of Nursing Program
Blinn College
Bryan, Texas

Sandy Sánchez, PhD
Professor and BSN Coordinator
University of Texas-Pan American
Edinburg, Texas

Regina Smeltzer, RN, MSN
Assistant Professor, Coordinator of RN to BSN Program
Francis Marion University
Darlington, South Carolina

Diane L. Smith, RN, MSN
Assistant Professor
College of the Ozarks
Point Lookout, Missouri

Gale A. Spencer, PhD, RN
Distinguished Teaching Professor, Decker Chair in Community Health
Decker School of Nursing, Binghamton University
Binghamton, New York

Lori R. Steffen, RN, MA
Assistant Professor
Gustavus Adolphus College
St. Peter, Minnesota

Kathleen Walker, MS, BA, AAS, RN, BCCHN
Associate Professor of Nursing
Roberts Wesleyan College
Rochester, New York

Marlene Wilken, PhD, RN
Associate Professor
Creighton University School of Nursing
Omaha, Nebraska

Cathy H. Williams, DNP, RN
*Associate Professor, Department of Nursing Program
  Director*
Albany State University
Albany, Georgia

Acknowledgments

This book would not have been possible without the contributions of experts in the field. We are grateful for their dedication and assistance in presenting public health and nursing in a clear manner within the context of the real world. They have our sincere gratitude.

We thank our developmental editors Shirley Kuhn and Robin Levin Richman and Content Project Manager Victoria White, along with the staff at F.A. Davis who helped make this book a reality.

We are grateful to our families for their support and patience and to our students for the inspiration they provided for the writing of this book.

Table of Contents

Appendix *652*

Chapter 1

Public Health and Nursing Practice

LEARNING OUTCOMES

After reading this chapter, the student will be able to:

1. Describe public health in terms of current frameworks and organization from a local to a global perspective.
2. Compare and contrast the terms commonly used within the context of public health.
3. Discuss current issues related to health promotion and health protection.
4. Investigate the role of environment and culture in the health of populations.
5. Describe the practice of public health nursing from a historical perspective.
6. Identify the key roles and responsibilities of public health nurses (PHNs).

KEY TERMS

Aggregate
Community
Core functions

Determinants of health
Health
Population

Population health
Population-focused care
Public health

Public health nursing
Public health science

▮ Introduction to Public Health

Public health science provides nurses with the skills and knowledge needed to answer questions related to the health of populations and communities. **Public health science** is the scientific foundation of public health practice and brings together other sciences including environmental science, epidemiology, biostatistics, biomedical sciences, and the social and behavioral sciences.[1,2] Sometimes we identify a health problem that affects an individual and his or her family, and sometimes we see a problem in the community. Our first step is to ask, "What can we do about it?" This requires that we understand the underlying risk and protective factors related to the problem, some of which are individual based and some that are population based.[3] Understanding these risk factors from both perspectives allows us to develop nursing interventions that incorporate the full continuum of health from individuals to populations, and, it is hoped, to contribute with each intervention to the overarching goal of the

World Health Organization (WHO): to improve health and well-being for the global population.[4] The WHO is the public health arm of the United Nations (UN).

According to Issel,[5] individuals do not achieve health at the individual level through uninformed, individualistic actions. Instead, individual health occurs within the context of the population and the environment surrounding the individual. Therefore, all nurses need skills and knowledge related to the informed actions taken by individuals within the context of the health of their community. During the last century and into the 21st century, public health science has been the backbone of the nursing interventions we provide to individuals, families, and communities. Standard care, such as flu vaccinations, lead poisoning screening, and prevention programs, comes from work done using the principles of public health science. As nurses, we must be sufficiently competent to understand the basics of this science and apply it daily in our care. After all, it is our heritage, with the modern founder of our profession, Florence

Nightingale, recognized as an early pioneer in epidemiology and public health science.

What Is Public Health?

Although **public health** has contributed significantly to the health of the nation over the past century, it is often difficult to define. In 1920, a respected public health figure, C.E.A. Winslow, defined public health as

> the science and art of preventing disease, prolonging life and promoting health and efficiency through organized community effort for the sanitation of the environment, the control of communicable infections, the education of the individual in personal hygiene, the organization of medical and nursing services for the early diagnosis and preventive treatment of disease, and for the development of the social machinery to insure everyone a standard of living adequate for the maintenance of health, so organizing these benefits as to enable every citizen to realize his birthright of health and longevity.[1]

Winslow's definition actually reflects what public health is, the scientific basis of public health, and what it does, and it remains relevant to this day.[2]

In 1988, the Institute of Medicine (IOM), in its report *The Future of Public Health,* added clarity to the term by defining public health as what society does collectively to assure the conditions for people to be healthy.[6] It identified three **core functions** that encompass the purpose of public health. These include (1) assessment, (2) policy development, and (3) assurance. *Assessment* focuses on the systematic collection, analysis, and monitoring of health problems and needs. *Policy development* refers to using scientific knowledge to develop comprehensive public health policies. *Assurance* relates to assuring constituents that public health agencies provide services necessary to achieve agreed-upon goals.

In 1994, the Public Health Functions Steering Committee, a group of public and private partners, added further clarification to the definition by establishing a list of essential services. It developed the list of essential services through a consensus process with federal agencies and major national public health agencies[7] (see Box 1-1).

Although the government is likely to play a leadership role in ensuring that the essential services are provided, public, private, and voluntary organizations are also needed to provide a healthy environment and are a part of the public health system.[8] This is best depicted in the U.S. Department of Health and Human Services' *Healthy People 2020* explanation of the key components of the public health infrastructure[9] (see Box 1-2).

BOX 1-1 Ten Essential Public Health Services

The 10 essential public health services provide the framework for the National Public Health Performance Standards Program (NPHPSP). Because the strength of a public health system rests on its capacity to effectively deliver the 10 Essential Public Health Services, the NPHPSP instruments for health systems assess how well they perform the following:

1. Monitor health status to identify community health problems.
2. Diagnose and investigate health problems and health hazards in the community.
3. Inform, educate, and empower people about health issues.
4. Mobilize community partnerships to identify and solve health problems.
5. Develop policies and plans that support individual and community health efforts.
6. Enforce laws and regulations that protect health and ensure safety.
7. Link people to needed personal health services and assure the provision of health care when otherwise unavailable.
8. Assure a competent public health and personal health-care workforce.
9. Evaluate effectiveness, accessibility, and quality of personal and population-based health services.
10. Research for new insights and innovative solutions to health problems.

Source: American Public Health Association, http://www.apha.org/programs/standards/performancestandardsprogram/resexxentialservices.htm.

BOX 1-2 *Healthy People 2020:* Public Health Infrastructure

Public health infrastructure is fundamental to the provision and execution of public health services at all levels. A strong infrastructure provides the capacity to prepare for and respond to both acute (emergency) and chronic (ongoing) threats to the Nation's health. Infrastructure is the foundation for planning, delivering, and evaluating public health. Public health infrastructure includes 3 key components that enable a public health organization at the Federal, Tribal, State, or local level to deliver public health services. These components are:

A capable and qualified workforce
Up-to-date data and information systems
Public health agencies capable of assessing and responding to public health needs
These components are necessary to fulfill the following 10 Essential Public Health Services

Sources: http://www.healthypeople.gov/2020/topicsobjectives2020/overview.aspx?topicId=35.

Public Health Frameworks: Challenges and Trends

Public health in the 21st century is facing new challenges and trends that are likely to demand different frameworks for its practice today. The events that brought this fact to the forefront were two disasters: the attacks of September 11, 2001, and Hurricane Katrina. On September 11, 2001, 2,998 people in the United States were killed in terrorist attacks. Before this event, few would have thought that such an event could happen on American soil. The world changed that day. The United States, along with the rest of the world, recognized the existence of new public health concerns, biological warfare, chemical weapons, and nuclear and radiological weapons.

In contrast, Hurricane Katrina, which savaged the Gulf Coast of the United States in the summer of 2005, was a natural disaster. A horrified public watched as the emergency systems in New Orleans collapsed, leaving people to suffer and die, not only from the destruction of the hurricane, but also from a lack of water, food, sanitation, and medical attention. After Katrina and the attacks of September 11, 2001, the country acknowledged the need to strengthen the public health infrastructure, with an increasing emphasis on disaster preparedness and emergency response.

The lessons of September 11, 2001, and Katrina and its aftermath have extended to the global community. Any disaster can quickly escalate from direct injuries and deaths to indirect illness and death because of the destruction of the public health infrastructure and the denial of public health resources to vulnerable populations. Therefore, from a global perspective, public health systems in developed and developing countries deserve international public health resource monitoring.[10]

Globalization is another challenge for public health in the 21st century. Globalization is defined as "the process of increasing economic, political, and social independence and integration as capital, goods, persons, concepts, images, ideas, and values cross state boundaries."[11] It is associated with increased travel, trade, economic growth, and diffusion of technology, resulting sometimes in greater disparities between rich and poor, environmental degradation, and food security issues.[12] It has also resulted in greater distribution of products such as tobacco or alcohol. With globalization, there is also an emergence or reemergence of communicable diseases, including human immunodeficiency virus (HIV), acquired immunodeficiency syndrome (AIDS), severe acute respiratory syndrome (SARS), hepatitis, malaria, diphtheria,

cholera, measles and Ebola virus. Planning for communicable disease outbreaks such as a pandemic will require new ethical frameworks to guide decision making regarding appropriate action with limited resources.[13] The world needs new regulations to strengthen national and global surveillance capabilities.[14]

Public health also needs ethical frameworks to address the advancement of scientific and medical technologies.[12] The increasing use of genomics, for example, raises questions of how to protect against discrimination. Another challenge is the aging and more diverse population. With aging, there is an increase in noncommunicable (chronic) illness. Noncommunicable illness, in turn, occurs in part owing to lifestyle behaviors such as smoking and nutrition. In 1926, Winslow discussed the need for new methods to address heart disease, respiratory diseases, and cancer.[15] We still need frameworks to help improve noncommunicable disease outcomes and, from a global perspective, to address how international collective action becomes essential to combating the tobacco epidemic.[16]

Emerging Public Health Frameworks

In 2003, the IOM produced a report, *The Future of the Public's Health in the Twenty-First Century,* as an update of the 1988 IOM report.[6,8] In this report, the IOM presented the ecological model as the basis not only for understanding health in populations but also for assuring conditions in which populations can be healthy.[17] The committee built on an ecological model created by Dahlgren and Whitehead,[18] and based its model on the assumption that health is influenced at several levels: individuals, families, communities, organizations, and social systems (Fig. 1-1). The model is also based on the assumptions that:

- There are multiple determinants of health.
- A population and environmental approach is critical.
- Linkages and relationships between the levels are important.
- Multiple strategies by multiple sectors are needed to achieve desired outcomes.[19]

Conventional public health models such as the epidemiological model of the agent, host, and environment recognize this ecological approach (Chapter 3). However, this newly defined ecological model reflects a deeper understanding of the role not only of the physical environment but also of the conditions in the social environment creating poor health, referred to as an "upstream" approach.[8,20] *Upstream* refers to determinants of health that

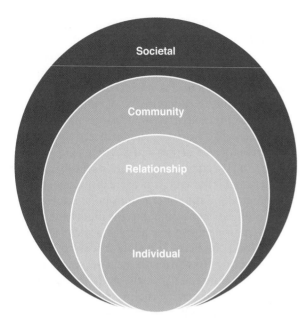

Figure I-I The Social-Ecological Model. *(Adapted by CTLT by Dahlgren and Whitehead, 1991, Worthman, 1999.)*

are somewhat removed from the more "downstream" biological and behavioral bases for disease. These upstream determinants include social relations, neighborhoods and communities, institutions, and social and economic policies.[21]

Community Partnerships

One of the recommendations of the 2003 IOM report is the need for multisectored engagement in partnerships with the community. In the past, the community's role in health programs had often been that of a passive recipient, beneficiary, or research subject, with the active work carried out by public health experts. There is a growing commitment to collaboration now in promoting the health of communities. There is evidence that benefits of such efforts increase effectiveness and productivity, empower the participants, strengthen social engagement, and ensure accountability.[8]

Community collaborations are really vehicles for bringing participants together. It might be a local coalition working to stop tobacco use in restaurants. It might be an advocacy group for the mentally ill working with legislators to write a policy for better health coverage. It might be a school collaborating with the health department to start a school-based clinic. It might be nongovernmental agencies in one country working with the American Red Cross to address disaster needs.

Public Health Organization and Management

Under the larger umbrella of public health, governments have instituted public health departments, also known as boards of public health. The previous section of this chapter covered the broader public health field. In this section, you will learn about the governmental bodies that are concerned with the protection of the public's health. Even though these governmental bodies do not encompass the entirety of the field, they are a key component and are responsible for oversight in relation to the public health infrastructure in the United States.

The U.S. Constitution provides for a two-layer federal system composed of the federal level and the state level. However, the Constitution did not make any specific provisions for the management of public health issues at the federal level with the intent that health would come under state authority.[22] Congress addressed the issue of protection of the public over the rights of the individual through the amendment process. After ratification of the 14th Amendment, states were required to provide protections to their own citizens, which helped to legalize activities of local health departments to take such actions as imposing quarantines.

State Public Health Departments

States independently decide how they will structure their local and state health departments. Often there is no direct provision for public health within the state constitution; rather, the state constitution empowers either the legislative or executive branch to make decisions related to the public health such as setting up a statute, regulation, or executive order related to the establishment of a state board of health.[22]

This has resulted in variations across states in relation to the organization and management of formal public health systems. The variation stems, in part, from how the state government has directed the establishment of public health boards or departments and from the variation in state jurisdictional structure. For example, some states such as Pennsylvania use a town/city (municipality), township, or county system, and other states such as Massachusetts divide their entire state into municipalities. Finally, some states such as Alaska have territories as well as municipalities because they have smaller populations spread across a larger land mass. Sovereign American Indian nations within their borders present another challenge in the structuring of public health departments for Alaska and other states in the United States.

Local Public Health Departments

The basic mandate of the local public health department is to protect the health of the citizens residing in their county, municipality, township, or territory. However, how public health departments implement this protection varies across states. This results in variability in the services offered and the public health activities of the local health departments. As a result of federal mandates, public health departments uniformly perform certain activities. These include surveillance, outbreak investigation, and quarantine as well as mandated reporting of specific diseases and cause of death to state health departments and the Centers for Disease Control and Prevention (CDC). This allows the federal government to track the incidence and prevalence of disease from a national perspective.

In addition to these mandated activities related to disease, local health departments also oversee public sanitation and the safety of the water supply. They accomplish this through laboratory testing of water samples, inspection of sewer systems, and health-related mandates such as the boiling of water when they have identified a potential threat to health. For some health departments, this oversight includes the actual provision of these services, but not always. Private water companies still exist in the United States. Public health departments also oversee food safety and carry out inspections of restaurants and food retailers.

What else do local health departments do aside from monitoring disease and sanitation in their community? Some also provide direct health care. For example, some local health departments manage public health clinics that provide direct care aimed at health promotion for their residents, including vaccinations, prenatal care, and well-baby visits. Other health departments provide care at the individual level such as home health nursing services.

In 1988, the IOM identified assessment of the community as a core function of public health. This requires that public health departments base their activities on a planned methodological assessment of the community they serve.[6] After the IOM published *The Future of Public Health,* models of community assessment emerged (see Chapter 4), some from within the public health system and some from the healthy communities movement. The healthy communities movement used a grass roots approach aimed at mobilizing communities to come together and promote health within their community. All of the models were collaborative and required that community members and stakeholders actively participate in the process. This process shifted public health departments from pure governmental top-down structures to collaborative entities that joined with their communities in an inclusive process as described in the first section of this chapter.

Since September 11, 2001, health departments have taken on major responsibilities related to the disaster preparedness and emergency response needs that were discussed earlier. For many public health departments, traditional public health programs and health priorities have become secondary to this new mandate.[23] Health departments have become involved in setting policy and securing funds that will help to improve the ability of their department and their communities to respond to natural and man-made disasters. The challenge for health departments is to keep the needs of disaster preparedness in perspective in relation to the community they serve. The ability to do this requires a new application of the assessment process mentioned earlier. What is the likelihood of a terrorist attack? How likely is the community to experience an outbreak of a communicable disease such as SARS (Fig. 1-2)? For some communities, the risk is much higher, but determining the level of risk requires gathering the facts related to a specific community. In some cases, local health departments can only determine the risk by joining forces with other local health departments or by initiating the effort from the state level, as evidenced by large-scale earthquake disaster drills in California because of the widespread risk of earthquakes across that state (Fig. 1-3).

Another serious issue for health departments is securing funds. It is difficult for a health department to balance

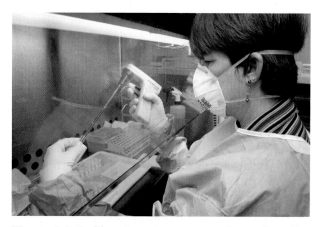

Figure 1-2 Sudden acute respiratory syndrome (SARS) epidemic: Deborah Cannon of the Special Pathogens Branch of the Centers for Disease Control and Prevention processing SARS specimens. *(From the Centers for Disease Control and Prevention, courtesy of Anthony Sanchez. Photographer, James Gathany, 2003.)*

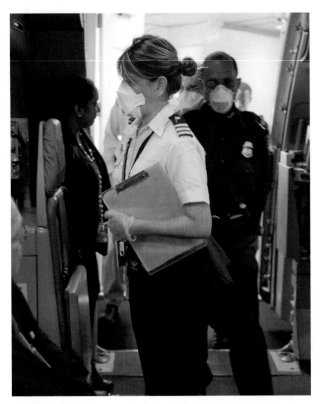

Figure 1-3 October 2008: Preparedness exercise involving a number of federal and local agencies, including the Centers for Disease Control and Prevention (CDC).

the need for vaccine programs, well-baby visits, and restaurant inspections with the cost of putting in place a disaster preparedness program, especially in an economy of shrinking tax revenue. The public health infrastructure needs economic support.

To bring more uniformity to the operation of health departments, the CDC, in collaboration with other groups, identified three core department components: (1) the public health workforce capacity and competency; (2) information, data, and communication systems; and (3) organizational and systems capacity.[24] In addition, the CDC laid out 10 essential public health services, which are listed in Box 1-1. These functions and services directly relate to the ability of a public health department to:

- Prevent epidemics and the spread of disease.
- Protect against environmental hazards.
- Prevent injuries.
- Promote and encourage healthy behaviors.
- Respond to disasters and assists communities in recovery.

- Assure the quality and accessibility of health services.[24]

So infrastructure includes all the parts of public health departments related to these 10 essential services and three core functions.[7]

National Public Health Departments: The Centers for Disease Control and Prevention

The CDC, which was founded on July 1, 1946, grew out of the wartime effort related to malaria control.[26] In the beginning, the CDC employed approximately 400 people, including engineers and entomologists (scientists who study insects). Only seven employees functioned as medical officers.

Activities of the CDC: From this humble beginning, the CDC has grown into one of the major operating components of the Department of Health and Human Services (DHHS) and is an integral part of the public health system in the United States. The CDC's goal is to be the premiere health promotion, prevention, and preparedness agency in the United States and a global leader in public health. The scope of the agency's efforts includes the prevention and control of communicable and noncommunicable diseases, injuries, workplace hazards, disabilities, and environmental health threats. In addition to health promotion and protection, the agency also conducts research and maintains a national surveillance system. It also responds to health emergencies and provides support for outbreak investigations. According to the CDC, it is distinguished from its peer agencies for two reasons: the application of research findings to people's daily lives, and its response to health emergencies.[27]

The surveillance and outbreak investigation arm of the CDC is far reaching. The CDC collaborates with state and local health departments in relation to surveillance and outbreak investigations, including bioterrorism. It sets standards for the implementation of disease prevention strategies and is the repository for health statistics. Health statistics are available to health providers, health departments, and the public. Web sites of interest to nurses needing population level information include CDC WONDER, FASTSTATS, and VITALSTATS (see Box 1-3 for details).

Healthy People 2020: A central component to the work of the CDC and the United States Department of Health and Human Services (USDHHS) is *Healthy People 2020 (HP 2020)*. This initiative builds on four decades of work goals, indicators, and objectives. The four main goals are to (1) eliminate health disparities and achieve health equity, improving health for all groups; (2) attain

---

BOX 1–3 Centers for Disease Control and Prevention Web Resources

CDC WONDER provides online data sources (AIDS public use data, births, cancer statistics); environment (daily air temperature, land service temperatures, fine particulate matter, sunlight and precipitation); mortality (detailed mortality, infant deaths, online tuberculosis information systems); population (bridged population, census); sexually transmitted morbidity, vaccine adverse event reporting.
Source: http://wonder.cdc.gov/.
FASTSTATS provides statistics on topics of public health importance.
Source: http://www.cdc.gov/nchs/fastats/.
VITALSTATS is a Web site that provides users with the ability to access and use vital statistics and population data interactively. Vital statistics products include tables, data files, and reports.
Source: http://www.cdc.gov/nchs/vitalstats.htm.

BOX 1–4 *Healthy People 2020* Leading Health Indicator Topics

1. Access to Health Services
2. Clinical Preventive Services
3. Environmental Quality
4. Injury and Violence
5. Maternal, Infant, and Child Health
6. Mental Health
7. Nutrition, Physical Activity, and Obesity
8. Oral Health
9. Reproductive and Sexual Health
10. Social Determinants
11. Substance Abuse
12. Tobacco

Source: *Healthy People 2020* http://www.healthypeople.gov/2020/LHI/default.aspx.

---

high-quality longer lives free of preventable disease, disability, injury, and premature death; (3) create healthy social and physical environments; and (4) promote quality of life, healthy development and healthy behaviors across all stages.[28]

The CDC chose and organized the main goals around four focus areas: (1) General Health Status, (2) Health-Related Quality of Life and Well-Being, (3) Determinants of Health, and (4) Disparities.[27] *HP 2020* outlines the agenda for 10 years with specific indictors and specific objectives. From the objectives listed under each goal, the CDC selected leading health indicators organized around 12 topics (Box 1-4). The CDC chose these health indicators because they would motivate action, provide data to monitor progress toward the objective related to the indicator, and would represent broad public health issues.[28]

■ HEALTHY PEOPLE 2020
Leading Health Indicators

HP 2020 provides a comprehensive set of 10-year national goals and objectives for improving the health of all Americans. *HP 2020* contains 42 topic areas with nearly 600 objectives (with others still evolving), which encompass 1,200 measures. A smaller set of *HP 2020* objectives, called Leading Health Indicators, has been selected to communicate high-priority health issues and actions that can be taken to address them. The Leading Health Indicators are composed of 26 indicators organized under 12 topics.[29]

Global Public Health: The World Health Organization (WHO)

Not only does the CDC collaborate with state and local health departments, it also collaborates with public health entities across the world and has personnel stationed in 25 foreign countries. An organization the CDC collaborates with extensively is the WHO. On April 7, 1948, the WHO's constitution was enacted. That date is now World Health Day. One of the WHO's initial goals, as it was for the CDC, was the eradication of malaria. Other initiatives included maternal–child health, malnutrition, communicable diseases, and the establishment of public health infrastructure to address sanitation and support environmental health.

The WHO is the world health authority under the auspices of the UN. Both the WHO and the CDC have six core functions: (1) global leadership in health; (2) health research; (3) setting norms and standards for health; (4) establishing ethical and evidence-based policy; (5) providing technical support, working toward change, and sustaining health services capacity; and (6) conducting disease surveillance and monitoring health trends.[27,30] Membership in the WHO includes 193 countries and three associate members. The WHO employs more than 8,000 health experts who operate out of 147 country offices, six regional offices, and the WHO headquarters in Geneva, Switzerland. The office for the region of the Americas is located in Washington, DC.[4]

In 1978, the WHO shifted its focus from such things as malaria control to the development of basic health services.[30] In that year, the WHO held a conference in Alma-Alta (now Almaty), Kazakhstan, that supported the resolution that primary health care was the means for

BOX 1–5	**World Health Organization Core Functions**

Core functions of the WHO are to:
- Provide leadership on matters critical to health and engage in partnerships where joint action is needed.
- Shape the research agenda and stimulate the generation, translation, and dissemination of valuable knowledge.
- Set norms and standards and promote and monitor their implementation.
- Articulate ethical and evidence-based policy options.
- Provide technical support, catalyze change, and build sustainable institutional capacity.
- Monitor the health situation and assess health trends.

Source: See reference 30.

BOX 1–6	**The Eight Millennium Development Goals**

- Goal 1: Eradicate extreme poverty and hunger.
- Goal 2: Achieve universal primary education.
- Goal 3: Promote gender equality and empower women.
- Goal 4: Reduce child mortality.
- Goal 5: Improve maternal health.
- Goal 6: Combat HIV/AIDS, malaria, and other diseases.
- Goal 7: Ensure environmental sustainability.
- Goal 8: Develop a global partnership for development.

Source: See reference 33.

attaining health for all. Though criticized for being too broad and optimistic, the WHO adopted primary health care as the means to attain health for all by 2000.[31] This effort has resulted in an increase in accessible health services throughout the world.

In the early 21st century, the WHO faces new challenges. The WHO based its adoption of the primary care model on the health-care problems of the 1970s: acute infections and malnutrition. With the advent of AIDS and the increased globalization of populations, some experts are concerned that the model is no longer relevant because of the increase in chronic communicable diseases and chronic noncommunicable diseases. At the beginning of the first decade in the 21st century a new model emerged of integrated services that respond to both of these threats to health.[32] The WHO has expanded to include emergency response and disaster preparedness initiatives (see Chapter 25). Another key initiative was the institution of International Health Regulations (IHRs) that countries must follow in response to disease outbreaks. To increase the ability of the WHO to respond to public health emergencies brought on by natural or manmade disasters such as the tsunamis in Southeast Asia in 2004 and in Japan in 2010, or the 2010 earthquake in Haiti, the WHO has a strategic health operations center.[4]

In 2000, 191 countries met and set the millennium development goals (MDGs) aimed at improving the health of all populations by 2015. There are eight MDGs (Box 1-6). The initial goal of maternal–child health set by the WHO in 1948 remains in Goals 4 and 5. Goal 6 also stems from the early work of the WHO, which is to combat communicable diseases. Despite efforts to eradicate malaria in the early years, communicable diseases continue to threaten populations. The final two goals build on the Alma Alta initiative related to primary care

and focus on public health infrastructure that goes beyond access to care.[30,33]

Public Health as a Component of Nursing Practice Across Settings and Specialties

Nursing practice requires the application of knowledge from multiple sciences, including public health. Health is not just a result of individual factors such as biology, genetics, and behavior; it is also a product of an individual's social, cultural, and ecological environment. To meet our obligation to maximize health on all levels, we must incorporate public health science into our nursing care.

Introduction to Population Health and Population-Focused Care

What is a population and what is health? According to Caldwell,[34] a population is a mass of people that make up a definable unit to which measurements pertain. The WHO defined **health** as "the state of complete physical, mental and social well-being and not merely the absence of disease or infirmity."[35] Does this mean that we can define **population health** by combining these two terms or is population health something more?

Because individuals make up populations, let us first start with the nursing care of individuals and personal health. Much of the curricular content in nursing programs pertains to acquiring the knowledge and skill the nurse needs to deliver nursing care to individuals. The nurse learns to apply the nursing process to help set up a plan of care for an individual that often pertains to a single episode of care. When the nurse delivers care to an individual, the outcomes of interest are at the individual level. The goal is to implement nursing interventions that contribute to the individual's ability to achieve a maximum health state. However, achieving a complete state of health and well-being usually extends beyond the interventions that nurses and other health-care professionals provide on an individual level during a single episode of care. Though the nursing interventions help to move the person toward a state of health, the full range of actions needed requires an inclusion of the individual's mental, social, and economic needs as well as the immediate health needs addressed during this point in time. To take in this wider scope of influences on the person's health, the nurse must consider the individual as a part of a greater whole, which includes the social, mental, and economic health needs that depend on the individual's interactions with other individuals and groups. This requires placing the individual within his or her socioecological context.

The first step is to go beyond the individual and consider what populations include this individual. Now the individual's health takes on a broader context. The foundation of health care is not only to promote the health of individuals, but also to provide the means for a population to achieve maximum health. Allen, Stanley, Crabtree, and Werner[36] stressed that clinical prevention and population health activities are central to the goal of improving the health status of the nation and stated that these activities have the potential to reduce leading causes of death and improve quality of life across diverse populations. The activities mentioned by Allen et al. require a sound foundation in public health science and an ability to link the nursing interventions provided at the bedside to nursing interventions provided to populations.

Health From a Population Perspective

When a nurse is looking to acquire a foundation in public health science, the best place to start is to understand that health and disease occur within the context of the social, economic, cultural, and environmental influences on populations and, thus, on individuals. Elements directly related to the health of populations include air quality, access to adequate supplies of food, sanitation, and safe water. Populations with healthy environments thrive. The rise of ancient civilizations illustrates the importance of these components. For example, ancient Egypt developed along the Nile where crops flourished, water was plentiful, and the weather was mild. A question then arises: Are these environmental elements related to health relevant to nursing? The construction and maintenance of sewer systems and the delivery of public water come under the umbrella of public health but not necessarily public health nursing, because nurses do not typically deliver these public health interventions. However, understanding the importance of sanitation and water becomes quite relevant during a natural disaster

when nurses join forces with other public health officials to prevent cholera, dehydration, and starvation.

In 2004, the tsunami that struck Southeast Asia left whole populations without safe drinking water and food (Fig. 1-4). In 2010, a tsunami in Japan, a natural disaster, precipitated the threat of nuclear fallout from the compromising of a nuclear power plant. Closer to home, Hurricane Katrina resulted in a complete breakdown of the water and sanitation capacity of a modern U.S. city (Fig. 1-5). In 2012, Hurricane Sandy left thousands homeless.

Therefore, knowledge of environmental science is one of the foundational sciences in the broader field of public health science. In addition, there are five other scientific

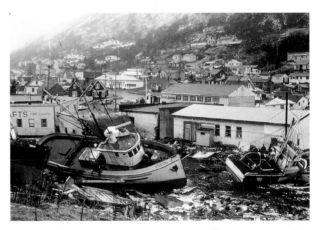

Figure 1-4 Tsunami in Southeast Asia; aerial photo of Kalutara Beach, Sri Lanka, taken on December 26, 2004. *(From the Federal Emergency Management Association, 2005.)*

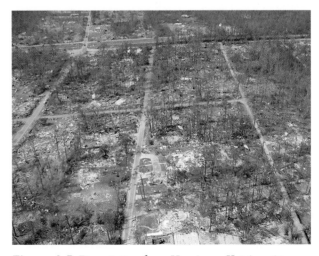

Figure 1-5 Devastation from Hurricane Katrina. *(From NOAA's National Weather Service [NWS] Collection, 2005.)*

disciplines that provide the foundation of public health science, including epidemiology, biostatistics, biomedical sciences, social sciences, and behavioral sciences.[2,37] With individuals, nurses always start their care with an assessment. This requires knowledge of the biomedical social and psychological sciences. When providing **population-focused care**, nurses need a basic knowledge of the different scientific disciplines that make up public health science, so when nurses assess a community and/or a population they use their knowledge of epidemiology and biostatistics to help identify priority health issues at the population level. Some terms relevant to a discussion of public health—*aggregate*, *population*, and *community*—are sometimes used interchangeably, but there are differences among them (see Box 1-7 for detailed definitions).[38,39] All of these interventions, grounded in public health science, when framed beyond the individual ultimately improve the health of **aggregates, populations,** and **communities.**

Public Health Science and Nursing Practice

In 2010, the IOM published a report on the future of nursing.[40] The stated goal was to have 80% of all registered nurses prepared at the baccalaureate of science in nursing (BSN) level or higher. The rationale for this goal was that BSN programs emphasize liberal arts, advanced sciences, and nursing coursework across a wide range of settings, along with leadership development and exposure to community and public health competencies. In addition, the authors emphasized that entry-level nurses need to be able to transition smoothly from their academic preparation to a range of practice environments, with an increased emphasis on community and public health settings.[40]

Health Promotion, Risk Reduction, and Health Protection

Health promotion activities are an essential component of nursing practice.[41] Health promotion interventions occur from the individual level to the population level.

Again, authors use various terms in relation to reducing the occurrence or severity of disease in a population and enhancing the capacity of a population to achieve optimal health. These terms include *health promotion, risk reduction,* and *health protection*. Brubaker[42] defines *health promotion* as the provision of care directed toward the attainment of a high level of wellness through environmental or behavioral change. As defined by the WHO, *health promotion* is the process of enabling people to increase control over, and to improve, their health. *Risk reduction* refers to actions taken to reduce a person's risk for disease.[30] Lately, authors use the term *health protection* more often than *risk reduction*, switching the emphasis to increasing the person's ability to protect against disease. An example of a health promotion intervention is the institution of an exercise program in an elementary school; an example of a health protection, risk reduction program is a vaccination outreach program. The first intervention promotes a healthy behavior and the second increases the ability of the immune system to protect against a communicable agent, thus reducing risk.

BOX 1–7 Definitions for *Aggregate*, *Population*, and *Community*

For this book these terms are defined within the context of public health building on standard dictionary definitions and definitions used in the literature.

Aggregate: In public health this terms represents individual units brought together into a whole or a sum of those individuals. In public health science, the term aggregate often refers to the unit of analysis, that is, at what level the health-care provider analyzes and reports data.

Population: Refers to a larger group whose members may or may not interact with one another but who share at least one characteristic such as age, gender, ethnicity, residence, or a shared health issue such as HIV/AIDS or breast cancer. The common denominator or shared characteristic may or may not be a shared geography or other link recognized by the individuals within that population. For example, people with type 2 diabetes admitted to a hospital form a population but do not share a specific culture or place of residence and may not recognize themselves as part of this population. In many situations, the terms *aggregate* and *population* are used interchangeably.

Community: Refers to a group of individuals living within the same geographical area, such as a town or a neighborhood, or a group of individuals who share some other common denominator, such as ethnicity or religious orientation. In contrast to aggregates and population, individuals within the community recognize their membership in the community based on social interaction and establishment of ties to other members in the community, and often join collective decision making.

Sources: See references 38 and 39.

In nursing, health promotion often focuses on individual-level interventions, which may be defined as health education interventions.[43] This approach is not unique to nursing. According to O'Donnell's[44] suggested revised definition, health promotion is both a science and art that helps people change their lifestyles to achieve optimal health. From O'Donnell's perspective, health promotion remains rooted in individual behavioral change. However, looked at from a broader perspective, health promotion at the individual level also encompasses activities taken to promote health that require changes other than behavioral changes, such as facilitating the individual's ability to improve the health of his or her environment. Facilitating the individual's ability to access resources needed to promote health, such as good nutrition or a safe place to exercise, is another example.

O'Donnell's definition also lacks a consideration of health promotion at the population health level, also known as *ecological health promotion*. Ecological health promotion targets environmental change through the empowerment of community members to initiate and implement the changes.[45] The changes occur at multiple levels and utilize various strategies including educational, policy, economic, and environmental strategies. Another term used to describe population-level health promotion is *community health promotion*. Racher and Annis[46] base population-level health promotion on the belief that the individuals that make up a community can as a group identify and solve their problems. This approach shifts away from health education focused on lifestyle and behavioral change at the individual level toward community empowerment, political change, and environmental enhancement.[46]

This illustrates that health promotion can occur across a continuum.[47] If it is indeed an essential component of nursing care, then nurses must recognize that it occurs at more than the individual level and requires more than health education interventions. However, providing health promotion across the continuum requires an understanding of the context in which health occurs. Therefore, the next step in the process is to examine this context.

The Context of Health

Protecting and promoting health requires the consideration of the geographical, social, economic, and cultural context of where the person lives, not just identifying and treating specific diseases and injuries. This section introduces the context of health in relation to two areas: population diversity and environment. Both diversity and environment have significant impacts on the health of populations; the success of interventions depends on an understanding of these important factors directly related to the health of a population.

Population and Diversity

The first step in understanding the context of health is to acknowledge the diversity of populations within our country and across the globe. *Diversity* is a term used frequently within the health-care field. What does it really mean? According to Issel,[5] diversity reflects the fact that groups and individuals are not all the same but differ in relation to culture, ethnicity, and race. At first glance, culture, ethnicity, and race may seem to reflect the same idea. However, while they overlap, they are different.

Culture refers to beliefs, values, and norms shared across a group of people. To better understand the term, Spector equates it to a set of luggage that a person carries that contains such things as beliefs, habits, norms, customs, and rituals that are handed down from one generation to the next through both verbal and nonverbal communication. Spector goes on to state, "All facets of human behavior can be interpreted through the lens of culture."[48] Thus, nurses must have an appreciation for cultures represented within the population they are caring for while acknowledging and understanding their own cultural views of the world, also known as *cultural lenses*.

Next, consider *ethnicity*. Is it not the same as *culture*? Once again, multiple definitions exist for the term. Commonalities across definitions include shared geographical origin, language or dialect, religious faith, folklore, food preferences, and culture. O'Neill[49] includes physical characteristics as well and suggests that we use *ethnicity* in two distinct ways:

1. To classify people who may have no specific cultural traditions in common into a loose group
2. To classify groups that have a shared language and cultural traditions

For example, to classify an ethnic group under the name *Native American* results in grouping together people who are actually diverse in both culture and language. However, if the ethnic group is a specific Native American tribe, such as the Navaho, then the group does share specific cultural traditions, beliefs, and language that are not shared with other Native American tribes such as the Inuit. Therefore, care is required when using the term *ethnicity* because of the variation in its use. Identifying the ethnicity of a group of people, which only takes into account broad shared characteristics, may miss key cultural differences within the group.

Geographical differences also play a part in diversity across groups and can result in shared cultural traditions that extend across ethnic groups within that geographical region. In the United States, cultural differences exist within specific regions, such as New England, the South, and the West Coast. These three regions differ in dialect, accepted protocol for social interactions, and food preferences.

Cultural differences also exist between regions of the United States. For example, the "Down-Easters" in the state of Maine differ from people residing in Boston in dialect and protocols for social interaction. These differences extend across the ethnic groups residing in these two different geographical areas within the larger New England region.

Finally, there is the term *race*. Race categorizes groups of people based on superficial criteria such as skin color, physical characteristics, and parentage. In the United States, we continue to use racial categories with increasingly less accuracy as more and more people within our country marry across ethnic groups. The U.S. Census Bureau acknowledges that the use of racial categories is limited, especially because some people may classify themselves as belonging to more than one category.[50,51] As the field of genetics grows, so does the evidence that there is no scientific basis for placing an individual into one racial group. A classic article in *Newsweek*, "What Color Is Black?"[52] challenges the myth of race and concludes that it is not a legitimate method for classifying groups of people. Scientists found that people with very dissimilar racial characteristics such as skin color and facial features were in some cases more closely related genetically than groups with similar skin color. However, race continues to be used to identify groups. Traditionally, scientists report epidemiological data using racial categories as a means of identifying disparity between racial groups, especially in relation to health outcomes and access to care. Following the U.S. 2010 Census, the ability to group people using racial categories is increasingly difficult as these categories expand to include individuals who identify themselves as biracial and multiracial.

So what does this all mean? How important is it to include diversity as a major factor in the delivery of nursing interventions to populations? If a nurse plans an intervention without taking into account the cultural and ethnic diversity within the population, failure to achieve the goals of the intervention may result from violation of ethnic and cultural values or beliefs. If the nurse only views the intervention through his or her cultural lens, and if that lens differs from those who will receive the intervention, then a key piece is missing. Does the population view the intervention as culturally relevant? Is the desired health outcome valued? For example, if a nurse develops an intervention aimed at increasing the number of women who breastfeed their infants, the first step is to evaluate the cultural view of breastfeeding. If the target population includes all the women giving birth at a large urban hospital, the population is probably diverse and may include cultures with different practices related to breastfeeding. If the nurse fails to acknowledge this fact and incorporate possible cultural differences into the assessment and planning stage (Chapter 5, pg. 122), the intervention may not succeed with women who have different cultural beliefs surrounding breastfeeding.

The nurse must take into account another key issue: understanding the importance of including the population as an active partner in improving health. Interventions planned *for* communities rather than *with* communities ignore the point made by Murphy[53] that communities interpret their own health. In addition, Murphy states that communities themselves can come up with ways to improve their health. From a population health perspective, collaboration and community participation are essential when developing interventions.[53] Engagement with the community can occur only within the context of culture and ethnic heritage and the community's own perception of what constitutes optimal health.

Environment and Resource Availability

Health also occurs within the context of the environment. As mentioned earlier, the abundance of water and food supplies correlates with the rise of ancient civilizations. The health of an environment is driven by the availability of clean air, abundant and potable water, and adequate food supplies. For much of humankind's existence, the health of a population was concerned with the short-term survival of that population and centered on food sources, predators, and pestilence. This changed dramatically during the industrial revolution as populations moved from rural communities to urban areas. As large groups of people congregated in these urban areas, new issues arose related to sanitation, food supplies, and water. The science of epidemiology, the study of the occurrence of disease in humans centered on environment as a key factor contributing to morbidity and mortality, emerged in the 19th century in response to these new challenges brought by the industrial revolution. Though early epidemiologists did not understand that microscopic pathogens caused disease (the germ theory), they firmly established the role that environment plays in the health of humans. Efforts during the last half of the

19th century and into the 20th century focused on the introduction of sanitary measures, including management of sewage and providing clean water and adequate ventilation.[54]

Aspects of the environment first studied by epidemiologists related to sanitation as evidenced by the classic investigation of a cholera outbreak conducted in the Soho area of London in 1854 by John Snow.[55] Snow mapped out cholera deaths block by block and found that they clustered around the Broad Street pump, leading him to conclude that the pump was the source of the contamination. He even examined the water under a microscope and identified "white, flocculent particles" that he thought were the causative agents. Though other authorities dismissed his evidence of a microscopic agent, he convinced others of the link between the disease and the water pump. He was successful in getting the water company to change the pump handle.[55] Snow's work brought attention to the importance of safe water. The measures taken did not require a change in individual behavior, but rather a change in how the water company delivered water to the populace.

Initial public health efforts focused on the development of a public health infrastructure related to sanitation and delivery of safe water supplies. In the late 19th and early 20th centuries, large metropolitan areas initiated the development of underground sewerage systems and water pipes that are still in service today. The implementation of similar systems in towns and rural areas occurred later, with outhouses still in use in the 1950s. In the United States, long before antibiotics were available, addressing these two major issues directly reduced the spread of communicable diseases such as infantile diarrhea and cholera. In undeveloped countries without this public health infrastructure, these two diseases continue to contribute to the morbidity and mortality of their populations.

To survive, humans need adequate water and food supplies, shelter from the elements, and protection from pestilence and disease. In modern developed societies, geopolitical groups come together to supply adequate potable water and sewerage. Agricultural businesses provide food. In most developed societies, individuals and families have the means to purchase adequate shelter and the health care needed to protect them from both communicable and noncommunicable diseases. In some societies, government-based programs provide the means for obtaining health-care resources aimed at protection from pestilence and disease, and in other societies individuals purchase the health care either directly or indirectly through health insurance. Governments and individuals need adequate money to provide these resources; thus, obtaining adequate resources to promote the health of a population depends on a population's economic health. When the economy is healthy, the majority of the population has the means to obtain adequate water, food, and shelter. However, an economy in jeopardy results in a reduced ability to meet these basic needs. In all societies, the nurse must be aware of the environment in which the patient resides. Does the patient live in a community with a healthful environment? Is there adequate water? Is food available, affordable, and nutritionally beneficial? Is the economy strong enough to provide access to needed health-care resources? Environment is one of the main determinants of health for individuals, populations, and the communities they live in.

Health Behavior and Health Determinants

Determinants of health include a range of personal, social, economic, and environmental factors.[56] Before developing an intervention to improve health outcomes in a population, a nurse must first identify these determinants of health. MacDonald[54] explains that earlier models related to population health were built on the assumption that patterns of disease and health occur through a complex interrelationship between risk and protective factors. This resulted in a focus on biological and behavioral risk factors that require change at the individual level. Multiple examples exist of health promotion activities that focus on changing individual behavior to reduce risk, such as smoking cessation, healthy eating, and increased exercise. Some success has occurred with this approach. However, there have also been successful efforts at the macrosocioecological level. This level focuses on the whole population within its ecological context. These interventions focus on population behavioral change that then trickles down to the individual. Population behavioral change addresses population-level risk factors that affect the whole population, such as provision of potable water to prevent cholera. The underlying assumption is that the population level of risk affects health outcomes independent of individual/family-level risk factors.

Take, for example, lung cancer. One of the well-documented determinants of this disease is the use of tobacco. Efforts to reduce this risk factor focus on changing individual behavior. Theories have emerged that help to explain behavior, such as the Transtheoretical Model of Change.[57] This model theory helps a health-care provider determine in what stage of change a person is and helps the provider to put together a plan of care that fits the individual's readiness to quit smoking. However, many of the inroads made in smoking cessation in this country began with a broader population health approach, including media campaigns related to smoking cessation and governmental nonsmoking policies that resulted in a cultural shift within our society. Once researchers made the case for the hazards of secondary smoke, tolerance of smoking within the community dramatically decreased. The population's exposure to tobacco smoke as a whole has decreased because the cultural view of tobacco use has changed, as has the willingness of communities to implement policies that reduce the community's risk. In turn, the reduced prevalence of smoking is largely due to a cultural shift in the tolerance of smoking in public places and the ostracism experienced by smokers.

Healthy behaviors remain a key issue in the health of populations. The Institute for the Study of Healthcare Organizations & Transactions[58] exemplifies the standard approach to health determinants and health behavior. It frames health behaviors as those that occur while a person is well. The organization attempts to expand the concept to family, provider, and institutional behaviors, but it still leaves out the healthy (or risky) behaviors of populations. Keller, Strohschein, Lia-Hoagberg, and Schaffer[59] stress that health determinants include factors from the individual level to the population level. Warnecke et al.[3] state that collaborations already exist across the United States that incorporate a population-level approach and stress that the next step is to develop interventions that take this population health approach to health. They provide a model for the analysis of population health and health disparities that combines individual health determinants with population health determinants. This broader approach allows for both individual and family behavioral changes as well as change in health behaviors at the population level. Viewing health determinants across a continuum from the individual to the population level provides the nurse with more opportunity for intervening. That said, how does a nurse who is not a specialist in public health nursing participate in the national and global effort to improve the health of populations?

Population-Focused Care Across Settings and Nursing Specialties

Nurses provide population-focused care every day, in every setting. For a staff nurse working in an urban hospital, the population of interest is the patients who come to that hospital for care. The population may include various subpopulations based on shared geographical residence, age group, primary diagnosis, culture, and ethnic group. Staff nurses in an acute or community-based setting take care of patients on an individual level, often serving as the member of the health-care team that delivers the interventions and evaluates the effectiveness of those interventions. Nurses actively participate in reviewing how well the team is delivering care to the patient population as a whole. Over time, the health-care team begins to group patients based on diagnosis or other identifying characteristics to provide better care. This may occur when nurses are engaged in performance improvement activities, the development of a care map, or in response to changes in the population.

For example, over a period of 60 days, a nursing team identifies that there is an increase in patients admitted with a diagnosis of community-acquired pneumonia. The job of the team is to get at the who, what, when, where, how, and why of the situation so they can provide optimal care to the individuals admitted to their unit. Who has pneumonia? What is the common pathogen causing the pneumonia? When did these patients acquire pneumonia? Where do the patients reside in the community? How is the pathogen transmitted? Based on this information, can you determine why there is an increase? The answers to these questions provide the basis for what actions need to be taken. The answers help in the development of improved discharge planning relevant to the population they are seeing so that they may reduce readmissions. Finally, this approach leads to collaborating with other stakeholders and the community to develop a prevention strategy to reduce the number of new cases, such as promoting the provision of pneumonia vaccine to the population most at risk.

The purpose of this book is to provide nursing students with the knowledge needed to successfully answer the "who, what, when, where, why, and how" of health problems within the context of populations. This requires obtaining knowledge and skills related to public health science that the nurse then applies across practice settings. The provision of individual care alone after disease has occurred is an essential part of what nurses do. However, failure to place that care within the larger context of health as defined by the WHO reduces the profession's contribution to the promotion of optimal health for the global population. In a sense, all nurses are PHNs because our mandate is not only to provide state-of-the-art care to individuals, but also to safeguard the public's health and actively participate in the optimizing of health for all populations.

Public Health Nursing as a Specialty

Public health nursing (PHN) as a specialty is the practice of promoting and protecting the health of populations using knowledge from nursing, social, and public health sciences.[60] It is population focused, with the goals of promoting health and preventing disease and disability for all people through partnering with communities and advocating for system-level changes.[61] If we think about Winslow's classic definition of public health,[1] which focuses on prevention and promotion of health and organized community efforts, it is clear that specific educational preparation in nursing, social, and public health sciences is critical to attaining basic-level competencies. Public health nursing distinguishes itself from other nursing specialties by its adherence to eight principles outlined in an unpublished white paper by the Quad Council in 1997[62] and cited in the several editions of *Public Health Nursing: Scope and Standards of Practice*.[61] (See Box 1-8.) These principles define the client of public health nursing as the population and further delineate processes and strategies used by PHNs.

BOX 1–8	The Eight Principles of Public Health Nursing

1. The client or unit of care is the population.
2. The primary obligation is to achieve the greatest good for the greatest number of people or population as a whole.
3. The processes used by PHNs include working with the client as an equal partner.
4. PRIMARY prevention is the priority in selecting appropriate activities.
5. Public health nursing focuses on strategies that create healthy environmental, social, and economic conditions in which populations may thrive.
6. A PHN is obligated to actively identify and reach out to all who might benefit from a specific activity or service.
7. Use of available resources must be optimal to assure the best overall improvement in the health of the population.
8. Collaboration with a variety of other professions, populations, organizations, and other stakeholder groups is the most effective way to promote and protect the health of the people.

Source: Quad Council of Public Health Nursing Organizations. (1997). The tenets of public health nursing. Unpublished white paper. Cited in American Nurses Association. (In press). *Public health nursing scope and standards.* Silver Spring, MD: Nursebooks.org.

Public Health Nursing as a Core Component of Nursing History

History not only provides us with an understanding of the role of PHNs in improving the health of populations, but also gives us direction for the future. As with any other specialty in nursing, public health nursing must be seen within the historical context of the time. Health policy decisions, in particular, have a special relevance to the development of the field.

The roots of public health nursing lie in the work of women who provided comfort, care, and healing to individuals during the Middle Ages. During that time, nuns, deaconesses, and women of religious orders provided comfort and care to the sick in their homes.[63,64] In the 1500s, for example, women occupied a significant role in promoting and preserving the health of many Londoners by delivering nursing, medical, pharmaceutical, and surgical services throughout the city as a part of an organized system of health care.[65] These women were often hired by parishes, hospitals, and private individuals. Charitable nursing services in the United States were also provided by nonreligious groups, such as benevolent or ethical societies, beginning in the 1700s.[63] Untrained nurses were managed by a local board, often wealthy philanthropic ladies, who wanted to provide relief to the poor. The immediate precursor to public health nursing was district nursing, which began in England. The contributions of home visiting to improving health outcomes were recognized in 1859 by William Rathbone, a philanthropist and merchant from Liverpool. He employed a nurse to care for his wife during her terminal illness and after this experience realized that home visiting to the sick poor could benefit society. This resulted in the development of district nursing, under which towns were divided into districts and health visitors provided nursing care and education to the sick poor within those districts. In 1861, Rathbone wrote Florence Nightingale to request the development of a training school for both infirmary and district nursing, which eventually resulted in trained nurses in 18 districts of Liverpool.[66,67]

Florence Nightingale: A Health Reformer

Public health nursing owes much of its early development to Florence Nightingale, who was born in 1820 into a rich upper class British family. She is well known for the creation of a school for nursing education at St. Thomas Hospital, which established nursing as a profession. She is less known for her work as a sanitarian and social reformer.[67] She was concerned about the care of the sick poor and the quality of their homes and workhouses. She is also widely known for her work during the Crimean War, during which she kept impeccable statistical records on the living conditions of the soldiers and on the presence of disease.[67-69]

Nightingale was a promoter of health reform. She wrote extensively about nursing systems that she studied in France, Germany, Austria, and Italy.[67-70] She was instrumental in the development of district nursing and its expansion to other cities. Her writings also provide us with insight into her health-care reform efforts, which were focused on reforming workhouse infirmaries in England and on sanitary reform in India. She recognized the need for legislative changes to truly affect the health of the general population.[67]

Nightingale was also an agent of individual reform, which is perhaps evident when one views the theme of poverty in her writings.[67] She recognized the role of the nurse in depauperizing the poor, which for her was changing the state of mind of the poor.

Beginnings of Public Health Nursing in the United States

Public health nursing in the United States evolved from district nursing in England. In 1877, the New York City Mission hired Francis Root to make home visits to the sick. Other sites followed suit, and visiting nurse associations were set up in Buffalo (1885), followed by Boston and Philadelphia (1886). Trained nurses cared for the sick poor and provided instruction on improving the cleanliness of their homes. Originally these associations bore the name District Nursing Services with the Boston association referred to as the Boston Instructive District Nursing Association. Eventually they all changed their names to Visiting Nurse Associations.[71] Visiting nurse services grew, and in the beginning of the 20th century many cities, including Washington, Baltimore, and Los Angeles, provided these services through charitable agencies as well as through health departments. They were often supported by wealthy lady philanthropists, who acted as managers and provided oversight.[72,73] The evolution of visiting nurse associations from charitable organizations to that of businesses was a natural progression over time.[73]

Henry Street Settlement and Lillian Wald: In 1893, Lillian Wald and Mary Brewster established a district nursing service called the Henry Street Settlement on the Lower East Side of New York. It was here that Lillian Wald coined the term *public health nurse*.[74] Henry Street was an experiment that led to the formalization of public health nursing in the United States. It also advocated for reform. Henry Street was modeled after other settlement houses, such as Hull House in Chicago where Jane Adams led the crusade for social reform.[75]

Lillian Wald was born in 1867 in Cincinnati, Ohio, and like Florence Nightingale she grew up in a well-to-do family. She entered the New York Hospital School of Nursing and upon graduation in 1891 worked in the New York Juvenile Asylum. Discouraged with this position, she decided to teach a home nursing course for new immigrants on New York's Lower East Side, where she encountered what she described as her "baptism by fire."[76] She was led up the steps of a tenement house on Ludlow Street where she found a woman who was hemorrhaging after childbirth.[78,79] With the help of philanthropists Jacob Schiff and Mrs. Solomon Loeb, the Henry Street Settlement was purchased in 1893. This allowed Wald and Mary Brewster, her friend and colleague, to establish the Visiting Nurse Service. In her work, Wald emphasized the role that social and economic problems played in illness and developed unique programs to address the health needs of the immigrant population. "Wald's vision resulted in nursing practice that went beyond simply caring for families during illness to encompass an agenda of reform in health, industry, education, recreation, and housing."[76]

Lillian Wald's accomplishments were many and often carried out through partnerships. She collaborated with the Metropolitan Life Insurance Company, which decided to provide home nursing to its policyholders. On the basis of high absenteeism in schools, Wald talked the Commissioner of Health in New York City into trying a school nurse demonstration project that allowed a school nurse, Lina Rogers, to work in the schools, thus leading the way for the development of school nursing.[80] She collaborated with the American Red Cross to provide public health nursing in small towns and rural districts, resulting in nearly 3,000 American Red Cross public health nursing service locations during the 1920s.[76]

The success of Wald in her work is attributed to her effective leadership, assertive management, and knowledge of power structures.[79] Poverty was increasingly seen as a cause of social problems and poor health in communities. Wald believed that environmental and social conditions were the causes of ill health and poverty.[78,82] In the early 1900s, social reform was viewed as an attack on institutions and structures. For Lillian Wald and her colleagues, efforts of social reform were focused on civil rights for minorities, voting rights for women, the prevention of war, child labor laws, and unsafe working conditions.[63] Wald and colleagues were successful at influencing the development of the federal Children's Bureau, which was founded in 1912 to fund and support child welfare services. In addition, the Sheppard-Towner Act was passed in 1921, which actually provided the federal funds for maternal and infant care.

Public Health Nursing in the 20th Century

Wald's accomplishments were the background for the development of the public health nursing specialty. At the turn of the 19th century, the average life expectancy in the United States was 47.3 years. In 2010, the life expectancy was 78.7 years; Hispanic females had the longest life expectancy (83.6 years), followed by non-Hispanic white females (81.1), Hispanic males (78.8), white males (76.4 years), and black males (71.4 years)[83,84] (Figs. 1-6 and 1-7). In 1950, the infant mortality rate was 29.8 per 1,000 births. By 2011, it had dropped to 6.1 per 1,000 births[84] (see Chapter 18). These extraordinary achievements in population health are largely the result of public health efforts, especially the reduction in the incidence of acute communicable diseases. Public health efforts taken in the early part of the 20th century made

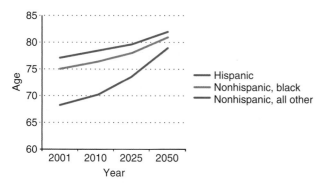

Figure 1-6 Life expectancy in the United States, 2001 to 2050, for males by race. *(From the National Vital Statistics System, Mortality, Centers for Disease Control and Prevention.)*

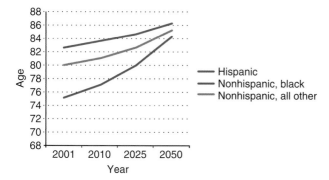

Figure 1-7 Life expectancy in the United States, 2001 to 2050, for females by race. *(From the National Vital Statistics System, Mortality, Centers for Disease Control and Prevention.)*

great strides in reducing disease, especially owing to advances related to the provision of potable water, regulations around food and milk supply, removal of garbage, and disposal of sewage. However, authorities realized that they needed to implement other programs to work on improving health education among those most at risk, especially the poor. PHNs filled this need and provided care to the sick while educating families on personal hygiene and healthy practices.[73]

The visiting nurse movement, with a focus on caring for the sick poor, joined forces with public health to focus on prevention. According to Buhler-Wilkerson, "By 1910, the majority of the large urban visiting nurse associations had initiated preventive programs for school children, infants, mothers, and patients with tuberculosis."[73] In the United States, Dr. William Welch singled out public health nursing as the America's greatest contribution to the public health movement.[71] Winslow described this provision of direct services to the impoverished as "the Health Center Movement." He described it as the provision "of free public services for the examination of well people or of people who suspect the presence of disease, for their hygienic instruction and for the administration of preventive medical treatment or reference to private physicians or to institutions where such treatment can be secured."[15] This included conducting prenatal clinics, infant welfare stations, school services, tuberculosis clinics, venereal disease clinics (sexually transmitted infections), mental hygiene clinics, heart clinics, and cancer clinics. These endeavors continued until the 1990s, when managed care organizations assumed responsibilities for many of these populations and duties.

Two methods of funding new programs existed in the 19th century and at the beginning of the 20th century. Joint ventures between nursing associations and voluntary agencies were created in which nursing associations provided the nurses and the voluntary agencies provided the money for projects. The other method was a demonstration project, in which the nursing agencies initiated a project on a small scale using their own money, hoping to prove its value. School nursing is the best illustration of this.[73]

The initiation and growth of health departments took place in the latter part of the 19th century. In fact, by 1900, 38 states had established health departments.[85] Local governments, state governments, and boards of health hired more nurses and by 1924, 54% of all PHNs worked for official or government agencies.[86] With time, there was a growing number of services being offered by both voluntary and "official" government agencies, leading to some conflict and confusion about roles. As a consequence of these divisions, sick nursing became the sole domain of the voluntary organizations, while the teaching of prevention became the responsibilities of official agencies.[73]

Public health nursing continued to grow with the expansion of the federal government. During the 1930s, the hiring of local PHNs increased.[87] The Social Security Act of 1935 provided funding for expanded opportunities in health protection and promotion, resulting in the employment of PHNs, increased education for nurses in public health, the establishment of health services, and research. World War II accelerated the need for nurses both for the war effort and at home.

In the 1960s, health policy had a strong impact on the development of the field. In 1965, Congress revised the Social Security Act, resulting in the passage of Medicare and Medicaid. Medicare is the U.S. government's health insurance program for people age 65 or older, while Medicaid is funded by the federal and state governments and pays for medical care for those who cannot afford it. This content can be found online at http://www.investorwords.com/3032/Medicaid.html.

These regulations actually resulted in many local and state health departments changing their policies to allow agencies to provide reimbursable home care for existing illness, often resulting in a reduction in the delivery of interventions aimed at health promotion and disease prevention.[87]

In the 1960s and 1970s, there were also many social changes addressing poverty and concern for various aspects of preventive health. These resulted in increased funding for neighborhood health centers, Head Start programs, mental health agencies, mental retardation assistance programs, maternal–child health programs, and community health training. By the 1980s, however, there was a shift again in funding to more acute services, medical procedures, and long-term care. The use of health maintenance organizations was encouraged. By the latter part of the 1980s, public health as a whole had declined and the percentage of PHNs working as government employees had dropped to 40%.[87,88]

Public Health Nursing Today

During the 20th century, nursing played a significant role in the evolution of public health practice and the health achievements that occurred in the United States As noted by the CDC, the public often views public health as the provision of care to the underserved. In reality, public health's overarching goal relates to the promotion of optimal health in populations. In 1926, C.E. Winslow described the achievements of public health from 1875 to 1925.[15] During this 50-year span, the fundamental public health problems were communicable diseases and environmental health. In 1875, the leading causes of death were pulmonary tuberculosis, acute respiratory diseases, infant diarrhea, and diphtheria and croup. Public health efforts focused on sanitary engineering, bacteriology, and personal hygiene.

In 1999, the Centers for Disease Control and Prevention[89] reported on the 10 great public health achievements over the past century (Box 1-9). These included immunizations, fluoridation of water, and workplace safety. The implementation of childhood vaccination programs resulted in the eradication of smallpox and the banishment of mumps and chickenpox from schools in the United States. Without an active public health infrastructure, the marked increases in life expectancy in the 20th century would not have occurred. The public health achievements of the 20th century establish the necessity of a strong public health infrastructure. However, public health cannot rest on its laurels.

Based on a report completed by the Health Resources and Services Administration on the registered nurse population in the United States, PHNs were the third largest category of workers in nursing after hospitals and ambulatory care.[90] In 2008, it was estimated that 7.8% of all nurses in the United States worked in public or community health settings, a drop from 10.7% in 2004. By 2012, only 2% of nurses surveyed worked in a community/public setting.[91] Settings included state or local health departments, community-based home health agencies, various types of community health centers, student health services, and occupational health services. Of these, the majority were employed in home health and school health, followed by state and local health departments. In home care, the focus is on providing care to ill, injured, or disabled individuals, in contrast to an emphasis on prevention and populations.

BOX 1–9	**Top 10 Public Health Achievements**

1. Immunizations
2. Motor vehicle safety
3. Workplace safety
4. Control of communicable diseases
5. Declines in deaths from health disease and stroke
6. Safer and healthier foods
7. Healthier mothers and babies
8. Family planning
9. Fluoridation of drinking water
10. Tobacco as a health hazard

Source: See reference 89.

There are many challenges overall for the public health workforce. Public health practice is influenced by legislative and environmental factors that influence the political will to support the public health infrastructure. Following September 11, 2001, for example, heightened attention to emergency preparedness stimulated an increase in funding for workforce preparedness and training, resulting in an increase in the funding for emergency preparedness.[92] The challenge remains, however, in the production and retention of the workforce. In fact, the Quad Council of Public Health Nursing Organizations, an alliance of four national nursing organizations including the American Nurses Association (ANA), Association of Community Health Nurse Educators (ACHNE), American Public Health Association—Public Health Nursing Section (APHA), and the Association of Public Health Nurses (APHN) (formerly the Association of State and Territorial Directors of Nursing) published a report in 2007 outlining the impact of the nursing shortage on the public health system.[93] In 1980, the number of PHNs made up 39% of the public health workforce; by 2000, that percentage had decreased to 17.6%.[92] The trends pointing to more shortages include:

- A rapidly aging workforce whose average age is 46.6 years
- Public health retirement rates as high as 45%
- Current vacancy rates up to 20% in some states
- Public health employment turnover rates of 14% in some parts of the country

PHNs face other challenges as well, including emerging and reemerging infections, the organization of health care, and how to work more effectively for social betterment.[85] Within the nursing profession, there has been a great deal of controversy about the concept of advanced community/public health nursing, because most state nurse practice organizations do not include population skills in their definition of advanced practice.[94] This has resulted in a redefining of the advanced public health nursing role. The most important challenge, though, is that of improving the health of people and communities overall, which of course requires more preventive actions and a focus on providing health promotion and primary prevention within the community, not merely interventions focused on secondary or tertiary levels of care. Close to a decade ago, Robertson wrote about the role of advanced PHNs: "Societal trends and predicted needs of the health care system indicate that there will be increasing demands for health care professionals who can effectively manage the health needs of populations and communities."[94] Based on our history and visionary leaders, there is no better group to do this than PHNs.

Now in the 21st century, we face new challenges in the public health infrastructure. As a result of advancements in transportation and information technology, we are now a global society. With these technological advancements, terrorist activities span the globe. New infectious agents such as HIV/AIDS are easily shared across national borders and oceans. With national economies tied to one another, the economic stability of one nation no longer stands alone. Finally, changes in the earth's climate occur globally, affecting the quality of the air we breathe, the food we eat, and the water we drink.

Public Health Nursing Scope and Standards of Practice

The development of the specialty of public health nursing is reflected not only in its history but also in the development of standards of practice. The standards, functions, and qualifications for PHNs were first prepared in 1931 by the Subcommittee on Functions of the National Organization for Public Health Nursing.[72] Many revisions have occurred since then, but the latest is *Public Health Nursing: Scope and Standards of Practice*, an ANA document published in 2013, which outlines the expectations of the professional role of the PHN and sets the framework for public health nursing practice in the 21st century.[61] This document is the result of a volunteer work group of public health nursing stakeholders who revised the 2007 *Scope and Standards of Public Health Nursing Practice* and is adapted from the template language of *Nursing: Scope and Standards of Practice*.[95] The document clearly reflects the work of PHNs in improving health by focusing on populations.

Public Health Nursing Standards

There are six standards of practice that describe a competent level of care using the nursing process (Box 1-10): (1) Assessment, (2) Population Diagnosis and Priorities, (3) Outcomes Identification, (4) Planning, (5) Implementation, and (6) Evaluation. Specific standards related to implementation include the coordination of care, health teaching and health promotion, consultation, and regulatory activities. These standards of practice are differentiated for the PHN and the advanced PHN. There are 11 Standards of Professional Performance (see Box 1-10).

Public Health Nursing Competencies

The *Scope and Standards of Practice* delineates competencies for practice and these competencies are based on the ANA nursing framework assuring that public health nursing fits as a recognized nursing specialty. In addition, the Council of Linkages Between Academia and Public Health Practice, a coalition of organizations concerned with the public health workforce, produced

BOX 1–10	**Standards of Public Health Nursing Practice**

Standard 1. ASSESSMENT
The PHN collects comprehensive data pertinent to the health status of populations.
Standard 2. DIAGNOSIS
The PHN analyzes the assessment data to determine the diagnoses or issues.
Standard 3. OUTCOMES IDENTIFICATION
The PHN identifies expected outcomes for a plan specific to the population or situation.
Standard 4. PLANNING
The PHN develops a plan that prescribes strategies and alternatives to attain expected outcomes.
Standard 5. IMPLEMENTATION
The PHN implements the identified plan.
Standard 5A. COORDINATION OF CARE
The PHN coordinates care delivery.
Standard 5B. HEALTH TEACHING AND HEALTH PROMOTION
The PHN employs multiple strategies to promote health and a safe environment.
Standard 5C. CONSULTATION
The PHN provides consultation to influence the identified plan, enhance the abilities of others, and effect change.
Standard 5D. PRESCRIPTIVE AUTHORITY
The advanced practice registered nurse *practicing in the public health setting* uses prescriptive authority, procedures, referrals, treatments, and therapies in accordance with state and federal laws and regulations.
Standard 5E. REGULATORY ACTIVITIES
The PHN participates in applications of public health laws, regulations, and policies.
Standard 6. EVALUATION
The PHN evaluates progress toward attainment of outcomes.

Standard 7. ETHICS
The PHN practices ethically.
Standard 8. EDUCATION
The PHN attains knowledge and competence that reflect current nursing practice.
Standard 9. EVIDENCE-BASED PRACTICE AND RESEARCH
The PHN integrates evidence and research findings into practice.
Standard 10. QUALITY OF PRACTICE
The PHN contributes to quality nursing practice.
Standard 11. COMMUNICATION
The PHN communicates effectively in a variety of formats in all areas of practice.
Standard 12. LEADERSHIP
The PHN demonstrates leadership in the professional practice setting and the profession.
Standard 13. COLLABORATION
The PHN collaborates with the population, and others in the conduct of nursing practice.
Standard 14. PROFESSIONAL PRACTICE EVALUATION
The PHN evaluates her or his own nursing practice in relation to professional practice standards and guidelines, relevant statutes, rules, and regulations.
Standard 15. RESOURCE UTILIZATION
The PHN utilizes appropriate resources to plan and provide nursing and public health services that are safe, effective, and financially responsible.
Standard 16. ENVIRONMENTAL HEALTH
The PHN practices in an environmentally safe, fair, and just manner.
Standard 17. ADVOCACY
The PHN advocates for the protection of the health, safety, and rights of the population.

Source: See reference 61.

a document in 2001 that has been used as a framework for the development of additional public health nursing competencies. The Quad Council, developed the first version of these competencies in 2004[96] and in 2011 updated them to align better with the public health competencies from the Council on Linkages.[97] The 2011 revised version of the PHN Core Competencies incorporates three tiers of practice: Basic or generalist (Tier 1); Specialist or mid-level (Tier 2); and Executive and/or multisystem level (Tier 3). In addition, there are eight domains that include:

1. Analytic assessment
2. Policy development/program planning
3. Communication
4. Cultural competency
5. Community dimensions of practice
6. Basic public health science
7. Financial planning and management
8. Leadership and systems thinking

These competencies are intended to reflect the standards for public health nursing practice.

In addition to the public health nursing competencies published by the Quad Council, other competencies exist for specific roles in public health or public health nursing. Preparing public health professionals for emergency response, for example, has received much attention with the growing attention to bioterrorism and emerging communicable diseases.[98-100]

Public Health Nursing Roles and Responsibilities

Ruth Freeman, a public health nursing leader in the 1970s, claimed that the role of the PHN is dependent on perceptions of the role and specifically what the professional organizations deem appropriate for the role.[101] The Subcommittee on Functions from the National Organization for Public Health Nursing outlined the functions, standards, and qualifications of PHNs in 1931. This was subsequently revised in 1955 to include (1) Functions relating to public health nursing care to individuals, families, and groups; and (2) functions relating to the development and operation of the agency, school, and community health program.[72]

The 2013 *Standards and Scope of Practice of Public Health Nursing* clearly outlines the functions of PHNs in relationship to populations. Selective standards are highlighted to provide further insight into the roles of PHNs.

Coordination, Consultation, and Leadership: A PHN is responsible for coordinating programs, services, and other activities to implement an identified plan.[60] The recognition of the need for a coordinated system of care to follow up medical health problems of adolescents admitted to juvenile services is an example. The advanced PHN provides the leadership to actually integrate the delivery of services and possibly initiate public policy changes to assure health.

A PHN acts as a consultant when he or she is able to work with community organizations or groups to develop a local health fair or is able to provide the latest information about a communicable disease outbreak to the community. At the advanced level, a PHN provides expert testimony at the federal or state level about a health promotion program. Evidence of leadership is exemplified in a variety of ways. For example, a PHN can serve as the leader in coalition-building efforts around a health issue such as teen smoking prevention or promoting healthy community and work environments.

Advocacy: Advocacy is concerned with the unique responsibility of all PHNs to act as spokespeople for those who have no voice or are unable to address their own health-care concerns.[61] Assisting families living in poverty to access appropriate services is one example of an important role of PHNs. Another example of advocacy is engaging in strategies to affect policy at the local, state, or national level. Strategies that PHNs use to address structural inequities and to promote change often include community discussions about poverty and its effect on families, putting the issues of poverty on the agenda of professional associations, working for the development of policies that decrease poverty, and empowering the community with information and resources to challenge the causes of poverty.[102]

Health Education and Health Promotion: The PHN uses many strategies to promote health, prevent disease, and ensure a safe environment (e.g., appropriate health education efforts and services for populations). This includes selecting teaching and learning methods, presenting the information in a culturally competent manner, implementing the health education program and evaluating the effectiveness of the program by and collecting feedback from participants. For example, PHNs developed material on how to reduce exposure to West Nile virus and distributed it to the public. At an advanced level, the PHN provides the leadership to plan and implement these programs and services.

Regulatory Activities: Since the beginnings of public health nursing, health policy has been an important aspect of practice. Responsibilities include identifying, interpreting, and implementing public health laws, regulations, and policies.[61] Activities include monitoring and inspecting regulated entities such as nursing homes. It also includes educating the public on relevant laws, regulations, and policies. At an advanced level, it includes revising public health laws or by actually participating in the development of new laws. At the state level, nurses in roles of chief nurse or nursing director take part in health policy debates.[103]

Ongoing Education and Practice Evaluation: Standard 8 of *Public Health Nursing: Scope and Standards of Practice.* states that the PHN attains knowledge and assures competency in nursing practice. PHNs are responsible for maintaining and enhancing their knowledge and skills necessary to promote population health. This requires PHNs to take the initiative to seek experiences that develop and maintain their competence as PHNs. Standard 6 states that PHNs evaluate their own practice using practice standards, guidelines, statutes, rules, and regulations.[61] This requires that PHNs engage in self-evaluation, seek feedback about performance, and implement plans for accomplishing one's own goals and work plans.

Professional Relationships and Collaboration: The establishment of effective partnerships is the mechanism for moving the public health agenda forward. This requires collaborating with populations/communities, organizations, and health and human service professionals.[61] An example of an effective partnership is that of nurses in a health department joining with other human service providers to develop an effective method for promoting cancer prevention through public service announcements. Another example is that of PHNs providing information to health-care providers in primary care related to prevention of flu transmission to share with their patients. PHNs seek collegial partnerships with peers, students, and colleagues as a means of enhancing public health interventions.

Public Health Nursing Ethics

Public health nursing is grounded in both nursing ethics and public health ethics. PHNs apply the *Code of Ethics for Nurses With Interpretive Statements* to practice.[104] The principles guiding any ethical discourse in nursing include autonomy, dignity, and rights of individuals. Assuring confidentiality and applying ethical standards are critical in advocating for health and social policy. Equally important to any discussion of public health ethics is the fact that public health is concerned with the public good, which can override individual rights. This is evident in the enforcement of laws that are aimed at the whole population, (e.g., immunizations, disease reporting, or quarantines).[105] Social justice is the basis of public health and public health nursing practice and is defined in the *Scope and Standards of Public Health Nursing* as

> the principle that all persons are entitled to have their basic human needs met, regardless of differences in economic status, class, gender, race, ethnicity, citizenship, religion, age, sexual orientation, disability, or health. This includes the eradication of poverty and illiteracy, the establishment of sound environmental policy, and equality of opportunity for healthy personal and social development.[61]

Serious disparities in health exist in the United States and at the global level, which can be seen by comparing life expectancies between high-income countries and low-income countries. For example, estimated life expectancy in 2014 in Monaco was 89.6 years, whereas in Chad it was 49 years.[106] To address these disparities public health as a science is shifting from the traditional way of addressing bioethics as it related to population health that focused on dramatic cases to a focus on existing disparities and the underlying social determinants of health, such as poverty.[107]

For example, although decent affordable housing is often overlooked, it is the building block of healthy neighborhoods and shapes the health of individuals, families, and communities.[108]

The mission of public health is to assure and protect the health of the public. This underscores the inherent moral imperative of public health that carries with it certain responsibilities. According to one authority, "It [public health] carries with it an obligation to care for the well-being of others and it implies the possession of an element of power in order to carry out the mandate. The need to exercise power to ensure health and at the same time to avoid the potential abuses of power are at the crux of public health ethics."[24]

Discussions among our legislators in Washington, DC, often include the term *moral imperative*. The call to address the 47 million people who were uninsured in our country resulted in the passing of the Affordable Care Act in 2010. There are other policy-level efforts that aim at addressing the health needs of children at the national and global levels. For example, there are efforts being made to address the public health effects of global climate change. The WHO reports that the change in global climate "has the potential to affect human health in a number of ways, for instance by altering the geographical range and seasonality of certain communicable diseases, disturbing food-producing ecosystems, and increasing the frequency of extreme weather events, such as hurricanes."[109] Understanding that the health of individuals is closely tied to the health of populations is key to the success of the work that nurses do as a key component in the promotion of optimal health for all.

Thus, public health encompasses efforts to improve the health of populations from the local level all the way to the global level. Gone are the days when each community could independently decide how it would work to ensure the health of its own population. Increasingly, our own health is dependent on the health of not only our direct neighbors, but also on the health of all. Public health provides us with the means to build a healthy environment and respond to threats to our health from nature and to those that are manmade. Nursing is a key component within public health, whether the nurse works directly for a public health department or not. The goal of nursing is to help people achieve optimal health, which ultimately requires understanding the health of the population because no one's health is totally under the control of the individual.

■ Summary Points

- Public health encompasses efforts to improve the health of populations from the local level all the way to the global level.
- Public health provides us with the means to build a healthy environment and respond to threats to our health from nature and from those that are man-made.
- Public health nursing has a rich history and has contributed to the overall health of populations.
- Nursing is a key component within public health, whether or not the nurse works directly for a public health department.
- The goal of nursing is to help people achieve optimal health, which ultimately requires understanding the health of the population because no one's health is totally under the control of the individual.

▲ CASE STUDY
Smoke-Free Ordinances and Heart Attacks
Learning Outcomes

The case study and problem-based learning activity will help the student:

- Gain understanding of the science of public health from a local to a global perspective
- Describe the role of environment and culture in the health of populations
- Define the practice of public health nursing

In 2009, the CDC reported that a smoke-free ordinance resulted in a reduction in acute myocardial infarction (AMI) admissions to hospitals in Pueblo, Colorado. In addition to the initial reduction in AMIs, the decrease in AMI admissions continued over time. Based on these findings, the CDC recommended that smoke-free policies are an important component of interventions to prevent heart disease morbidity and mortality. Access the *MMWR* article at http://www.cdc.gov/mmwr/preview/mmwrhtml/mm5751a1.htm and then answer the following questions:

1. Is this an example of an individual-, family-, community-, or population-level intervention and why?
2. At what level is this intervention feasible: local, state, national, and/or global?
3. A PHN in your city or town decides to get involved in implementing a similar intervention. What role would the nurse play and how does it fit into the public health nurse scope of practice?

REFERENCES

1. Winslow, C.E.A. (1920). The untilled field of public health. *Modern Medicine, 2,* 183-191.
2. Turnock, B.J. (2004). *Public health: What it is and how it works.* Sudbury, MA: Jones & Bartlett
3. Warnecke, R.B., Oh, A., Breen, N., et al. (2008). Approaching health disparities from a population perspective: The national Institutes of Health Centers for Population Health and Health Disparities. *American Journal of Public Health, 98*(9), 1608-1615.
4. World Health Organization. (2014). *About WHO.* Retrieved from http://www.who.int/about/en/.
5. Issel, L.M. (2008). *Health program and evaluation: A practical, systematic approach for community health* (2nd ed.). Sudbury, MA: Jones & Bartlett. .
6. Institute of Medicine. (1988). *The future of public health.* Washington, DC: National Academies Press.
7. Centers for Disease Control and Prevention, National Public Health Performance Standards Program (NPHPSP). (2013). *The public health system and ten essential public health services.* Retrieved from http://www.cdc.gov/od/ocphp/nphpsp/essentialphservices.htm.
8. Institute of Medicine. (2003). *The future of the public's health in the twenty-first century.* Washington, DC: National Academies Press.
9. US Department of Health and Human Services, Healthy People 2020. (2014). *Public health infrastructure.* Retrieved from http://www.healthypeople.gov/2020/topicsobjectives2020/overview.aspx?topicId=35.
10. Burkle, F.M., & Greenough, P.G. (2008). Impact of public health emergencies on modern disaster taxonomy, planning, and response. *Disaster Medicine Public Health Prep, 293,* 192-199.
11. Yach, D., & Bettcher, D. (1998). The globalization of public health, I. Threats and opportunities. *American Journal of Public Health, 88*(5), 735-738.
12. Institute of Medicine, Hernandez, L.(Ed) (2003). *Who will keep the public healthy? Workshop summary.* Washington, DC, National Academies Press.
13. Thompson, A.K., Faith, K., Gibson, J.L., & Upshur, R.E. (2006). Pandemic influenza preparedness: An ethical framework to guide decision-making. *BMC Medical Ethics, 7,* E12.
14. Baker, M.G., & Fidler, D.P. (2006). Global public health surveillance under new international health regulations. *Emerging Infectious Diseases, 12*(7), 1058-1065.
15. Winslow, C.E. (1926). Public health at the crossroads. *American Journal of Public Health, 89*(11), 1075-1085. Reprinted in *American Journal of Public Health, 89*(11), 1645-1648.
16. Shibuya, K., Ciecierski, C., Guindon, E., Bettcher, D.W., Evans, D.B., & Murray, C. (2003). WHO framework convention on tobacco control: Development of an evidence based global public health treaty. *BMJ, 327,* 154-157.
17. American Nurses Association. (2007). *Public health nursing: Scope and standards of practice.* Silver Spring, MD: Nursesbooks.org.

18. Dahlgren, G., & Whitehead, M. (1991). *Policies and strategies to promote social equity in health.* Stockholm, Sweden: Institute for the Futures Studies.

19. Institute of Medicine (2003) *The Future of the Public's Health in the 21st Century.* Washington, DC: National Academies Press.

20. Bauer, G., Davies, J.K., Pelikan, J., Noack, H., Broesskamp, U., & Hill, C. (2003). Advancing a theoretical model for public health and health promotion indicator development: Proposal from the EUHPID consortium. *European Journal of Public Health, 13*(3s), 107-113.

21. Institute of Medicine. (2000). *Promoting health: Intervention strategies from social and behavioral research.* Washington, DC: National Academies Press.

22. Fallon, L. F., & Zgodzinski, E.J. (2005). *Essentials of public health management.* Sudbury, MA: Jones & Bartlett.

23. Rowitz, L. (2006). *Public health for the 21st century: The prepared leader.* Sudbury, MA: Jones & Bartlett.

24. Public Health Leadership Society. (2002). *Principles of ethical practice of public health.* Retrieved from http://www.apha.org/NR/rdonlyres/1CED3CEA-287E-4185-9CBD-BD405FC60856/0/ethicsbrochure.pdf.

25. Stover, G.N & Bassett, M.T. (2003). Practice is the purpose of public health. *American Journal of Public Health, 93*(11), 1799-1801.

26. Spencer, D.J. (2006). CDC's 60th anniversary: Director's perspective. *Morbidity and Mortality Weekly Report, 55*(27), 745-749.

27. Centers for Disease Control and Prevention. (2014). *About CDC: Mission goal and pledge.* Retrieved from http://www.cdc.gov/about/organization/mission.htm.

28. United States Department of Health and Human Services Healthy People 2020. (2014). *About Healthy People 2020.* Retrieved from http://www.healthypeople.gov/2020/about/default.aspx.

29. United States Department of Health and Human Services, Healthy People 2020. (2014). *Leading health indicators.* Retrieved from http://www.healthypeople.gov/2020/LHI/default.aspx.

30. World Health Organization. (2014). *The role of the WHO in public health.* Retrieved from http://www.who.int/about/role/en/index.html.

31. Cueto, I.M. (2004). The origins of primary health care and selective primary health care. *American Journal of Public Health, 94*(11), 1864-1874.

32. Hoosen-Coovadia, R.B. (2008). From Alma-Alta to Agincourt: Primary health care in AIDS. *The Lancet, 372,* 866-868.

33. World Health Organization. (2014). *Health in the millennium development goals.* Retrieved from http://www.who.int/mdg/goals/en/print.html.

34. Caldwell, J. (1996). Demography and social science. *Population Studies, 50,* 1-34.

35. World Health Organization (1948). *The WHO definition of health.* Preamble to the Constitution of the World Health Organization. Retrieved from http://who.int/about/definition/en/print.html.

36. Allen, J.D., Stanley, J., Crabtree, M.K., & Werner, K.E. (2005). Clinical prevention and population health curriculum framework: The nursing perspective. *Journal of Professional Nursing, 21*(5), 259-267.

37. Schneider, M.J. (2011). *Introduction to public health.* Sudbury, MA: Jones & Bartlett.

38. MacQueen, K.M., McLellan, E, Metzger, D.S., Kegeles, S., Strauss, R.P., Trotter, R.T. (2001). What is community? An Evidence-based definition for participatory public health. *American Journal of Public Health, 91*(12), 1929-1938.

39. Kindig, D., & Stoddart, G. (2003). What is population health? *American Journal of Public Health, 93*(3), 380-383.

40. The Institute of Medicine. (2010). *The future of nursing: Leading change, advancing health.* Retrieved from http://www.iom.edu/Reports/2010/The-Future-of-Nursing-Leading-Change-Advancing-Health.aspx#.

41. Whitehead, D. (2006). Health promotion in the practice setting: Findings from review of clinical issues. *Worldviews on Evidenced-Based Nursing, 4th Quarter, 3*(4), 165-184.

42. Brubaker, B.H. (1983). Health promotion: A linguistic analysis. *Advances in Nursing, 2,* 1-14.

43. Casey, D. (2007). Nurses' perception, understanding and experiences of health promotion. *Journal of Clinical Nursing, 16,* 1039-1049.

44. O'Donnell, M.P. (2008). Evolving definition of health promotion: What do you think? *American Journal of Health Promotion, 23*(2), iv.

45. Kok, G., Gottlieb, N.H., Commers, M., & Smerecnik, C. (2008). The ecological approach to health promotion programs: A decade later. *American Journal of Health Promotion, 22*(6), 437-442.

46. Racher, F. E., & Annis, R.C. (2008). Community Health Action Model: Health promotion by the community. *Research and Theory for Nursing Practice: An International Journal, 22*(3), 182-191.

47. Irvine, F. (2007). Examining the correspondence of theoretical and real interpretations of health promotion. *Journal of Clinical Nursing, 16*(3), 593-602.

48. Spector, R.E. (2004). *Cultural diversity in health and illness* (6th ed.). Upper Saddle River, NJ: Pearson.

49. O'Neill, D. (2006). The nature of ethnicity. Retrieved from http://anthro.palomar.edu/ethnicity/ethnic_2.htm.

50. Humes, K.R, Jones, N.R, Ramirez, R.R. (2011). *Overview of race and Hispanic origin: 2010. 2010 Census Briefs.* Retrieved from http://www.census.gov/prod/cen2010/briefs/c2010br-02.pdf.

51. U.S. Census Bureau. (2013). *What is race?* Retrieved from http://www.census.gov/population/race/.

52. Morganthau, T. (1995, February 13). What color is black? *Newsweek,* 62-69.

53. Murphy, N. (2008). An agenda for health promotion. *Nursing Ethics, 15*(5), 697-699.

54. MacDonald, M.A. (2004). From miasma to fractals: The epidemiology revolution and public health nursing. *Public Health Nursing, 21*(4), 380-381.

55. Sommers, J. (1989). *Soho—a history of London's most colorful neighborhood* (pp 113-117). London, England: Bloomsbury.

56. Diem, E., & Moyer, A. (2005). *Community health nursing projects: Making a difference.* Philadelphia, PA: Lippincott Williams & Wilkins.

57. Prochaska, J.O., & Velicer, W.F. (1997). The transtheoretical model of health behavior change. *American Journal of Health Promotion, 12,* 38-48.

58. Institute for the Study of Healthcare Organizations & Transactions. (2004). *Health and behavior.* Retrieved from http://www.institute-shot.com/health_and_behavior.htm.

59. Keller, L.O., Strohschein, S., Lia-Hoagberg, B., & Schaffer, M.A. (2004). Population-based public health interventions: Practice-based and evidence-supported, part 1. *Public Health Nursing, 21*(5), 453-468.

60. American Public Health Association. Public Health Nursing Section. (2013). *The definition and practice of public health nursing: A statement of the Public Health Nursing Section.* Washington, DC: Author.

61. American Nursing Association. (2013). *Public health nursing: Scope and standards of practice.* Silver Spring, MD: Nursesbooks.org.

62. Quad Council of Public Health Nursing Organizations. (1997). *The tenets of public health nursing.* Unpublished white paper.

63. Bekemeier, B. (2007). A history of public health and public health nursing. In L. Ivanov & C. Blue (Eds.), *Public health nursing: Leadership, policy, and practice* (pp 2-26). Clifton Park, NY: Thomson Delmar Learning.

64. Fissell, M.E. (2008). Introduction: Woman, health, and healing in early modern Europe. *Bulletin of the History of Medicine, 82*(1), 1-17.

65. Harkness, D. E. (2008). A view from the streets: Women and medical work in Elizabethan London. *Bulletin of the History of Medicine, 82*(1), 52-85.

66. Brainard, A.M. (1922). *The evolution of public health nursing.* New York, NY: Garland.

67. Monteiro, L.A. (1985). Florence Nightingale on public health nursing. *American Journal of Nursing, 75*(2), 181-186.

68. Malpas, P. (2006). Florence Nightingale: Appreciating our legacy, envisioning our future. *Gastroenterology Nursing, 29*(6), 447-452.

69. Gill, C.J., & Gill, G.C. (2005). Nightingale in Scutari: Her legacy reexamined. *Clinical Infectious Diseases, 40*(12), 1799-1805.

70. Dock, L.L., & Stewart, I.M. (1925*). A short history of nursing: From the earliest times to the present day.* New York, NY: G.P. Putnam's Sons.

71. Doona, M.E. (1994). Gertrude Weld Peabody: Unsung patron of public health nursing education. *Nursing & Health Care, 15*(2), 88-94.

72. Hanlon, J. (1964). *Principles of public health administration.* Saint Louis, MO: C.V. Mosby.

73. Buhler-Wilkerson, K. (1989). *The rise and decline of public health nursing—1900–1930.* New York, NY: Garland.

74. Buhler-Wilkerson, K. (1985). Public health nursing: In sickness or in health? *American Journal of Public Health, 75,* 1155-1161.

75. Brodie, B. (1994). From charity to business: Community health nursing, 1900–1926. *Nursing Connections, 7*(1), 35-43.

76. Buhler-Wilkerson, K. (1993). Bringing care to the people: Lillian Wald's legacy to public health nursing. *American Journal of Public Health, 83*(12), 1778-1786.

77. Brown, V.B. (2001). Jane Adams. In Schultz, R.L., & Hast, A. (Eds.), *Women building Chicago 1790–1990: A biographical dictionary.* Bloomington: Indiana University Press.

78. Jewish Women's Archive. (2009). *JWA—Lillian Wald—introduction.* Retrieved from http://jwa.org/womenofvalor/wald/.

79. Frachel, R.R. (1988). A new profession: The evolution of public health nursing. *Public Health Nursing, 5*(2), 86-90.

80. Silverstein, N.G. (1985). Lillian Wald at Henry Street, 1893–1895. *Advances in Nursing Science, 7*(2), 1-12.

81. Vessey, J.A., & McGowan, K.A. (2006). A successful public health experiment: School nursing. *Pediatric Nursing, 32*(3), 255-256.

82. Reisch, M., & Andrews, J. (2001). *The road not taken: A history of radical social work in the United States.* Philadelphia, PA: Brunner-Routledge.

83. Centers for Disease Control and Prevention. (2012). *NCHS data brief: Death in the United States 2010.* Retrieved from http://www.cdc.gov/nchs/data/databriefs/db99.htm#How.

84. Hoyert, D.L., & Xu, J. (2012). Death: Preliminary data for 2011. *National Vital Statistics Report, 61*(6) 1-51. Retrieved from http://www.cdc.gov/nchs/data/nvsr/nvsr61/nvsr61_06.pdf.

85. Hanlon, J.J., & Pickett, G.E. (Eds.). (1984). *Public health: Administration and practice* (8th ed.). St. Louis, MO: Mosby.

86. Tattershall, L. (1926). Census of public health nursing in the United States. *Public Health Nurse, 18,* 266.

87. Dieckmann, J. (2008). History of public health and public and community health nursing. In M. Stanhope & J. Lancaster (Eds.), *Public health nursing: Population-centered health in the community* (pp 22-45). Toronto, Ontario, Canada: Elsevier.

88. Smith, C. (2009). Origins and future of community/public health nursing. In F. Maurer & C. Smith (Eds.), *Community/public health nursing practice* (pp 31-54). Toronto, Ontario, Canada: Elsevier.

89. Centers for Disease Control and Prevention. (1999). Ten great public health achievements in the 20th century. *Morbidity and Mortality Weekly Report, 48,* 241-243.

90. U.S. Department of Health and Human Services, Health Resources and Services Administration. (2010). *The registered nurse population: Initial findings from the 2008 National Sample Survey of Registered Nurses.* http://bhpr.hrsa.gov/healthworkforce/rnsurveys/rnsurveyfinal.pdf

91. AMN Healthcare (2012). *2012 survey of registered nurses.* Retrieved from http://www.amnhealthcare.com/uploadedFiles/MainSite/Content/Healthcare_Industry_Insights/Industry_Research/AMN%202012%20RN%20Survey.pdf.

92. Centers for Disease Control and Prevention, Office of Public Health Preparedness and Response. (2013). *Funding and guidance for state and local health departments.* Retrieved from http://www.cdc.gov/phpr/coopagreement.htm.

93. Quad Council of Public Health Nursing Organizations. (2007). *The public health nursing shortage: A threat to the public's health.* Retrieved from http://www.apha.org/NR/rdonlyres/D3EB89A3-9727-45B9-9C83-5596626BCA74/2484/QCPHNShortage207.pdf.

94. Robertson, J.F. (2004). Does advanced community/public health nursing practice have a future? *Public Health Nursing, 21*(5), 495-500.

95. American Nurses Association. (2010). *Nursing: Scope and standards of practice.* Silver Spring, MD: Nursesbooks.org.

96. Quad Council of Public Health Nursing Organizations. (2004). Public health nursing competencies. *Public Health Nursing, 21*(5), 443-452.

97. Quad Council of Public Health Nursing Organizations. (2011). *Quad Council competencies for public health nurses.* Retrieved from http://quadcouncilphn.org.

98. Markenson, D., DiMaggio, C., & Redlener, I. (2005). Preparing health professions students for terrorism, disaster, and public health emergencies: Core competencies. *Academic Medicine, 80*(6), 517-526.

99. Polivka, B.J., Stanley, S.A.R., Gordon, D., Taulbee, K., Kieffer, G., & McCorkle, S.M. (2008). Public health nursing competencies for public health surge events. *Public Health Nursing, 25*(2), 159-165.

100. Gebbie, K., & Merrill, J. (2002). Public health worker competencies for emergency response. *Public Health Management, 8*(3), 73-81.

101. Freeman, R.B. (1970). *Community health nursing.* Philadelphia, PA: W.B. Saunders.

102. Cohen, B.E., & Reutter, L. (2007). Development of the role of public health nurses in addressing child and family poverty: A framework for action. *Journal of Advanced Nursing, 60*(1), 96-107.

103. Robert Wood Johnson Foundation. (2008). *Charting nursing's future.* Retrieved from www.rwjf.org.

104. American Nurses Association. (2001). *Code of ethics for nurses with interpretive statements.* Washington, DC: Author.

105. Easley, C.E., & Allen, C.E. (2007). A critical intersection: Human rights, public health nursing and nursing ethics. *Advances in Nursing Science, 30*(4), 367-382.

106. Central Intelligence Agency. (2014.). *The world factbook.* Retrieved from https://www.cia.gov/library/publications/the-world-factbook/rankorder/2102rank.html.

107. Dwyer, J. (2003). Teaching global bioethics. *Bioethics, 17*(5-6), 432-446.

108. Welch, D., & Kneipp, S. (2005). Low-income housing policy and socioeconomic inequalities in women's health: The importance of nursing inquiry and intervention. *Policy Politics and Nursing Practice, 6*(4), 335-342.

109. World Health Organization. (2013). *Climate change.* Retrieved from http://www.who.int/topics/climate/en/.

Chapter 2

Optimizing Population Health

LEARNING OUTCOMES

After reading this chapter, the student will be able to:

1. Describe the National Prevention Strategy.
2. Describe public health in terms of current frameworks guiding prevention efforts from a local to a global perspective.
3. Apply public health prevention frameworks to specific diseases.
4. Compare and contrast different levels of health promotion, protection, and risk reduction interventions.
5. Identify health education strategies and chronic disease self-management within the context of prevention frameworks.
6. Describe components of screening from a population and individual perspective.
7. Identify public health methods used to evaluate the outcome and impact of population-based prevention interventions.

KEY TERMS

Attributable risk
Behavioral prevention
Clinical prevention
Downstream approach
Environmental prevention
Health literacy
Health prevention
Health promotion
Health protection/risk reduction
Indicated prevention
Intervention Wheel
Multiphasic screening
Natural history of disease
Prevalence
Prevalence pot
Prevented fraction
Prevention
Primary prevention
Reliability
Secondary prevention
Selective prevention
Sensitivity
Specificity
Tertiary prevention
Universal prevention
Upstream approach
Validity
Yield

Introduction

The vision of *Healthy People 2020 (HP 2020)* is that of "a society in which all people live long, healthy lives."[1] Health promotion and prevention of disease are the underlying activities required to achieve this vision of health for all. The major objective of nursing practice is the provision of interventions that require multiple levels of prevention along the entire spectrum of health and disease. To provide the best possible care requires not only an understanding of the pathophysiology of disease but also the concepts of health promotion, risk reduction, and underlying frameworks of prevention that help guide the intervention(s). These frameworks are not unique to nursing and for the most part come from the public health sciences.

■ HEALTHY PEOPLE 2020
Optimizing Population Health
Vision
A society in which all people live long, healthy lives.
Mission[1]
To improve health through strengthening policy and practice, *Healthy People* will:

- Identify nationwide health improvement priorities;
- Increase public awareness and understanding of the determinants of health, disease, and disability and the opportunities for progress;
- Provide measurable objectives and goals that can be used at the national, state, and local levels;
- Engage multiple sectors to take actions that are driven by the best available evidence and knowledge;
- Identify critical research and data collection needs.

On June 16, 2011, the National Prevention Strategy, authorized by the Affordable Care Act, released a comprehensive plan whose purpose is to increase the number of Americans who are healthy at every stage of life.[2] In June 2012, the National Prevention Council Action Plan emphasized the federal commitment to the vision, goals, priorities, and recommendations of the prevention strategy.[3] There are four broad strategic directions fundamental to this prevention strategy: (1) building healthy and safe community efforts; (2) expanding quality preventive services in both clinical and community settings; (3) empowering people to make healthy choices; and (4) eliminating health disparities (Fig. 2-1). There are seven priorities: (1) tobacco-free living, (2) preventing drug abuse and excessive alcohol abuse, (3) healthy eating, (4) active living, (5) injury- and violence-free living, (6) reproductive and sexual health, and (7) mental and emotional well-being.

Increasing the number of healthy Americans at all stages of their life requires purposive and well-planned prevention on the part of nurses. The goal of this chapter is to provide the reader with an understanding of health promotion, disease prevention, selected public health prevention frameworks, and a nursing model focused on interventions at multiple levels to promote population health. In addition the chapter covers screening, health education, and evaluation of the effectiveness of disease and injury prevention programs.

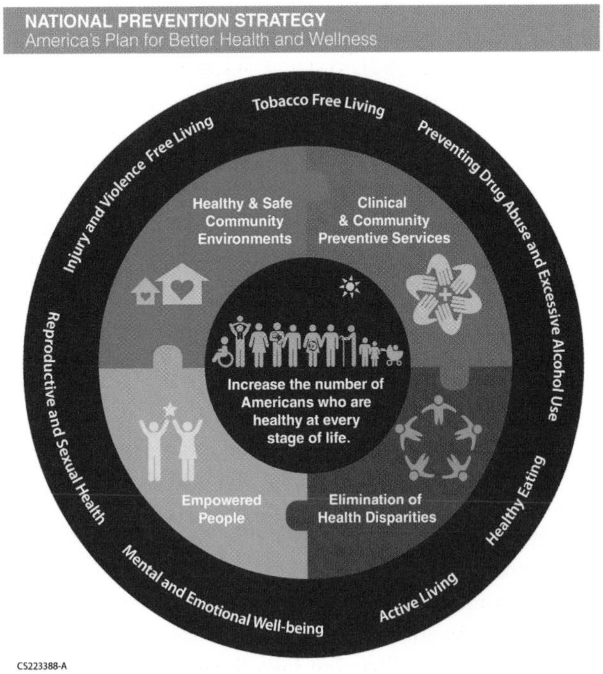

Population Health Promotion, Health Protection, and Risk Reduction

The ecological model of health introduced in Chapter 1 is the basis for understanding health promotion and prevention efforts key to the achievement of the National Prevention Strategy. The ecological model incorporates the physical and social environments as components of health.[4,5] These determinants of health are different from the individual-level biological and behavioral determinants of disease that are the usual focus of health prevention interventions. Including the ecological model in the discussion of health promotion, health protection, and risk reduction requires the inclusion of social relations, neighborhoods and communities, institutions, and social and economic policies in the development of prevention strategies.[6] This chapter builds on the information provided in Chapter 1 related to the ecological model as the primary focus. This approach is different from the more traditional individual-based health promotion, health protection, and risk reduction approaches learned when caring for individuals and families. The health issue of obesity is used in this chapter to help illustrate the importance of these three prevention interventions from a population perspective.

Health Promotion

As defined in Chapter 1, **health promotion** at the individual and family level helps people make lifestyle changes aimed at achieving optimal health.[7] These prevention interventions are implemented in various ways and often focus on behavioral change. In relation to obesity, health promotion activities focus on diet and exercise. Health-care providers deliver these interventions to individuals in their care. These interventions are also delivered to populations via health education programs, media campaigns, or in the workplace. The goal of these health promotion programs is to achieve change at the individual level based on the biological and behavioral issues related to developing disease due to obesity. The assumption is that the promotion of healthy behaviors will reduce risk and thereby reduce the prevalence of morbidity and mortality related to obesity.

The ecological model, however, provides a broader view of community health promotion. The ecological model incorporates what is referred to as an **upstream approach** in contrast to a **downstream approach** to these efforts.[8] These two terms are important in understanding

Figure 2-1 National Prevention Strategy Priorities. (*From National Prevention Council, 2012.*)

health promotion efforts today to address the four strategic directions of the National Prevention Strategy. Let's take obesity as an example. With a downstream approach, a health provider may focus primarily on nutritional health teaching based on nutritional patterns, portions, and choices without taking into consideration the environmental factors influencing choices within a community. If there are no supermarkets within a community, it is difficult to make healthy choices. In contrast to a downstream approach, an upstream approach to obesity might include interventions focused on agriculture subsidies, transportation policies, and urban zoning. It might also involve interventions restricting television advertising of food to children, creating national nutrition standards for meals served in childcare settings, or working with the private sector to introduce healthier options in restaurants and local markets

An upstream approach to health promotion related to the obesity epidemic is to examine the environmental factors that contribute to the epidemic and institute prevention interventions that target environmental change. Using the first and third strategic directions of the National Prevention Strategy as examples, this can occur through empowering community members to initiate and implement the changes to create a healthy community.[9] For example, to promote healthy eating behaviors in children, a school system in Kentucky took action and eliminated all fried foods that had been offered on the school menu. Other communities have eliminated all vending machines in schools that offer unhealthy beverages and food. A new national law, the National School Lunch and School Breakfast Programs, was implemented in 2012 that changed the school lunch programs, calling for larger portions of fruits and vegetables, less sodium, and no *trans* fats. It also placed a cap on the number of calories for the school lunch at 650 for grades K through 5, 700 calories for grades 6 through 8, and 850 calories for grades 9 through 12. Milk can be at most 1% fat and flavored milk must be fat free.[10] These are examples of community health promotion and are based on the assumption that the individuals who make up a community can as a group identify and solve their problems.[11] Such an approach to health promotion requires that the planners for the health promotion intervention take into account the context of the healthy behavior they hope the population will adopt. If the focus is only on having the schoolchildren change their eating habits without taking into account the food available to them in their total environment, then that kind of health promotion program will likely fail.

Health Protection and Risk Reduction

In contrast to health promotion, which focuses on the promotion of a healthy lifestyle and environment, **health protection/risk reduction** interventions protect the individual from disease by reducing risk. These terms are often used interchangeably, but are in actuality distinct. A good example of health protection is the use of vaccines. When an individual is vaccinated, the body develops immunity to the infectious agent and is therefore protected from the disease. The use of a vaccine has in effect reduced the risk of developing disease. Risk reduction, conversely, encompasses more than biological protection and can involve removing risk from the environment or reducing the level of risk, for example, by reducing hazardous chemical emissions produced at industrial plants. Health protection and risk reduction activities are an important component of our national effort to prevent disease.

Much of the health protection and risk reduction activities currently used in our health-care system focuses on influencing behavioral change at the individual level. The focus is to have individuals adopt protective health activities, even if the prevention program is offered to groups or populations. For example, policies related to the recommended childhood vaccines are population based and aimed at reduction risk for the development of childhood communicable disease. However, the actual delivery of the vaccine requires an individual response.

Thus risk reduction and health promotion must take into account the broader concept of risk for development of disease by incorporating environmental and social risk factors associated with the development of disease that may not be amenable through individual-level interventions. For example, protection from lead poisoning requires an environmental approach aimed at eradicating lead paint in the environment. Thus the risk factor, lead paint, cannot be eliminated solely at the individual level and often requires a systems or community approach related to allocation of funds, development of public policy, and follow-through with the removal of lead paint from older buildings in the community.

Prevention Frameworks

Prevention is a word used often in health care, but what does it mean and how does it work? From a simplistic standpoint, *prevention* refers to stopping something from happening. From a health perspective, **health prevention** refers to the prevention not only of disease and injury, but also to the slowing of the progression of the disease as well as the prevention of the sequelae of diseases and injury, such as the prevention of blindness related to type 1 diabetes. Health prevention is accomplished through the institution of public health policies, health programs, and practices with the goal of improving the health of populations, thus reducing the risk for disease, injury, and subsequent disability and/or premature death.

Health promotion and protection are fundamental concepts for nursing practice and are based on prevention frameworks in use in the public health field.[12,13] Prevention frameworks help nurses shape prevention interventions within a particular context. In the fall of 2009, a major public health issue was the H1N1 flu pandemic. Preventing the spread of the disease was the main focus of the public health interventions taken by the Centers for Disease Control and Prevention (CDC) and the World Health Organization (WHO). These activities included behavioral, environmental, and clinical interventions. People were asked to modify their behavior by changing how they coughed in public places and how they washed their hands. Those working in health-care settings changed their environment by supplying hand sanitizers and having employees implement personal protective equipment. Clinically, populations at greatest risk were given the vaccine. Institutions put policies in place related to restricting ill people from coming to work, closing schools, and eliminating the requirement of having a physician's note when absent from work. How do these interventions relate to the natural history of disease and how do they fit into current public health prevention frameworks?

Natural History of Disease

Having an understanding of the natural history of disease is an essential basis for the discussion of current prevention frameworks that follows. The **natural history of disease** provides the foundation for the public health frameworks currently in use, especially the most widely used framework of primary, secondary, and tertiary prevention. The natural history of disease depicts the continuum of disease from the disease-free state to resolution. The four stages are (1) susceptibility; (2) the subclinical phase after exposure when pathological changes are occurring without the person being aware of them; (3) clinical disease with the development of symptoms; and (4) the resolution phase in which the final outcomes are cure, disability, or death.[14] The subclinical phase is also sometimes referred to as the incubation period for communicable diseases and latency period for noncommunicable illness (Fig. 2-2).

This traditional presentation of the natural history of disease with four stages is at first glance linear. For some diseases such as influenza, this linear model works well. In some disease processes an individual may go from a subclinical stage to a clinical stage and then back to a subclinical stage. For example, in human immunodeficiency virus (HIV) infection, during the initial subclinical stage an infected individual has no clinical symptoms that meet the criteria for a diagnosis of acquired immunodeficiency syndrome (AIDS). As the infection progresses, the person may develop one or more clinical diagnoses, thus placing the individual in the clinical stage of the disease. However, with the treatments now available for treating AIDS, an individual may recover from a clinical episode and return to being asymptomatic but there has been no resolution of the disease; instead, that individual has reverted to a subclinical stage.

Figure 2-2 also depicts the outcome of a particular disease. Following the development of clinical disease, an individual recovers completely (cure), is disabled by the disease (disability), or dies. Some diseases, both communicable and noncommunicable, have no endpoint except death. HIV/AIDS is an example of a communicable disease with no cure. Those who become infected will remain infected for the rest of their lives. An example of a

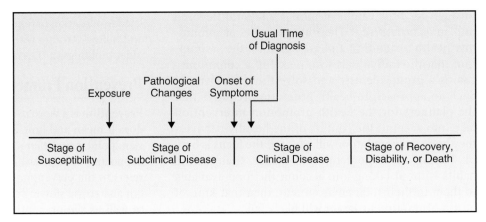

Figure 2-2 The natural history of disease timeline. *(From Centers for Disease Control and Prevention. [1992]. Principles of epidemiology [2nd ed.]. Atlanta, GA: U.S. Department of Health and Human Services. Retrieved from http://www.cdc.gov/osels/scientific_edu/ss1978/lesson1/Section9.html.)*

communicable disease without a cure is type 1 diabetes. A person diagnosed with this type of diabetes does not at some point in time revert to producing insulin at normal levels.

To further illustrate, examine the prevalence of a disease and the prevalence pot. **Prevalence** is basically the number of total cases of disease (numerator) divided by the total number of people in the population (denominator) and reflects the total number of cases of a disease in a given population. A **prevalence pot** is a way of depicting the total number of cases of the disease in the population that takes into account issues related to duration of the disease and the incidence of the disease (Fig. 2-3). For some communicable diseases with a short incubation period such as H1N1 flu, cases rapidly move in and out of the prevalence pot, but for long-term chronic diseases with no known cure, the prevalence pot can grow over time (e.g., HIV infection). If the definition of a case is infection with the HIV virus, then individuals who are subclinical and those who have evidence of clinical illness that meets the criteria for an AIDS diagnosis would all be in the prevalence pot. During the early years of the epidemic there were few treatment options. Once diagnosed, an individual often died within a short period of time. As treatment has improved and the survival rate for those infected with HIV has greatly improved, the number of AIDS-associated deaths has declined. However, the HIV/AIDS prevalence pot has grown, because the only way out of the prevalence pot is through death. In developing countries where treatment for HIV/AIDS is less available, the prevalence pot has not grown as rapidly, even with a higher number of cases, because the life span of those with HIV/AIDS remains short.

Mapping out a disease using the natural history of disease model helps to identify where on the continuum prevention efforts are needed. The prevalence pot helps to identify those health conditions that may have an increasing number of cases over time if the development of new cases is not prevented. In the case of H1N1, laying out the natural history of this strain of flu helps to determine where the primary focus should be. In the beginning of September 2009, the majority of the U.S. population was free of disease. As the next few months progressed, more and more people became infected, and some of them died. Because of the potential of death, a nationwide large-scale prevention effort was instituted. That effort was aimed at vaccinating populations at greatest risk, resulting in a focus on those without disease.

How does the natural history of the disease and the prevalence pot help public health officials focus on interventions? In the case of H1N1 flu epidemic in 2009, the incubation period, that is, the time interval between infection and the first clinical signs of disease (Chapter 9), was short, with those infected rapidly developing symptoms. In addition, the course of the disease was also short. People infected with H1N1 are able to infect others from 1 day before getting sick to 5 to 7 days after getting sick. Those who become infected with the H1N1 flu virus rapidly developed clinical symptoms including fever, cough, and in some cases gastrointestinal symptoms. New cases that entered the prevalence pot in the fall of 2009 left the pot for the most part within 7 days. Most recovered completely, some experienced long-term effects such as coma and/or respiratory problems, and some died.

Using the natural history of disease model, the nurse can lay out the progression of H1N1 (see Fig. 2-2). The preclinical phase is very short (1 to 2 days) and there are no interventions available that would prevent the progression from this phase to clinical disease. Once the patient is in the clinical phase there are limited options for intervention because the causative agent, the H1N1 flu virus, does not respond to antibiotics. However, early recognition in certain patients, such as pregnant women, and treatment with antiviral medication helped to reduce the risk of adverse consequences to mother and the fetus. Because of the limited ability of antiviral medication to prevent adverse consequences in at-risk populations and the short period of time between phases, the best approach was to focus on preventing disease from occurring in the first place. The natural history of H1N1 provided the basis for the nationwide public focus on primary prevention through the development, distribution, and administration of the H1N1 vaccine with the hope

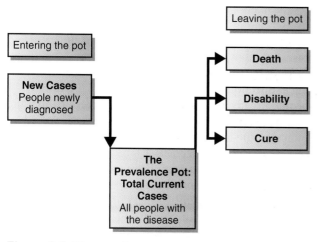

Figure 2-3 The prevalence pot.

of keeping the majority of the population disease free because of the limited ability to provide effective secondary or tertiary prevention interventions.

The natural history of a disease also allows the nurse to identify who is at greatest risk for developing the disease. For H1N1, early evaluation of the prevalence of the disease by age groups revealed that those who were over the age of 60 were less apt to become ill. The CDC concluded that the H1N1 flu caused a greater disease burden on those under the age of 25.[15] Unlike in other flu outbreaks, those who were younger, were immune compromised, or pregnant were at increased risk of death. This led to the speculation that the virus was related to earlier strains and those in late adulthood had immunity due to earlier exposure. Thus, the older members of the population had natural biological protection, whereas those under the age of 60 did not. With limited vaccine available in the fall of 2009, decisions were made to provide the vaccine to those at highest risk. This included pregnant women, household and caregiver contacts of children younger than 6 months of age, health-care and emergency medical services personnel, people from 6 months through 24 years of age, and people aged 25 through 64 years who had medical conditions associated with a higher risk of influenza complications.

In contrast, the natural history of disease in relation to type 1 diabetes is quite different. The etiology, or cause, of the disease is usually genetic rather than due to an infectious agent. There is no known prevention for developing the disease, but early detection that determines whether a person has the disease during stage one can lead to early diagnosis and treatment. However, identifying the disease early will not prevent the development of clinical disease, which lasts for a lifetime because the body is unable to produce insulin. Thus, there is no cure. This places the majority of the focus on treatment of the patient in the clinical stage to prevent premature death and disability. Another key distinction between the natural history of these two diseases is that H1N1 is population based, that is, the disease can be spread from one person to another. Interventions are required to protect the entire population at risk. In contrast, a disease such as type 1 diabetes is individual based and the risk is usually tied to a genetic trait passed down in families.

Public Health Prevention Frameworks

The natural history of a disease and the difference between population-based risks and individual-based risks form the basis for two main prevention frameworks used in public health science. The first framework is the traditional public health prevention model of primary,

secondary, and tertiary prevention.[16] The second is the Institute of Medicine (IOM) framework of universal, selected, and indicated prevention based on work done by Gordon.[17] Both use a health promotion and health protection approach and employ the three types of interventions—clinical, behavioral, and environmental. The best place to start is with the traditional primary, secondary, and tertiary prevention model, because it has been in use since the 1950s and the newer IOM framework was not used widely until it was mandated by the Centers for Substance Abuse Prevention (CSAP), a branch of the U.S. federal Substance Abuse and Mental Health Service Administration (SAMHSA), in 2004.[18]

Levels of Prevention

The traditional public health approach to prevention focuses on health prevention based on the natural history of disease and includes three levels of prevention—primary, secondary, and tertiary. **Primary prevention** interventions are conducted to prevent development of disease or injury. The focus is on people at risk for developing the disease or injury. Activities include promoting healthy behaviors and building the ability of populations and individuals within that population to protect themselves against disease. Many health policies are aimed at primary prevention such as banning smoking in public places, which is aimed at reducing the development of diseases secondary to exposure to secondhand smoke. The goal is to reduce risk factors for a health problem. If the risk for developing disease or sustaining an injury can be reduced, then the incidence (occurrence of new cases) of a disease will be reduced. **Secondary prevention** interventions include those aimed at early detection and initiation of treatment for disease, thus reducing disease-associated morbidity and mortality. If early intervention results in cure from the disease, with or without disability, screening can contribute to the reduction of the prevalence of a disease (total number of new and old cases), thereby reducing the size of the prevalence pot. Secondary prevention can include screening or case finding in infectious disease outbreaks by seeking contacts of people already ill. The focus of **tertiary prevention** is the prevention of disability and premature death and when indicated the initiation of rehabilitation for those diagnosed with disease. It includes interventions aimed at preventing secondary complications related to disease such as the prevention of bedsores.[16]

Primary Prevention: Primary prevention is a central part of nursing practice. Nurses engage in the delivery of primary prevention across settings, including the acute care setting where on first glance it looks as though the nurse is only providing tertiary prevention interventions. Because this approach is based on the natural history of disease, what types of primary prevention does a nurse provide in an acute care setting when every patient admitted has a diagnosis of clinical disease? A prime example is the activities nurses do to prevent hospital-acquired infections. All nurses must follow hospital policy related to the use of personal protective equipment, isolation precautions, and personal hygiene. These activities prevent the spread of infection from a patient with disease to a patient or health-care workers without disease. Nurses also participate in primary prevention from a health protection perspective. All nurses must comply with hospital policy related to vaccinations. In this way the members of the health-care workforce who are free of disease take steps to build their immunity to disease, thus preventing the spread of disease to patients and fellow workers who are free of disease. All these activities are population based.

Nurses also apply the principles of primary prevention on an individual level to individuals through health education, vaccination, and other activities aimed at promoting and protecting the health of their patients and increasing the patients' ability to protect themselves from disease. Patients receiving nursing care in acute care settings who are receiving care for one clinical disease may be at increased risk for other disease or injury. Nurses often include primary prevention in their plan of care, such as altering the environment to prevent falls and teaching basic fall prevention strategies to patients and their families that can be implemented on discharge. Health education begins with primary prevention, teaching patients to reduce risk for disease (e.g., teaching patients to increase exercise, reduce caloric intake, and perform proper hand hygiene). Nurses working in the community provide primary prevention through provision of health education, promotion of breastfeeding, and working with communities to reduce hazards such as lead paint.

The H1N1 pandemic depended on nurses as frontline workers in the nationwide primary prevention efforts to reduce the incidence of the disease and prevent premature death. Public health departments across the country mobilized nurses and student nurses to administer the vaccine at schools, health clinics, and other community settings. Because of the need for nurses to deliver the vaccine to large groups of at-risk individuals, nurses were often the first to receive the vaccine when it became available. Primary prevention is an essential part of nursing care to individuals and populations across all settings.

Secondary Prevention: Nurses also regularly participate in secondary prevention interventions in all settings. Screening is one aspect of secondary prevention and is an essential component of the nursing assessment focused on early detection of problems in asymptomatic individuals who already have certain risk factors. It is also targeting conditions that are not yet clinically apparent for purposes of earlier detection to improve morbidity and mortality. In acute, community, and long-term care settings nurses regularly screen patients of all ages for the possible existence of a number of conditions. Screening for developmental delays is an example of secondary prevention in children, whereas encouraging mammograms is an example of a secondary prevention intervention for adults. The goal of mammograms is to detect early stage breast cancer. Some activities done by nurses can serve as both secondary prevention and tertiary prevention. For example, the simple taking of blood pressures at a blood pressure clinic held in a local senior center can be seen as an illustration of screening when conducted with older adults who have not been identified previously as having hypertension. At the same clinic, taking an individual's blood pressure reading may function as a method for monitoring the health status of an older person who has already been diagnosed with hypertension.

Through early detection, nurses can implement interventions that will alter the natural history of the disease. For example, on admission to long-term care facilities, elderly patients are routinely screened for skin integrity. If there is any evidence of skin breakdown, nursing interventions are immediately put in place to halt the progression of a stage 1 pressure ulcer (bed sore) to a stage 2. In stage 1 the skin is reddened but there is no break in the skin. Without intervention, the patient is at greatly increased risk for skin breakdown and rapid development of a stage 2 to a stage 3 pressure ulcer.

There are many diseases that benefit from early detection and initiation of treatment prior to the development of clinical disease. Public health efforts to prevent premature death due to cancer include media campaigns for mammography screening, colonoscopies, and prostate screening. Screening is also conducted for behavioral health issues such as excessive alcohol use. There has been a nationwide campaign to have all health-care providers screened for problem alcohol use.[19] Screening for syphilis and early treatment can prevent serious disability, reduce the incidence of syphilis infection in newborns, and prevent premature death. Nurses participate in these efforts through the direct provision of screening as well as through health education with patients to encourage participation in screening.

Health education is done with a secondary prevention focus. For example, a nurse participating in a blood pressure screening health fair will include secondary prevention health education for seniors 60 years and older with a blood pressure reading greater than or equal to 150/90. For those whose blood pressure reading is between 120/80 and 150/90 lifestyle modifications are important. For adult patients with diabetes or chronic kidney disease with a blood pressure reading greater than 140/90, the nurse will give instructions on following up with their primary care provider for further care.[20] These seniors usually come to the screening clinic with no symptoms present and are unaware that their blood pressure is above the normal limits. Early intervention through lifestyle changes and medical intervention can reduce the development of life-threatening conditions such as stroke or myocardial infarction.

Tertiary Prevention: The primary focus of nursing interventions in most acute care settings is tertiary prevention. Once an individual has been diagnosed with clinical disease, prevention aims at reducing disability, promoting the possibility of cure when possible, and preventing death. Efforts are made to interrupt the natural progression of the disease or to reduce the impact of the injury through multiple strategies including medical, environmental, and psychosocial.

Health education is a key tertiary prevention activity for the nurse. For those with chronic diseases, a disease self-management approach is often used that puts the individual in charge of managing his or her disease with the goal of reducing disability and preventing premature death. The nurse serves as the teacher/facilitator by helping the individual to identify the key strategies needed to manage disease, such as regular foot care and blood sugar monitoring in patients with diabetes. The use of disease self-management is effective in reducing

health-care utilization in general populations, improving perceived self-efficacy, and improving perception of health status.[21,22]

Universal, Selected, and Indicated Prevention Models

The traditional public health framework consisting of the levels of prevention was introduced in the 1950s and still has utility today, especially for diseases in which the natural history and causal pathways for development of the disease are well understood. It is also useful when the early clinical and subclinical signs of the disease are known and the disease is actually preventable. On the flip side, the framework has limitations because of the underlying linear approach to diseases with a clear etiology. The framework is difficult to adapt to diseases or disorders (see Chapters 11 and 12) with complex risk factors; a curvilinear progression; and broad health outcomes that encompass not only physical outcomes but also psychological, social, and economic outcomes. It also limits the majority of the prevention efforts to interventions conducted by health-care providers and is not as readily applicable to the broader interdisciplinary field of public health.

An alternate approach using a continuum-of-health framework, was proposed by the IOM in the 1990s and has been adopted by the Substance Abuse and Mental Health Services Administration (SAMHSA).[18] This model divides the continuum of care into three parts: prevention, treatment, and maintenance (Fig. 2-4). Under prevention there are three categories: universal, selected, and indicated. This model was first adopted by the behavioral health field because there is less distinction in mental disorders and substance use disorders between the traditional levels of prevention that were developed based on the natural history of

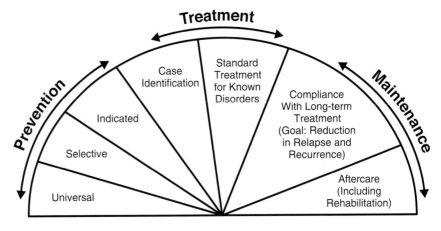

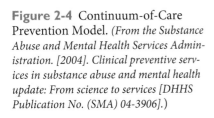

Figure 2-4 Continuum-of-Care Prevention Model. *(From the Substance Abuse and Mental Health Services Administration. [2004]. Clinical preventive services in substance abuse and mental health update: From science to services [DHHS Publication No. (SMA) 04-3906].)*

disease—primary (stage of susceptibility), secondary (subclinical stage), and tertiary (clinical stage).[17]

A **universal prevention** intervention is one that is applicable to the population as a whole and is not based on individual risk. The intervention is aimed at the general population. The purpose is to deter the onset of a health issue within the population. Public health media campaigns use a universal approach by targeting everyone in the population with such things as a billboard anti-smoking campaign or TV ads aimed at preventing drunk driving. All individuals in the population are provided with the information and/or skills necessary to prevent disease regardless of risk. Often the intervention is passive, as in media campaigns, in that nearly all of the population is exposed to the intervention. The intervention often does not include participation on an individual level. However, universal vaccination programs are not passive and require active participation by individuals. This is an appropriate approach when the entire population is at risk and would benefit from prevention programs.

Selective prevention interventions are aimed at a subset of the population that has an increased level of risk for developing disease. This can be based on demographic variables such as age, gender, or race, or it can be based on other risk factors such as genetic, environmental, or socioeconomic risk factors. An example of selective prevention interventions are efforts to screen women for breast cancer who have a known family history of breast cancer, or providing community education programs to prevent lead poisoning in older urban neighborhoods. This level of prevention targets everyone in the subgroup regardless of risk. For example, everyone in a neighborhood with older buildings is included in the selective lead poisoning intervention whether or not they have already removed the lead from their own residence. Once again a selective intervention can be passive or have an active component on the individual level.

Indicated prevention interventions are provided to populations with a high probability of developing disease. The purpose of indicated interventions is to intervene with individuals with early signs of disease or subclinical disease to prevent the development of a more severe disease. It is similar to secondary prevention. The difference is that the individuals included in the intervention have already been identified as being at greater risk for the disease. This approach is used in the substance abuse field to develop programs for individuals with early warning signs such as falling grades, at-risk alcohol use, and use of gateway drugs such as marijuana. Only those individuals with specific risk factors for developing the disease but who do not yet meet

the diagnostic criteria for the disease are included in the intervention. The purpose is to reduce behavioral risk factors that contribute to the development of disease and to delay onset of disease or severity of disease. The level of intervention provided is more intensive and is often multilevel. It always requires individual participation. An example of an indicated prevention program is that of a weight-loss program for adolescents who are obese and are showing signs of hyperglycemia but who have not been diagnosed with type 2 diabetes. Such an intervention would probably include case management, health education, nutritional counseling, and an individualized exercise plan. If the program is effective, participants may not only delay the onset of type 2 diabetes, but may also reverse the hyperglycemia and not develop the disease.

Delivery of Public Health Prevention Strategies

The delivery of prevention services includes the use of three basic strategies—clinical, behavioral, and environmental. **Clinical prevention** strategies are those that use a one-to-one delivery method between the health-care provider and the patient and usually occur in traditional health-care settings. These can include health protection activities such as vaccinations, as well as screening, and early detection of disease. **Behavioral prevention,** often focused on health promotion strategies, are aimed at changing individual behavior such as exercise promotion, smoking cessation, or responsible drinking. **Environmental prevention** often focuses on health protection by improving the safety of the environment such as fluoridating water, banning smoking in public places, enacting laws against drunk driving, enforcing clean air acts, and building green spaces for recreation.[16]

In an effort to standardize clinical prevention strategies through the application of evidence-based prevention practices, the Agency for Healthcare Research and Quality created the U.S. Preventive Services Task Force.[23] This task force is made up of a panel of experts in primary care and prevention. These experts systematically review the evidence found in published research related to the effectiveness of prevention strategies and then develop recommendations for clinical interventions. These recommendations are helpful in the development of a clinical prevention program.

The earlier example of type 2 diabetes illustrates how to apply both frameworks to a serious national health issue. Globally, many health issues contribute to premature death. The CDC provides yearly updates on the top 10 causes of death in the United States (Box 2-1).[24] This is based on the classification of the death or injury using

BOX 2-1   **Number of Deaths for Top Ten Leading Causes of Death, 2013**

- Heart disease: 611, 105
- Cancer: 584, 881
- Chronic lower respiratory diseases: 149, 205
- Accidents (unintentional injuries): 130, 557
- Stroke (cerebrovascular diseases): 128, 978
- Alzheimer's disease: 84, 767
- Diabetes: 75, 578
- Influenza and Pneumonia: 56, 979
- Nephritis, nephrotic syndrome, and nephrosis: 47, 112
- Intentional self-harm (suicide): 41, 149

Source: See reference 24. Centers for Disease Control and Prevention (2015). Faststats: Leading Causes of Death. Retrieved from http://www.cdc.gov/nchs/faststats/leading-causes-of-death.htm

accepted codes that are entered in the death registry for each death. This information is sent to the U.S. Department of Health and Human Services, which then sends the information to the CDC. The cause of death listed on the death certificates at the local level is the basis for the aggregate statistics related to mortality rates at the state and national levels. Though this provides important information, the underlying risk factors provide the information needed to build health promotion, protection, and risk-reduction interventions.

Not only is cause of death classified by disease or injury, but it is also further classified by risk factor, that is, the underlying cause of death. In 2011 in the United States, four health at-risk behaviors, lack of exercise or physical activity, poor nutrition, tobacco use, and drinking too much alcohol, were the underlying cause for illness and premature death.[25] Based on this information, the CDC identified key indicators for chronic disease surveillance.[26] In other words, it is important not only to track the causes of actual deaths, but also to track the occurrence of preventable risk factors to help predict whether efforts to prevent these deaths are working. This information helps to guide major prevention efforts aimed at reducing both morbidity and mortality in populations.

Each death can also be classified in quantitative terms using attributable risk and prevented fraction. **Attributable risk** is the measure of the proportion of the cases or injuries that would be eliminated if a risk factor was not present. Epidemiologists begin by determining the theoretical limit of the impact of prevention aimed at removing the risk factor. That is, if the risk factor did not exist, how many cases would be eliminated? For example, if no one smoked, how many cases of lung cancer would be eliminated, or if no one drove while intoxicated, how many motor vehicle crashes would not occur? It is

calculated using the population attributable risk (PAR), which is based on the strength of the risk factor and the prevalence of the risk factor in the population. The strength of the risk factor is based on the relative risk (Chapter 3). If these pieces of the equation are known, that is, the relative risk and the prevalence, then the PAR can be calculated.[16]

Those who wish to implement a prevention program can use the PAR to calculate the cost benefit and cost effectiveness of the prevention program. However, the PAR is population based and operates on the assumption that the risk factor is removed from the entire population being targeted. The prevented fraction provides the information on what can be accomplished based on the intervention actually being delivered at the community level. The **prevented fraction** is defined as a measure of what can actually be achieved in a community setting and includes the proportion of the population at risk that actually participates and the number of cases prevented. This approach takes into account the number of participants in a program who will actually succeed in eliminating the risk factor. For example, how many obese children participating in an after school activity program will actually reduce their weight to a normal body mass index?

Prior to implementing an intervention aimed at prevention, it is important to understand the underlying risk factors. The top three risk factors for preventable death in the United States—tobacco use, improper diet and physical inactivity, and alcohol use—relate to behaviors.[25] At first glance, it appears that a behavioral intervention is the best approach. However, other interventions are also helpful, including environmental and policy-based interventions. For example, alcohol-related motor vehicle crashes (MVCs) can occur with just one episode of heavy episodic drinking. The teenage driver who has consumed alcohol for the first time at high levels and then drives home may become involved in an MVC that results in the death of people who are not consuming alcohol. The teen did not have an alcohol use disorder but instead had engaged in at-risk alcohol use. Thus the natural history of disease does not fit this health-related issue, yet prevention of alcohol-related MVCs is an important issue. The questions become:

- What types of interventions will work to prevent disease or injuries?
- Is it primary, secondary, or tertiary prevention?
- Can it occur using a clinical, behavioral, or environmental approach?
- In designing this approach, should it be addressed as a universal, selected, or indicated preventive intervention?

In answering these questions it is important to have a better understanding of some potential public health nursing interventions as well and a framework that guides public health nursing practice.

The Intervention Wheel

Conceptual frameworks and models guide the practice of public health nurses (PHNs). One of the most recent models is the **Intervention Wheel,** which illustrates how

PHNs improve the health of the individuals, families, communities, and systems.[27-29] (Fig. 2-5). The model evolved from the practice of public health nurses in Minnesota and consists of several components. The first component is the population basis of all interventions. This component illustrates that the focus of all interventions is concerned with population health. The second component consists of the three levels of care: individual/family, community, and systems. Care can be provided at all three levels of working with individuals, the community

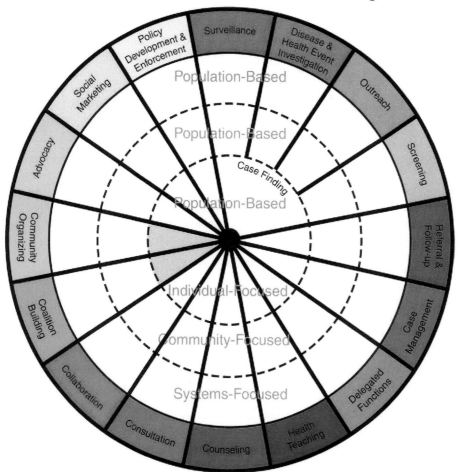

Public Health Interventions
Applications for Public Health Nursing Practice

March 2001

Minnesota Department of Health
Division of Community Health Services
Public Health Nursing Section

Figure 2-5 Components of the Intervention Wheel. *(From Minnesota Department of Health, Division of Community Health Services, Public Health Section. [2001]. Public health interventions: Applications for public health nursing practice.)*

as a whole, or with systems. Individual level practice focuses on knowledge, attitudes, practices, beliefs, and behaviors of individuals. A public health nurse's home visit to a new mother is an example of individual-level practice. In the visit the public health nurse provides anticipatory guidance about the value of breastfeeding.

Community-level practice is focused on changing community norms, attitudes, practices, awareness, and behaviors. An example of community-level practice is the development of a faith-based program focused on smoking cessation. Systems-level practice is concerned with policies, laws, organization, and power structures within communities. For example, a coalition of several senior housing sites could be formed to address pest control and improvement of overall environmental conditions, or a group of parents could come together to build a safe playground for the children.

The third component consists of 17 public health interventions (Box 2-2). Three of these interventions—health education, screening, and case management—are discussed in this chapter as they relate to levels of prevention, and the other interventions are discussed in other chapters.

A Primary Prevention Approach: Health Education

The purpose of health education is to positively change behavior through increasing knowledge about health and disease. Health education is an important nursing intervention and it is important in changing behavior at all levels of prevention. The Joint Committee on Health Education and Promotion Terminology defined *health education* as "any combination of planned learning experiences based on sound theories that provide individuals, groups, and communities the opportunity to acquire information and the skills needed to make quality health decisions."[30] The WHO defines *health education* as "consciously constructed opportunities for learning involving some form of communication designed to improve health literacy, including improving knowledge, and developing life skills which are conducive to individual and community health."[31] The WHO *Glossary* points out that health education is not just concerned with teaching but also with encouraging and giving confidence to people to take the necessary action to improve health, which includes making changes in social, economic, and environmental determinants of health.

An example of the application of this expanded definition of health education took place in rural Uganda. In Uganda, the fertility rate was one of the highest in the world at 6.9 births per 100 women of childbearing age

in 2000.[32] In one small rural village the fertility rate had not decreased, even after several community teaching sessions. A group of Ugandan nursing students, under the supervision of Dr. Sara Groves, in their public health clinical experience worked together with the community to develop and implement a teaching plan that used new teaching strategies. They visited each household and gave private, individualized instruction to extended families on family planning, allowing a safer environment in which to ask questions and for the family to acknowledge their lack of understanding of family planning. The students discreetly provided condoms if the family wanted them, role-played with the women about how they could discuss contraception with husbands, and gave them detailed direction on how and when to access family planning at the local Ministry of Health Clinic. They offered to meet individually with women at the clinic should they want additional support. As a result of this education program and teaching new life skills, 10 women from the village sought out and received family planning for the first time (S. Groves, personal communication, September 10, 2011).

Theories of Education

Health education involves teaching; therefore, understanding how people learn is essential to effective teaching. There are multiple theories of learning.[33] As our knowledge increases about how we learn from both a physiological and social basis, the theories change and expand. The theories tend to be grouped under:

- Behaviorism
- Cognitivism
- Constructivism
- Humanism

Behaviorism is the theory of classical conditioning. In this framework, the behavior change is what is important, and it is achieved with an environmental stimulus that results in a response. The focus is only on the observed behavior change and not on the mental activity. Learning is based on reward and punishment by conditioning (e.g., when a monkey learns to push a button for a reward of food).[33]

The cognitive framework focuses more strongly on inner mental activity. It is more rational than it is on reflexively responding to an external stimulus. There is behavior change as a result of knowledge that has changed thought patterns. It frequently occurs as a result of varied sensory inputs with repetition. The social learning theory of Bandura is rooted in both the behavior and cognitive frameworks, emphasizing that understanding, in addition

BOX 2–2 | Public Health Interventions

Advocacy pleads someone's cause or act on someone's behalf, with a focus on developing the community, system, individual, or family's capacity to plead their own cause or act on their own behalf.

Case finding locates individuals and families with identified risk factors and connects them with resources.

Case management optimizes self-care capabilities of individuals and families and the capacity of systems and communities to coordinate and provide services.

Coalition building promotes and develops alliances among organizations or constituencies for a common purpose. It builds linkages, solves problems, and/or enhances local leadership to address health concerns.

Collaboration commits two or more people or organizations to achieve a common goal through enhancing the capacity of one or more of the members to promote and protect health. (Henneman, Lee, & Cohen. [1995]. Collaboration: A concept analysis. *Journal of Advanced Nursing, 21*, 103-109.)

Community organizing helps community groups to identify common problems or goals, mobilize resources, and develop and implement strategies for reaching the goals they collectively have set. (Minkler, M. [Ed.]. [1997]. *Community organizing and community building for health* [p 30]. New Brunswick, NJ: Rutgers University Press.) Delegated functions are direct care tasks that a registered professional nurse carries out under the authority of a health-care practitioner as allowed by law. Delegated functions also include any direct care tasks that a professional registered nurse entrusts to other appropriate personnel to perform.

Consultation seeks information and generates optional solutions to perceived problems or issues through interactive problem-solving with a community, system, family, or an individual. The community, system, family or individual selects and acts on the option best meeting the circumstances.

Counseling establishes an interpersonal relationship with the community, a system, the family, or an individual intended to increase or enhance their capacity for self-care and coping. Counseling engages the community, a system, family, or an individual at an emotional level.

Disease and other health event investigation systematically gathers and analyzes data regarding threats to the health of populations, ascertains the source of the threat, identifies cases and others at risk, and determines control measures.

Health teaching communicates facts, ideas, and skills that change knowledge, attitudes, values, beliefs, behaviors, and practices of individuals, families, systems, and/or communities. (Adapted from American Nurses Association [2010]. *Nursing's social policy statement: The essence of the profession.* [2010]. Silver Springs, MD; American Nurses Publishing.)

Outreach locates populations-of-interest or populations-at-risk and provides information about the nature of the concern, what can be done about it, and how services can be obtained.

Policy development places health issues on decision makers' agendas, acquires a plan of resolution, and determines needed resources. Policy development results in laws, rules and regulations, ordinances, and policies.

Policy enforcement compels others to comply with the laws, rules, regulations, ordinances, and policies created in conjunction with policy development. (Minnesota Department of Health, Division of Community Health Services, Public Health Section. [2001]. *Public health interventions: Applications for public health nursing practice.* Retrieved from http://www.health.state.mn.us/divs/opi/cd/phn/docs/0301wheel_manual.pdf.).

Referral and follow-up assist individuals, families, groups, organizations, and/or communities to identify and access necessary resources to prevent or resolve problems or concerns.

Screening identifies individuals with unrecognized health risk factors or asymptomatic disease conditions in populations.

Social marketing uses commercial marketing principles and technologies for programs designed to influence the knowledge, attitudes, values, beliefs, behaviors, and practices of the population-of-interest.

Surveillance describes and monitors health events through ongoing and systematic collection, analysis, and interpretation of health data for the purpose of planning, implementing, and evaluating public health interventions (Centers for Disease Control and Prevention. [2012]. CDC's vision for public health surveillance in the 21st century. *Morbidity and Mortality Weekly Report, S61*.)

Source: See reference 27.

to behavior and environment, are all interrelated. He stresses imitation of a behavior and reinforcement in learning.[34] An example of Bandura's theory of social learning is television commercials. An action is portrayed, eating a certain food or using a certain cleaning product, and the audience, seeing it as desirable, is encouraged to model or imitate that behavior.

Constructivism is a learning theory that reflects on our own experiences.[33] We actively construct our own world as we increase our experience and knowledge. It is a process that builds knowledge within our own unique framework. A good example is problem-solving learning. To learn, students are actively involved in integrating new knowledge in their own frameworks with guidance from the teacher. For example, children can learn about what happens to their heart rate with exercise by experimenting with different types of exercise and counting pulse rates. They experience the concept of a heart rate rather than merely having it verbally explained to them. Humanism learning uses feelings and relationships, encouraging the development of personal actions to fulfill one's potential and achieve self-actualization.[33] It is self-directed learning, examining personal motivation and goals. This is also a theory of adult learning.[35] As an example, an individual diagnosed with elevated cholesterol purchases books, seeks out articles, talks with knowledgeable people, in general informs him- or herself about the problem and actions to take to solve the problem and then self-initiates these activities to improve health.

All of the learning theories influence how we teach. The identified teaching methods based on these theories are varied but include the need to be developmentally appropriate with children in particular as well as adults with varying levels of education. Many of the more recent theories provide a more balanced learning; encourage experiential learning; and solve real problems in real places by using role playing, visual stimuli, service learning, interpersonal learning, and the promotion of complex higher-order thinking.

Adult Learning

Pedagogy (pedagogical learning) is the correct use of teaching strategies to provide the best learning. *Andragogy* is similar but is specifically the art and science of helping adults learn using the correct strategies.[35] In nursing we are often teaching adults, as it is adults who generally develop the chronic diseases, are in a position to promote health, and care for the children. In the 1950s Malcolm Knowles, using humanism learning theory, suggested that adults learn differently from children and that the role of the instructor is quite different. Adults bring a great deal of experience to the learning situation and this experience influences what education they receive and how they receive it.[36] They are active learners and need to see applications for the new learning. Knowles identified six suppositions for adult learning:

1. The adult needs to know why he or she is learning something.
2. The adult's own experiences are an important part of the learning process.
3. Adults need to participate in the planning and evaluation of their learning.
4. Adults learn better if the information has immediate relevance.
5. Adults like problem-centered approaches to learning.
6. Adults respond better to internal rather than to external motivation.

The role of the teacher in this situation is to direct the learner.[36]

To be an effective educator the nurse needs to be flexible. Nurses organize the learning experience by first assessing the individual's or population's learning needs. They then select the best learning format, create the best possible learning environment, and send a clear message. The learning should be participatory and include evaluation and feedback.

Health Literacy

One of the first considerations before planning health education is to consider the health literacy of the individual client, the group, or the population. In conjunction with literacy, culture and language should also be included. **Health literacy** is defined as "the degree to which individuals have the capacity to obtain, process, and understand basic health information and services needed to make appropriate health decisions."[37] The IOM built on this definition and added key issues related to the individual receiving information. They stated that health literacy is something that "emerges when the expectations, preferences, and skills of individuals seeking health information and services meet the expectations, preferences, and skills of those providing information and services. Health literacy arises from a convergence of education, health services, and social and cultural factors."[38]

According to the CDC, approximately 9 out of 10 Americans have difficulty reading health information.[39] The majority of the written health related materials far exceeded the reading level of most adults. The lack of health literacy was greatest in older Americans, especially those with limited education. There is evidence of a causal relationship between health literacy and health outcomes. Individuals with low health literacy had less knowledge of chronic disease management, performed fewer health promotion activities, had poorer health status, and were less likely to use any preventive services. There is an association between low health literacy, low utilization of the health-care system, and high health-care costs. In 2007, several economists projected the cost of health illiteracy to the health-care delivery system escalating from $106 to $238 billion, enough to provide health insurance to all those who were uninsured. They also projected that with no intervention the future cost to the system in 30 to 40 years would be $1.6 to $3.6 trillion.[40]

Shame and stigma of having low health literacy have been found to be major barriers to seeking care. The IOM committee found that health education occurred in most primary and secondary schools but there was no universal sequencing, and only about 10% of teachers were qualified health educators. One of the most telling of the IOM findings was that health professionals had limited training in patient/population education and had few opportunities to develop skills to improve a patient's health literacy. The IOM gave multiple suggestions on how to improve health literacy and points of intervention (Fig. 2-6). Some of the most relevant to nursing included:

- Improve K through 12 basic health education.
- Help individuals learn how to assess the credibility of what they see and read about health.
- Provide clear communication, allow ample time to give this information, and encourage questions from the patient.[38]

In the past few years, considerable research has been done that brings better understanding to the magnitude and consequences of the health literacy problem. One of the issues is how to assess correctly and rapidly the level of health literacy in a patient/population. The Test of Functional Health Literacy in Adults (TOFHLA) is a common tool and easily accessible. The TOFHLA consists of a 50-item reading comprehension and 17-item numerical ability test, takes up to 22 minutes to administer, and

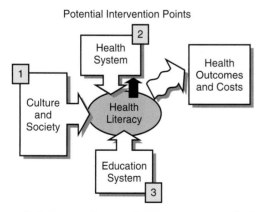

Potential Intervention Points

Figure 2-6 Potential points for intervention in the health literacy framework. *(From Nielsen-Bohlman, L., Panzer, A., & Kindg, D. [2004]. Health literacy: A prescription to end confusion [IOM Report].)*

is available in English and Spanish. There is also a shorter form that takes 7 to 10 minutes to administer. The TOFHLA is a valid, reliable indicator of patient ability to read health-related materials. Data suggest that a high proportion of patients cannot perform these basic reading tasks.[41] Jeppesen, Coyle, and Miser recognized the clinical importance of identifying diabetic patients whose health literacy was low. They attempted to pinpoint what screening demographic questions might be reliable, valid, and quicker to administer than the TOFHLA. They found that they could accurately predict patients with low health literacy by asking three short questions. The patients who reported a low educational level, a low self-rated reading ability, and a frequent need for help in understanding health materials had correspondingly low TOFHLA scores that predicted low health literacy.[41] Another tool, the Rapid Estimate of Adult Literacy in Medicine (REALM), has also been used to assess reading skills of patients. It is a 66-item medical word pronunciation recognition test that takes about 3 minutes and is available only in English.[42]

Weiss and colleagues developed a new tool, the New Vital Signs (NVS), in Spanish and English that is a reliable and an accurate measure of health literacy with high sensitivity, and appropriate to use in the primary care setting. It is a six-item test based on the ability to read and apply information from a nutrition label, and it takes about 3 minutes to complete.[43] If you wish to use the tool, there is no fee or need for permission. The TOFHLA and REALM are good predictors of low reading and numeric understanding but they still do not meet all the criteria discussed by the IOM in examining health literacy. Health literacy not only improves reading and using numbers but it also increases the individual's capacity to use the information effectively. The NVS is an attempt to assess whether an individual can both read and then apply the information correctly.

Solutions to low health literacy come from many directions. In New Jersey, a literacy volunteer organization worked individually with clients to teach them new skills such as reading a thermometer, filling out health forms, reading medication labels, and learning how to communicate with their health-care provider. The organization does a lot of role-playing to help clients increase their comfort in communicating. The organization also encouraged providers to use plain language and not words such as *cardiologist* and acronyms such as *EKG*.[44]

Staff in Southern California assessed their congestive heart disease and coronary heart disease clinic population in a large, urban, safety-net hospital, and found the health literacy was low. The staff's solution was to prioritize the development and implementation of low-literacy educational materials, programs, and services.[45] It is important for nurses to carefully review all written material used with patients before it is distributed. First the nurse should be certain that the content is correct, appropriate, and what the organization supports. If the well-baby clinic supports exclusive breast- or bottle feeding for the first 6 months of life, then the written information given to the new mother should not suggest the introduction of cereal at 4 months. The written material should also be the appropriate culture and language for the population who will receive it. Using the Suitability of Assessment of Material (SAM) framework created by Doak, Doak, and Root will help with a complete evaluation of written health information for content, literary demand, graphics, layout and type, learning stimulation and motivation, and cultural appropriateness. This is a simple and also accessible tool, and can be used to assess a variety of written materials.[46]

Develop a Teaching Plan

Writing a teaching plan for the individual or population is important for two reasons. It clearly defines what will be taught and it provides a structure for evaluation (Box 2-3). The teaching plan has many similarities to a program plan (see Chapter 6 for more details on writing a program plan). As part of the nursing process the nurse's first step in developing the teaching plan is to review the assessment of the learning needs. What does this individual or population need to learn or would benefit from learning to promote health, prevent disease, or help manage an identified health problem? Next, the nurse assesses the type of learner or learners who will receive the education. The nurse should keep in mind that health literacy is low in the United States and that by definition both health education and health literacy encourage not only providing information but also developing new skills on how to utilize the information, how to change behaviors, and how to best interact with the health-care system.

Health literacy/health learning fosters client participation in the health system. Access to education and information is essential to achieving effective participation and the empowerment of people and communities. If the client has not been evaluated for health literacy and it is determined that there might be a problem, the most appropriate of the tools above should be used. If the intended audience is children, their developmental level and their learning style for this topic should be assessed first. For adults, the Knowles suppositions[36] for their learning should be considered and used to determine how best to direct the lesson. It is also important to understand the culture of the learners and adapt the plan if there are different languages.

Next, identify the goal, that is, the overall desired outcome of the teaching. This is best done in collaboration with the learners, and is essential if the nurse is teaching adults. Likewise the specific objectives should be written in partnership with the learners. Even very young children can participate in helping to identify what to include in the teaching plan. This is an opportunity to assess what the learners already know so the nurse can build on student knowledge or take the information the students have and help them apply or analyze it.

To develop appropriate learning objectives, it is helpful to refer to the work of Benjamin Bloom who, in the 1950s with a group of other educational psychologists, identified three learning domains:[47]

1. Cognitive
2. Affective
3. Psychomotor

Within the cognitive domain Bloom identified six levels of cognitive learning from the simple knowledge recall to the more abstract and higher-level synthesis and evaluation. Each level, especially the first three, builds on the next. This is referred to as Bloom's Taxonomy, and this classification is useful in looking at levels of learning, outcomes, and the correct action verbs to be used when writing specific-level learning objectives (Box 2-4). The first level of learning is knowledge, which refers to remembering or recalling specific information that has been taught. Comprehension is the second level and requires some demonstration of really understanding what was learned. Application, the third level, requires using the knowledge

---

| BOX 2–3 | **Steps in Developing a Health Education Teaching Plan** |

1. Identify the health education need in the selected population (individual/family/community).
2. Assess the learner; include health literacy, culture, language, age, and learning style.
3. Write a goal for the teaching intervention.
4. Write specific, measureable objectives for the teaching intervention (consider Bloom's Taxonomy).
5. Identify materials and resources needed for the teaching plan; include the appropriate teaching environment and the length of the lesson.
6. Describe the lesson; include key concepts.
7. Write out the procedure step by step for teaching the lesson using a variety of teaching methods.
8. Have a plan for the evaluation.

BOX 2–4	Bloom's Taxonomy of Learning*				
Knowledge	Comprehension	Application	Analysis	Synthesis	Evaluation
Define	Discuss	Interpret	Distinguish	Plan	Judge
Repeat	Recognize	Apply	Calculate	Design	Appraise
List	Explain	Use	Test	Assemble	Value
Name	Interpret	Practice	Compare	Invent	Assess
Tell	Outline	Demonstrate	Question	Compose	Estimate
Describe	Distinguish	Solve	Analyze	Predict	Select
Relate	Predict	Show	Examine	Construct	Choose
Locate	Restate	Illustrate	Compare	Imagine	Decide
Write	Translate	Construct	Contrast	Propose	Justify
Find	Compare	Complete	Investigate	Devise	Debate
State	Describe	Examine	Categorize	Formulate	Verify
Arrange	Classify	Classify	Identify	Create	Argue
Duplicate	Express	Choose	Explain	Organize	Recommend
Memorize	Identify	Dramatize	Separate	Arrange	Discuss
Order	Indicate	Employ	Advertise	Prepare	Rate
	Locate	Practice	Appraise	Propose	Prioritize
					Determine

Source: See reference 47.

*Active verbs represent each level.

in real situations such as problem-solving. The next level is analysis, wherein the acquired knowledge is broken down by its organization and such things as making inferences and looking for motives or causes. The last two are synthesis and evaluation. In synthesis, the acquired knowledge is used creatively to produce something new. Evaluation provides a way to judge the end product. In addition to cognitive learning, Bloom also identified affective and psychomotor learning. The affective domain looks at a growth in feelings, values, and attitudes. Psychomotor learning is the development of manual or physical skills, a domain frequently taught by nurses.

Once the objectives are clearly written, using action verbs in a measureable format, the nurse then needs to reflect on what materials and resources will be needed for effective teaching. The learner's needs are determined based on the length of the lesson, where it will be taught, what activities will promote the best learning, and how much time will be needed to prepare the lesson. It is helpful to write out a description of the lesson including the key concepts and the learning domain of knowledge, attitude, and/or practice.

The final two steps are to write out the detailed procedure for the teaching plan, carefully outlining each activity, and, if appropriate, the follow-up for these activities. The final component is how an evaluation will be made of whether the intended learning took place. The evaluation plan should reflect the learning objectives and be in place before teaching begins to anticipate how to measure the outcomes.

Methods of Instruction

There are many ways to learn the same information, and each of us has a preference for how we like to learn. There are lists of different teaching methods that include formal presentations, small-group work, field trips, role playing, written assignments, and Internet activities, to identify a few. Usually, experiential learning is most effective for adults. Lecture format rarely appeals to an adult who wants guided interactive learning. If people can feel it, handle it, see it, taste it, smell it, and discuss it, they can better integrate it into their own life experiences. A group concerned with nutrition and being overweight may be told that Ritz crackers, potato chips, corn chips, and cheeseburgers are high in fat and also high in calories. The group can be given numbers of calories and grams, but it is not easily integrated into their life experiences. However, if the portion size of four

Ritz crackers, 10 potato chips, and 1 ounce of corn chips, all having 8 to 9 grams of fat, are demonstrated, it is easier for people to put it into the context of their own lives.

Using real-life scenarios to teach how to solve health problems has also been quite effective. Giving new mothers a vignette in which a family is having difficulty getting adequate sleep at night because their 4-month-old infant is awake all night allows for group discussion and problem-solving that can be relevant at the moment. This is information these women can take home and apply immediately. Telling children the importance of exercise by using videos, Internet, and PowerPoint slides can be entertaining and provide basic knowledge. Helping children form walking groups and joining them for their walks can help them apply this knowledge and start to change behavior. Written material can help enforce oral discussion but the material must be appropriate for literacy, content, culture, and language.

Regardless of the teaching method, it is always important to emphasize the benefits of the proposed behavior change and to personalize the message. A good strategy is to apply the intended new behavior within the context of the individual's lifestyle and needs. Help clients weigh the cost and the benefit of the new health behavior. Key points should be emphasized during teaching and new information provided in small increments. Most people can absorb only one or two new pieces of information in an encounter. Learners are the best source of information about what they want to learn and if the teaching method is meeting their needs. Feedback should be frequently sought from learners.

The environment should not be neglected in a teaching plan. The physical environment is important and should be maximized as much as possible even when many things in a community setting may be outside of one's control. A space should be the right size, have a comfortable temperature, adequate places to sit, the necessary resources for the planned lesson, and a place where, as appropriate, the learners can receive and share confidential information. However, one also needs to create an environment conducive to learning in which the learner has space to be an active learner and to learn from real situations with someone to assist with guidance and direction to master the material. It should be a place in which individuals feel free to voice opinions, experiment with new ideas, and identify what they do not know, a place in which there is enthusiasm for learning in a nonthreatening environment.

Evaluation

Successful learning changes behavior. Deciding how to evaluate whether this learning has occurred requires referring back to the specific objectives for the level of learning that was to take place and the specific outcomes expected. If the first stage of teaching was to increase knowledge, an appropriate method is needed to measure whether the knowledge did increase. If the objective was for the mother to explain how the different childhood immunizations will keep her child healthy and prevent disease, the mothers should be asked to repeat back the information they have just received, or play a game in which they have to know the answers to specific factual questions. If the objective was to help individuals apply knowledge, the applied learning should be evaluated in a different way. For application one can provide a scenario at the end of the teaching session, then note how students solve the problems utilizing the information just taught. A follow-up discussion with the group may be held after they have had time to apply their new knowledge. If the objective was for the mother to practice primary prevention by having her child fully immunized by 2 years of age, the mother's behavior may be observed after the teaching to determine whether the knowledge has been applied and the child has been fully immunized.

There are several tools that can be used to evaluate health education. It is always a good idea to ask for verbal reaction to the teaching at the end of a teaching session. This is useful in planning for future health education sessions. To measure an increase in knowledge, a classic pre- and post-test should be used, or a pre- and post-interview/observation. Using a formal testing method is frequently not well liked by adult learners, especially those who have limited literacy skills. They respond better to the oral interview but this is more difficult to carry out. To assess change, one can observe and interview over a specific time period, especially to note the sustainability of the change. These tools need to be thoughtfully developed to provide objective, reliable data. Likewise, long-term effects of the teaching may be evaluated through the use of objective pre-designed tools (for more complete discussion of evaluation, see Chapter 6).

Health education forms the basis for many health prevention programs aimed at improving the health of individuals as well as of families. Nurses learn this skill first with individuals, then families, and finally with populations and communities. It operates under the assumption that improving health literacy is central to improving health. In addition to health education, other activities regularly performed by nurses, such as screening, contribute to building the health of communities. Often these activities require the use of health education as a strategy to improve full participation in the prevention activity.

Screening and Early Identification

Just as health education is the basis of many primary prevention programs, screening is central to secondary prevention. The classic definition of *screening* is the presumptive identification of unrecognized disease or defect by the application of tests, examinations, or other procedures that can be applied rapidly to sort out those with a high probability of having the disease from a large group of apparently well people.[48] Screening is not diagnostic and only indicates who may or may not have a disease or a risk factor for disease.

Screening is often done by the nurse across healthcare settings. This type of intervention clearly fits within the secondary prevention phase of the traditional public health prevention model. This allows for early identification and treatment and, it is hoped, prevents adverse consequences and/or premature death due to the disease. A good example is blood pressure screening. If those with hypertension are identified prior to development of clinical symptoms, the institution of behavioral and clinical interventions such as diet modification and the use of a diuretic can bring the individual's blood pressure back to within the normal range and prevent adverse health consequences associated with hypertension, such as stroke.

Screening is also conducted to detect risk factors in people without disease, such as screening for heavy/at-risk drinking as recommended by the National Institute on Alcohol Abuse and Alcoholism (NIAAA). This type of screening is aimed at distinguishing those with a higher risk for disease from those with low risk. For example, screening for heavy/at-risk drinking not only identifies those who may have an alcohol use disorder, but also identifies those with a current drinking pattern that puts them at risk for developing an alcohol use disorder and/or for developing alcohol-related adverse consequences or experiencing alcohol-related injury.

When using the traditional public health model, screening clearly falls into the category of secondary prevention. The purpose is to identify within a group of apparently well people those who probably have the disease. For those with complex risk factors and a less clear natural history of disease, the traditional model has less utility. This is true with mental health, substance use disorders, and injury. In these cases, screening is done for the purpose of detecting risk for disease or injury prior to the occurrence of disease as well as the detection of disease in those who are apparently well. It can be classified as both primary and secondary prevention.

Using a continuum of health approach to prevention provides a broader context for understanding the role of screening as a prevention intervention. Screening includes identification of those with risk factors for disease or injury as well as those with subclinical disease. In the first case, the assumption is that early identification and treatment of those with disease will result in reduction of the morbidity and mortality associated with the disease. In the second case the assumption is that early detection of risk and delivery of risk reduction interventions will reduce disease or injury from occurring. This allows for screening for the purpose of preventing disease or injury from occurring in the first place (primary prevention) as well as preventing adverse health consequences that can be avoided with early detection and treatment of disease (secondary).

Most diseases are associated with a complex set of risk factors and often do not progress in a linear fashion. In addition, the broader continuum health model takes into account not only adverse physical outcomes, but also psychological, social, and economic outcomes. An example of screening that reflects primary prevention is the approach being used to prevent childhood obesity. Screening for risk factors such as inactivity and high caloric intake can help to identify children without disease who would most benefit from an intervention. Thus, the screening process is conducted in a population without disease to separate those with a high probability for developing disease or sustaining an injury from those with low or no risk factors for the disease or injury.

Diagnosis, Screening, and Monitoring

The difference between diagnosis, screening, and monitoring is often blurred. For example, taking blood pressure readings at a blood pressure screening event that only includes people who have not been diagnosed with hypertension is clearly screening, detecting probable disease in a population of apparently well people. Taking a blood pressure reading for a patient every 4 hours on a medical-surgical unit in the hospital is done to monitor the patient's vital signs and detect possible changes in the patient's status and it is not a screening activity. Taking blood pressure readings at a booth at a health fair where many of the participants come to the booth and state that they have hypertension and need to know how they are doing is a combination of screening and monitoring, because many of the participants have already been diagnosed. The nurse practitioner or physician takes a blood pressure reading during a physical work-up to assist in establishing a differential diagnosis for hypertension. The same activity is done to screen, monitor, or assist in obtaining a diagnosis.

For each of these activities, there are set parameters for the measure. In the case of monitoring the patient, the nurse compares the most recent blood pressure reading with the patient's baseline reading and the readings over the admission to determine whether there has been a change in the patient's status. The blood pressure reading is part of a larger nursing assessment and, if the reading reflects a change in the patient's status, the nurse may change the plan of care for either a positive or negative change. When using the blood pressure reading from a diagnostic standpoint, there are specific guidelines for the clinician and the blood pressure levels are is based on the average of two or more readings. These readings are taken during the course of two or more visits.[20] Using the guidelines the clinician can make a diagnosis of stage 1 or stage 2 hypertension or classify the patients as prehypertensive (Box 2-5). The guidelines have been revised based on growing evidence related to both hypertension and the development of a new category of risk, prehypertension, and are evidence based.

The guidelines state that the process for diagnosing hypertension occurs after an initial screening. So how does the screening differ from the diagnostic stage since the same measurement is taken—a blood pressure reading using standard equipment? In this case, the main difference is that the screening is based on one reading rather than two or more blood pressure readings over a number of visits, and the purpose of taking the blood pressure reading is to identify those who may be hypertensive and are in need of further assessment and possible treatment. The clinician conducting the screening will refer the individual whose blood pressure meets the cutoff for probable hypertension to a clinician who is qualified to conduct the needed assessment and able to make a differential diagnosis.

Sensitivity and Specificity

For all of these activities—screening, monitoring, and diagnosis—the clinician must have a clear understanding of the reliability and validity of the measure chosen to screen for risk and/or probability of disease. Understanding the reliability and validity of a screening tool provides the clinician conducting the screening with the guidelines for deciding what is a positive screen and what is a negative screen, that is, who most probably has the disease and who most probably does not. Or in the case of screening for risk, it provides the guidelines for deciding what is considered high risk and what is considered low risk. In the case of blood pressure screening, the screening is done for the most part using the same basic instrument used to diagnose disease and monitor physical status, but for other health issues, the screening tool is different from the diagnostic tool. Determining the validity of the instrument for screening uses different criteria than for diagnosis or for monitoring status.

In screening, the reliability and validity of the instrument is crucial. **Reliability** is defined as the ability of the instrument to give consistent results on repeated trials. **Validity** is defined as the degree to which the instrument measures what it is supposed to measure. For screening instruments the two aspects of validity that are the main concerns are the sensitivity and the specificity of the instrument. **Sensitivity** is defined as the ability of the screening test to give a positive finding when the person truly has

BOX 2–5	**Cutoff Points for Hypertension**

Blood Pressure Levels

The classifications in the table below are for people who are not taking antihypertensive (blood pressure–lowering) drugs and who are not acutely ill. When a person's systolic and diastolic pressure readings fall into different categories, the higher category is used to classify the blood pressure status.

Classification of Blood Pressure for Adults Aged 18 to 59.			
Category	Systolic (mm Hg)		Diastolic (mm Hg)
Normal*	Less than 120	and	Less than 80
Prehypertension	120–139	or	80–89
Hypertension			
Stage 1	140–159	or	90–99
Stage 2	160 or higher	or	100 or higher

*Unusually low readings should be evaluated for clinical significance.

Source: See reference 20.

the disease, or true positive. **Specificity** is defined as the ability of the screening test to give a negative finding when the person truly does not have the disease, or true negative.

● APPLYING PUBLIC HEALTH SCIENCE
The Case of the Silent Killer
Public Health Science Topics Covered:
- Screening
- Population assessment
- Health planning

Choosing a screening instrument requires understanding the importance of both sensitivity and specificity. For example, a team of nurses at a large urban hospital noticed that there had been an increase in admissions of African American men with a diagnosis of cardiovascular disease secondary to hypertension. They wanted to put in place a large-scale blood pressure screening program for the African American men in their city to improve early detection of hypertension and potentially reduce the need for hospitalization. Prior to implementing the program they wanted to make sure that the method they used to screen for hypertension was valid. This was important for two reasons. First, they did not want to have too many false negatives. In other words, they wanted to identify as many men as possible with hypertension because there was such a high morbidity and mortality rate for untreated hypertension in the male African American population. Second, they did not want too many false positives, because this population had limited resources to pay for care. Unnecessary visits to the physician could result in reduced participation in the program, especially because an accurate diagnosis requires more than one visit to a health-care provider. Too many false positives could result in unnecessary utilization of health-care resources.

Prior to initiating a full-scale screening program, the nurses conducted a pilot with 250 African American men who had not been diagnosed with hypertension, who were not taking antihypertensive (blood pressure–lowering) drugs, and who were not acutely ill. To do the screening, they used a standard blood pressure cuff and stethoscope and measured the blood pressure in millimeters of mercury (mm Hg). The cutoff point for a positive screen was a blood pressure reading greater than or equal to 140 systolic (mm Hg) and greater than or equal to 90 diastolic. To evaluate the sensitivity and specificity of the screening, all the participants were asked to complete three follow-up visits with a primary care physician

to establish whether or not the participants had hypertension. Because this was a pilot study, the nurses obtained written consent from the participants and followed the Internal Review Board process required by their institution.

Once they had obtained approval, the nurses conducted the pilot study with 250 participants. First the nurses screened the participants for possible hypertension by obtaining a blood pressure reading. They then obtained follow-up data on all 250 in relation to whether or not they were diagnosed with hypertension based on the current classification of hypertension for adults age 18 years and older. A diagnosis of hypertension is based on the average of two readings greater than or equal to 140 systolic (mm Hg) and greater than or equal to 90 diastolic.[47] The nurses then calculated basic frequencies on their data and found that 55 of the participants screened positive for hypertension and, on follow-up, 55 were diagnosed with hypertension. On the surface, it looked as though their screening instrument was 100% sensitive as they correctly identified all who had the disease, but that was not the case.

To determine the sensitivity and specificity of the method they used to screen for hypertension, the nurses constructed a two-by-two matrix using screening and diagnostic data (Fig. 2-7). They determined the number of

Screening for stage 1 or 2 hypertension with 250 persons

A = True positives (screened positive and had the disease)

B = False positive (screened positive and did not have the disease)

C = False negatives (screened negative and had the disease)

D = True negatives (screened negative and did not have the disease)

Disease (+ = BP ≥ 140/90)			
Screening Results	**Yes**	**No**	**Total**
Yes	40 A	15 B	55
Yes	15 C	180 D	195
Total	55	195	250

Figure 2-7 Sensitivity and specificity matrix.

participants that belonged in each box of the matrix. Each box of the matrix corresponds to four different categories of participants: (1) those who were true positives, that is, they screened positive and the physician diagnosed them with hypertension, box A; (2) those who were false negatives, that is, they screened negative but the physician diagnosed them with hypertension, box C; (3) those who were false positives, that is, they screened positive and the physician did not diagnose them with hypertension, box B; and (4) those who were true negatives, that is, they screened negative and the physician did not diagnose them with hypertension, box D.

Using these numbers the nurses examined the sensitivity of their instrument. They took the total of all positive screens with disease and divided it by the total number of people with the disease and multiplied this by 100. Another way to express this formula is to use the letters in the lower right-hand corner of two of the boxes in the matrix, boxes A and C. The total number of true positives, or A, is 40, and the total number with disease (true positives plus false negatives) equals 55, or A + C. Thus the formula for sensitivity is (A/A + C) × 100. In this example the sensitivity is

$$(40/55) \times 100, \text{ or } 72.7\%$$

They then determined the specificity of their instrument. To do this, they repeated what they had done with sensitivity, but now they were concerned with the relationship between those who were true negatives and the total number who screened negative. Again, the letters in the lower right-hand corner of the boxes are used to construct the formula, but this time the boxes of interest are boxes B and D. The total number of participants who are true negatives, or D, is 180, and the total number without disease equals 195, or D + B. The formula for specificity is (D/B + D) % 100. In this example the specificity is

$$(180/15 + 180) \times 100 = 92.3\%$$

In this example the specificity of the screening test is higher at 92.3% than the sensitivity that is 72.7%. More than 25% of the participants who had hypertension would have been missed if the participants relied on screening alone, but less than 10% of those without disease were incorrectly identified as possibly having hypertension when they actually did not have the disease (see Fig. 2-5). The nurses had met one of their requirements for the program (high specificity), but not the other requirement of high sensitivity. How could they address these issues?

First, they could look at the reliability of the instrument they were using to obtain the blood pressure reading. Because the method of measurement for screening and diagnosis in this case is the same, the reliability could be a concern. There are two possible issues: variation in the method and observer variation. Observer variation has been known to happen when taking blood pressures using the standard method owing to observer variation in hearing acuity and experience in taking blood pressures. The nurses actually addressed this issue prior to conducting the pilot study. They did both inter-rater and intra-rater reliability, testing at baseline for the nurses who would conduct the screening. For the inter-rater reliability they had different nurses take the blood pressure on the same individual to determine the variation between each rater's blood pressure reading. For intra-rater reliability, they compared one nurse or rater's measure of repeated blood pressures on the same person. They initially found low inter- and intra-rater reliability between the nurses. They then conducted a blood pressure training workshop for all the nurses who participated in the screening. Following training, the reliability of the measure was high.

Because the nurses felt confident that they had been using a reliable instrument, they considered adjusting their cutoff point. They had used the diagnostic criteria for hypertension to choose their cutoff point. Adjusting the cutoff point to a lower value could improve the sensitivity of the screening process, but it would result in reducing the specificity. So which is more important? Making this decision is done by comparing the consequences of a false negative with the consequences of a false positive. In this case, a false positive would result in extra visits to the physician, whereas a false negative would result in untreated disease. Missing more than a quarter of the population being screened is a serious problem. Hypertension is known as the silent killer, that is, the disease has few if any clinical symptoms until damage has occurred. A person with the disease often does not know he or she has it until damage has already occurred.

The nurses plotted the blood pressure readings on a chart to help determine the cutoff point for 100% sensitivity and 100% specificity to help decide whether a lower cutoff point would increase sensitivity while still maintaining adequate specificity. Plotting out the normal distribution of the blood pressure values in those with hypertension and those without hypertension helped to illustrate what would happen if they changed the cutoff value (Fig. 2-8). If they changed the value to 130/85, they would have 100% sensitivity, but their specificity would drop to nearly 50%. If they shifted the cutoff point to 145/95, they would achieve 100% specificity but decrease their sensitivity to less than 70%. Choosing a cutoff value is always a compromise. In this case, the nurses decided to use a cutoff value of greater than or equal to 135 systolic and greater than or equal to 90 diastolic as their cutoff point. This increased their sensitivity to over 80% while the specificity decreased only a small amount to a little less than 90%.

Armed with the information on the reliability and validity of their screening method, the nurses were ready to present a proposal to their hospital for conducting the hypertension screening program as a citywide outreach program for the hospital. They approached the director of the community outreach department with their information, sure that they would be able to proceed. The director asked them questions to which they could not respond, so they went back to obtain more information.

The first question the director posed was, "What is the expected yield of the screening program?" The nurses were not sure what this meant. They found that the **yield** is defined as the number of previously undiagnosed cases of disease that result in treatment following screening. They already had a crucial piece of information, the sensitivity of the screening program they proposed. The higher the sensitivity is, the greater the potential yield will be. The next issue related to yield is the prevalence of undetected disease. This depends on the duration of the disease, the duration of the subclinical phase of the disease, and

the level of available care. The natural history of disease (see Fig. 2-2) was a helpful guide for the nurses. They went back to their original literature review related to hypertension and once again found clear evidence that the duration of the subclinical phase (stage 1) can be long and that early treatment can have significant effects on reducing morbidity and mortality. They also reviewed the statistics on access to care for the low-income African American population with high levels of poverty in their city. Owing to a recent economic downturn, access to care was limited and African American males were less likely to have regular physical checkups. The nurses also charted out the current national estimates on the prevalence of undiagnosed hypertension in African American males. They found that the prevalence of hypertension among African American males was as high as 39%[49] and that hypertension was often not diagnosed in this population until individuals became symptomatic.

The nurses concluded that because of the high sensitivity of their screening method and the high prevalence in the target population, the potential yield was high. However, they had not reviewed the availability of medical care. Because they needed to determine whether treatment was available for those who screened positive, they did a review of all the primary care clinics in the area. They also reviewed their pilot data on the resources used by the participants to identify which primary care clinics were most frequently used. They then contacted these clinics to determine whether the clinics would be able to handle a large influx of potentially new clients following the screening. The nurses were able to establish that the existing primary care system was sufficient and that the majority of clinics and primary care offices were willing to put in writing their support for the project.

The second question the director asked had to do with **multiphasic screening,** defined as administering multiple tests to detect multiple conditions during the same screening program. The nurses had not considered this idea, but felt it had merit and reviewed the current information on health and African American males. They found that colorectal cancer and high cholesterol were two other serious health problems for African American males. However, conducting colorectal cancer screening would require a different approach owing to the complexity of the screening procedure. Though combining blood pressure screening with screening for high cholesterol was promising, it was

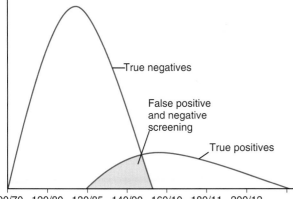

100/70 120/80 130/85 140/90 160/10 180/11 200/12

Figure 2-8 Distribution of blood pressure readings in those with and without hypertension.

more invasive and would require purchasing more supplies, possibly using more personnel. The nurses also did not have pilot data to provide information on the sensitivity and specificity of screening with a sample from the target population, so they would have to rely on national data.

The director had also asked about the cost benefit of the program. Because they were asking the hospital to fund this program, the director wanted to know the possible benefits of the program related to cost, simplicity of administration, safety, and acceptability of the population. The nurses mapped out the actual budget of the proposed program. Because no new equipment was needed, the majority of the cost was in staff time. To reduce costs, the nurses had collected a pool of nurse volunteers willing to participate in the program. The taking of blood pressures is safe and noninvasive and takes little time to complete. This helps to reduce cost because the time needed to conduct the screening per individual is short.

When reviewing the acceptability of the program, they were careful not to make the assumption that because blood pressure clinics are common, the population they wished to engage would come to theirs. They had asked the participants in their pilot study for feedback on the best site for conducting the screening and they also enlisted the help of members of the community in identifying the right sites and means of advertising the program. They also reviewed the literature for evidence of other successful screening programs with African American males. Though some of the participants had mentioned schools or churches as good sites, the site that was mentioned most and also supported in the literature was the local barbershop.

The nurses shared their data with the director and reported that the blood pressure screening program they proposed had a potentially high yield and the cost would be low given the availability of volunteers. They suggested that the screening program be conducted in the local barbershops, but recommended that further work be done to develop a partnership with the owners of these shops prior to implementing the program. They then discussed the possibility of developing a multiphasic screening program by combining blood pressure screening with other screenings such as cholesterol but cautioned that this would require additional funding and time investment.

The director then challenged them to describe how they would evaluate the success of the program.

In response they shared with him the hospital discharge data that had initially sparked their interest in doing the screening. They felt that this would provide sufficient baseline data to help evaluate the outcome of the screening program. The director asked them to clarify what their programmatic outcome would be. They were not sure so the director asked them to come back when they had a clear idea of how they would evaluate the success of the program (for more on evaluation, see Chapter 5). After reviewing basic models for program evaluation they decided on a short time span for their evaluation and chose simple measures to evaluate the impact of the program. They chose to measure the number of people who attended the program, the number of positive screens, and the number of positive screens who accepted information related to referral for treatment. They went back to the director and stated that owing to the limited resources for the targeted population there were three clinics that were most often used by residents in the targeted community. The nurses felt it would be practical to track individuals post screening. To do this, they proposed to first keep a record of how many men attended the screening. They then would contact each of the clinics and ask them to track the number of men who said they had been referred by the screening program. Based on all the information provided, the director finally approved their request and the nurses were able to institute the screening program (Fig. 2-9).

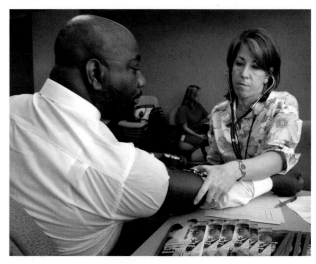

Figure 2-9 Blood pressure screening. *(From Centers for Disease Control and Prevention, James Gathany, 2005.)*

Criteria for Screening Programs and Ethical Dilemmas

Screening is performed on a regular basis across populations and settings and is often taken for granted as a worthwhile endeavor. Prior to implementing a screening program, it is important to determine whether the screening program meets certain criteria. There are serious ethical considerations that must be addressed. For the majority of screening the core assumption is that the screening program will reduce disease-associated morbidity and mortality. The other major assumption is that all those who screen positive from probable disease have access to appropriate assessment and treatment services. These assumptions form the basis of the criteria used to determine whether a screening program should be implemented.

Criteria for Screening Programs

The first criterion is to be certain that the screening test has high specificity and sensitivity. This is complex. There is always a trade-off between specificity and sensitivity. When planning a screening program it helps to review the impact of missing true cases versus falsely identifying a person with the disease as having the disease. For example, if the disease being screened has a high mortality rate, it may be more important to identify as many individuals with the disease as possible; that is, it should have a high sensitivity. That way there is a good chance of detecting disease, even if the specificity is low and the percentage without disease that ends up going through diagnostic testing is high. However, those who screen positive and do not have disease may unnecessarily experience a high level of stress while waiting to find out whether they do indeed have the disease. On the opposite end, if the mortality for the disease is lower and the cost and inconvenience of diagnostic testing is high, high specificity may be more important than high sensitivity. The best-case scenario is to have a test with both high specificity and high sensitivity. There is always a trade-off.

The next important criterion is that the test needs to be simple to administer, inexpensive, safe, rapid, and acceptable to patients. Screening that can be done quickly with minimal time and effort has a higher likelihood of success. It also needs to be safe. Some screening tests are invasive and may carry some risk. For example, a colonoscopy requires some anesthesia with its associated risk. A paper-and-pencil questionnaire is noninvasive and carries minimal risk. Also, a simple one-page paper-and-pencil screening tool is rapidly administered, whereas a colonoscopy requires a minimum of 24 hours including preparation for the test, the administration of the test, and recovery from the test. Acceptability of the screening test is often dependent on cost, time, safety, and ease of administration, which are reasons that it is harder to get individuals to have the recommended colonoscopy screening than it is other screening tests.

Even paper-and-pencil tests should be reviewed for simplicity. Many screening tests take too long to administer, decreasing the chance that a person will complete a test. Consider the difference between screening for possible depression using a 10-item questionnaire that can be inserted into a regular health assessment versus a 32-item questionnaire. A 10-item test is simpler. It is also easier to learn and perform and can be delivered by nonmedical personnel. A good example of a measurement tool for depression with high sensitivity, specificity, and reliability is the 10-item Center for Epidemiologic Studies Short Depression Scale (CES-D 10).[50,51] The original screening tool was 20 items long and took longer to learn and administer. The shorter form is easier to administer and more acceptable to patients.

The next criterion is that the disease be sufficiently serious to warrant screening. The purpose is to prevent the adverse consequences associated with the disease. In the case of colonoscopy, the screening test does not meet the rapid, simple, inexpensive, and acceptable criteria. However, the severity of the disease outweighs the inconvenience and cost of the screening test. Colorectal cancer (CRC) is the third leading cause of cancer-related deaths in the United States.[52] Screening and early detection of CRC increase the chance of cure in a disease with a high mortality rate when treated in its late stages[52,53] because screening often leads to the identification of precancerous lesions (i.e., adenomas), which can be removed, thus preventing CRC. The next criterion addresses the issue of whether the treatment for disease is easier and more effective when the disease is detected early. This is not the case for all diseases and is the reason that there is ongoing scientific inquiry into the utility of screening tests. If screening is done, will it reduce the disease-associated morbidity and mortality through initiation of early treatment and to what extent? If there was a screening test for Parkinson's disease, what type of early treatment exists? Because there is no known cure and treatment is confined to reducing symptoms, early detection does not serve to reduce the disability associated with the disease. Conversely, mammography has the potential of identifying breast cancer in the early stages, thus increasing the potential survival rate.

This then raises the issue of the acceptability of the available diagnostic services and treatment. If screening is done, will those who screen positive seek further assessment and will those with a positive diagnosis engage in treatment? This issue was raised over the issue of using a reliable instrument to screen for drug abuse. There is no evidence that screening resulted in subsequent assessment and treatment. Those who screened positive were not likely to follow up with the next steps related to the screening. Based on this, the National Quality Forum's (NQF) publication on evidence-based treatment for substance abuse does not recommend that health-care providers screen for drug abuse as a standard practice in general populations.[54] When screening will not result in the needed follow-up, the screening program will not result in reduced disease-related morbidity and mortality.

Another criterion for implementing a screening program is to determine whether the prevalence of a disease is high in the population to be screened. Despite the NQF's recommendation that drug abuse screening not be conducted in the general population, it is applicable in a population in which the prevalence of drug abuse is high, such as an inner-city program for adolescent males with failing grades. The prevalence is higher, and the program staff can be trained to provide health education along with the screening, thus improving the acceptability of subsequent referral and possible treatment by the boys in the program who screen positive.

This criterion is also helpful when deciding whom to target when putting together a screening program. The IOM continuum health prevention model referenced above[18] provides a framework for deciding whom to include in the screening program. A universal approach would include everyone in the population regardless of age, gender, or other characteristic. A screening program that uses a selected approach would focus on those at higher risk. Making these decisions is based on prevalence and risk for disease. For example, breast cancer screening through mammography is not done using a universal approach. Instead, age, gender, and risk factors are used to determine who should get a mammogram and how often.

The final and ethically the most important criterion is that resources are available for referral for diagnostic evaluation and possible treatment. In our example of putting together a screening program for hypertension in African American men, the team must first ascertain whether there are available resources to handle those with a positive screen. The main issues to address are economic access, physical access, and capacity to treat. Economic access refers to the ability to pay for care. Will all those who attend the screening program be able to receive follow-up diagnostic services and possible treatment? If the answer is yes, will they have physical access to the clinics providing the care? For example, what type of transportation is available to get to the clinics providing services and will everyone

who attends the screening have adequate transportation in terms of time, utility, and cost? Finally, if a large-scale screening program is done, does the existing health-care system have the capacity to provide diagnostic and treatment services for the anticipated increase in individuals needing these services? This last criterion is rarely addressed and can result in serious consequences.

Ethical Considerations

The criteria discussed raise serious ethical questions related to screening. It is unethical to conduct screening if treatment is not available. Screening programs are often done without thinking through the consequences. A serious ethical question is, what will be done with the positive screens? Availability of treatment is not just related to the existence of health-care resources that provide the treatment, but also to the ability of those participating in the screening to access those resources. What if nurses conducted blood pressure screening with a homeless population in a neighborhood where the nearest hospital was three bus rides away; the nearby clinics required a minimal co-pay of $50.00; there were no pharmacies in the area that provided medications to those without the ability to pay; the soup kitchens in the area served donated food that was high in salt, fat, and sugar; and there were limited public toilets? What would they do with the homeless person who had a positive screen? Even if they managed to get him to see a physician who then prescribed a salt-free diet and a powerful diuretic, how would that person be able to fill the prescription and follow the diet? If the person were able to fill the prescription, how would the person handle the frequent need to urinate without getting arrested for urinating in public? The primary question is, did the screening program result in reduced morbidity and mortality in this population? Was it ethical to conduct the screening without ensuring first that a system was in place to provide the needed health-care services?

Another example involves the American Cancer Society's eagerness to provide free breast exams and mammography to poor Hispanic and African American women in a Midwestern city. The organization engaged several partners to provide the service (at a time before most states provided free screening to poor women). The director of one of those clinics agreed to see a specific number per week for free (one criterion was no health insurance). However, the director insisted that the clinic would do this only if the American Cancer Society had a plan in place for diagnosing and treating any woman who screened positive for the cancer. The ethical and moral question that the planners then addressed was what to do if they told a participant in the screening program that she had cancer and then had no way for her to receive treatment. The planners were able to contract with three physicians and two hospitals that agreed to provide care. The screening program began and the first woman screened was positive for breast cancer, requiring major surgery. She had no insurance and no resources to pay for the surgery. To be eligible for Medicaid, she would have had to give up her home, a resource for which she had spent a lifetime saving. Because of the preplanning, this woman and the four other women participating in the program who were diagnosed with cancer all received the needed surgery. Without the generosity of the physicians and hospitals, they would not have been able to have the surgery and the planners of the screening program would have been left with a serious ethical dilemma.

Another ethical issue has been raised by the possible use of genetic screening as a means of identifying those who are genetically at risk for developing disease. For example, with our increased knowledge related to genetically linked disease, genetic screening can help determine whether a well person without disease is at risk for developing disease. A woman's risk of developing breast and/or ovarian cancer is greatly increased if she inherits a deleterious (harmful) *BRCA1* or *BRCA2* mutation. Men with these mutations also have an increased risk of breast cancer. Both men and women who have harmful *BRCA1* or *BRCA2* mutations may be at increased risk of other cancers. Should genetic screening be done and if so, what interventions should occur related to positive results? There are no easy answers. Consider the woman who screens positive for a *BRCA1* or *BRCA2* mutation. Should she consider removing her healthy breasts prior to the development of disease?

Tertiary Prevention and Noncommunicable Disease

Secondary prevention attempts to reduce morbidity and mortality through early detection and treatment. Tertiary prevention is another powerful prevention approach that can also reduce the burden of disease. During the past 100 years, as the life span of populations has increased, the prevalence of chronic disease has also increased, creating a growing burden of noncommunicable chronic disease in the United States and across the world.[55] Almost half of the population in the United States has been diagnosed with at least one noncommunicable chronic disease and four in every five health-care dollars are spent on the care of noncommunicable disease. Though the U.S. health system is built on an acute care model, the vast majority of the care provided is for the management of noncommunicable chronic diseases.[56]

A chronic disease is defined as a disease that lasts a year or more, requires medical attention over time, and/or limits the ability to perform activities of daily living (ADLs).[56] Once it has been identified, how does chronic disease fit into the prevention frameworks presented above? Using the traditional public health model, tertiary prevention is the logical choice. The goal of the tertiary prevention interventions is to prevent premature mortality and adverse health consequences related to the chronic disease. For some diseases, such as hypertension, tertiary prevention efforts can result in the person returning to a normal state; that is, a combination of behavioral changes and pharmaceutical interventions can result in the patient's blood pressure returning to normal limits. In other diseases, the prevention strategies are aimed at slowing the progression of the disease and reducing the likelihood of adverse consequences related to the disease. With pharmaceutical interventions, patients with Parkinson's disease can improve their gait and reduce the tremors. This reduces their risk of falls and other injuries while improving their ability to perform ADLs, but they are not returned to a normal state.

Tertiary prevention appears at first glance to be individual based rather than population based. However, the burden of noncommunicable chronic diseases affects the whole population, and movement toward more population-level interventions is gaining momentum. The WHO released a report calling for "urgent action to halt and turn back the growing threat of chronic diseases."[57] In that report, the WHO stresses that population interventions can be done related to reducing the burden of already diagnosed chronic diseases. One of these strategies is to improve access to care.

Two main strategies associated with tertiary prevention of noncommunicable chronic disease are case management and chronic disease management. These strategies are discussed in more detail in Chapter 9. Chronic disease self-management (CDSM) is defined as an ongoing process by which an individual with a chronic illness or condition engages in management of medications, management of symptoms, and promotion of health.[58,59] This approach has proved to be effective in helping patients and their caregivers in improving their health status and their health-related quality of life.[60,61] Nursing case management is defined as the process for coordinating health care by planning, facilitating, and evaluating intervention across levels of care. It is a well-established intervention aimed at improving health outcomes and decreasing cost for those with chronic disease.[62,63] These two strategies focus on behavioral and clinical interventions that require interventions with individuals and families. However, the WHO report includes environmental and policy strategies that truly use a population-based approach to the management of chronic disease with the goal of reducing the burden of chronic disease not only on individuals but also on populations.

More detail related to noncommunicable disease is presented in Chapter 9. The main issue here is that prevention models can be used to help develop interventions related to reducing the burden of chronic diseases. As the cost of medical care increases, the need for population-level prevention across the continuum of disease is needed.

Emerging Opportunities for Population Health Interventions

As the global community becomes increasingly connected through technology and the Internet, new opportunities are emerging for improving the health of populations. The emergence of the worldwide Web (WWW) in 1969 changed how the world communicates. Forty years after the initiation of the WWW, almost 25% of the world population was connected to the Internet and 75% of North America was connected.[64] Cell phone usage across the globe continues to increase with more than 50% of the world population now connected via cell phone. These two methods of instant communication and dissemination of information have changed how health information is spread and have provided healthcare providers with innovative methods for the development of health promotion and protection interventions.

The challenge is that the iterative process intrinsic to these technologies leaves the originator of the intervention with minimal control. Once information has been released through these technologies, the information can be altered, added to, and disseminated in ways not foreseen by the originator of the information.

Social Networking and Twitter

Social networking sites and Twitter provide a venue for rapid dissemination of information. This process follows no clear path and depends on individuals to pass on the information they have received to others. The opportunities presented by this technology have yet to be fully explored. As demonstrated by the 2009 Iranian elections and Arab Spring movement in 2011, this method of disseminating information across the Internet and cell phones allowed citizens in a highly regulated society to communicate with the global community, thus overriding governmental control. The potential for using this technology for the management of disasters, rapidly disseminating critical health information, and promoting health policies is enormous.

Health Web Sites

Health Web sites represent a more traditional use of the Internet to disseminate health information. WebMD is a well-known site that provides information on most diseases, including health promotion activities to help prevent a certain disease, screening that can be done for secondary prevention, and a review of evidence-based treatments. The institutes and agencies under the umbrella of the U.S. Department of Health and Human Services have Web sites with a great deal of the space dedicated to providing key health information to the public. Where social networks and Twitter are examples of interactive and active information dissemination, health Web sites use a passive approach, posting key information that can be used by health-care providers and laypeople, but do not usually actively engage the user. However, with the emergence of more interactive technologies, these Web sites are adopting new methods to engage the user such as providing the means to complete a pencil-and-paper screening test in one's own home using Web-based survey technology.

In the business world, the term *disruptive technology* is technology that disrupts the marketplace in an unanticipated way. These emerging technologies have the potential to "disrupt" the health promotion marketplace through the provision of health information at no cost to those who may not have ordinarily had access to the information. Unfortunately, health-care providers have much less control over this technology and misinformation is a real risk; that is, some Web sites may provide health information that is not evidence based and can potentially result in unintended consequences. For example, the debate over the association between autism and childhood vaccines has not only hit the media but has also been disseminated via the WWW on such sites as the National Vaccine Information Center that provide information that is not necessarily evidenced based The controversy was supported in part by evidence from one study published in 1998 that has since been retracted.[65] Subsequent studies have failed to replicate the findings and no causal link has been established.[66–68] In 2011, *The Lancet* retracted the article because of serious scientific misconduct related to the study. Despite the retraction and the lack of scientific evidence, the controversy continues. Based on a recent national survey, 13% of parents followed an alternative vaccination schedule with more than 50% of these parents refusing or delaying vaccines. This is having the unintended effect of increasing the prevalence of childhood communicable diseases as evidenced by the measles outbreak in 2015. It is an exciting new world of health promotion that combines technology with a growing awareness that health for individuals depends on the promotion of societies and environments that promote the health of the whole. Yet dangers exist in the proliferation of health information on the Web as well as Facebook, Twitter, and other social media formats that is unsupported by scientific evidence that can place the health of the population as a whole at risk.

◼ Summary Points

- Health promotion and protection are major emphases of national and global health organizations.
- The new ecological model of health promotion uses an upstream approach that includes the social, environmental, and economic contexts of healthy populations.
- The health of a population is greater than the sum of the health of each individual in the population.
- Health prevention frameworks provide guidance for the development of prevention interventions.
- Health education and health literacy are key to improving the health of populations.
- Screening for possible disease has the potential to reduce disease-related morbidity and mortality but has serious ethical issues that must be addressed.
- Tertiary prevention can help to reduce the burden of chronic diseases.
- Emerging technologies offer potential innovative strategies for improving health.

▲ CASE STUDY

Screening for Colorectal Cancer

Screening for colorectal cancer (CRC) raises the issue of which screening method to use. There are three methods that can be used to screen for CRC, including the fecal occult blood test (FOBT) done at home by the patient, flexible sigmoidoscopy done in a physician's office, and colonoscopy usually done with sedation in the office of a gastroenterologist. You have been assigned the task to come up with a recommended screening protocol for your medical center related to these three screening methods that will result in the highest reduction in morbidity and mortality related to CRC. Begin with the current mortality rates for the counties served by your medical center and compare them with state and national rates. Then determine the sensitivity and specificity of each of the screening methods based on available published information on the screening instruments. A valuable Web site for completing this plan is the National Cancer Institute's interactive CRC screening Web site located at http://cisnet.cancer.gov/projections/colorectal/.

REFERENCES

1. Centers for Disease Control and Prevention. (2009). *Healthy People 2020*. Retrieved from http://www.healthypeople.gov/hp2020/advisory/PhaseI/summary.htm#_Toc211942896.
2. National Prevention Council. (2011). *National Prevention Strategy*. Washington, DC: U.S. Department of Health and Human Services, Office of the Surgeon General. Retrieved from http://www.surgeongeneral.gov/initiatives/prevention/strategy/report.pdf.
3. National Prevention Council. (2012). *National Prevention Council Action Plan*. Retrieved from http://www.surgeongeneral.gov/initiatives/prevention/2012-npc-action-plan.pdf.
4. Bauer, G., Davies, J.K., Pelikan, J., Noack, H., Broesskamp, U., & Hill, C. (2003). Advancing a theoretical model for public health and health promotion indicator development: Proposal from the EUHPID consortium. *European Journal of Public Health, 13*(3s), 107-113.
5. Institute of Medicine. (2003). *The future of the public's health in the twenty-first century*. Washington, DC: National Academies Press.
6. Institute of Medicine. (2000). *Promoting health: Intervention strategies from social and behavioral research*. Washington, DC: National Academies Press.
7. O'Donnell, M.P. (2008). Evolving definition of health promotion: What do you think? *American Journal of Health Promotion, 23*(2), iv. doi: 10.4278/ajhp.23.1.iv.
8. Blue Cross and Blue Shield of Minnesota. (2006). *Moving upstream: Working together to create healthier communities*. Retrieved from http://www.docstoc.com/docs/120735357/Moving-Upstream-Working-To-Create-Healthier-Communities.
9. Kok, G., Gottlieb, N.H., Commers, M., & Smerecnik, C. (2008). The ecological approach to health promotion programs: A decade later. *American Journal of Health Promotion, 22*(6), 437-442.
10. McClellan, J. (2012). New school lunch guidelines: Fewer calories, more fruits, veggies. *The Arizona Republic*. Sept. 17, 2012 02:32 PM. Retrieved from http://www.azcentral.com/arizonarepublic/news/articles/2012/09/17/20120917new-school-lunch-guidelines-fewer-calories-more-fruits-veggies.html.
11. Racher, F.E., & Annis, R.C. (2008). Community Health Action Model: Health promotion by the community. *Research and Theory for Nursing Practice: An International Journal, 22*(3), 182-191.
12. Morgan I.S., & Marsh, G.W. (1998). Historic and future health promotion contexts for nursing. *Image: Journal of Nursing Scholarship, 30*(4), 379-383.
13. Pender, N., Murdaugh, C.L., & Poarsons, M.A. (2006). *Health promotion in nursing practice*. Upper Saddle River, NJ: Prentice Hall.
14. Dicker, R., Coronado, F., Koo, D. & Parish, G. (2011). *Principles of epidemiology in public health practice, 3rd edition*. Atlanta, GA, Centers for Disease Control and Prevention.
15. Centers for Disease Control and Prevention. (2009). *Novel H1N1 flu facts and figures*. Retrieved from http://www.cdc.gov/h1n1flu/surveillanceqa.htm.

16. Centers for Disease Control and Prevention. (1992). A framework for assessing the effectiveness of disease and injury prevention. *Morbidity and Mortality Weekly Report, 41*(RR-3).
17. Gordon, R. (1987). An operational classification of disease prevention. In J.A. Steinberg & M.M. Silverman (Eds.), *Preventing mental disorders* (pp 20-26). Rockville, MD: Department of Health and Human Services.
18. Substance Abuse and Mental Health Services Administration. (2004). *Clinical preventive services in substance abuse and mental health update: From science to services* (DHHS Publication No. [SMA] 04-3906). U.S. Department of Health and Human Service, Rockville, MD.
19. National Institute on Alcohol Abuse and Alcoholism. (2007). *Helping patients who drink too much: A clinician's guide* (2nd ed.). Rockville, MD: U.S. Department of Health and Human Services.
20. James, P.A., Oparil S., Carter B.L., Cushman, W.C., Dennison-Himmelfarb C., Ortiz E., et al. (2014). 2014 evidence-based guideline for the management of high blood pressure in adults: report from the panel members appointed to the Eighth Joint National Committee (JNC 8). *JAMA, 311*(5):507-20. doi: 10.1001/jama.2013.284427.
21. Barlow J.H., Wright, C.C., Turner, A.P., & Bancroft, G.V. (2005). A 12-month follow-up study of self-management training for people with chronic disease: Are changes maintained over time? *British Journal of Health Psychology, 10,* 589-599.
22. Lorig K.R., Ritter, P., Stewart, A.L., Sobel, D.S., William Brown, B., Bandura, A., et al. (2001). Chronic disease self-management program: 2-year health status and health care utilization outcomes. *Medical Care, 39*(11), 1217-1223.
23. U.S. Preventive Health Services Task Force (2014). Home. Retrieved from http://www.uspreventiveservicestaskforce.org/Page/Name/home.
24. Centers for Disease Control and Prevention (2015). *Faststats: leading causes of death.* Retrieved from http://www.cdc.gov/nchs/fastats/leading-causes-of-death.htm.
25. Centers for Disease Control and Prevention. (2014). *Chronic disease prevention and health promotion.* Retrieved from http://www.cdc.gov/chronicdisease/overview/.
26. Centers for Disease Control and Prevention. (2004). Indicators of chronic disease surveillance. *Morbidity and Mortality Weekly Report, 53*(RR11), 1-6.
27. Keller, L.O., Strohschien, S., Lia-Hoagberg, B., & Schaffer, M. (2004). Population-based public health interventions: Practice-based and evidence-supported, part 1. *Public Health Nursing, 21,* 453-468.
28. Minnesota Department of Health, Division of Community Health Services, Public Health Section. (2001). *Public health interventions: Applications for public health nursing practice.* Retrieved from http://www.health.state.mn.us/divs/opi/cd/phn/docs/0301wheel_manual.pdf.
29. Cross, S., Block, D., Josten, L., Reckinger, D., Keller, L. O., Strohschein, S., Rippke, M., & Savik, K. (2006). *Development of the public health nursing competency instrument.* Public Health Nursing, 23(2), 108-114.
30. Joint Committee on Health Education and Promotion Terminology. (2001). Report of the 2000 Joint Committee on Health Education and Promotion Terminology. *American Journal of Health Education, 32*(2), 89-103.
31. World Health Organization. (1998). *Health promotion glossary.* Retrieved from http://www.who.int/hpr/NPH/docs/hp_glossary_en.pdf.
32. Index Mundi. (2011). *Total fertility rate Uganda.* Retrieved from http://www.indexmundi.com/g/g.aspx?c=ug&v=31.
33. Shunk, D.H. (2012). *Learning theories: An educational perspective, 6th edition.* Boston: Pearson.
34. Bandura, A. (1977). *Social learning theory.* New York: General Learning Press.
35. Hughes, N. & Schwab, I. (2010). *Teaching adult health literacy: principles and practice.* Berkshire, England; McGraw Hill.
36. Knowles, M.S. (1990). *The adult learner: A neglected species, 4th edition.* Houston, TX: Gulf.
37. Ratzan S.C., & Parker, R.M. (2000). Introduction. In C.R. Selden, M. Zorn, S.C. Ratzan, & R.M. Parker (Eds.), *National Library of Medicine current bibliographies in medicine: Health literacy* (NLM Pub. No. CBM 2000-1). Bethesda, MD: National Institutes of Health, U.S. Department of Health and Human Services.
38. The Institute of Medicine, Committee on Health Literacy, Board on Neuroscience and Behavioral Health. (2004). *Health literacy: A prescription to end confusion.* Washington, DC: The National Academies Press.
39. Centers for Disease Control and Prevention. (2011). *Health literacy: Learn about health literacy.* Retrieved from http://www.cdc.gov/healthliteracy/learn/.
40. National Patient Safety Foundation. (2007). *New report estimates cost of low health literacy between $106 – $236 billion dollars annually.* Retrieved from http://www.npsf.org/updates-news-press/press/new-report-estimates-cost-of-low-health-literacy-between-106-236-billion-dollars-annually/.
41. Jeppesen, K., Coyle, J., & Miser, W. (2009). Screening questions to predict limited health literacy: A cross-sectional study of patients with diabetes mellitus. *Annals of Family Medicine, 7*(1), 24-31.
42. Parker, R.M., Baker, D.W., Williams, M.V., & Nurss, J.R. (1995). The test of functional health literacy in adults: A new instrument for measuring patients' literacy skills. *Journal of General Internal Medicine, 10*(10), 537-541.
43. Weiss, B., Mays, M., Martz, W., Castro K., DeWalt, D., Pignone, M., et al. (2005). Quick assessment of literacy in primary care: The newest vital sign. *Annals of Family Medicine, 3*(6), 514-522.
44. Literacy Volunteers Association (2014). *Health literacy.* Retrieved from http://www.lvacapeatlantic.com/health-literacy.html.
45. Cordasco, K., Asch, S., Franco, I. & Mangione, C. (2007). *Health literacy and English language comprehension among elderly inpatients at an urban safety-net hospital.* Paper presented at the annual meeting of the Robert Wood Johnson Clinical Scholars, Fort Lauderdale, FL.

46. Practice Development Inc. (2008). *SAM, Suitability of Assessment of Material.* Retrieved from http://www.beginningsguides.net/pdfs/SAM-for-Beginnings.pdf.

47. Bloom, B.S. (1956). *Taxonomy of educational objectives: Handbook 1. The cognitive domain.* New York, NY: David McKay.

48. Commission on Chronic Illness. (1951). *Chronic illness in the United States* (Vol. 1, p 45). Cambridge, MA: Harvard University Press, Commonwealth Fund.

49. Ferdinand, K.C., & Welch, V.L. (2007). An update on hypertension among African Americans. *Proceedings of the American Society of Hypertension, Twenty-Second Annual Scientific Meeting and Exposition, 4*(1):81-4

50. Radloff, L.S. (1977). The CES-D scale: A self-report depression scale for research in the general population. *Applied Psychological Measurement, 1,* 385-401.

51. Andresen, E.M., Malmgren, J.A., Carter, W.B., & Patrick, D.L. (1994). Screening for depression in well older adults: Evaluation of a short form of the CES-D (Center for Epidemiologic Studies Depression Scale). *American Journal of Preventive Medicine, 10,* 77-84.

52. National Cancer Institute. (2008). *A snap shot of colorectal cancer.* Retrieved from http://www.cancer.gov/aboutnci/servingpeople/colorectal-snapshot.pdf.

53. National Cancer Institute, NIH, DHHS. (2007). *Colorectal cancer mortality projections, Bethesda, MD.* Retrieved from http://cisnet.cancer.gov/projections/colorectal/.

54. National Quality Forum. (2007). *National voluntary consensus standards for the treatment of substance use conditions: Evidenced-based treatment practices.* Washington, DC: Author.

55. Abegundi, D., & Stanciole, A. (2006). *An estimate of the economic impact of chronic noncommunicable disease in selected countries.* Geneva, Switzerland: World Health Organization, Department of Chronic Disease and Health Promotion. Retrieved from http://www.who.int/chp/working_paper_growth%20model29may.pdf.

56. Center for Disease Control and Prevention (2014). *Chronic disease prevention and health promotion.* Retrieved from http://www.cdc.gov/chronicdisease/overview/.

57. The World Health Organization. (2009). *Preventing chronic diseases: A vital investment.* Retrieved from http://www.who.int/chp/chronic_disease_report/en/.

58. Lorig, K.R., Ritter, P., Stewart, A.L., Sobel, D.S., William Brown, B., Bandura, A., et al. (2001). Chronic disease self-management program: 2-year health status and health care utilization outcomes. *Medical Care, 39,* 1217-1223

59. Lorig, K.R., & Holman, H.R. (2003). Self-management education: History, definition, outcomes and mechanisms. *Annals of Behavioral Medicine, 26,* 1-7.

60. Bodenheimer, T., Lorig, K., Holman, H., & Grumbach, K. (2002). Patient self-management of chronic disease in primary care. *Journal of the American Medical Association, 288,* 2469-2475.

61. Marks, R., Allegrante, J.P., & Lorig, K. (2005). A review of the synthesis of research evidence for self-efficacy-enhancing interventions for reducing chronic disability: Implications for health education practice (part 1). *Health Promotion Practice, 6,* 37-43.

62. Zander, K. (2002). Nursing case management in the 21st century: Intervening where margin meets mission. *Nursing Administration Quarterly, 26,* 58-67.

63. Taylor, P. (1999). Comprehensive nursing case management: An advanced practice model. *Nursing Case Management, 4,* 2-13.

64. Miniwatts Marketing Group. (2009). *Internet usage statistics.* Retrieved from http://www.internetworldstats.com/stats.htm.

65. Wakefield, A. J., Murch, S.H., Anthony, A., Linnell, J., Casson, D.M., Malik, M., et al. (1998). Ileal-lymphoid-nodular hyperplasia, non-specific colitis, and pervasive developmental disorder in children. *The Lancet, 351*(9103), 637-642.

66. Hornig, M., Briese, T., Buie, T., Bauman, M.L., Lauwers, G., Lipkin, W.I., et al. (2008). Lack of association between measles virus vaccine and autism with enteropathy: A case control study. *PLoS ONE, 3*(9), e3140. doi:10.1371/journal.pone.0003140. Retrieved from http://www.ncbi.nlm.nih.gov/pmc/articles/PMC2526159/pdf/pone.0003140.pdf.

67. Dempsey, A.F., Schaffer, M.A., Singer, D., Butchart, A., Davis, M., & Freed, G.L. (2011). Alternative vaccination schedule preferences among parents of young children. *Pediatrics.* doi:10.1542/peds.2011-0400. Retrieved from http://pediatrics.aappublications.org/content/early/2011/09/28/peds.2011-0400.full.pdf+html.

68. Centers for Disease Control and Prevention. (2012). *Vaccine safety. Measles, mumps, rubella and varicella vaccine.* Retrieved from http://www.cdc.gov/vaccinesafety/Vaccines/MMRV/Index.html .

Chapter 3

Epidemiology and Nursing Practice

LEARNING OUTCOMES

After reading this chapter, the student will be able to:

1. Describe aspects of person, place, and time as they relate to epidemiological investigation.
2. Explain the epidemiological triangle.
3. Apply the epidemiological constants to an investigation.
4. Identify sources of epidemiological data.
5. Apply basic biostatistical methods to analyze epidemiological data.

6. Differentiate cohort and case-control study design and select appropriate measures of effect.
7. Explain behavioral, environmental, and genetic factors that have an impact on health.

KEY TERMS

Agent
Analytical epidemiology
Attack rate
Biostatistics
Causality
Demography

Descriptive epidemiology
Environment
Epidemiology
Host
Incidence
Infectivity

Morbidity
Mortality
Percent change
Prevalence
Prospective
Rate

Retrospective
Secondary attack rate
Web of causation

◼Introduction

The term **epidemiology** is the combination of three Greek words: *epi,* translated as "upon"; *demos,* translated as "people"; and *logy,* or "the study of something."[1] Epidemiology is a natural fit for the nursing profession as nursing, unlike many of the health-related professions, extends well beyond the one-on-one patient clinician mode of operation engaging groups of people where they live, work, and play. Public health nursing has traditionally blended health promotion, disease prevention, health education, and population-based initiatives in an effort to maximize the health and wellness of individuals through population-level strategies. As 21st-century health professionals, nurses are now more than ever required to demonstrate both competency and proficiency in the principles of epidemiology. Today the curriculum in accredited colleges of nursing is shifting toward the inclusion of epidemiology as core content. The historical development of epidemiology is replete with references

to the same women who carved out the nursing profession. Public health nursing and population-based health and wellness are observed in the pioneering efforts of Florence Nightingale, Lillian Wald, Clara Barton, Mary Breckinridge, and Dorothea Dix. Each of these legendary women initiated public health efforts from a population health perspective toward the reduction of disease and promotion of health within populations.

What Is Epidemiology?

Epidemiology has been defined many ways. Traditionally, it is the study of the distribution of disease and injury in human populations. More recently, broader definitions of the term move beyond the study of disease and include the examination of factors that affect the health and illness of populations, thus providing the basis for interventions aimed at improving the health and well-being of populations. The focus of epidemiology is populations rather than individuals. Epidemiology takes an analytical investigative approach to this study of health and disease and is built on three central elements:

- Person: Which groups of individuals are affected?
- Place: Where is the health issue occurring, i.e., what geographically defined region?
- Time: Over what specified period of time is the health issue occurring?

These three elements of person, place, and time are the bricks of epidemiology. The mortar cementing these bricks is made up of the methods of quantitative comparison used by epidemiologists when studying patterns of disease and health. The tools used by epidemiologists are best described as comparative, numeric, and analytical. To effectively quantify illness and disease, accurate data are requisite. Epidemiological data sources vary widely. Some of the more frequently used data sources include data from hospitals, community-based clinical practices, health departments, workplaces, schools, and health insurance reimbursement claims. The capacity for an epidemiologist to effectively analyze and present data is inextricably linked to the network of health care–related workers throughout an array of health and human service–related industries. Nurses are pivotal to the accurate assessment and timely reporting of health-related data upon which epidemiology is grounded.

Historical Beginnings

John Snow is celebrated as the founder of modern epidemiology just as Florence Nightingale is recognized as the founder of modern nursing (see Chapter 1). John Snow's watershed work, *Snow on Cholera*, introduced methods of epidemiological investigation and methods through which contemporary epidemiological methods are founded.[2] His work laid the foundation for investigation of disease in populations based on his use of the epidemiological strategy now defined as disease mapping to study the incidence of cholera deaths reported in London, England. The Lambeth Company provided residents of London with drinking water collected from the Thames river.[3] Snow's enumeration and subsequent investigation of cholera deaths reported for residents living in the vicinity of the Lambert Company's Broad Street water pump is heralded as the defining event upon which all future epidemiological methods are founded. Snow developed a frequency distribution of the number of human deaths by placing a hash mark on a city street map. Upon visual inspection of the map it became clear to Snow that there were residential patterns of deaths. He demonstrated that greater numbers of cholera deaths were clustered within the vicinity of

a specific public water source, the Broad Street water pump. The number of cholera deaths in the vicinity of the Broad Street pump far exceeded the deaths in other areas of London (Fig. 3-1).

Snow's work illustrated the three central elements related to his investigation: person, place, and time. The person variable can be defined as the number of human cholera deaths. Place is visually demonstrated by the street mapping method Snow used to count human deaths by street of residence. Finally, the time variable in Snow's study was the 5-year period between 1849 and 1854 when the Lambeth Company drew community water from the contaminated source, the Thames river. In the 150 years since Snow's community disease mapping, epidemiologists have developed more effective and timely measures for disease investigation using contemporary 21st-century methods. The three elements of person, place, and time are as central to an epidemiological investigation now as they were in the time of Snow and they form the building blocks for modern-day epidemiological investigations.

Since the time of Snow's work, epidemiology has gone through various phases. The first phase is referred to as the *sanitary phase*. It was based on the miasma theory that illness was related to poisoning by foul emanations from soil, air, and water. During this phase, public health efforts focused on improving sanitation. This approach to illness prevailed until the discovery of microscopic organisms that were linked to disease, which led to the germ theory and the *infectious disease phase* of epidemiology. This phase led to the examination of single causes for a disease and worked well in a world where infectious diseases were the number one killers. With the emergence of antibiotics and the reduction of infectious disease, the life expectancy of populations increased, especially those in developed countries. This resulted in the emergence of noncommunicable diseases and a new phase in epidemiology, the *risk factor phase*. This phase of study is still a mainstay of epidemiological investigations. It relies on the linking of exposures to the occurrence of injury or disease and helps us to identify risk factors that when reduced may result in a subsequent reduction in morbidity and mortality. The most recent phase in epidemiology is the ecological model as proposed by Susser and Susser in the 1990s,[4,5] This helps to move the science of epidemiology to a broader perspective and, as explained in Chapter 1, reflects not only the biological and behavioral influences on health but also a deeper understanding of the role of the physical environment and the underlying conditions in the social environment that create poor health.

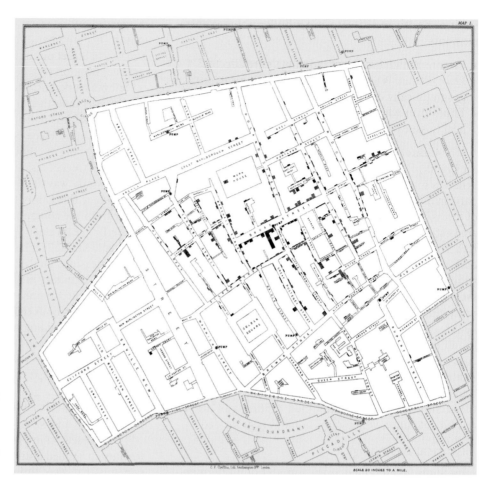

Figure 3-1 Snow map. *(Published by C.F. Cheffins, Lith, Southhampton Buildings, London, England, 1854. Snow, J. On the mode of communication of cholera [2nd ed.]. John Churchill, New Burlington Street, London, England. Retrieved from 1855. http://www.ph.ucla.edu/epi/snow/snowmap1_1854_lge.htm.)*

Epidemiological Frameworks

There are several frameworks guiding the field of epidemiology such as the epidemiological triangle, the web of causation, and the ecological model. The latter two frameworks evolved from the epidemiological triangle framework. Public health professionals continue to use these and other frameworks to assist in better understanding health phenomena.

The Epidemiological Triangle

The classic model used in epidemiology to explain the occurrence of disease is referred to as the epidemiological triangle. There are three main components to the triangle: agent, host, and environment (Fig. 3-2). In communicable diseases the model helps the epidemiologist map out the relationship between the agent or the organism responsible for the disease and the host (person) as well as the environmental factors that enhance or impede transmission of the agent to the host.

Though this model is ideally suited for explaining the transmission of an infectious agent to a human host, it is now applied to noncommunicable diseases, such as lung cancer, with a specific exposure, such as cigarette smoke, representing the agent or causative factor. The agent can be viewed as the causative factor contributing to noninfectious health problems or conditions. The **agent** may be biological (organism), chemical, (liquids, gases), nutritive (dietary components or lack of dietary components), physical (mechanical force, atmospheric such as an earthquake), or psychological (stress). The **host** is the susceptible human or animal, whereas the **environment** is all of the external factors that can influence the host's vulnerability to the risk factors related to the disease.

The value of this model lies in the fact that it helps in the development of interventions. For example, in the case of the H1N1 outbreak, epidemiologists first worked at isolating the agent. Based on the type of agent, a flu virus, it was clear that the environment needed for transmission was both the breathing in of air droplets that contained the virus and coming in contact with the virus via a *fomite,* that is, an inanimate object such as a water

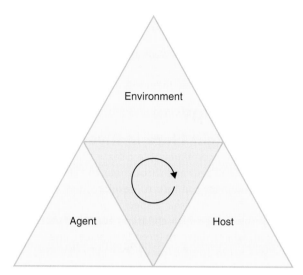

Figure 3-2 Epidemiological triangle.

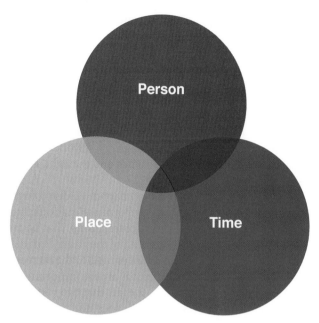

Figure 3-3 Epidemiological constants.

faucet. Based on this information, three prevention interventions were instituted. The initial approach focused on the environment. To reduce exposure of people to the virus in the environment, all those with signs and symptoms of H1N1 were asked to stay home and to cough into their arms rather than their hands. Uninfected individuals were also instructed to use hand sanitizers. The second approach was aimed at the protecting the host (person) through the development and distribution of the H1N1 vaccine. The use of a vaccine reduced the susceptibility of hosts to the agent, which, in turn, reduced further introduction of the virus into the environment. In this example, no interventions were aimed at the agent because no viable options were seen to eradicate the agent directly.

The Epidemiological Constants of Person, Place, and Time

In addition to the epidemiological triangle there are three constants that are the foundation for any epidemiological investigation: person, place, and time (Fig. 3-3). The *person* aspect typically includes demographic variables including age, gender, and ethnicity. *Place* considerations include such variables as city resident, office building user, or downhill skier. Finally, the third constant, *time*, is a critical dimension of consideration. Conditions in one location with the same subset of individuals can change substantially as a product of the passage of time. It is important to keep in mind that this model is the foundation upon which our understanding of illness and disease are built and can help guide investigations into a health issue in a population.

Who, What, When, Where, Why, How, and How Long: To further understand the use of the epidemiological triangle and the constants of person, place, and time, seven questions have been used to conduct an epidemiological investigation. These questions have most often been used to examine the epidemiology of infectious diseases. The *who* question relates to the person, the *place* question to where, the *when* and *how long* questions to time, the *what* to the causative agent, and the *why* and *how* to the mechanism for acquiring disease such as the mode of transmission in infectious diseases. The use of these seven questions provides an effective model by which illness can be analyzed at the population level for purposes of developing interventions that will improve health and/or prevent disease. This approach is an example of naturalistic experimentation, a study that occurs in the natural world and not in a controlled laboratory environment.

Causality

Although the seven questions help the investigator learn about the occurrence of disease, that knowledge only begins to provide a broader understanding of the multiple factors that could be related to the occurrence of the disease. Epidemiologists investigate possible causes of disease to better understand how to prevent and treat disease. The term *cause* is traditionally used to indicate that a stimulus or action results in an effect or outcome. For example, if you turn on a light switch, the observed effect is that the lightbulb lights up. When it comes to epidemiology, **causality** refers to determining whether a cause-and-effect relationship exists between a risk factor and a health effect. In health a cause can include a number of things related to person, place, and time. Using the light switch example again, it may be first assumed that the singular cause for lighting the bulb is the physical act of flipping the switch. In actuality, there are other factors involved, including the presence of a source of electrical energy, a working electrical connection between the switch and the light, and a lightbulb that is not burned out.

As presented throughout this chapter, epidemiological studies typically report measures of associations that are based on population-based correlations; that is, an increase or decrease in the amount of the risk factor and the frequency of the risk factor are parallel to the increase or decrease of the health issue. It is always important to keep in mind that correlation, the fact that two variables are correlated with one another, does not necessarily mean that one factor causes the other. For example, heavy smokers often have a yellow stain on the fingers that hold the cigarette. Though the presence of yellow stains on the fingers may be correlated with lung cancer, the yellow stain is not the cause of lung cancer.

To examine the possibility of causality, the first step is to determine whether there is a statistical relationship between the risk factor and the health issue. In other words, can the association between the two be attributed to chance alone—does the association between the two occur at a frequency that is higher than what could be attributed to chance? After determining that the relationship does not occur by chance alone, the next step is to determine whether the relationship is causal. In some cases the relationship between two variables is statistically significant but the relationship is noncausal. For example, in a group of schoolchildren height may be statistically correlated with grade level; that is, the higher the grade level the taller the children, but grade level is not the causal factor for the increase in height.

A causal relationship is present when there is a direct or indirect relationship between the two factors. If it is a direct relationship, then the factor causes the disease. For example, the mumps virus directly causes mumps. A nondirect relationship exists when the factor contributes to the development of the disease through its effect on other variables. Being overweight does not directly cause disease, but it adversely affects the body, thus increasing the risk of cardiovascular disease and diabetes, for example.

Results from studies conducted in the field can be limited because sources of error might be present. These errors most likely relate to assumptions of causality. For example, error can occur when deciding who was actually exposed to a potential risk factor and who was not. There can be errors in how some important variable was measured and errors relating to who received a vaccine and who did not.

▲ CASE STUDY

Asthma Right Here in River City

Asthma is a noncommunicable disease that affects individuals of all ages and throughout the life span. An epidemiologist can help to develop a better understanding of asthma within a specific pediatric population by examining which children have the disease (person), where these children live (place), and when they have acute attacks (time). This information is then used to develop community-specific health improvement initiatives that target those children at greatest risk for asthma. The first step in the investigation of any illness is to begin with inquiry. Ask questions across the seven areas of who, what, when, where, why, how, and how long.

Jane Paterson is a public health nurse employed by the Children's Medical Center of River City, a midwestern city with a population of 75,000 and a mix of urban and suburban residents. One of the primary objectives of Jane's job is to develop community-based health promotion and disease prevention initiatives targeting area youth diagnosed with asthma. According to the most recent U.S. Census data available, there are 3,000 urban and 7,000 suburban River City residents aged birth to 18 years. Of the 3,000 urban residents in this age-group, 1,500 are defined as asthmatic. Of the 7,000 nonurban residents in this age-group, 1,000 are asthmatic. Jane has been instructed that she is to have a community youth asthma intervention plan ready to roll out by the end of this year based on data from the current U.S. Census.

The Chief Financial Officer (CFO) of River City's Children's Medical Center has expressed a significant concern with the number of patients presenting in the emergency room (ER) with asthma attacks, because they are admitted to the hospital as uninsured or underinsured. The majority of these youths are eligible for the State Children's Health Insurance Program (SCHIP), a federal/state-funded health insurance program for uninsured children, but many of their parents have failed to complete required SCHIP enrollment paperwork. Though Jane recognizes that the CFO's primary goal is related to the fiscal bottom line, she is able to use the potential cost benefit as an incentive for funding her program aimed at reducing the burden of asthma-related illnesses in children.

The hospital administration would like to see a 10% reduction in asthma admission by the end of next year and a 25% reduction within the next 5 years. Jane must first have solid baseline information on childhood asthma in the population the hospital serves. She begins by answering the seven questions:

1. Who is the population of interest?
   Answer: Residents of River City aged birth to 18 years, including both asthmatic and nonasthmatic youth
2. What is it we want to do?
   Answer: Develop community-based interventions targeting youths with asthma
3. When are these health promotional initiatives being developed?
   Answer: Currently, with an asthma program or intervention to be operational by the end of the year
4. Where is this being developed?
   Answer: River City—somewhere in the Midwest
5. Why is this being developed?
   Answer: To reduce the number of low and non-compensated patients presenting at the ER and subsequently being admitted to the Children's Medical Center for treatment of uncontrolled asthma
6. How is this being developed?
   Answer: As a community-based health promotion and disease prevention initiative of the medical center
7. How long does Jane have to study and roll out a program?
   Answer: Until the end of the year to develop community interventions and support her programs with evidence based on data collected—she has been asked to reduce asthma admission by 10% next year and 25% during the next 5 years.

Web of Causation

The difficulty for Jane is to determine which risk factors for asthma in children are of priority concern for River City. Multiple factors are correlated with asthma in children, including environmental risk factors both internal and external, lack of access to care, obesity, gender, and race. Untangling the risk factors to determine what type of intervention should be developed is a challenge. To help understand the multiple factors that contribute to the development of disease, epidemiologists use a framework called the **web of causation.** This framework or model can be used to illustrate the complexity of how illness, injury, and disease are determined by multiple causes and are at the same time affected by a complex interaction of biological and sociobehavioral determinants of health (Fig. 3-4).[6-8] It helps health-care providers develop more comprehensive strategies to reduce disease- and injury-related morbidity and mortality through primary and secondary prevention measures.

The term *web* is used because the model acknowledges the complexity related to occurrence of disease[6]. Simply stated, the spider is the reason the fly is caught in the web. What are the factors that converged, resulting in the ill-fated fly being caught in the web? The fly selected the path that led him to the web, he was ill equipped to extract himself from the web once entangled, the spider selected that specific location to construct his web . . . the list of predetermining factors is endless. The fact is for both the fly caught in the spider's web as well as for humans there is frequently no one single cause for an undesirable outcome but a convergence of circumstances, actions, inactions, and behaviors.

Ecological Model

The ecological model has been used in recent years to design health promotion efforts and understand health behavior. The terms *health promotion* and *health behavior* have been used during the past 25 years to help understand the interventions that can be done to help maintain

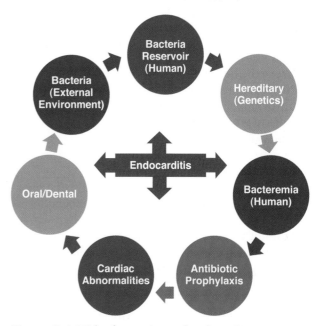

Figure 3-4 Web of causation and endocarditis.

and improve health (health promotion) and the behaviors that contribute either positively or negatively to overall health (health behaviors). The ecological model provides a formal theoretical foundation on which public health nursing has established a professional identity and knowledge base.

Ecological studies use groups, not the individual, as the unit of analysis.[9] Conclusions from ecological studies should be considered with caution. The classic notion of the stork bringing the baby to new parents is a contemporary manifestation of what one might suggest could have been an ecological study, demonstrating the ecological fallacy discussed later in this chapter. Anchored in the pagan belief that storks brought babies to expecting mothers, the arrival of storks in northern Germany coincided with the storks' spring and the increase in the number of human births. The increased birth rates in spring might have something to do with the 9-month elapsed time between summer and normal human gestation. Analyses of health-related behaviors at the group level are carried out by epidemiologists, providing the evidence by which practice-based health-care providers can begin the development of interventions using the ecological model approach. An effective ecological model defines, understands, changes behavior, and ultimately promotes population-level health and wellness.

◼ Tools of Epidemiology: Demography and Biostatistics

The science of epidemiology requires the use of particular tools to help epidemiologists study health and wellness as well as determine which interventions will help improve the health of populations. Among these tools are demography and biostatistics. Understanding how to apply demography and biostatistics helps nurses in all settings to provide better care and promote the health of the populations they serve.

Demography

Demography is the population-level study of person-related variables or factors. The field of demography has been around since the early 20th century. Warren Thompson, an early pioneer, developed the demographic transition model used today to explain the shift from high birth and death rates to low birth and death rates within populations.[10] Warren Thompson is to the field of demography as Florence Nightingale is to nursing and John Snow is to epidemiology. Establishing methods for tracking populations over time adds to the methods of

tracking disease established by John Snow. Public health and health-related disciplines use demography and associated methods to better understand population-level patterns related to health phenomena.

Typically, person-related variables are compared over two or more time periods to establish trends within the population of interest. Comparing demographic data from time 1 to time 2 is fundamental to the promotion and establishment of relevant prohealth environments, policies, and behaviors across time. For example, comparing the percentage of the population below the poverty level in a particular community from 2000 to 2010 can help identify changes in the population that may affect access to health care. Another example is to put together a visual depiction of demographic data using the demographic transition model (Fig. 3-5). This model refers to population change over time, especially in relation to birth and death rates.

The study of trends across time results in interventions including policy reform, re-engineering, educational initiatives, and enforcement of standards and laws to assure the health of the public. Public health is a dynamic interdisciplinary field that is associated with other fields such as political science, sociology, criminology, and psychology. Ultimately the sociobehavioral determinants of health contributing to the health of individuals are affected substantially by subsystems such as political, social, and environmental factors.[11]

Obtaining Population Data

A challenge for public health professionals is obtaining current and accurate population data. There are various sources of data from the local to the international level. Data are obtained initially through various routes

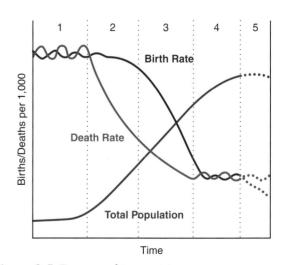

Figure 3-5 Demographic transition.

including surveys, mandatory health data reports, independent research, and hospital data, to name a few. Some of the data are available on the Internet, whereas other data are protected and special permission is needed to obtain them.

Census Data: Census data are extremely useful sources of demographic data. These public domain data are available on both the official U.S. Census Bureau Web site (see Web Resources on Davis*Plus*) as well as in multiple formats upon special request. It is advised that public health researchers, health promotion planners, and other professionals charged with developing and implementing health promotion and disease prevention initiatives access and review local regional and state-level data provided in the U.S. Census. Accessing U.S. Census data related to a population located in a specific geographical area is a very effective starting point when seeking to quantify a health-related phenomenon. Demographic variables include gender, race, housing, economic level, age, and other relevant data. However, census data reflect populations within a specific geographical area. The census data are available from the national level down to the neighborhood or census block level and are useful if the population of interest is defined based on a geographical community. The data can be viewed based on ZIP code, town, county, or state. Accessing the Web site provides a mechanism for exploring a town or county to determine what the population is, how many housing units are rented or owned and how many people living in the town or county have an income below the poverty level.

Community Data: More typically, public health professionals are asked to address community-level health issues. Community data are valuable resources with both strengths and limitations. Before addressing sources of community data, it would be useful to review the discussion of community in Chapter 1. Which of the following is representative of a community—residents in Portland, Oregon, diabetics in the tri-state area, women above age 65 years, or gay men in Houston, Texas? An answer of "all of the above" would be correct. Community data are not limited to simply a geographical location but can take on additional characteristics such as disease status (diabetes), lifestyle (gay, lesbian, bisexual), and demographical considerations (race, ethnicity, and age). Examples of typical opportunities for public health nurses and other health-related professionals to use community data include hospital-based initiatives, health plan initiatives, nonprofit agency initiatives, special interest groups, and local/state/federal initiatives.

Some examples of community data relating to the health of residents in cities, states, and territories include the Behavioral Risk Factor Surveillance Study (BRFSS) found at the Centers for Disease Control and Prevention Behavioral Risk Factor Surveillance System Frequently Asked Questions at its Web site. Disease-specific data and health-planning and education resource materials can be found at the American Diabetes Association Web site as well as at local area health-care agencies (see Web Resources on Davis*Plus*). As mentioned above, if the community is a geographical community, the U.S. Census data can be used to focus on demographic information such as the number of women older than age 65 years. More challenging might be tapping community-level data on variables such as lifestyle. Challenges in estimating lifestyle variables (e.g., number of gay men living in Houston, Texas) are difficult to overcome as there is a lack of accurate and reliable data sources on these types of variables. Data relating to these more complex variables can and often are generated through original data collection at the community level.

The Nurses' Health Study, now more than 30 years old, is of special interest to nursing professionals. Information on this study can be found on a Harvard University Web site (see Web Resources on Davis*Plus*). This study provides community-level data that have been generalized to women's health in the general population. By seeking to better understand community-level data, such as women's health, a more complete understanding of the factors influencing health and appropriate proactive measures toward the improvement of women's health can be successfully achieved. Community data can relate to person, place, and time variables and a myriad of interactions between these three broad categories. Responsible investigators should always take a critical look at the sources of data and remain cognizant that error likely exists within any data to be used in the development of community health programming. Potential sources of error should not halt efforts to promote the health of the public but should be carefully considered and reported openly.

Biostatistics

Biostatistics reflects the analysis of data related to human organisms. Biostatistics is used in public health science and other biological sciences. It examines variation between biological organisms (people, mice, cells). Thus, it is a core part of public health science.

Mean, Median, and Mode

Demographers use descriptive statistics as well as advanced inferential statistical methods to describe the size, structure, and distribution patterns of populations and subpopulations within geographically defined regions. These measures include the computation of the mean, median, mode, quartiles, and interquartile ranges. Demographers also compute the percent change in populations over time as well as estimate population counts for the future. These come under the umbrella of descriptive data analysis.

Descriptive data analysis is regarded by most epidemiologists as the initial step in analysis of demographic data. However, the analysis of data at the descriptive or inferential level of analysis is only as good as the accuracy of the data being used. Though the accuracy of data and the methods by which data are gathered go beyond the scope of this text, there are many useful references that should be consulted in developing original data collection protocols (see Web Resources on DavisPlus).

Determining the mean, the median, and the mode uses basic math skills. All three are measures of central tendency. The mean is what is commonly considered the average, as it is the mathematical average of a set of numbers. The *mean* is calculated by summing the total of all values and dividing by the total number of values in the set. The *median* is the middle value in a set of values. For example, if you have 20 individual patient blood pressures, the 10th occurrence in an ordered set from lowest to highest is the median. The *mode* is the value that occurs more times within a data set than any other occurrence. To help you understand these basic concepts complete the question in Box 3-1.

Percent Change

It is useful to have a time 1 and time 2 estimate to estimate a **percent change** related to a demographic variable or health statistic. The time 1 measure is often referred to as the baseline and can be used to establish the proportion or percentage of illness or disease within the population. This is often used to evaluate changes in a population over time and is calculated by taking the new number (B) and subtracting the original number (A) and dividing the resulting number by the original number A (Box 3-2). This information is quite valuable when completing community assessments (see Chapter 4), because it explains shifts in population that may have an impact on the health of the community or the type of interventions needed. For example, if there has been a positive 20% change in the population who are over the age of 85, then the community may have increased health needs related to aging, but if the opposite has occurred, a negative 20% change in those over the age of 85 and a 20% increase in those aged 1 to 5 years, there may be less need for interventions aimed at the very old and more interventions needed to support infant health.

BOX 3–1 Calculating Population Mean, Median, and Mode

Methods Review

Mean, Median, Mode, Quartiles, and Interquartile Range
  Twenty students have been admitted to the dual degree MSN/MPH degree program. You have been asked by the Dean of the College to report the average age of these students.

Data Set [Not real persons]:

Name	Gender	Age in Years
1. Angela Jones	F	23
2. Bill Baker	M	32
3. Connie Clark	F	22
4. Dennis Daniels	M	24
5. Emily Edwards	F	56
6. Frank Fitzgerald	M	23
7. Georgia Grant	F	24
8. Herald Hall	M	22
9. Ingrid Israel	F	22
10. James Jennings	M	24
11. Kelly Karr	F	22
12. Lawrence Lee	M	35
13. Melissa Martin	F	22
14. Nelson Newman	M	21
15. Olivia Owen	F	22
16. Paul Pierce	M	31
17. Quinn Queen	F	27
18. Robert Reynolds	M	23
19. Sarah Salzman	F	22
20. Timothy Tucker	M	22

Q1: The mean, median, and mode are all measures of central tendency—averages. You should report all three.
A: Mean = 25.96
A: Median = 23
A: Mode = 22

BOX 3–2 Calculating PercentChange [Not from an actual data set]

Formula

(Time B–Time A)/Time A × 100 = percent change

Population City A	2000 Time A	2010 Time B	Percent change
Hispanic	1,512	1,955	29.3%
85 years of age or older	215	92	−57.2%

Rates

To help in understanding the distribution of disease in a population, epidemiologists calculate rates. In understanding the magnitude of a health-related phenomenon, epidemiologists need both a numerator and a denominator. What does this statement mean? Imagine that a health educator in Columbus, Ohio, reports that there are 12,500 smokers in his city and a health educator in the Columbus, Indiana, health department reports that there are 11,800 smokers in his city. Based on these two estimates, it is fair to say that smoking is a greater problem in Columbus, Ohio, than it is in Columbus, Indiana, correct? It is clear that there are 700 more smokers in the Ohio city than there are in the Indiana city. However, the denominator is missing in this equation. By going to the U.S. Census Bureau and learning what the city population estimate was, we can effectively establish a denominator. It is always advised to use the same source when possible so that comparable population estimates and associated collection methods are assured in establishing estimates. If the estimated population for Columbus, Ohio, is 730,657 and for Columbus, Indiana, it is 39,059, then it is possible to calculate the percentage. Now the facts are that 1.7% of the population in Columbus, Ohio, smokes compared with 30.2% in Columbus, Indiana!

Using these data from the two towns, we just calculated the rate of smoking in each population. To further illustrate how a rate is determined, consider being the health commissioner of Petersburg, Oregon, population 5,000. Of the total population, 1,250 people report that they are current cigarette smokers. The health department receives a weekly report on the number of influenza cases reported in the city in the month of January (Table 3-1).

One should assume that these data are accurate and that no reporting error exists.

Given the data in Table 3-1 and the information on how many people live in the city, we can construct population rates of influenza cases across the two classifications of smoker and nonsmoker. First, using the data in the table calculate the rate of influenza in smokers during week 1. To do this divide 50 by 1,250, which illustrates a rate of 4%, or 4 in every 100 smokers came down with the flu in week 1. In comparison less than 1% of nonsmokers came down with the flu in week 1 (1 in 100). If one considers the total population percentages by week, there was a spike in cases during the third week of January. However, by breaking the data out by smoking status it is clear that there are variations in the monthly pattern across the two groups. Therefore a **rate** represents the proportion of a disease or other health-related event such as mortality within a population at a certain point in time. It is the basic measure of disease used by epidemiologists and other health professionals to describe the risk of disease in a certain population over a certain period of time.

How to Calculate: Calculating rates is a relatively simple mathematical procedure, that is, assuming that one can secure an accurate estimate of disease or illness in the population to use as the numerator and an accurate total population estimate to serve as the denominator (Box 3-3). Again, using the data in Table 3-1, focus on the first cell corresponding to week 1 by smokers with influenza. The numerator is 50 (week 1 influenza cases) and the denominator is 1,250 (smokers residing in Petersburg, Oregon). The number 100 represents a constant, in this case per 100 smokers. The constant could be 1,000 or 10,000 depending on the frequency of the disease in the

TABLE 3–1	Fabricated Data—Influenza in Anytown, USA		
Week	Influenza Smoker *Number of New Cases*	Influenza Nonsmoker *Number of New Cases*	Total Influenza *Number of New Cases*
1	50 (4.0%)	20 (0.5%)	70 (1.4%)
2	40 (3.2%)	25 (6.8%)	65 (1.3%)
3	80 (6.4%)	50 (1.35%)	130 (2.6%)
4	700 (56.0%)	100 (2.7%)	800 (16.0%)
	1,250 (Smokers)	3,700 (Nonsmokers)	5,000 (Total Population)

BOX 3–3   Calculating Rates

Using the data in Table 3-1, focus on the first cell corresponding to week 1 by smokers with influenza.

The rate of influenza was calculated using the following formula:

(Number of cases [numerator] ÷ population [denominator]) × a constant = rate per 100; 1,000; 10,000; or 100,000.

For this case

$$(50 \div 1,250) \times 100 = 4.0\%$$

---

population. This approach allows for the presentation of rates based on various constants. For example, one may express it in terms of 1,000 or 10,000 rather than 100 if the number of cases is small. Infant mortality rate is expressed as the number of infant deaths for infants less than age 1 year per 1,000 live births.

Types of Rates: Mortality and morbidity are two commonly used rates in epidemiology as well as within the health-care professions. **Mortality** refers to the number of deaths within a given population. To calculate the mortality rate take the number of deaths within a specified time period and divide it by the total number of individuals within the same populations during the same time period. A commonly used mortality rate is the infant mortality rate, as this measure is considered an effective metric by which to gauge the health-care "systems" of a nation. To calculate the infant mortality rate, take the number of infant deaths among those age birth to 365 days and divide by the total number of live births during the same 365-day period. To establish a rate include a multiplier that represents the constant mentioned above (e.g., × 1,000). **Morbidity** refers to the number or proportion of individuals experiencing a similar disability, illness, or disease. Examples of conditions and diseases that are reported using morbidity are the number of infants within a county with pertussis ("whooping" cough), the number of new mothers delivering at St. Ann's in 2010 experiencing postpartum depression, the number of returning service men and women experiencing post-traumatic stress disorder (PTSD), and the number of adults in the United States living with diabetes. Note that the challenge in reporting these conditions as rates is in accurately establishing the denominator or the total number of individuals at risk for the condition in question.

Attack rates are calculated by placing the number of ill or diseased people in the numerator and dividing by the total number of ill plus well people (in the susceptible population) in the population of interest, then multiplying by a given multiplier (e.g., 100,000). The **secondary attack rate** can be calculated by taking the number of new cases of a disease or illness among the contacts of the initial (primary) cases dividing by the number of people in the population at risk and multiplying by a given multiplier (e.g., 100,000).

Prevalence, Incidence: Prevalence and incidence rates are used by epidemiologists to demonstrate the burden of disease or illness within the population of interest. However, these practitioners must carefully consider when and how to report these rates, as they can be misleading. What is the difference between prevalence and incidence? **Incidence** can be best understood as the number of new cases of a disease or illness at a specific time or over a specific period of time. **Prevalence** is the total number of accumulated cases of a disease or illness both new and preexisting at a given time.

Imagine that you are a public health official and that you have been serving the people of New York City for the past 25 years. In 1994, the total number of newly diagnosed cases of HIV was 2,500 and the total number of existing or prevalent cases in 1994 was 5,000. In 2009, 15 years later, the number of newly diagnosed cases of HIV is 1,000 and the total number of existing or prevalent cases is 50,000. The change in annualized new HIV cases went from 2,500 to 1,000 and the prevalence went from 5,000 to 50,000 over the 15-year period. This 15-year change shows a decrease in new cases, whereas the prevalence rate comparing the difference across the 15-year period is a 10-fold increase. Given these data, would it be fair for a reporter from the *New York Times* to feature a headline of "HIV in New York City Drastically Increases Fifteen Times Since the Mid-1990s!" or "HIV in NYC Decreases After 15 Years of Prevention Education"? Both headlines are accurate, yet neither is a fair nor accurate account of the state of HIV in the city.

A **prevalence** rate is basically the number of existing cases (numerator) divided by the total number of persons in the population (denominator). The rate calculated using the information in Table 3-1 can be understood as a point prevalence or the number of ill people divided by the total number of people in the population "group" at a specific point in time. An associated measure, referred to as the *period prevalence*, is calculated as the number of people ill divided by the estimate of the average number in the population during a specified time period. An application of period prevalence might be the number of people living with a chronic disease within a given population during a specified time, such as a year. Asthma is a chronic disease that might be effectively presented using a period prevalence.

In addition to prevalence there are other rates reported by epidemiologists that are important to understand and use appropriately (Table 3-2). They are incidence rate, attack rate, and secondary attack rate. An **incidence** rate can be calculated by placing the number of new cases diagnosed in a given period of time by the total number at risk in the population over that same time period and multiplying by a given multiplier (e.g., 100,000). For example, the incidence of H1N1 in a school during a specified period of time would be the number of new cases of H1N1 divided by the denominator, those children in the school who had not had H1N1 in the past. Those children who had had H1N1 would be removed from the denominator to indicate those children at risk.

A good way to examine the difference between the incidence and prevalence rate is the *prevalence pot* (Fig. 3-6), defined in Chapter 2. The prevalence pot represents all the current cases of a disease in a population. Entering into the pot are the new cases reflected by the incidence rate. Exit from the prevalence pot occurs by one of three events: death, cure, or disability. For some diseases such as HIV/AIDS the only way a case leaves the prevalence pot is through death. For other diseases such as polio, all three options occur. The size of the prevalence pot depends both on the incidence rate and on the duration of the disease. Over time the prevalence pot for HIV/AIDS in the United States has grown not because of dramatic increases in the incidence of HIV/AIDS, but because of the pharmaceutical interventions that have extended life spans. For other serious health threats such as the 2009–2010 H1N1 virus, the prevalence pot grew rapidly with the increase in incidence, but dropped rapidly once incidence rates dropped because of the short duration of the disease.

The incidence and prevalence rates are affected by factors such as the number of people being screened for the disease and the number of people surviving with a positive

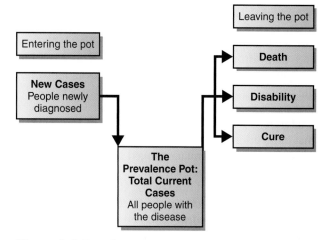

Figure 3-6 Prevalence pot.

HIV status. During the early 1980s and into the 1990s, few people survived a positive diagnosis for more than a few years. Thus, the absence of effective medical treatment options would have resulted in higher death rates and subsequently lower prevalence rates. As screening tests became more widely available and stigmatizing labels began to be reduced, more people became willing to be screened for HIV. What is missing from the presentation is the number of people tested who were not positive for HIV. The lesson to be learned is that data reporting does not necessarily result in effective interpretation. Careful, cautious, and intentional epidemiological data reporting is a critical task of the public health information officer.

Comparing Dependent and Independent Rates: Data in Table 3-1 provide a useful illustration of independent and dependent rates. The weekly influenza rates independent of smoking status for the month of January are 15.0, 12.5, 26.0, and 16.0 per 100 persons, respectively. Simply stated, these weekly rates are independent of the smoking status of the individuals within the

TABLE 3–2	Differentiating Rates		
Measure	Numerator	Denominator	Multiplier
Point prevalence	Number ill	Population	e.g., 100,000
Incidence rate	Number of new cases over specified time	Total number at risk during time period	e.g., 100,000
Attack rate	Number of new cases during an epidemic period	Total number in population at start of epidemic period	e.g., 1,000
Secondary attack rate	Number of new cases among contacts of known cases	Total number of population at risk	e.g., 1,000

population. The converse is true for dependent rates where the rates of influenza by smoking status by week range from approximately 40% to 32%, spiking to 64%, and finally dropping to 56%. The week 3 spike pattern is also reflected in the nonsmoking population. However, the proportion of nonsmokers with influenza is consistently 25% to 50% lower than that estimated for smokers. Therefore, a public health official might accurately state that influenza rates (independent of smoking) for Petersburg, Oregon, for January ranged between 12.5% and 26%. In addition, dependent rates adjusted for smoking status for the city and time period demonstrated a substantially greater proportion of influenza among smokers.

The terms *independent rates* and *dependent rates* are also used to describe rates that are independent or not independent of each other. For example, if you were concerned with the infant mortality rate in city Y compared with the infant mortality rate in city X, the two rates would be independent of each other. In contrast, if you wanted to compare the rates between city Y in state X and the rate in state X, the rates are dependent; that is, all of the cases in city Y are included in the count of cases in state X because the city is in state X.

■ Descriptive and Analytical Epidemiology

Now that we have examined the basic demographics of the population of interest, what else can be done to learn about the specific health issue? There are three broad categories of epidemiological studies that help to answer questions about the health of populations: descriptive, analytical, and experimental studies. The vast majority of epidemiological investigations, particularly community-based public health investigations, are defined as either descriptive or analytical. In descriptive case control and cohort studies, the investigator has no control over the exposure or nonexposure status of subjects. In contrast, experimental epidemiology consists of the research methodology whereby the investigator has direct control over the subject's assignment to exposure status. Clinical trials fall into the latter classification. Experimental studies tend to fall under the authority of clinical research scientists and are housed in academic research centers, federal agencies, or private research and development agencies, such as pharmaceutical companies.

Descriptive Epidemiology

Descriptive epidemiology refers to the analysis of population and health data that are already available. It includes the calculation of rates (e.g., mortality) and an examination of how they vary according to demographic variables (e.g., gender, race, socioeconomic status).[12] Similar to the concepts discussed relating to demography, descriptive epidemiology provides an understanding of the general features of the population of interest. In contrast to demography, the epidemiologist shifts from a broad population demographic representation to one that illustrates aspects of health, wellness, and/or disease considerations within the population.

Analytical Epidemiology

Analytical epidemiology involves examining health-related data to determine the association between risk factors and the occurrence of a health phenomenon. In descriptive epidemiology the epidemiologist can use the findings to formulate a hypothesis about possible causes for the health phenomenon. In analytical epidemiology the purpose is to test the hypothesis. There are three basic types of studies that use analytical epidemiology methods: the case-control study, the cohort study, and the clinical trial. The study may use a cross-sectional study design that reports health-related information for a specific point in time. Or the study may use a prospective, retrospective, or longitudinal design related to data collected in more than one time period.

Cross-Sectional Studies

Cross-sectional studies or surveys examine risk factors and disease using data collected at the same point in time. It is easy to remember that a cross-sectional study provides an estimate of the disease status or frequency at one point in time; thus, it is truly a cross section of the disease or illness within the population of interest at a given moment in time. It is also called a prevalence study. For example, numerous health surveys are conducted by the National Center for Health Statistics as a means of determining the prevalence of disease at a given point in time. They are relatively easy to administer and the data can be collected in a rather short period of time. However, because they are cross-sectional, they do not provide a temporal, or time-related, sequence of events. For example, if nurse Jane in River City wanted to determine how many school-age children in River City had asthma, she might conduct a survey of all parents through the school system and ask whether their child had ever been diagnosed with asthma. Jane might also ask whether they are current smokers. Because Jane collected data at one point in time, she cannot with confidence assert that parental smoking preceded the diagnosis of asthma. However, the data can provide valuable information on which children are at greatest risk for asthma.

The cross-sectional design methods are not limited to the study of disease or even illness factors. For example, satisfaction with health care–related services within a community can be and are evaluated using this research design methodology.

Case-Control Studies and Odds Ratio

The case-control study design allows the epidemiologist to compare the ratio of disease in those exposed to a risk factor with those who were not exposed to the same risk factor. Using the case-control method the epidemiologist has a specified number of people with a disease or illness. These individuals who are defined as diseased or ill are the "cases." The epidemiologist then must seek to establish as the controls a representative group of people without the disease or illness. Then both the cases and controls are measured related to a specific exposure or multiple exposures.

A standard two-by-two table is used to divide individual-level or person-specific data into disease status (yes/no) and exposure status (yes/no). The odds ratio (OR) is defined as the odds of having a disease or condition among the exposed in comparison with the odds of those who were not exposed. The calculation of the OR is a relatively simple mathematical procedure. The OR is mathematically expressed as [OR = AD/BC] (Box 3-4). The epidemiologist then determines whether the OR for those with disease to have experienced the exposure is significantly greater than the controls by calculating confidence intervals and *p*-values for each OR point estimate. This calculation goes beyond the introductory nature of this text. Intermediate and advanced epidemiology textbooks can and should be consulted to gain depth of understanding of these calculations.

Take, for example, individuals with oral cancer of the gums. The researcher hypothesizes that people who use or have a history of using smokeless tobacco (chewing tobacco) are at greater risk of developing oral cancer. The researcher now needs a group of individuals to serve as the controls. To construct the two-by-two table and establish the risk of oral cancer from chewing tobacco, she needs a group of individuals who have not been exposed to chewing tobacco. The cases are the individuals with oral cancer, who are asked to report on exposure variable and use of chewing tobacco. The challenge is to find a fair representative group that fits into the control or "no disease" category. Often studies of this nature are conducted using controls at the same health-care facility with a different disease or illness. In this scenario, skin cancer patients will be used as controls. The biological plausibility of developing skin cancer as a result of using chewing tobacco is unlikely, but could indeed be a confounder, that is, a variable that can cause the disease being studied and is also associated with the exposure of interest. Confounders can make it difficult to establish a clear causal link unless adjustments are made for their effects. Confounders are potential limitations in all epidemiological studies; methods of controlling for confounders are addressed in advanced epidemiological textbooks.

Case-control studies have limitations. There can be effects from multiple determinants of health, the complexity of additive and/or interactive exposures on health. There are also potential problems related to the representativeness of the cases and the controls, that is, how well they reflect the target population. Another issue is accurately determining exposure. Case-control studies are done **retrospectively;** that is, disease has already occurred in the cases. For both cases and controls, determining whether individuals had been exposed requires obtaining a history from the individuals rather than through direct observation of the exposure. See Box 3-5 for a case-control study of the asthma cases in River City.

BOX 3–5 **Case-Control Study for River City**

Set up a two-by-two table for children aged birth to 18 years with residency (urban/non-urban) on one axis and asthma status (yes/no) on the other axis.
Answer:

	Asthma (Yes)	Asthma (No)	Totals
Urban	1,500	1,500	3,000
Non-urban	1,000	6,000	7,000
Totals	2,500	7,500	10,000

Calculate the appropriate measure of association. HINT: Either relative risk or odds ratio.
Answer: Odds ratio — AD ÷ BC = 1,500 × 6,000 ÷ 1,500 × 1,000 — [OR = 6.0] Interpretation: River City youth between the ages of birth to 18 years living in the urban district have six times the risk of presenting to the ED with asthma-like symptoms as compared with nonurban children.

BOX 3–4 **Calculating Odds Ratio**

	Disease Status (Yes)	Disease Status (No)
Exposure status (Yes)	A	B
Exposure status (No)	C	D

Cohort Studies and Relative Risk

Cohort studies are studies that follow a specific population, subset of the population, or group of people over a specified period of time. Cohort studies can be effective in generating a wealth of data relating to the population of interest. The epidemiologist has substantial control over the data collection process; therefore, cohort studies have strong validity. This validity comes with high costs that include actual direct costs in personnel as well as costs in time from data collection to the generation of findings and conclusions. Three types of cohort studies are found in application:

- Prospective
- Retrospective
- Historical

Two Web links are provided below. The first directs you to the Fels Longitudinal Study established in 1929, the longest-running continuous human life span and development study in the world. This longitudinal study is housed at the Wright State University Boonshoft School of Medicine in Dayton, Ohio, and can be accessed at http://www.med.wright.edu/lhrc/fels. The second is to the Framingham study, a commonly referenced cardiovascular health study established in 1948. Both studies are longitudinal and provide useful data to researchers on human populations over time. Information on the Framingham study can be accessed at http://www.framinghamheartstudy.org.[13]

The *relative risk* is the measure of association used for cohort studies. Relative risk is determined by comparing the incidence rate in the exposed group with the incidence rate in the nonexposed group. This measure is calculated by dividing the number of people in the yes/yes (cell A) divided by the row total divided by the number of people in the yes/no (cell C) divided by the row total (Box 3-6).

For example, if we were interested in exploring the risks of using oral birth control pills and stroke (these are fabricated data), we could follow 500 women from age 18 to 25 during a specific time period. We would divide these women into two groups: those taking an oral birth control pill (250) and those using alternative birth control or none (250). We find that after following these 500 women during the 32-year study, among those who were taking the pill, 100 suffered a stroke and 150 had no stroke, whereas among those not taking the pill, 24 had stroke and 225 had no stroke. How would the relative risk be calculated?

Confounder WARNING: Of the 100 women taking oral contraception 90 were cigarette smokers. What additional information is needed to establish a confounder effect based on tobacco use? As explained earlier, a confounder is another variable that may actually account in whole or in part for the relationship between the observed variable (taking the pill) and the outcome (stroke).

Most cohort studies use a **prospective** longitudinal approach that requires following a group over a long period of time, which can be 30 years or more. An example is the Nurses' Health Study that began in 1976. The purpose of the study was to examine the long-term effects of oral contraceptives.[14] The researchers have added to this important study with the Nurses' Health Study II in 1989 and the Nurses' Health Study III in 2008. Data are collected from participants every 2 years with a sustained 90% response rate. Clearly, this type of design is limited in application because waiting more than 30 years to establish conclusive results can be problematic. In addition, the notion of confounders, or factors affecting the outcome other than the factor of interest, is a limitation. Despite these challenges, data from large cohort studies have contributed greatly to our understanding of risk factors related to disease. The Framingham heart study is still ongoing today, spanning three generations.[13] Prior to the study the common belief was that cardiovascular disease was part of the aging process. The information obtained in the study changed the approach to the prevention and treatment of cardiovascular disease and continues to contribute to our understanding of cardiovascular disease today.

There are times when a cohort study is done retrospectively. Imagine a situation in which 500 women today are asked to report on their past 32 years of history. Specifically, data are collected on all 500 women relating to oral contraception usage and stroke. Note: In this retrospective study design, you can add a variable such as cigarette smoking. This design methodology provides the researcher with the opportunity to report findings in the present relating to the variables of interest. Sources of error in this design include accuracy of reporting by the subjects, subject attrition or discontinued participation, a concern known as *right censoring*, which is beyond the scope of this introductory text, confounding, and other issues related to following a large cohort over a long period of time.

BOX 3–6	Calculating Relative Risk		
HINT: $(A \div [A + B]) \div (C \div [C + D])$			
	Stroke	No Stroke	Total
Oral pill	100	150	250
No oral pill	25	225	250

Finally, the combination of both the retrospective and prospective methods above is referred to as *historical prospective*. In this design, we seek past information as well as future data to establish our data set. This is a useful method as it provides the opportunity to reduce the length of time necessary to establish results while at the same time giving the researcher the opportunity to gather future data from subjects. This method can be used to gather data quickly but is open to errors in accuracy. Nurses in clinical practice settings collect patient histories, which are good examples of these data. Recall is often a problem with any study design that seeks to collect data from the subjects based on their recall regardless of the recall period. Often an individual can't remember what he or she ate for breakfast a week ago, or what his or her last fasting blood sugar was. Imagine how much error might be present in collecting health behavior data from the general population.

Clinical Trials and Causality

Clinical trials represent a special type of epidemiological investigation and the research methods relating to clinical trials are a special subset. Clinical trials vary widely in their methods. Clinical trials have a control and an experimental group and require random assignment to either the control or the experimental group. The control group is not exposed to a treatment, medication, or therapy, whereas the experimental group is exposed to the treatment or intervention of interest. The two groups are then compared to evaluate whether there are statistically significant differences in outcomes between the two groups. Clinical trials are more likely to result in findings that lend themselves to causal statements of relationships. Cohort and case-control studies can demonstrate an association between two variables, but a clinical trial gets much closer to establishing causality. That said, causality is always a challenging goal to attain and causal assumptions within clinical research trials should be carefully considered.

■ Outbreak Investigations

Outbreak investigation is fundamental to field epidemiology and pivotal to the role of epidemiologists, public health nurses, and public health workers. As previously confirmed, epidemiology is truly an applied science. It uses quantitative data analysis methods at the population level to better understand health-related circumstances within communities. The unit of analysis is groups of people, not the individual. It is critical to remain cognizant of the risk of committing an *ecological fallacy*. The fallacy refers to the erroneous assumption that one can draw conclusions for individuals based on group findings, which occurs when the researcher draws conclusions at the individual level based solely on the observations made at the group level. An example of an ecological fallacy can be illustrated based on a study of obesity in women in two cities. Consider that the women in City A had a higher body mass index (BMI) on average than the women in City B. It would be a fallacy to conclude, just based on these averages, that a randomly selected woman from City A would have a higher BMI than a randomly selected woman from City B. Since the BMI reported in the study reflected an average and not a median, there is no information about the distribution of BMI values in the two cities, and a randomly selected individual woman from City A may actually have a lower BMI than a randomly selected woman from City B.

While much of the work of public health nurses and public health workers is focused on implementing initiatives that prevent disease or illness, the outbreak investigation is in response to elevated levels of a disease or illness within the defined population. The outbreak investigation is one of the more commonly recognized applications of epidemiology by the general public. Examples of commonly recognized outbreak investigations include foodborne illness investigations resulting from salmonella, gastroenteritis illness investigations at community daycare centers resulting from *Shigella,* communities with elevated numbers of pediatric asthma emergency room visits and subsequent hospitalization, health-care providers with unusually high numbers of patients with uncontrolled type 2 diabetes, employees with elevated levels of asbestosis, and communities with unexpectedly high numbers of infants with elevated blood lead levels. Outbreak investigations are an important application of epidemiology because of the truly applied nature of the inquiry. The investigation is not simply an academic exercise but an opportunity to initiate disease or illness investigation, analyze data collected within the community or workplace, interpret data, implement health promotion and risk reduction interventions, and evaluate short- and long-term health and the effects of wellness on the population. Precipitating factors relating to person, place, and time are essential as is an awareness of disease or illness etiology. Outbreak investigations can occur in relation to infectious diseases, chronic disease, and exposure to toxic agents.

Investigation strategies are dependent on the type of agent resulting in illness, the communicability of the illness, the virulence of the agent, and the **infectivity** of the agent, defined as the proportion of persons exposed to an infectious agent who become infected by it and the specific route of infection. As presented earlier in this chapter, three key aspects of tracking disease within a population and developing strategies to reduce the spread and severity of outbreaks are contingent on person, place, and time considerations. The importance of effective surveillance of disease and illness is vital in establishing expected levels of illness within the population. The Centers for Disease Control and Prevention (CDC) maintains publically reportable data on a number of diseases.

Illnesses such as influenza and pertussis have seasonal variations and can be substantially reduced through preventive vaccination. The number of reported influenza cases typically spikes annually from December through March. Public health community-wide vaccination campaigns are initiated in autumn each year in an attempt to prevent disease through targeted immunization at the population level. A vaccine for the prevention of pertussis was developed in the 1940s and aggressive public health childhood immunization initiatives resulted in a low number of reported cases nationally in the mid-1970s. Unfortunately, the number of pertussis cases has increased during the past 30 years with an increasing proportion of cases among the adult and older segments of the U.S. population.[15]

Communicable Disease Outbreaks

Communicable diseases can be the result of a point source or a common source followed by secondary spread within the population. Typically, person-to-person spread is observed. However, communicable diseases such as the West Nile virus are spread through vectors, specifically insect to human. The 21st century has witnessed a substantial reduction of diseases as a result of improved environmental conditions and sanitation systems. Person-to-person spread of communicable disease continues to present substantial challenges to professions charged with promoting health and reducing the burden of disease at the population level. Unlike systems, which can be reengineered to eliminate risks of exposure, strategies addressing person-to-person transmission of disease can be daunting. Global public health and disease prevention initiatives such as hand hygiene education and safe sex practices are initiatives seeking to address person-to-person spread of communicable diseases. See Chapter 10 for further information on how to investigate a communicable disease outbreak.

Noncommunicable Disease Outbreaks

In the latter decades of the 20th century, chronic diseases have replaced communicable diseases as the major disease classification in high-income countries. Simply stated, as a result of aggressive interventions during the past 100 years, the mortality rate from communicable diseases has dramatically declined, contributing to higher life expectancy. With this increased life expectancy more people are surviving long enough to develop noncommunicable diseases that occur later in life such as cardiovascular disease. Often referred to as lifestyle diseases, illnesses related to poor diet, a lack of exercise, and tobacco and alcohol use have become epidemic. Some typically diagnosed noncommunicable diseases include heart disease, stroke, type 2 diabetes, cancer, and chronic obstructive pulmonary disorder (COPD). Initiatives including tobacco cessation programs, balanced nutrition education, and exercise/fitness programs have been and continue to be developed to combat the negative impact of noncommunicable diseases.

Although not necessarily demonstrative of traditional outbreak investigation, noncommunicable diseases can be studied with epidemiological methods comparing risk factors such as tobacco use and BMI and the presence or absence of disease states. Unlike communicable diseases in which there exists a direct cause-and-effect relationship between the exposure and the onset of disease, noncommunicable diseases are usually connected to multiple risk factors and it can be harder to demonstrate a direct cause and effect. This presents challenges in both demonstrating direct causes of disease and changing destructive behaviors within the population that compromise health.

Exposure to Toxins

Similar to noncommunicable diseases, exposure to toxins has emerged as a substantial risk to human health and wellness. As with noncommunicable diseases a direct cause-and-effect relationship is difficult to prove. In fact, toxic substances often have thresholds below which exposures do not present human health risks but above which can prove to have adverse and at times fatal consequences. The movement during the past 40 years has been to advance the study of risk exposure to potentially toxic substances. Organizations including the Environmental Protection Agency (EPA), National Institute for Occupational Safety and Health (NIOSH), CDC, and the Agency for Toxic Substances and Disease Registry (ATSDR) have made substantial gains in research and policy to reduce toxic risks adversely affecting the health of the public.

■ Risk Factors

The field of epidemiology is focused on the study of disease and illness within groups or populations of people. It is vital to consider three categories of risk factors that place individuals and groups at increased hazard for illness and disease:

- Behavioral
- Environmental
- Genetic

These three broad epidemiological categories within the pyramid model roughly align with the three risk factors presented in these final sections of our epidemiological focus.

Person-related aspects are certainly aligned with the behavioral risk factors. Place-related considerations are effectively illustrated by the environmental risk factors. It is important to think broadly about environment within the context of health risk and exposure. Finally, genetic risk factors loosely align with the time component; that is, genetic risk is associated with the biological makeup of individuals that provides protective factors or risk factors for the development of disease. The genetic component is the most challenging aspect of this triad to disaggregate. Consider that epidemiology uses groups of people as the unit of analysis. Is there an easy way to study genetic considerations at the group level? Likely not. Research into the human genome has made remarkable advances in our understanding of genetic markers of disease. Efforts to better understand genetic risk factors have been under way since the early 1990s through the Human Genome Project. This emerging and rapidly expanding area of epidemiological study is truly the 21st-century frontier within epidemiology. As research into the study of human health expands into the realm of genetic variation and predispositions, a new generation of epidemiologists and health promotion professionals will begin to affect the health of populations through individual-level approaches aimed at maximizing the health of the public. Behavioral, environmental, and genetic risk factors follow.

Behavioral Risk Factors

The CDC began the now nationwide Behavioral Risk Factor Surveillance System (BRFSS) in 1984. This human health behavioral survey is the largest telephone survey assessment in the world. The BRFSS provides timely health behavior data for policy makers in all 50 states as well as the District of Columbia, Puerto Rico, U.S. Virgin Islands, and Guam. These data are effective in providing health-related trend analysis and serve to guide and direct local, state, and national pro-health initiatives. Figure 3-7 presents national-level trended data on tobacco use. The BRFSS can be used to present population-level trend data related to many behavioral risk factors. For community-based health educators these data are an effective resource to assist in planning community health interventions.

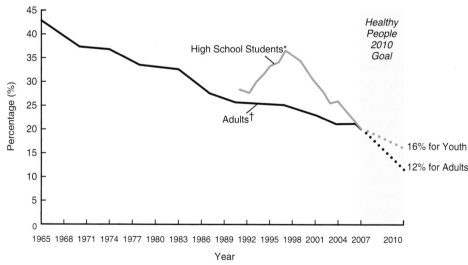

Trends in Current Cigarette Smoking Among High School Students* and Adults,† United States, 1965–2007

*Percentage of high school students who smoked cigarettes on 1 or more of the 30 days preceding the survey. Data first collected in 1991. (Youth Risk Behavior Survey, 1991–2007).
†Percentage of adults who are current cigarette smokers (National Health Interview Survey, 1965–2007).

Figure 3-7 Trends in tobacco use by high school students and adults. *(From Centers for Disease Control and Prevention. [n.d.]. Smoking and tobacco use. Retrieved from http://www.cdc.gov/tobacco/data_statistics/tables/trends/cig_smoking/index.htm.)*

Environmental Risk Factors

Is it possible that the community in which one lives and/or works puts one at an increased or decreased risk for developing a given illness or disease? Yes, it does. The Agency for Toxic Substances and Disease Registry (ATSDR) Web site provides useful information on adverse health effects linked to health-related environmental risk from exposure ranging from arsenic to zinc and everything in between (see Web Resources on Davis*Plus*). Often, increased environmental risk for residents of communities is related to specific industries located in and around the community. By mapping industries related to hazardous waste it is possible to identify populations at greater risk for disease at the local and state levels. The federal government has set aside funds referred to as the Superfund to clean up uncontrolled hazardous waste sites across the country through the Environmental Protection Agency (EPA). The states with the greatest number of Superfund cleanup sites include New Jersey, Pennsylvania, and New York, with more than 100 Superfund sites per state. The EPA Web site at http://www.epa.gov/superfund/ provides information on identifying possible industry-related environmental hazards.

Public health professionals working within the environmental health professions often focus on three critical areas in assuring the health of the public: safe air quality conditions, safe water supplies, and safe soils throughout the nation's agricultural industry. The majority of the human health risks are associated with what we breathe and ingest. It is important to keep in mind that the environmental risks affecting humans are indeed vast, including issues such as automobile safety, seatbelt use, and safe conditions throughout public recreational facilities. Public health professionals use a combination of education, engineering, and enforcement to achieve our mandated goals and objectives.

Genetic Risk Factors (Genomics)

The field of genetic epidemiology otherwise known as *genomics* seeks to understand and explain heritability of factors that have an impact on the development of illness and disease. The past two decades have witnessed the expansion of research into genetic markers for disease. We will likely see a transformation in the evaluation, assessment, and tools surrounding genetically relevant strategies at the population level as a result of emerging individual-level genetic knowledge.

Application of genomics to population health poses some practical and ethical dilemmas. First, at the population level the purpose is to develop interventions relevant to the population that will result in a general improvement of health at the population level. Genetic testing is done at the individual level and usually results in individual decision making related to potential risk for development of disease. For diseases such as cerebral palsy that are related to one gene, genetic testing can help with early identification and treatment for those born with the disease and may assist parents make childbearing decisions prior to conception. However, most diseases occur owing to multiple factors and are linked to more than one gene as well as numerous other risk factors. Evidence on the benefit of genetic screening for most diseases is limited. In addition, genetic testing can be costly.

A good example of the controversy over the benefits of genetic testing is the issue of *BRCA1* and *BRCA2*. These are human genes referred to as tumor suppressors. Based on recent research it is apparent that mutation of these genes is associated with hereditary breast and ovarian cancers.[16] The company that developed the screening test for *BRCA1* and *BRAC2* initiated an advertising campaign encouraging women to have the genetic screen. Though the National Cancer Institute lists possible options for managing cancer risk for those with a positive screen, it acknowledges that the evidence concerning the effectiveness of these strategies is limited. Testing can cost up to $3,000 for those who do not know their family history. The high cost raises the ethical question of taking a universal approach to screening all women for this genetic risk factor, especially as less than 10% of all breast cancers are genetically related and the direct benefit of the testing in reducing cancer rates is not known. Genomics is a growing field with the potential benefit of better understanding the role individual genetic makeup plays in an individual's health. However, as the *BRCA1* and *BRAC2* screening example illustrates, the applicability of genomics to population-level interventions from a practical and ethical standpoint has still not been determined.

▪ Summary Points

- Epidemiology provides the scientific basis for understanding the occurrence of health and disease.
- An epidemiological investigation revolves around person, place, and time.
- The two-by-two table is a principle pertaining to epidemiological investigation and analysis.
- Epidemiological investigations include descriptive and analytical epidemiology.
- An understanding of risk factors for disease from an individual and ecological perspective is essential for the development of effective interventions.

REFERENCES

1. Friis, R.H., & Sellers, T.A. (2014). *Epidemiology for public health practice* (5th ed.). Boston, MA: Jones & Bartlett.
2. Snow, J. *Snow on cholera.* (1965). Cambridge, MA: Harvard University Press.
3. Lilienfeld, A.M., & Lilienfeld, D.E. (1980). *Foundations of epidemiology* (2nd ed.). New York, NY: Oxford University Press.
4. Susser, M., & Susser, E. (1996a). Choosing a future for epidemiology: I. Eras and paradigms. *American Journal of Public Health, 86*(5), 668-673.
5. Susser, M., & Susser, E. (1996b). Choosing a future for epidemiology: II. From black boxes to Chinese boxes and eco-epidemiology. *American Journal of Public Health, 86*(5), 674-677.
6. Krieger, N. (1994). Epidemiology and the web of causation: Has anyone seen the spider? *Social Science Medicine, 39*(7), 887-903.
7. Diez Roux, A.V. (2007). Integrating social and biological factors in health research: A systems review. *Annals of Epidemiology, 17*(7), 569-574.
8. Shapiro, S. (2008). Causation, bias and confounding: A hitchhiker's guide to the epidemiological galaxy, part 2. Principles of causality in epidemiological research: Confounding, effect modification and strength of association. *Journal of Family Planning and Reproductive Health Care, 34*(3), 185-190.
9. Reifsnider, E., Gallagher, M., & Forgione, B. (2005). Using ecological models in research on health disparities. *Journal of Professional Nursing, 21*(4), 216-222.
10. Lee, P.R., & Estes. C.L. (2003). *The nation's health* (7th ed.). Burlington, MA: Jones & Bartlett.
11. Szklo, M., & Nieto, F.J. (2012). *Epidemiology: Beyond the basics* (3rd ed.). Boston, MA: Jones & Bartlett.
12. Babbie, E. (2012). *The practice of social research* (13th ed.). New York, NY: Wadsworth.
13. National Heart, Lung and Blood Institute, Boston University. (2015). *Framingham heart study.* Retrieved from http://www.framinghamheartstudy.org/.
14. *The Nurses' Health Study.* (n.d.). Retrieved from http://www.channing.harvard.edu/nhs/index.php/history/.
15. CDC. (2014). Pertussis (whooping cough). Retrieved from http://www.cdc.gov/pertussis/surv-reporting.html.
16. National Cancer Institute. (2015). *BRCA1 and BRCA2: Cancer risk and genetic testing.* Retrieved from http://www.cancer.gov/about-cancer/causes-prevention/genetics/brca-fact-sheet.

Chapter 4

Introduction to Community Assessment

LEARNING OUTCOMES

After reading this chapter, the student will be able to:

1. Define a community assessment.
2. Describe six approaches to conducting an assessment (comprehensive community assessment, population focused, setting specific, problem focused, health impact, rapid needs assessments).
3. Describe two assessment frameworks (MAPP, CHANGE).
4. Use secondary data to identify health characteristics of a community.
5. Describe qualitative and quantitative methods to collect primary data for conducting an assessment.

6. Describe the use of new techniques and tools (geographic information system [GIS], PhotoVoice) to conduct community assessments.
7. Discuss the usefulness of community assessments.
8. Use the frameworks in conducting a hypothetical assessment of a community.
9. Analyze primary and secondary data to identify strengths and needs of a community.

KEY TERMS

Assets
Census tract
Community
Community-based
  participatory research
  (CBPR)
Community Health
  Assessment aNd Group
  Evaluation (CHANGE)

Focus group
Geographic information
  system (GIS)
Health impact assessment
Inventory of resources
Kinship/Economics/
  Education/Political/
  Religious/Associations
  (KEEPRA)

Key informant
Mobilizing for Actions
  Through Planning and
  Partnerships (MAPP)
PhotoVoice
Population
Population pyramid
Primary data
Qualitative data

Quantitative data
Rapid needs assessment
Secondary data
Windshield survey

■ Introduction

Assessment, the first step in the nursing process, is focused on determining the health status and needs of an individual. In public health practice, a **community health assessment** is a strategic plan that describes the health of a community by collecting, analyzing, and using data to educate and mobilize communities; develop priorities; obtain resources; and plan actions to improve health.[1,2] Assessment is one of the three core public health functions established by the Institute of Medicine (IOM)[3] in 1988 (see Chapter 1) and is critical to the work of public health, especially as it relates to the other core functions, policy development and assurance.[3] Public

health nurses (PHNs) conduct community assessments to develop policies, programs, and interventions to assure the health of a community or population. Think for a moment about a PHN working within a neighborhood with a large population of older adults. Based on health statistics and the sociodemographic characteristics of the surrounding community, the PHN identifies a need for an elder wellness clinic.[4] In this case, a community assessment provides the rationale for the development of the clinic based on the sociodemographics of the community and preventive health concerns that arise in the comprehensive assessment.

  In another situation, a PHN conducts an assessment of a specific target population, children with asthma, to provide the data needed to support the development of a new preventive program related to secondhand smoke.

An assessment can be focused on a health problem such as lead poisoning. In this case, a PHN conducts an assessment to design appropriate interventions to reduce lead poisoning among low-income toddlers by identifying the prevalence of lead poisoning within the community and the risk factors associated with it.[5] A school nurse conducts an assessment of a school and identifies environmental safety concerns on the playground or a congregational nurse serving a local church conducts an assessment of the congregation to discover the most prevalent health conditions in her congregation.

Just as an individual nursing assessment requires special skills, a community assessment also requires a unique set of skills to systematically examine the health status, needs, perceptions, and assets or resources of a community. Some of the skills or competencies needed to conduct such an assessment include selecting health indicators, using appropriate methods for collecting data, evaluating data, identifying gaps, and interpreting and using data. In May 2010, the core assessment competencies for public health professionals were revised and adopted by the Council on Linkages Between Academia and Public Health Practice (Box 4-1).[6]

Definitions of Community and Community Health

Defining the concepts of community and community health is critical in thinking about a community assessment. A community is commonly defined by its geographical boundaries, which may be an urban neighborhood or a rural town. Two communities with very different characteristics (racial, socioeconomic, cultural characteristics) may exist side by side within an urban setting and have very different health statistics and needs. A community can also be defined as a group of people who share common interests or goals. A group of nursing students attending a certain school and a group such as Alcoholics Anonymous are examples of such communities.

A **community** as defined in Chapter 1 refers to a group of individuals living within the same geographical area, such as a town or a neighborhood, or a group of individuals who share some other common denominator, such as ethnicity or religious orientation. In contrast with aggregates and population, individuals within the community recognize their membership in the community based on social interaction, establishment of ties to other members in the community, and often collective decision making.[7]

BOX 4-1	Core Assessment Competencies for Public Health Professionals Analytic/Assessment Skills—Tier One

1. Describes factors affecting the health of a community
2. Identifies quantitative and qualitative data and information
3. Applies ethical principles in accessing, collecting, analyzing, using, maintaining, and disseminating data and information
4. Uses information technology in accessing, collecting, analyzing, using, maintaining, and disseminating data and information
5. Selects valid and reliable data
6. Selects comparable data
7. Identifies gaps in data
8. Collects valid and reliable quantitative and qualitative data
9. Describes public health applications of quantitative and qualitative data
10. Uses quantitative and qualitative data
11. Describes assets and resources that can be used for improving the health of a community
12. Contributes to assessments of community health status and factors influencing health in a community
13. Explains how community health assessments use information about health status, factors influencing health, and assets and resources
14. Describes how evidence is used in decision making

Source: See reference 6.

There is a great deal of media interest in the health of communities, which is evidenced by the identification of the healthiest cities in our country using various indices such as mental wellness, lifestyle behaviors, fitness, health status, and nutrition. Public health agencies also focus on defining the health of a community. At the national level the Centers for Disease Control and Prevention (CDC) promotes healthy communities through its Healthy Communities Program. This program is focused on engaging communities in preventing noncommunicable diseases and seeks to promote collaboration between communities and national resources.[8]

In defining the health of a community, three characteristics of importance are health status, structure, and competence. Selected biostatistics provide vital information about leading health issues in a community. Statistics commonly used when doing a community assessment that are related to health and disease are covered in Chapters 3 and 9. These statistics include such indicators as mortality rates and morbidity rates (the incidence and prevalence of disease). Mortality is often depicted by crude rates or age-adjusted rates. Next there is the structure of a community, which includes the demographics of the community as well as the services and resources available in the community. The demographic data include such indicators as age, gender, socioeconomic indicators, racial/ethnic distributions, and educational levels. The community health services and resources include information about the resources available in the community as well as service use patterns, treatment data, and provider/client ratios.

Finally, the health of a community may be conceptualized as effective community functioning, a concept developed by Cottrell in the 1970s and expanded by Goeppinger and Baglioni in the 1980s.[9,10] Conditions and select measures of community competence include commitment to the community, conflict containment, accommodation (working together), participant interaction, decision making, management of the relationships with society, participation (use of local services), self–other awareness, and effective communication. A competent community is able to identify its needs, achieve some goals and priorities, agree on ways to implement those goals, and collaborate effectively.[10] The establishment of a Neighborhood Watch program to address growing crime in a community is an example of effective functioning in which the community comes together, works to come up with a solution to a problem, and promotes a higher level of functioning by pulling together to address an issue.

Types of Community Health Assessment

Assessments are done for the purpose of gathering information and identifying areas for improving the health of communities and populations. Assessment is the first step in the process of health planning and provides essential data needed to decide where best to allocate community resources. Assessments also provide baseline data. For example, if the community is concerned about the health of infants and mothers, a community assessment can provide the data needed to determine what the actual status of maternal and infant health (MIH) is for the community; whether problems exist for the community as a whole; or whether there is a disparity in MIH based on socioeconomic status, ethnicity, or geographical location in the community. Baseline data on premature births, infant mortality, and vaccination rates help health planners determine during the evaluation phase of health planning (Chapter 5) whether the intervention had an impact. The key is to understand what type of assessment is the best approach. There are several types of community health assessments:

- Comprehensive assessment
- Population-focused assessment
- Setting-specific assessment
- Problem- or health-issue-based assessment
- Health impact assessments
- Rapid needs assessment

Comprehensive Assessment

Since the 1988 IOM report, *The Future of Public Health,* improving health in populations or communities has been linked to performing comprehensive assessments.[3] There is a mandate for public health agencies to regularly and systematically collect, assemble, analyze, and make available information on the health of the community, including statistics on health status, community health needs, and epidemiological studies of health problems.[11] In addition the Affordable Care Act now requires that nonprofit hospitals conduct community health assessments.[12] Data regarding demographic and health characteristics of the entire population are collected in these assessments. A **comprehensive community assessment** is defined as the collection of data about the populations living within the community, an assessment of the assets within a community such as the local health department capacity, and identification of problems and issues in the community (unmet needs, health disparity) and opportunities for action.[13,14]

Since 1992, the CDC has guided communities in conducting assessments, making health decisions, and developing policy. Most recently it has published an action guide for using the **Community Health Assessment aNd Group Evaluation (CHANGE)** tool that includes a process for conducting a comprehensive assessment of a community.[15] In addition, guidelines, resources, and tool kits for conducting assessments are often found on state or university Web sites. Examples of community or county profiles can also be found on Web sites of state and local health departments (Table 4-1).

Population-Focused Assessment

A **population** as defined in Chapter 1 refers to a larger group whose members may or may not interact with one another but who do share at least one characteristic such as age, gender, ethnicity, residence, or a shared health issue such as HIV/AIDS or breast cancer. The common denominator or shared characteristic may or may not be a shared geography or other link recognized by the individuals within that population. For example, persons with diabetes type 2 admitted to a hospital form a population but do not share a specific culture or place of residence and may not recognize themselves as part of this population. In many situations, the terms *aggregate* and *population* are used interchangeably. An assessment can be

Name of Web Site	URL	Description
Community Health Assessment aNd Group Evaluation (CHANGE): Building a Foundation of Knowledge to Prioritize Community Needs	http://www.cdc.gov/nccdphp/dch/programs/healthycommunitiesprogram/tools/change.htm	The CHANGE tool provides a guide to community-based teams related to conducting an assessment and developing a community action plan. The tool helps to structure the assessment process so that it leads to the identification of health priorities.
Community Tool Box: Community Assessment University of Kansas Community Tool Box	http://ctb.ku.edu/en/More_Information_About_CTB.aspx	Promotes community health and development by connecting people, ideas, and resources. Includes 46 chapters with 300 different sections providing practical, step-by-step guidance in community-building skills.
Florida Community Health Assessment Resource Tool (CHARTS) & Compass	http://www.doh.state.fl.us/planning_eval/CHAI/index.htm	Provides information about health planning in Florida. The Compass guide has the Florida MAPP guide to doing assessments.
North Carolina's Community Health Assessment 2014	http://publichealth.nc.gov/lhd/cha/	Aims to provide local health jurisdictions with the tools and training needed for effective community health assessment.
Intervention MICA (Missouri Intervention Community Assessment)	http://health.mo.gov/data/interventionmica/index.html	Contains three primary tools: (1) *Data* MICA—data and statistics for needs assessment; (2) *Priorities* MICA—facts and figures to guide priority setting; (3) *Intervention* MICA—information, tools, and resources for intervention design, implementation, and evaluation.
The Community Health Assessment Clearinghouse	http://www.health.state.ny.us/nysdoh/chac/index.htm	Provides community health practitioners with tools, ideas, resources, and a platform for dialogue toward a common goal of developing effective health assessments.

TABLE 4–1 Resources Focused on Conducting Community Assessments

focused on a specific population for purposes of planning and developing intervention programs. A population-focused assessment, for example, might focus on pregnant women or immigrants living within a community. One community assessment was conducted to examine the health needs especially in relation to nutrition that focused on Hispanic immigrants. The findings were used to help develop an intervention aimed at reducing obesity.[16]

A population-focused assessment can also focus on a certain age range or a population with a specific health characteristic that may put the group at risk (e.g., children or specifically children with disabilities). In health departments, nurses are often involved with writing grants to serve the needs of mothers and children (see Chapter 18). The components needed for these grants consist of the collection and analysis of information on health needs of children and mothers to guide program planning.[17] The identification of the health indicators of

interest is a beginning step in the process of conducting this type of assessment. For example, the World Health Organization (WHO) identified 11 maternal child health indicators (Box 4.2).[18] These indicators provide insight into the health of this population as well as provide a mechanism for tracking accomplishment in improving these indicators over time.

Setting-Specific Assessment

Assessments can also be focused on a specific setting. Assessments of this nature may focus on identifying strengths and weaknesses of an organization or policies and programs within an organization. Not unlike other assessments, a setting-specific assessment requires a clear understanding of the purpose of the assessment in order to proceed in an organized manner. An assessment of an industry will most likely consist of a description of the company, the working population, the health programs, and stressors present at the work site. The same

BOX 4–2 The WHO 11 Indicators of Maternal, Newborn, and Child Health

1. Maternal mortality ratio
2. Under-5 child mortality, with the proportion of newborn deaths
3. Children under 5 who are stunted
4. Proportion of demand for family planning satisfied (met need for contraception)
5. Antenatal care coverage (at least four times during pregnancy)
6. Antiretroviral prophylaxis among HIV-positive pregnant women to prevent HIV transmission and antiretroviral therapy for [pregnant] women who are treatment-eligible
7. Skilled attendant at birth
8. Postnatal care for mothers and babies within 2 days of birth
9. Exclusive breastfeeding for 6 months (0–5 months)
10. Three doses of combined diphtheria-tetanus-pertussis immunization coverage (12–23 months)
11. Antibiotic treatment for suspected pneumonia.

Source: See reference 18.

principles apply in assessing a school setting. The PHN must identify indicators that are relevant to the setting. Health indicators relevant to an industrial setting might include work-related injury or days absent. At a school setting the assessment would most likely begin with a description of the school, the history, policies, support services, the actual school building from an environmental perspective, the population (teachers, staff, and students), and the existing programs with an emphasis on health. There are many additional tools that can be used to assess components of school health. The School Health Index,[19] a tool available through the CDC, addresses physical activity, healthy eating, tobacco use prevention, unintentional injury, violence prevention, and asthma rates within a school system (see Chapter 19).

This type of health assessment treats the setting as the community and takes into account the population that is located in the setting. Thus a setting assessment combines components of a comprehensive assessment and a population assessment. Taking the example of a health assessment conducted at an industrial work site by an occupational health nurse (see Chapter 21) it would be helpful to collect and analyze data relevant to the environment, the resources available to promote health, and health statistics specific to the population. According to the CDC, a workplace assessment involves obtaining information related to the health of employees within the

workplace setting, including protective and risk factors for the purpose of identifying opportunities to improve the health of the workers.[20]

Problem- or Health-Issue-Based Assessment

Assessments can also focus on a specific problem or health issue. In many cases, assessments and tool kits for specific health issues can be found on the Internet. For example, obesity is a growing problem in the United States and communities are identifying the need to promote an understanding of the policies, practices, and environmental factors that contribute to the nutrition and physical activity choices within a community. An assessment can help a community to identify physical activity and nutrition policies, practices, and environmental conditions within the local community at large work sites, school systems, and the health-care delivery system. Assessments can help to identify specific issues related to the health issue and can also be population and/or setting specific, as in the assessment done by Kong et al.[21] Often assessments related to a specific health issue include analysis of data to help determine who is at risk for the disease, such as the use of a case control study (see Chapter 3).

Health Impact Assessment

There are two other types of assessments: **health impact assessment** and rapid needs assessment. The WHO notes that there are a number of definitions of health impact assessments. The main definition it has adopted is based on a 1999 European Centre for Health Policy definition of a health impact assessment as "a combination of procedures, methods and tools by which a policy, program or project may be judged as to its potential effects on the health of a population, and the distribution of those effects within the population."[22] A growing awareness of the multiple determinants of health, with a particular focus on the environment, has resulted in an increased focus and utilization of health impact assessments throughout the world. Health impact assessment methods are used to evaluate the impact of policies and projects on health, and a successful health impact assessment is one in which its findings are considered by decision makers to inform the development and implementation of policies, programs, or projects.[23,24]

Health impact assessments are often associated with assessments of the environment or assessments focused on the social influences of large projects. Zoning laws, for example, may increase the availability of walking paths that in turn may help to reduce the prevalence of obesity in a community. An example is the Eastern Neighborhoods Community Health Impact Assessment that was conducted by the San Francisco Department of Public Health to evaluate the health benefits and burdens of rezoning and community planning in three neighborhoods.[25] A health impact assessment provides advice to a community on how to optimize the health of the community,[26] is conducted prior to implementing a community-level intervention, and includes specific steps (Box 4-3).

Rapid Needs Assessment

Another type of assessment is a **rapid needs assessment,** a tool that helps establish the extent and possible evolution of an emergency by measuring the present and potential public health impact of an emergency, determining existing response capacity, and identifying any additional immediate needs.[27] This type of assessment was first used in international settings during the 1960s to assess for immunization coverage, morbidity from diarrheal and respiratory diseases, and service coverage. In the 1970s, it was used in the smallpox eradication program in West Africa and was then adapted by the WHO for the Expanded Program of Immunization to assess immunization coverage in the 1980s.[28] At the national level the CDC, the Federal Emergency Management Agency, and the U.S. Public Health Service (USPHS) have all adopted a rapid needs assessment format when responding to a disaster. For example, following the earthquake in Haiti in 2010, a rapid needs assessment quickly established the impact the earthquake had on the potable water supply in the country, especially in its capital, Port au Prince (Fig. 4-1).

A rapid needs assessment is an effective use of limited resources and in general involves a straightforward collection of data. There are four basic steps: (1) review existing information, (2) conduct a visual inspection,

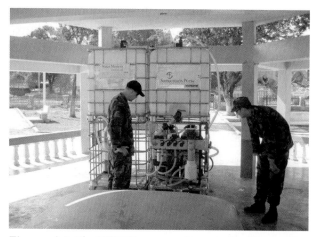

Figure 4-1 The USPHS personnel overseeing the supply of fresh water and inspecting a drinking water purifier that had been set up in a Haitian town shortly after the country's devastating earthquake in January 2010. *(Photograph by Lt. Cmdr. Gary Brunette, USPHS.)*

(3) interview key informants, and (3) conduct rapid surveys.[26] It is one form of surveillance conducted during an emergency and can provide valuable data as evidenced by the rapid needs assessments done during the aftermath of Hurricane Katrina.[29,30]

Concepts of Relevance to Community Assessments

There are two important concepts relevant to conducting a community assessment discussion: needs versus assets and community-based participatory research initiatives. These issues reflect the importance of working with a community while maximizing the strengths of the community rather than focusing on deficits within the community. In the past community assessments were done by outsiders and for the most part highlighted where the health gaps were without acknowledging assets within the community or including the community as a partner.

Needs Assessments Versus Asset Mapping

Initially, community assessments were based on the premise that the purpose of a community health assessment was to identify needs. In 1995, Witkin and Altschuld defined a needs assessment as "a systematic set of procedures undertaken for the purpose of setting priorities and making decisions about program or organizational improvement and allocation of resources. The priorities are based on identified needs."[31] A need was considered a discrepancy or a gap between what is and what should be.[31]

BOX 4–3	**Major Steps in Conducting a Health Impact Assessment (HIA)**

- Screening (identifying plans, projects or policies for which an HIA would be useful),
- Scoping (identifying which health effects to consider),
- Assessing risks and benefits (identifying which people may be affected and how they may be affected),
- Developing recommendations (suggesting changes to proposals to promote positive health effects or to minimize adverse health effects),
- Reporting (presenting the results to decision-makers), and
- Monitoring and evaluating (determining the effect of the HIA on the decision).

Source: See reference 26.

In contrast with this view of community health assessments, Kretzmann and McKnight published a landmark book that made the argument that an assessment should focus on the positive **assets** of a community rather than on its deficits. Assets are useful qualities, persons, or things. They combined this concept of assets with the concept of mapping, that is, exploring, planning, and locating, and proposed that community assessments should include asset mapping. Some of their ideas grew out of the plan to rebuild troubled urban communities based on capacity building.[32] According to Kretzmann and McKnight, a needs approach views communities as a list of problems, makes resources available to service providers instead of residents, contributes to a cycle of dependence, and focuses on maintenance and survival strategies instead of development plans.[32] In contrast, an asset mapping approach focuses on effectiveness instead of deficiencies, builds on interdependencies of people, identifies how people can give of their talents, and seeks to empower people.[33]

The assets approach, based on Kretzmann and McKnight's work, is based on constructing a map of assets and capacities. Three aspects of a community can be included in an asset map: (1) people, (2) places, and (3) systems.[33] People include individuals and families living within the community; places include the resources within the community such as schools, businesses, recreational facilities, and health-care resources. Systems include both formal systems such as government and churches as well as informal systems within the community such as neighborhood organizations. These systems are not always discrete and separate but, rather, influence each other.

Although these approaches of needs and assets appear diametrically opposed, the reality is that comprehensive community assessments consist of the identification of both weaknesses and strengths. Identifying the strengths as well as the problems is critical in the analysis of data.

Community-Based Participatory Research (CBPR)

The second concept of particular relevance to assessment is that of community engagement in the process of the assessment. There are various terms used to describe this approach including *community engagement, citizen engagement, public engagement, translational science, knowledge translation, campus-community partnerships, and integrated knowledge translation.*[34] For the purposes of this book the term **community-based participatory research (CBPR)** is used. The definitions related to this approach all include engagement of members of the community as full partners in the process of assessment.

The idea is to use a collaborative approach that combines the knowledge and interest of the community members with the expertise of the professionals. The end goal is to achieve change aimed at improving the health of the community.[34–36]

CBPR emphasizes the essential principles of capacity building, shared vision, ownership, trust, active participation, and mutual benefit.[37] A benefit of this approach is that it is a colearning process wherein the researchers and community members contribute equally and achieve a balance of research and action. In addition, it is a way of providing culturally competent care. For the PHN working with the community, it is important to be aware of the principles of CBPR. One of the first steps in the community assessment is to engage partners in the process and to develop a common vision.[35]

The engagement of communities in the community assessment process using CBPR methods has become an accepted method for not only engaging the community in the process but also engaging the end users in the action that will be taken to improve health.[34] When using CBPR methods, it is important to evaluate the possible ethical issues that can arise. These include issues of power, fairness, appropriate selection of representatives, obtaining consent, upsetting community equilibrium, and issues of dissemination of sensitive data.[35,38–41]

Assessment Models/Frameworks

Models or frameworks provide the structure and guidance for actually conducting an assessment. PHNs can choose from a number of models based on what best fits the type of assessment that is being conducted. Examples of models that can help guide a comprehensive community health assessment are the CHANGE tool[15] and the **Mobilizing for Actions Through Planning and Partnerships (MAPP)** strategic model.[42]

Community Health Assessment and Group Evaluation (CHANGE)

The CDC created the CHANGE tool built on the socioecological model (see Chapter 2) to help communities build an action plan based on identified assets and areas for improvement. The stated purpose of the CHANGE tool is "to enable local stakeholders and community team members to survey and identify community strengths and areas for improvement regarding current policy, systems, and environmental change strategies."[15] The process provides a community with the foundation for conducting a program evaluation. The idea is to start with the end in mind and include evaluation in the beginning of the assessment process.[15] This tool includes a set of Microsoft Office Excel spreadsheets that communities can use to manage the data they collect. The tool provides a guide to doing a community assessment and helps with prioritizing areas for improvement.

CHANGE utilizes an eight-step process for conducting the assessment (Table 4-2). The first three steps focus on gathering and educating the team. Steps 4 through 6 involve gathering, inputting, and reviewing data from the assessment. The last two steps are the development of an action plan. CHANGE is a tool to help a community complete an assessment that not only provides a diagnosis but also ends with the presentation of an action plan. The idea is to create a living document that the community can use to prioritize the health needs of the community and provide a means for structuring community activities around a common goal.[15]

The National Association of County and City Health Officials in cooperation with the Public Health Practice Program Office, CDC, developed a planning tool for improving community health. The tool was developed with input from a variety of organizations, groups, and individuals who made up the local public health system between 1997 and 2000 (Fig. 4-2). The vision for implementing MAPP is for "communities [to achieve] improved health

TABLE 4–2	Best Practice Approach to Public Health Assessment: Comparison of MAPP With CHANGE
MAPP	**CHANGE**
Phase 1: Partnership	Action Step 1: Assemble the community.
	Action Step 2: Develop a team
Phase 2: Visioning	Action Step 3: Review community sectors.
Phase 3: Assess residents, public health system, community health, and forces of change	Action Step 4: Gather data from each sector.
	Action Step 5: Review data and reach consensus.
	Action Step 6: Enter data.
Phase 4: Identify strategic issues	Action Step 7: Analyze data and assign ratings to each sector.
Phase 5: Formulate goals and strategies	Action Step 8: Build an action plan.
Phase 6: Action cycle	

Sources: See references 15 and 42.

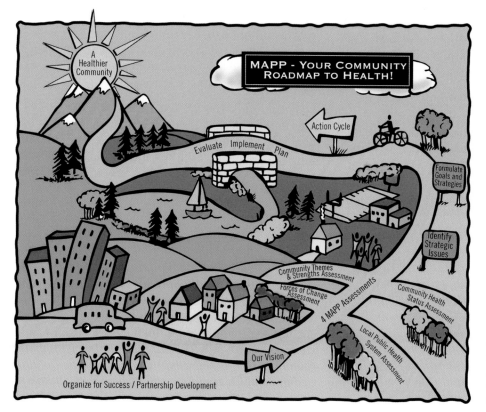

Figure 4-2 Mobilizing for Action Through Planning and Partnerships (MAPP). *(Source: National Association of County and Community Health Officials. [2013]. Retrieved from http://www.naccho.org/topics/infrastructure/MAPP/index.cfm.)*

and quality of life by mobilizing partnerships and taking strategic action."[42]

The MAPP assessment model was based on earlier models used by public health departments such as the Assessment Protocol for Excellence in Public Health (APEX*PH*), which was released in 1991.[43] Building on the concepts included in the APEX*PH* model, MAPP strengthened the community involvement component of assessment and aligned the model with the 10 essential public health services (see Chapter 1).[42] The MAPP tool includes the full scope of health planning including assessing, diagnosing, developing an intervention, implementing the intervention, and evaluating the effectiveness of the intervention. In contrast, CHANGE focuses on assessment and diagnosis with evaluation built in as the goal (see Table 4-2). MAPP has been used by communities and public health departments across the country; because it includes an action phase, it provides a comprehensive approach to improving the health of a community.

The focus of the first five phases of MAPP is the process involved in working with the community on strategic planning and conducting four separate assessments. The MAPP handbook[42] contains access to the tools, resources, and technical assistance needed to conduct the assessment, including a toolbox to provide an explanation and the many examples of assessments that have been conducted. The MAPP process has six phases: (1) organizing for success and partnership development, (2) visioning, (3) performing the four assessments, (4) identifying strategic issues, (5) formulating goals and strategies, and (6) moving into the action cycle (Box 4-4).

Phase 1: Organizing for Success and Partnership Development

This phase is focused on identifying who should be involved in the process and developing the partners who will participate in the process.

BOX 4-4	The Six Phases of the MAPP Process

Phase 1: Organize for Success and Partnership Development
Phase 2: Visioning
Phase 3: Four Assessments
1. Community Themes and Strengths Assessment
2. Local Public Health System Assessment (LPHSA)
3. Community Health Status Assessment.
4. Forces of Change Assessment
Phase 4: Identify Strategic Issues
Phase 5: Formulate Goals and Strategies
Phase 6: Action Cycle

Source: See reference 42.

Phase 2: Visioning

This phase is done at the beginning of the assessment process and is focused on mobilizing and engaging the broader community. An advisory committee guides the effort by conducting visioning sessions, resulting in a vision and values statement. The following are some sample questions that can guide the brainstorming during this phase:

- What does a healthy community mean to you?
- What are the important characteristics of a healthy community for all who live, work, and play here?
- How do you envision the local public health system in the next 5 or 10 years?

Phase 3: Performing the Four Assessments

Four assessments form the core of the MAPP process. The assessment phase results in a comprehensive picture of a community by using both quantitative and qualitative methods and consists of the following.

Community Themes and Strengths Assessment: This provides important information about how the residents feel about issues facing the community. It also provides qualitative information about residents' perceptions of their health and quality of life concerns. Some questions to guide this assessment include:

- What is important to your community?
- How is quality of life perceived in your community?
- What assets do you have that can be used to improve community health?

Local Public Health System Assessment (LPHSA): This focuses on all of the organizations and entities that contribute to the public's health. It is concerned with how well the public health system collaborates with other public health services. The LPHSA answers the following questions:

- What are the components, activities, competencies, and capacities of your local public health system?
- How are the essential services being provided in your community?

Community Health Status Assessment: The community health status assessment is largely focused on quantitative data about many health indicators. These include the traditional morbidity and mortality indicators, quality of life indicators, and behavioral risk factors resulting in a broad view of health.

Forces of Change Assessment: This is an analysis of the external forces, positive and negative, that have an impact on the promotion and protection of the public's health. It is concerned with legislation, technology, and other impending changes that can influence how the public health system can work. It answers questions such as:

- What is occurring or might occur that affects the health of our community or the local public health system?
- What specific threats or opportunities are generated by these occurrences?

Phase 4: Identifying Strategic Issues

During this phase, the assessment data are used to determine the strategic issues the community must address to reach its vision. Some questions to help the community in determining the important strategic issues include the following:

- How large a public health issue is the item?
- Can we do it?
- Is it reasonable, feasible, and financially cost effective?
- What happens if we do nothing about it?

Phase 5: Formulating Goals and Strategies

Goals and strategies are formulated for each of the strategic issues. A community health improvement plan is often created during this phase.

Phase 6: Moving Into the Action Cycle

This is the phase in which the actual planning, implementing, and evaluating of the strategic plan takes place. Phases 5 and 6 are described in more detail in Chapter 5, which is focused on health planning.[42]

A Comprehensive Community Health Assessment

MAPP and CHANGE are examples of frameworks that provide the blueprint for how to go about conducting a community health assessment. Regardless of which framework is chosen, engagement of partners in the process is the first step. As described in the CHANGE tool, this first action step involves assembling a diverse and representative community team. The team then establishes the purpose of the assessment. This begins with a clarification of how the community is being defined. Is the community being defined in relation to a clear geopolitical community such as a city or a county or is the community a neighborhood that may not have clear geopolitical boundaries? For example, a group of researchers was conducting a focused assessment of maternal and infant care in subsidized housing in Winton Hills, Ohio, a neighborhood located within the Cincinnati, Ohio, metropolitan area. It had no political standing (it was designated as a town or city but did not have governmental systems in place). Instead, it was a neighborhood that roughly matched a designated ZIP code, so for the purposes of the assessment the community was defined based on a specific ZIP code.[44]

Once the community has been defined it is important to identify the indicators one is looking at and to identify the sources of data for those indicators. This step often involves a discussion of the history of the community and the proposed project. Through these efforts the team can identify sources of data that are already in existence. In some cases, previous surveys have been conducted that can provide good baseline data to help understand trends and changes in the community. Other data can be obtained from national-level surveys; the U.S. Census Bureau; and sources of local data, such as reports on crime, motor vehicle accident, and fire.

Next the team can develop a timeline to help guide the assessment. A timeline helps the team to decide at what point each step in the assessment will take place, the estimated time for completing each of the steps, and who will be responsible for each step. If the team is using the CHANGE model, the members will try to understand the total picture and will include assessment of five sectors of the community: (1) the community-at-large sector, (2) the community institution/organization sector, (3) the health-care sector, (4) the school sector, and (5) the work site sector. Once this is complete, the team will then begin to gather data for each sector and evaluate the quality of the data. Different methods can be used to collect data, including obtaining secondary data available from other sources, as noted above, and collecting their own data using both quantitative and qualitative methods. Under step 4 in the CHANGE model, the different **primary data** collection methods listed that can be used include doing a windshield survey, PhotoVoice, doing a walkability audit, conducting focus groups, and administering a survey to individuals.

Windshield Survey

A **windshield survey** is an example of primary data collection that can help the team get an initial understanding of the community and is sometimes viewed as part of a preassessment phase. The windshield survey is what it sounds like—a drive through or walk through the community to observe the community. The idea is to actually observe the community prior to conducting a more formal assessment of the community to help in understanding the community.

A windshield survey is the first step in taking the pulse of the community. The questions a windshield survey can begin to answer include:

- Are there obvious health-related problems?
- What is the perspective of the media in relation to the community?
- What does the community look like? Just by driving around, key issues related to the environmental health of the community can be observed, such as the number of for-sale signs, the amount of green space, the number of bars, the number of churches, the number of open (or closed) businesses and the general upkeep of the community. Clean streets, well-kept parks, busy grocery stores, and religious places of worship with multiple services offered are signs of a healthy community. In contrast, trash in the streets, vacant lots, multiple bars, vacant places of worship, boarded-up businesses, and a lack of grocery stores are all visual indicators of a community that may have some serious health challenges.

A windshield survey can also provide information on the demographics of a community. Observations made while driving through (or walking around) can provide a beginning understanding of the age groups in the community simply by observing how many children, older adults, or young people are on the street. This can be time-dependent. For example, in the early morning young mothers and children may be observed as the children walk to the school. Later in the morning older adults may be observed. One approach to observing formal institutions within a community is to use the **Kinship/Economics/Education/Political/Religious/Associations (KEEPRA)** acronym. It provides a list of categories to consider while collecting observational related data:

- *Kinship*—What observations can you make about family and family life?
- *Economics*—Does the community appear to have a stable economy or are there signs of economic decline or economic growth?
- *Education*—What observations can you make related to schools and other educational institutions such as libraries and museums?
- *Political*—Is there evidence of political activity in the community such as signs supporting someone's candidacy for elected office?
- *Religious*—Are there any mosques, churches, or synagogues in the community?
- *Associations*—What evidence do you see of neighborhood associations? Business associations? What other resources are present such as recreation centers?

Using the CHANGE list of sectors is another possible approach to conducting an observational review of the formal institutions in a community:

- *Community-at-Large Sector* includes community-wide efforts that have an impact on the social and built environments such as improving food access, walkability or bikeability, tobacco use and exposure, or personal safety.
- *Community Institution/Organization Sector* includes entities within the community that provide a broad range of human services and access to facilities such as childcare settings, faith-based organizations, senior centers, boys and girls clubs, YMCAs, and colleges or universities.
- *Health-Care Sector* includes places where people go to receive preventive care or treatment, or emergency health-care services such as hospitals, private doctors' offices, and community clinics.
- *School Sector* includes all primary and secondary learning institutions (e.g., elementary, middle, and high schools, whether private, public, or parochial).
- *Work Site Sector* includes places of employment such as private offices, restaurants, retail establishments, and government offices.[15]

Secondary Community Health Data Collection

Once the windshield survey is complete it is often helpful to review secondary data prior to collecting more primary data. **Secondary data** are data that were collected for a purpose other than the current assessment such as census data, crime report data, or national health survey data. These sources of community data are often accessible via the Internet.

An essential component of a community health assessment is the review of sociodemographic data. From a geographical perspective, the team can access census data relevant to their community from the U.S. Census Bureau. These data provide the team with information on the number of people in their community; the number of households; and information related to age, gender, marital status, occupation, income, education, and race/ethnicity. Census data in the United States are collected every 10 years by the U.S. Census Bureau. The data are reported at the aggregate level based on geopolitical perspective. Aggregate data are obtainable at the national, state, county, metropolitan area, city, town, census track, or census block. According to the U.S. Census

Bureau a **census tract** is a relatively permanent statistical subdivision of a county that averages between 2,500 and 8,000 inhabitants and that is designed to be homogeneous with respect to population characteristics and economic status. A *census block* is an area that is bounded on all sides by visible features. Examples of boundaries provided by the U.S. Census Bureau include visible boundaries such as roads, streams, and railroad tracks, and by invisible boundaries such as the geographical limits of a city or county. Typically, it is a smaller geographical area, but in some rural areas a census block may be large.[46] The data provide a snapshot of the population every 10 years. In between those years changes may occur and local data may be needed to supplement census data especially toward the end of a decade.

Another source of secondary health data at the aggregate level about a community can be obtained from a public health department. Examples of public health information related to morbidity and mortality in a community include the crude mortality rate, the infant mortality rate, motor vehicle crash rate, and the incidence and prevalence rates of communicable and noncommunicable diseases. To get a better understanding of the rates, it helps to obtain age-specific mortality rates for leading causes of death and age-adjusted, race-, or sex-specific mortality rates. An example of Web-based sources of health-related aggregate data at the county level is the Web site maintained by the University of Wisconsin Population Health Institute and sponsored by the Robert Wood Johnson Foundation. It provides information on health indicators at the county level with comparative statistics at the state and national levels.[47] Another source of data is vital statistics. These statistics provide information about births, deaths, adoptions, divorces, and marriages. These data are available through state public health departments.

Information on the health of a community can also be obtained from surveys that are conducted routinely at the national level and often at the regional level. The National Center for Health Statistics (NCHS), a division of the CDC, provides data about the prevalence of health conditions in the United States. The NCHS manages surveillance systems including the National Health Interview Survey (NHIS) and the National Health and Nutrition Examination Survey (NHANES). The NHIS is conducted every year and surveys approximately 35,000 households annually. The survey focuses on a core component of health questions including health status and limitations, injuries, health-care access and use, health insurance, and income and assets. In addition, a supplement is used each year to respond to new public health

data needs as they arise.[48] The NHANES is an annual survey that began in the 1960s and combines an interview with medical, dental, and lab tests and physiological measures.[49] The Behavioral Risk Factor Surveillance System (BRFSS), administered by the CDC, is a telephone survey of 350,000 adults in 50 states, the District of Columbia, Puerto Rico, the U.S. Virgin Islands, and Guam. It has been conducted on an annual basis since 1984 and it collects information on health risk behaviors, preventive health practices, and health-care access primarily related to chronic disease and injury.[50] The CDC also publishes the *Morbidity and Mortality Weekly Report,* which reports infectious diseases and health concerns by states with each publication providing current state-and city-level incidence data on reportable diseases. Other examples of aggregate health data include the annual report to Congress and other reports to Congress on health-related issues such as alcohol and drug use (see Chapter 11). Other sources of health data include cancer registries and the National Institute of Occupational Safety and Health (NIOSH). The National Cancer Center of the National Institutes of Health maintains 11 population-based cancer registries. They provide data on the number of individuals diagnosed with cancer during the year. NIOSH monitors exposures to environmental factors in work settings.

Secondary data are also available that are not specific to individuals, that is, data related to the environment. The Environmental Protection Agency (EPA) collects data on environmental pollutants and the Department of Transportation collects data on the number of vehicles using the roads. Another example is information obtained and maintained by the U.S. Department of Agriculture (USDA), which includes information on farmers markets, the Food Access Research Atlas, and the Food Desert Locator, an online map highlighting thousands of areas where, the USDA says, low-income families have little or no access to healthy fresh food.[51] Secondary sources of local data also exist but may not be readily available in aggregate form on the web. These include information on the organizations within the community such as hospitals, schools, and police department information. Gathering the data from various local organizations (minutes, reports) may be helpful in relation to the different sectors included in the CHANGE model such as information about the schools. Although these records may be helpful to some extent, there are limitations. Records of any nature often have documentation limitations since the records may not be complete, may not be in a usable format, or the keepers of the data may not be willing to provide the information to the community assessment team. The list of available secondary data is long and interesting and should be reviewed as the first step to avoid the more costly process of having the team collect the data.

Primary Community Health Data Collection

When the review of the available secondary data is complete, the next step is to determine gaps in the data and decide on what further data needs to be collected by the team. The CHANGE model provides a list of a number of possible methods and suggests that multiple methods should be used (two or more).[15] These data are then combined with the secondary data to determine needs and assets.

Inventory of Resources

The agencies and organizations present in a community often have a significant effect on health. The CHANGE handbook has sample organizational questionnaires that can be used for each of the five sectors to help collect data on different organizations such as health-care organizations and schools.[15] The use of these questionnaires can help the team gather essential information about the resources within the community.

Quantitative Data: Surveys

When gaps in data are identified, one method for obtaining the missing data is to conduct a survey for the purpose of collecting community level quantitative data. **Quantitative data** are data that can be assigned numerical values such as the number of new cases of tuberculosis or the assigning of a number to a categorical variable such as ethnic group.

A first step in conducting a community health survey is to outline the purpose of the survey. The team decides on the information needed, then decides on the target population and the method for obtaining a representative sample of the population and the survey delivery method. For example, a hypothetical community assessment team in county X found that the members did not have enough information on the health-related quality of life (HRQoL) of older adults living in their community. The county had just completed a telephone health survey and this population was underrepresented. After careful consideration they decided that their target population was in fact those older than age 65 who were not currently residing in a health-care facility. The use of an e-mailed survey seemed to pose even more problems related to response rate than did a telephone survey. So they decided that a face-to-face approach was best to deliver the survey. The team members decided they needed

to reach those living in different areas of the county as well, so they put together a sampling process that would help them to include older adults living in different areas of the county. This example demonstrates that conducting a survey can be complex and may include issues related to time, which requires careful planning. The advantages of surveys include their cost-effectiveness and ability to make inferences about a population based on the representativeness of the sample. A survey allows for the collection of a large amount of information from a large number of individuals.

Defining the Sample: There are several approaches to defining the sample. Defining the community or target population is once again the critical step. If the focus of the assessment is on adolescents within a specific school, sampling will be based on the adolescents in that school; however, if the purpose of the assessment is to say something about adolescents in the city, a different sampling approach is needed.

Sampling Approaches: Once the target population is defined, there are several types of sampling approaches. A simple random sample involves a list of the eligible individuals and then selection is made based on a random selection, possibly based on using a list of random numbers. Convenience sampling is a common approach that takes into consideration the availability of participants. Some different types of convenience sampling include quota sampling, which involves a fixed number of subjects; interval sampling, which is the selection of subjects in a sequence (i.e., every eighth person); or snowball sampling, which starts with a small group of participants and then uses those participants to identify other participants. One other type of sampling used with large numbers is systematic sampling, in which a list of the possible participants is presented and the number needed for the sample is divided into the total population. For example, from that point, n, every nth person is chosen.

Methods for Conducting a Survey: There are also several methods for conducting a survey. A survey can be mailed, done by telephone, given in certain settings as a written document or by computer, or conducted through a face-to-face interview. The format for the survey is determined based on consideration of cost, resources, and preference. In some cases, the choice of the format may be determined by the study participants, as noted in the example above of the survey conducted with the older adults in the county.

Deciding Items to Be Included in a Survey: Choosing and developing the items to be included in a survey is another decision to be made as one plans for the actual assessment. The majority of healthy surveys use a quantitative approach; that is, the questions are closed-ended and can be entered into a database using statistical software to help with analysis. Some surveys also include open-ended questions that allow respondents to provide information not asked in the survey questions.

Evidence-Based Tools for Community Assessment: There are several health status, evidenced-based instruments available for conducting a community health assessment. For example, the CDC has developed a 14-item HRQoL questionnaire.[52] The advantage of using the CDC questionnaire is that it allows for comparison of the community sample with national benchmarks.

The *Speak to Your Health* community survey is an example of a project of the Genesee County Community Board of the Prevention Research Center of Michigan. This county board used the biennial survey to shape policy changes and guide strategic planning at the county health department, which, in turn, informs local health intervention programs. For example, the board used these survey data to map estimated diabetes cases and identify risk factors. They found that areas in the county with the greatest risk for diabetes had only moderate rates of diabetes screening. They also used findings from the survey to develop local physical activity promotion campaigns to address sedentary lifestyles.[53]

Qualitative Data

Although quantitative data can provide a wealth of information, other approaches to data collection provide an opportunity to gather more in-depth information about the health of a community. One approach to achieving this is to gather **qualitative data,** that is, data that cannot be assigned a value and represent the viewpoint of the person providing the information. These data are not generalizable to a large population but can provide insight into the how, why, what, and where of the phenomenon being studied. In this case, the phenomenon in the health status of a community.

Focus Groups: The most commonly used method for collecting data when conducting a community assessment is the focus group(s). A **focus group** is the process of conducting a group interview with a group of people with similar experiences or backgrounds who meet to discuss a topic of interest.[54] A focus group typically includes six to eight participants, with a facilitator who guides the group discussion by designing an interview guide that has unstructured open-ended questions for purposes of discovering opinions, problems, and solutions to issues. The interview generally lasts for 1 to 2 hours. Once the focus group has been conducted, an analysis of either the transcribed tape recording or notes from the group session consists of examining the data for patterns that emerge, common themes, new questions that arise, and conclusions that can be reached.

Key Informants: Another approach to gathering more in-depth data is to conduct individual interviews with key informants. A **key informant** is often represented as a gatekeeper, one who comes closest to representing the community. Although interviews can be time consuming, interviews with one or more key informants can provide a wealth of information about the opinions, assumptions, and perceptions of others about the health of a community. The interview can be conducted face-to-face or over the telephone, and the tool to conduct the interview can be structured, semistructured, or unstructured. A structured interview is more formal, with specific identical questions being asked of each person interviewed. A semistructured interview is less structured, with a list of questions that guide the interview but with time for a more relaxed conversation. An unstructured interview is conducted by asking questions that seem appropriate for the person being interviewed.

The next consideration is whom to interview. This really depends on the purpose of the assessment and the purpose of the interview. If a PHN wants to learn more about the resources for adolescents in a community, the nurse will want to interview personnel in health clinics and recreation centers, school nurses, parents, and adolescents about their perceptions of resources and needs in the community. If there is a need to learn about the needs of the older adults living in the community, the sites for identifying key informants may now shift to health clinics, senior citizen centers, nursing homes, long-term care sites, seniors themselves, and organizations representing them. If it is a comprehensive assessment, it is important to make sure that everyone is represented. It is important to include business representatives, government employees, and members of voluntary organizations. Another issue is to examine the makeup of the community by ethnicity to make sure that each group's members have had a chance to voice their opinions. For example, during a community assessment conducted in Lancaster County, Pennsylvania, the team realized they would have a zero response rate on the telephone health survey for residents in the county who belonged to the Amish community because they do not use telephones. To address this issue, the team conducted focus groups with both the women and the men in the community.[55]

Determining the type of interview to conduct with a key informant, face-to-face or by telephone, requires some thought about the advantages and disadvantages of both formats. Some of the advantages of face-to-face interviews are flexibility, ability to probe for specific answers, ability to observe nonverbal behavior, control of the physical environment, and use of more complex questions. The telephone interview needs to be shorter but allows for the ability to interview people who do not have the time to meet face-to-face. It is important to summarize the interview immediately, especially if it is not being recorded. An analysis of the interview data is similar to the analysis of focus group data. The community health assessment team reads the notes or transcripts from the interviews and identifies common themes between key informants as well as specific issues for the group they represent. To help verify the information provided by a key informant, it is helpful to use triangulation, a technique that allows the interviewer to verify the information with another source.

PhotoVoice: **PhotoVoice** is another qualitative methodology used to enhance community assessments. It is based on the theoretical literature on education for critical consciousness, feminist theory, and community-based approaches to document photography.[56,57] PhotoVoice involves having community members photograph their everyday lives within the context of their community, participate in group discussions about their photographs, and have an active voice in mobilizing action within the community. When using this technique in a community assessment, residents can be provided with disposable cameras and asked to take pictures that reflect family, maternal, and child health assets and concerns in the community. From these photographs, the participants' concerns will be highlighted and concerns such as developing safe places for recreation and making improvements in the community environment can emerge.

Additional Tools and Strategies

Community Mapping: Community mapping is another step during the assessment phase that can be used in the initial windshield survey, during the inventory data collection, during interviews, and in more advanced analyses of both assets and problems in a community. The advantages of actually mapping assets are that the strengths of the community are outlined and can be used then in developing an action plan. Mapping allows the community assessment team to visualize the community and to study concentrations of disease, to identify at-risk populations, to better understand program implementation, to examine risk factors, or to study interactions that affect health. It is a process of collecting data through direct observation and to use secondary data sources to describe the physical characteristics of a neighborhood or community, the location of institutions and resources, and the social and demographic characteristics of a community.[58] In the study by Aronson and colleagues, primary data were collected by walking through the community with residents noting categories of interest. Secondary data collected included housing inspection data, liquor license data, crime reports, and birth certificates. The purpose of this assessment was to study the community context and how it might contribute to infant mortality, with an evaluation of Baltimore City Healthy Start, a federally funded infant mortality prevention project. The Healthy Start Program was an initiative whose purpose was to reduce infant mortality by providing comprehensive services to women and their children and partners and at the same time to contribute toward a neighborhood transformation. The researchers mapped vacant houses, liquor stores, and crime data. The data showed that participation in the prevention program was higher in lower risk census blocks. Changes were made to obtain better penetration of the program based on these findings.[59]

Geographic Information System (GIS): A **geographic information system (GIS)** is a tool that is increasingly used in public health. GIS is a computer-based program that can be used to collect, store, retrieve, and manipulate geographical or location-based information.[60] GIS databases consist of both spatial and nonspatial data. Nonspatial data include demographic or socioeconomic data that can be identified by geographical boundaries, whereas spatial data are assigned by exact geographical location by geocoding, or address matching.[61,62]

In a recent study, GIS was used to display environmental risk factors and associated health risks. The target population was patients attending a clinic in an urban setting who were asked to complete an environmental health basic exposure survey. The researchers combined these data with Toxic Release Inventory information, which is a publicly available EPA database that contains information on toxic chemical releases and waste management activities reported annually by certain industries as well as federal facilities.[63] The Toxic Release Inventory Program run by the EPA uses GIS to examine air emission sites from the Aerometric Information Retrieval System/AIRS Facility Subsystem database, which is a computer-based repository for information about air pollution in the United States.[63]

Analysis of the Data

Once the data have been collected, it is important to analyze them. The CHANGE model includes three action steps related to this phase of the assessment: (1) review the data, (2) enter the data, and then (3) review the consolidated data. Reviewing the data refers to having the team brainstorm, debate, and reach consensus on the meaning of the data. Entering the data is the process of transcribing the data into a software program such as Excel to help with the analysis and interpretation of the data. Data are then rated by all researchers. Reviewing the data includes four steps: (1) create a CHANGE summary statement, (2) complete a sector data grid, (3) fill out the CHANGE strategy worksheets, and (4) complete the Community Health Improvement Planning template. Doing so provides the foundation for the final step in CHANGE, building the community action plan.[15]

Making sense of the collected data is done a variety of ways. One of the most important points to consider is what changes over time, or noticeable trends. Sociodemographic comparisons include changes from one census data collection period to another. The time period for comparing disease trends varies by the prevalence of disease. A communicable disease outbreak may be monitored on a weekly or monthly basis, while trends in heart disease might require a trend analysis during a 5-year period. Trends can help to identify improvements or declines in health indicators in the community over time, such as the infant mortality rate, or they can be used to determine whether there have been changes in the demographics of the population over time. For example, is the population aging or have there been changes in home ownership?

The health indicators and the demographics of the community can be compared with other populations such as similar local jurisdictions, the state, and ultimately national data. The data can also be compared within the community. Do disparities exist on key health indicators such as prevalence of disease or access to needed resources? These analyses allow the team to interpret the statistics to identify the important health issues for the community. It is a complex process that involves combining the information obtained from all sources and coming to conclusions. The CHANGE handbook provides an excellent guide for a team to use to complete the analysis. It often requires having a member of the team who not only is familiar with software but who also has a background in statistical analysis so that the team can compute rates and complete a meaningful presentation of the data.

Postassessment Phase: Creating, Disseminating, and Developing an Action Plan

In the final action step outlined in the CHANGE model, the community assessment team builds a community action plan. This requires the development of a project period with annual objectives and should reflect the data that were collected. The end result of a community health assessment should include a brief narrative describing the adequacy of services currently provided in relation to the overall needs of the community. It should highlight the areas of need in the community that are not met and list any additional resources that could be developed to meet any unmet needs in the community.

Evaluating the Assessment Process

Evaluating assessments is as important as conducting assessments to better understand their impact. The effectiveness of a community assessment is defined by Solet and colleagues as those assessments that support the development of data-informed policies, environmental changes, systems changes, or other interventions that promote health and prevent disease.[58] Myers and Stato identified 21 criteria for assessing the usefulness of comprehensive health assessments.[64] These criteria included content-related issues (clear goals, appropriate comparisons of data, focus on assets as well as problems, documentation of process and methods), the format of the document (organization, summary, and detailed versions), and impact of the community health assessment (serving as a resource for plans, writing grants, and guiding health promotion). More recently, Friedman and Parrish identified a series of measures that can be used for evaluating the outputs and outcomes of community health assessments as a means of identifying successful assessments.[65]

● APPLYING PUBLIC HEALTH SCIENCE

The Case of the Sick Little Town

Public Health Science Topics Covered:

- Assessment
- Epidemiology and biostatistics

The nurse managers on three of the medical-surgical units in a regional hospital noticed that there was an increase in patients, many of whom with limited insurance, who were being admitted from Smalltown USA, a small town served by the regional hospital. There did not seem to be any pattern to the admissions related to diagnosis, age, or gender. The medical center had just launched its "We are community!" campaign. The nurse managers approached the vice president responsible for community outreach services, pointed out the increase to him, and suggested that a community assessment might help to identify what was behind the increased admissions. The vice president stated that this matched the medical center's "We are community!" campaign and asked the nurses whether they would be willing to form a task force to conduct an assessment of the community to uncover the reason for the increase in admissions, better understand the health issues and strengths within the community, and at the same time build a better bridge to the community. The vice president had been examining the hospital admissions records and had confirmed their information on the increase in hospital admissions from Smalltown USA, especially among the uninsured and underinsured. He had also conducted a cost analysis and found that there was an increase in unreimbursed care and that the use of the emergency department (ED) for nonurgent care by residents of Smalltown USA had also increased. He felt that the assessment was important and authorized that a certain part of their workload should include participating in the assessment project.

The next day the nurses met and at first were not sure where to start. They tried to remember what they had learned about community assessments in their undergraduate program and one of them remembered that it was important to start with a model to guide the assessment. Another one remembered the importance of including members of the community from the beginning of the process. The third nurse remembered doing a windshield survey for her community health project in school and stated she had driven through Smalltown USA only once and had never actually driven around in it. After much discussion they decided to start by inviting a PHN who worked for the health department to join them to discuss their concerns. When the PHN joined them, they learned that the public health department was actually in the planning stages of an assessment, so the concerns of the hospital nurses were in line with efforts just beginning at the health department. The health department was using CHANGE[15] to guide the process. The PHN conveyed the health concerns of the hospital nurses to the health officer and the officer expressed support for the PHN to work with the nurses from the hospital on conducting an assessment as a part of the overall comprehensive assessment for the county.

The small team of nurses and health department personnel got back together and began putting together their core support team, a list of those who should be a part of the CHANGE committee, and planning how to get broad community involvement.

They used the guidelines outlined by CHANGE in thinking through their process. A nurse who lived in the community and the PHN were able to guide the process. The former knew some key stakeholders in the community and the PHN knew people with expertise who could help them with data collection and analysis. The PHN asked the county public health department epidemiologist whether he could assist with the data collection and analysis and he agreed and became a part of the core team. The nurse from the community stated that there was a visiting nurse who not only lived in the community but also provided home care to the residents of the community. She, too, joined the core team.

The core team then began building a CHANGE committee that could help broaden community involvement. When completed, the preliminary CHANGE committee consisted of four residents of the community, the school nurse, the director of the community recreation center, a member of the police force, the CEO of the hospital, the director of the health department, and the publisher of the town newspaper.

The CHANGE committee and the core team next began to work on developing the team strategy process included in the CHANGE model. They decided to form subgroups to help make the assessment more manageable. The PHN explained that the CHANGE model would be useful for getting the community behind this project and would help provide a framework for the project that the community could own. One of the nurse managers was worried that this would mean that the project was no longer under the control of the medical center. The PHN explained that having the assessment come from the community rather than the hospital would truly support the medical center's "We are community!" campaign. Further, she explained that the CHANGE model would conclude with a community action plan. She explained that having a clear picture of the health of Smalltown USA required buy-in from multiple constituents within the community.

The core team expanded to make sure there was diverse representation from the community. The team talked with the town historian to find former community initiatives and built statement communication strategies for keeping the community informed by writing an article for the weekly newspaper, seeking input and suggestions. After running the article, the editor reported getting many e-mails for or against the campaign or with suggestions for information that the team should include. The committee worked to bring all this input together and came up with a final vision statement: "Smalltown USA, the place to be for healthy living." In the case of the Smalltown USA assessment, the purpose was to identify needs and assets to better understand the health of the population. In this beginning phase it is important to understand as much as possible about the population under study.

Next they mapped out the town borders using local maps. Smalltown USA is located in the state of Massachusetts. It has a town center built next to a small river. The town includes a total of 75 square miles and is a 35-minute drive from the medical center. Four towns border Smalltown USA, three of which have a smaller population than Smalltown USA. The town with the slightly higher population is to the east of the town and can be reached by a main road that goes through Smalltown USA. It takes 20 to 25 minutes to drive from the center of Smalltown USA to the center of the other four towns. Most of the population lives in the center of town. The outskirts of town are wooded and include a small state park.

Collect Secondary Data: Sociodemographic Data

The town was initially settled by descendants from the *Mayflower* and their contemporaries. That gives a starting point for the original culture—English and Puritan. They moved west to farm, but this area was difficult to farm because of the terrain. However, the river provided a source of power for mills. These families formed the owner and merchant classes for the town. Although the first wave of workers was Irish, the majority of the workforce came from French Canada, as the territory once belonged to French Canada. Many of the residents' last names are French. By World War I the Irish section of town was small and was seen as the lowest rung of the social classes. The church with the largest congregation is the Catholic church, since this was a town of few owners and many workers, almost all of whom were Catholic. Thus, Smalltown USA has had a firm class structure as well as three major ethnic groups—English, French Canadian, and Irish—for most of its history.

In the 1970s, when the town was the recipient of state funds to build subsidized housing for families on welfare, there was an influx of families into the town who were at or below the poverty level, all of whom were white and most of whom were single mothers. They became the new lowest rung on the class ladder. Now there is an increasing number of Hispanic families in the town, once again changing the town's cultural and class structure.

Knowing the history, the team's next step was to complete a demographic assessment of the town. The team members began with specific demographic indicators that were available from the U.S. Census Bureau including gender, age, race, home ownership, and income. They collected data from the current census and from the census conducted 10 years earlier so that they could determine what changes might have occurred in the population. From this they constructed a **population pyramid** related to the age of the population for 2010 (Fig. 4-3A) and compared it with the population of the United States (Fig. 4-3B).[66]

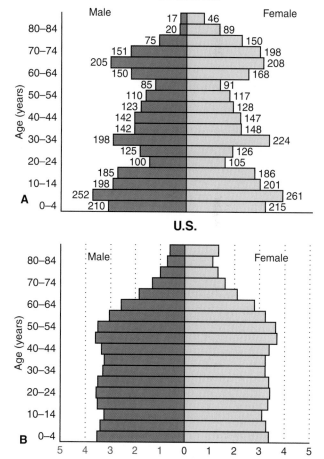

Figure 4-3 A&B Population pyramids, 2010: Smalltown, compared with the United States. *(Source: A, Data from Centers for Disease Control and Prevention [2010]. Community Health Assessment aNd Group Evaluation [CHANGE] action guide: Building a foundation of knowledge to prioritize community needs. Atlanta, GA: U.S. Department of Health and Human Services; B, Data from U.S. Census Bureau, Population Division.)*

A population pyramid is an effective way to visually compare a population based on a particular demographic variable, in this case age. The pyramid can tell you a lot about a population. If the pyramid has a broad base and a small top it is an example of an expansive pyramid in which there is most likely a rapid rate of population growth. A population pyramid with indentations that even out from top to bottom indicates slow growth. A stationary pyramid has a narrow base, with equal numbers over the rest of the age groups and tapering off in the oldest age groups. A declining pyramid is one that has a high proportion of people in the higher age groups. In 2000, the population pyramid for North America met the definition of a slow growth pyramid. The projected 2050 pyramid for North America is a classic example of a stationary pyramid. In contrast,

the population pyramid for Somalia in 2000 demonstrated a clear example of an expansive pyramid, indicative of rapid population growth. However, it also indicated that the longevity of the population was lower than in North America. By 2050 the population pyramid for Somalia is projected to match the 2000 pyramid for North America, indicating that population growth is projected to slow (Fig. 4-4).[66]

The team examined their population pyramid (Fig. 4-3A) and compared it with the U.S. data (Fig. 4-3B). Based on the pyramid, they made some conclusions about the population in Smalltown USA. What would they be? How does Smalltown USA compare with the United States? They then wanted to know whether the population in Smalltown USA had changed over time. The epidemiologist from the

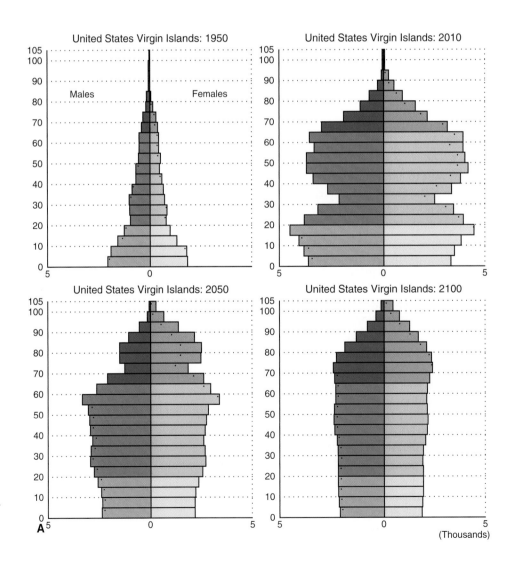

Figure 4-4 United States populations pyramids compared with population pyramids of Somalia. A, United States; B, Somalia. *(Data from the United Nations Department of Economic and Social Affairs.)*

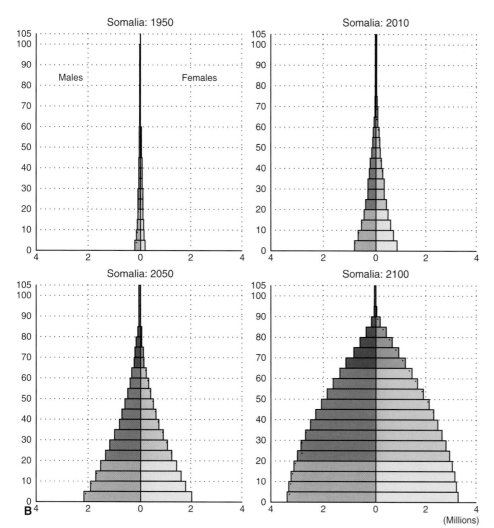

Figure 4-4—cont'd

(Millions)

county public health department recommended that they track the population based on age and race and determine the percent change from 2000 to 2010 using census track data. Percent change (see Chapter 3) represents the change in a variable from one point in time to another. They were surprised at the simplicity of the math required to calculate the percent change. The epidemiologist explained that they should subtract the old value from the new value. They then would divide this by the old value. Then when they multiplied the result by 100, they had the percent change. He showed them how to set it up in an Excel file so that they could enter all the population numbers they were interested in, set up the formula, and then have a table ready for distribution to the committee (Box 4-5, Table 4-3).

BOX 4–5	**Percent Change**

New value minus the old value divided by the old value times 100 equals the percent change.

Example:

If the town's population in 2000 was 2,000 and in 2010 it grew to 2,520, the percent change is 26%:

$$2{,}520 - 2{,}000 = 520$$

$$520/2{,}000 = 0.26 \times 100 = 26\%$$

Percent change can tell a lot about a population. In the case of Smalltown USA, the percent change in the Hispanic population showed a shift in the town. In 2000 almost 97% of the population was white. In 2010, only

TABLE 4–3	Percent Change for Demographic Characteristics in Smalltown USA, 2000–2010		
	2000	2010	% Change
Total	9,611	10,164	6%
Male	4,766	5,039	6%
Female	4,845	5,125	6%
White	9,223	9,018	–2%
Black	77	122	58%
American Indian	29	33	14%
Asian	60	45	–25%
Other	98	101	3%
Two or more races	124	152	23%
Hispanic	195	693	255%
Vacant housing units	213	189	–11%
Population 25 years or older	6,056	6,591	9%
High school graduates	4,974		
Bachelor's degree or higher	848		
Mean travel time to work	29.5		
Median household income	$43,750.00		
Families below poverty level	171		

These data are collected every 10 years, the decennial census, to compile information about the people living in the United States. These data provide the federal government with the information needed for the apportionment of seats in the U.S. House of Representatives. The U.S. Census Bureau also conducts many other surveys and is a rich source of secondary population data. The Census Bureau provides these data in aggregate format and by law cannot release data in a way that could identify individuals.[67] In this case, the team went to the American FactFinder section of the U.S. Census Bureau's Web site and were able to print out a sheet that included the Census 2010 demographic profile highlights.[67] These included a number of demographic categories including general, social, economic, and housing characteristics. Under economic characteristics they found that in Smalltown USA 67% of the population older than age 16 were in the workforce and the median household income was $42,625. The fact sheet also listed comparative percentages for the United States so that they could compare Smalltown USA with the nation. Smalltown USA's statistics were comparable to the national statistics on all of the economic indicators except poverty. In Smalltown USA 10.2% of the families lived below the poverty level compared with 9.2% of the U.S. population. They were also able to print out fact sheets for the county, the state, and the surrounding towns, thus comparing Smalltown USA with its neighbors. The economic indicators between the neighboring towns and Smalltown USA differed in relation to income, with Smalltown USA having a somewhat higher median household income ($42,625 compared with $40,328), although the poverty level statistics were approximately the same. However, compared with the state, the town had a lower median income ($42,625 compared with $50,502).

The team then reviewed the other demographic categories. A few facts were noted as possibly being important. First, the median value of the houses in Smalltown USA was lower than in the rest of the state ($108,500 versus $185,700) and the percentage of the population older than age 25 with a bachelor's degree or higher was lower than in the state (14% versus 33%). Based on the review of the demographics, a picture was beginning to emerge of the town. What would your impressions be? What further data would you need if you were on this team? Demographics give a surface view of a community and helped to guide this team, but they needed to collect further data to

89% of the population was white. This information can also help to estimate changes in the population in the future. If the current trend continues with a 2% decline in the white population and a 255% increase in the Hispanic population during the next 10 years, what would the population look like in 2020?

A demographic assessment can include numerous variables. The team looked at gender, age, and race. Other areas the team decided to include were home ownership, poverty level, crime, and fire safety. The Census Bureau data provided a great secondary source of data for their assessment. As discussed earlier in the section Secondary Community Health Data Collection, secondary data are collected for a different purpose from the current study or assessment. In this case, census data were collected by the federal government.

develop a deeper understanding of the town and discover its assets to promote a healthy community.

Health Status Assessment Using Secondary Data

At this point, one of the nurses on the team wondered about the actual health of the town. She reminded the team that this project was started because of the increased admissions to the hospital and the increased use of the ED. She suggested that the team look at some health indicators that they could review using secondary data. The PHN suggested that they look at the Massachusetts Department of Health Community Health Profile that included a health status indicator report for Smalltown USA. This report provided information on a number of health indicators and reduced the need for the team to find these data themselves. This report used secondary sources of data collected by public health departments, referred to as vital records. These include data on death certificates, reportable diseases, hospital discharges, and infant mortality. Once again, the report provides aggregate rather than individual data so that individuals cannot be identified.

The health status indicators chosen by the Massachusetts Department of Health included perinatal and child health indicators, communicable diseases, injury, chronic disease, substance abuse, and hospital discharge data. The core group brought the published information to the larger community group for discussion. One of the members of the community group noted that at the top of the report was a section on small numbers and wanted to know what that meant. The epidemiologist explained that the numbers of cases for each indicator are placed in a cell in a table. Sometimes the numbers in these cells for smaller towns contain small numbers. The general rule of thumb, he explained, is that if there are fewer than five observations (or cases) then the rates are usually not reported. If they are reported, then rates based on small numbers should be interpreted very cautiously, because there are not enough cases to create a base from which to draw conclusions.

The perinatal and child health indicators included births, infant deaths, and other perinatal and postnatal data from 2010. They found a small numbers problem right away with only one infant death in 2010. However, Smalltown USA had a higher low-birth-weight rate than the state (9.4 per 100 live births versus 7.9 per 100 live births). They also found that the rate of births to teenage mothers was 2.5 times higher than the rate

for the state (16% versus 6.4%). There were no differences in prenatal care in the first trimester or the percentage of mothers receiving publicly funded prenatal care compared with the rate for the state.

When the group reviewed the other indicators, they found that Smalltown USA had lower or similar rates to the state on most of the other indicators. The rates that were higher than the state rates were the rates for cardiovascular deaths (397 per 100,000 deaths versus 214 per 100,000 deaths) and for hospital discharges related to bacterial pneumonia (495.3 per 100,000 deaths versus 329.6 per 100,000 deaths). The team also noted that some of the rates were age adjusted and wanted to know more about the process. The county epidemiologist explained that crude rates may not be as good an indicator because populations may differ on a characteristic, in this case age, which accounts for some of the difference between the rates in two populations. For example, if death rates for cardiovascular disease in a city in Florida with a high proportion of retirees in the community were compared with the rates in a town that has a younger population, the crude death rate would most likely be higher in the Florida community. Adjusting the rate based on age allows for comparing rates in such a way that controls for the age variance between the two populations. The age-adjusted rate is the total expected number of deaths divided by the total standard population times 100,000, which is why the rate is expressed as per 100,000 deaths. The epidemiologist referred the group to a Web site for the Pennsylvania Department of Health that provided more information on how to calculate the age-adjusted rate (see Web Resources on DavisPlus).

Comparing Rates

The team concluded from these health indicators that there was a difference between Smalltown USA and the state in relation to low birth weight, teen births, bacterial pneumonia, and cardiovascular disease–related deaths. A member of the team living in the community wanted to know whether these differences should cause concern. The public health nurse explained that there are statistical methods that can be used to compare rates to see whether they are statistically significant. The epidemiologist agreed to compare the town's rates with the rates of the state and the four towns adjacent to Smalltown USA to help determine whether the differences were significant, that is, the difference could not be attributed to chance. He also explained that he would use a different approach to compare the rates between Smalltown USA and Massachusetts than he would when comparing the town with the rates of the other four towns. When comparing the rates between the town and the state, the rates are dependent, that is, the cases in the town are included in the total number of cases for the state. But when comparing the different towns with one another they are independent rates, because the cases in one town are not included in the number of cases in the other town. When he was done with his calculations he stated that all of the rates were significantly higher than the state rates. However, only three rates—bacterial pneumonia, teen births, and cardiovascular disease–related deaths—were significantly higher than the rates in the adjoining towns.

The team was also interested in gathering secondary data regarding behavioral risk factors. One of the members reminded the group that the BRFSS was available for the community. Since 1984, the BRFSS has been tracking health conditions and risk behaviors. The assessment committee was interested in lifestyle factors affecting premature mortality. The lifestyle risk factors that they were particularly interested in were tobacco use, alcohol use, exercise, and nutritional patterns. Some of these findings can be seen in Table 4-4. What do you conclude from these data?

Health Status Assessment Using Primary Data

At this point, one of the members of the community who regularly attended the meetings stated that this information was good but it was all just numbers and rates and did not really capture how the individuals in the town viewed their own health. Others agreed and they asked whether there was a way to collect data from people living in the town about how healthy they thought they were. The PHN stated that there were

several approaches they could take, including one commonly used approach, conducting a survey.

In addition, the committee members realized they needed to complete an **inventory of resources.** They decided to begin by doing the inventory first to have a better idea of the resources within the community. They divided the community up and identified common resources in which they were interested. In particular, they wanted more information about school, recreation centers and activities, neighborhood associations, churches, health-related clinics, hospitals, and agencies. They used the CHANGE handbook to help guide their data collection related to these organizations.[15]

Health Status Surveys

When this was complete, it was time to begin the survey. The PHN explained that a survey can be constructed to collect health-related information from individuals by using a paper-and-pencil method . Unlike the secondary data they had been reviewing, a survey relies on self-report in which individuals respond to the survey designed for a specific purpose in the assessment rather than using data collected for other reasons such as vital statistics or a census. She further explained that a health survey is quite useful when doing a comprehensive community health assessment, because the researchers can decide ahead of time what information they need and provide information missing from the secondary data sets. The PHN also told them that they did not have to reinvent the wheel; in other words, different surveys were available for them to review and adapt to their own community.

The team decided they wanted to proceed with a health survey in the community. The PHN showed them a survey that had been used by another town in Massachusetts. She explained that the survey included questions related to specific health indictors including HRQoL, protective health practices (see Chapter 3), and behavioral health issues. It also had space at the end for open-ended questions.

The community team members wanted to know more about the part of the survey that measured HRQoL. The PHN explained that HRQoL is a multidimensional construct that relates to a person's perception of the impact his or her physical and emotional health has on his or her quality of life. On the sample survey the questions numbered 1 through 14 were based on the CDC HRQoL survey tool.[52] Another

TABLE 4–4	BRFSS Adult Data for Smalltown USA	
Health Behavior	Prevalence in Smalltown USA	Prevalence in Massachusetts
Current smoking 2005–2009	19%	18%
Binge drinking (2005–2009)	18%	17%
Overweight	67%	54%
Leisure-time activity	68%	74%

advantage, she explained, was that when the scores are converted to standardized scores they can be compared with national norms.

As the team members looked over the sample survey, they realized that the items included would provide information on the health of the community that the secondary data had not provided. The members of the team who were residents of the community began making suggestions on how to improve the survey. The member who worked in the fire department thought that questions should be added about safety, and one of the other community members wanted to know whether people were using the recreation center or the new playground. As the discussion continued, the team built a survey that included other key health issues that the team decided were important—safety, recreation, nutrition, and number of hospitalizations in the past year. They also addressed issues related to the cultural relevance of the survey and the language used (see Chapter 23). The final survey was four pages long and was approved by the members of the committee who lived in the community as being culturally appropriate.

Modifying the survey took some time, but the PHN explained that it was better to take the time now rather than rush, then find out they had missed a key piece of information. Once the survey had been modified, the team had to decide how to deliver it. Should they do a telephone survey with a random sample of households, as is frequently done with national surveys or should they try a different method? They seriously considered the telephone survey approach, but someone pointed out that many households in the town no longer had a landline, especially younger families. The editor of the town newspaper offered to distribute the survey in an issue of the paper (an example of a convenience sample); however, the problem with getting people to return the survey was raised. Another approach for conducting the survey was discussed: taking the survey door to door and having members of the community administer it. This approach seemed the most feasible. The PHN explained that they could do a stratified random selection of households. Stratification would allow them to include different types of households based on home ownership. According to the Census Bureau data, Smalltown USA had 3,660 housing units, of which 68% were owner occupied, 26% were renter occupied, and 5.8% were vacant. The team members decided they wanted to attempt to get a minimum of 10% of the households to respond to the

survey in the two strata. Then someone else spoke up and said that the community was split, with the growing Hispanic population living in one part of town in less expensive housing. They turned to the epidemiologist, who helped them come up with a strategy to include an adequate sample based on both ethnic group and home ownership. Once they identified the strata and their actual representation in the population, random sampling was then used to select the households. The final number of households that needed to be surveyed was approximately 400. The community members of the committee formed a subcommittee to recruit volunteers in the community to administer the survey. The PHN said she would like to train the volunteers in the administration of the survey.

Obtaining data through the health survey provided the committee with much needed information about the health status of the community. With the help of the epidemiologist they analyzed the data and prepared a report on the survey for the community (Box 4-6). The editor of the paper included the report as an insert in the weekly paper. They now had further information on their community that they could add to the secondary data they had obtained. The core members of the team met to discuss where they were with the MAPP model that they were using. They decided that they had been mainly focused on the Community Health Status Assessment and they now had data on the traditional morbidity and mortality indicators, quality of life indicators, and behavioral risk factors.

The team members then decided to review how to create their CHANGE summary statement as outlined by the CHANGE model. The selectperson or the community leader suggested that they use the town hall format to have an open town forum on the health of the community. He said that the current town governance structure lent itself to obtaining this more qualitative data from the community and could also serve as a way to reengage the community in the work they had been doing. The committee went back to their vision of "Smalltown USA, the place to be for healthy living" and began to plan a town forum. They enlisted the help of the town moderator and the town selectperson to help run the meeting. The members of their committee who represented different sections of the community, such as the Hispanic member and the member living in the senior housing complex, agreed to encourage their neighbors and friends to attend.

On the day of the forum more than 900 members of the community attended, more than triple the

BOX 4-6   Sample Report on Findings From a Health Survey Health Survey Report

Smalltown USA, Massachusetts

Vision: "Smalltown USA, the place to be for healthy living"

To help provide information about the health of Smalltown USA and to obtain recommendations from the community, a health survey was conducted. This report includes the findings from this survey.

Methods

A random sample of households was selected to complete a door-to-door survey. The survey included items designed to measure HRQoL, access to care.

Findings

Of the 400 surveys that were completed, a total of 396 were included in this analysis. Four were not included because they contained incomplete data. The majority (80%) of the respondents were female, 95% identified themselves as white. The mean age was 52 with a range from 27 years of age to 95. Twenty-two percent of the respondents were older than 64. Only 8% of the respondents lived alone, with 56% reporting that there were three or more in their households. Forty-three percent reported that a child younger than 18 years of age lived in their household. Ninety-five percent reported that they had health insurance and 60% reported having dental insurance.

Health-Related Quality of Life: The majority of respondents reported that their general health was good, very good, or excellent (see the following figure on general health). In relation to the two questions related to physical function, 15% of respondents stated that they were limited physically "a lot" on the first question and 13% on the second. In relation to the two questions related to physical role, 9% responded all or most of the time they accomplished less and/or were limited in the work they could do.

The responses on the next two sections of the SF-12, vitality and pain, had interesting results. Only a little more than half of the respondents (52%) reported having energy (vitality) all or most of the time, and 23% reported that pain at least moderately interfered with their activities. Thirty-two percent reported that their physical and/or emotional health interfered with their social activities.

The last section of the SF-12 relates to emotional health. More than a quarter of the respondents reported that they felt downhearted or depressed at least some of the time (see the following figure on mood) and 8% felt calm only a little or none of the time. In relation to the two questions related to emotional health and their role, 11% responded all or most of the time that they accomplished less than they would like and 6% were limited in the work they could do.

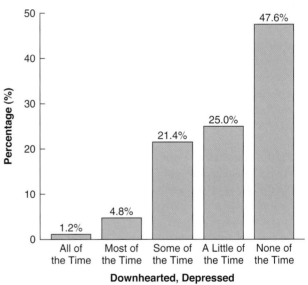

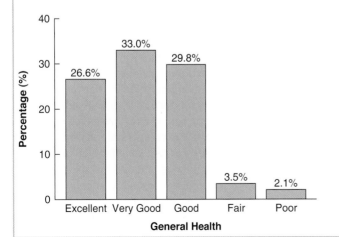

Access to Care and Health Practices: The majority of respondents (84%) reported that they had had a checkup in the past year. However, 30% reported that they did not get care when they needed it, with the majority of these respondents reporting that the reason was lack of money or insurance. The majority of respondents received screening in the past year, with 95% reporting they had had their blood pressure checked, 75% had their cholesterol checked, and 67% had their blood sugar checked. Less than half (48%) had received a flu shot.

Half of the respondents (51%) stated they had a medical condition and the majority of these (40%) reported a cardiovascular-related diagnosis. Only 7.5% of respondents

BOX 4–6   Sample Report on Findings From a Health Survey Health Survey Report—cont'd

reported that they were current smokers and almost half (48%) reported that they did not drink alcohol at all. Of those that reported alcohol use, 25% were daily drinkers.

Obesity: Of the 94 respondents, height and weight information was available for 89 respondents. Using the standard calculation, a body mass index (BMI) was computed for each respondent. Using the national guidelines, 55% of the respondents were overweight or obese. One-quarter of respondents met the criteria for obesity.

Conclusions

There is a match between one of the findings of the health survey and the suggestions given by the respondents. With the majority of the respondents having a BMI greater than 25, the suggestions to develop nutrition and exercise programs would address this issue. However, although respondents rated their general health at the high end, a large percentage reported issues having to do with depression, pain, and the negative impact of both their emotional and physical health on their daily role and ability to function. Suggestions were made to address some of these issues, but only two respondents mentioned mental health in the open-ended questions. Also, although most respondents indicated that they had health insurance, insurance and access to care were listed in the open-ended questions section. Finally, there were numerous suggestions to include support programs for various health issues. Suggestions ranged from new moms, to seniors, to reaching out to those who were homebound and/or ill.

Recommendations

1. Develop a healthy eating and physical exercise program.
2. Review models for support programs for seniors, new moms, and families experiencing illness and adapt for this community. Include links to existing programs such as Meals on Wheels.
3. Put together an informational packet on existing health services in the community with a focus on helping those with limited or no health insurance.

---

number that usually attended town hall meetings. The town moderator opened the meeting with one question: "How healthy a community is Smalltown USA?" During the next 2 hours the community engaged in a lively debate over how healthy the community was and what health problems they thought the town had. The talk began with the lack of health care. The plant in the neighboring town had closed 6 months earlier and many of the people no longer had health insurance. Some people were now threatened with foreclosure. The cost of gas had gone up, making it more problematic to get to the doctor.

Another mother brought up the issue of the rise in teen births and wanted to know why there was not a family planning clinic is town. This brought opposition from several people. The town moderator demonstrated his skills in working with the community. He carefully brought the discussion back to the vision of healthy living and away from the more polarizing issue of family planning. People then shared opinions about the difficulty of obtaining prenatal care and well-child services because none was located in the town. Even the federally subsidized program for Women, Infants, and Children that provides supplemental foods to women and children at nutritional risk no longer had an office in town. Finally, one person stood up and said that the air seemed to be thicker. Someone else volunteered that there were too many wood stoves burning as a result of the high cost of heating oil, and that was why the air was hard to breathe. Others chimed in and stated they had to keep their thermostats down because they could not afford the oil, and that their children had more colds in winter.

After the forum ended, committee members compared their notes and came to the conclusion that for the members of the community access to care was a major concern. They discussed the heated debate that occurred when teen pregnancy was raised. The members of the committee who lived in the community reminded everyone that Smalltown USA has a large population of French Canadians and Hispanics who had opposed family planning clinics in the past. The committee acknowledged that for this community to be successful the issue of teen pregnancy would need to be addressed within the culture of the community. They were also interested in looking into the issue of heating and possible reduction in air quality. They concluded that the town forum had added additional information to their assessment. An interesting finding was the value of the town moderator and it was suggested that he be added to the committee.

The use of the sector approach to the assessment included in the CHANGE model helped to guide the team in including an examination of the components, activities, capacities, and competencies of the local public health system. By this time, the momentum for the assessment had raised a certain amount of enthusiasm in the community. There was a need to form a local public health department subcommittee. New members were eager to join the activities. The subcommittee consisted of the health department director, the PHN, the local fire department representative, a local physician in the community, and the vice president of the hospital who met to discuss how the Ten Essential Public Health Services were being provided in the community. Not everyone in the group was aware of the essential services, so all participants were oriented to each of the services. Organizations within the community providing the services were then identified and gaps were noted. The results of the assessment revealed that many organizations in the community were providing more than one of the essential services. In particular, the essential services that received the most attention by several agencies were service #1, monitoring health status to identify community health problems; service #3, informing, educating, and empowering people about health issues; and service #7, linking people to needed personal health services and assuring the provision of health care.

Weaknesses of the public health system included a need to develop better use of technology such as GIS to better understand vulnerabilities. In addition, another weakness was the need for more activities and resources for the provision of services to teens, especially those teens who were pregnant. With a recent economic downturn, there was some concern about the adequacy of the workforce. The recent budgetary cuts in public health prevented the public health system from exploring new and innovative solutions to health problems.

The team now came together to reach consensus in relation to the data collected. The broad categories that the committee considered important to consider were (1) trends or patterns over time; (2) factors that are discrete elements such as a change in a large ethnic population; and (3) events of a one-time occurrence. The core steering committee helped to lead the brainstorming sessions. At the end of the discussion the committee identified three major trends in the community:

1. Changing demographics
2. Emerging public health issues—teen pregnancy in particular

3. Shifting funding streams within the health department, particularly a loss of a grant that focused on maternal child issues

The core team members now realized that they needed to begin to bring all of the data together to determine the priorities and build the community action plan. The analysis of the data consisted of examining trends over time, comparing statistics in different jurisdictions, and identifying high-risk populations. It was clear that the primary data corroborated the secondary data in several areas. These included the health problems identified—cardiovascular health, teen pregnancies, and bacterial pneumonia. Information from secondary data and the survey supported the finding of a problem with a lack of insurance. The BRFSS data and the survey data supported the need to address some lifestyle behavior issues. The additional assessments supported the need to examine the resources both within the community and the local health department, including the lack of support for young teens in the community and the local health department.

The team used the forms suggested by CHANGE to outline the strengths and problems identified both through secondary data and primary data. The data were presented at another town meeting. This was followed by the core committee and steering committee prioritizing the problems based on the criteria of magnitude of the problem, seriousness of the problem, and feasibility of correcting the problem. In the case of Smalltown USA, the assessment process informed the county of the need for a program to address teen pregnancy. This seemed to be a primary concern of most people in the community. This was followed by the need for additional resources to address the needs of older adults, especially as they related to increased cardiovascular health needs, bacterial pneumonia, and growing problems with being overweight. The issue of the increasing numbers of uninsured, the issue that sparked the concerns of the hospital, was highlighted. The downturn in the economy and the changing workforce were important issues. The importance of providing resource information to those experiencing difficulties was highlighted. The assessment was followed by the development of the final report and the beginning development of an action plan.

■ Summary Points

- The purpose of an assessment is to provide an accurate portrayal of the health of a community to develop priorities, obtain resources, and plan actions to improve health.
- There are seven different approaches to assessment, varying from comprehensive assessments to more specific narrow assessments focused on a health problem, a specific health issue, or population. Other types of assessments include health impact assessments and rapid needs assessments.
- Frameworks or models can be used to guide the community assessment process. Two models include MAPP and CHANGE.
- Assessment data consist of both secondary and primary data.
- Qualitative methods of data collection include focus groups and key informant interviews. Quantitative methods often include surveys.
- Newer techniques of collecting data include the use of GIS and PhotoVoice.
- In interpreting the level of health of a community, it is important to join secondary data with the primary data. One needs to consider trends or changes over time, comparison of local data with data from other jurisdictions, and an identification of populations at risk.
- Prioritization of health issues is based on several criteria: magnitude of the problem, seriousness of the consequences, feasibility of correcting, and other criteria as determined by the community assessment team.

▲ CASE STUDY
EXPLORING YOUR TOWN

Many of us think we know a lot about our town, but we do not know the particulars such as how many residents own their home and how many are renters. How many vacant homes are in our town? Has the population gotten older, poorer, richer? The U.S. Census Bureau has already aggregated much of the data that answer these questions and more. It is possible to drill down right to your own neighborhood if you know your census tract. To obtain census tract data, you must first identify the census tract number. This can be identified by a street address or by consulting a census tract map. If you have a street address, use the street address search.

1. Go to American Factfinder at http://factfinder.census.gov.

2. Enter the name of a town in which you are interested. What information can you find about the percentage of families living in poverty? What is the mean income?
3. Identify census tract information.
4. If you have a street address, use the Select Geographies drop down box to determine in which census tract a family lives in. What does this information tell you about the neighborhood?
5. If you do not have an address, use the reference map feature by selecting maps from the left menu, and then reference maps.
6. Select a state from the map and zoom so that you can see census tract boundaries. Determine the correct tract number.
7. Switch to search (on the top menu) and select the Geography tab.
8. Show more selection methods and more geographical types.
9. Change the search boxes with the name of the state, county, and tract number.
10. Search for the map of the census track to determine the population.

A good resource for learning about using census data can be found at the U.S. Census Bureau fact finder webpage.[67] It is also possible to gather data by ZIP codes.

Sources

U.S. Census Bureau. (n.d.). American Factfinder. Retrieved from http://factfinder2.census.gov/faces/nav/jsf/pages/index.xhtml.

University of Delaware Library. (2014). Research Guides: U.S. Census Bureau. Retrieved from http://www2.lib.udel.edu/subj/census/resguide/small.htm.

U.S. Census Bureau. (n.d.). Zipcode statistics. Retrieved from http://www.census.gov/epcd/www/zipstats.html.

REFERENCES

1. New York State Department of Health. (2006). *Findings.* Retrieved from http://www.health.state.ny.us/statistics/chac/usefulcha/findings.htm.
2. Turnock, B. (2009). *Public health: What it is and how it works.* Boston, MA: Jones & Bartlett.
3. Institute of Medicine. (1988). *The future of public health.* Washington, DC: National Academies Press.
4. Shellman, J. (2000). Promoting elder wellness through a community-based blood pressure clinic. *Public Health Nursing, 17*(4), 257-263.

5. Polivka, B.J. (2006). Needs assessments and intervention strategies to reduce lead-poisoning risk among low-income Ohio toddlers. *Public Health Nursing, 23*(1), 52-58.

6. Council on Linkages Between Academia and Public Health Practice. (2014). *Core competencies for public health professionals.* Retrieved from http://www.phf.org/resourcestools/Documents/Core_Competencies_for_Public_Health_Professionals_2014June.pdf

7. MacQueen, K.M., McLellan, E., Metzger, D.S., Kegeles, S., Strauss, R.P., Scotti, R., Blanchard, L., & Trotter, R.T. (2001). What is community? An evidence-based definition for participatory public health. *American Journal of Public Health, 91*(12), 1929-1938.

8. Centers for Disease Control and Prevention. (2012). *CDC's Healthy Communities Program.* Retrieved from http://www.cdc.gov/healthycommunitiesprogram/overview/index.htm.

9. Cottrell, L.S. (1976). The competent community. In B.H Kaplan, R.N Wilson, & A.H. Leighton (Eds.), *Further explorations in social psychiatry* (pp 195-209). New York, NY: Basic Books.

10. Goeppinger, J., & Baglioni, A.J. (1985). Community competence: A positive approach to needs assessment. *American Journal of Community Psychology, 13*(5), 507-523.

11. Honoré, P.A., & Scott, W. (2010). *Priority areas for improvement of quality in public health.* Washington, DC: Department of Health and Human Services. Retrieved from http://www.hhs.gov/ash/initiatives/quality/quality/improvequality2010.pdf.

12. National Association of County and City Health Officials. (2013). *Community benefit.* Retrieved from http://www.naccho.org/topics/infrastructure/mapp/chahealthreform.cfm.

13. National Association for State and Community Programs. (2011). *A community action guide to comprehensive community needs assessments.* Retrieved from http://www.nascsp.org/data/files/CSBG_Resources/Train_Tech_Assistance/Needs_Assessment_FINAL_-_8.22_print_to_pdf.pdf.

14. Byrne, C., Crucetti, J.B., Medvesky, M.G., Miller, M.D., Pirani, S.J., & Irani, P.R. (2002). The process to develop a meaningful community assessment in New York State. *Journal of Public Health Management Practice, 8*, 45-53.

15. Centers for Disease Control and Prevention. (2010). *Community Health Assessment and Group Evaluation (CHANGE) action guide: Building a foundation of knowledge to prioritize community needs.* Atlanta, GA: U.S. Department of Health and Human Services.

16. Castellanos, D.C., & Abrahamsen, K. (2014). Using the PRECEDE-PROCEED Model to assess dietary needs in the Hispanic population in northeastern Pennsylvania. *Hispanic Health Care International, 12*(1), 43-53. doi:10.1891/1540-4153.12.1.43.

17. Health Resources and Services Administration. (n.d.). *Title V maternal and child health block grant program assessment.* Retrieved from http://mchb.hrsa.gov/programs/needsassessment/index.html.

18. World Health Organization. (2013). *Indicators of maternal, newborn and child health.* Retrieved from http://www.who.int/woman_child_accountability/progress_information/recommendation2/en/.

19. Centers for Disease Control and Prevention. (2012). *Adolescent and school health: School health index.* Retrieved from http://www.cdc.gov/healthyyouth/shi/index.htm.

20. Centers for Disease Control and Prevention. (2011). *Workplace health promotion: Assessment.* Retrieved from http://www.cdc.gov/workplacehealthpromotion/assessment/index.html.

21. Kong, A.S., Farnsworth, S., Canaca, J.A., Harris, A., Palley, G., & Sussman, A.L. (2012). An adaptive community-based participatory approach to formative assessment with high schools for obesity intervention. *Journal of School Health, 82*(3), 147-154. doi:http://dx.doi.org/10.1111/j.1746-1561.2011.00678.x.

22. World Health Organization. (2013). *Health impact assessments (HIA): Definition of HIA.* Retrieved from http://www.who.int/hia/about/defin/en/index.html.

23. Davenport, C., Mathers, J., & Parry, J. (2006). Use of health impact assessment in incorporating health considerations in decision making. *Journal of Epidemiology Community Health, 60*, 196-201.

24. Dannenberg, A.L., Bhatia, R., Cole, B.L., Cora, C., Fielding, J.E., Kraft, K., et al. (2006). Growing the field of health impact assessment in the United States: An agenda for research and practice. *American Journal of Public Health, 96*(2), 262-270.

25. Farhang, L., Bhatia, R., Scully, C., Corburn, J., Gaydos, M., & Malekafzali, S. (2008). Creating tools for healthy development: Case study of San Francisco's eastern neighborhoods community health impact assessment. *Journal of Public Health Management Practice, 14*(3), 255-265.

26. Centers for Disease Control and Prevention. (2013). Healthy places: *Health impact assessment.* Retrieved from http://www.cdc.gov/healthyplaces/hia.htm.

27. North Carolina Center for Public Health Preparedness–the North Carolina Institute for Public Health. (2009). Rapid Needs Assessments and GIS. *Focus on Field Epidemiology, 5*(3), 1-5.

28. Connolly, M.A. (2005). *Communicable disease control in emergencies: A field manual.* Geneva, Switzerland: World Health Organization. Retrieved from http://www.who.int/hac/techguidance/pht/communicable_diseases/field_manual/en/.

29. Centers for Disease Control and Prevention. (2006). *Illness surveillance and rapid needs assessment among Hurricane Katrina evacuees—Colorado, September 1–23, 2005. Morbidity and Mortality Weekly Report, 55*(9), 244-247.

30. Horney, J., Snider, C., Gammons, L., & Ramsey, S. (2008). Factors associated with hurricane preparedness: Results of a pre-hurricane assessment. *Journal of Natural Disease, 3*(2), 143-149.

31. Witkin, B., & Altschuld, J.W. (1995). *Planning and conducting needs assessments.* Thousand Oaks, CA: Sage.

32. Kretzmann, J.P., & McKnight, J.L. (1993). *Building communities from the inside out: A path toward finding and mobilizing a community's assets.* Evanston, IL: Institute for Policy Research.

33. Community Outreach of Our United Villages. (n.d.). *Community asset mapping workbook.* Retrieved from http://ouvcommunityoutreach.org/resources/community-building-tool-packets/.

34. Newman, S.D., Andrews, J.O., Magwood, G.S., Jenkins, C., Cox, M.J., & Williamson, D.C. (2011). Community advisory boards in community-based participatory research: A synthesis of best processes. *Preventing Chronic Disease, 8*(3), A70. Retrieved from http://www.cdc.gov/pcd/issues/2011/may/10_0045.htm.

35. Savage, C.L., Xu, Y., Lee, R., Rose, B., Kapesser, M., & Anthony, J.S. (2006). A case study in the use of community-based participatory research in public health nursing. *Public Health Nursing, 23*(5), 470-476.

36. Flicker, S., Travers, R., Guta, A., McDonald, S., & Meagher, A. (2007). Ethical dilemmas in community-based participatory research: Recommendations for institutional review boards. *Journal of Urban Health, 84*(4), 478-493.

37. Seifer, S.D., & Sisco, S. (2006). Mining the challenges of CBPR for improvements in urban health. *Journal of Urban Health, 83*(6), 981-984.

38. Israel, B.A., Krieger, J., Vlahov, D., Ciske, S., Foley, M., Fortin, P., et al. (2006). Challenges and facilitating factors in sustaining community-based participatory research partnerships: Lessons learned from the Detroit, New York City and Seattle urban research centers. *Journal of Urban Health, 83*(6), 1022-1040.

39. Minkler, M. (2005). Community-based research partnerships: challenges and opportunities. *Journal of Urban Health, 82*(Suppl. 2), 83-ii3-ii12.

40. Freeman, E.R., Brugge, D., Bennett-Bradley, W., Levy, J.L., & Carrasco, E.R. (2006). Challenges of conducting community-based participatory research in Boston's neighborhoods to reduce disparities in asthma. *Journal of Urban Health, 83*(6), 1013-1021.

41. Israel, B.A., Eng, E., Schulz, A.J., & Parker, E.A. (2005). *Methods in community-based participatory research for health.* San Francisco, CA: Jossey-Bass.

42. National Association of County and Community Health Officials. (2013). *Mobilizing for action through planning and partnerships (MAPP).* Retrieved from http://www.naccho.org/topics/infrastructure/MAPP/index.cfm.

43. National Association of County and Community Health Officials. (n.d.). *APEXPH.* Retrieved from http://www.naccho.org/topics/infrastructure/APEXPH/index.cfm.

44. Savage, C.L., Anthony, J.S., Lee, R., Rose, B., & Kapesser, M. (2007). The culture of pregnancy and infant care African American women: An ethnographic study. *Journal of Transcultural Nursing, 18*(3), 215-223.

45. Moyer, A. (2005). Starting well: Beginning a small-scale project. In E. Diem & A. Moyer (Eds.), *Community health projects* (pp 57-82). Philadelphia, PA: Lippincott Williams & Wilkins.

46. U.S. Census Bureau. (2012). *Geographic definitions.* Retrieved from http://www.census.gov/geo/www/geo_defn.html#CensusTract.

47. University of Wisconsin Population Health Institute. (2013). *County health ratings.* Retrieved from http://www.countyhealthrankings.org/.

48. Centers for Disease Control and Prevention. (2013). *National health interview survey.* Retrieved from http://www.cdc.gov/nchs/nhis.htm.

49. Centers for Disease Control and Prevention. (2013). *National health and nutrition examination survey.* Retrieved from http://www.cdc.gov/nchs/nhanes.htm.

50. Centers for Disease Control and Prevention. (2013). *Behavioral risk factor surveillance survey.* Retrieved http://www.cdc.gov/brfss/index.htm.

51. U.S. Department of Agriculture. (2013). *Food access research atlas.* Retrieved from http://www.ers.usda.gov/data-products/food-access-research-atlas/go-to-the-atlas.aspx.

52. Centers for Disease Control and Prevention. (2013). *Health-related quality of life: Methods and measures.* Retrieved from http://www.cdc.gov/hrqol/methods.htm.

53. Kruger, D.J., Shirey, L., Morrel-Samuels, S., Skorcz, S., & Brady, J. (2009). Using a community-based health survey as a tool for informing local health policy. *Journal of Public Health Management Practice, 15*(1), 47-53.

54. Urden, L.D. (2003). Don't forget to ask: Using focus groups to assess outcomes. *Outcomes Management, 7*, 1-3.

55. Savage, C.L. (Ed.). (1996). *Health of Lancaster County.* Lancaster, PA: Lancaster Health Alliance.

56. Wang, C.C., & Pies, C.A. (2004). Family, maternal, and child health through PhotoVoice. *Maternal and Child Health Journal, 8*(2), 95-102.

57. Skovdal, M. (2011). Picturing the coping strategies of caregiving children in western Kenya: From images to action. *American Journal of Public Health, 101*(3), 452-453.

58. Solet, D., Ciske, S., Gaonkar, R., Horsley, K., McNees, M., Nandi, P., et al. (2009). Effective community health assessments in King County, Washington. *Journal of Public Health Management Practice, 15*(1), 33-40.

59. Aronson, R.E., Wallis, A.B., O'Campo, P., & Schafer, P. (2007). Neighborhood mapping and evaluation: A methodology for participatory community health initiatives. *Maternal Child Health Journal, 11*, 373-383.

60. Croner, C.M., Sperling, J., & Broome, F.R. (1996). Geographic information systems (GIS): New perspectives in understanding human health and environmental relationships. *Statistics in Medicine, 15*, 17-18, 1961-1977.

61. Kazda, M., Beel, E.R., Villega, D., Martinez, J.G., Patel, N., & Migala, W. (2009). Methodological complexities and the use of GIS in conducting a community needs assessment of a large U.S. municipality. *Journal of Community Health, 34*, 210-215.

62. Choi, M., Afzal, B., & Sattler, B. (2006). Geographic information systems: A new tool for environmental health assessments. *Public Health Nursing, 23*(5), 381-391.
63. Environmental Protection Agency. (2013). *Toxic Release Inventory Program.* Retrieved from http://www.epa.gov/TRI/.
64. Myers, S.S., & Stoto, M.A. (2006). *Criteria for assessing the usefulness of community health assessments: A literature review.* Santa Monica, CA: RAND. Retrieved from http://www.rand.org/pubs/technical_reports/2006/RAND_TR314.pdf.
65. Friedman, D.J., & Parrish, R.G. (2009). Is community health assessment worthwhile? *Journal of Public Health Management Practice, 15*(1), 3-9.
66. U.S. Census Bureau. (n.d.). *U.S. Population Projections.* Retrieved from http://www.census.gov/population/projections/data/regdivpyramid.html.
67. U.S. Census Bureau. (n.d.). *American FactFinder.* Retrieved from http://factfinder2.census.gov/faces/nav/jsf/pages/index.xhtm.

Chapter 5

Health Program Planning

LEARNING OUTCOMES

After reading this chapter, the student will be able to:

1. Discuss the use of *Healthy People 2020* in health program planning.
2. Identify components of different health planning models.
3. Describe the steps in writing a community diagnoses.
4. Explain the importance of evidence-based practice in program planning.
5. Describe the process of writing goals, objectives, and activities for a health program.
6. Discuss the different types of program evaluation and their value.

KEY TERMS

Community capacity
Community diagnosis
Community organizing
Formative evaluation
Goal

Health program planning
Impact
Objective
Outcome
Output

Process evaluation
Program evaluation
Program implementation
Resources
SMART objectives

Social justice
Summative evaluation

■ Introduction

We all want to live in healthy communities. A healthy community is a place where children are safe to play and learn, a place where there are educational and employment opportunities, a place with safe, affordable housing, and a neighborhood with good communication and support. In a healthy community, when teenagers use alcohol, older adults have difficulty accessing health care, or the percentage of obese adults increases, the community works together with other collaborative partners to solve the problem. Program planning can lead to increased community capacity to solve these problems and create healthier communities.

Community program planning is the process that helps communities to understand how to move from where they are to where they would like to be.[1] **Health program planning** is defined as "a multi-step process that generally begins with the definition of the problem and development of an evaluation plan. Although specific steps may vary, they usually include a feedback loop, with findings from program evaluation being used for program

improvement."[2] Planning occurs at the local level with both public and private agencies, at the state and federal levels, and also as part of strategic planning for the public's health at the global level (see Chapter 13). Today public health program planning is one of the 10 essential public health services that should be undertaken in all communities.[3] Program planning is most successful when the community is a collaborative partner, bringing together community resources to achieve agreed upon goals and increasing community capacity. **Community capacity** refers to the ability of community members to work together to organize their assets and resources to improve the health of the community. It is the ability of a community to recognize, evaluate, and address key problems. Building community capacity can increase the quality of the lives of individual community residents; it can promote long-term community health and increase community resilience. The community as a whole can become self-reliant in identifying root causes of health problems and achieving identified outcomes. It can be quite self-sustaining when community members are empowered to make their own decisions about interventions and outcomes. Community capacity building is about working in partnerships and supporting community members in their decision making.[4]

Health program planning utilizes a four step process that includes assessment (see chapter 4), development of interventions, implementing interventions, and evaluating the effectiveness of interventions. It is the same basic steps of the nursing process that is applied to populations rather than individuals. It begins with the assessment phase covered in Chapter 4. Based on the assessment, the collaborative community partners arrive at a community diagnosis. They then decide what action would be most productive to improve the health of the community and begin to plan a program or programs aimed at addressing the priority health issues identified. Once the plan is in place they act (implement the plan). The final stages are to evaluate how well the plan addressed the priority issue and, if it works, how best to sustain the program.[4] The program could involve such things as policy change, health education, or the creation of new public health services. Frequently it means putting in place a program aimed at addressing the community health diagnosis with the goal of improving health outcomes for the population and reducing the risk of disease and/or minimizing the impact of the disease. Program planning follows the same process for the population level as the nursing process uses with individuals, and is similar to the development of a care plan in the nursing process and the evaluation of the effectiveness of the intervention.

National Perspective

Program planning has been an integral part of public health practice since its conception and has received a lot of attention in the past 25 years. In 1988, the Institute of Medicine (IOM) published a landmark report focusing on the future of public health (see Chapter 1). In this document public health practice was recognized as population and not individual focused, health planning was recognized as important at the local level, and the core public health functions of assessment, policy development, and service assurances were identified.[5] The IOM report of 2002 further defined public health practice and the shift from the individual to populations with the essential engagement of the community and diverse partners in the practice of public health,[6] and the 2012 IOM report strongly advocated for increased funding of public health and population-level interventions.[7] Public health nurses (PHNs) today

embrace this population focus with their community-based assessments, their health planning, population-based program designs and interventions, program evaluation, and policy development.[8] Both PHNs and nurses who work in other settings need skills related to engaging community partners in these program efforts and how to make successful programs sustainable. Keller and her colleagues have been instrumental in identifying within the Intervention Wheel Practice Model (Chapter 2) the areas of community organizing, coalition building, collaborating, social marketing, and policy development.[9,10] All of these are useful in health planning and program design, implementation, and evaluation.

Healthy People 2020

A key federal effort that provides a tool for community public health planning in the United States is *Healthy People 2020 (HP 2020),* a national compilation of disease prevention and health promotion goals and objectives for better health (see Chapter 1). *Healthy People* during the past three decades has become a part of health planning at the local, state, and federal levels. *HP 2020* provides a guide to communities wishing to implement *HP 2020* guidelines.[11] The guide uses MAPIT (Mobilize, Assess, Plan, Intervene, and Track progress) to help communities set targets and indicators of success (Box 5-1).

In addition, one of the *HP 2020* topics is educational and community-based programs.[12] Thus, *HP 2020* recognizes the need for health planning at the community level and provides clear objectives and strategies for population-based health programs.

BOX 5–1	*Healthy People 2020*

Implementing *HP 2020* MAPIT: A Guide to Using *HP 2020* in Your Community

Healthy People is based on a simple but powerful model that helps to
- Establish national health objectives
- Provide data and tools to enable states, cities, communities, and individuals across the country to combine their efforts to achieve them
  Use the MAPIT framework to help
- Mobilize partners
- Assess the needs of your community
- Create and implement a plan to reach *HP 2020* objectives
- Track your community's progress

Source: See reference 11.

■ HEALTHY PEOPLE 2020
Health Planning and Evaluation

Targeted Topics: Educational and Community-Based Programs

Goal: Increase the quality, availability, and effectiveness of educational and community-based programs designed to prevent disease and injury, improve health, and enhance quality of life.

Overview: Educational and community-based programs play a key role in:

• Preventing disease and injury
• Improving health
• Enhancing quality of life

Health status and related health behaviors are determined by influences at multiple levels: personal, organizational/institutional, environmental, and policy based. Because significant and dynamic interrelationships exist among these different levels of health determinants, educational and community-based programs are most likely to succeed in improving health and wellness when they address influences at all levels and in a variety of environments/settings.

Source: See reference 12.

Healthy People goals and objectives were first presented in 1979, and they have continued to influence the nation, not just to assess health status but also to project improved status with outcome measurement (see Chapter for 1). The *Healthy People* document in 1979 established for the first time national health objectives and provided the structure for the development of state and community health plans. The first 10-year plan had five goals, each established for distinct age groups, and 226 objectives.[13] The success of the first plan was limited. The reasons may have included too many goals, not enough significant interest generated in the public health and community arenas, and a lack of political support.[14]

The next 10-year plan, *Healthy People 2000* (1990–2000), replaced the first five goals with three new goals, 22 priority areas, and 319 objectives that included specific subobjectives to measure outcome with special populations experiencing health disparities. The goals included (1) increase the span of healthy life for Americans, (2) reduce health disparities among Americans, and (3) provide access to preventive health services for all Americans. These goals and objectives were influenced by the first 10-year plan, but they were also influenced by a concern for high-risk populations and the need to increase community organizing to better plan health. In the evaluation of the objectives at the end of the second decade of *HP,* there were some excellent outcomes, but there were situations in which health worsens.

The support for *Healthy People* as a planning tool grew and has now become part of the local, state, and national public health practice.[11] The *Healthy People 2010* (2000–2010) plan continued to build on previous *Healthy People* plans and refined the goals to two: (1) increase quality and years of life and (2) eliminate health disparity. It had more detailed objectives and 28 specific focus areas to help measure outcomes. *HP 2020* built on these previous efforts and now has 42 topics (Box 5-2).[15]

All health-related agencies are encouraged to use this document and its indicators, such as a school for its breakfast program and industry in its work site wellness programs. The current plan is continuing to foster change in health behavior, but it also looks at long-range planning and priority programs for target populations. The intention of *HP 2020* is to continue to guide efforts to plan, implement, and evaluate health promotion and disease prevention interventions for the nation. This is an important document to review and implement when planning health programs. It gives guidance in writing program objectives and identifying appropriate health indicators.

Overview of Health Program Planning

To provide population-focused care, it is necessary to have skill in health program planning and evaluation. Issel states the purpose of health program planning is "to ensure that a program has the best possible likelihood of being successful, defined in terms of being effective with the least possible resources."[16] To design appropriate programs, nurses who are part of a team must contribute to the completion of a reliable community assessment, participate in analyzing the community data, construct the community diagnoses, prioritize needs, and determine resource availability. Using this information, the nurses, other public health staff, community partners, and community members can begin the program planning process.

Health Program Planning Models

A number of models are available to assist with health program planning and evaluation. Program planning begins with a clear statement of the health problem.

BOX 5–2	*HP 2020's* 42 Topics

1. Access to Health Services
2. Adolescent Health*
3. Arthritis, Osteoporosis, and Chronic Back Conditions
4. Blood Disorders and Blood Safety*
5. Cancer
6. Chronic Kidney Disease
7. Dementias, including Alzheimer's Disease
8. Diabetes
9. Disability and Health
10. Early and Middle Childhood*
11. Educational and Community-Based Programs
12. Environmental Health
13. Family Planning
14. Food Safety
15. Genomics*
16. Global Health*
17. Health Communication and Health Information Technology
18. 30 Healthcare-Associated Infections*
19. Health-Related Quality of Life and Well-Being*
20. Hearing and Other Sensory or Communication Disorders

21. Heart Disease and Stroke
22. HIV
23. Immunization and Infectious Diseases
24. Injury and Violence Prevention
25. Lesbian, Gay, Bisexual, and Transgender Health*
26. Maternal, Infant, and Child Health
27. Medical Product Safety
28. Mental Health and Mental Disorders
29. Nutrition and Weight Status
30. Occupational Safety and Health
31. Older Adults*
32. Oral Health
33. Physical Activity
34. Preparedness*
35. Public Health Infrastructure
36. Respiratory Diseases
37. Sexually Transmitted Infections
38. Sleep Health*
39. Social Determinants of Health*
40. Substance Abuse
41. Tobacco Use
42. Vision

*Objectives for these topic areas are under development.
Source: http://www.healthypeople.gov/2020/default.aspx.

The assessment helps the team developing health programs to identify the priority health problems for the population and/or community. Following the establishment of the health priority, the team then works to understand the underlying factors that contribute to the problem. As explained by Issel, this is the first step in deciding what intervention(s) are the best choice for addressing the problem and ultimately improving the health of the population and/or community.[16]

Most program planning models use a systems approach and provide guidance on how to identify the problem and then systematically apply the best solution. These models all incorporate basic steps, and there are multiple resources that can be used to assist with each step (Table 5-1).

PRECEDE-PROCEED Model

Planning is essential to guarantee appropriate use of resources. One of the oldest models for program planning has come from Lawrence Green's well-researched PRECEDE-PROCEED model. Two other community health planning models in current use that can assist in program planning include Community Health Assessment aNd Group Evaluation (CHANGE) Action Guide and Mobilizing for Action Through Planning and Partnerships

(MAPP) (see Chapter 4). The CHANGE model (see Chapter 4) has eight phases and only the last phase, develop the community action plan, deals with program planning and MAPP's action cycle is the program planning phase.

Another model not discussed in Chapter 4 is the PRECEDE-PROCEED model, developed by Green, which gives insight into how to develop an educational program that will positively change health behavior. This model was first designed in 1968, and has generated evidence-based practice in many diverse areas of health education. Green started out with two ideas: (1) health problems and health risks are caused by multiple factors and (2) efforts to produce change must be multidimensional, multisectoral, and participatory.[17]

The PRECEDE component letters stand for **P**redisposing, **R**einforcing and **E**nabling factors, and **C**auses in **E**ducational **D**iagnosis and **E**valuation. When a community uses the PRECEDE process, it begins with a comprehensive community assessment process as described in Chapter 4. When the assessment phase is complete, the model provides guidance on how to examine the administrative and organizational issues that need to be dealt with before implementing a program aimed at improving the community's health.

TABLE 5–1	Steps in Health Program Planning

The types of steps that are generally used in program planning are listed here, along with selected resources that may be useful at each step.

Using Evidence-Based Resources for Program Design, Implementation, and Evaluation

Step	Description	Suggested Resources
1	Identify primary health issues in your community.	• Community Health Assessment aNd Group Evaluation (CHANGE) • County health rankings • National Public Health Performance Standards • MAPP (Mobilizing for Action Through Planning and Partnerships)
2	Develop measurable process and outcome objectives to assess progress in addressing these health issues.	• *HP 2020* Leading Health Indicators • HEDIS (Healthcare Effectiveness Data and Information Set) performance measures
3	Select effective interventions to help achieve these objectives.	• The Guide to Clinical Preventive Services • Health Evidence • National Guideline Clearinghouse
4	Implement selected interventions.	• Partnership for Prevention • CDCynergy
5	Evaluate selected interventions based on objectives; use this information to improve the program.	• Framework for Program Evaluation in Public Health • CDCynergy
1–5	All of the above	• The Community Health Promotion Handbook: Action Guides to Improve Community Health • Cancer Control P.L.A.N.E.T. (Plan, Link, Act, Network With Evidence-Based Tools) • Community Tool Box • Diffusion of Effective Behavioral Interventions (DEBI)

The final steps of this model are related to the design, implementation, and evaluation of a program. Evaluation includes examining data related to process, outcome, and impact objectives and indicators that were established during the development phase of the program planning.

Green felt that the more active and participatory the program interventions were for the recipients of the program, the more likely the recipients were to change behavior. Green also noted that for behavior change to take place recipients must be willing to work with the program, with the ultimate decision to change behavior up to the recipients. The second half of the model is the PROCEED component that was developed from the work with the PRECEDE component. PROCEED goes beyond the recipients of the interventions and reflects an effort to modify social environment and promote healthy life style, which evolved as a clear need. PROCEED involves **P**olicy, **R**egulatory, **O**rganizational Constructs in **E**ducation, and **E**nvironmental **D**esign.[17] This

model has served as the basis for other health program planning and assessment models such as MAPP and CHANGE (see Chapter 4).

Logic Model

Another model used by many program planners is the logic model. A logic model provides the underlying theory that drives the program design. This model guides a team in the careful planning of a well-thought-out program. A logic model approach to program planning can result in a plan that is clear to implement and evaluate; is based on theoretical knowledge; and includes a clear understanding of resources, time, and expected outcomes. Logic models are such useful tools for program evaluation that many grant agencies now require a logic model in their grant application.[18]

The concept of a logic model is that it logically moves like a chain of reasoning from the planned work to the intended results in five steps, starting with input and resources to program activities to outputs to outcomes to impact (Fig. 5-1). The model is read from left to right. The components are as follows:

1. **Resources** (inputs) are those items needed and available for the program. This includes human resources, financial resources, equipment, institutional resources, and community resources.
2. Next come the **activities** that produce the program intervention. It can involve processes such as health education, as well as tools technology or other types of activities that are classified as the intended intervention. These two components make up the planned work of the health program.[19]

The next three components of a logic model make up the intended results:

3. **Outputs** are the direct product of the activities of the program, for example, a class completed on family planning, immunization for tetanus, or a service from the dentist. This is the process component of program evaluation. Successful output occurs when the program's intended outcome is achieved.
4. **Outcomes** are the intended results or benefits of the planned intervention and are those items that the team plans to measure. This can include a change in knowledge, in skills, in behavior, or in an attitude. The outcomes should be reasonable, realistic, and significant. The short-term and medium-term outcomes are the objectives, which reflect the above characteristics. In program planning it is always important to think about what might be some unexpected or unintended outcomes if a program is implemented.
5. **Impact** is the program goal, producing long-term change in the community. This may often occur only after the program has been in effect for 5 to 8 years, and even after the program funding has ended.[19,20]

Although linear reasoning occurs in all logic models, the model can come in all sizes and shapes. Some organizations have added other components and complexities to the model to help with particular clarification of the program design. Two areas that can be added and can help in understanding the theory of the logic model are the assumptions the program planners have made, such as principles behind the program development, how and why a change in strategies will work, and any research knowledge and clinical experience. A second area is a listing of external factors (culture, economics, demographics, policies, priorities) that will affect both resources and the program activities (see Fig. 5-1). A logic model is built on the community assessment, a clear identification of the problem, and best solutions within the context of the community in which the program will take place.

A logic model is a good tool for everyone involved in the program to use to help them organize their thoughts

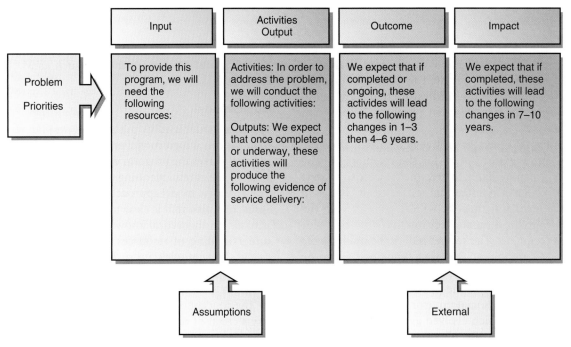

Figure 5-1 The basic logic model.

and ideas to work cooperatively for the same outcomes. It helps the program implementers understand why the activities are structured the way they are, helping to maintain the integrity of the program. The model is not static and can be adjusted and improved as need arises with good, ongoing review and evaluation. If you are entering the program as an implementer after the design has been established the logic model, read from left to right, offers you an excellent road map of *what* resources are available for implementation, *what* program is to be produced, with *what* results.

If you are entering the program as one of the stakeholders to help with the design, it is often best to start from what you hope the program will have as an impact (goal), move to the left identifying objectives (outcomes), and then determine which activities and output would help the community reach the intended objectives. Then you establish what resources are necessary to implement the intended activities.

In the program planning stage, you read a logic model from right to left. However, as noted above, there is nothing static in the program planning process. As you complete the different sections you may find that you need to rewrite objectives based on the best practices you have found in the literature about a particular activity you would like to implement. You may find you have fewer resources than what you need to implement a particular activity, which will change your intended outcomes. You can try various scenarios to determine which one is the best fit for the community and the organization, identifying strengths and weaknesses of the plan.

By the end of the process, the stakeholders will be able to see visually how the program goal(s) relate directly to the objectives that relate directly to the program activities and the resources available. An example of a logic model is presented for the Elwood Community (see case study page 118) incorporating the assessment data, goal, objectives, activities, and output (Table 5-2).

TABLE 5–2 Logic Model: Program to Create Social Integration Among Elmwood Residents

Resources	Activities	Outputs	Outcome	Impact
• Space in residential building including heat and electricity • Support (human and material) from the Primary Public School • Support from the community center (staff) at the residential site • PHN time, 8 hours per week for the program and other time for nursing care of the population • Residents of the facility • Support of time and resources from the two local churches • Additional community support	1. A senior outreach program to the public schools for 2 hours two times a week 2. A reading program for young children attending the Primary Public School 3. Creation and maintenance of a resident organization with one of its objectives being the improvement of communication among residents 4. Presentation/discussion groups twice a month with initial church leadership: suggested first topics include • safety in the community • celebrating differences in culture and ethnicity	• 15 seniors are working with 30 children at the Primary Public School • There is a reading session once a month with 10 seniors and 20 first grade children for 1 hour at the housing site • There is an Elmwood Community Association that has elected leaders and representatives from both buildings that meets regularly • There is a larger community organization that is meeting regularly to unite against crime in the community • The churches are working together to provide twice-monthly interactive programs at Elmwood	1. Establishment of a volunteer school program run by Elmwood residents to work with 50 children at the school and 25 children on site within 6 months 2. Development of consistent monthly programs in each building with a minimum of 40 resident attendees that foster social interaction by October 2017 3. Formation of a resident community organization	• Meaningful communication occurs among the elderly population in the two senior high-rise Elmwood residential buildings • Seniors are integrated into the community, feeling valued

Assumptions: (1) If residents of the Elmwood Buildings work together on programs and reach out to the community, the communication among themselves will increase. (2) If the residents feel their work is meaningful and interesting, then they will convey this to other residents, the program will expand, and there will be increased communication. (3) If the residents are offered interesting and appropriate programs in the building, they will attend, they will have more interaction, and communication will continue to increase.

The logic model is not the only tool available for program planning and, like all tools, has its drawbacks. In evaluating the use of the logic model, researchers have found that the emphasis on activities and outcomes has decreased the importance of understanding the rationale for the program choice.[20] Other tools such as concept mapping (a pictorial relation of concepts and relationships), a geographic information system (GIS, a computer-based program that can be used with geographical or location-based information; see Chapter 4), and community mapping (a visual map representation of resources and information corridors) are useful but are also limited. The University of Maryland, like many universities and organizations, developed Web-based tools that can assist in program development.[21] The tools are comprehensive and interactive, such as the Decision Support System (DSS), which is a step-by-step program planning series that gives on-screen feedback; Empower, which is based on the PRECEDE/PROCEED model; and the Outcome Toolkit, which facilitates planning and data analysis to make community improvement efforts measurable and accountable.

The logic model can serve several functions in addition to the actual program plan. Mulroy and Lauber described how their staff used it to plan their program evaluation for families at risk of homelessness.[22] It also helped the staff to discuss and specify assumptions they all held in common, for example, that within the community all families have strengths and that appropriate job training and related activities will prevent homelessness. This then helped them to better define their goal: to prevent homelessness and move families to self-sufficiency. Mulroy and Lauber were also able to limit their activities and more precisely determine immediate and intermediate outcomes. These authors agreed that logic modeling helped provide an analytical structure for better outcome development and better program management and evaluation.

In a breast health program designed for rural communities, Lane and Martin also found that the logic model was a useful guide for nurses in their program planning.[23] The nurses felt that the Logic Model was most helpful in providing a visual diagram that could be easily communicated to others. It became the heart of the program development and identified the future direction for the program.

Key Components of Health Program Planning

The important components of health program planning are:

- Active involvement of the community as a partner
- Skill and time to do a competent assessment

- Shared conclusions with the partners of the needed interventions
- Actual program planning, interventions, and evaluation[1]

Nurses at all levels of practice are involved in these processes and it is critical that nurses understand program planning in order to make significant contributions to the process.

As part of health program planning, nurses need to be involved in community organizing as this plays a pivotal role in successful planning as was recognized in the focus of *HP 2020* and in the Centers for Disease Control and Prevention (CDC) assessment and program model CHANGE (Chapter 4).[24] **Community organizing** is bringing people together to get things done. It is helping people to act jointly in the best interest of their community. Most frequently, community organizing occurs with poorer communities that are disenfranchised, uniting people to gain power and fight for social justice. The process is inclusive of everyone in the community and is a powerful tool in all communities for health planning and program design. The role of the nurse in community organizing is not one of leadership, but one of listener, facilitator, and developer of community leadership skills. It is to provide opportunities for the development of new relationships within the community.[1]

Inclusion of the community begins during the assessment phase (Chapter 4) and continues through the action and evaluation phases. The key is to assemble a representative team from the community to help develop, implement, and evaluate a community health program. The CHANGE manual provides a guide on how to begin to assemble a team (Box 5-3). The Community Tool Box (Fig. 5-2) out of the University of Kansas also stresses the importance of including the community, and provides extensive guidance and examples on how to accomplish this. This includes bringing together a diverse group, actively recruiting members, and developing a plan for engaging the larger community in the process.[1]

Social Justice

Another key concept central to the health program planning is **social justice.** Improving the health of everyone in the community often requires addressing social injustices. It is also a basic underlying concept of public health. Social justice dictates that society is based on the concepts of human rights and equality. The idea is that those who have plenty will be willing to share with those who do not have enough in order to provide for equality. In a just health-care system everyone should have the basic opportunities for a healthy life.

Action Step 1: Assemble the Community Team

Assembling a community team starts the commitment phase of the community change process. Representation from diverse sectors is a key component of successful teamwork, enables easy and accurate data collection, and enables data assessment, which is the next phase of the community change process. All members of the community team should play an active role in the assessment process, from recommending sites within the sectors to identifying the appropriate data collection method. This process also ensures the community team has equitable access to and informed knowledge of the process, thereby solidifying their support. Consider the makeup of the community team (10 to 12 individuals maximum is desirable to ensure the size is manageable and to account for attrition of members). Include key decision makers—the CEO of a work site or the superintendent of the school board—to diversify the team and use the skill sets of all involved.

Source: Centers for Disease Control and Prevention. (2010). *Community Health Assessment aNd Group Evaluation (CHANGE) action guide: Building a Foundation of Knowledge to Prioritize Community Needs.* Retrieved from http://www.cdc.gov/nccdphp/dch/programs/healthycommunitiesprogram/tools/change/pdf/changeactionguide.pdf.

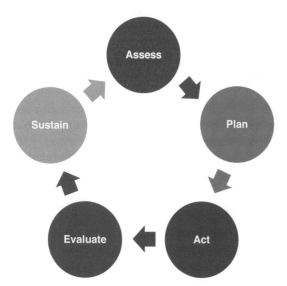

Figure 5-2 University of Kansas Community Tool Box: Health planning process. *(From Centers for Disease Control and Prevention. [2013]. National performance standards. Retrieved from http://www.cdc.gov/od/ocphp/nphpsp/EssentialPHServices.htm.)*

Poverty, illness, and premature mortality are a tragic waste of human resources and defy the dignity and inherent worth of the individual. Social justice dictates that everyone should have access to basic health services, economic security, adequate housing and food, satisfactory education, and a lack of discrimination because of race or religion. It is more often the distal social determinants (income, education, housing, racism) that are more important to changing the health status of individuals and populations than putting into place programs that change individual behavior in communities of very limited resources. Providing adequate education that leads to employment with a satisfactory income for housing and food can make more of an impact on health than teaching low-income individuals how to use their meager income for healthy foods or better housing. Communities with scant resources frequently organize around issues of disparity. As they build their skills in organizing and create change within the community, they build community capacity and work toward social justice. As the community capacity increases, the health of the community improves. Community members learn how to be independent in identifying their problems, the root causes, and the skills to solve these problems.

The nurse must always consider social justice in program planning. In making the decision about public health action, there is the consideration of equal distribution of benefits and burdens based on needs and contribution of the community. The community must decide the minimum goods and services required, how they can be acquired, and what programs will best serve the population with the available resources. Buchanan warns against public health paternalism where individual rights are limited for the greater public good. He argues that if communities are given freedom to make choices including the availability of those choices they will achieve good health.[25]

Working to ensure universal health care has great impact on health planning in the United States, and is a social justice action that is particularly important to the public health nurse. It was a major platform promise during President Obama's first campaign and resulted in the establishment of the Patient Protection and Affordable Care Act (ACA). Today these political and policy actions are important to the future functioning of our health-care system, and can have a major impact on the health of the entire population. The American Nurses Association has long been a supporter of health-care reform and supported the passing of the ACA.[26] Nurses can also advocate, support, and work for the distal social determinants of a better educational systems, better child welfare, better housing laws, and better occupational and environmental protection. These actions will help the nation to achieve the objectives set out in *HP 2020*, with people living longer and leading more active lives with less health disparity.

Community Diagnoses

Community diagnoses have been used in public health by multidisciplinary groups for many years, and evolved separate from nursing and medical diagnoses, which tend to focus on individual need. Community diagnoses represent the last phase of the community assessment process and the first phase of the health program planning process. A clear statement of the health problem and the causal reasons or theories for the health problem provides the basis for designing a health program that will actually improve the health issue. A **community diagnosis** is a summary statement resulting from the community assessment and the analysis of the data collected. The diagnosis guides the community team's thinking in how to design the program and what components are necessary. A community-specific diagnosis is needed because each community is unique in how the problems are manifested and solved. There are many types of community diagnoses and most share many parts in common, but the more detailed and complete the diagnoses, the easier it is to tailor them to an appropriate program.

Nursing community diagnoses generally contain four parts:[27] (1) the problem, (2) the population, (3) what the problem is related to (characteristics of the population), and (4) how the problem is demonstrated (indicators of the problem).[16,27]

▶ SOLVING THE MYSTERY

The Case of the Lonely Older Adults
Public Health Science Topics Covered:

- Assessment
- Community diagnosis

The PHN, Meghan, is working with a geriatric population in the Elmwood senior high-rise, publicly funded housing units. Her employer, the city health department, has allocated to the PHN one day a week for health programming in these two closely spaced buildings located in the inner city of a moderately large urban area. To determine what kind of programs would be most useful, Meghan enlisted community partners in the Elmwood community and the city housing authority to do an assessment to help identify community strengths and health needs.

During the assessment, residents of the buildings were interviewed, as were both formal and informal leaders. The assessment group toured the Elmwood buildings looking at the apartments and other resources that were part of the units. They spoke with community key informants including the employees in the neighborhood schools and local churches. The group evaluated community safety and resources within walking distance of the Elmwood buildings, which included supermarkets, pharmacies, banks, health-care facilities, social service resources, and local stores. They reviewed demographic data, vital statistics, and other community indicators for the neighborhood, and compared the data with the city and with other areas in the United States. The community partnership, with the help of the PHN as a member of the team, summarized their assessment findings. One of the identified problems, which was at the top of the list for many residents, was the lack of meaningful activities for the residents within their apartment buildings. The residents were justifiably concerned about safety outside their buildings and had many mobility issues, which resulted in boredom and isolation, without an avenue for social communication.

Meghan had initially imagined she would implement an educational program, for example, teaching the residents about the health benefits of eating vegetables, the correct way to take their medications, or the importance of a low-fat diet. This was based on the type of interventions she had already been doing in the buildings one-on-one with individual clients. However, she was more than willing to explore a community-specific program that would facilitate social interaction. To do this, with the help of her community partners she elaborated this problem in a community diagnosis (Box 5-4).

Meghan also decided to include mediating and moderating factors as part of her community diagnosis.[27] This allowed her not only to examine the health problem, the

| BOX 5–4 | **Community Diagnosis** |

Problem: Lack of meaningful social interaction resulting in social isolation.
Population: Older adult population in the two Elmwood senior residential buildings.

The isolation of the older adults was related to no formal programs in the building, limited social contact among residents, inadequate community safety, and residents' restricted mobility as indicated by residents being able to name only one other person in the building, the fact that no one spoke to others while waiting for the elevator, the neighborhood had the second highest crime rate in the city, 62% of residents complained of loneliness, and 59% of the residents had mobility problems.

Source: See reference 45.

population, indicators, and causal factors, but also how the problem was mediated by specific moderating factors and the presence of antecedent factors (those behaviors that existed prior to the health problem).[27] It is frequently important to know that some behaviors may cause the problem directly and others may be more indirect. Moderating factors can make the problem better or worse. Mediating factors occur between the causal factors and the outcomes and are significant to designing the program because they alter outcome. Increased details of the specific health problem can contribute significantly in determining the best program design.

Meghan noted in reviewing the analysis of the assessment that in the Elmwood senior buildings the housing authorities mixed two ethnic neighborhood groups that had been hostile to each other for the past 20 years. Also, 15 years ago two of the large churches in this community held different positions on several neighborhood political and religious issues and each congregation had united against the other with several harsh words spoken in public. The churches had subsequently left the decaying neighborhood, but many of the congregants were still living in the community. This antecedent information contributed to a better understanding of the current problem of limited communication among Elmwood residents that led to social isolation.

The assessment committee had also spoken with the community center 10 blocks from the Elmwood. The workers were frustrated at not attracting more senior clients for their multiple programs and expressed concern that they might have to discontinue these programs owing to lack of participation. They admitted they had done little marketing to the seniors at Elmwood, had no means to transport residents of the apartments to their center, and had little knowledge of the community dynamics, especially in relation to the senior population. They did provide escort services for the schoolchildren coming to the community center because of a recent outbreak of gang violence in the area. They had not considered that this might also have an impact on the seniors' decision not to come to the center.

The local churches confirmed that there had been community discord and that many of their current older members were still angry. This had caused some friction in the current churches, but the pastors were working on mediating these factors to create more united congregations and better sharing among the memberships. All of the local churches provided transportation to services on Sunday and Wednesday

evenings. They currently had no other outreach to the senior housing.

When visiting the primary school one block from the senior housing, all the teachers and the principal talked about a lack of resources in the school. They repeatedly mentioned the need for many of the children to have more one-on-one interactions to increase their basic skills of reading and writing. With this additional information, Meghan added to the community diagnosis, and she now had a clearer understanding of some of the origins of the problem and the mediating and moderating factors that could help design a program that not only would provide opportunity for more social interaction among the senior residents but could also enhance the health of the entire community (Fig. 5-3).

Having completed the community diagnosis, Meghan explained to the team that it was time to begin the program development phase. She explained that they would work together with all the stakeholders from all aspects of the identified community to determine how they could solve the problem of the lonely older adults. Meghan said that they first must decide who will receive the intervention. They needed to decide whether it would be individuals, families, communities, or a whole system. She cautioned that this was the time to consider carefully what interventions would be most appropriate and effective, and if there was evidence to confirm their decision. The team would together decide what immediate effects they would like this program to have and what long-term effects they might expect. All of this should be reflected from their community diagnosis, and would guide the community discussion.

Meghan stressed this approach because she knew that the clearer and more rational the explanation for solving the problem, the stronger the program would be. This was the time to discuss what kind of program activities the group would like to implement, and what evidence-based practices existed to help guide the development of a program. The team began with a review of the literature, looking not only for established approaches, but for new and innovative ones as well. Their discussion was tempered by resources, the nature of the community, the culture of the community, and other distal variables that influence receptivity to different types of programs. Much of the information gathered during their assessment helped them to think about what might work in their community.

The discussions were somewhat time intensive because of multiple agendas of the people at the table,

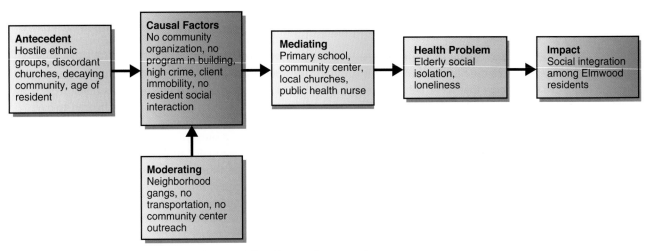

Figure 5-3 Diagram of community diagnosis for Elmwood Senior Housing.

different approaches to problem-solving, varied understanding of the process of program planning, different cultural and communication styles, and different expectations. Yet Meghan persevered and helped guide the discussion, allowing members to voice their opinions but then bringing them back to the task at hand. Because she had worked in the community for a long time, she was able to help interpret cultural and value differences, facilitate communication, and encourage the planning team to use the community diagnosis statement to guide the design.

Megan carefully considered who should participate in the discussion. Based on the community diagnosis, Meghan specifically invited leadership from the school, churches, and the community center. After she reviewed the community diagnosis with the group, the school representative immediately repeated the need for help with more one-on-one activity with the students at the school and mentioned several ways the seniors could participate. The school representative said they could provide on-site orientation at Elmwood for the seniors who would be willing to come to the school. He suggested first a 3-week training program, after which they would provide escorts to the school one block away on Tuesdays and Thursdays for the seniors to work 2 hours each of these days with the children. The Elmwood residents at the meeting asked whether the school could also bring some of the children to the Elmwood buildings once a month for story time with those seniors whose mobility was more limited. Several community members suggested that this could be accomplished by creating the Elmwood Community Action Committee, which could meet jointly

with school representatives to design the reading program. The community center offered to provide staff to help support these meetings. The community center saw this as an opportunity to get involved with a program the seniors would attend and were happy to do it at the Elmwood site. Other ideas included on-site, church-sponsored discussion groups about ways to decrease crime in the community and participatory cultural presentations (food, music, beliefs) from different ethnic groups in the community. At the end of the brainstorming meeting there were more than eight suggestions and several people agreed to research programs similar to these for more in-depth applications, successful outcomes, and identification of potential problems when applied to other communities.

Once the planning group reached consensus about the broad aspects of the program design, Meghan explained to them that the next step was to write the goals and objectives for the program. She pointed out that there were two important points to remember at this stage of the development of the program. The creation of a program is a process, and as a process the planning is fluid. She explained that the group might decide on an intervention, only to change it later as they start to write goals and objectives and identify indicators, and that this was all part of the process. Likewise, the goals and objectives might change as the group more carefully defined the program activities. However, she stressed that it was important in the final program design that the activities and outcomes correspond to the goals and objectives agreed on by the team and that this was again reflected in the process and outcome evaluation. She stated that members of the group would need to be responsible for monitoring the process and making sure the goals, objectives, activities, and evaluation all worked together. She volunteered to be part of this subgroup.

She then explained to the team that the second consideration was how best to write the goals and objectives and determine health indicators. She cautioned that a very large group discussion could be time consuming and result in poorly worded objectives. The team decided to appoint a smaller task force to write these up and present them back to the full group. They asked Meghan to be the facilitator for this task force.

When the task force had its first meeting Meghan began with an overview of how to write goals and objectives for the program plan and how they formed the framework of the plan. She explained that goals and objectives are very different and that each has a specific purpose. A goal is a broad statement of the impact expected by implementing a program, that is, a short general statement of the overall purpose of a program with a focus on the intention of the program. In most situations, it is a statement of outcome rather than activity, and frequently projects to a future situation, such as 5 years from program initiation. There are usually only a few goals for a program. There may be only one goal for a simple program and two or three for a more complex program. Because it is a general statement, there are usually no actual outcome measurements in it, but the goal should be realistic and reachable.

Meghan provided the team with examples. One example of a goal she provided was from a colleague of hers who was a high school nurse who developed a program to prevent teen pregnancies. The goal of that program was to prevent all teenage pregnancies at Reed High School. Another example she provided was from a community in Alabama concerned about the increase in obesity in all age groups. They designed a community-based fitness program with the goal of providing opportunities for all community residents to increase or maintain the necessary physical activities for them to be physically fit. After much discussion the task force decided that the goal for the program was the following:

> To increase meaningful communication among the older adult population in the two senior high-rise Elmwood residential buildings.

The next step for the task force was to come up with specific objectives for the program. Megan explained that **objectives** clarify the goal, are an

outcome measurement, and keep the program focused on the intended intervention. She knew that writing objectives is not easy, but understood that well-written and well-thought-out objectives were components for the success of the program and key in the process of program planning. Objectives include *who* will *achieve what* by *how much* by *when*. They are measureable, time limited, and action oriented. She suggested that they use an accepted approach to writing objectives first introduced in 1981 called **SMART objectives**. SMART stands for Specific, Measureable, Achievable, Realistic, and Time.[28] She explained that SMART objectives are action oriented and specify the goals and the desired results in a concrete, well-defined, and detail-focused statement. A specific objective answers the six "w" questions, who, what, where, when, which, and why. An objective that is measurable tells you the measurement criteria for when you have succeeded in meeting the objective, the most essential component of an objective. An objective that is achievable is one that can attain the desired outcome in the prescribed time frame. An objective that is realistic is one in which the resources (economic, manpower, skills) are available to implement the action. An objective that has defined time parameters indicates when this objective will be achieved and provides a deadline. All of these components working together in one objective can give you the clearest outcome measure.

The task force began to write up their objectives. They made sure there was an objective for every major program activity with a description and desired outcome that was clear to everyone. They hoped this would decrease confusion among stakeholders and the larger team when they presented it to them. They also realized it needed to be clear to those who would implement the program.

As they reviewed each objective, they examined how each would help guide the intended implementation of the program. They asked whether the objectives would work well taken all together and would reflect the goal for the program. Meghan explained that this program was somewhat complex. To help provide clarity, the group first added some level objectives that gave more detail. They also added process objectives to measure what the staff would do, how much they would do, and during what time period.

Meghan knew that she needed to become very familiar with the objectives and the indicators identified for this program as well as other programs she worked with for the health department. She was particularly concerned with ensuring the integrity of these programs when implemented, and ensuring that the right data were collected for the program evaluation phase. As the objectives were developed, Meghan identified indicators with which to measure the objectives chosen by the group and helped demonstrate how the program performed. She knew that good indicators are relevant to any health program, are scientifically defensible, when possible, are based on national benchmarks, are feasible to collect, are easy to interpret and analyze, and changes can be tracked over time.[29] The team developed clear and specific objectives and were then able to identify appropriate indicators to measure what was expected to change. The indicators they chose were practical and with specific steps in place to collect the necessary data.

The Elwood task force presented their final draft of the goals and objectives to the larger community team. The team accepted the draft and began to move into the implementation of the program.

Goal: To increase social communication among the older adult population in the two senior high-rise Elmwood residential buildings

Objectives:
1. *To establish a volunteer school program run by Elmwood residents to work with 50 children at the school and 25 children on site within 6 months*
2. *To develop consistent monthly programs in each building with a minimum of 40 resident attendees that foster social interaction by October 2017*

Cultural Considerations in Planning Programs

When assessing communities, analyzing data, and designing programs, the partnership must always consider the culture, ethnicity, and language of the community. It is important for staff and community members to feel secure asking questions and gaining information so they feel comfortable with the culture of the community the program serves. It is also important that organizations have clearly stated values that endorse cultural competency and sensitivity (see Chapter 23).

Although cultural competency is always an essential component in program planning, in some programs it takes on a central role. Aitato and colleagues in Hawaii noted in their assessment that cancer is the leading cause of death for Samoans in the United States.[30] They concluded that the design of a program aimed at decreasing

morbidity and mortality related to cancer for this population required a culturally relevant approach. When designing the program they linked the Samoan beliefs about health and illness with the need for early cancer detection. They reviewed the sociological and cultural literature to better understand appropriate interventions. Through their examination of the culture they found that most Samoans in response to cancer were fatalistic and passive. This was also observed in clinical settings. Aitato et al. also reported that church affiliation was exceptionally important for this immigrant group, especially because it provided them a community where they could practice their more traditional lifestyle. Based on this evidence, the program designers used a community-based participatory research method to gather information within the Samoan churches. As a community, through focus groups the Samoans determined the most appropriate programs, including the need to use the Samoan language, the serving of appropriate Samoan food, and the need to recognize a traditional leader.

Other examples of integrating cultural components into program planning include a perinatal program for urban Native Americans (NAs)[31] and a family education diabetes series for a Midwestern NA community.[32] The perinatal program emphasized the importance of staff cultural awareness and knowledge of the local community and customs to facilitate networking. The authors attributed the success of the perinatal program in part to the ability of the staff to understand the history of abuse of the NA women in the program and the ability of the staff to empathize with the culture even if they were not NAs.[31]

Evidence-Based Practice in Program Planning

It is important to use evidence-based practice (EBP) in all the steps of program planning. The development of a health program begins with a review of the literature for similar problems and the population-based approaches to solving the problem(s) and the evidence that the approach worked. Look at theory and rationales for these other programs and see how they relate to your program. Look for similar programs in similar communities and see whether your strategies are also similar. Note whether the strategies in these other communities produced their expected outcomes. If you want to try something unique, see whether there is anything in the literature that allows you to build your own rationale for the effectiveness of your selected approach. Arguments for using a specific intervention are strongest when there is demonstrated previous success with the method, and especially with a similar population.

■ EVIDENCE-BASED PRACTICE
Engagement of the Older Adult

Practice Statement: Social isolation poses a significant health risk for older adults.

Targeted Outcome: Engagement with the community

Evidence to Support: Intergenerational programs at schools that include older adults and young children are shown to have a beneficial impact on both (Fig. 5-4). The children receive additional attention and the older adults feel needed and appreciated. Specifically, researchers found that older adults had increased self-esteem and better health. Children at risk for failure did much better in these programs, and all the children had a more positive attitude toward older adults. Another finding was that the older adults had a calming effect on the classroom. In one study, the researchers compared two programs, one with a formal design with older adult receiving pretraining and one that accepted volunteers and integrated them into the classroom without any training. The final outcome of effectiveness was the same.

Sources

1. Kaplan, M. (2001). *School-based intergenerational programs. UNESCO Institute of Aging.* Retrieved from http://www.unesco.org/education/uie/pdf/school-basedip.pdf.
2. Kaplan, M., & Larkin, E. (2004). Launching intergenerational programs in early childhood setting: A comparison of explicit intervention with an emergent. *Early Childhood Educational Journal, 31*(3), 157-163.
3. The U.S. Environmental Protection Agency. (2011). *Aging initiative: Benefits of international programs.* Retrieved from http://www.epa.gov/aging/ia/benefits.htm.

Resources for Evidence-Based Programs

The Community Tool Box, created by the University of Kansas, offers additional suggested resources for information on promising evidence-based programs or programs with interesting new interventions.[1] A central suggestion in the Community Tool Box is networking with local and state agencies and checking public and private professional organizations or advocacy groups to see whether they have published information on evidence-based programs.

For example, in developing an obesity prevention and management program in a rural community, Hawley, Beckman, and Bishop explored previous EBP.[32] They acknowledged that according to the literature, merely gaining knowledge about nutrition and fitness frequently did not translate into behavior change. Based on their review of the literature, such things as goal setting, strengthening self-efficacy, and using theory of change had more success in actually changing behavior than just providing information. They also found that multifaceted community efforts have increased physical activities. With this evidence, they designed their program.

Determining whether a program has good evidence to support it can be accomplished using a few different approaches. First, examining both the quantitative and qualitative data from studies as well as the current program provides essential information. Even simple statistical analysis can help determine whether a program is thriving, whether participants are reaching their outcomes, and whether positive things are happening in the community. Good indicators that the community likes the program are the continued use of the program by participants and ongoing growth of a program. However, it is important to know whether there are outside factors that are contributing to the success that might make it difficult to duplicate the program in other communities or with other groups. Another issue may be that the outcomes are really measurement of behavior change and not real outcomes. When reviewing program data it is important to

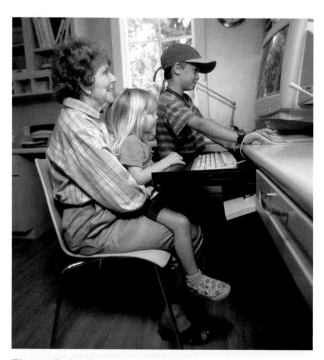

Figure 5-4 Adopt a Grandparent. *(From the Centers for Disease Control and Prevention, Richard Duncan, MRP, Sr. Proj. Mngr, North Carolina State University, the Center for Universal Design, 2000.)*

note whether there is a researched theoretical framework to support the intervention, whether the statistical analysis is clear, whether there are enough participants to make conclusions, whether the target outcomes are appropriate, and whether the program reached these targets. In reviewing the program it helps to evaluate whether the indicators seemed appropriate and whether the tools were well designed. It also helps to think about the usefulness of the indicators of the program. Did the intervention reach the intended population, and is this population similar to or different from the intended population? It is also important to be aware of what resources were used and compare the amount of resources available for your program. In the 1990s Lisbeth Schorr, a well-known social analyst, identified seven characteristics of highly effective programs that are still relevant today.[33] Although they are focused on programs aimed at improving the health of children, they can be applied to other populations. Effective programs:

- Are comprehensive, flexible, responsive, and persevering
- See children in the context of their families
- Deal with families as parts of neighborhoods
- Have a long-term, preventive orientation, a clear mission, and continue to evolve over time
- Are well managed by competent and committed individuals with clearly identifiable skills
- Have staff who are trained and supported to provide high-quality, responsive services
- Operate in settings that encourage practitioners to build strong relationships of mutual trust and respect

Many of these attributes are part of effective program planning, implementation, and evaluation, and include looking at communities and not just individuals, being flexible and persevering, having clear goals, forming partnerships and working collaboratively, and having passion on the part of staff for the work and for social justice. In successful programs, the staff is nurtured and supported and the program is well managed.

Program Implementation

After the program has been designed and the logic model solidified, it is time to implement the program. **Program implementation** encompasses the resources needed to provide a program as well as the mechanism for putting the program in place. Prior to putting a program in place it is important to map out exactly how this will be done. For example, when implementing a screening program it is important to know how many participants are anticipated, how many screening tools/how much equipment will be needed, how many personnel are needed, and what the flow for participants from arrival through the screening and referral process will be. Nurses are frequently part of the implementation team and assist in adding the necessary detail to the actual program activities. Ervin identified five stages related to program implementation:[27]

1. Community acceptance of the program
2. Specifying tasks and estimating needed resources
3. Developing specific plans for program activity
4. Establishing a mechanism for program management
5. Putting the plan into action

Partnering with the community from the beginning of the planning process facilitates community interest and ownership of the program, which should be culturally and politically specific and acceptable. Although adequate resources to implement the program were identified in the planning, it is important to confirm that the resources are available and adequate, and how these resources are to be used in the program activities and evaluation.

The implementation team needs to make certain that the indicators for the outcomes are identified and a mechanism is in place to collect the data. Everyone needs to know the steps of the program. It may be necessary to write protocols and procedures for the intervention. If additional staff members are needed, they need to be hired and to undergo orientation. There may also be a need for additional staff training. Several program evaluations have stressed the importance of pilot testing the program or components of the program and the planned evaluation before implementation of the complete program. Littleton and her colleagues noted several lessons they learned while implementing a community health program.[34] The first was the importance of establishing a personal working relationship with the community. They also suggested that the program leader strive to build partnerships by listening, observing, and integrating the experiences between the program and the community. They also found it was best to be flexible and emphasized simplicity when implementing community activities.

Program Evaluation

Project management and program evaluation are inextricably linked whether in public health programs or a health program in an acute care setting implemented by the nurse manager.[35] **Program evaluation** is the systematic collection of information about the activities, outputs, and outcomes to enhance the program and its effectiveness. Evaluation is defined as the systematic acquirement and analysis of information to provide useful feedback. Evaluation is essential to good management and to good program design, and evaluation strategy should be developed prior to the project management and programs being implemented. Evaluation is used to evaluate the effectiveness of the program, and, provide information to guide any needed improvement of the program. Through evaluation you strengthen the project. Programs need to be evaluated for multiple reasons. You need to know whether your objectives and goals are being met. From the evaluation you can determine whether the:

- Activities are implemented as they were designed
- Program is cost effective
- Intervention and program theories are correct
- Time line is appropriate
- Program should be expanded or duplicated in another location

Evaluation helps with program planning, program development, and program accountability. Frequently the PHN works with comprehensive collaborative community interventions that are complex to evaluate, as there may be no clear cause and effect with multiple interventions. Often the program operates within the unique local political issues and circumstance of the community that demand a customized evaluation to really understand what is happening. PHNs and other local providers can help interpret this information for the interior or exterior evaluators or as part of an evaluation team.

Percy provided a good example that underscores the necessity for program evaluation.[36] She described a school health program in one school district that was so busy providing good health care to the schoolchildren that the district failed to design and implement an evaluation plan. Without an evaluation of the program, the district was unable to determine whether the program was effective. Because the program required a registered nurse (RN) in each school, the lack of evaluation data resulted in the inability to demonstrate the need for the added cost of the school nurses. The city council members had budget constraints and needed to cut programs. Without the evaluation data, the nurses could not show the council members the importance of this nursing distribution. To have a more cost-effective budget, the city council replaced the nurses with nursing assistants. When the city tried to extend this cost savings to another school district, the nurses in the second school district had been evaluating their program routinely and had excellent outcome data to demonstrate the effectiveness of having a RN in each school. Their program did not get cut.

Evaluation of family and individual care, community services, and programs has grown over the past several decades as a response to the stakeholders, especially the funders, who to know whether the nurse and colleagues from other disciplines are successful in improving health and are doing so in a cost-effective manner. Most grant agencies that fund these types of interventions now make evaluation mandatory.

Evaluation Models

Formative Evaluation

There are several models for program evaluation. One model is to divide the evaluation into either formative or summative or both. **Formative evaluation** occurs during the development of a program, while the activities are forming and being implemented for the first time. It is an ongoing feedback on the performance of the program, identifying aspects that need improvement and providing opportunity to offer corrective suggestions. Formative evaluation is concerned with the delivery of the program, the organizational context including structure and procedures. This is an opportunity to examine what happens in the reality of the implementation, and allows the opportunity to see whether the program outputs can really create the change necessary to meet the objectives and goals. Usually a formative evaluation is internal and ongoing, with the staff constantly asking what are the strengths, weaknesses, barriers, and unexpected opportunities that these new program activities offer. The activities and outputs are the dynamic part of the program and lend themselves to formative evaluation. The program can positively respond to the evaluation and change interventions, change the way outcome measurements are collected, or change other parts of the program designed to better meet the program goals and objectives. It is appropriate to change things if the program is not working as well as possible.

Process Evaluation: **Process evaluation** is a type of formative evaluation that investigates the process of delivering the program or technology, including alternative delivery procedures. The main concern with process evaluation is to document to what extent the program has been delivered and whether the delivery was what was defined in the program design. There should be detailed information on how the program actually worked (the program operations), any changes made to the program, and how those changes have had an impact on the program. It is also important for an evaluator to be aware of any outside environmental events or intervening events that might have influenced the

program activities. These type of data can be collected by noting actual numbers related to the interventions, such as the number of people attending a class, the number of pamphlets handed out, and the number of screening tests performed. Qualitative data methods can include, among others, direct observation, in-depth interview, focus groups, and review of documents.

The importance of formative evaluation should not be underestimated. It is a strong tool in helping to improve the activities and output of a program and for determining whether the theoretical understanding of how the program will influence change is accurate and appropriate.

Summative Evaluation

Summative evaluation occurs at the end of the program and is the evaluation of the objectives and the goal. It is judging the worth of the program at the end of the activities and discovering whether the program achieved the intended change. It looks at outcome and impact of the benefits the selected population has received by participating in the program. It looks at the causal relationship and the theoretical understanding of the planned intervention. It can also examine the cost of the program, looking at cost-effectiveness and cost benefit.[37] When conducted on well-established programs, it allows funders and policy makers to make major decisions on the continuation of the program and how the outcomes could influence policy at the local to the national level.

As more hospitals strive for magnet status, baccalaureate nurses are being called on to initiate health programs in acute care settings and to evaluate their effectiveness. In public health settings, the PHN is often responsible for managing community-based programs in which evaluation is essential to the sustainability of the programs. Several nonprofit funding agencies and the CDC offer suggestions on how to do internal evaluations and when to seek external evaluator assistance.

Nine Steps of Program Evaluation

The W.W. Kellogg Foundation identified nine steps in developing a program evaluation that is useful for both smaller programs and for the complex multi-activity community program interventions that many organizations implement (Box 5-5).[37] The first four steps occur in the program planning stage, the next three in the implementation of the program, and the last two after the program evaluation is complete. Program evaluation is an integral part of the program design and the program evaluation plan should be in place before the program is initiated. **Step 1:** Step 1 is completed before the program begins. It identifies among the stakeholders the people who

---

BOX 5–5 Nine Steps in Developing a Program Evaluation

Program
1. Select the evaluation team.

Planning Stage
2. Develop the evaluation questions.
3. Have a budget in place for the evaluation.
4. Decide whether to use an internal or external evaluator.

Program Implemented
5. Determine data collection methods.
6. Collect the data.
7. Analyze and interpret the results.

Evaluation Complete
8. Communicate findings.
9. Improve the program.

---

should be included on the evaluation team, staff representation, and what community representation and participants are needed in the program.

Step 2: In step 2, evaluation questions are created. All participants need to help phrase questions that will be useful in reflecting the program theory, improving the program, and determining effectiveness. These questions can include the following: What data do you need to collect? What kind of information is needed? What do we want to accomplish? What do we need to know about the program? How will we know when we have accomplished our goal? Where do we find the data and what indicators do we need? The questions will also involve how this information is communicated to others: Who is the audience for the results? What kind of information should we tell them?

Step 3: Step 3 is the creation of a budget. The amount of the budget varies depending on several components such as the size of the program, the number of staff needed to carry out the evaluation, the need for other resources such as software for data entry and analysis, and the length of time needed to complete the evaluation.

Step 4: In step 4, a decision must be made about whether the evaluation will be internal or will have an external evaluator. If you decide on an external evaluator, it is good to identify that person so the evaluator can be a part of the program planning process from the beginning. These are all components of the planning and occur as the program is designed.

Step 5: Steps 5 through 7 occur during the program implementation phase. In step 5, data collection methods are determined.

Step 6: In step 6, data are collected.

Step 7: In step 7, the results are analyzed and interpreted.

Step 8: After the completion of the evaluation, in step 8 the findings and new perceptions of the program are communicated to the stakeholders. It is important that the appropriate information is communicated to the identified audiences.

Step 9: In step 9, evaluation information is used to prove or improve the program. The better informed we are, the better we are at making good program decisions. This may be in sharing with funding agencies to receive more funding for the successful program; it may be to change some of the program activities and outputs to improve outcomes; or it may be to refine the population served, to help change policy, or to discontinue the program (Box 5-5).

When developing the process for health program evaluation it is important to be as objective as possible. Some of the ethical dilemmas that can emerge during program evaluation include:

- Pressure to slant the finding in the direction wanted by key stakeholders
- Compromised confidentiality of data sources
- Response on the part of the evaluator to one interest group more than to others
- Misinterpretation or misuse of the findings by the program stakeholders
- Evaluator using a familiar tool to collect data rather than a more appropriate one

The team can use these points to examine the methods chosen to evaluate a program as a means of eliminating as much bias as possible.

Through successful programs, communities can better their health. These programs can be synergistic in creating positive change and can lead to new policies with an even wider influence on health. The purpose of health programs is to strive for a community in which everyone is safe, environments support health, actions are taken to prevent and control acute and chronic disease, and individuals and families can thrive.

Summary Points

- Health planning occurs across health-care settings including public health settings, primary care, acute care, and schools with the focus on improving the health of the populations served.

- *HP 2020* provides a framework of goals and indicators that can help in creating health programs for our communities.
- All models of program planning include the community as a partner, and it is important that the community is involved in every step of the process.
- Health planning includes community assessment, community diagnoses, program design, program implementation, and program evaluation.
- Using logic modeling can help create a well-structured program with clear indication of how to do both process and outcome evaluation of the program.
- Every program should be evaluated and evaluation begins when you start designing the program.
- Formative, process, and summative evaluations each provide important information about the program and how to make it more effective.

▲ CASE STUDY

Program Evaluation at Elmwood

The Elmwood Senior Housing program was designed to increase social integration and has been in place for 9 months. The activities include residents working in the public schools in an intergenerational program, the first and second graders each coming to Elmwood once a month for a 2-hour reading program, the solidification of an Elmwood community organization, and weekly discussion and activity programs at the center with assistance from the community center and the local churches. The PHN and other members of the team have been doing ongoing process evaluation and are now meeting to discuss the implementation of their outcome evaluation plan.

To answer the following questions, use the established goal, outcomes, and output in the logic model (Fig. 5-1) that was developed by the community group. You can also reference the Community Tool Box from the University of Kansas (http://ctb.ku.edu/en/table-contents/), Part J: Evaluating Community Programs and Initiative, Chapters 36–39.

1. What data would you collect as part of the process evaluation? How would these data help you in the formative process of your program? Would you change activities based on these data?
2. What would have been the steps in setting up the evaluation plan? What might be your evaluation questions? What would be your indicators? What kind of data should you collect? How would you specifically know whether your program has been successful?

REFERENCES

1. Work Group for Community Health and Development. (2013). *The community tool box, University of Kansas.* Retrieved from http://ctb.ku.edu/en/TakingActionInTheCommunity.aspx#plan.
2. U.S. Department of Health and Human Services. (2013). *The guide to community preventive services: Program planning resource.* Retrieved from http://www.thecommunityguide.org/uses/program_planning.html.
3. Centers for Disease Control and Prevention. (2015). *National public health performance standards (NPHPS).* Retrieved from http://www.cdc.gov/nphpsp/index.html.
4. Fawcett, S.B., Francisco, V.T., Hyra, D.S., Paine-Andrews, A., Schultz, J.A., Russos, S., et al. (Eds.). (2013). *Our model of practice: Building capacity for community and system change, University of Kansas.* Retrieved from http://ctb.ku.edu/en/tablecontents/sub_section_main_1002.aspx.
5. Institute of Medicine. (1988). *The future of public health.* Washington, DC: National Academies Press.
6. Institute of Medicine. (2002). *The future of the public's health in the 21st century.* Washington, DC: National Academies Press.
7. Institute of Medicine. (2012). *For the public's health: Investing in a healthier future.* Washington, DC: National Academies Press.
8. American Public Health Association: Public Health Nursing Section. (2015). *Public health nursing.* Retrieved from http://apha.org/apha-communities/member-sections/public-health-nursing.
9. Keller, L.O., Schaffer, M., Lia-Hoagberg, B., & Strohschein, S. (2002). Assessment, program planning, and evaluation in population-based public health practice. *Journal of Public Health Management and Practice, 8,* 30-43.
10. Keller, L.O., Strohschein, S., Lia-Hoagberg, B., Schaffer, M. (2004) Population-based public health interventions: Practice-based and evidence-supported. Part I. *Public Health Nursing, 21*(5), 453-468.
11. U.S. Department of Health and Human Services. (2013). *Implementing Healthy People 2020: MAP-IT a guide to using Healthy People 2020 in your community.* Retrieved from http://healthypeople.gov/2020/implement/MapIt.aspx.
12. U.S. Department of Health and Human Services. (2013). *Educational and community based programs.* Retrieved from http://healthypeople.gov/2020/topicsobjectives2020/overview.aspx?topicid=11.
13. Public Health Service. (1979) *"Healthy People": The Surgeon General's report on health promotion and disease prevention.* Washington, DC: U.S. Government Printing Office, DHEW.
14. Chrvala, C., & Bugar, R. (Eds.). (1999). *IOM report. Leading health indicators for "Healthy People 2010": Final report.* Washington, DC: National Academies Press.
15. U.S. Department of Health and Human Services. (2015). *Healthy People 2020.* Retrieved from http://www.healthypeople.gov/2020/default.aspx.
16. Issel, L. (2014). *Health program planning and evaluation.* (3rd ed.) Sudbury, MA: Jones & Bartlett.
17. Green, L.W., & Kreuter, M.W. (2005). *Health program planning: An educational and ecological approach* (4th ed.). New York, NY: McGraw-Hill Higher Education.
18. W.K. Kellogg Foundation. (2004). *Logic model development guide.* Battle Creek, MI: Author. This guide is also available at www.wkkf.org/Pubs/Tools/Evaluation/Pub3669.pdf.
19. University of Wisconsin. (2002). *Enhancing program performance with logic model.* Retrieved from http://www.uwex.edu/ces/lmcourse/interface/oop_M1_Overview.htm.
20. Garrett, K., & Kaplan, S.A. (2005). The use of logic models by community-based initiatives. *Evaluation and Program Planning, 28,* 167-172.
21. University of Maryland. (2009). *Program planning public health informatics.* Retrieved from http://www.phi.umd.edu/what/progplantools.html.
22. Mulroy, E., & Lauber, H. (2004). A user-friendly approach to program evaluation and effective community interventions for families at risk of homelessness. *Social Work, 49*(4), 573-586.
23. Lane, A., & Martin, M. (2005). Logic model use for breast health in rural communities. *Oncology Nursing Forum, 32*(1), 105-110.
24. Centers for Disease Control and Prevention. (2015). *Community Health Assessment aNd Group Evaluation (CHANGE) action guide.* Retrieved from http://www.cdc.gov/healthycommunitiesprogram/tools/change/downloads.htm.
25. Buchanan, D. (2008). Autonomy, paternalism, and justice: Ethical priorities in public health. *American Journal of Public Health, 98,* 15-21.
26. American Nurses Association. (2015). *Policy and advocacy: Health care reform.* Retrieved from http://www.nursingworld.org/MainMenuCategories/Policy-Advocacy/HealthSystemReform.
27. Ervin, N. (2002). *Advanced community health nursing practice.* Upper Saddle River, NJ: Prentice Hall.
28. Doran, G.T. (1981). There's a S.M.A.R.T. way to write management's goals and objectives. *Management Review, 70*(11), 35-36.
29. UNFPA. (2004). *Programme manager's planning monitoring & evaluation toolkit.* Retrieved from http://www.unfpa.org/monitoring/toolkit/tool6.pdf.
30. Aitato, N., Braun, K., Dang, K., & So'a, T. (2007). Cultural considerations in developing church-based programs to reduce cancer health disparities among Samoans. *Ethnicity and Health, 12*(4), 381-400.
31. Prater, S., & Davis, C. (2001). A perinatal intervention program for urban American Indians. Part 2: The story of a program and its implications for practice. *Journal of Perinatal Education, 11*(2), 23-32.
32. Hawley, S., Beckman, H., & Bishop, T. (2006). Development of an obesity prevention and management program for children and adolescents in a rural setting. *Journal of Community Health Nursing, 23*(2), 69-80.
33. Schorr, L. (1997). *Common purpose: Strengthening families and neighborhoods to rebuild America.* New York, NY: Anchor Books.

34. Littleton, M., Cornell, C., Dignan, M., Brownstein, N., Raczynski, J., Stalker, V., et al. (2002). Lessons learned from the Uniontown Community Health Project. *American Journal of Health Behavior, 26*(1), 34-42.

35. DeSilets, L., & Dickerson, P. (2008). The role of the nurse planner. *Journal of Continuing Education in Nursing, 39*(4), 149-150.

36. Percy, M. (2007). School health. Quality of care: or why you HAVE to evaluate your program. *Journal for Specialists in Pediatric Nursing, 12*(1), 66-68.

37. W.K. Kellogg Foundation. (1998) *W.K. Kellogg Foundation evaluation handbook*. Battle Creek, MI: Author. The guide is also available at http://www.wkkf.org/Pubs/Tools/Evaluation/Pub770.pdf.

Chapter 6

Environmental Health

KEY TERMS

Air Quality Index (AQI)
Ambient air
Ambient air standard
Area sources
Bioaccumulation
Built environment
Community environmental health assessment
Criteria air pollutants
Environmental exposure
Environmental health
Environmental justice
Environmental sustainability
Exposure
Gene-environment interaction
Half-life
Integrated pest management
International building codes
Latency period
Mobile sources
Point sources
Risk assessment
Routes of entry
Safe Drinking Water Act
Toxicity

■ Introduction

In the spring of 2010, one of the worst American environmental disasters unfolded in the waters of the Gulf of Mexico. When an oil rig exploded, the first concern was for the workers involved in the explosion. In the following days, there was increasing concern about the amount of the oil spillage from the damaged rig. With reassurances from the British Petroleum corporate headquarters, the initial estimation of the amount of oil that was leaking following the explosion remained low. Unfortunately, those initial estimations failed to warn us of the enormous amount of oil that would eventually spill into the Gulf or of the long-term effects that oil would have on the environment.

The health of our environment has everything to do with our own health and the health of the patients and communities we serve. The pollution of the Gulf directly disturbed the animals and plants living in and near the Gulf, thus affecting the region's food supply.[1-4] The loss to the fishing industry and the oil industry influenced the ability of the population to maintain employment and, thus, disrupted the economic health of a region already affected by a devastating hurricane 4 years earlier. The workers hired to clean up the spill were exposed to toxins from both the oil and the materials used to disperse and clean the oil.[2] Thus, this oil spill affected the quality of the air, the water, recreational facilities, employment, and the habitat of a major food source, seafood. Pollution of the Gulf waters will continue to have an impact on the environment for decades at all these levels, and has the potential to have negative impacts on the health of individuals particularly susceptible to exposure to the toxins released by the spill.[4] The spill illustrates the close relationship between the health of the environment we live in and our own health.

Hardly a day goes by without a report in the media that links environmental conditions to human health. High rates of childhood asthma, industrial explosions, hurricanes and other natural disasters, as well as reports of polluted water and air remind us of the many ways we are affected by the world around us and how the health of individuals and communities strongly depends on environmental determinants. In addition to the adverse environmental impact of human-made and natural disasters such as the Gulf oil spill and the Japanese tsunami[5] (Chapter 25) are the day-to-day aspects of the environment in which we live, work, and play that can cause immediate or long-term harm.

The World Health Organization (WHO) defines **environmental health** as follows:

> *Environmental health addresses all the physical, chemical, and biological factors external to a person, and all the related factors impacting behaviors. It encompasses the assessment and control of those environmental factors that can potentially affect health. It is targeted towards preventing disease and creating health-supportive environments. This definition excludes behaviour not related to environment, as well as behaviour related to the social and cultural environment, and genetics.[6]*

This perspective of environmental health extends beyond food, air, water, soil, dust, and even consumer products and waste. It includes all aspects of our living conditions, the use and misuse of resources, and the overall design of communities. The ecological models of health promotion (see Chapter 1) encompass the environment in which we live. Using an ecological approach requires an understanding that individuals/populations interact with their environment.[7] All of these factors play a role in the health of the individuals and populations living in the environment.

The broad scope of environmental determinants of health is obvious with the inclusion of 24 objectives under the *Healthy People 2020 (HP 2020)* topic of environmental health.[8]

■ HEALTHY PEOPLE 2020
Environmental Health

Targeted Topic: Environmental Health
Goal: Promote health for all through a healthy environment.
Overview: Humans interact with the environment constantly. These interactions affect quality of life, years of healthy life lived, and health disparities. The WHO defines *environment*, as it relates to health, as "all the physical, chemical, and biological factors external to a person, and all the related behaviors."[1] Environmental health consists of preventing or controlling disease, injury, and disability related to the interactions between people and their environment.

The *HP 2020* Environmental Health objectives focus on six themes, each of which highlights an element of environmental health:

1. Outdoor air quality
2. Surface and groundwater quality
3. Toxic substances and hazardous wastes
4. Homes and communities
5. Infrastructure and surveillance
6. Global environmental health

Creating health-promoting environments is a complex process and relies on continuing research to understand more fully the effects of exposure to environmental hazards on people's health. **Exposure** is defined as any contact with a hazardous substance that occurs within an environmental context.[9]

The WHO's 10 facts on environmental health illustrate the importance of environmental health.[8] First, 13 million deaths could be prevented worldwide if the environment was healthy. Establishing safe household water would result in a 94% reduction in diarrheal deaths, one of the top three causes of death in children worldwide. The WHO advocates for increasing the safety of buildings; safe use and management of toxins both at work and at home; better road safety; and promotion of better water resource management (see Chapter 13).[10]

The Role of Nursing in Environmental Health

Nurses in a variety of settings, but particularly those in the field of public health, play a significant role in preventing harm from occurring and in restoring well-being to all who face hazardous conditions in their environment. Nurses are among the environmental health professionals with the responsibility to detect and assess the presence of environmental hazards as well as the health risks they pose, and to take action to protect the health of populations.[11]

In 2007, the American Nurses Association (ANA) published a report titled *ANA's Principles of Environmental Health for Nursing Practice With Implementation Strategies.*[11] According to the report, registered nurses play a critical role in both assessing environmental health issues and addressing them. The report included 10 principles (Box 6-1) for healthy safe environments that are applicable across settings.

Armed with an appreciation for the complexities of the interaction of environment and health, nurses can be

BOX 6-1 ANA's Principles of Environmental Health for Nursing Practice

1. Knowledge of environmental health concepts is essential to nursing practice.
2. The Precautionary Principle guides nurses in their practice to use products and practices that do not harm human health or the environment and to take preventive action in the face of uncertainty.
3. Nurses have a right to work in an environment that is safe and healthy.
4. Healthy environments are sustained through multidisciplinary collaboration.
5. Choices of materials, products, technology, and practices in the environment that impact nursing practice are based on the best evidence available.
6. Approaches to promoting a healthy environment respect the diverse values, beliefs, cultures, and circumstances of patients and their families.
7. Nurses participate in assessing the quality of the environment in which they practice and live.
8. Nurses, other health care workers, patients, and communities have the right to know relevant and timely information about the potentially harmful products, chemicals, pollutants, and hazards to which they are exposed.
9. Nurses participate in research of best practices that promote a safe and healthy environment.
10. Nurses must be supported in advocating for and implementing environmental health principles in nursing practice.

Source: See reference 11.

leaders in defining and encouraging solutions. As experts in educating individuals and communities and appreciating the value of leading by example, nurses can be catalysts in improving the health of the environment, thus improving health. Issues emerge from the ANA report specific to nursing practice: (1) knowledge of the role environment plays in the health of individuals, families, and populations; (2) ability to assess for environmental health hazards and make appropriate referrals; (3) advocacy; (4) utilization of appropriate risk communication strategies; and (5) understanding of policies and legislation related to environmental health. The ANA principles were designed to help support the nurse in the role of environmental health activist.[11]

Approaches to Environmental Health

A useful framework to use in examining human-environment interactions and their potential impact on health of individuals, families, and communities is the well-established epidemiological triangle, which describes the relationship between an agent (exposure), host

(human), and environment (the complex setting in which agent and host come together) (see Chapters 3 and 8). In actuality, the epidemiological triangle is a simplistic model and must be placed in the context of the real world to better appreciate the importance of the triangle point—environment—that brings agent and host together in the places we live, that is, housing, schools, workplaces, recreational spaces, communities, and, ultimately, the world (Fig. 6-1).

The approach in the United States for handling environmental health in the past was usually at the state and local health departments rather than at the federal level. Local health departments focused on sanitation and waste management as a way to provide potable (safe, drinkable) water. However, maintaining healthy air and reducing pollutants in water, air, and soil became an issue that crossed state borders. In 1970, the U.S. Environmental Protection Agency (EPA) was formed with the mission to protect human health and to safeguard the natural environment—air, water and land—by writing and enforcing regulation based on laws passed by Congress.[12] The EPA is a regulatory body that performs environmental assessments, does research, educates, and sets and enforces national environmental standards. Since the early 1970s there have been multiple federal laws passed by Congress. This legislation includes the Clean Air Act, the Occupational Health and Safety Act, the National Institute

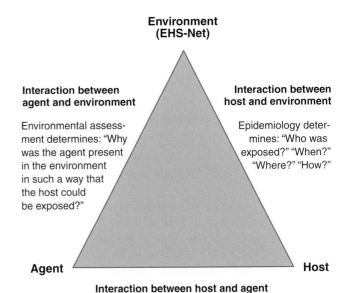

Figure 6-1 Environmental health specialists and the epidemiologic triangle.

of Occupational Safety and Health, the Clean Water Act, and Comprehensive Environmental Response, Compensation, and Liability Act, also known as the Superfund, among others. The growing concerns among the American people about the environment have created pressure to increasingly monitor and regulate the environment.

In the United States, there is a network of environmental health specialists housed in the Centers for Disease Control and Prevention (CDC) National Center for Environmental Health that, using the epidemiological triangle (Chapter 3), works collaboratively with the Environmental Health Services Network to identify and prevent environmental factors that can produce disease. Their stated purpose is to help identify underlying environmental factors, assist with improving prevention efforts, train environmental health specialists, and help to strengthen the collaboration among different disciplines and services involved in improving environmental health.[13] Key issues include the built environment, toxic materials, air and water quality, and environmental stability.

The Built Environment

The **built environment**, the human-made surroundings created for the daily activities of humans, reflects the range of physical and social elements that make up a community.[14] Scientists are examining how the structure and infrastructure of a community facilitate or impede health. Poor communities often have a built environment with limited resources, higher pollution, poorer maintenance of buildings, fewer options for outside activities, a smaller selection of goods (including groceries), and limited transportation, all leading to poorer health (e.g., lead poisoning, asthma, cancer). There is considerable interest in examining how communities can modify their built environment to promote the health of the community residents.

The Prevention Institute has highlighted 11 examples of how working together, low-income communities in partnerships with others were able to alter their built environment and improve the health of their residents.[14] Some of these activities included designing a safe 1.5 mile walking/jogging trail in a Hispanic community; over a 5-year period bringing a full-service grocery store to a community without any food stores; minimizing soil lead exposure in people's yards in a community with high lead levels; and in another community closing liquor stores, whose presence increased crime in the community. An example of the relationship between the built environment and health is obesity. There is strong evidence that aspects of the built environment such as food availability and access to recreational opportunities

are associated with obesity.[10] Many programs have been instituted to help reduce the epidemic of obesity in the United States.

■ EVIDENCE-BASED PRACTICE
Obesity and the Built Environment

Practice Statement: An increasing number of studies have documented that obesity, which has reached epidemic proportions in the United States, is related to several aspects of the built environment.[15–20]
Targeted Outcome: Reduction in prevalence of obesity.
Evidence to Support: The same risk factors that promote weight gain in individuals—increased caloric intake and decreased physical activity—apply on a larger scale to populations. Several measures have been used to describe the risk factors for obesity, but the evidence continues to point to the influence of the built environment on diet and activity. For example, physical activity is associated with community attributes such as road connectivity, presence of sidewalks, availability of safe play areas, and residential density. Dietary influences include the number and proximity of fast-food restaurants, availability of healthy food choices, and the cost of food. Specific risk factors may differ between urban and suburban settings, but the relationship between the built environment and obesity persists in both.[17]

The CDC recently initiated a project called the Common Community Measures for Obesity Prevention Project (the "Measures Project"). An expert panel identified 24 strategies for preventing obesity and complementary measures that can be used to monitor progress within a community over time. Nurses are well positioned to initiate and promote these strategies in the course of their practice as they work with communities and community members.[18]

The following is a list of selected prevention strategies that were identified in the Measures Project and that can be applied as nurses work with communities to attack the risk factors that promote higher rates of obesity. A guide to implementing these strategies is available from the CDC.[21]

To address factors related to diet and the built environment, communities should:

1. Improve availability of affordable healthier food and beverage choices in public service venues
2. Improve geographical availability of supermarkets in underserved areas
3. Improve availability of mechanisms for purchasing foods from farms

4. Provide incentives for the production, distribution, and procurement of foods from local farms
5. Discourage consumption of sugar-sweetened beverages

To address factors related to physical activity and the built environment, communities should:

1. Increase opportunities for extracurricular physical activity
2. Improve access to outdoor recreational facilities
3. Enhance infrastructure supporting walking
4. Support locating schools within easy walking distance of residential areas
5. Improve access to public transportation
6. Enhance traffic safety in areas where people are/could be physically active

Hazardous Substances

The probability that individuals will be adversely affected by a hazardous substance depends on three major factors: (1) its inherent **toxicity,** that is, ability to cause harm to humans; (2) whether it enters the body and reaches susceptible organs; and (3) the amount that is present. Toxicologists are fond of summarizing the teaching of Renaissance alchemist Paracelsus with the phrase "the dose makes the poison." In other words, it is very important to recognize that the mere presence of an agent, even if it is known to have toxic properties, does not necessarily mean there is a risk to health. For example, we know that lead can harm several organ systems (as presented in an example later in this chapter). However, it must first be ingested or inhaled or it will not reach the organs that are sensitive to its effects. When an x-ray technician uses a lead apron for protection from radiation, lead is actually serving a helpful function and will not cause toxicity to the gastrointestinal, nervous, or hematological system because it is not in a form that allows it to be absorbed. However, if lead is heated and the fumes are inhaled, or if chips of lead paint are ingested, then there is a definite risk of lead poisoning. Many other substances, such as solvents, can enter the body through skin contact. These three pathways or **routes of entry**—ingestion, inhalation, and dermal absorption—differ in their importance according to the specific substance. Also, do not be fooled into thinking a substance is not hazardous just because its effects are not seen immediately. Cancer, for example, often develops many years after an exposure occurs. These time lags, known as **latency periods,** can interfere with our ability to identify cause-and-effect links and hamper our ability to anticipate and prevent negative health effects.[22]

Exposure Risk Assessment

The process that is used by policy makers and other regulators to evaluate the extent to which a population may suffer health effects from an environmental exposure is called **risk assessment.** Risk assessment involves four steps: (1) *hazard identification* (described in more detail below); (2) *dose-response assessment* (based on experiments that look for a correlation between an increase in harmful effects and an increase in quantity of a substance); (3) *exposure assessment* (consideration of the level, timing, and extent of the exposure); and (4) *risk characterization.* This last step brings together the information from the first three steps to guide a judgment about the risk of health problems to those who are exposed. That judgment is never without its uncertainties.

Types of Exposures

Environmental exposures can be broadly categorized as chemical agents, biological agents, physical hazards, and, perhaps less commonly recognized, psychosocial factors. To identify a hazard, we are interested not only in what agents are present, but also whether (and how) they can affect human health.

Chemical Agents

Examples of chemicals are easily named, and many are well known for their dangers to human health. For example, carbon monoxide is produced by combustion and is typically encountered in automobile exhaust and home-heating emissions. Specific metals and pesticides affect many body systems, sometimes accumulating in the body and, owing to their release over time, perpetuating their effects over a long period of duration. Lead, for example, is stored in the bone, where it can slowly release over time to cause deleterious health effects long after the actual exposure has occurred. As a final example, environmental cigarette smoke contains thousands of chemicals, some of which are associated with cancer.

While we have knowledge of the actions of some of the chemicals that are in current use, these represent only a minor proportion of those that might be toxic. There are more than 80,000 chemicals in use worldwide, some natural and some made by humans. The Agency for Toxic Substance and Disease Registry (ATSDR) provides detailed information on chemicals. Using their portal you can search out information on chemicals and how they may affect health.[23]

Biological Agents

The category of biological agents clearly includes infectious agents that are well known to nurses, such as bacteria, viruses, and other organisms such as rickettsia (Chapter 8). However, there are many others. Some molds are known to have effects on the respiratory system and possibly other more systemic outcomes. Also, there are many documented hazards associated with plant and animal contact. Toxic plants and fungi such as poisonous mushrooms and inedible plants are not always thought of as environmental hazards. Likewise, allergens such as dust mites, cockroaches, and pet dander are serious but often unrecognized sources of biological hazards.

Physical Agents

Even more varied are the hazards classified as physical agents, defined as those responsible for the injurious exchange of energy. Examples include heat and cold, all forms of radiation, noise, and vibration. Other physical forms of environmental risk for bodily injury include events such as falls, vehicle crashes, and crush injuries, as well as hazards associated with violence, such as knife or gunshot wounds (see Chapter 12). These are environmental hazards that nurses and the public health system work to prevent and mitigate.

Psychosocial Factors

Finally, psychosocial factors form a less commonly acknowledged category of environmental risk to health that is not generally included in a formal environmental risk assessment. However, it is important to recognize that communities and individuals that live in fear or experience stress, panic, and anxiety associated with real or perceived threats are subject to psychosocial conditions that affect not only health and safety but also overall well-being. These must be considered in a comprehensive assessment of environmental determinants of health.

Mixed Exposures

Rarely do the environmental hazards exist independently. Almost all scenarios that pose environmental risks to health combine more than one threat to health, and these combinations often act synergistically to raise the level of danger. Chemicals usually exist as mixtures, as is the case with cigarette smoke, which contains more than 50 carcinogens.[24] Interaction and a subsequent increase in hazard may also occur when different agents are combined. For example, noise (a physical hazard) in the presence of some chemicals may be more likely to cause hearing loss.[25] Asbestos, a fiber used for insulation and other purposes, causes, among other diseases, lung cancer, but that risk increases for individuals who smoke.[26] An additional example is the danger related to combining household products. Mixing cleaning agents that contain ammonia with others containing chlorine leads to the production of chloramines, which are much more toxic chemicals than is ammonia or chlorine alone.

The Environmental Health History

Understanding environmental exposures and the detrimental health effects they can cause is only one step along the way to protecting the health of individuals, families, and communities. That knowledge must then be applied to strategies to effect change. While the community assessment focuses on environmental health risks at the population level, the experiences of individuals vary according to the proximity of where they spend their time to environmental hazards including the home, recreational facilities, and the workplace. The Agency for Toxic Substances and Disease Registry (ATSDR) has designed a systematic process for reviewing an individual's potential environmental exposures across all locations, current and past. It also serves as a reminder of the actions a nurse can take to protect a client from environmental exposures and their health effects. The systematic areas of inquiry are guided by set of questions that form a mnemonic, I PREPARE (Box 6-2).[27]

These questions are only guidelines and should prompt further questions when appropriate. For example, the exploration of alternative healing or certain cultural practices may require further probing, depending on the client's background and lifestyle. Actions required to address environmental health hazards often raise the ethical question of when to choose the public good over individual rights. For example, in the case of lead poisoning should homeowners and landlords be required to pay for the cost of lead abatement? Another example is the ban on smoking in public places. The ban reduces the population's exposure to the harmful effects of secondary smoke while limiting the rights of individual smokers.

When taking a history of environmental exposures, past and current, it is important to take into consideration the client's cultural background. This may reveal a new universe of possible sources of toxic exposures. The discovery of potential exposures associated with cultural practices has implications not only for risk assessment but also for culturally appropriate communication.

Here are some examples of behaviors and practices that may be overlooked in a traditional environmental history:

- Kohl, a form of eye makeup that is sometimes used, particularly in the Middle East, is high in lead content and a proven risk for lead toxicity.[28]

BOX 6–2 | **A Systematic Environmental Exposure History: I PREPARE**

I—Investigate Potential Exposures

Investigate potential exposures by asking: Have you ever felt sick after coming in contact with a chemical, pesticide, or other substance? Do you have any symptoms that improve when you are away from your home or work?

P—Present Work

At your present work: Are you exposed to solvents, dusts, fumes, radiation, loud noise, pesticides, or other chemicals? Do you know where to find Material Data Safety Sheets on chemicals that you work with? Do you wear personal protective equipment? Are work clothes worn home? Do coworkers have similar health problems?

R—Residence

When was your residence built? What type of heating do you have? Have you recently remodeled your home? What chemicals are stored on your property? Where does your drinking water come from?

E—Environmental Concerns

Are there environmental concerns in your neighborhood (i.e., air, water, soil)? What types of industries or farms are near your home? Do you live near a hazardous waste site or landfill?

P—Past Work

What are your past work experiences? What is the longest job held? Have you ever been in the military, worked on a farm, or done volunteer or seasonal work?

A—Activities

What activities and hobbies do you and your family engage in? Do you burn, solder, or melt any products? Do you garden, fish, or hunt? Do you eat what you catch or grow? Do you use pesticides? Do you engage in any alternative healing or cultural practices?

R—Referrals and Resources

Use these key referrals and resources:
Agency for Toxic Substances & Disease Registry
    www.atsdr.cdc.gov
Association of Occupational & Environmental Clinics
    www.aoec.org
Environmental Protection Agency www.epa.gov
    Material Safety Data Sheets www.hazard.com/msds
Occupational Safety & Health Administration
    www.osha.gov
Local Health Department, Environmental Agency,
    Poison Control Center

E—Educate (A Checklist)

Are materials available to educate the patient? Are alternatives available to minimize the risk of exposure? Have prevention strategies been discussed? What is the plan for follow-up?

Source: ASTDR (2008) I PREPARE. Available at http://www.atsdr.cdc.gov/asbestos/site-kit/docs/IPrepareCard.pdf.

- Lead from improperly glazed pottery can leach into food or drink, especially when contents are acidic, and become sources of lead poisoning. These dishes are frequently manufactured outside the United States but pose a danger in any region to which they are exported.[29]
- Herbal supplements and nontraditional medicines have led to various forms of poisoning, including cardiac and gastrointestinal symptoms.[30]
- Religious or secular practices may incorporate the use of toxic substances such as mercury, which is believed by some to promote health, good fortune, or protection from evil.[31]

● APPLYING PUBLIC HEALTH SCIENCE

The Case of the Peeling Paint

Public Health Science Topics Covered:

- Screening
- Case finding
- Advocacy
- Policy

Jane, a nurse working at the county health department based in a large, urban midwestern city, was asked to participate in the county lead-screening program to identify families exposed to lead in their environment. The goal of this secondary prevention screening program was twofold: (1) to identify current cases and initiate medical management and (2) to identify what measures should be taken to prevent further harm to children in these families and other community members. The health department established the program in response to the recommendation from the CDC that all children whose families are eligible for Medicaid be screened for lead poisoning at 12 and 24 months of age.[32] Because of the high lead levels in previous child-screening programs, the county extended their screening program to all 1- and 2-year-old children in this urban county. In the case of lead, a well known hazard to children, screening in this program consisted of measuring the concentration of lead in the blood to estimate the amount of lead that had been absorbed into the body, and at the same time providing all the parents with health education information about lead.

Jane used the 2012 CDC recommendations on childhood lead poisoning prevention guidelines in relation to the blood lead level (BLL) that would require initiation of prevention measures. The prior BLL that triggered interventions was 10 to 14.9 micrograms per deciliter (mcg/dL) but was changed to a BLL value of 5 mcg/dL based on evidence that even lower levels of exposure increase the risk for adverse health outcomes in children (Fig. 6-2). Jane found that eliminating lead poisoning in children was one of the *HP 2020* environmental health objectives listed under Toxics and Waste.[8]

Jane then reviewed evidence-based interventions needed to prevent the adverse health effects associated

with lead in the body.[33] She decided to implement a home visiting approach. In this program, parents of children screened with a blood level at or above 5 mcg/dL received a home visit from the public health nurse (PHN) and were provided with an environmental assessment of their home, education regarding dietary and environmental actions to reduce the lead poisoning, and help with lead abatement in their homes if needed. The home visit also included providing the parents with information on their legal rights as tenants/homeowners. They were also provided with follow-up BLL monitoring for their child.

Jane's role in the screening program was to conduct the home environmental assessments for all children who screened positive for lead poisoning. Based on the findings of her assessment, Jane recommended and sometimes coordinated abatement efforts and educated parents and others about the control and prevention of

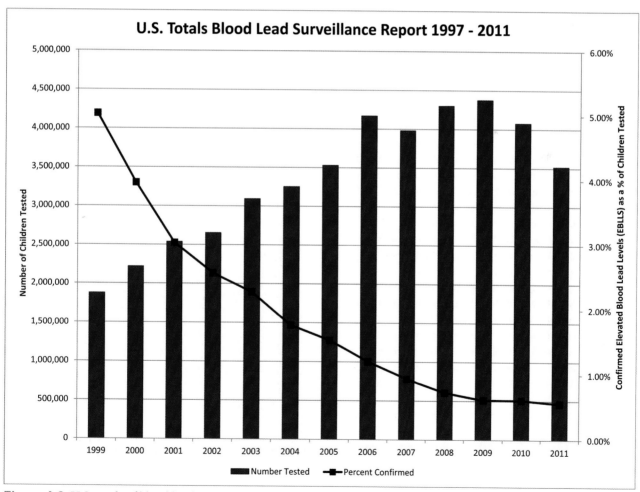

Figure 6-2 U.S. totals of blood level surveillance report, 1997–2011. Comparison of the number tested with the percentage confirmed. *(From the Centers for Disease Control and Prevention, retrieved from http://www.cdc.gov/nceh/lead/data/StateConfirmedByYear_1997_2011.pdf.)*

lead exposure. She also was responsible for educating the community about lead poisoning and the actions the community could take to eliminate lead exposure, the much preferred primary prevention.[34] With extensive interventions the health department would be able to eradicate lead poisoning in the community.

Prior to making her first home visit, Jane reviewed the pathophysiology of lead poisoning in children. She found that young children are at greater risk because they are more likely to ingest materials containing lead and absorb more of the lead when it is ingested. A child or fetus is especially vulnerable to the effects of lead and many other toxic substances because their developing organ systems are at high risk of damage. Toddlers are more likely to put items contaminated with lead, such as paint chips, in their mouths, making screening most useful at 1 and 2 years of age. Ingestion of lead, the most common route, can have an irreversible negative effect on the child's developing central nervous and hematopoietic systems. Thus, children exposed to lead can have lifelong health issues. Even with low levels (5 mcg/dL) a child's cognitive and behavioral development can be slowed, resulting in learning disabilities.[33] Children with high BLLs are at increased risk for serious effects such as encephalopathy marked by seizures and even coma. These effects can lead to long-term, sometimes irreversible damage. In contrast, the more mature central nervous system of adults is better protected from the effects of lead so that damage to peripheral nerves, rather than the central nervous system, is more likely. Inhalation rather than ingestion is the more common route for lead poisoning in older children and adults.[35]

Jane was assigned a home visit to a family with a 2-year-old child with a BLL of 13 mcg/dL to investigate possible environmental risks in the home. The child, Bobby, lived in an older building in one of the poorest sections of the city. As she was greeted at the door by Bobby's mother, Sharon, Jane noticed a cockroach skittering away from under a chair. She noted that the apartment was in need of major maintenance. She recognized that she would have to assess the home for potential environmental hazards as well as lead. She began with a focus on lead. Sharon told Jane that she had rented the home for a little more than a year and lived there with her three children—an infant, 2-year-old Bobby, whose blood lead level was elevated, and another child in first grade. Sharon held Bobby in her lap for the first half of the interview, but Bobby got restless and slid off of her lap to play on the carpet. Jane asked Sharon whether she would take her on a tour of the house to see where the lead might originate.

Jane used her knowledge of environmental risks associated with lead poisoning in children to guide her assessment. In the United States, leaded gasoline and paint were both banned around the same time in the early 1970s. Thanks to these policy interventions, average blood lead levels in children have been steadily dropping since.[36] Jane's question was, How did Bobby become poisoned with lead despite the new regulations? Lead poisoning is a good example of environmental risks in the built environment. Though lead paint has been banned, buildings built before 1978 often contain lead paint. Many cities have initiated lead abatement programs to remove this paint. This population-based policy approach to the problem is one of the best examples of how legislation can improve public and environmental health.[35] However, not all cities have successfully removed all lead paint from city residential buildings and it is especially problematic in the poorer neighborhoods where older buildings are not well maintained.

Jane learned that Bobby played with his toys on the floor of a room in which the paint was peeling from the windowsills. Suspecting that lead-based paint was largely responsible for the child's elevated levels, she noted the condition of all of the house's painted surfaces and found that many of them were chipping, especially on the baseboards and windowsills, and marred with tooth marks. Paint in older homes is known to be high in lead content, and its availability to a child is a strong indication that the paint is a major source of exposure. Even children who do not directly ingest the peeling paint are at major risk of exposure from lead dust that sloughs from the painted surfaces and contaminates floors and toys that through the common hand-mouth behavior of children are ingested or inhaled.

In response to her findings, Jane explained to Sharon how lead was probably ingested by Bobby. She shared with Sharon the recommendations from the CDC on doing home repairs (Fig. 6-3). In particular Jane explained that precautions are needed when doing any removal or work on painted surfaces in homes built before 1978. Taking precautions will reduce paint chips and airborne particulates. Jane also explained that ventilation is important as well as wearing personal protective apparel such as goggles, respirator, and gloves, and in this case, child safety, if applicable. Reading the safety panel of the paint containers would dictate the appropriate precautions that needed to be followed.

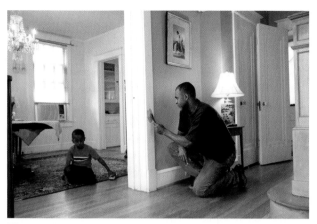

Figure 6-3 Home repair hazards. *(From the Centers for Disease Control and Prevention, courtesy of Dawn Arlotta, photograph by Cade Martin, 2009.)*

Jane helped Sharon set up an appointment with technicians from the health department who would come to the home to verify and measure the lead content of the paint and help Sharon identify sources for assistance with the removal of lead from her home. Depending on the state of the home, Jane explained that it might be necessary to physically abate the exposure by entirely removing the paint, which means moving the family either temporarily or permanently to a more suitable, lead-free living environment. Jane explained that there were resources through the county public health department and the housing authority to help the family if this step was necessary.

Jane asked Sharon about Bobby's health. Sharon reported that he did complain occasionally of stomach pain, but she was surprised by the elevated lead because she had seen no real symptoms of lead poisoning. Jane explained that frequently there are no signs of the poisoning and that the results of the poisoning take time to manifest. That is why the screening is so important. Jane suggested that Sharon take Bobby for a full checkup at the county's child health clinic or with the child's local provider, and that Sharon and the other children should also be screened for lead poisoning. Pregnant women with high lead levels can transmit lead to their unborn children because it crosses the placental barrier, and lead can also be transmitted in breast milk, affecting both mother and unborn child. Jane also explained that stomach pain can be a sign of lead poisoning and urged Sharon to tell the doctor about Bobby's complaints. Jane helped Sharon set up these appointments and worked with her to develop a plan that set mutual goals and a time line for managing the lead poisoning.

At this point, Jane noticed that Sharon seemed worried. When prompted, Sharon said she had heard about lead poisoning but did not understand what it meant to her and her children. Jane went over in more detail the relationship between lead in the home environment and children's health and explained to Sharon that Bobby's blood level was of concern and that the trip to the clinic would provide her with more information on Bobby's health status. Jane commended Sharon for having Bobby screened and explained that early intervention can help to mitigate the effects of lead poisoning.

Sharon said that she had talked with the landlord about the apartment because of what she had seen on the news about lead poisoning, and was assured that there were no problems. She also explained that her sister lived in the same building. Jane realized that finding an elevated lead blood level in one child had uncovered an environmental hazard that could affect all of the tenants in the building, especially the children. The affordability of the apartments and proximity to the school resulted in the building being home to many young families, especially single mothers. Jane was aware that the environmental hazard also extended to mothers in the building who were pregnant or breastfeeding their babies.

Jane went on to explain steps that Sharon could take now to protect her family from further lead poisoning. She went over cleaning methods that included mopping hardwood floors with a weak bleach dilution to remove the dust, frequently wiping window sills with a damp cloth, vacuuming with high-efficiency particulate air (HEPA) filters, and ensuring that the children were kept away from areas with active chipping and peeling paint.

Jane also reviewed with Sharon a secondary prevention strategy that she could use to reduce the amount of lead a child absorbs and increase the amount excreted by providing a calcium-rich, high-iron, vitamin C–containing diet. Jane was aware that this may be more difficult for some families than for others. Impoverished areas, which represent low-income residents and poor social conditions, can be thought of as "food deserts" where access to affordable healthy food is greatly limited.[37] Sharon confirmed that Jane was enrolled in the local Women, Infants, and Children (WIC) supplemental nutrition program and had access to the foods needed to implement this strategy.

Bobby's lead exposure illustrates the way in which toxins enter the body and ultimately cause harm to health. Lead was present in the ambient environment—primarily in paint and dust. It was also in a form that resulted in ingestion as the most probable route of exposure, especially given the hand-mouth behavior of a small child.

As she was working in the program, Jane became very interested in primary prevention for lead poisoning. It was clear that although screening was important it would be much better to prevent the problem in the first place. She became interested in the wider issue of the health of the built environment and found the U.S. Department of Housing and Urban Development is an excellent resource on the broader spectrum of health risks in homes.[38]

Jane found that the main primary prevention approach is lead abatement, which is removal of lead-based paint in the home or workplace. As of April 22, 2010, a federal law went into effect that required that all contractors doing renovations, repair, or painting that disturbed more than 6 square feet in homes, schools, and childcare centers must be certified in lead abatement. In addition, landlords are required to inform renters about potential hazards related to lead-based paint.[39] Jane found multiple state and municipal regulations that focused on reducing exposure to lead paint, lead paint dust, and soil contaminated from exterior lead-based paint.

Despite all the regulations, Jane discovered that one of the big stumbling blocks to starting a successful lead abatement program in her county was cost. Because of the seriousness of exposure to lead, the federal government and states have in place strict lead abatement regulations that result in labor-intensive measures and the use of specialized equipment in accordance with lead abatement regulations. The high cost of abatement raises the question of whether or not the cost outweighs the benefit and illustrates a common public health ethical issue of determining whether the benefits of a costly abatement program outweigh the rights of the individual homeowner or landlord to choose not to remove lead paint from a building.

In addition to the interventions Jane conducted with this family and the community education she provided, she also worked with her colleagues in the health department to initiate interventions at the aggregate level. In particular she was concerned about Sharon's story that the landlord had assured her that there were no environmental problems in the apartment. It is against federal law for landlords to withhold information on environmental hazards in their buildings. She was also concerned about the other children living in the building, because this was the only child in the building who had been screened. This resulted in two different levels of action. First, from an advocacy perspective, Jane reported the landlord for failure to disclose the fact the apartment contained lead paint and began to explore alternative housing for the young families living in the building.

Second, she implemented her role of case finding. She asked the mother whether she would introduce her to her sister and her neighbor and help get all the families in the building screened. She was able to screen all of the children in the building and identified several other children with elevated BLLs.

Environmental Justice

Disadvantaged populations—whether as a result of low income, racial or cultural differences, age, health status, or other social indices of susceptibility—are frequently at greatest risk of exposure to environmental hazards. Such populations face barriers such as substandard housing, lack of access to health care, diminished resources such as nutritious food and safe places to play, poor working conditions, and absence of clean air and water. Even those who are employed tend to be in the most risky jobs. Disadvantaged communities tend to be located near industrial areas, highway, and rail transportation routes where dangerous cargo and exhaust pose dangers and where hazardous waste disposal sites exist.[40,41] **Environmental justice** refers to fair distribution of environmental burdens.[40] According to the EPA, it also refers to fair application of environmental laws, policies, and regulations regardless of race, color, national origin, or income.[42] Social disadvantage can result in increased exposure to environmental risks as well as an increased susceptibility to the risks.[40,41] The EPA has taken the lead to promote environmental justice through specific programs and the coordination of the Federal Interagency Working Group on Environmental Justice.[41–43] The latter is a body of federal agencies and White House offices that strives to integrate environmental justice principles into federal programs; identify opportunities for collaboration; and share information and experiences.[43]

▶ SOLVING THE MYSTERY
The Case of the Hazardous House
Public Health Science Topics Covered:

- Assessment
- Health planning
- Program evaluation

Jane's work on the lead screening program resulted in an expansion of the program to include reducing home environmental risk factors associated with childhood asthma in the same neighborhood where she had had the most positive lead screenings. She helped to initiate a county health department safe home program focused on asthma and developed in collaboration with the local school department, the local Parent-Teacher Association (PTA), and the county pediatric hospital. The program was initiated because of increased prevalence of childhood asthma, lost school days by asthmatic children, and the increased emergency department (ED) visits for acute asthma attacks.

First, the PTA and the school conducted a campaign to promote the benefits of having Jane visit the homes of children with asthma to provide an environmental assessment, additional health education, and linkages to resources. The program contained three steps: (1) referral, (2) home inspection, and (3) the development of a home safety plan. All students with asthma were referred to Jane, who then contacted the parents of the children. She offered to provide an environmental assessment for possible pollutants in the home. When invited, Jane conducted a home visit that focused on residential health. She began by explaining to family members that she was using an assessment tool specifically designed to identify health hazards in the home. She showed the family how the assessment was based on a set of comprehensive reference and inspection manuals available from the CDC[44] that have been developed for systematically reviewing residential health and safety risks. She invited them to participate in the review of their home as full partners and encouraged them to ask questions.

Jane started each home visit by asking parents what concerns they had. She worked at developing a partnership with parents to help build an intervention specifically targeted to maximize the use of available resources to help improve the health of their home environment. Jane worked to develop a relationship with the parents that was nonjudgmental and that would help empower the parents with the knowledge and access to resources they would need to address possible risk factors for childhood asthma.

On one visit Jane met a family with a 7-year-old boy, Joshua, who had repeated asthma attacks, multiple absences from school, and an increasing number of ED visits. The family lived in a three-bedroom apartment in a 300-unit building in an inner-city neighborhood in New York State. There were other children in the home not in school: a 4-year-old, a 2-year-old, and a newborn. The mother, Betsy, reported that the 4-year-old was also being treated for asthma and that the other two children had frequent colds. With Betsy, Jane conducted an inspection of the home to help identify environmental risk factors that could be addressed,

beginning with the kitchen. Under the sink they found cockroaches and evidence of mice. Jane noted that pesticides and cleaning products were stored in that location and that a dripping faucet had resulted in an accumulation of a small amount of water in the space under the sink along with some mold. Betsy also kept the kitchen wastebasket under the sink where she disposed of food scraps. Betsy stated that she was constantly trying to deal with the cockroaches and the mice but had not been successful. She had not realized that the black smudges were actually mold.

When Jane asked Betsy about whether anyone smoked in the home, she learned that both parents smoked. Jane also noted that there was worn wall-to-wall carpeting throughout the apartment. When they went into Joshua's room that he shared with his 4-year-old brother, Jane noted the large number of stuffed animals. With Betsy, Jane examined Joshua's bed. Betsy explained that there was no money for mattress protectors or pillow covers. She also stated that with four children it was difficult to get to the Laundromat to wash the sheets so she only did them once every 3 to 4 weeks. Jane also asked Betsy about the use of medications she was using to treat Joshua's asthma. Betsy confirmed that Joshua needed to administer his inhaler frequently and stated that she was careful about giving him his medications on time and regularly.

After completing the overview of the home environment, Jane discussed her findings with Betsy. Jane complimented Betsy on her adherence to the medication plan for Joshua. Jane explained that medications are less effective if there continue to be triggers in the environment such as cigarette smoke, dust mites, and allergens related to vermin.[45] She provided the mother with further information on risk factors for asthma, pulling up the CDC Web site on her tablet so Betsy could see a review of environmental risk factors. The main risk factors mentioned by the CDC were tobacco smoke, dust mites, outdoor air pollution, cockroaches, pets, and mold. The only home environmental risk factor that was not present was pets, since the family had none.

Jane and Betsy discussed actions the family could take to help reduce the risk. Jane began with the problem of secondhand smoke. She explained that this might also explain the frequent colds experienced by the infant.[46] Jane asked Betsy whether either she or her husband, both of whom have state-funded health insurance, would be interested in getting help to quit smoking. Betsy stated that they would consider this if it would improve the health of their children, especially Joshua.

Jane gave Betsy information on resources such as local clinics that offer services for smoking cessation. She also encouraged Betsy and her husband to smoke only outside the apartment in a space that was not near where the children played or by an open window.

Jane then discussed with Betsy the issue of cockroaches and mice as serious health risks to families.[45] Aside from producing allergens that can exacerbate asthma, they both carry a host of bacteria and viruses that are dangerous to people, including staphylococcus, streptococcus, *Escherichia coli,* and salmonella. Another hazard associated with pest infestation has to do with the types of chemicals and poisons that are used to fight them, such as aerosol spray insecticides and poisoned pellets, all of which put children at risk for poisoning. Serious health outcomes associated with pesticides include skin disorders, damage to the nervous system, poisoning, endocrine disruption, respiratory illness, cancer, and death. Jane described methods other than pesticides that Betsy could use for controlling pest within the apartment, beginning with removing food and standing water. Jane described how to use a separate container for food scraps with a tight lid that would provide a barrier to roaches and mice. She also explained about how to store food in the pantry in plastic containers with tight lids rather than bags or cardboard containers.

Jane again used her tablet to refer Betsy to the New York State Health Department's Web site on the landlord and tenant's guide to pest control. Together they reviewed steps Betsy could take and what steps her landlord could take for addressing the rodent and cockroach issue (Box 6-3). Jane also explained to Betsy that she could contact her local cooperative extension service for assistance with pest control.

The practice described on the New York State Health Department's Web site is known as **integrated pest management,** a program that includes caulking and sealing cracks and holes larger than a 16th of an inch, eating in one place in the home to consolidate the area that must be cleaned, getting rid of clutter where pests hide, storing food in containers with locking lids, preventing the accumulation of grease, and disposing of the trash nightly.[47,48] Jane also explained about better chemical methods for fighting pests, such as the use of bait stations and gels that do not contaminate surfaces or the air, rather than poisons. She gave Betsy some mice snap traps to be used in place of the poisoned pellets, explaining that mice carry the poison from seemingly safe locations and drop it in places

Proper Pest Management Practices for Landlords and Tenants:

Integrated Pest Management is geared toward long-term prevention or elimination of pests that does not solely rely on pesticides. Integrated Pest Management follows the principles of preventing entry, inspecting, monitoring, and treating pests on an as-needed basis. These principles help manage pests by using the most economical means, and with the least possible hazard to people, property, and the environment. Pests thrive in environments where food, water, and shelter are available. If an undesirable environment is created, pests can be prevented, reduced, or eliminated.

Using Integrated Pest Management:

- Reduce pest problems by keeping the house, yard, and garden free from clutter and garbage. Food should not be left uncovered on counters. Food should be stored in tightly sealed containers or in the refrigerator.
- Keep pests outdoors by blocking points of entry. Quality sealant or knitted copper mesh can be used along baseboards, pipes, drains, and other access points to seal cracks and repair holes.
- If a pest problem arises, identify the pest and the extent of the infestation. Your local branch of Cooperative Extension office can offer assistance.
- Use methods with the least hazard to people and pets, such as setting traps/bait, using a flyswatter or fly ribbon paper. Bait and traps should be kept out of the reach of children and pets.
- Remove trash on a regular basis and always use trash cans with tight fitting lids. If pests can get in garbage, they will return repeatedly to get food.
- If a certified pesticide applicator is needed, be sure that (s)he understands and follow Integrated Pest Management principles and practices.

Source: See reference 47.

easily accessible to her young children. Jane also handed Betsy a brochure from the local poison control center with a magnet for the refrigerator and a child safety lock for the cabinets under the sink. The lock was for immediate short-term use, until chemicals were moved to a safer site. Poisons, solvents, cleaners, and other types of household products should always remain in their original container so information contained on the label will be available to inform emergency care or calls to a poison control center.

Betsy stated that her sink has been leaking for some time, but her landlord was unresponsive to her request for its repair. The same was true of her furnace. Jane provided her with a copy of the New York State Tenants' Rights Guide[49] and told Betsy that she would write up a housing code violation report that should result in the landlord making these repairs.

With Betsy's permission, Jane's assessment of the home expanded to included risk factors beyond those associated with childhood asthma. In the utility room, Jane inspected the furnace and water heater and noted that the water heater was set to 140° Fahrenheit. She told Betsy that she should always make sure the heater is set below 120°F to prevent scalding, and demonstrated how to lower the temperature. Jane also observed that the vent connecting the water heater to the furnace was not sealed, thereby allowing the release of combustion products, such as carbon monoxide. Jane explained to Betsy that, just like the gas stove upstairs, water heaters, dryer vents, and furnaces should be regularly maintained, and the level of carbon monoxide should be monitored. She provided Betsy with a carbon monoxide detector with an alarm that emits a warning sound when carbon monoxide levels are too high. Assuring good ventilation, such as turning on the fan when cooking or making sure that a window is open, are other actions that families can take to make sure that the air their families breathe is as healthy as possible.

While still on the topic of alarms, Jane asked whether the family had working smoke alarms, windows that could be opened on each floor, and a fire escape plan. Betsy showed Jane the smoke detector in the living room and then led Jane down the hall to see the other one, which she thought needed new batteries. Jane noticed that there was an extension cord running along the hall floor. While Jane helped Betsy change the batteries in the smoke detector she mentioned to Betsy the hazards associated with extension cords, including fire, tripping, and strangulation. Betsy explained that some of the outlets in the back rooms were not working. Jane went over how Betsy could address this with the landlord.

The final two areas that Jane and Betsy discussed were the problems related to dust mites and mold. Jane suggested that Betsy add repair of the kitchen faucet to her request to the landlord. Meanwhile, Betsy could clean under the sink using a solution of 1/10 bleach to 9/10 water, thus eliminating existing mold. Betsy also explained that there were multiple sources

of dust mites in the apartment including the carpets, the stuffed animals, and the bedding. Removal of the carpets should be added to the landlord requests. Removal of stuffed animals might be more difficult if the children were attached to them, but Betsy felt the boys were growing out of the stuffed animal phase and that she would be able to remove most of them and would regularly wash the others. Betsy explained that she had limited money to spend on pillow case covers and mattress covers. Together they searched the department store Web sites on Jane's tablet and located stores with reasonably priced mattress protectors and pillow covers that Betsy felt she could afford.

When the visit was completed, Jane and Betsy had developed an action plan that included actions Betsy could take on her own, steps that she would need to take with help from the landlord, and the identification of available resources in the community. Betsy was encouraged by the resources that were available and the assistance that Jane had provided. Jane agreed to follow up with Betsy in 2 weeks to determine whether she was in need of further assistance.

Over the course of 6 months, word spread among the parents of the school about how helpful Jane's visits were. Prior to starting the home visits, Jane and the school nurse, Edward, had developed an evaluation plan for the program (Chapter 5). They had collected baseline data on the key outcome indicators for children with asthma in the school including numbers of days absent, use of inhalers, number of acute asthma attacks during school, and the number of pediatric ED visits related to asthma for children living in the school district. They also kept track of the number of visits Jane made and the time each visit took. Based on these data they found a significant improvement for all of the key outcome indicators and a significant drop in ED use for severe asthma episodes. These data helped them demonstrate that the cost of Jane's home visits were offset by the savings in health-care costs, the reduction in costs related to truancy, and overall improved health outcomes for the children.

Environmental Health and Susceptible Populations

As described in Chapter 24, some populations have increased vulnerability to health risks. This also holds true for environmental health risks. This is especially true for children and older adults.

Children

Physiological and behavioral characteristics increase vulnerability at each step of early development. Children playing on the ground and floor may spend their time in the most contaminated areas. For example, outdoor soil is often contaminated with heavy metals and pesticides, and hand-to-mouth behavior promotes ingestion of both seen and unseen agents. Children near parents who are washing work clothes may be playing amid toxins that have been carried home as particles from the workplace. Even toys may pose a risk for exposure to toxins including lead and cadmium.[50,51] Children have ingested substances from unlabeled food containers that have been repurposed to hold chemicals or were located in an easily accessible place such as under the sink.

Compared with adults, children have faster rates of absorption of most toxic substances and, once in the body, the toxic action can be more deadly owing to a higher metabolic rate, faster rate of cell growth, and less developed immune and neurological systems. There are equally grave concerns for the fetus, which may be the ultimate target of exposures to a pregnant woman. Body systems are selectively more vulnerable according to their stage of development and the timing of exposure. Although women are increasingly aware of the risks associated with alcohol and environmental tobacco smoke during pregnancy, they are often less informed about the dangers of other environmental exposures. In addition, a pregnancy may not be recognized in time to avoid or minimize exposures. This is especially a concern during the first trimester, when the earliest differentiation of organ systems begins. For example, carbon monoxide, which is easily transported across the placental barrier, is potentially devastating to the developing fetus because of its sensitivity to hypoxia. Other substances that cross the placenta may accumulate in fetal tissue, leaving the newborn to begin life with a body burden of a toxin. In addition, breast milk can constitute an ongoing source of ingested toxins.

It is also important to recognize the influence of environmental factors with regard to injury risk in children. In urban settings, there are often limited spaces where children can play, and they may be fraught with hazards such as faulty playground equipment, soil contaminated by previous commercial use of the property, or threats of violence (Chapter 12). Without designated places to play safely, these children may turn to more dangerous sites such as streets and alongside roadways. In agricultural settings, children and adolescents are at risk of injuries from farm equipment and vehicles, often as a result of operating them without training or supervision.

A set of resources that can be used for reference as well as health education on the environmental health risks to children has been compiled as the *Pediatric Environmental Health Toolkit for Primary Health Care Providers & Patients.*[52] The materials that make up the toolkit are useful for learning more about environmental exposures and children's health and can be used to share with families and others who care for children.

There is clearly a need for community education and assistance in identifying alternative, safer environmental conditions for children. The safety of children is an emotionally charged issue and one that can galvanize a community and spur it to action, whether it is by committing or redistributing resources, enacting policy changes, or seeking other solutions. Nurses who understand the vulnerabilities of children can be partners and change agents in this process.

Older Adults

At the other end of the life span, faced with a different set of physical and behavioral characteristics from children and midlife adults, are older adults (Chapter 20). The EPA has developed 10 initiatives for older adults aimed at addressing environmental health issues facing them and improving environmental stewardship (Box 6-4).[53] The EPA is also helping to develop a national agenda aimed at identifying priority environmental health hazards for older adults. The process includes an examination of environmental health issues as well as engagement of communities in developing plans to address these issues.

In addition to changes in physical and mental functioning that are associated with age, older adults also experience increased rates of chronic health conditions, accounting for increased vulnerability to environmental health issues. Some age-related changes that increase risk from environmental hazards include hearing and vision loss, respiratory disease, increased fragility of

| BOX 6-4 | **EPA's Initiatives for Older Adults** |

- Age Healthier, Breathe Easier
- Building Healthy Communities for Active Aging
- Carbon Monoxide Poisoning Prevention
- Diabetes and Environmental Hazards
- Effective Control of Household Pests
- Environmental Hazards Weigh Heavy on the Heart
- Health Effects of Ultraviolet Radiation
- "It's Too Darn Hot"—Planning for Excessive Heat
- Water Works
- Women and Environmental Health

Source: See reference 53.

skin, decreased rates of metabolism, and disorders such as osteoporosis and heart disease.[53] Older adults also have higher body burdens of chemicals that have been absorbed over their lifetimes. Some substances accumulate over time in the body, a process known as **bioaccumulation.** These toxic substances are commonly retained in tissues such as bone or adipose (fat) and can become a long-term cause of poor health outcomes including cancer, organ damage (in particular, to the kidneys, heart, and liver), cardiac disease, increased chance of stroke, and neurological, immunological, and hematopoietic disorders. For example, lead is stored in the bone with a **half-life** (time over which only half of the amount is excreted) of more than 20 years. Its slow release over time is reflected by high blood lead levels (BLLs) that reach and damage target organs.[54] Those whose organ systems are already compromised are at higher risk. For example, individuals with cardiac disease will be more quickly and more seriously affected in oxygen-deprived atmospheres. In addition, many older adults tend to spend a greater amount of their time indoors, where indoor air pollutants and issues related to climate control may be an issue.

Older adults are also more vulnerable to weather conditions. In the summer of 1995 a heat wave in Chicago claimed the lives of more than 700 people, especially older adults living in low-income areas of the city.[55] To understand how the environment plays a role, consider a hypothetical Chicagoan, Mr. Roberts, age 78, who in 1995 lived on the ninth floor of an 18-story high-rise apartment building for low-income older adults and disabled community members. His wife had died the year before, and his children lived three states away. There were two elevators to serve the 180 occupants, but one of them regularly broke down. Mr. Roberts had worked most of his life as a carpenter. When he was 62, he fell off a roof, sustaining a hip injury that ended his working career. Following the injury he began to use a walker and developed failing eyesight. Because of his exercise limitations, he gained weight and developed type 2 diabetes. He tried to be adherent to therapy by checking his blood glucose, but his limited fixed income, travel distance to the closest supermarket, and solitary cooking situation stood in the way of eating healthy foods. Because of these problems, as well as fear of robbery by strangers who sometimes lurked in his building, he rarely went outdoors. Mr. Roberts mainly kept to himself, did not mix with his neighbors, and simply enjoyed his air-conditioned apartment with its pretty view of the city.

When the temperatures soared above 110°F, Chicago started to experience brownouts, then power outages, resulting in a 3-day loss of power in Mr. Roberts's building. The temperature inside began to climb, particularly in the afternoon. Two days later, a neighbor of Mr. Roberts called the building's management to complain that the television in Mr. Roberts's apartment had been on for days, and she wanted Mr. Roberts to turn it down. The maintenance person came to check, but after getting no answer to his knock, he assumed Mr. Roberts had gone away with family and left his television on loudly as a deterrent for would-be burglars. He left a note, the scope of his authorization, because, as in many municipalities, landlords are required to give 24-hour notice to a tenant before they can enter without the owner's permission. Sadly, when the maintenance man entered the apartment the next day, he discovered that Mr. Roberts had died during the heat wave.

This scenario is typical of stories that pepper the news each summer in the United States. Mr. Roberts died of heat stroke, a direct result of an environmental hazard amplified by his age, health, and the built environment. Another issue for Mr. Roberts was his social isolation, a factor that may explain why more older men than women died in the Chicago heat wave.[55] A heat wave is an example of a natural disaster (Chapter 25), but the built environment often increases the risk of morbidity and mortality, especially for the older adult.

One of the contributing environmental factors that increase the vulnerability of older adults to heat waves is the lack of adequate cooling through fans or air-conditioning. With age, the ability to regulate body temperature becomes diminished; thus, external mechanical methods are needed to reduce the surrounding temperature. Unfortunately, this susceptibility often combines with other risk factors for heat injuries, particularly in urban settings. Seniors, who are more likely to stay indoors, often live in relative isolation with few social contacts, and those whose incomes cannot support telephones or sophisticated air-conditioning systems are at greater risk for heat-related illnesses. In several extraordinary heat waves, death rates from heat stroke were highest among the oldest age groups. For example, a severe heat wave in France for 3 weeks during August 2003 resulted in 14,800 deaths, mainly among women older than age 75. These deaths, especially when they occur in developed nations, are preventable, and as a result France set up a Heat Health Watch Warning system as well as prevention plans.[56] Some of these actions were also instituted in the United States, resulting in lower mortality rates in the 2006 heat wave compared with the 1995 Chicago heat wave.[57] Thus the environment—adequate cooling, adequate availability of water for hydration, and an effective method of communication—are key components to interventions aimed at reducing environmental issues faced by older adults who are caught in a heat wave.

Nurses may have intervened at a number of points to prevent the death of Mr. Roberts, beginning with those at the office of his primary care provider. Help with contacting the city's social services department could have initiated home visiting care. Many older people and others with disabilities are unaware of their eligibility for such services, and many others might be aware of these services but they need assistance with applications. Nurses bear a part of developing emergency preparedness and disaster management plans (Chapter 25). Such plans should include the establishment of warning systems and emergency cooling centers, monitoring of older adults and isolated persons, and improving communication and awareness among city officials and emergency medical services. Outreach by PHNs to tenant organizations in buildings such as the one in which Mr. Roberts lived is a means of informing community members about available public health services, fostering better networking and communication among residents, and helping to strategize about safety concerns.

Many issues also arise in cold climates concerning home heating. In addition to cold injuries and death that can result from lack of heat, many people use space heaters that use fuel such as kerosene. This type of space heater presents a serious fire hazard, as do other makeshift forms of sustaining home heat. Deaths have been caused not only by fire, but also from carbon monoxide poisoning when fuels such as charcoal or wood have been burned indoors. There are programs in many locales to assist low-income or older clients. Power companies can provide information about these and, in most locations, cannot abruptly discontinue service before taking a number of required steps.

In addition, landlords must also abide by housing codes.[49] For example, when it comes to heating spaces, most housing codes dictate a minimum temperature that must be achievable if the space is to be legally rented. There are many codes that apply to rental properties as illustrated in Solving the Mystery: The Case of the Hazardous House. You should know how to access the code in the community where you work and live and, if it is insufficient, advocate for adoption of the **international building codes** that are being used increasingly across the United States.[58]

Gene-Environment Interaction

There is growing evidence that genetic factors may be responsible for some degree of individual variability in susceptibility to toxic exposures. **Gene-environment interaction** is defined as "an influence on the expression of a trait that results from the interplay between genes and the environment."[59,60] In other words, genes interact with the environment either positively or negatively in a way that influences development of disease. Often it involves a complex interaction between multiple genes and the environment. There is a growing body of research that identifies an increased risk for disorders such as diabetes, pulmonary disease, breast cancer, and other diseases when individuals with a specific genetic makeup encounter environmental exposures. In addition, some genes are thought to be protective and thus responsible for a decreased risk of environment-related health outcomes. This knowledge may someday be useful in identifying individuals who are at higher risk and intervening by controlling their exposures. In 2006, the National Institute on Environmental Health Sciences established a 5-year genes and environment initiative in an effort to increase our understanding of the interaction between environment and genes with a focus on asthma, diabetes, and cancer. The efforts of this initiative have resulted in an increased understanding of the interaction between genes and environment and helped to develop better ways to measure environmental exposures.[61]

Community Environmental Health Assessment

Although the environmental assessments discussed thus far have focused on individuals or families, a community assessment focuses on environmental health risks at the population level. The **community environmental health assessment** is a means by which public health and environmental health professionals and agencies partner with community members, organizations, and each other to identify, prioritize, and address environmental health issues.[62] One of the most widely used community assessment methodologies is the Protocol for Assessing Community Excellence in Environmental Health (PACE EH), developed in partnership between the National Association of County and City Health Officials (NACCHO) and the CDC.[63] Communities that have implemented PACE EH consider it to be a successful tool for expanding the capacity of health agencies in essential environmental health services; engaging the community in problem-solving; and implementing action plans that use community resources to reduce health risks.[64-66]

According to the PACE EH guidebook (pp ix, x), PACE EH is intended for use domestically and internationally and is being used in numerous locales to take a "collaborative community-based approach to generating an action plan that is based on a set of priorities that reflect both an accurate assessment of local environmental health status and an understanding of public values and priorities."[63,65] It outlines a series of tasks, shown in Box 6-5, to accomplish this goal. Implementation of the PACE EH process is supported by several resources that are available from NACCHO, including guidebooks in English and Spanish, other publications, a toolbox with a number of materials and resources, and online and regional training. In addition to PACE EH methodologies, there are a number of additional approaches to community assessment in current use, one of which is to conduct a health impact assessment (HIA). These assessments allow communities to examine the impact of city planning related to land use and policy on the health of the community.[66,67] HIAs are being implemented at a growing rate throughout Europe as a way to effectively gauge the health impacts of land use planning and policy decisions.[66]

Natural Disasters and Environmental Health

Natural and man-made disasters (Chapter 25) have an impact on the health of an environment. Public health efforts to address all forms of large-scale disasters are called all-hazards preparedness. In December 2006, Congress passed and the President signed the Pandemic and All-Hazards Preparedness Act, Public Law No. 109-417, that provided new authority for a number of programs, including the advanced development and acquisitions of medical countermeasures and called for the establishment of a quadrennial National Heath Security Strategy.[68] Planning for such events must take place at the community, family, and individual levels, and should involve

---

| BOX 6–5 | **Steps in PACE EH Methodology*** |

This methodology guides communities and local health officials in conducting community-based environmental health assessments. PACE EH draws on community collaboration and environmental justice principles to involve the public and other stakeholders in:
- Identifying local environmental health issues,
- Setting priorities for action,
- Targeting populations most at risk, and
- Addressing identified issues.

*PACE EH = Protocol for Assessing Community Excellence in Environmental Health

Source: See reference 63.

---

nursing input when emergency operations plans are developed.

In assessing the risks to a community, a PHN can take advantage of the work that has already been done and the information that has already been compiled to develop a community response plan, which has been developed to comply with the Emergency Planning and Community Right to Know Act (EPCRA). Superfund Amendments and Reauthorization Act of 1986 created EPCRA, a statute designed to improve community access to information about chemical hazards and to facilitate the development of chemical emergency response plans by state/tribe and local governments.[69] Information that has been assembled within that plan can be used as a guide for other purposes. For example, by designating major industries and transportation routes where hazardous substances are employed, the plan can suggest areas where air, water, or soil contamination may be an issue during nonemergency times. Knowledge of the major area industries can give clues as to what substances might be carried into the home on workers' clothing or items from work, as well as explain health conditions of unknown origin.

Air

All animals depend on an adequate supply of oxygen to maintain life. A healthy environment requires not only air with an adequate supply of oxygen, but also air that is free from pollutants. Air pollution has long been an issue, but with the arrival of the industrial revolution the quality of the air we breathe has changed drastically. Industry and the need for energy have resulted in the emission of toxic chemicals into the air (Fig. 6-4). The famous London fog is not a natural weather phenomenon, but rather arrived on the heels of the Industrial Revolution. Cities with high dependence on motor vehicles for transport, such as Los Angeles, have struggled with severe smog due to emissions from automobiles. In the 21st century, the quality of the air is a major public health concern.

Ambient Air

Ambient air is defined as the air surrounding a place or structure and is also referred to as outdoor air. Poor ambient air quality is associated with increased mortality rates from pulmonary and cardiovascular disease.[70,71] Sources of air contaminants occur because of the emissions of pollutants into the atmosphere at consistent concentrations over time, such as the emissions from factories. Scientists devised a mechanism to evaluate the

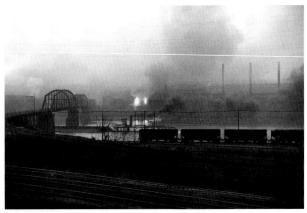

Figure 6-4 Industrial pollution in 1946 prior to EPA policies on emissions. This historical image was captured during a U.S. Public Health Service field study, and depicts the air-polluted landscape of an American city. *(From the Centers for Disease Control and Prevention, courtesy of Barbara Jenkins, NIOSH Historic Photo Collection. Photographer, Roy Perry.)*

current air quality called the **ambient air standard.** This refers to the highest level of a pollutant in a specific place over a specific period of time that is not hazardous to humans. It is computed as the number of parts per million per hour that are considered the limit for safety. For some countries such as China, the amount of air pollution is a serious concern (Fig. 6-5).

Variability in air quality often reflects the surrounding built environment. Populations located in the shadow of chemical plants and next to large equipment, railroad tracks, trailer trucks, and dusty access roads are often made up of lower socioeconomic groups, because the property values of homes located next to these sources of pollution are lower. Thus, the population is disproportionally

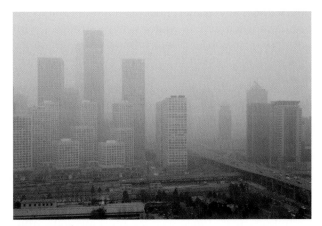

Figure 6-5 Smog in Beijing. *(©iStock.)*

vulnerable to all types of hazardous exposures that come with living in an industrial area. In addition to the risks associated with chemicals emitted in industrial areas, these residents face the social strain brought on by these circumstances.

Many outdoor air contaminants originate from major stationary sources, known as **point sources,** which include chemical plants, power plants, refineries, and incinerators. Alternatively, pollutants may be generated by transportation sources such as buses, trucks, and cars (on-road) and ships, planes, and construction equipment (off-road), all referred to as **mobile sources.** A third type, **area sources,** defines smaller sources of emission such as gas stations, dry cleaners, commercial building heating and cooling systems, railways, and waste disposal facilities such as landfills and wastewater treatment operations.[72]

In 1970, the United States promulgated the Clean Air Act, which was reauthorized in 1990. The Clean Air Act, enforced by the EPA, specifies allowable limits, known as the National Ambient Air Quality Standards, for industrial emission of a set of major air pollutants called the **criteria air pollutants.**[73] These are carbon monoxide; nitrogen dioxide; ozone; particulate matter; lead; and sulfur dioxide. Ground-level ozone and particulate matter are felt to be the greatest threats to human health. Because particulate matter varies in size, separate standards are set for all particles less than 10 micrometers (μm) in size (PM_{10}) and for those less than 2.5 μm ($PM_{2.5}$). The size of a particle determines the site of its deposition in the respiratory system. Particles less than 10 μm (less than the width of a human hair) are considered to be respirable; that is, they are not removed in the upper airways, as are larger particles. Increased levels of PM_{10} air pollution appear to affect the lung function and symptoms in asthma patients of all ages.[73] The subset of particles that are less that 2.5 μm enter the alveoli and are associated with lung cancer and cardiovascular death.[73] Vehicle traffic, in particular, diesel exhaust, is an important source of particulate matter. Note that dust masks that can be purchased from hardware stores do not protect the lungs from the effects of small particles. The EPA has established criteria regarding air pollutants (Box 6-6).

One way to evaluate the degree of air pollution in a specific area is the **Air Quality Index (AQI)** (Box 6-7).[74] The AQI is computed by the EPA based on measures of the five criteria for air pollutants. While the calculation of the AQI results in values on a scale of 0 to 500, these are generally reported to the public as levels that are described in six categories: good, moderate, unhealthy for sensitive groups, unhealthy, very unhealthy, and hazardous. They are also denoted by colors that range from

---

BOX 6–6 **Criteria Air Pollutants**

Description of Common Ambient Air Pollutants

Carbon monoxide (CO): An odorless and colorless gas produced by incomplete combustion of fuels in vehicles, heating systems, lawn mowers, and other motorized machinery.
Health effects: Reduces the oxygen carrying capacity of blood, deprives tissues of oxygen to potentially aggravate heart disease, harms fetuses, and damages oxygen-sensitive organs.

Nitrogen Oxides (NO_x): Levels are usually low in the United States. Plays a role in the production of ozone. Sources are vehicles, waste disposal systems, power plants, silage on farms.
Health effects: Lung irritant, aggravates asthma, and lowers resistance to infection; pulmonary edema at high concentrations; pulmonary fibrosis at long-term lower concentrations.

Sulfur Oxides (So_x): Sources are metal smelters and processes that burn sulfur-containing coal and oil, such as power plants and industrial boilers. Creates "acid rain" and smog.
Health effects: Bronchoconstriction, aggravates and triggers asthma, long-term exposure pulmonary fibrosis and possibly lung cancer.

$PM_{2.5}$ and PM_{10}: Sources are vehicles, wildland and other types of fires.
Health effects: Dangerous to those with heart and lung disease, causing shortness of breath, arrhythmias, angina, and myocardial infarction. Long-term, exposures may be related to chronic obstructive lung disease (COPD), lung cancer, and cardiovascular disease.

Lead: A widely used metal present in smelting operations, paint in old housing, water distribution systems, solder, painted items such as some toys, and many others. Organic lead compounds were once used in gasoline, accounting for 81% of transportation emissions in 1985. This quantity has been reduced substantially since lead was banned from this use. Lead often contaminates air, water, food and soil, and bioaccumulates.
Health effects: Damage to renal, gastrointestinal, reproductive, hematopoietic and nervous system. Affects development and learning ability of children.

Ozone: In the stratosphere, 6 to 30 miles above the earth, ozone is beneficial because it blocks the sun's harmful ultraviolet rays. At ground level, ozone is a dangerous component of urban smog, produced by sources such as power plants, refineries, and chemical plants.
Health effects: Irritates the respiratory system, aggravates and triggers asthma.

Source: See reference 71.

BOX 6–7 **Air Quality Index**

The features of the AQI include:
- A category that provides specific warnings for sensitive groups, such as children with asthma and others with special respiratory conditions
- Detailed warnings about how all people should protect themselves and their families from harmful levels of air pollution
- Warnings based on the most up-to-date scientific information on the known health effects of air pollution levels

Source: See reference 73.

---

green to maroon. A value of 100 or less, corresponding to the levels of "good" and "moderate" (green and yellow), is the level set by EPA to protect public health. As the index increases, the health hazards associated with air pollution increase, first affecting the most sensitive individuals at levels of 101 to 150, and at higher levels, everyone. As levels above those classified as yellow (index of 100) are reached, individuals should reduce their levels of exertion and outdoor activities accordingly. The EPA provides a daily updated forecast of the AQI and more information about air pollutants on its Web site Air Now. This Web site provides the current AQI for areas around the country and includes information that can be used for teaching clients.[75] The EPA has also published a helpful guide to the AQI for the public, which is available online.[76] One issue now being addressed by the EPA is the impact of the mixture of air pollutants in ambient air. The current approach used to evaluate the air quality examines each pollutant separately. An emerging framework uses a multipollutant approach that includes the impact mixtures of air pollutants.[77] Significant advances have been made in reducing ambient air pollution during the past 60 years. Continued efforts to improve the health of ambient air will require collaborative efforts within and across nations.[77]

Indoor Air Pollution

With the exception of laws that ban smoking in public places and Occupational Safety and Health Administration standards for workplace exposures, there is little regulation of indoor air contaminants. Several of these have been mentioned previously in this chapter in the discussion of the home evaluation. These included environmental tobacco smoke, animal dander, cockroaches, and the spores of molds that grow in damp environments. Each of these agents can cause allergic reactions, and all are recognized triggers for asthma.

Many of these pollutants exist in the home in the form of house dust, which may also be composed of heavy metals, pesticides, gram-negative bacteria, and chemicals such as phthalates. The very young are especially at risk owing to their greater ingestion of dust and greater physical susceptibility to toxins. Home cleaning methods, which can easily be taught to families and reinforced by home visits, significantly reduce dust exposures over time periods as short as 1 week when practiced by motivated individuals. Effective interventions combine the use of vacuum cleaners with dirt finders, HEPA filters, allergy-control bed covers, and quality doormats.[78]

Chemicals such as formaldehyde that are associated with the materials used to build homes are another concern. Formaldehyde was found to be emitted from materials inside the trailers used to house victims of Hurricane Katrina.[79] Newer buildings that are well insulated, are tightly sealed for efficient climate control, and lack windows that can be opened by occupants are more likely to retain indoor air pollutants, especially if the ventilation systems provide infrequent air exchanges per hour.

Potable Water

Just as all animals need oxygen to survive, all living things need water. The availability of potable water has since ancient times dictated where humans settle. Humans need water to sustain their own bodies and also to sustain their crops and livestock. Water has also played a key role in commerce and the generation of hydroelectrical power. Water has become an important issue in the United States in areas that have less access to water, especially in the Southwest and in Southern California. The lack of water contributed to the depth of the Depression of the 1930s, creating the dust bowl on the Great Plains and one of the worse environmental disasters in the 20th century. The drought that hit the Midwest wiped out farmers economically and reduced the availability of food, resulting in 3 million leaving their farms and half a million migrating to other states.[80] The quality of the water is a major determinant of the health of a population. Both organic and inorganic contaminates are associated with adverse outcomes.[81]

Inorganic Water Contaminants

In the United States, there are National Primary Drinking Water Regulations, or primary standards, that set the standards for the safety of public drinking water. They are legally enforceable. The purpose is to protect the public health through a reduction in the contaminants in the water used for public consumption. As with air quality standards, the EPA has a list of the safe levels of contaminants.[82]

▶ SOLVING THE MYSTERY
The Case of the Contaminated Aquifer
Public Health Science Topics Covered:

- Assessment
- Epidemiology
  - Rates
  - Surveillance
  - Case Control study

In a suburban county, the community association of a residential section that sits on a river running into Chesapeake Bay learned that radium was found in the well water of some homes. The association knew that the water contained significant amounts of iron and sulfur compounds, both easily identified by the taste and smell of the water plus the evidence of yellow stains on clothing washed in untreated well water. Most residents had installed small water treatment systems in their homes to remove the iron and neutralize the sulfur odor. The finding of radium occurred by chance when the county tested regional water for other chemicals. Not to be confused with the gas *radon*, which is its decay product, radium is a carcinogenic metal with radioactive properties that falls into the category of physical exposures. Because radium has properties that are similar to those of iron, the home water treatment systems that remove iron also remove radium. Community members wondered whether the high rates of lung cancer in their area were due to the radium and they demanded that the county take action.

The county health officer, a nurse, reviewed the results of the well testing and readily saw a pattern of positive tests that corresponded to one aquifer that ran across the county at a depth of about 100 feet. This was one of two aquifers underlying the region and was the one being used for recent and current wells. The deeper aquifer traversed the county at about 200 to 300 feet, and was very expensive to reach by drilling.

Three issues now faced the health officer: (1) how to further assess the risk to the community; (2) how to control exposures if the risk were elevated; and (3) what to communicate to the community members. The nurse relied on several experts in her health department to assist in her approach including a preventive medicine physician, and an environmental hygienist epidemiologist. Together they began by comparing rates of cancer within the county with rates in other counties, the state, and the nation. They accessed the State Health Department registry that provides data on county-by-county cancer rates by type (see Chapter 9), but the surveillance data were not broken down by specific communities within the county. At the county level, there was a significantly higher rate of lung cancer compared with other counties in the state. However, one possible explanation for the difference in rates was the higher rates of tobacco use. Because tobacco use is a strong risk factor for lung cancer, it was not possible for them to conclusively link the higher rates of lung cancer in the county to the use of well water. As is often the case, the question of causality cannot be answered without conducting a formal study to obtain further data. The team decided to conduct a case control study to compare those with lung cancer with controls without lung cancer in relation to exposure to well water while controlling for tobacco use (see Chapter 3). Based on their findings, the team concluded that those exposed to well water had a one-and-one-half time greater odds for having lung cancer than those who were not exposed.

The next step was complicated for the team. The quality of well water used in a household did not fall within the jurisdiction of federal, state, or local government.[83] The team recommended that the county public health department develop an education program for residents using well water. A town hall meeting was held with interested community members and health department representatives to discuss the findings and possible courses of action. At the meeting, the county environmental hygienist, whose expertise was exposure measurement, presented the map of wells that were tested and the levels that were found. The levels of radium in the well water were slightly above the standard set by the EPA, which sets standards for 90 contaminants that may be found in water.[82] These contaminants include biological agents such as bacteria and viruses as well as organic and inorganic chemicals and radionuclides such as radium. Although some of these are naturally occurring, as is radium, many are from industrial, agricultural, household, and other uses related to human activities.

The health officer used basic risk communication strategies to facilitate the community meeting (Chapter 25). Rather than lecturing to the residents, their feedback was sought, particularly with regard to perceived concerns, actions that should be taken, and ways to reach and communicate with the entire community. The health officer ensured that technical terms

were limited or explained. She made sure she took concerns seriously and explained honestly that she might not have the answer to certain questions such as the causal relationship between the water and the risk for lung cancer. She acknowledged that matters were not handled perfectly, such as getting the water testing results sooner to the community.

As part of the discussion the health officer provided comparisons between the levels of radium found in the well water and the EPA standards. The effectiveness of home water systems for the removal of radium was also explained. The county made well water testing available at a nominal cost for a range of contaminants, including radium and lead. Community members who were aware and concerned about the issue were engaged in the process of communicating with the community at large, educating them about the water testing findings, precautions such as home treatment systems, and the availability of testing services. The community newsletter and a mailing to residents were used for this purpose, and section representatives alerted those who were less likely to attend to written communication or Internet sites. The health department Web site provided the same information and links to other resources. On a regulatory level, the county did have the ability to mandate well water testing and disclosure of findings to the purchaser at the time of sale of a property. Probably the most effective regulation enacted, although not one that pleased all residents, was the requirement to dig new wells to the deepest aquifer. This added additional costs to building new homes and replacing failed wells, but was deemed a necessary step because of the unknown relationship between well water exposure and cancers.

Municipal drinking water does fall under the jurisdiction of EPA and must comply with the standards. Local governments and private water suppliers are responsible for ensuring that those standards are met. The **Safe Drinking Water Act** sets the legal criteria and procedures for assuring a safe supply of drinking water from public systems.[84]

Safe Water From a Global Perspective

The major global issue related to potable water is organic contaminates that increase the risk for communicable diseases (Chapter 8).[81] According to the WHO, diarrheal disease accounts for 4.1% of the *daily* global burden of disease, with unsafe water accounting for 88% of the burden and the greatest impact on children in low-income countries.[85]

It is estimated that 1.1 billion people worldwide do not have access to safe drinking water[86] (Fig. 6-6).

The main barriers to the provision of safe drinking water include setting it as a priority, financial capacity, sustainability of the water supply, sanitation, and hygiene behaviors. The main actions recommended by the WHO include increasing the supply of safe water, increasing the number of facilities for the sanitary disposal of excrement, and implementing safe hygiene practices.[87]

In May 2013, the WHO released a report on the progress made on improving sanitation and increasing access to safe water. They concluded that despite efforts at the global level, we are "off-track" in meeting the Millennium Development Goal (MDG) (Chapter 13) related to sanitation. They estimated that 2.4 billion people worldwide lacked necessary sanitation. The good news in the report is that the world met the MDG in relation to water despite the fact that regional disparities continue.[88] The safety of drinking water remains a serious environmental health issue.

Environmental Sustainability

The issue of **environmental sustainability** is thought by many to be the most important emerging public health issue. It reflects the rates in which renewable resources are harvested, the depletion of nonrenewable resources, and the creation of pollution that can continue for an indefinite period of time. If the rates cannot be continued indefinitely, then the environment is not sustainable. Nurses and other public health professionals can play a critical role in the world's response to maximize sustainability from the

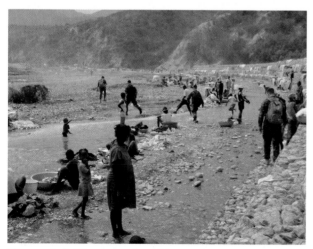

Figure 6-6 Water supply in Haiti. *(From the Centers for Disease Control and Prevention, courtesy of Lt. Cmdr. Gary Brunette, 2010.)*

local to the global environment.[89] Increasing attention has been given to this issue and it is now a global priority. The detrimental human actions that threaten our environment include our use of finite energy resources, waste disposal, land use, and food production. The immediate impact on health is clear, but the long-term effects are predicted by some to be devastating and a threat to human survival. The problem of scarce and diminishing resources has even been linked to violence and war.[89] The first step that nurses can take is to inform themselves about the many aspects of environmental sustainability in their own communities and to recognize the interconnections between human behavior and health outcomes.

Climate Change

The impact of climate change is becoming more apparent and is associated with increases in atmospheric carbon dioxide and ozone, and a steadily rising surface temperature of the earth. As described earlier in this chapter, heat waves cause direct injury, such as heat exhaustion and heat stroke, which are devastating to those who are most susceptible, for example, older adults and the very young. Changes in atmospheric and weather conditions are related to increased or exacerbated cardiovascular and pulmonary disease. But there are also more indirect effects on health and well-being. Climate-related redistribution of vectors for diseases, such as mosquitoes, allows infections to reach new and broader populations, who are often the least immune. Decreased yield of crops brought about by droughts, floods, or other impacts on the natural environment will add to the current billion people in the world who have inadequate nutrition. In addition, changes in sea level are projected to cause displacement of populations when their living spaces are destroyed.[90]

Based on a survey conducted by Polvika, Chaudry, and Crawford, PHNs demonstrated clear knowledge of the effects of climate change on health and that it was a responsibility of public health to address climate change but felt that they had access to limited resources to address the problem.[91] The CDC is taking the lead to track climate change as well as be ready to respond to and manage health risks that are associated with climate change.[92] This requires that nurses and public health agencies at the state and local levels incorporate into their programs systems to track and manage the adverse health effects of climate change. In addition, PHNs should advocate for their communities by supporting policies that will not only allow for better tracking of climate change and management of risk but also for supporting policies that seek to prevent the underlying causes of climate change.

■ Summary Points

- Nursing plays a crucial role in the promotion of optimal environmental health.
- The built environment contributes to the health of individuals, families, and populations.
- Environmental conditions that are associated with human-made and natural disasters are the source of serious health threats to populations and individuals.
- Assessment and management of environmental threats to a community must involve community members at all stages.
- There is an interaction between genetics and the environment.
- Characteristics of populations, such as age and health status, can increase susceptibility to negative health effects from environmental agents.
- Air and water pollution contribute significantly to the global burden of disease.
- Environmental sustainability must be a priority for all nurses.

▲ CASE STUDY
A Contaminated Town
Learning Outcomes

At the end of this case study, the student will be able to:

- Describe the effects of an environmental toxin on the health of a population
- Discuss polices related to environmental hazards
- Apply primary, secondary, and tertiary prevention approaches to an environmental health issue

Since the early 1900s, the major industry in the town of Libby, Montana, was the mining of vermiculite, a material used to insulate buildings. A contaminant of vermiculite is asbestos, which is well known for causing serious lung diseases, including cancer. Concerns about health problems among the town residents, not only the miners, began to surface when a reporter revealed the population's high rate of asbestosis and related diseases. Contaminated soil was considered to be the major source of asbestosis around town—near homes, schools, and many public places that included athletic fields—and the dust made its way indoors on vehicles such shoes, pets, and workers' clothes. The mine was closed in 1990, but by then a large proportion of the townspeople had been exposed, with ongoing exposure because the asbestosis remained in the soil. In 2002, the EPA placed Libby on its National Priority List, thereby identifying the town as a site that appeared to warrant remedial action and leading to the testing and inspection of almost 5,000 residential and commercial properties. Cleanup operations began throughout the town. In 2009, the EPA declared the town of Libby a public health emergency. This status mobilizes funds to conduct further home-to-home cleanup and install health-care resources for those with asbestos exposure.

1. What type of hazardous agent is asbestos, what is the typical route of exposure, and what are its major health effects? Are there government standards that regulate the permissible amount of asbestos?
2. List the agencies that would partner to address this extensive environmental disaster.
3. What primary, secondary, and tertiary preventive actions can be applied to protect the public's health?
4. A useful starting place for researching this problem is http://www.epa.gov/libby/background.html.

REFERENCES

1. Centers for Disease Control and Prevention. (2010). *Emergency preparedness and response: Health surveillance.* Retrieved from http://emergency.cdc.gov/gulfoilspill2010/2010gulfoilspill/health_surveillance.asp.
2. Centers for Disease Control and Prevention. (2012). *Deepwater Horizon response: Gulf of Mexico oil cleanup.* Retrieved from http://www.cdc.gov/niosh/topics/oilspillresponse/.
3. Solomon, G.M., & Janssen, S. (2010). Health effects of the Gulf oil spill. *Journal of the American Medical Association, 304*(10), 118-119.
4. Diaz, J.H. (2011). The legacy of the Gulf oil spill: Analyzing acute public health effects and predicting chronic ones in Louisiana. *American Journal of Disaster Medicine, 6*(1), 5-22.
5. Larsson, L.S., & Butterfield, P. (2002). Mapping the future of environmental health and nursing: Strategies for integrating national competencies into nursing practice. *Public Health Nursing, 19*(9), 301-308.
6. Ratnapradia, D., Conder, J., Ruffing, A., & White, V. (2012). The 2011 Japanese earthquake: An overview of environmental health impacts. *Journal of Environmental Health, 74*(6), 42-50.
7. World Health Organization. (2013). *Environmental health.* Retrieved from http://www.who.int/topics/environmental_health/en/.
8. U.S. Department of Health and Human Services. (2013). *Healthy People 2020 topics: Environmental health.* Retrieved from http://www.healthypeople.gov/2020/topicsobjectives2020/objectiveslist.aspx?topicId=12.
9. Richard, L., Gauvin, L., & Raine, K. (2011). Ecological models revisited: Their uses and evolution in health promotion over two decades. *Annual Review Public Health, 3*, 307-326.

10. World Health Organization. (2013). *10 facts on prevention of disease through healthy environments.* Retrieved from http://www.who.int/features/factfiles/environmental_health/environmental_health_facts/en/.

11. American Nurses Association. (2007). *ANA's principles of environmental health for nursing practice with implementation strategies.* Retrieved from http://nursingworld.org/MainMenuCategories/WorkplaceSafety/Healthy-Nurse/ANAsPrinciplesofEnvironmentalHealthforNursingPractice.pdf.

12. Environmental Protection Agency (EPA). (n.d.). *About EPA.* Retrieved from http://www.epa.gov/aboutepa/index.html.

13. Centers for Disease Control and Prevention. (n.d.). *Environmental Health Services.* Retrieved from http://www.cdc.gov/nceh/ehs/EHSNET/.

14. Aboelata, M. (2004). *The built environment and health: 11 profiles of neighborhood transformation.* Retrieved from http://www.preventioninstitute.org/index.php?option=com_jlibrary&view=article&id=114&Itemid=127.

15. Papas, M.A., Alberg, A.J., Ewing, R., Helzlsouer, K.J., Gary, T.L., & Klassen, A.C. (2007). The built environment and obesity. *Epidemiologic Reviews, 29,* 129-143. doi:10.1093/epirev/mxm009.

16. Frank, L.D., Andresen, M.A., & Schmid, T.L. (2004). Obesity relationships with community design, physical activity, and time spent in cars. *American Journal of Preventive Medicine, 27*(2), 87-96. doi:10.1016/j.amepre.2004.04.011.

17. Lopez, R.P., & Hynes, H.P. (2006). Obesity, physical activity, and the urban environment: Public health research needs. *Environmental Health, 5,* 25. doi:10.1186/1476-069X-5-25.

18. Khan, L.K., Sobush, K., Keener, D., Goodman, K., Lowry, A., Kakietek, J., et al., & Centers for Disease Control and Prevention. (2009). Recommended community strategies and measurements to prevent obesity in the United States. *Morbidity and Mortality Weekly Report, 58*(RR-7), 1-26.

19. Sallis, J.F., & Glanz, K. (2006). The role of built environments in physical activity, eating, and obesity in childhood. *The Future of Children / Center for the Future of Children, the David and Lucile Packard Foundation, 16*(1), 89-108.

20. Jackson, R.J. (2003). The impact of the built environment on health: An emerging field. *American Journal of Public Health, 93*(9), 1382-1384.

21. Centers for Disease Control and Prevention. (2013). Division of Nutrition. *Physical activity and obesity: Resources and publications.* Retrieved from http://www.cdc.gov/nccdphp/dnpao/publications/index.html.

22. Levy, B.S. (2006). *Occupational and environmental health: Recognizing and preventing disease and injury* (5th ed., pp 269-310). Philadelphia, PA: Lippincott Williams & Wilkins.

23. Agency for Toxic Substances and Disease Registry. (2012). *ATSD Toxic substances portal.* Retrieved from http://www.atsdr.cdc.gov/substances/index.asp.

24. Shields, P.G. (2000). Epidemiology of tobacco carcinogenesis. *Current Oncology Reports, 2*(3), 257-262.

25. Hoet, P., & Lison, D. (2008). Ototoxicity of toluene and styrene: State of current knowledge. *Critical Reviews in Toxicology, 38*(2), 127-170. doi:10.1080/10408440701845443.

26. Lee, P.N. (2001). Relation between exposure to asbestos and smoking jointly and the risk of lung cancer. *Occupational and Environmental Medicine, 58*(3), 145-153.

27. Parazino, G.K., Butterfield, P., Nastoff, T., & Ranger, C. (2005). I PREPARE: Development and clinical utility of an environmental exposure mnemonic. *American Association of Occupational Health Nursing Journal, 53*(1), 37-42.

28. Al-Ashban, R.M., Aslam, M., & Shah, A.H. (2004). Kohl (surma): A toxic traditional eye cosmetic study in Saudi Arabia. *Public Health, 118*(4), 292-298. doi:10.1016/j.puhe.2003.05.001.

29. Vallejos, Q., Strack, R.W., & Aronson, R. E. (2006). Identifying culturally appropriate strategies for educating a Mexican immigrant community about lead poisoning prevention. *Family & Community Health, 29*(2), 143-152.

30. Barrueto, F., Jr., Jortani, S.A., Valdes, R., Jr., Hoffman, R S., & Nelson, L.S. (2003). Cardioactive steroid poisoning from an herbal cleansing preparation. *Annals of Emergency Medicine, 41*(3), 396-399. doi:10.1067/mem.2003.89.

31. Riley, D.M., Newby, C.A., & Leal-Almeraz, T.O. (2006). Incorporating ethnographic methods in multidisciplinary approaches to risk assessment and communication: Cultural and religious uses of mercury in Latino and Caribbean communities. *Risk Analysis, 26*(5), 1205-1221. doi:10.1111/j.1539-6924.2006.00809.x.

32. Centers for Disease Control and Prevention. (2000). Recommendations for blood lead screening of young children enrolled in Medicaid: Targeting a group at high risk. *Morbidity and Mortality Weekly Report, 49*(RR14), 1-13.

33. Centers for Disease Control and Prevention. (2010). *CDC response to Advisory Committee on Childhood Lead Poisoning Prevention recommendations in "Low level lead exposure harms children: A renewed call of primary prevention."* Retrieved from http://www.cdc.gov/nceh/lead/acclpp/cdc_response_lead_exposure_recs.pdf.

34. American Academy of Pediatrics Committee on Environmental Health. (2005). Lead exposure in children: Prevention, detection, and management. *Pediatrics, 116*(4), 1036-1046. doi:10.1542/peds.2005-1947.

35. Bellinger, D.C., & Bellinger, A.M. (2006). Childhood lead poisoning: The torturous path from science to policy. *Journal of Clinical Investigation, 116*(4), 853-857. doi:10.1172/JCI28232.

36. Centers for Disease Control and Prevention. (2013). *Blood levels in children aged 1–5 years—United States 1999–2010.* Retrieved from http://www.cdc.gov/mmwr/preview/mmwrhtml/mm6213a3.htm.

37. Morland, K., Wing, S., Diez Roux, A., & Poole, C. (2002). Neighborhood characteristics associated with the location of food stores and food service places. *American Journal of Preventive Medicine, 22*(1), 23-29. doi:10.1016/S0749-3797(01)00403-2.

38. U.S. Department of Housing and Urban Development. (n.d.). *Healthy homes for healthy families.* Retrieved from http://www.hud.gov/offices/lead/healthy homes/index.cfm.

39. U.S. Environmental Protection Agency. (2013). *Lead.* Retrieved from http://www2.epa.gov/lead.

40. Hilmers, A., Hilmers, D.C., & Dave, J. (2012). Neighborhood disparities in access to healthy foods and their effects on environmental justice. *American Journal of Public Health, 102*(9), 1644-1654.

41. Hicken, M.T., Gee, G.C., Morenoff, J., Connell, C.M., Snow, R.C., & Hu, H. (2102). A novel look at racial health disparities: The interaction between social disadvantage and environmental health. *American Journal of Public Health, 102*(9), 2344-2351.

42. U.S. Environmental Protection Agency. (2013). *Environmental justice.* Retrieved from http://www. epa.gov/compliance/environmentaljustice/.

43. U.S. Environmental Protection Agency. (2013). *Federal Interagency Work Group on Environmental Justice.* Retrieved from http://www.epa.gov/ Compliance/environmentaljustice/interagency/ index.html.

44. Centers for Disease Control and Prevention, U.S. Department of Housing and Urban Development. (2006). *Healthy housing reference manual.* Atlanta, GA: U.S. Department of Health and Human Services.

45. Centers for Disease Control and Prevention. (2013). *Asthma: Basic information.* Retrieved from http:// www.cdc.gov/asthma/faqs.htm.

46. Centers for Disease Control and Prevention. (2013). *Smoking and tobacco use: Health effects of secondhand smoke.* Retrieved from http://www.cdc.gov/tobacco/ data_statistics/fact_sheets/secondhand_smoke/ health_effects/.

47. New York State Department of Health. (2013). *The landlord and tenant guide to pest management—the key to safe pest control is teamwork.* Retrieved from http://www.health.ny.gov/publications/3204/index.htm.

48. U.S. Environmental Protection Agency. (2012). *Integrated pest management in schools.* Retrieved from http://www.epa.gov/opp00001/ipm/.

49. New York State Attorney General. (2008). *Tenants' rights guide.* Retrieved from http://www.housingnyc. com/html/resources/attygenguide.html.

50. Centers for Disease Control and Prevention (2009). *Lead: Toys.* Retrieved from http://www.cdc.gov/ nceh/lead/tips/toys.htm.

51. Agency for Toxic Substances and Disease Registry. (2011). *Cadmium.* Retrieved from http://www.atsdr. cdc.gov/substances/toxsubstance.asp?toxid=15.

52. Physicians for Social Responsibility. (n.d.). *Pediatric environmental health toolkit.* Retrieved from http://www.psr.org/resources/pediatric-toolkit. html.

53. Environmental Protection Agency. (2013). *Aging initiative.* Retrieved from http://www.epa.gov/aging/.

54. Levy, B.S. (2006). *Occupational and environmental health: Recognizing and preventing disease and injury* (5th ed., pp 214-215). Philadelphia, PA: Lippincott Williams & Wilkins.

55. Kleinberg, E. (2002). *Heat wave: A social autopsy of disaster in Chicago.* Chicago, IL; University of Chicago Press.

56. Pirard, P., Vandentorren, S., Pascal, M., Laaidi, K., Le Tertre, A., Cassadou, S., et al. (2005). Summary of the mortality impact assessment of the 2003 heat wave in France. *Euro Surveillance: Bulletin European sur les Maladies Transmissibles, 10*(7), 153-156.

57. Fouillet, A., Rey, G., Wagner, V., Laaidi, K., Empereur-Bissonnet, P., Le Tertre, A., et al. (2008). Has the impact of heat waves on mortality changed in France since the European heat wave of summer 2003? A study of the 2006 heat wave. *International Journal of Epidemiology, 37*(2), 309-317. doi:10.1093/ije/dym253.

58. ICC—International Code Council. (2010). Retrieved from http://www.iccsafe.org/Pages/default.aspx.

59. National Institute of Environmental Health Sciences. (2013). *Gene environment interaction.* Retrieved from http://www.niehs.nih.gov/health/topics/science/ gene-env/index.cfm.

60. National Human Genome Research Institute. (2013). *Talking glossary of genetic terms.* Retrieved from http://www.genome.gov/glossary/index.cfm?id=72.

61. National Institute of Environmental health Sciences. (2011). *The genes and environmental health initiative.* Retrieved from http://www.genome.gov/19518663.

62. Tillman, L., & Waltz, T. (2003). Pursuing environmental health through community assessment. *Northwest Public Health,Spring/Summer 2003,* 6-9.

63. Centers for Disease Control and Prevention. (2013). *PACE EH—Protocol for Assessing Community Excellence in Environmental Health.* Retrieved from http://www.cdc.gov/nceh/ehs/CEHA/ PACE_EH.htm.

64. Orians, C., Rose, S., Hubbard, B., Sarisky, J., Reason, L., Bernichon, T., et al. (2009). Strengthening the capacity of local health agencies through community-based assessment and planning. *Public Health Reports, 124*(6), 875-882.

65. Higman, K., Servatius, C., Webber, W.L., & McDonald, T. (2007). Using the PACE EH model to mobilize communities to address local environmental health issues—a case study in Island County, Washington. *Journal of Environmental Health 70*(1), 37-41, 63.

66. Dannenberg, A.L., Bhatia, R., Cole, B.L., Heaton, S.K., Feldman, J.D., & Rutt, C.D. (2008). Use of health impact assessment in the U.S.: 27 case studies, 1999–2007. *American Journal of Preventive Medicine, 34*(3), 241-256. doi:10.1016/j.amepre.2007.11.015.

67. National Association of County and City Health Officials. (2013). *Health impact assessment.* Retrieved from http://www.naccho.org/topics/environmental/ landuseplanning/HIA.cfm.

68. U.S. Department of Health & Human Service. (n.d.). *Pandemic and All-Hazards Preparedness Act (PAHPA)*. Retrieved from http://www.hhs.gov/aspr/opsp/pahpa/index.html.

69. Environmental Protection Agency. (n.d.). *Emergency Planning and Community Right-To-Know Act (EPCRA)*. Retrieved from http://www.epa.gov/oecaagct/lcra.html#Summary of Emergency Planning And Community Right-To-Know Act.

70. World Health Organization. (2011). *Air quality and health*. Retrieved from http://www.who.int/mediacentre/factsheets/fs313/en/.

71. Centers for Disease Control and Prevention. (2013). *Air pollution and respiratory health*. Retrieved from http://www.cdc.gov/nceh/airpollution/.

72. Good Guide. (2011). *Definitions of air pollution source categories*. Retrieved from http://scorecard.org/env-releases/def/air_source.html.

73. U.S. Environmental Protection Agency. (2006). *List of lists: Consolidated list of chemicals subject to the Emergency Planning and Community Right-to-Know Act (EPCRA) and section 112(r) of the Clean Air Act*. Retrieved from http://emergencymanagement.wi.gov/EPCRA/forms/EPA_List_of_Lists1.pdf.

74. U.S. Environmental Protection Agency. (2011). *Air Quality Index*. Retrieved from http://www.epa.gov/reg3artd/specprog/AQI/Aqi.htm.

75. U.S. Environmental Protection Agency. (n.d.). *AIRNow air quality index (AQI): Local air quality conditions and forecasts*. Retrieved from http://airnow.gov/.

76. U.S. Environmental Protection Agency. (2003). *Air quality index: A guide to air quality and your health*. Retrieved from http://www.enviroflash.info/assets/pdf/AQI_2003_9-3.pdf.

77. Johns, D.O., Stanek, L.W., Walker, K., Benromdhane, S., Hubbell, B., Ross, M., et al. (2012). Practical advancement of multi pollutant scientific and risk assessment approaches for ambient air pollution. *Environmental Health Perspectives, 120*(9), 1238-1242.

78. Roberts, J.W., Wallace, L.A., Camann, D.E., Dickey, P., Gilbert, S.G., Lewis, R. G., et al. (2009). Monitoring and reducing exposure of infants to pollutants in house dust. *Reviews of Environmental Contamination and Toxicology, 201*, 1-39. doi:10.1007/978-1-4419-0032-6_1.

79. Maddalena, R., Russell, M., Sullivan, D P., & Apte, M. G. (2009). Formaldehyde and other volatile organic chemical emissions in four FEMA temporary housing units. *Environmental Science & Technology, 43*(15), 5626-5632.

80. Egan, T. (2006). *The worst hard time*. Boston, MA: Houghton Mifflin.

81. World Health Organization. (2013). *Water quality*. Retrieved from http://www.who.int/water_sanitation_health/dwq/en/.

82. U.S. Environmental Protection Agency. (2013). *Drinking water contaminants*. Retrieved from http://water.epa.gov/drink/contaminants/index.cfm.

83. U.S. Environmental Protection Agency. (2013). *Private drinking water wells*. Retrieved from http://water.epa.gov/drink/info/well/.

84. U.S. Environmental Protection Agency. (2012). *Safe Drinking Water Act*. Retrieved from http://www.epa.gov/ogwdw/sdwa/.

85. World Health Organization. (2013). *Water sanitation health: burden of disease and cost effectiveness estimates*. Retrieved from http://www.who.int/water_sanitation_health/diseases/burden/en/index.html.

86. World Health Organization. (2013). *Water sanitation health: Water supply, sanitation and hygiene development*. Retrieved from http://www.who.int/water_sanitation_health/hygiene/en/.

87. World Health Organization. (2014). *Millennium development goals*. Retrieved from http://www.who.int/topics/millennium_development_goals/en/.

88. World Health Organization. (2013). *Water sanitation and health*. Retrieved from http://www.who.int/water_sanitation_health/hygiene/en/.

89. Schwartz, B S., Parker, C., Glass, T.A., & Hu, H. (2006). Global environmental change: What can health care providers and the environmental health community do about it now? *Environmental Health Perspectives, 114*(12), 1807-1812.

90. Brenner, S.A., & Parker, C.L. (2010). *Health effects of global climate change: How health professionals can be part of the solution*. Retrieved from http://cme.medscape.com/viewprogram/19115.

91. Polvika, B., Chaudry, R.V., & Crawford, J.M. (2012). Public health nurses knowledge and attitudes regarding climate change. *Environmental Health Perspective, 120*(3), 321-325.

92. Centers for Disease Control and Prevention. (2011). *CDC policy on climate and health*. Retrieved from http://www.cdc.gov/climateandhealth/policy.htm.

Community Health Across Populations: Public Health Issues

Chapter 7

Health Disparities

LEARNING OUTCOMES

After reading this chapter, the student will be able to:

1. Compare and contrast the concepts of health disparity, inequity, and inequality.
2. Discuss the magnitude of health disparities both in the United States and internationally.
3. Describe the role of *Healthy People 2020* in eliminating health disparities.
4. Identify different actions nurses can take to alleviate health disparities within the health-care system.
5. Understand the reasons why health disparities continue in the United States.
6. Define and explain the role of the social determinants of health in contributing to health disparities.
7. Discuss solutions to decreasing health disparity caused by the social determinants of health, specifically how nurses can be part of the solution.

KEY TERMS

Disparity

Equity

Health disparity

Inequality

Social determinants of health

Universal health care

▮ Introduction

Whenever there is interest in health-care reform in the United States, the issue that recurs is why our health care comes with an exorbitant cost yet results in poor health outcomes, especially when measured against other industrialized countries that spend considerably less per person on health care. The differences in these health outcomes are not universal for all Americans. They are significantly worse for those who have less income; people who are African American, Latino, or from other racial and ethnic minorities; and people who have no health insurance.

Health providers and policy makers in the United States have been aware of these persistent differences for many years. The 1985 *Report of the Secretary's Task Force on Black and Minority Health* revealed large, continuing gaps in health status among Americans of different racial and ethnic groups.[1] This resulted in the creation of the Office of Minority Health (OMH) in 1986 by The U.S. Department of Health and Human Services. The Web site for the OMH provides profiles with extensive health data for the different minority groups, guides and information on cultural competency, minority profiles, and other useful data on U.S. minority populations.[2] The Centers for Disease Control and Prevention (CDC) created its own Office of Minority Health in 1988, now known as the Office of Minority Health and Health Equity (OMHHE). Its mission is "to accelerate CDC's health impact in the U.S. population and to eliminate health disparities for vulnerable populations as defined by race/ethnicity, socio-economic status, geography, gender, age, disability status, risk status related to sex and gender, and among other populations identified as at-risk for health disparities."[3] Two years after the CDC established the OMHHE, Congress passed the Disadvantaged Minority Health Act of 1990 to improve the health status of underserved populations, including racial and ethnic minorities.[4]

As a result of the documentation of these persistent differences, *Healthy People 2010* selected as one of its two goals in 2000 to eliminate health disparities in the United States. This goal remains one of four overarching goals in *Healthy People 2020 (HP 2020)* and is one of the four foundational health measures that serve as indicators of progress toward achieving these goals.[4] Another result, prompted by a request from Congress, was a detailed report from the Institute of Medicine (IOM) that reviewed health disparities and offered interventions to reduce these disparities. In 2003, the IOM report *Unequal Treatment: Confronting Ethnic and Racial Disparity in Health Care* responded to identified racial and ethnic differences in health outcomes among Americans.[6] The organization found disparity at two levels:

1. The health-care system and the environment level in which the system functions
2. The individual patient-provider level

Examples of these provider-level disparities included differences in the treatment of heart disease, the quality of treatment for HIV/AIDS, different cancer diagnostic testing, different treatment of diabetes, and the different treatment of end-stage renal disease for people of different racial and ethnic backgrounds and economic levels.[6]

Elimination of disparities has been declared a priority in our current health-care system, yet Orsi, Margellos-Anast, and Whitman found that the elimination of health disparities in the United States, and specifically in Chicago, remains problematic. The authors found that even with intense attention to the issues of reducing health disparities at the local, state, and national levels the impact was negligible.[6]

In *HP 2020,* the format has been changed to become more interactive, but the goals still are focused on more equitable health:

- Eliminate preventable disease, disability, injury, and premature death.
- Achieve health equity, eliminate disparities, and improve the health of all groups.
- Create social and physical environments that promote good health for all.
- Promote healthy development and health behaviors across every stage of life.[4]

Definitions

The term **health disparity** reflects differences in incidence, prevalence, and severity of health conditions among subpopulations that are socioeconomically disadvantaged as well as medically underserved in both rural and urban communities. It is not always clear when a difference in health becomes a disparity and what measures are used to identify and monitor the disparity. The IOM report in 2003 defined health disparity somewhat narrowly as "racial or ethnic differences in the quality of health care that are not due to access-related factors or clinical needs, preferences and appropriateness of intervention."[6] *HP 2020* explained that "if a health outcome is seen in a greater or lesser extent between populations, there is disparity. Race or ethnicity, sex, sexual identity, age, disability, socioeconomic status, and geographic location all contribute to an individual's ability to achieve good health."[8] The World Health Organization (WHO) expanded the definition to include the concept of equity: "differences in health which are not only unnecessary and avoidable but, in addition, are considered unfair."[9] The term health disparity is used regularly in the United States, but other countries more frequently talk about inequality and inequity in health care. This chapter uses the broader WHO definition and provides an in-depth look at health disparity where the difference is inequitable, meaning that it is unjust, unfair, avoidable, and unnecessary.

The term **equity** means "fairness." Health inequities are defined as unfair, unjust, and avoidable causes of ill health.[10] This is an ethical or moral judgment that generally reflects the belief that everyone has a right to health care. The WHO defines equity in health as "all people [having] an equal opportunity to develop and maintain their health, through fair and just access to resources for health."[10] There are unequal health opportunities when there are unequal opportunities to access health care, to have nutritious food, and to have safe housing. The government of any nation is the first entity responsible for the equity of health in a country. Inequities in the health of populations are often the consequence of inequities in life opportunities such as having a low level of education or living in poverty.

The *Universal Declaration of Human Rights* adopted by the General Assembly of the United Nations in 1948 is the framework for equity in health. The *Declaration* consists of 30 articles that serve as a standard of achievement for all nations to measure compliance to human rights and fundamental freedoms. Article 25 states, "Everyone has the right to a standard of living adequate for the health and well-being of himself and of his family, including food, clothing, housing and medical care and necessary social services, and the right to security in the event of unemployment, sickness, disability, widowhood, old age or other lack of livelihood in circumstances beyond his control."[11] Articles 22 to 27 are most specific to equity in health care examining economic, social, and cultural rights (Box 7-1).

In 1978 at the International Conference on Primary Care, the Alma-Ata Declaration affirmed these human rights. The goal was to see the provision of primary health care to every individual by the year 2000, thus achieving the goal of health care for all. The second section of the Alma-Ata Declaration stated, "The existing gross inequality in the health status of the people particularly between developed and developing countries as well as within countries is politically, socially and economically unacceptable and is, therefore, of common concern to all countries."[12]

Jones stated that disparity is morally wrong because it reflects and continues historical injustices based on race, ethnicity, and social class. The consequence of disparity is also morally wrong. Many who suffer from health disparity have been disenfranchised by past laws and past health-care practices.[13] Who is to decide what is unfair, unjust, and avoidable? To identify health differences as inequitable demands an ethical judgment as well as an epidemiological one.

Inequality, conversely, is the condition of not being equal. It does not necessarily mean that the situation is unjust or unfair. Disparity can mean inequality as well as inequity. **Disparity** is generally defined as the state of being unequal where there is a difference in some aspect of a thing or situation. Therefore, as noted above health disparity is a difference or inequality in some aspect of health, such as a disparity in the infant mortality rate between two groups.

BOX 7–1   The *Universal Declaration of Human Rights*, WHO, 1948

Article 22

Everyone, as a member of society, has the right to social security and is entitled to realization, through national effort and international co-operation and in accordance with the organization and resources of each State, of the economic, social and cultural rights indispensable for his dignity and the free development of his personality.

Article 23

(1) Everyone has the right to work, to free choice of employment, to just and favorable conditions of work and to protection against unemployment.
(2) Everyone, without any discrimination, has the right to equal pay for equal work.
(3) Everyone who works has the right to just and favorable remuneration ensuring for himself and his family an existence worthy of human dignity, and supplemented, if necessary, by other means of social protection.
(4) Everyone has the right to form and to join trade unions for the protection of his interests.

Article 24

Everyone has the right to rest and leisure, including reasonable limitation of working hours and periodic holidays with pay.

Article 25

(1) Everyone has the right to a standard of living adequate for the health and well-being of himself and of his family, including food, clothing, housing, and medical care and necessary social services, and the right to

security in the event of unemployment, sickness, disability, widowhood, old age or other lack of livelihood in circumstances beyond his control.
(2) Motherhood and childhood are entitled to special care and assistance. All children, whether born in or out of wedlock, shall enjoy the same social protection.

Article 26

(1) Everyone has the right to education. Education shall be free, at least in the elementary and fundamental stages. Elementary education shall be compulsory. Technical and professional education shall be made generally available and higher education shall be equally accessible to all on the basis of merit.
(2) Education shall be directed to the full development of the human personality and to the strengthening of respect for human rights and fundamental freedoms. It shall promote understanding, tolerance and friendship among all nations, racial or religious groups, and shall further the activities of the United Nations for the maintenance of peace. (3) Parents have a prior right to choose the kind of education that shall be given to their children.

Article 27

(1) Everyone has the right freely to participate in the cultural life of the community, to enjoy the arts and to share in scientific advancement and its benefits.
(2) Everyone has the right to the protection of the moral and material interests resulting from any scientific, literary or artistic production of which he is the author.

Source: See reference 11.

Margaret Whitehead, Chair of Public Health at the University of Liverpool and Head of the WHO Collaborating Centre for Policy Research on the Social Determinants of Health, specifies seven determinants of health disparity:

1. Natural biological variation
2. Health-damaging behavior that is freely chosen (playing football, bungee jumping)
3. Transient health advantage of one group over the other when one group is first to adopt a health-promoting behavior (a community passes a city ordinance that taxes high sugar beverages, decreasing the consumption of these beverages)
4. Health-damaging behavior where the degree of choice of lifestyles is severely restricted (lack of fresh fruits and vegetables at a reasonable cost in the inner city)
5. Exposure to unhealthy, stressful living and working conditions (living in a segregated community with a high violent crime rate)
6. Inadequate access to essential health services and other basic services (no primary care facility within a 40-mile drive in a rural community)
7. Health-related social mobility involving the tendency for sick people to move down the social scale (loss of job and their related insurance benefits due to recurring illness)[14,5]

Whitehead states that the first three determinants of health disparity result in inequality but are not necessarily unjust or inequitable. The last four determinants are unjust and, thus, inequitable.

Magnitude of the Problem

Health disparity is a global problem. The problem does look quite different between the industrialized and non-industrialized countries, between those with a universal national health-care system and those with inequitable distribution of health-care services, and between countries with unequal distribution of national income and resources.

There is health disparity between countries. For example, a comparison of infant mortality rates between countries demonstrates the gap between high and low income countries. In 2012, the infant mortality rate for Sierra Leone was 117 per 1000 live births while for Sweden it was 2 per 1000 live births.[16] Life expectancy is another marker for disparity. For example life expectancy at birth for females born in Sweden in 2012 was 38 years greater for a girl born in Sweden where the life expectancy was 84 years than it was for a girl born in Sierra Leone where the life expectancy was 38 years.[17] There is

also health disparity within countries. These disparities are frequently seen as a health gradient wherein there are series of progressively increasing or decreasing differences. For example, in Uganda, in the richest 20% of households for children under age 5, the death rate is 106 per 1,000 live births, and in the poorest 20% of households for children under age 5, the death rate is 192 per 1,000 live births. In Bolivia, a child born to a mother with no education has a 10% chance of dying, whereas a child born to a Bolivian mother with at least a secondary education has a 0.4% chance of dying. In each of these examples, there is a gradient so that as education or income improves, the statistics improve on a continuum. In Australia, males of European ancestry are likely to live 17 years longer than Aboriginal Australian males.[18] In the United States, ethnic differences in life expectancy persist; 886,202 deaths would have been averted between 1991 and 2000 if African Americans died at the same rate as non-Hispanic whites.[19]

According to the CDC, data show that there are significant differences in health outcomes between racial and ethnic groups in the United States. The infant mortality rate is more than twice as high for African Americans as it is for non-Hispanic whites, and the American Indian/Alaskan Native infant mortality rate is almost as high as that of African Americans. Heart disease is 40% higher and prostate cancer is double the rate for African Americans than it is for non- Hispanic whites. Non-black Hispanics are twice as likely to die of diabetes, with more obesity and high blood pressure, than are whites. American Indian/Alaskan Natives have twice the rate for diabetes than do non-Hispanic whites.[2,19,20]

In discussing the difference between inequality and inequity in health care, a valid social justice argument can be made that ethically inequitable health disparities must be eliminated. LaVeist, Gaskin, and Richard[21] supported that argument, but demonstrated that there was also a strong positive economic argument to eliminate inequities among racial and ethnic groups in the United States; that is, social justice is cost effective. In this study, commissioned by the Center for Economic and Political Studies, LaVeist et al. found that direct medical costs were higher for racial and minority populations because the individuals were sicker. They also found that there were indirect costs to U.S. society as a result of the individual's loss of productivity and lost wages. They concluded that the magnitude of the economic burden is enormous. LaVeist et al. found that between 2003 and 2006:

- Combined cost of health inequalities and premature death in the United States was $1.24 trillion

- Eliminating health disparities for minorities would have reduced direct medical care expenditures by $229.4 billion
- For African Americans, Asians, and Hispanics 30.6% of direct medical care expenditures were excess costs owing to health inequalities
- Eliminating health inequalities for minorities would have reduced indirect costs associated with illness and premature death by more than $1 trillion[21]

Researchers in Michigan[17] found the same outcomes with preterm births. A preterm birth is defined as a birth before the completion of 37 weeks of gestation, and occurs on average 11% of the time for non-Hispanic whites and 18% of the time for African Americans. If preterm births were the same rate in Michigan in 2003 for African Americans as they were for non-Hispanic whites, 1,184 preterm births and preterm deaths would have been avoided. Not only does this have significant impact on health outcomes for the preterm child and the family, but it also has an impact of an additional cost of $329 million across the life span of these children in associated hospitalizations, productivity, and major disabilities.[22] Where could the dollars be better spent—preventing the health disparity or treating it once it occurs?

Goal to Eliminate Health Disparities

Healthy People is committed to the achievement of optimal health for all people in the United States.[5] *HP 2020* reaffirmed its commitment to reducing health disparities with the following statement:

> During the past 2 decades, 1 of *Healthy People's* overarching goals has focused on disparities. In *Healthy People 2000,* it was to reduce health disparities among Americans. In *Healthy People 2010,* it was to eliminate, not just reduce, health disparities. In *Healthy People 2020,* that goal was expanded even further: to achieve health equity, eliminate disparities, and improve the health of all groups.[23]

■ HEALTHY PEOPLE 2020
Health Disparities

Disparities

Although the term "disparities" often is interpreted to mean racial or ethnic disparities, many dimensions of disparity exist in the United States, particularly in health. If a health outcome is seen in a greater or lesser extent between populations, there is disparity. Race or ethnicity, sex, sexual identity, age, disability, socioeconomic status, and geographic location all contribute to an individual's ability to achieve good health. It is important to recognize the impact that social determinants have on health outcomes of specific populations. *Healthy People 2020* strives to improve the health of all groups. [23]

The Agency for Health Care Research and Quality has regularly distributed a report on health-care quality and disparities. Based on 2011 data, improvements in disparities were identified in some areas. Areas in which disparity worsened included the disparity between African Americans and non-Hispanic whites in relation to the maternal mortality rate and breast cancer being diagnosed at an advanced stage. In addition, disparities worsened in relation to access to care for those with a low income compared with those with a high income.[24] To help address persistent disparities in our country the CDC implemented its Racial and Ethnic Approaches to Health program, aimed at funding community-based initiatives that address disparity. Their specific goal is to support efforts aimed at eliminating racial and ethnic disparities in health. Funded programs must be community based and culturally tailored to ethnic or racial groups currently experiencing disparity in health.[25]

Reflection of Health Disparities in Health Outcomes

In 2003, the focus of the IOM report *Unequal Treatment* was to assess the extent of racial and ethnic differences in health care that were not attributed to known factors such as access to care. The members of the task force looked at differences, disparity, and racial ethnic discrimination in health care from both the operation level of the health-care delivery system and the individual patient-clinician relationship level. This included individual biases, prejudice, stereotyping, and uncertain communication between patients and health-care providers.[6]

The IOM report paid particular attention to the discrimination that occurred in health-care providers' direct care to patients. They found that the racial and ethnic disparities existed and were associated with worse health outcomes, and that they occurred within the context of a broader historical and contemporary social and economic inequality. The committee reviewed a large body of research that documented these disparities and offered several recommendations. A summary of selected recommendation on how to decrease these disparities is found in Box 7-2.

The lack of access to health care also has had a negative impact on health outcomes. One cause for lack of access or diminished access is a lack of health insurance or inadequate insurance. In 2011 48.2 million Americans younger than age 65 did not have health insurance.[26] In 2008, uninsured

BOX 7–2	Recommendation to Decrease Health Disparity From the IOM Report

Unequal Treatment

- Strengthen the stability of patient-provider relationship in publicly funded health plans.
- Increase the proportion of racial and ethnic minority health professionals.
- Promote consistency and equity of care through evidence-based guidelines.
- Support the use of interpretation services.
- Provide financial incentives to health care practices that reduce barriers to providing quality care.
- Support the use of community health workers.
- Implement multidisciplinary treatment and preventive care teams.
- Implement patient education to increase knowledge of how to best access and utilize the health care system.
- Integrate cross-cultural education into the training of health care workers.
- Collect and monitor data on health care disparities.
- Conduct further research on all aspects of health disparities.

Source: See reference 6.

patients with breast cancer had a 30% to 50% higher mortality than those who were insured, and uninsured accident victims had a 37% higher mortality than those with insurance.[27] According to a Harvard study in 2008, 45,000 unnecessary deaths were linked to lack of health insurance.[28] With the introduction of the Affordable Care Act the hope is that access to care will improve for ethnic minorities. The act includes provision for improving access to care for minority populations such as American Indians and Native Alaskans. Whether or not these provisions will result in improved access is still under debate.[29]

In addition to access to adequate level of health insurance, there are other financial concerns. Many cannot afford care even with insurance if they are responsible for a copayment, purchasing medicine, or paying for procedures that are not included in the coverage. Many Americans are underinsured and have severe limitations in their coverage, such as limited primary care, and steep deductibles that must be paid before the insurance carrier will pay for service. For this and other reasons families may not have a regular source of care, relying on episodic health visits at clinics or the hospital emergency department. These families do not have a traditional medical home where they repeatedly see the same health-care provider. Instead they receive episodic care from a variety of providers with little or no primary prevention, which all contributes to poorer quality of health.

One mechanism for addressing disparity in access to health care is **universal health care.** Universal health care is defined as the provision of access to care without financial hardship through governmental policies. In 2005, the World Health Assembly passed Resolution 58.33 that affirmed that everyone should have access to health services without financial hardship. In 2010, the WHO concluded that "on both counts, the world is still a long way from universal coverage."[30] There are two main approaches to providing universal health care:

1. Government provision of health care
2. Government mandates that require citizens to obtain health insurance

For example, Britain and Canada use a centralized health-care system to provide care to all citizens without charge. Other countries such as Germany have laws that mandate that all citizens must have health insurance.

The United States was the last developed country to address the issue of universal health care. The Affordable Care Act (ACA) was passed by Congress and became law in 2010. This bill mandates that all Americans have health insurance coverage. It also provides mechanisms to assist persons to obtain health insurance who may not have the resources to do so. This bill encompasses four broad areas of health care, including rights and protections, insurance choices, issues for those aged 65 years or older, and employers (Box 7-3). The bill expands coverage to 32 million Americans.[31]

BOX 7–3	Key Features of the Affordable Care Act

The health-care law offers clear choices for consumers and provides new ways to hold insurance companies accountable. The most important parts of the law are broken into groups below.

Rights and Protections

- Summary of Benefits and Coverage (SBC) and Uniform Glossary
- Consumer Assistance Program
- Appealing Health Plan Decisions
- Preventive Care
- Patient's Bill of Rights
- Children's Pre-Existing Conditions
- Doctor Choice & ER Access
- Grandfathered Health Plans
- Curbing Insurance Cancellations

Insurance Choices

- Pre-Existing Condition Insurance Plan (PCIP)
- Young Adult Coverage
- Affordable Insurance Exchanges
- Co-Op Insurance Plans

Insurance Costs
- Value for Your Premium Dollar: 80/20 Rule and MLR
- Lifetime and Annual Limits
- Flexible Spending Account Changes Rate review

Source: See reference 31.

Having adequate health insurance coverage is only one issue related to disparity and access to care. A lack of personal transportation linked with poor public transportation can make seeing a practitioner costly in both time and money. It can make it difficult for people to access care, especially older people and families with small children. Other difficulties in seeking care are the frequent long waits in getting an appointment in clinic systems that do not have enough primary care providers. Once at the health-care facility, a person may experience additional delays in seeing a provider, even with an appointment.

Other specific components of the U.S. delivery system that foster health disparities include the following:

- There is a lack of primary health-care providers and specialists in some parts of the county, particularly in rural areas and inner cities (see Chapter 17). This poor ratio of provider to patient will universally increase as more people are insured under the ACA and will seek out primary health services. This will increase the wait time for an appointment and decrease the amount of time a provider can spend with an individual patient unless the number of primary care physicians increases and more nurse practitioners are educated.[32,33]
- There is a lack of racial and ethnic diversity among health workers. An increase in diversity can assist in providing quality and culturally competent care, mitigating some of the factors that increase health disparity. Minority populations account for about 34% of the U.S. population and within the next few decades will account for 50% of the population. Of the nurses practicing in the United States, only 16.8% were from a minority background.[34] In September 2004, the landmark Sullivan Commission on Diversity in the Healthcare Workforce stated that the lack of diversity in the workforce alienates minorities who feel distant and uncomfortable with people who are vastly different from themselves, and that this lack of diversity may account for more disparity than the lack of health insurance.[34]

- A universal problem with low health literacy (see Chapter 2), a first language other than English, and a lack of cultural sensitivity by the care providers (see Chapter 23) make communication and making informed decisions more difficult. Optimal patient communication is essential for quality care. There are several studies that show patients, regardless of race/ethnicity, are more likely to follow through on prevention and treatment if the health-care provider can communicate the importance of these health actions.[35,36] A lack of cultural competence by health-care providers can make it difficult to correctly diagnose health problems, and correctly communicate that diagnosis to guarantee optimal follow-up of the health problem.

Kagawa-Singer and colleagues examined the role of culture as a causal pathway for health disparities in the whole cancer care continuum. They found that cultural and ethnic groups were equally adaptive to the diagnosis of cancer, but many had very different worldviews, goals, and strategies for coping. The researchers urged health-care providers to be careful about labeling behavior as adaptive or maladaptive before they thoroughly understand their patients' culture. In much of our health care, Eurocentric beliefs and values are assumed. The authors encouraged health-care providers to incorporate cultural sensitivity to augment their clinical skills, to improve communication, and to develop trust and rapport with the patient and the family. They believed this would provide more equitable care across all economic and social groups and better decision making about treatment and treatment options.[37]

Many health-care providers may have no experience and feel uncomfortable caring for a diverse patient group, including same-gender couples. At times, health-care providers (consciously or unconsciously) provide different care to different racial or ethnic groups, generally providing less choice and fewer options for minority populations, which may include, for example, providing less pain medication and fewer kidney transplants.

● APPLYING PUBLIC HEALTH SCIENCE

The Case of the Doctorless Children

Public Health Science Topics Covered:
- Community assessment
- Health planning

Emily is working as a school nurse for the department of public health in a large community-based public elementary school in a very diverse urban neighborhood. The city is not large, but the lower-income, working-class community where this school is located has many first generation immigrants. There are 15 languages spoken at the school, and communicating with parents is a challenge for Emily. New immigrants from Asia, Africa, and South America make up 20% of the students; African Americans, 40%; Hispanics, 30%; and whites, the remaining 10%.

Emily reviewed the health statistics for the population at her school at the beginning of the school year. In this school she found disparities in disease/illness rates compared with those in other schools in the district:

- 32% were not completely immunized compared with 3% at other schools.
- 51% had not received the required physical exam.
- There was a higher than average rate of failure for the vision and hearing screening tests.
- There was a higher absenteeism rate.
- 67% had not seen a dentist compared with 31% at the other schools.
- 24% of the children were overweight but not much more than the children in the other community schools.
- Children between 5 and 8 years old had a higher rate of asthma than in other schools in the same district.

Emily was very concerned about these health indicators and wondered if health disparities were contributing to the differences. She knew access to care can be a strong contributor to health disparity. When she continued to assess the situation at her school, she found that:

- Few children had a primary care physician, and many are underinsured or had not accessed all the health benefits available
- Both parents worked and few owned cars

Emily gathered more data from the parents to find out why the children had received less health care than children in the other schools in the district, especially preventive care. The parents reported that the only primary care clinics were located outside the neighborhood and required taking two to three buses with time-consuming transfers. They said the clinics were very crowded and then you spend less than 10 minutes with the care provider. The parents reported that going to the clinic had little value since no one tells them anything about what the doctor has found, nothing about prevention, and no explanation of the prescriptions, if given. Most of the parents used the urgent care clinic in the community, but only when someone was really ill.

The parents mentioned that the department of public health provides free immunization clinics and school physicals for a nominal charge, but they pointed out that both parents are working and they cannot afford to miss a day of work without pay to bring the children. They regreted the clinics do not meet on Saturday or in the evenings. The English-speaking children of parents who do not speak English told Emily that their parents state that none of the clinics had a translator and only one clinic had a Spanish-speaking nurse and another clinic had one physician who speaks Chinese.

Emily analyzed this new information and identified several factors in the health-care system that contributed to the health-care disparity at her school:

- Limited access to care
- Lack of primary care practitioners in the overburdened clinics
- No primary health care in the immediate neighborhood
- Health department clinics that meet at hours inaccessible to the working population in the community
- Poor public transportation
- Inadequate cultural competency
- Low health literacy among the parents
- Inadequate racial and ethnic diversity of the health-care staff
- Lack of translators at the clinics

She invited parents, teachers, and staff to attend a meeting to strategize about how some of these factors could be mitigated to reduce the disparity. She held the meeting in the early evening at the school so the working parents could attend with easy access by walking. Several of the teachers and the school counselor saw this as an important component of school health and also agreed to attend. Emily suggested that the parents who do not speak English try to find someone who can translate for them and that the translators can also participate. She encouraged the families to bring others from the community. She pointed out that it is really a community issue and not just a school issue. Emily valued the time of all these stakeholders and tried to be organized to help them arrive at some clear outcomes by the end of the meeting.

At the community meeting parents of the diverse ethnic/racial groups attended, and several brought bilingual friends who facilitated communication. The group had three meetings. Participants offered suggestions and concrete plans to be implemented, some to be done at the school and others in the community. These suggested collaborative actions included the following:

- Improve access to care.
- With the partnership of the local public health department, provide an immunization clinic and school physicals one evening a month (or on Saturday) at the school.
- Negotiate with one of the primary care clinics outside the community and the board of education to provide a satellite comprehensive clinic at the school, developing school space that is underutilized.
- Provide information at the school about the insurance and other health program eligibilities for children of low-income working parents.
- Bridge cultural/literacy gaps.
- Develop evening English as a Second Language (ESL) classes for the parents, coordinated by one teacher at the school, a local social service agency, and volunteers from the local university.
- Start monthly cultural programs organized by the school Parent-Teacher Association to showcase all of the cultures at the school and facilitate more communication among the parents.
- Create information tools that can be used by people with low health literacy to gain information on common childhood illnesses, health promotion and disease prevention actions, and new skills the families can use even with limited resources to navigate the U.S. health-care system. Offer to share these information tools with the local primary care clinics.
- Communicate with the clinics about the need to provide required translation services either with trained, certified volunteers including university students, or with a telephone translation service.

With the assistance and support of the community, Emily and the planning group were ready to design actions to implement some of these changes. Emily had received some small grants to assist with some of the initial planning and program implementation and everyone felt optimistic that most of these actions can be implemented without many additional resources.

Actions to Reduce Health Disparities

There are many actions that nurses can implement to reduce health disparities in the health-care delivery system, whether it is in a community or a hospital setting. As illustrated in the case study, the following actions are usually most successful when incorporating the community and other stakeholders, and frequently do not take huge resources:

- Increase cultural awareness and sensitivity.
- Initiate cultural assessment of the individual, community, or population with appropriate interventions to minimize health inequities. Take care not to display judgmental and inappropriate action. Cross-cultural communication skills are essential.
- Promote training of health-care providers to develop culturally sensitive and empathetic communication skills.
- Increase the diversity of the health-care staff.
- Work with national nursing organizations to support the education of minority students.
- Make sure patients receive equitable health-care services.
- Take on the role of the patient advocate. One must be careful not to be paternalistic, but rather to be helpful in assisting and working together with individuals, families, and community to obtain appropriate and adequate health care.
- Always use a translator when the patient has a different language and is not fluent in English. Use a trained translator; if one is not available within your agency, access other resources such as phone-based translators.
- Recognize that nurses and other care providers are discriminatory. Everyone needs to take the time to examine his or her own behavior, and make certain that when working with individuals, families, and communities people are not treated differently because of their race, religion, gender, appearance, or economic level. The actions may be very subtle, and we may not be consciously aware of them without continuous self-examination.

Health Disparities Have Not Been Solved

The more these areas within the health-care system are examined and positive changes made, the more questions arise because there have been limited results at closing the health disparity gap. Since 2000 it has become clear that the health care provided or not provided is not the only thing that contributes to health disparities. Woolf and colleagues noted that even though the government and private industry have annually invested billions of dollars on new pharmaceutical products and devices, there was little change in the overall mortality rate in the United States. Using U.S. vital statistics for 1996 to 2002, these researchers compared the maximum number of deaths averted with new medical technology with the number of deaths that could have been averted if mortality rates among adults with less than a college education were the same as those with a college education. They found that medical advances averted a maximum of 178,193 deaths. If the disparity in education in the United States had been corrected, the corrected mortality rate would have saved 1,369,335 people in the same period, a ratio of 8:1. According to these authors a better investment for the health of the nation would be equitable education, with the probable outcome of people living longer and healthier lives.[38] With minimal success at decreasing health disparities by changing how we deliver health care, there has been increased focus on examining the social determinants of health.

Social Determinants of Health, Health Disparity, and Social Justice

The **social determinants of health** are the social and environmental conditions in which people live and work. These determinants not only have an impact on infectious and chronic health conditions, but also play a strong role in community violence, individual abusive behavior, drug addictions, and other major population-based public health issues. These social determinants include housing, nutrition, and meeting basic needs, as well as community resources that promote health such as safety, exercise, social relationships, and meeting cultural and religious needs (Fig. 7-1). Raphael's definition provides more depth:

Social determinants of health are the economic and social conditions that shape the health of individuals, communities, and jurisdictions as a whole. Social determinants of health are the primary determinants of whether individuals stay healthy or become ill (a narrow definition of health). Social determinants of health also determine the extent to which a person possesses the physical, social, and personal resources to identify and achieve personal aspirations, satisfy needs, and cope with the environment (a broader definition of health). Social determinants of health are about the quantity and quality of a variety of resources that a society makes available to its members.[39]

International Recognition of Social Determinants of Health

Social determinants of health are major contributing factors to health disparities. We need to look "upstream" for the causes of these disparities. The report of the WHO Commission on Social Determinants of Health clearly states, based on a synthesis of a multitude of global sources, that there is a line of causality from impoverished environment to poor health outcomes.[40] The commission clearly points out the need for economic redistribution and illustrates the consequences of how poverty and social inequality affect the health of the world. Using poverty as a determinant, there is a clear social gradient of health that is seen in communities in the United States and duplicated in industrialized countries such as England and less developed regions such as

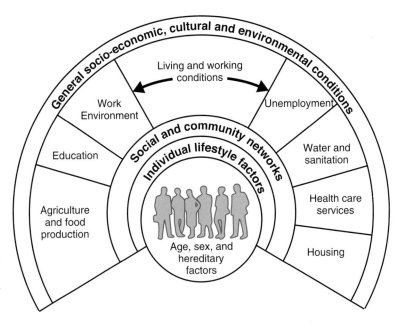

Figure 7-1 What are the social determinants of heath? *(PAHO. [2008]. Introduction to social determinants, unit 1. Retrieved from http:// dds-dispositivoglobal.ops.org.ar/curso/cursoeng/ unidad1B.html.)*

Uganda and Peru. The poorest quarter of the population has the worst health outcomes, the next quarter has better health outcomes than the bottom quarter but not as good as the quarter above, and the top income quarter of the population definitely has the best health outcomes. We need to be careful not only to compare the very poor with the very rich, or the illiterate with the college educated, but also to look across the whole spectrum of determinants such as income and education. The social gradient shows a continuing worsening of health as the income and education decrease, which clearly points out that all of us fall somewhere on this continuum and all of us experience the social determinants of health.

There are stark differences between racial and ethnic groups in the United States, with about twice as many African Americans and Hispanics reporting having fair or poor health as non-Hispanic whites. If the population is looked at using socioeconomic standards, it is even more significant; almost five times as many adults in poverty report fair or poor health compared with those with the highest incomes. Income inequality has been increasing during the past 30 years in the United States, with those at the bottom losing their buying power but with a significant increase in buying power for those at the top. [41]

Several organizations (the WHO, Social Determinants National Conference, the Canadian government, Australian Medical Association, Robert Wood Johnson Foundation) have identified different determinants of health. They have looked at which are the most significant and subject to new policy development:

- Poverty
- Economic inequality
- The state of the economy
- Income and social status
- Transportation
- Stress
- Early life experiences
- Education (early childhood development, number of years completed, health literacy)
- Social exclusion (race/ethnicity, gender, religion, same-sex relationships)
- Employment/working conditions and job security
- Community
- Social support (social safety net)
- Food security
- Life skills
- Personal health practices and coping skills
- Housing

There is evidence that suggests that social determinants of health are equal to or more important than people's behavioral choices such as the use of tobacco, high-fat and high-caloric diets, and a sedentary lifestyle. Raphael noted that current research is demonstrating that socioeconomic circumstances during early childhood are a better predictor of cardiovascular disease and diabetes than lifestyle behaviors. He also noted that social determinants actually structure lifestyle choices.[42] It is interesting to compare national health outcomes between countries who take very seriously providing income, food, and housing security and minimizing wealth inequality (Sweden), compared with countries whose attitude toward these determinants is much more laissez-faire (United States, Canada).

Role of Race

It was thought for a long time that race served as an etiological factor in the high prevalence of type 2 diabetes in African Americans (50% to 100% more likely than in non-Hispanic whites), and in Native Americans who were thought to have a genetic susceptibility (one estimate is that 50% of the Pima Indians have the disease). Geneticists today believe that there are no genetic markers unique to race for diabetes. Sinorello and colleagues investigated whether race accounted for the disparities that exist in type 2 diabetes between African Americans and non-Hispanic whites. These researchers found that the differences between the two races were most probably tied to known nongenetic risk factors that include living in impoverished communities. They found almost equal rates of diabetes in populations (African American and non-Hispanic white) that have the same socioeconomic status.[36] An Indian Health Service report, with no mention of genetic causes, states, "Lower life expectancy and the disproportionate disease burden exist perhaps because of inadequate education, disproportionate poverty, discrimination in the delivery of health services, and cultural differences."[43] The report notes that the disparities in health status could have resulted from the disparities in wealth and power that have endured since colonization.

Researchers today are pondering the role of race in examining health disparities. Race is a social construct with no biological foundation (see Chapter 23). Based on current genetic knowledge, it is understood that race is not a useful clinical marker for disease. However, there are clearly poorer health outcomes among African Americans, American Indian/Alaska Natives, and Hispanics in several disease areas.[43,44] If we do not use race, how do we identify and measure the factors that do contribute to these health disparities? One possibility is to use social class as the real determinant of health. In many European countries, class rather than race is recorded in their national databases and frequently used as the marker. This is also true in several of low income countries. They all verified that those in the lower classes have poorer health outcomes than those in the upper classes. In the past, the United States has not nationally recorded class, and without class data the United States has used race as a proxy for class. However, poverty is not necessarily related to race since 42% of those living in poverty in 2011 were white.[45]

There is a complicated web of causation between race and poor health outcomes (see Chapter 3). Racial housing segregation has been looked at as one part of the web that results in lower socioeconomic status among African Americans. Residential segregation, created out of institutional racism, leads to segregated elementary and high schools that have fewer resources to support learning, decreased opportunities for decent employment, limited access to quality resources to maintain health, and a cascade of other effects such as lack of space for physical activity, poor sources of nutritious food, and limited social interactions/networks. Several researchers have suggested that inattention to eliminating racial housing segregation or the consequences of it may limit the work done to eliminate health disparity.[46-48]

Role of Income and Education

Generally, within the same racial group the social class determines the amount of health disparity. Middle-class and upper-income African Americans have better health outcomes than those African Americans living in poverty, and in an incremental manner. However, this is not always true. African American women who are better educated and in a higher social class are more likely to have lower-birth-weight babies than lower-class African American women. Race may have an independent influence (i.e., personal experience of discrimination and lifestyle) that is divergent from poverty.[41] Current research suggests that race, social class, and education are significantly interrelated but also have independent health influences.[49, 50]

Utilizing 11 health indicators of public health importance to children and adults, a group of researchers in the United States examined socioeconomic disparities.[50] They found a striking social gradient of health using income and education. The richer you were, the healthier you were. This did not hold only for the very poor and the very rich. From the working poor to the middle class to those in the upper income, the more money you had, the better your health. This was also true of education: the more years of education you had, the better your health. However, they also noted that on several indicators,

African Americans did worse than whites at each income and education level. For example, in looking at heart disease, both racial groups had less heart disease as they earned more money and had more years of education. However, with many diseases including heart disease, whites did better than African Americans at each economic level and each educational level.[50] Krieger and colleagues found that the decrease in breast cancer in 2002 was only in white rich women and not in women of color. It was an economic issues and not a racial issue, because the disease decreased only in the group of women who previously could afford to use hormonal replacement therapy and had stopped. All of these authors caution that it is important to examine both socioeconomic and racial/ethnic disparities together.[51] See the following Evidence-Based Practice box for further details.

■ EVIDENCE-BASED PRACTICE
Social Determinants of Cardiovascular Disease Risk Factors

Practice Statement: Identifying social determinants can help health-care providers decrease risk factors for cardiovascular disease.

Targeted Outcome: Minimize cardiovascular risk factors for men, paying particular attention to those with social determinants that indicate higher risk factors.

Evidence to Support: This study found that social determinants of health are associated with cardiovascular disease in men in both urban and rural settings, with black men being more affected. Lower education, unemployment, lower income, and increased stress were the significant health determinants. Rural men were twice as likely to have two risk factors.

Recommended Approaches: To decrease cardiovascular disease it is important for the health providers to address the social determinants with the individual patient. It is also important to take these determinants into consideration when doing program planning and implementation to ensure effectiveness. Nurses might also think of ways they can be successful in changing policies specifically to minimize differences in education and employment in the greater community.

Reference: Quarells, R.C., Liu, J., & Davis, S.K. (2012). Social determinants of cardiovascular disease risk factor presence among rural and urban black and white men. *Journal of Men's Health, 9*(2), 120-126.

Health is not synonymous with health care. Social determinants dictate how individuals are exposed and respond to threats to health, how they utilize primary prevention measures such as vaccinations to decrease health risks, how they manage their illness, and how well they recover. These social determinants are an essential part of the nursing assessment in the community (see Chapter 4). The assessment must acknowledge how these determinants affect the population, the families, and the individuals living in the communities in which the public health nurse (PHN) practices. This knowledge directs choices of program interventions and how these interventions are implemented. It also directs the nurse to advocate and help implement policy changes that affect the community determinants of health.

Solutions to Health Disparities

Despite the challenges, there is some progress, especially in programs that look at all the factors that restrict equitable health care. The *HP 2020* action model reflects an emphasis on the determinants of health by including family and community and looking at the broader picture of income, education, sex, race/ethnicity, geographical location, and access to health care. Also of concern are the natural environments, those that already exist without human intervention, such as a geological area, and the built environments, those that are made by humans, such as cities (Fig. 7-2). For example, poorer urban populations often live in built environments that are poorly maintained and

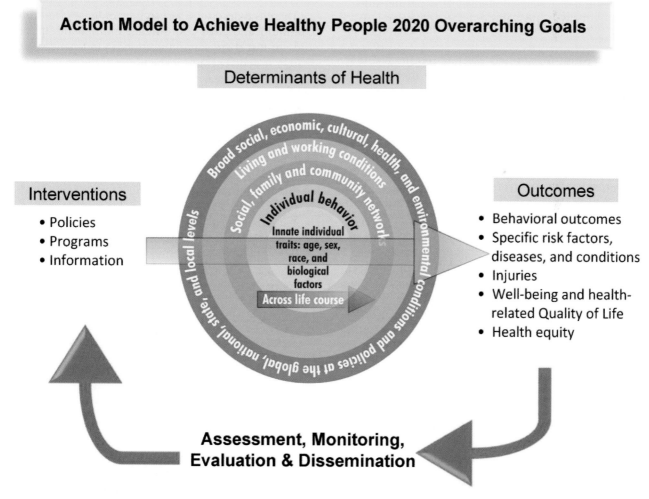

Figure 7-2 Action model to achieve *Healthy People 2020* overarching goals. (*U.S. Department of Health and Human Services. [2008]. Developing Healthy People 2020, executive summary. Retrieved from http://healthypeople.gov/2020/about/advisory/PhaseI.pdf.*)

present significant environmental hazards such as lead paint, whereas wealthier urban populations live in healthier sections of the city that contain more green space.

Office of Minority and Health

In 2012, the CDC's Office of Minority Health (OMH) convened the Science of Eliminating Health Disparities: integrating science policy and practice summit. The summit called for a multipronged approach to advancing the science, policy, and practice related to eliminating health disparities. The session built on the general conclusions from the 2008 summit that health disparity research should focus on:

- Social determinants
- Collaboration and promotion of community engagement
- Promotion of sustainable and effective partnerships
- Media outreach and communication of research findings

The need for the summit was built on the fact that there was no historical model of how to approach this problem nationally and globally. With the acknowledgment of the importance of the social determinants of health, there needs to be interdisciplinary work on the solutions. It requires transformational change to stop health disparities. The National Institutes of Health has recognized the need for research and program implementation in the areas of science, policy, and practice.[52,53] The OMH continues to help to decrease health disparity by maintaining its current levels of programming for minorities, including Native Americans on reservations. The OMH is also supporting and conducting assessment, research, education, and intervention with public and private collaborative partners as suggested by the summit.[2]

The OMH has generated a logic model to assist in better examining the issues of health disparity as a community issue (see Chapter 5). The model, "A Strategic Framework for Improving Racial/Ethnic Minority Health and Eliminating Racial/Ethnic Health Disparity" (Fig. 7-3), can be used by health-care providers, policy makers, community stakeholders, and researchers to move the process along in a unified way.[54] The goal is to create interventions that change outcomes and decrease racial and ethnic disparities. The five purposes of the model are to:

1. Provide policy makers and others concerned with health disparities a better appreciation of the issues
2. Understand better the interrelationship of all the variables
3. Provide a research format and direction for data input

4. Give building blocks to the community stakeholders so they can contribute input and improve structure
5. Improve the systematic planning of data collection, interventions, and evaluation[45]

Paradigm Shift

Leaders in the area of health disparity research and program implementation are proposing the need for a paradigm shift.[53] In relation to research, we need to transform the way we study health disparity, moving from detection and correlation studies to causation and intervention studies. With health disparities there is also a need to focus on translational research. Translational research takes the evidence from controlled randomized trials and tests the findings in real-world settings. These types of studies provide the knowledge needed to choose the best interventions to prevent or correct health disparities.

There is a need for a research team to be clear in its communication and acknowledge multiple disciplines and not just share communication on independent research. A good example is the use of community-based participatory research in which the community and other stakeholders are full partners in conducting the research. This approach requires full collaborative partnership with the community during the research process. It also encourages interdisciplinary studies so that researchers who used to stay within the confines of their own discipline come out of their "silos" and begin partnering with other disciplines. This provides opportunities to examine a problem from more perspectives and perhaps create new theories. With this restructuring we will have the opportunity to approach health disparities differently and create positive change.[53] In addition to changing how we study health disparity, how we address it will also benefit from this paradigm shift.

▶ SOLVING THE MYSTERY
The Case of the Vanishing Buses
Public Health Science Topics Covered:

- Program planning and implementation
- Partnership

James and Rose are two PHNs working in a poor inner-city neighborhood with very mixed ethnic and racial groupings. James works with the teens in the community to increase their knowledge of their own health, teaching them how to make positive decisions and how to set future goals, especially continuing their education. He works in two community centers and has been able to help many of the students to get part-time and summer jobs and internships in different

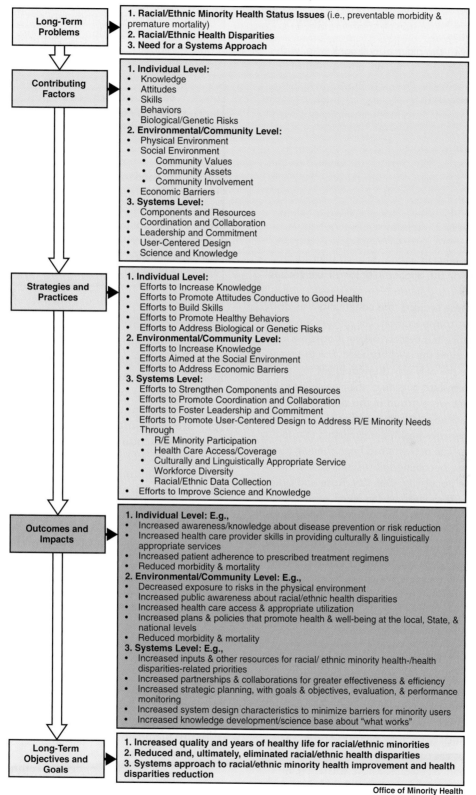

A Strategic Framework For Improving Racial/Ethnic (R/E) Minority Health & Eliminating R/E Health Disparities

Long-Term Problems
1. **Racial/Ethnic Minority Health Status Issues** (i.e., preventable morbidity & premature mortality)
2. **Racial/Ethnic Health Disparities**
3. **Need for a Systems Approach**

Contributing Factors
1. **Individual Level:**
   - Knowledge
   - Attitudes
   - Skills
   - Behaviors
   - Biological/Genetic Risks
2. **Environmental/Community Level:**
   - Physical Environment
   - Social Environment
     - Community Values
     - Community Assets
     - Community Involvement
   - Economic Barriers
3. **Systems Level:**
   - Components and Resources
   - Coordination and Collaboration
   - Leadership and Commitment
   - User-Centered Design
   - Science and Knowledge

Strategies and Practices
1. **Individual Level:**
   - Efforts to Increase Knowledge
   - Efforts to Promote Attitudes Conductive to Good Health
   - Efforts to Build Skills
   - Efforts to Promote Healthy Behaviors
   - Efforts to Address Biological or Genetic Risks
2. **Environmental/Community Level:**
   - Efforts to Increase Knowledge
   - Efforts Aimed at the Social Environment
   - Efforts to Address Economic Barriers
3. **Systems Level:**
   - Efforts to Strengthen Components and Resources
   - Efforts to Promote Coordination and Collaboration
   - Efforts to Foster Leadership and Commitment
   - Efforts to Promote User-Centered Design to Address R/E Minority Needs Through
     - R/E Minority Participation
     - Health Care Access/Coverage
     - Culturally and Linguistically Appropriate Service
     - Workforce Diversity
     - Racial/Ethnic Data Collection
   - Efforts to Improve Science and Knowledge

Outcomes and Impacts
1. **Individual Level: E.g.,**
   - Increased awareness/knowledge about disease prevention or risk reduction
   - Increased health care provider skills in providing culturally & linguistically appropriate services
   - Increased patient adherence to prescribed treatment regimens
   - Reduced morbidity & mortality
2. **Environmental/Community Level: E.g.,**
   - Decreased exposure to risks in the physical environment
   - Increased public awareness about racial/ethnic health disparities
   - Increased health care access & appropriate utilization
   - Increased plans & policies that promote health & well-being at the local, State, & national levels
   - Reduced morbidity & mortality
3. **Systems Level: E.g.,**
   - Increased inputs & other resources for racial/ ethnic minority health-/health disparities-related priorities
   - Increased partnerships & collaborations for greater effectiveness & efficiency
   - Increased strategic planning, with goals & objectives, evaluation, & performance monitoring
   - Increased system design characteristics to minimize barriers for minority users
   - Increased knowledge development/science base about "what works"

Long-Term Objectives and Goals
1. **Increased quality and years of healthy life for racial/ethnic minorities**
2. **Reduced and, ultimately, eliminated racial/ethnic health disparities**
3. **Systems approach to racial/ethnic minority health improvement and health disparities reduction**

Office of Minority Health

Figure 7-3 Logic model of a strategic framework for improving health disparities. *(CDC, Office of Minority Health. [2008]. A strategic framework for improving racial/ ethnic minority health and eliminating racial/ethnic health disparities [Chart]. Retrieved from http://minorityhealth.hhs.gov/images/78/PrintFramework.htm.)*

businesses, exposing them to new and different professional opportunities.

Rose works with the older populations who, with their limited fixed incomes, had become quite isolated, had difficulty accessing primary health care, and had found it increasingly difficult to shop for fresh groceries when the two supermarkets in the community closed. The older adults, feeling vulnerable, were reluctant to walk very far because of their fear of street crime. Rose has created two safe sites for the older men and women to meet, providing both educational and social opportunities, a primary care clinic once a week with a local physician, and a food co-op of fruits and vegetables delivered every 2 weeks by a group of local farmers. One group of the older women was working to increase the co-op participation through their local churches, providing the opportunity for all age groups to participate.

For both of these projects, the community was dependent on public transportation. The seniors were able to get reduced-price bus passes, making it possible for them to move around the neighborhood. For the teens, these buses were the only way they could get to the new jobs and internships outside of their neighborhood.

Rose and James were proud of the success of their projects, and saw these activities as possible solutions to some of the negative health determinants that led to health disparities. The projects had been running for about a year, were becoming self-sustaining, and had both increased in popularity. One day, Rose and James both noticed that they were having fewer participants and that people were often late to arrive. When questioned, both the teens and the older adults were very angry. They said the buses were running less frequently and it seemed that some of the routes had completely disappeared. Everyone knew the city had financial problems that needed to be solved. On further inquiry, it seemed that one solution implemented was to severely cut back on buses, especially in the inner city. The city council, whose members did not ride the buses, had thought this would be the most economic and fair thing to do, a better budgetary solution than cutting education expenditures.

The buses had disappeared from the streets of Rose and James's community. The adults and the project teens had difficulty commuting to their jobs. The seniors could not get to the centers; no one could buy the fresh fruits and vegetables. There was again increased disparity for this already marginalized group. The two PHNs called a community meeting at which they encouraged the community to talk about the impact of the city's decision to limit buses and what they could do about it. The people saw this as unjust and inequitable.

They discussed several options but recognized a need to convince the city council that severely limiting bus service was not the best decision. They sought and got a hearing on the transportation issue. Working together, the two groups were able to demonstrate with program data from Rose and James and from their own survey the need for the bus service and the positive outcomes that resulted from the service. They got media and other community group support, and they worked with some community-based researchers from the local university to look at the broader issues of social determinants. By doing this, they were successful at restoring the public transportation system.

International Solutions

EURO Health for All policy specifies that by 2020 the health disparity gap between European countries and between socioeconomic groups within the countries will be reduced by at least 25%. Understanding the multiple determinants that have an impact on health, they are examining all policy areas at the national, regional, and local levels for their effects on health. The following *EURO Health for All* policy recommendations are being implemented in member countries of the European Union and various other neighboring countries, providing a useful model for similar action in other regions:

- Establish national health inequity targets by identifying and advocating relevant national and regional health targets and by tackling health determinants to reduce health inequalities.
- Work at the local level by supporting community development approaches and the integration of local services, multidisciplinary approaches, and partnerships.
- Reduce barriers to ensure access to and use of effective health-care and prevention services by socially disadvantaged and vulnerable groups.
- Develop indicators and systems for monitoring health inequalities, including systems for collecting data on structural factors and determinants of health, such as social class, gender, and ethnicity.
- Assess health impact by developing and applying procedures, methods, and tools by which policies, programs, and projects may be judged as to their

potential effects on the health of a population and the distribution of those effects within the population.

- Evaluate financial and human resources to ensure sufficiency and to increase knowledge on how to effectively tackle health inequities.
- Create and support opportunities to disseminate models of good practice and evidence-based approaches to tackle health inequalities, including databases of successful interventions.[55]

After a 3-year study, the WHO Commission on Social Determinants of Health identified three overarching recommendations that speak to solutions for the removal of health inequities and creation of universal social justice for all countries:

1. Improve the daily living conditions from before birth to old age, especially among the very young.
2. Increase the equitable distribution of power, money, and resources encouraging social and economic development that also responds to climate change. Be aware of the urban and rural shifts and protect the rights of the rural workers to keep their livelihood and remain healthy. Provide full, fair employment and decent work, and universal health-care coverage that is publicly funded with good primary care.
3. Monitor local, national, and global health inequities, develop policies to decrease these inequities, and provide training of all health professionals in the social determinants of health.[56]

The WHO commission argues that we can decrease health inequities within the span of one generation if we work from multiple angles, from the top down, and from the grassroots up. We can work not only within the health-care system at local and national government levels, but also in other areas to improve education, social planning, transportation, employment, and all the other sections that have been shown to affect the social determinants of health.[56] Sir Michael Marmot, chair of the commission, said, "The key message of our report is that the circumstances in which people are born, grow, live, work, and age are the fundamental drivers of health and health inequity. We rely too much on medical interventions as a way of increasing life expectancy. A more effective way of increasing life expectancy and improving health would be for every government policy and program to be assessed for its impact on health and health equity and to make health and health equity a marker for government performance."[57]

Economic development is frequently thought to be good for the health of the population, but not all economic development is equitable. It is important that the resources from development be invested in increasing the standard of living for everyone, especially for the lowest quarter of the population. Likewise, the money needs to be invested in the national systems such as in health, education, and transportation to have an impact on health disparities.

National Solutions

Another approach is to implement interventions that create the most positive outcome. For example, selecting a chronic disease such as type 2 diabetes as a targeted health issue requires advocating in the United States for better access to primary care. In primary care, the majority of the prevention and treatment has a direct effect on the reduction of morbidity and mortality associated with a chronic disease. If primary care is linked with strengthening consumer and environmental protections laws, that creates an even more powerful model to decrease premature morbidity and mortality and, in the process, decrease health disparity. Freudenberg and Olden suggested that this would provide a cost-effective way to start to achieve equity. They argue that by addressing a common level of causation, the health of all Americans will be affected. It will also be easier to institute public policy and promote social solidarity. They also argue that by focusing on primary care and consumer protection policies and law, there will be a greater emphasis on primary prevention, which has the biggest impact on health and therefore on reducing health disparities.[58]

Others have looked at the Special Supplemental Nutrition Program for Women, Infants, and Children (WIC) program to see whether it is a positive public health intervention to improve health outcomes and decrease racial disparities. Khanani and his colleague at the Cincinnati Health Department looked at prenatal use of WIC by residents in Hamilton County, Ohio, from 2005 to 2008. They found that for African Americans, participation in the program was associated with a significant improvement in infant mortality rates, a decrease in preterm deliveries, and a reduction in racial disparity between African Americans and white participants.[59]

The Robert Wood Johnson Foundation Commission to Build a Healthier America also identified several interventions based on the known determinants of health. The commission's approach was a little different. It identified choices that would optimize federal investments but go beyond the health-care delivery system when decreasing disparities. These interventions are feasible within the current economic climate and pay particular attention to children, in whom the longest-lasting impact will occur. Their very practical interventions include the following:

- Ensure that all children receive high-quality early developmental support including educational and childcare services.
- Fund WIC and Food Stamp programs to provide nutritious food.
- Create public-private partnerships to open and sustain full-service grocery stores in communities without nutritious food.
- Feed children healthy foods in school.
- Require all school-age children to engage in physical activity every day in school.
- Be a smoke-free nation.
- Create "healthy community" demonstrations to evaluate health-promoting policies and programs.
- Develop a "health impact" rating of housing and infrastructure projects.
- Integrate safety and wellness into every aspect of community life.
- Build health into all public and private policies and practices providing policy makers with the needed reliable data.[60]

Nurses Are Part of the Solution

There are several actions that nurses can take in addition to acting directly within the health-care delivery system. These actions focus more on local and national policy, monitoring, and research. However, all of us all of the time should be cognizant of how to increase social justice in our daily practice in the following ways:

- Speak out on the health inequities in communities and in politics. Encourage debates on these issues.
- Advocate for change to decrease inequities for individuals, families, communities, populations, and systems.
- Initiate or support policies to increase physical education in the schools and eliminate all but healthy foods from the lunch and breakfast school menus.
- Contribute to collecting data for indicators of health inequities, and data to change policies.
- Help design clinical guidelines that reduce inequities and support the needs of vulnerable populations.
- Support culturally designed prevention and intervention programs. Programs such as those that support Afrocentric values that encourage relationship building, communalism, respect for elders, and other components can help to decrease stress.[61]
- Understand and communicate that population health is integrated, multilevel, and heavily influenced by

social determinants. This will expand the understanding of disease causation beyond the individual and the core medical sciences. Without this understanding nurses will not be able to appreciate the causes of health disparities and take action to correct or prevent them.
- Share the actual facts of social disparity with health workers and with the community to provide knowledge to hasten change and take informed action.
- Reinvest in the concepts of social justice

A World Without Health Disparities

Health disparities are not natural phenomena. Currently, most of the world's population fails to reach their full health potential. The disparity arises out of inequity and unnatural causes. The development of a country can be judged by the quality of the health of its population, the equal distribution of health across all the social classes, and the availability of a safety net for people who have significant health needs. Everyone—from the local community, including the business community, to the whole government—must be involved in ensuring equity for health. The actual health sector is just one part of all the sectors necessary to create programs and policies to ensure the disappearance of health disparities. A quality health system demonstrates equity at the population level at which everyone has a right to health care, and at the individual level at which everyone regardless of individual characteristics such as race, or age, or sex receives the same quality of care.[62]

■ Summary Points

- Elimination of heath disparities in the United States has been declared a priority and reflected in the goals of *Healthy People 2010* and *Healthy People 2020*.
- Health disparity is the difference in some aspect of health between two or more groups of people. The difference is inequitable, meaning that the difference is unjust, unfair, avoidable, and unnecessary.
- Health disparity is a global problem and is reflected between and within countries.
- In the United States, there are significant differences in the health outcomes of minorities (African Americans, Hispanics, Native Americans) compared with the majority.
- There are documented differences in health care provided at both the health system level and by individual practitioners that include biases, prejudice, stereotyping, poor communication, lack of access to care, and a lack of cultural sensitivity.

- Social determinants of health also help explain health disparities and may be more influential than the health-care delivery system. Social determinants include the social and environmental conditions in which people live and work.
- Several new models have been developed both to study and to implement change using social determinants of health to diminish health disparity. One is to examine all policy as it could relate to health; another is the importance of early childhood development; and another reviews the impact of the built environment on health and community.
- Nurses are an important part of the solution in both providing equal health care and in participating in changing policy that could decrease inequities in the social determinants of health.

▲ CASE STUDY
Community-Level Disparities
Leaning Outcomes

At the end of this case study, the student will be able to:

- Identify the social determinants of health that have the biggest impact in the United States, and in a specific self-identified region in the United States
- Gather data on health disparities for self-identified region
- Examine the impact of public policies, including spending policies, on the social determinants of health

You have just started working in your local community. One of the first things you need to do is make a community assessment. As part of this assessment, you want to collect data to determine the impact of the social determinants of health on health disparities in your community. Identify the community you will assess. Respond to the following questions in preparation for the assessment, as you conduct the assessment, and as you interpret your local data.

1. What are the national characteristics of the United States that influence the type and magnitude of inequities and inequalities?
2. Which social determinants have the biggest impact in your own community? How can you observe or record these differences?
3. Is local public spending oriented to help close some of the gaps?
4. Are their examples of local policies that affect the social determinants of health?

REFERENCES

1. U.S. Department of Health and Human Services. (1985). *Black & Minority Health. Report of the Secretary's Task Force.* Washington, DC: Author.
2. Office of Minority Health. (2011). *About OMH.* Retrieved from http://minorityhealth.hhs.gov/templates/browse.aspx?lvl=1&lvlID=7.
3. Centers for Disease Control and Prevention. (2012). *Office of Minority Health & Health Equity mission.* Retrieved from http://www.cdc.gov/minorityhealth/OMHHE.html.
4. The Library of Congress. (n.d.). *Bill summary and status, 101st Congress (1989–1990), H.R. 5702.* Retrieved from http://thomas.loc.gov/cgi-bin/bdquery/z?d101:H.R.5702.
5. U.S. Department of Health and Human Services, Healthy People.gov. 2020 (2012). *About Healthy People.* Retrieved from http://www.healthypeople.gov/2020/about/default.aspx.
6. Smedley, B., Stith, A., & Nelson, A. (2003). *IOM report: Unequal treatment confronting ethnic and racial disparity in health care.* Washington, DC: National Academies Press.
7. Orsi, J., Margellos-Anast, H., & Whitman, S. (2009). Black-White white health disparities in the U.S. and Chicago: A 15-year progress analysis. *American Journal of Public Health, 100*(2), 349-356.
8. U.S. Department of Health and Human Services. (2014.). Healthy People.gov. 2020: *Health disparities.* Retrieved from http://www.healthypeople.gov/2020/about/disparitiesAbout.aspx.
9. Carter-Pokras, O., & Baquet, C. (2002). What is a "health disparity"? *Public Health Reports, 117,* 426-434.
10. World Health Organization. (1998). *Health promotion glossary.* Retrieved from http://www.who.int/hpr/NPH/docs/hp_glossary_en.pdf.
11. World Health Organization. (1948). *The Universal Declaration of Human Rights.* Retrieved from http://www.un.org/en/documents/udhr/.
12. World Health Organization. (1978). *Declaration of Alma-Ata, International Conference on Primary Care.* Retrieved from http://www.who.int/hpr/NPH/docs/declaration_almaata.pdf.
13. Jones, C. (2010). Why should we eliminate health disparities? *American Journal of Public Health, 100*(Suppl. 1), s47S47-S51.
14. Whitehead, M. (1991). *2000: The concepts and principles of equity and health.* World Health Organization: Regional Office for Europe, Copenhagen, Denmark: World Health Organization, Regional Office for Europe.
15. Hebert, P., Sisk, J., & Howell, E. (2008). When does a difference become a disparity? Conceptualizing racial and ethnic disparities in health. *Health Affairs, 27*(2), 374-382.
16. World Health Organization. (2014). *Global Health Observatory Data Repository: Data by country: MDG 4: Child health: Infant mortality.* Retrieved from. http://apps.who.int/gho/data/view.main.200?lang=en.
17. World Health Organization. (2014). *Global Health Observatory Data Repository: Life expectancy: Data*

by country. Retrieved from http://apps.who.int/gho/data/node.main.688?lang=en.

18. World Health Organization. (2008). *Inequities are killing people on grand scale, reports WHO's Commission.* Retrieved from http://www.who.int/mediacentre/news/releases/2008/pr29/en/index.html.

19. Centers for Disease Control and Prevention. (2014). *Minority Health: Black or African American Populations.* Retrieved from http://www.cdc.gov/minorityhealth/populations/REMP/black.html#Disparities.

20. Centers for Disease Control and Prevention. (2014). *Minority Health: American Indian & Alaska Native Populations.* Retrieved from http://www.cdc.gov/minorityhealth/populations/REMP/aian.html# Disparities.

21. LaVeist, T., Gaskin, D., and & Richard, P. (2011). The economic burden of health inequalities in the U.S. *International Journal of Health Services.* 41(2):231-8.

22. Xu, X., Girgorescu, V., Siefert, K., Lori, J., & Ranson, S. (2009). Cost of racial disparity in preterm births: Evidence from Michigan. *Journal of Health Care for the Poor and Underserved.* , 20, 729-747.

23. U.S. Department of Health and Human Services, Healthy People 2020.gov. (2014). *Disparities.* Retrieved from http://www.healthypeople.gov/2020/about/DisparitiesAbout.aspx.

24. Agency for Healthcare Research and Quality. (2012). *2011 National healthcare quality and disparities report.* Retrieved from http://www.ahrq.gov/research/findings/nhqrdr/nhqrdr11/qrdr11.html.

25. Centers for Disease Control and Prevention. (2013). Racial and Ethnic Approaches to Health REACH program. Retrieved from http://www.cdc.gov/reach/.

26. Centers for Disease Control and Prevention. (2012). *Health insurance coverage.* Retrieved from http://www.cdc.gov/nchs/fastats/hinsure.htm.

27. Agency for Healthcare Research and Quality. (2009). *2008 National healthcare quality and disparities report.* Retrieved from http://www.ahrq.gov/qual/qrdr08.htm.

28. Wilper, A.P., Woolhandler, S., Lasser, K.E., McCormick, D., Bor, D.H., & Himmelstien, D.V. (2009). Health insurance and morality in US adults. *American Journal of Public Health,* 99(12), 2289-2295.

29. Henry J. Kaiser Family Foundation. (2013). The Impact of the Coverage Gap in States not Expanding Medicaid by Race and Ethnicity, *Issues Brief.* December, 2013. Retrieved from http://kff.org/disparities-policy/issue-brief/the-impact-of-the-coverage-gap-in-states-not-expanding-medicaid-by-race-and-ethnicity/.

30. World Health Organization. (2010). *The world health report—health systems financing: The path to universal health care.* Retrieved from http://www.who.int/whr/2010/en/index.html.

31. HealthCare.gov. (2013). *The health care law and you.* Retrieved from http://www.healthcare.gov/law/index.html.

32. Schwartz, M.D. (2012). The US primary care workforce and graduate medical education policy. *Journal of American Medical Association* 308(21), 2252-2253. doi:10.1001/jama.2012.77034.

33. Auerbach, D.I. (2012). Will the nurse practitioner workforce grow in the future? *Medical Care, 50*(7), 606-610.

34. The Sullivan Commission. (2004). *Missing persons: minorities in the healthcare professions.* Retrieved from www.sullivancommission.org.

35. Health Resources and Services Administration. (2013). *Culture, language and health literacy.* Retrieved from http://www.hrsa.gov/culturalcompetence/index.html.

36. Katz, M., James, A., Pignone, M., Hudson, M., Jackson, V., and & Campbell, M. (2004). Colorectal cancer screening among African American church members: A qualitative and quantitative study of patient-provider communication. *BMC Public Health, 4,* doi:10.1186/1471-2458-4-62.

37. Kagawa-Singer, M., Dadia, A., Yu, M., & Surbone, A. (2010). Cancer, culture and health disparities: Time to chart a new course? *CA: A Cancer Journal for Clinicians, 60,* 12-39.

38. Woolf, S., Johnson, R., Phillips, R., & Philipsen, M. (2007). Giving everyone the health of the educated: An examination of whether social change would save more lives than medical advances. *American Journal of Public Health, 97*(4), 679-683.

39. Raphael, D. (2008). Introduction to the social determinants of health. In D. Raphael, D. (Ed.), *Social determinants of Health: Canadian Perspectives: 2nd Edition.* Toronto, Ontario, Canada: Canadian Scholars' Press.

40. WHO Commission on Social Determinants of Health. (2008). *Closing the gap in a generation: Health equity through action on the social determinants of health. Final report of the Commission on Social Determinants of Health.* Geneva, Switzerland: WHO, 2008 World Health Organization. Retrieved from www.who.int/social_determinants/final_report/en/index.html.

41. Adler, N., & Stewart, J. (2010). *Health disparities across the lifespan: Meaning, methods, and mechanisms.* Annals of New York Academy of Sciences. ISSN 0077-8923.

42. Raphael, D. (2003). Addressing the social determinants of health in Canada: Bridging the gap between research findings and public policy. *Policy Option, 3,* 35-40.

43. Signorello, L., Schlundt, D., Cohen, S. Steinwandel, M., Buchowski, S., McLaughlin, J., Hargreaves, M., & Blot, W. et al. (2007). Comparing diabetes prevalence between African Americans and whites of similar socioeconomic status. *American Journal of Public Health, 97*(12), 2260-2267.

44. Jones, D. (2006). The persistence of American Indian health disparities. *American Journal of Public Health, 96*(12), 2122-2134.

45. U.S. Census Bureau. (2012). *Income, poverty and health insurance coverage in the U.S. 2011.* Retrieved from http://www.census.gov/prod/2012pubs/p60-243.pdf.

46. Williams, D., & Collins, C. (2001). Racial residential segregation: A fundamental cause of racial disparity. *Public Health Report, 116,* 404-416.

47. Schulz, A., Williams, D., Israel, B., & Lempert, L. (2002). Racial and spatial relations as fundamental determinants of health in Detroit. *The Milbank Quarterly, 20*(4), 677-707.

48. Landrine, H., & Corral, L. (2009). Separate and un-equal: Residential segregation and black health dispar-ities. *Ethnic Disease, 19*(2), 179-184.

49. Kiwachi, I., Daniels, N., & Robinson, D. (2005). Health disparity by race and class: Why both matter. *Health Affairs, 24,* 343-352.

50. Braveman, P., Cubbin, C., Egerter, S., Williams, D., & Pamuk, E. (2010). Socioeconomic disparities in health in the U.S.: What the patterns tell us. *American Jour-nal of Public Health, 100*(Suppl. 1), S186-S196.

51. Krieger, N., Chen, J., & Waterman, D. (2010). Decline in US breast cancer rates after the women's health ini-tiative: Socioeconomic and racial/ethnic differentials *American Journal of Public Health, 100*(Suppl.1), S132-S139.

52. Dankwa-Mullan, I., Rhee, K., Williams, K., Sanchez, I., Sy, F., Stinson, N., Ruffin, J. et al. (2010). The science of eliminating health disparities: Summary and analy-sis of the NIH summit recommendations. *American Journal of Public Health, 100*(Suppl. 1), S12-S18.

53. Dankwa-Mullan, I., Rhee, K., Stoff, D., Pohihaus, R., Sy, F., Stinson, N., Ruffin, J. et al. (2010). Moving to-ward paradigm-shifting research in health disparities through translational, transformational, and transdis-ciplinary approaches. *American Journal of Public Health, 100*(Suppl. 1), S19-S24.

54. U.S. Department of Health and Human Services, Office of Minority Health. (2011). *A strategic framework for improving racial/ethnic minority health and eliminating racial/ethnic health disparities.* Retrieved from http://minorityhealth.hhs.gov/templates/content.aspx?lvl=1&lvlid=44&id=8844.

55. Casas-Zamor, J.A., & Ibrahim, S.A. (2004). Confronting health inequity: The global dimension. *American Journal of Public Health, 94*(12), 2055-2058.

56. World Health Organization. (2012). *Social determi-nants of health.* Retrieved from http://www.who.int/social_determinants/en/.

57. BBC News. (2008). *Social factors to ill health.* Re-trieved from http://news.bbc.co.uk/2/hi/7584056.stm.

58. Freudenberg, N., & Olden, K. (2010). Finding synergy: Reducing disparities in health by modifying multiple determinants. *American Journal of Public Health, 100*(Suppl. 1), S25-S30.

59. Khanai, I., Elam, J., Hearn, R., Jones, C., & Maseu, N. (2010). The impact of prenatal WIC participation on infant mortality and racial disparity. *American Journal of Public Health, 100*(Suppl. 1), S204-S209.

60. Robert Wood Johnson Foundation. Commission to Build a Healthier America. (2009). *Beyond health care: New direction to a healthier America.* Recommenda-tions. Retrieved from http://www.commissionon-health.org/Report.aspx?Publication=64498.

61. Gilbert, D., & Goddard, L. (2007). HIV prevention targeting African American women. *Family and Com-munity Health, 30,* 109-111.

62. Koh, H., Oppenheimer, S., Massin-Short, S., Emmons, K., Getter, A., & Viswanath, K. (2010). Translating re-search evidence into practice to reduce health dispari-ties: A social determinants approach. *American Journal of Public Health, 100*(Suppl. 1), S72-S80.

Communicable Diseases

■ Introduction

Four communicable diseases made national headlines in just 1 month—August 2012. There was an outbreak of West Nile virus requiring both on-the-ground and aerial applications of pesticide across a large section of affected areas to kill mosquitoes, the main source of transmission of the virus. The Centers for Disease Control and Prevention (CDC) reported that by the end of August there was a total of 1,590 cases of West Nile virus disease and 65 deaths across 48 states.[1] Another outbreak of a food-borne infectious disease, salmonellosis, caused by the bacteria of the genus *Salmonella*, resulted in a national alert from the CDC to discard cantaloupes grown on a particular farm in Indiana, the identified source of the bacteria. The outbreak affected 204 people in 22 states,

resulting in two deaths.[2] An outbreak of hantavirus pulmonary syndrome was linked to a campsite in Yosemite National Park that resulted in three cases—one probable case and two deaths. This resulted in a national effort to notify all those who had stayed at the campsite of the risk and possible need for treatment.[3] The Ebola outbreak in West Africa that began in March 2014 and extended to May 2015 became a global concern due to the high fatality rate and the spread by air and land to other countries (see Chapter 13).[4] In addition to these outbreaks, during the same month the CDC released a new recommendation that all baby boomers (those born between 1946 and 1966) be screened for the hepatitis C virus because of the high undetected infection rate in this population and the effectiveness of early intervention in the prevention of serious liver disease.[5] These August 2012 headlines demonstrate the very real threat of communicable diseases in today's world as a result of both acute outbreaks and the long-term adverse effects of chronic infection.

Communicable diseases have plagued humankind throughout their existence. As recently as the first part of the last century, communicable diseases were the leading causes of death. In the 1950s and 1960s, chickenpox, measles, and mumps were endemic in school-age children. With the advent of antibiotics and vaccines, communicable diseases were no longer the primary killer of humans with a resulting increase in life expectancy. In the 1980s, the effectiveness of vaccines and antibiotics led some health-care providers to predict that communicable diseases would be eliminated in many sections of the world, especially after the successful eradication of smallpox worldwide.[6] While these pronouncements were being made, a new infectious disease emerged, AIDS caused by HIV. During this period, other diseases emerged such as those caused by the Ebola family of viruses. At the same time the predicted decline in the incidence of other communicable diseases such as tuberculosis (TB) did not occur.

In the 21st century, communicable diseases are a main reason for morbidity and mortality in the United States and the world. In the United States, acute respiratory infections, including influenza and pneumonia, are listed in the top 10 leading causes of death.[7] The mortality rate linked to communicable diseases remains high in low-income countries, accounting for almost 40% of all deaths (Table 8-1).[8] For middle-income countries 4 of the top 10 leading causes of death are related to communicable diseases. For high-income countries only acute respiratory diseases are on the list of the top ten causes of death.[8]

A major responsibility of public health officials from the local to the global level is to conduct surveillance so that action can be taken to determine whether there is a communicable disease epidemic that threatens the health of populations. The term **epidemic** is the combination of two Greek terms, *epi* (upon) and *demos* (people), and has the same roots as the term *epidemiology* (see Chapter 3). At first the term *epidemic* was used to describe a collection of illnesses based on their characteristics such as diarrhea or cough, but with the arrival of the Black Death (bubonic plague) in Europe the word was used to describe the increased occurrence of a single disease.[9] In the 21st century, the term *epidemic* is used when there is a significant increase in cases that would normally occur. **Endemic** refers to the usual number of cases of a disease that occur within a population. At the other end of the spectrum, **pandemic** describes epidemics that are occurring across the globe.

Communicable Diseases and Nursing Practice

Communicable diseases are a public health issue and an important issue for all nurses working in the community and in acute care settings. Nurses are confronted with communicable diseases on a constant basis, and not only provide care to patients with a communicable disease disease, but also are required to incorporate preventive

TABLE 8–1	Top 10 Leading Causes of Death Linked to Communicable Disease by Country Level of Income		
Cause of Death	Low Income	Middle Income	High Income
Lower respiratory disease Percentage of deaths	Number 1 11.3%	Number 4 5.4%	Number 5 3.8%
Diarrheal diseases Percentage of deaths	Number 2 8.2%	Number 5 4.4%	–
HIV/AIDS Percentage of deaths	Number 3 7.8%	Number 6 2.7%	–
Malaria Percentage of deaths	Number 5 5.2%	–	–
Tuberculosis Percent deaths	Number 7 4.3%	Number 8 2.4%	–
Neonatal infections	Number 10 2.6%	–	–
Total Percentage of Deaths	**39.4%**	**14.9%**	**3.8%**

Source: See reference 8.

measures in their practice, such as the use of personal protection equipment (PPE) and proper cleaning of patient areas to prevent transmission of these diseases to themselves, coworkers, and other patients. These practices protect individuals and populations. For the practicing nurse, an understanding of communicable diseases at both an individual level and a population level is essential. If the nurse only focuses on caring for the patient with a communicable disease without taking into account the implications for the population, the care falls short and potentially endangers others.

The key to all these activities is to understand the infectious agents that cause disease, the environment relevant to the transmission of disease from one person to another, and who is at risk for becoming infected. Professional nurses back up their interventions related to the prevention and treatment of communicable diseases with knowledge of the public health science behind these interventions. In the same way that nurses do not dispense medications without understanding the pharmacokinetics behind the medications, nurses cannot intervene in relation to communicable diseases without understanding the science behind these diseases.

Public health science provides the basis for understanding how communicable diseases have an impact on the health of humans. Professional nurses armed with the scientific knowledge related to infectious agents are able to intervene in ways that reduce the risk for not only their individual patients and themselves but also the larger population they serve, with prevention the primary goal.

Communicable Disease and the Burden of Disease

Twenty-first-century improvements in technology and transportation have brought populations closer together and eliminated geographical barriers to transmission of disease. This increases the possibility of spreading communicable diseases that in the past may have been contained in one geographical area. Chapter 13 covers a number of communicable diseases in more depth from a global perspective. This chapter provides an overview of the communicable diseases that are leading causes of death with a focus on incidence and prevalence in the United States.

Infectious Respiratory Disease

A number of infectious agents are associated with respiratory disease (Box 8-1). These diseases are either bacterial or

| BOX 8–1 | **Respiratory Communicable Diseases that can Infect the Respiratory System** |

Chickenpox
Diphtheria
Group A *Streptococcus*
Haemophilus influenzae type b
Influenza
Legionnaire's disease
Measles (rubeola)
Mumps
Pneumococcal meningitis
German measles (rubella)
Tuberculosis
Whooping cough (pertussis)
Anthrax
Hantavirus pulmonary syndrome
Plague

viral. Many of these diseases can be prevented through vaccination. All children are required to receive vaccination for many of the communicable respiratory diseases prior to attending public school, such as vaccines for prevention of chickenpox, diphtheria, and rubella. A new policy for most health-care settings is to require that all employees receive an annual flu vaccine. Because of vaccination programs across the United States and other countries, the incidence of many of these diseases is declining. Despite these advances, respiratory disease caused by infectious agents continues to be a major public health issue. Some of these diseases are seasonal, for example, influenza (flu). Many have a higher morbidity and mortality rate in vulnerable populations, such as older adults and children.

A major public health concern in relation to infectious respiratory disease is the flu. Flu is seasonal, with a peak in early December and a peak in February. Because of the higher mortality rate in vulnerable populations such as children, older adults, and those who are already ill, many hospitals require that all employees receive a flu vaccination. The CDC publishes a report titled *FluView* that follows trends in flu across the year. Trends in flu vary from year to year. In 2009–2010, there was a pandemic outbreak of H1N1 influenza that peaked earlier in October, which resulted in an estimated midrange of 61 million cases, 240,000 hospitalizations, and 12, 470 deaths. In contrast, the 2011–2012 flu season was the mildest season on record (Fig. 8-1).[10]

Malaria

Malaria is a subtropical disease caused by a parasite, the intraerythrocytic protozoa of the genus *Plasmodium*

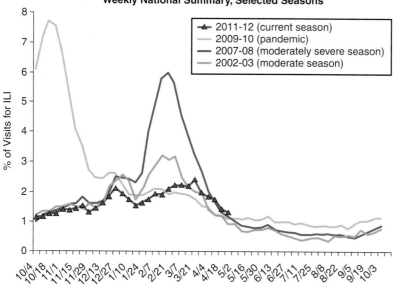

Percentage of Visits for Influenza-Like Illness (ILI) Reported by the U.S. Outpatient Influenza-Like Illness Surveillance Network (ILINet), Weekly National Summary, Selected Seasons

†There was no week 53 during these seasons, so the week 53 data point is an average of weeks 52 and 1.

Figure 8-1 Flu trends. *(Centers for Disease Control and Prevention. [2012]. 2011–2012 flu season draws to a close. Retrieved from http:// www.cdc.gov/flu/spotlights/2011-2012-flu-season-wrapup.htm.)*

transmitted through the bite of an infected mosquito.[11] About half of the world's population is at risk for malaria. According to the World Health Organization (WHO), in 2010 an estimated 655,000 deaths, mostly African children, were caused by malaria. The estimated number of cases in 2011 was 216 million. In comparison, in 2009 in the United States, there were 1,484 cases of malaria with four fatalities.[11,12] Malarial infections in the United States are primarily the result of exposure that occurred during travel abroad. In addition, these travelers had not adhered to recommended malaria prophylaxis. Malaria is a preventable disease and much is being done globally to eradicate it (Chapter 13). The economic and social burdens affect both individuals and governments in terms of the cost of care, lost work, and burial expenses. The cost just for treatment is estimated at $12 billion annually.[13]

Human Immunodeficiency Virus (HIV) and Acquired Immune Deficiency Syndrome (AIDS)

HIV impairs and destroys the immune cells in the infected person's body, affecting the ability to fight off infection. A person infected with HIV may not develop AIDS until 10 to 15 years after the initial infection. AIDS is diagnosed when a person infected with HIV develops cancer, infections, or other clinical symptoms associated with HIV infection. HIV has killed 25 million

people over the past three decades.[9] In 2011, an estimated 34.2 million people were living with HIV/AIDS worldwide.[14] In the United States, an estimated 1.2 million people are living with HIV/AIDS, approximately 50,000 persons become infected each year, and nearly 20% of those infected with HIV are unaware they are infected.[15]

The prevalence of HIV and AIDS is higher among persons in the 25- to 44-year-old age group, those who are African American and Hispanic, and in men. Racial disparity is especially apparent in children, with 80% of all pediatric cases being African American or Hispanic. HIV infection is also on the rise among older adults.[16] Certain behaviors increase the risk for transmission of HIV, including men having sex with men, those engaging in injection drug use, and those engaging in unprotected sex.[15] There is also variation in the distribution of cases geographically, with the majority of cases (55%) coming from New York, California, Florida, Texas, and New Jersey.[17] Prevalence is also growing in the older population because of increased longevity of those living with HIV as well as an increase in risky behaviors in this age group.[18]

Healthy People 2020 (HP 2020) has a separate topic related to HIV. The objectives related to the topic not only address disparity but also prevention, screening, and treatment.

■ HEALTHY PEOPLE 2020
HIV

Goal: Prevent HIV infection and its related illness and death.

Overview: The HIV epidemic in the United States continues to be a major public health crisis. An estimated 1.1 million Americans are living with HIV, and 1 out of 5 people with HIV does not know he or she has it. HIV continues to spread, leading to about 56,000 new HIV infections each year.[2]

In 2010, the White House released a National HIV/AIDS Strategy. The strategy includes three primary goals:

1. Reducing the number of people who become infected with HIV
2. Increasing access to care and improving health outcomes for people living with HIV
3. Reducing HIV-related health disparities[19]

Diarrheal Disease

Diarrhea is defined by the WHO as the passage of three or more loose or liquid stools per day. There are approximately 2 billion cases of diarrheal disease worldwide each year.[20] In low-income countries, it is a leading cause of death among children below the age of 5. The most common route for transmission of diarrheal disease is the fecal-oral route. Good hand hygiene, especially hand washing, and soap alone can reduce the incidence of diarrheal disease by as much as 48%.[21] Efficient sanitary systems and safe drinking water also play a huge role in prevention of diarrheal diseases.

Pathogens that cause diarrheal disease include viruses, bacteria, and protozoa. Transmission is usually waterborne (e.g., cholera), foodborne (e.g., *Escherichia coli* [*E. coli*]), or through person-to-person contact, and pathogens can infect the small bowel, the colon, or both. Worldwide, rotavirus is the most common cause of diarrheal disease among children, accounting for almost 40% of all cases of infant diarrhea, and is responsible for half a million deaths in children under 5 years old.[21,22] Until recently, infections with rotavirus among children under the age of 5 resulted in up to 70,000 hospitalizations and 60 deaths annually. In 2006, a vaccine was introduced that has helped reduce the incidence of this disease. There are now two vaccines available for use with infants, and subsequent to their introduction the incidence of rotavirus-associated diarrheal infections in children has declined.[21]

Emerging and Reemerging Communicable Diseases

The WHO defines an emerging disease as "one that has appeared in a population for the first time, or that may have existed previously but is rapidly increasing in incidence or geographic range."[23] Through public health efforts, some communicable diseases are close to eradication, for example, polio mellitus and dracunculiasis (guinea worm disease), or have been eradicated, as in the case of smallpox. Yet at the same time new communicable diseases have emerged such as severe acute respiratory syndrome (SARS) and West Nile virus infection, while other diseases such as malaria, TB, and bacterial pneumonias, are remerging in forms that are resistant to drug treatments, for example, multidrug resistant tuberculosis (MDRTB).[23,24] New diseases are emerging at a rate of one per year. In the first decade of the 21st century, emerging communicable diseases made global headlines such as SARS and the H1N1 flu virus as the incidence rate hit pandemic proportions. Response to such diseases results in a burden on the economic, social, and health-care systems of countries. Pandemics such as the SARS outbreak and epidemics within countries such as the West Nile virus epidemic in the summer of 2012 require a coordinated early response across political entities such as countries or states.

Tuberculosis

TB is an infectious disease caused by the *Mycobacterium tuberculosis*. TB in the past was referred to as the "white death," and has been part of the history of humankind. It has been called many names, from the great white plague to consumption. The word *consumption* is even found in the Bible. It wasn't until the end of the 19th century that the disease received the name *tuberculosis* after the agent that caused the disease was identified. In 1889, the National Tuberculosis Association (now the National Lung Association) realized that TB was preventable and not inherited. Since that time, prevention efforts have resulted in a steady downward trend in the incidence and prevalence of TB, so much so that 100 years later, in 1998, a TB elimination project was initiated in the United States with the target date of 2010 for TB elimination. Though this has not occurred, the downward trend in TB incidence and prevalence is encouraging. Continued efforts are needed to address the disparity between U.S.-born and foreign-born individuals as well as between whites and minorities.[25]

Back in 1988, infection control experts were optimistic that the elimination of TB was a realistic goal. Unfortunately, at the same time reports began to emerge of hospital-acquired MDRTB outbreaks. Between 1988 and 1992 five clusters of TB cases appeared in six hospitals. Four occurred in New York City, one in Florida, and one in New York State. What stood out about these cases was that the agent *M. tuberculosis* had mutated (changed) and was now resistant to drugs used to treat active TB. Surveillance was initiated that identified more patients who met the case definition of MDRTB. Upon investigation, a number of issues emerged. First, most of the patients were also infected with HIV. With HIV, TB does not always present in the classic manner and diagnosis was delayed in these cases. In addition, recognition of drug resistance was hampered by the length of time it took to complete the drug susceptibility tests. The **case fatality rate (CFR)** was high. A CFR is determined by taking the number of fatal cases and dividing it by the total number of cases. Within 16 weeks of diagnosis, 72% to 89% of patients had died.[26] Since that time, dramatic changes have taken place in acute care setting including strict Occupational Health and Safety Administration (OSHA) guidelines.

Globally in 2010, there was a total of 8.8 million cases of TB and 1.1 million TB deaths in HIV-negative persons. There were an additional 0.35 million deaths due to HIV-associated TB. In 2010 in the United States, there were 11,181 reported cases of TB. Overall, both the prevalence and incidence of TB are decreasing.[27] The number of new cases in 2010 in the United States was the lowest since 1953. However, the national goal to eliminate TB (less than 0.1 case per 100,000 population) was not met.[25] In the United States, TB rates in 2010 were 11 times higher in foreign-born residents than in U.S.-born residents. Also, among U.S.-born residents the rate for non-Hispanic blacks was seven times higher than that for non-Hispanic whites.[25]

The story of TB rates in the United States illustrates the importance of following trends of communicable diseases. As mentioned earlier, many communicable diseases must be reported to the health department. This information is electronically forwarded from all 50 states and the District of Columbia to the CDC. The CDC follows these trends of data over time. On the surface this is a simple process in that the total number of cases is followed by year. However, just knowing the number of cases does not provide the CDC with additional information needed to protect the health of the public. Through careful surveillance of TB, the CDC is able to determine who is at greatest risk based on numerous factors such as race, age, geographical location, and place of birth. The CDC can then examine whether the goal of eliminating TB is being met, and if not, where it needs to concentrate its efforts to meet the goal of TB's elimination.

▶ SOLVING THE MYSTERY
The Case of the Wandering Patient

In February 2002, a 42-year-old man with HIV and schizophrenia was admitted twice to one hospital for fever and unproductive cough. Chest radiographs were read as normal and a sputum culture was negative for *M. tuberculosis*. In April, he was admitted to another hospital with similar symptoms, treated with antibiotics, and released. Three days later he was readmitted and treated for suspected pneumonia. However, his stool culture came back positive for *M. tuberculosis*. A subsequent acid-fast bacillus (AFB) smear test was 4+, indicating that he was highly infectious. Despite the fact that he was placed in isolation, he continued to have contact with other patients and hospital personnel owing to a lack of vigilance on the part of the staff to observe strict isolation procedures, with serious consequences.[28]

The investigation into this case started with identifying the **index case,** that is, the first case identified in a particular outbreak. Because the normal mode of transmission is airborne from person to person, identifying the index patient provides the investigators with the starting point for their investigation. The investigators working on this case identified this 42-year-old man as the index case.

Their next step was to identify **secondary cases,** that is, patients who were diagnosed with active TB and who had contact with the index patient. Five secondary cases were identified; one had diabetes and HIV, one had diabetes, two had end-stage renal disease, and one was a phlebotomist. The first two steps of the investigation were now complete, identifying the index patient and secondary patients, but the investigation did not stop there. Because the index patient's sputum came back with a 4+ AFB smear, there was a high level of infectivity, that is, anyone who came in contact with the patient was probably exposed to a high level of the *M. tuberculosis* bacillus. If that were the case, then everyone who came in contact with the patient would be at risk.

The next step in the investigation was to identify all contacts. With some agents, once humans are infected with an agent the incubation period prior to the occurrence of symptoms is short and can last less than a week. In others, it might be a little longer and last up to 3 months, as with syphilis. With TB, a person can become infected and show no sign of disease for decades. This is known as latent TB. The investigators identified a total of 1,045 contacts, both patients and employees of the hospital. They were able to test close to two-thirds of all these contacts. Eleven percent of the tested employees tested positive and 23% of the tested patients tested positive. Those who tested positive were provided appropriate interventions to prevent development of disease.[28]

This case illustrates the challenges faced in identifying the presence of an active infection and the urgency of taking measures to prevent further spread of the infection. The investigation focused on three stages: (1) identification of the index patient; (2) finding secondary cases; and (3) investigation of contacts. The report included recommendations for hospital infection control programs.[28] The patient had been placed in isolation and the investigators established that the isolation room was in accordance with appropriate isolation procedures. However, the patient came into contact with other patients, so the possibility is raised that the patient did not remain in his room.

This case highlights the issue of isolation procedures in health-care agencies (see Chapter 15). The type of isolation is based on the cycle of transmission. Nurses are required to institute appropriate isolation procedures based on the known or suspected agent. These procedures are public health interventions aimed at preventing the spread of disease in three populations (other patients, employees, and community visitors). For airborne agents such as the bacterium that causes TB, isolation procedures involve preventing the spread of the agent through the hospital ventilation system, thus the need for negative pressure rooms. A negative pressure room is used in hospitals when respiratory isolation is needed. The ventilation system uses negative pressure so that air can come into the room but does not go back out into the building but is instead ventilated to the outside. Choosing the right level of isolation requires knowing how the agent is transmitted to humans (person-to-person, airborne, etc.).

Infectious Agents and the Cycle of Transmission

Public health departments are charged with protecting the population at large from the spread of infection. This requires understanding the cycle of infection. The key components of the cycle of infection begin with the epidemiological triangle, which includes the three main constructs needed for disease to occur in humans, the agent, the environment, and the host (see Chapter 3,

Fig. 3-2). In communicable diseases, the epidemiological triangle is expanded to help understand the cycle of transmission of the infectious agent from the reservoir to the host (Fig. 8-2).

Agent Characteristics

The term **agent** or **pathogen** is used in reference to the infectious organism that causes the disease such as a virus or a bacteria. Knowledge of agent characteristics begins with a review of the six general categories of pathogens based on the biological properties of the pathogens (Table 8-2). The categories include bacteria, rickettsia, viruses, mycoses (fungi), protozoa, and helminths. Also grouped with these agents are arthropods, parasitic insects that in themselves do not cause disease but transmit disease (e.g., ticks, fleas, and mosquitoes). This category also includes head, body, and pubic lice, though only body lice are known to transmit disease. The other two types of lice are included, because scratching from lice can result in a secondary bacterial infection of the skin and lice are transmitted from human to human.

Once the class of the pathogen is known, the specific characteristics of the category provide further necessary information. For example, if the pathogen is a helminth, it is a parasitic worm. This relates directly to the biological characteristics of the group of pathogens. Knowing the class of pathogen can help with the care of the individual patient. For example, because general antibiotics work with bacteria but not with viruses, knowing the class of the pathogen can

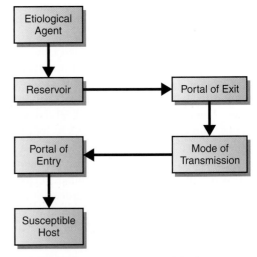

Figure 8-2 The cycle of communicable disease transmission.

TABLE 8–2	Types of Infectious Agents	
Category	Type of Agent	Examples of Diseases
Bacteria:	Microorganism, unicellular Either gram-positive or gram-negative	Bacterial meningitis Anthrax Bubonic plague Tuberculosis Streptococcal infections
Rickettsia:	Though in a separate class, they are a genus of bacteria that grows in cells. They are structurally similar to gram-negative bacteria	Typhus Rocky Mountain spotted fever
Viruses:	A submicroscopic organism with a protein coat that are a piece of genetic material (RNA or DNA) are microorganisms. They are unable to grow or reproduce outside a host cell.	HIV Common cold Influenza
Mycoses:	A disease caused by fungi	Candida Histoplasmosis Fungal meningitis
Protozoa:	Single-celled animals such as flagellates, amoeboids, sporozoans, and ciliates	Malaria *Giardia* Toxoplasmosis Trichomoniasis
Helminths:	Parasitic worm-like organisms that feed off living hosts	Hookworm Pinworm Trichinosis
Anthropods:	Insects that act as vectors and transmit the agent from its reservoir to its host.	Malaria Dengue fever Lyme disease Bubonic plague

Source: Friss, R.H, & Sellers, T.A. (2014). *Epidemiology for public health practice* (5th ed.). Burlington, MA: Jones & Bartlett.

help to determine whether the patient should receive an antibiotic or an antiviral.

In addition to the class of the agent, other characteristics of the agent are helpful to understand. The first characteristic is the **infectivity** of the agent. This reflects the capacity of an agent to enter and multiply in the host. Some agents have low infectivity, meaning either they have a decreased capacity to enter a human host and/or they have a decreased capacity to multiply once they are in the human host. The next characteristic of an agent is its **pathogenicity,** which is the capacity of the agent to cause disease in the human host. Not all infectious agents have the same capability to cause disease.

Toxigenicity is another key issue with an infectious agent and reflects the pathogen's ability to release toxins that contribute to disease within the human host. Not all agents release toxins. There is also variability between agents in relation to their resistance to survive environmental conditions. For example, HIV survives for only a short time outside its host (the human body), whereas anthrax can survive for decades in the soil or in warehouses where untreated animal hides have been processed.

Another important characteristic of the agent is the virulence of the agent. **Virulence** is defined as the ability of the pathogen to cause disease. Finally, agents differ on **antigenicity,** defined as the ability of the agent to produce antibodies in the human host. For example, prior to the arrival of vaccines, parents attempted to expose their children to infectious parotitis (mumps). Because a case of mumps usually results in the development of antibodies, the parents hoped their children would develop immunity to mumps during childhood because the disease can cause serious complications in adults. Thus, mumps virus has a high level of antigenicity.

Environmental Characteristics

Reservoir

The **environment** refers to the conditions external to the host and the agent associated with the transmission of the agent. The first of these is the **reservoir,** or where the agent resides. For the majority of communicable diseases, the reservoir is a human (the agent resides in an infected human). Another common reservoir is animals, and these communicable diseases are known as zoological diseases (e.g., Lyme disease and anthrax). For Lyme disease, the agent is a spirochete, *Borrelia burgdorferi,* and the reservoir is both animals and humans. For anthrax the reservoir is also animals, including elephants, hippopotami, cattle, sheep, and goats, and in spore form the reservoir is soil exposed to the feces of these animals. Reservoirs also include water (waterborne diseases), food (foodborne diseases), and the air (airborne diseases).

The human reservoir can be a person who is acutely ill or someone who is a **carrier,** which is defined as a human who is infected but who has no outward signs of disease. There are four main types of carriers: an incubating carrier, an inapparent carrier, a convalescent carrier, and a chronic carrier. An **incubating carrier** is someone who has been infected, but has not yet shown signs of the disease. An **inapparent carrier** is someone who is infected but does not develop the disease, yet continues to shed the agent, such as Typhoid Mary (Box 8-2). A **convalescent carrier** is a person who is infected but who no longer shows signs of acute disease. The **chronic carrier** remains infected with the agent with no sign of disease for a long period of time.

Mode of Transmission

The next consideration is the mode of transmission, the method through which the agent leaves its reservoir and enters its host. Transmission can occur through water, food, air, vectors, fomites, unprotected sexual contact, or penetrating trauma (Table 8-3). Vectors are usually insects that carry the disease from the reservoir to humans without becoming ill themselves. A fomite is an inanimate object. An infected host touches the object and sheds the agent onto the object. The agent is then transmitted to the next person who touches the object. Possible fomite transmission of the cold or the flu virus is used by marketers to sell their disinfecting products.

BOX 8–2   Typhoid Mary

Mary Mallon worked as a cook and had no idea that she was an inapparent carrier of typhus. She was the first identified "healthy carrier" of typhoid fever in the United States. She worked in several households between 1900 and 1907. During that time members in each household came down with typhus. She even nursed those who were sick, continuing to spread the disease. Though public health officials explained to her the reason she needed to be quarantined, she did not believe that she could spread the disease. Because of her disbelief, she escaped from her quarantine and went back to working as a cook. When she was once again apprehended she was taken to North Brother Island near New York City and remained there for 3 years. She was released when she promised not to work as a cook. She worked as a laundress for a period of time but the wages were low, so she changed her name and once again took a job as a cook, this time at New York's Sloane Hospital for Women. She infected 25 people and one died. She was apprehended again by authorities and spent the rest of her life on North Brother Island. Her name has become synonymous with the healthy carrier of disease.

Source: Leavitt, J.W. (1996). *Typhoid Mary: Captive to the public's health.* Boston, MA: Beacon Press.
For more information, watch the PBS special *The Most Dangerous Woman in America*: http://www.pbs.org/wgbh/nova/typhoid/.

Life Cycle of an Infectious Agent

The two aspects of the environment, reservoir and mode of transmission, are best illustrated through a review of the life cycle of an infectious agent. The life cycle provides essential information on the environment and how an agent goes from its normal reservoir to the host, known as the mode of transmission. Some agents have complex life cycles, such as the human hookworm (*Ancylostoma duodenale* or *Necator americanus*) (Fig. 8-3).[29] For other agents the life cycle of the vector is more important than the agent's own life cycle, as in the case of the agent responsible for Lyme disease, *B. burgdorferi*. A vector transmits the agent without becoming infected itself. The reservoir for *B. burgdorferi* includes mice, squirrels, and other small animals. This is where the agent resides. The blacklegged tick then transmits the agent among these animals to humans by biting an animal infected with the agent (the reservoir) and then biting a human. The blacklegged tick has a 2-year life cycle. This life cycle, rather than the life cycle of the agent, provides the environmental information needed to develop prevention programs. The tick feeds on small animals in the larval and nymphal stage and on deer in the adult stage. During the nymphal stage, the tick is most aggressive and more apt to bite the

TABLE 8–3	Types of Transmission	
Type of Transmission	Examples	Examples of Breaking the Cycle of Transmission
Fomite transmission: An inanimate object carries the pathogen from the reservoir to the host.	Transferring of viruses on the surface of inanimate surfaces such as a phone. Transferring of lice through exchange of clothing. Using a cutting board for meat products and then vegetables without cleaning the board in between use.	Decontamination of the fomite through the use of disinfectants or proper cleaning.
Aerosol or airborne transmission: The agent is contained in aerosol droplets and is transferred from one human to another or animal to human.	Transferring of the agent through the air, usually after the human host expels droplets into the air by coughing or sneezing.	Use of negative pressure rooms in hospitals and personal protective equipment such as face masks.
Oral transmission: The agent is transferred through food or water.	Ingestion of food or water contaminated with the agent such as cholera in untreated water and E. coli through the ingestion of contaminated beef	Eradication of the agent through cleaning of the water supply, implementation of food processing regulations, proper cooking of foods, hand hygiene.
Vectorborne transmission: An insect acquires the agent from an animal and transmits it to another.	Fleas, ticks, and mosquitoes are common vectors of agents to humans.	Eradication of the vector such as control of mosquito breeding grounds, use of insect repellent, and mosquito netting.
Zoonotic transmission: The agent is transmitted directly from animals to humans.	Dogs, sheep, pigs are common sources of direct transmission from animals to humans such as hookworm or rabies.	Vaccination of the animal.
Person-to-person transmission: The agent is transmitted through direct contact between persons, usually through contact with mucous membranes, blood, or saliva. It also occurs through venereal and in utero routes.		Vaccination such as the hepatitis B vaccine, use of personal protective equipment.

host. The tick's life cycle explains what seasons of the year humans can become infected and clarifies the mode of transmission.

The life cycle of the agent or the vector provides added information on the transmission of an infectious agent, including how the agent exits its reservoir (portal of exit), the mode of transmission (water, vector, fomite, etc.), and how the agent enters the host (the portal of entry). For example, the agent that causes TB, *M. tuberculosis*, primarily infects the lungs; thus, the portal of exit is through coughing. The action of coughing expels the agent from

the reservoir (human) into the air. The agent has now left its reservoir and is contained in the droplets expelled from the lungs. The mode of transmission is through the air, so TB is considered an airborne disease. The portal of entry for TB is almost always through the host's respiratory system (the host breathes in the droplets that contain the agent and inhales them into the lungs).

Host Characteristics

The final aspect of the cycle of transmission is the host. The **host** is the human who is at risk for disease due to

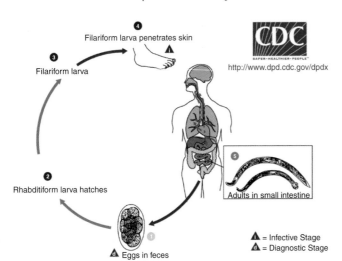

Figure 8-3 Life cycle of the hookworm.

exposure to the agent. The main characteristic is the **susceptibility** of the host, that is, the likelihood of becoming infected with the agent. This is expressed in terms of the host's **immunity,** or **resistance** to the disease.

Immunity

There are two types of immunity, humoral and cellular. **Humoral immunity** means that the host carries antibodies to the agent in the blood, and **cellular immunity** is specific to each type of cell. Immunity is passive or active. When a person has **passive immunity,** immunity is transferred from one individual to another. It can occur naturally or artificially and last for only a short time. Passage of immunity from the mother to her infant is an example of natural passive immunity. Artificial passive immunity involves the transfer of antibodies and can be done in various forms. **Active immunity** is acquired through exposure to the agent. It is long lasting and can last for life, as when a person who had mumps as a child remains immune for the rest of his life.

Inherent Resistance

Another measure of the host's level of susceptibility is **inherent resistance.** This is the ability of the host to resist the disease independent of antibodies. It can be inherited or acquired and is often linked to health status and is temporary rather than permanent. Even if exposed to the agent, the host does not become ill, owing to her own ability to resist the disease because of other factors that boost the body's ability to resist the disease, such as adequate nutrition.

Colonization

Another host characteristic is **colonization.** In this case, a person is infected with the agent but has no signs of infection. This term is mentioned frequently in acute care settings in relation to multiple drug resistant agents such as methicillin-resistant *Staphylococcus aureus.* Patients are admitted with no signs of infection but are colonized with a serious multidrug resistant pathogen. Colonized hosts are able to spread the disease despite not being apparently ill.

Breaking the Chain of Infection

When clinical signs and symptoms are present, the host is not only infected but disease has now occurred. The cycle of transmission is complete. The agent has traveled from the reservoir to the new host and has caused disease. For the nurse, understanding the cycle of transmission for a specific pathogen can guide the type of intervention that is developed to break the chain of infection. Interventions can be aimed at any point in the cycle of transmission. For example, with the outbreak of West Nile virus in Texas in the summer of 2012, the state attempted to break the cycle of infection by eradicating the reservoir, the mosquito, through application of pesticides. The use of mosquito nets in malaria-prone areas attempts to block the mode of transmission by placing a barrier between the portal of exit and the portal of entry.

One of the key components in breaking the chain of transmission is to reduce the susceptibility of the host. This is primarily achieved through vaccination. Because of the importance of this approach, the *HP 2020* topic related to communicable diseases includes a strong focus on immunization. The first objective under this topic is to "reduce, eliminate, or maintain elimination of cases of vaccine-preventable disease"[7] and has 10 vaccine-related targets with 4 out of 10 having a target of total elimination (no cases). The four communicable diseases targeted for elimination through vaccination include acute paralytic poliomyelitis, rubella, hepatitis B, and congenital rubella syndrome.[7]

■ HEALTHY PEOPLE 2020
Immunization and Communicable Diseases

Goal: Increase immunization rates and reduce preventable communicable diseases.

Overview: The increase in life expectancy during the 20th century is largely a result of improvements in child survival associated with reductions in infectious disease mortality because of immunization.[1] However, communicable diseases remain a major cause of illness, disability, and death. Immunization recommendations in the United States currently target 17 vaccine-preventable diseases across the life span.

HP 2020 goals for immunization and communicable diseases are rooted in evidence-based clinical and community activities and services for the prevention and treatment of communicable diseases. Objectives new to *HP 2020* focus on technological advancements and ensuring that states, local public health departments, and nongovernmental organizations are strong partners in the United States attempt to control the spread of communicable diseases. Objectives for 2020 reflect a more mobile society and the fact that diseases do not stop at geopolitical borders. Awareness of disease and completing prevention and treatment courses remain essential components for reducing infectious disease transmission.[7]

Outbreak Investigation

Despite efforts to prevent transmission of disease, outbreaks of infectious disease continue to occur. When they do, public health departments conduct outbreak investigations. An **outbreak investigation** related to communicable diseases involves conducting a systematic epidemiological investigation into the sudden increase in the incidence of a communicable disease. Conducting an outbreak investigation requires solving the mystery similar to what a detective does in solving a murder case, but with communicable diseases, solving the mystery always involves more than knowing "whodunit." In the game Clue, the winning player announces that it was Mrs. White who did it in the parlor with the lead pipe. Unlike in Clue, a communicable disease outbreak investigation requires much more. Investigators seek to identify who got sick, what made them sick, when they got sick, and at what point it happened. The public health team's goal is to gather enough information so that measures can be put in place to halt the spread of disease. These facts are essential to determining what is the best action to take to break the chain of transmission and prevent further spread of the disease to uninfected members of the population. Public health science provides the guide for answering these questions (see Chapter 3). Sometimes the investigation is completed more quickly, as in most foodborne disease outbreaks, but sometimes unraveling the mystery takes much more time and

detective work, especially if the disease is an emerging disease as was the case with HIV in the 1980s.

▶ SOLVING THE MYSTERY
The Case of the Halloween Cider
Public Health Science Topics Covered:
- Epidemiology
- Surveillance

Susan and Mary, the infection control nurses in two hospitals located in the same county, noticed an increase in positive laboratory results for *E. coli* 0157:H7 infections in their patients. On Monday, the laboratory informed Mary that there were two patients with positive results for *E. coli* 0157:H7. Mary called Susan to see whether her hospital had any cases. Susan called Mary back on Tuesday to report three cases; Mary had an additional seven cases. As required, they reported their findings to the county public health department. The public health nurse, Joe, asked them to join the investigation team. In any outbreak investigation, identifying the culprit, that is, the infectious agent responsible for causing the disease, is crucial.

Outbreak Investigation

The first thing Joe did was to determine whether there was an epidemic. He accomplished this through a review of the 10 reported cases at the time of Susan and Mary's first call. Most *E. coli* bacteria are harmless and are normal flora living in the intestines. However, Shiga toxin-producing *E. coli* (STEC) such as 0157:H7 are **pathogenic;** that is, they cause disease.[30] There are federal health regulations that require that certain diseases are designated as notifiable. *E. coli* 0157:H7 is one of these diseases. For each notifiable disease there is a CDC case definition.[31,32] To begin the investigation, they used the CDC guide to define what constituted a case. Case identification provides the investigators with information needed to plot the outbreak and helps to determine whether there is a common source.

Sometimes the agent is not known at the outset, so clinical parameters define a case until the pathogen is identified. When the pathogen is not known, a patient is considered a case if he or she manifests specific clinical symptoms such as fever, diarrhea, and vomiting, which the team determines based on review of the presenting cases. Because Mary and Susan had already identified the agent, a case was defined based on laboratory-confirmed *E. coli* 0157:H7. Much is known about the agent *E. coli* 0157:H7, which was isolated in the early 1980s. The CDC has published guidelines related to the case definition for *E. coli* 0157:H7 (Box 8-3).[32] In addition to the CDC guidelines, the team included in the case definition the date on which symptoms first occurred. This helped to confirm that the case occurred within a similar time frame as the other cases. The team members also extended their search outside of the county to determine whether there were any cases that had occurred within the same time frame, but diagnosed elsewhere.

Because the team members knew the identity of the agent, they also knew the usual reservoir and method of transmission. Because *E. coli* normally lives in the intestinal tracts of humans and animals, the normal route for transmission is the fecal-oral route. *E. coli,* therefore, is either water- or foodborne and has been traced in prior outbreaks to various types of produce,

such as spinach, as well as meats, such as undercooked hamburger. Thus, the team must determine whether there was a common source of infection and was it foodborne or waterborne. A **common source** of infection occurs when the pathogen is transmitted from a single source, such as cantaloupes grown on a particular farm or hamburgers served at a particular restaurant.

To help determine the severity of the outbreak, the team calculated a case fatality rate (CFR) using the total number of fatal cases divided by the total number of cases. In this outbreak, there was a total of 106 cases including 5 deaths. The CFR was 4.7%. Because of the CFR and the potential that this *E. coli* outbreak could be multistate, the county public health department worked in collaboration with the state health department and the CDC to help locate cases outside the county.

$$CFR = \frac{\text{Number of fatal cases}}{\text{Total number of cases}}$$

Once the team defined what constituted a case based on laboratory confirmation of infection with the agent, the members used basic epidemiology to help plan the next step. The team began to figure out the essential aspects of this potential outbreak and then plan the prevention efforts based on whether the intervention was aimed at the agent (eradicating the agent), the environment (interrupting transmission), or the host (reducing susceptibility). To do this they collected further data on each of the cases. This included onset of symptoms, place of residence, and information about where they were and what they ate, starting with the maximum exposure date. Because the range of incubation is 8 to 10 days, the team started with the day of onset of symptoms and worked backward to the maximum date of exposure. For example, for case number one symptoms began on November 7. The team worked backward to October 28 and collected data on where the person was and what he or she ate.

The team used the data to build an epidemic curve. An **epidemic curve** is constructed by plotting on a graph the number of cases (*y*-axis) based on the date of onset (*x*-axis). This requires making a graph that includes the number of new cases per day and month (Fig. 8-4). The graph helped to determine how much time elapsed between exposure to the pathogen and the beginning of clinical symptoms.

Because the incubation ranges from 8 to 10 days, the team could estimate what date(s) the exposure probably occurred.

BOX 8–3	*Escherichia coli* 0157:H7—CDC Clinical Description

Clinical Description

An infection of variable severity characterized by diarrhea (often bloody) and abdominal cramps. Illness may be complicated by hemolytic uremic syndrome (HUS) or thrombotic thrombocytopenic purpura (TTP); asymptomatic infections may also occur.

Laboratory Criteria for Diagnosis

- Isolation of *E. coli* 0157:H7 from a specimen, or
- Isolation of Shiga toxin-producing *E. coli* 0157:NM from a clinical specimen

Case Classification

Suspect: A case of postdiarrheal HUS or TTP (see HUS case definition)

Probable:
- Isolation of *E. coli* 0157 from a clinical specimen, pending confirmation of H7 or Shiga-like toxin, or
- Bloody diarrhea, HUS, or TTP that is epidemiologically linked to a confirmed or probable case

Confirmed:
- A case that is laboratory confirmed.

Comment

Confirmation is based on laboratory findings, and clinical illness is not required. Suspect, probable, and confirmed cases should be reported to local or state health departments.

Only confirmed cases are reported nationally.

Source: See reference 32.

New Cases

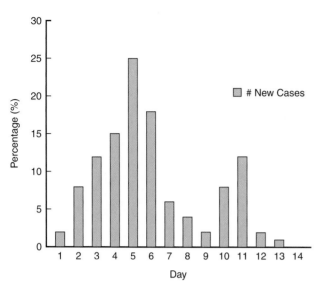

Figure 8-4 Plotting the epidemic curve.

The epidemic curve also helped to determine whether there was a **point source,** that is, the source of the exposure happened at one point in time; a **continuous source,** that is, the exposure is ongoing; or an **intermittent source,** that is, exposure comes and goes. After looking at the epidemic curve (see Fig. 8-4), Joe noted that after day five there was a decline in the number of cases but there was a subsequent increase in cases on days ten and eleven. This represented a bimodal curve that could be a result of two different point sources or to possible household exposure, because *E. coli* can be transmitted person to person. When the cases that occurred on the second curve were reviewed, all of them were family members of an earlier case. This led the team to conclude that there was a point source for the exposure.

Because it appeared to be a point source, team members then examined all the cases to determine whether there was a common source, that is, something that all of the cases ate, drank, or did that could have been contaminated with *E. coli.* The team also examined the data on where the patients were and whether there was a common restaurant or a food market where the people purchased food or drink.

The team next needed to determine how the cases come in contact with the agent. To help with this process, the team mapped out the cycle of transmission for *E. coli* 0157:H7. Mapping out this information

helped the team's investigation, because members needed to know the most likely places where patients may have come in contact with *E. coli.* Knowing something about the pathogen helped the team members develop a hypothesis for the source of the infection so they could begin to build an intervention to prevent further cases.

Generating a hypothesis about the sources of infection is a key step in outbreak investigations. The team began by reviewing the sources of infection in prior *E. coli* 0157:H7 outbreaks. There was an outbreak of *E. coli* 0157:H7 in Washington State in 1993 that resulted in 700 cases and 4 deaths. All of the fatalities were children. In 1999, there was an outbreak at the Washington State Fair. A total of 781 people were infected and 2 died.[33] An outbreak in 2007 resulted in only 12 cases, but caused the recall of 21.7 million pounds of ground beef and the closing of the Topps Meat Company.[34] In 2006, a much-publicized multistate outbreak occurred linked to fresh spinach.[35] The CDC reported on a group of 16 STEC *E. coli* national outbreaks. Of these, 11 were related to *E. coli* 0157:H7. Based on these cases, the team members developed the hypothesis that the outbreak was foodborne and began by examining the data to determine whether there were any commonalities among the cases. The data they examined included their survey of all the patients who met the definition of being a case. The infection control nurses, Susan and Mary, interviewed patients still in the hospital and Joe conducted phone interviews with those who were discharged or who were cared for at home. Based on information from Washington State and the CDC, cases were located outside the county and outside the state. The CDC and the state health department helped to coordinate the obtaining of data from these cases.

Based on the epidemic curve, the team narrowed the possible date of the initial exposure to a 5-day period that extended from October 28 to November 1. During that time, the county held a Halloween festival and all of the primary cases had attended the festival. At the festival there were multiple possible sources for exposure, including a petting zoo, the sale of apple cider from a local farm, a fresh fruit and salad stand, and a hamburger stand. With all the information gathered, the team then narrowed down possible sources based on the ones that the cases had in common. About half of the cases had gone to the petting zoo, a quarter of the cases had eaten fresh salads from the fruit and salad stand, and a third had consumed hamburgers. In contrast, all but four of the cases reported drinking cider. The team then calculated relative risk (see Chapter 3) for the disease based on the possible exposure to hamburgers, petting zoo, and cider. Based on their survey, they found that approximately 95% of the cases reported consumption of the apple cider sold at the food stand next to the kiddy rides. They then questioned the vendor and found that the cider came from a local farmer who made the cider just for the fair.

Management of the Epidemic

Now that the team had identified the probable source of the outbreak, the team had to isolate the source. In some of the E. coli 0157:H7 outbreaks, isolating the source had proved to be problematic. In an outbreak in 2006 associated with the consumption of fresh spinach, cases were distributed across 26 states.[35] In this hypothetical case, in order to manage the epidemic, the team located the farmer who supplied the cider to the stand at the fair. The cider was homemade and had not been pasteurized. Unpasteurized cider is one of the listed sources of E. coli 0157:H7.[36] If the cider had come from a commercial enterprise, the health department would want to intervene and make sure no further sale of the cider occurred. In this case, the public health department questioned the farmer about further sale of the product and discovered that the farmer had a vegetable stand. The county public health department closed the stand and all of the cider the farmer had was destroyed. The public health department also alerted the public to the threat of infection for those who had consumed the cider so that they could be screened for possible infection and provided with treatment if needed. A public service announcement was released advising the public to destroy any cider that had been purchased from this farm.

Managing an outbreak, especially in the case of a disease known to have an increased risk for mortality, requires prompt action on multiple levels. The key is to know how best to break the cycle of transmission. In this case, the reservoir was the target. The team focused on removal of the cider, the actual reservoir for the E. coli 0157:H7. The team also sought to eliminate further consumption of the Halloween cider. In this hypothetical case, a local intervention would work if the farmer who made the cider sold only to the vendor at the fair who then sold only single servings of the cider at the fair. Instead, the farmer owned a farm stand with cider products; therefore, a broader intervention was warranted.

Infectious Agents and Attack Rates

The Case of the Halloween Cider illustrates how humans become infected with an agent that can cause disease. A few other pieces of information are useful to have when conducting an outbreak investigation related to an infectious disease. First, transmission can occur from the reservoir directly or indirectly. Person-to-person contact is an example of direct transmission and occurs with sexually transmitted diseases (STDs). Indirect transmission occurs when the agent leaves the reservoir and is transferred to the human host through an indirect means such as a vector or in the case of fomite transmission.

Once transmission has occurred, disease is not necessarily immediately apparent. As mentioned earlier, inapparent infection is the subclinical phase during which there are no apparent clinical symptoms. From a public health perspective, it is often important to identify those with inapparent infection not only to provide early treatment but also to stop the spread of infection, as you will see in the next case. To help understand how long this inapparent infection phase can last, it is important to know the incubation period. This is the time interval between infection and the first clinical signs of disease. For E. coli, the incubation period is short, but for other pathogens it can be quite long. For example, persons infected with TB during childhood may not develop the disease until later in life.

As discussed in Chapter 3, time is a key issue in epidemiology. With communicable diseases, the incubation period for the pathogen is one example of time that must be considered when conducting an investigation of an outbreak and planning prevention. Another time aspect of infectious agents is the **generation time,** which is the interval between infection with the agent and the maximum time that the host is infectious, that is, the communicability of the host. Sometimes the incubation and generation time are the same. When symptoms appear, the host can no longer transfer the agent to other hosts, but that is not always the case. Generation time helps when dealing with the spread of agents that have a large number of subclinical cases.

Another issue related to infection at the population level is **community** or **herd immunity.** This refers to the immunity of a population to an agent. If a large portion of the population is immune (by vaccine or past infection), the spread of the disease to persons in the population who do not have immunity is prevented. There is usually a threshold of immunity that needs to be achieved to establish herd immunity. In other words, a certain percentage of the population must be immune to achieve herd immunity to a specific agent. With herd immunity, even if a few members of the community become infected, the population as a whole is protected from an outbreak.

In the hypothetical Case of the Halloween Cider, the team calculated a CFR. There are other rates that can be helpful in an investigation, including **attack rate** and **secondary attack rate.** An attack rate is actually a type of incidence rate (see Chapter 3 for more in-depth discussion). It is calculated using the number of persons who are ill divided by the total number of persons who are ill plus those who are well. This is multiplied by a constant (usually 100) and expressed over a certain time period. The attack rate can be calculated based on a particular risk factor. For example, suppose the team had narrowed down the possible risk factors at the county fair as the consumption of burgers at the burger stand, the petting zoo, and the cider. For each risk factor the team would calculate a separate attack rate for those exposed to the risk factor and those not exposed. Group A could be those who drank the cider and group B could be those who did not drink the cider. Once these two attack rates are calculated, the difference between the two attack rates would be determined. This process would then be repeated for the burgers and the petting zoo (Box 8-4). The risk factor with the greatest difference in attack rates may be your common source for the outbreak.

Another calculation useful in an outbreak investigation is the secondary attack rate. This reflects the spread of disease from those who contracted the disease from the initial source to others usually within the same household or other unit where people come in close contact with others. The secondary attack rate is calculated by dividing the number of new cases in a particular group minus the initial case(s) by the number of susceptible persons in the group minus the initial case(s) (see Box 8-4).

Sexually Transmitted Disease (STD)

Not all communicable disease outbreaks follow the course described in the Case of the Halloween Cider. In that case, the outbreak required public health officials to take action related to a food product and those who became ill were not aware of their risk. STDs, on the other hand, are related to behavior and much has been done to alert those who are sexually active to the risk involved in unprotected sexual activity.

In *HP 2020*, the topic "sexually transmitted disease" is a separate topic area from the topic "immunization and infectious diseases." Specific diseases targeted in the objectives are chlamydia, pelvic inflammatory disease (PID), gonorrhea, syphilis, and human papillomavirus.

■ HEALTHY PEOPLE 2020
Sexually Transmitted Diseases

Goal: Promote healthy sexual behaviors, strengthen community capacity, and increase access to quality services to prevent sexually transmitted diseases (STDs) and their complications.

Overview: Sexually transmitted diseases (STDs) refer to more than 25 infectious organisms that are transmitted primarily through sexual activity. STD prevention is an essential primary care strategy for improving reproductive health.

Despite their burdens, costs, and complications, and the fact that they are largely preventable, STDs remain a significant public health problem in the United States. This problem is largely unrecognized by the public, policy makers, and health-care providers. STDs cause many harmful, often irreversible, and costly clinical complications, such as:

- Reproductive health problems
- Fetal and perinatal health problems
- Cancer
- Facilitation of the sexual transmission of HIV infection[37]

BOX 8–4	**Rate Calculations**

$$\text{Attack Rate} = \frac{\text{Ill}}{\text{Ill} + \text{well}} \times 100 \text{ during a time period}$$

$$\text{Secondary Attack Rate (\%)} = \frac{\text{Number of new cases in group} - \text{initial cases}}{\text{Number of susceptible persons in the group} - \text{initial cases}} \times 100$$

Burden of Disease and Sexually Transmitted Diseases

STDs are caused by pathogens that are transmitted from human to human through sexual contact. The reservoir of the agent is the human body. These diseases can cause serious illness and disability and are preventable. There are three notifiable sexual diseases that have federally funded control programs including chlamydia, gonorrhea, and syphilis.[38]

The incidence rate of chlamydia (agent: *Chlamydia trachomatis*) has increased from 160.2 per 100,000 in 1990 to 426 per 100,000 in 2010 with the rate in women double the rate in men.[38] Chlamydia is associated with pelvic inflammatory disease (PID) and can be passed on to the infant during delivery. *Chlamydia trachomatis* is a bacterium and the disease is treatable with antibiotics. Unfortunately, for many women there are no symptoms and so often the disease goes undiagnosed. If the disease is not treated and PID develops, women can experience complications such as infertility, ectopic pregnancy, and chronic pelvic pain. As this is a treatable disease, public health efforts focus on screening and early treatment, as well as education and promotion of barrier use during intercourse.

Another serious STD is gonorrhea (*Neisseria gonorrhoeae*). After chlamydia, it is the most commonly reported STD in the United States. Though the incidence rate fell 75% from 1975 to 1997, the disease still poses a threat, especially to impoverished populations. Like chlamydia, it is a major cause of PID, infertility, and ectopic pregnancies. Again, the disease is treatable but serious health consequences occur if it is untreated. In addition, there is now widespread resistance to a class of antibiotics used to treat gonorrhea, the fluoroquinolones, resulting in a change in CDC guidelines for the treatment of gonorrhea with cephalosporins.[38]

The third STD under national surveillance is syphilis, a genital ulcerative disease caused by the bacterium *Treponema pallidum*. There are two classifications of syphilis during the acute phase, primary and secondary (P&S). The primary stage occurs between 10 and 90 days following infection and is evidenced by a sore or multiple sores at the site where the bacterium entered the infected person (Fig. 8-5). The sore or chancre often heals without treatment. If there is no treatment, then the disease enters the secondary phase. During the secondary stage, the person develops a skin rash and mucous membrane lesions can occur while the chancre is healing or shortly thereafter. It can be

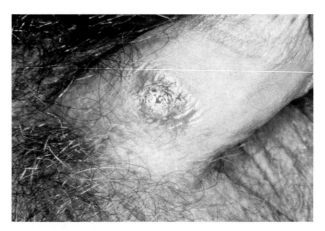

Figure 8-5 Chancre, located on the proximal penile shaft, which was diagnosed as a primary syphilitic infection. *(From the Centers for Disease Control and Prevention, courtesy Dr. Gavin Hart and Dr. N.J. Fiumara, 1976.)*

accompanied by various other symptoms such as fever or swollen lymph nodes, or the symptoms may be so mild that they are not noticed. These symptoms will also resolve with or without treatment. However, if no treatment is given it will progress to the late stage of latent syphilis, which begins when the symptoms of P&S syphilis disappear. This stage can last for years with symptoms emerging up to 20 years after the person was first infected. The consequences of late-stage syphilis are varied and can lead to death. They include damage to the internal organs including the brain, resulting in paralysis and dementia. Historical examples of people with late-stage syphilis include Al Capone and King George III of England, who was on the throne at the time of the American Revolution. In women, untreated syphilis leads to perinatal death in 40% of cases and can lead to infection of the fetus in approximately 80% of fetuses of mothers with untreated syphilis who were infected at least 4 years prior to pregnancy.[39]

Because of the concentration of syphilis in certain geographical areas and the steady decline in cases from 1990 to 2000, the CDC established a national plan to eliminate syphilis. The plan was updated in 2006 because incidence rates began to increase. In 2010, the incidence rate was higher in men than in women, with an increase in men from 3 cases per 100,000 in 2001 to 7.9 cased in 2010. In women, the number of cases per 100,00 increased slightly from 0.8 cases per 100,000 to 1.1 cases.[38]

Risk Factors

The main risk factor for STDs is unprotected sexual contact. The pathogens responsible for STDs are transmitted through the exchange of bodily fluids. Some groups are more at risk than others based not only on individual behaviors but also on ethnic group and access to care. The CDC includes in its analysis of surveillance data on STD cases a comparison of rates based on ethnic groups. The CDC concludes that racial disparities continue in the United States, with African Americans having disproportionate STD rates. For example, though African Americans represent only 12% of the population, they make up about 70% of all gonorrhea cases.[38] This may be owing in part to socioeconomic factors. For example, those with less health insurance coverage are more apt to seek care at public health clinics. Though STDs are reportable diseases, compliance with this law for reporting cases is higher in public clinics than it is in private physicians' offices. Access to care may also prevent early diagnosis and treatment.[38]

● APPLYING PUBLIC HEALTH SCIENCE

The Case of Syphilis in Baltimore City

Public Health Science Topics Covered:

- Health planning
- Community assessment

From 2003 to 2004 the prevalence of syphilis in Baltimore City increased by 40%. This rise resulted in an assessment of the data related to the new syphilis cases and the implementation of a population level intervention.[40] Since as noted above syphilis is a notifiable disease, all diagnosed cases in Baltimore are reported to the local public health department, which in turn reports the cases to the state health department. This information is then reported to the CDC. The case of syphilis in Baltimore City helps to illustrate the differences between a public health response to a foodborne infectious disease outbreak and an increase in the prevalence of an STD.

The first step for the team in Baltimore City was to determine whether the increase in cases was an epidemic. An excess of cases above the endemic levels in a specific community or region is considered an epidemic. To decide whether there is a need for action, public health officials examine the increase in

cases to determine whether the increase has reached an **epidemic threshold,** that is, the number of cases above the endemic rate associated with an increased risk for spread of the disease. The epidemic threshold is used to make decisions about whether to alert the public about a possible epidemic. Epidemic thresholds differ from disease to disease and the methods for determining the threshold can also vary. These calculations require a sophisticated approach, but they help guide public health officials in deciding when an epidemic alert is needed.[41,42] The choice of an epidemic threshold usually reflects the number of cases that exceeds a certain number per 100,000 population over a specified time period. Because the term *epidemic* is emotionally charged, public health officials use it with caution. When a general public alert is needed, the epidemic threshold can help the public health officials either assure the public that there is not an epidemic, or alert the public to a real risk.

The next question related to epidemics asks what the type of epidemic it is, which is related to the specific mode of transmission. The Case of the Halloween Cider fits the description of a common-source epidemic as do other water- and foodborne infections. There can also be a vectorborne epidemic such as the West Nile virus epidemic. In the case of syphilis, the disease has been endemic in the human population for thousands of years. Therefore, unlike an *E. coli* outbreak, the increase in syphilis cases in Baltimore City did not reflect a national epidemic or a pandemic, but rather a specific increase in one particular geographical area.

In this case, once the public health officials realized there was a dramatic increase in the number of cases, they first defined what constituted a case. They looked at the cases based on demographics and found that the increase in cases was occurring mainly in the Hispanic population. In that population, the incidence rate had increased by 73% from 2003 to 2004, compared with a 40% increase for the population in general. Another interesting detail also emerged in their review of cases. They found that the majority of all Hispanic cases were primary cases.[40]

Health Planning

Now the team was ready for action. Instead of a national media campaign and product recall as in the case of an *E. coli* 0157:H7 or *Salmonella* outbreak, a local program was put together, the Syphilis Elimination

Project. The Syphilis Elimination Project is an excellent example of how to plan a health program (see Chapter 5) to address an infectious disease epidemic. It is also a good example of incorporating both a primary and a secondary approach to prevention. In addition, they developed a prevention program that targeted a population at increased risk with a selected level of prevention based on the Institute of Medicine Model of prevention (Chapter 2).

The Syphilis Elimination Project had two goals. The first goal focused on knowledge, awareness, and decreasing incidence of syphilis in the Baltimore City Hispanic community and the second was to get those with syphilis into treatment. Under the first goal, the objective was to increase the number of Hispanics tested for syphilis by 50% from baseline.[40] This is an example of *case finding*. Case finding comes under the umbrella of secondary prevention. The purpose of finding cases is to identify those who are infected and get them into treatment. In STDs, the reservoir is humans. If there is an effective treatment for the disease, it is possible to eliminate the agent in the reservoir. Early treatment for the disease from a population perspective is therefore both a primary and a secondary prevention measure. Through case finding, public health officials can intervene in relation to the agent's reservoir.

For the Baltimore City Syphilis Elimination Project, there were specific challenges related to culture, stigma, and access to the population. Before the team members initiated their project, they had to address these challenges. In addition, skills related to cultural competency were needed to develop a program that would be accepted by the intended recipients (Chapter 23). The team members combined their efforts at case finding with a multimethod patient education campaign. Bilingual outreach workers conducted street outreach by providing education on syphilis in bars, stores, and on the street. Because there is no known method of reducing our biological susceptibility to syphilis, the Elimination Project could not reduce biological susceptibility of the host. Instead, they developed a culturally relevant educational program that provided the population at risk, Hispanics living in Baltimore City, with behavioral strategies to reduce their chances of becoming infected.

When there are no means available to reduce the biological susceptibility of the host, the focus of primary prevention in communicable disease becomes both the mode of transmission and the portal of entry. Through education, it is hoped that those who are not infected become educated on how the disease is transmitted and how it enters the body so that they can implement effective strategies to prevent becoming infected. In this case, an additional challenge was to reach the population most at risk, because the project fit the definition of a selective prevention program (see Chapter 2). The Syphilis Elimination Project team members had done their homework on who was getting infected and they had a good grasp of where this selected population resided. They designed a program that incorporated cultural and geographical issues related to the population. They used bilingual outreach workers who conducted their educational interventions during the evening hours and in the early mornings in high-traffic areas. They chose these times to try to reach the most people by targeting working and partying hours. By the end of 10 weeks they had met their first goal, with 2,825 Hispanics having received patient education and health information materials. Thus, by taking into consideration the role of culture and the importance of engaging the community, the project was successful in primary prevention (providing education to those not yet infected). They were also able to meet their second goal, screening (secondary prevention) and identifying those in need of treatment. Because the cases that were identified through screening were almost all primary infections, few needed tertiary interventions, that is, treatment of clinical disease as seen in secondary and latent syphilis.

Emerging Sexually Transmitted Diseases

Gonorrhea and syphilis are mentioned throughout history, whereas other STDs are new arrivals. In 1981, a new STD emerged that grabbed the attention of the world—HIV. Unlike gonorrhea and syphilis, there currently is no cure for this disease. When it was first identified, those with the infection had few treatment options and the CFR was high. Over the years, science has developed successful treatments and the diagnosis of HIV infection is no longer a death sentence in the United States. In 2009, it was estimated by the CDC that 1,148,200 persons aged 13 and older were living with HIV infection in the United States. This estimate included more than 200,000 (18.1%) persons with undiagnosed infection.[43]

The emergence of this STD changed how nurses provide care. Unlike other STDs, this virus could be transmitted through exposure to other bodily fluids, including blood. In the late 1980s, when surveillance data indicated that health-care workers were at increased risk for HIV infection through exposure to blood and other bodily secretions, a legal approach was taken to prevent the spread of this disease in health-care workers. OSHA put into law the requirement that health-care workers use PPE. As always, the prevention measures taken were based on the mode of transmission and targeted a population at risk for becoming infected. Following the institution of this law, the incidence rate of HIV in health-care workers with no other risk factors dropped dramatically. The use of PPEs has become routine in all health-care settings. This dramatic change in hospital-based infections control created as dramatic a shift in care as hand hygiene did after the discovery that germs caused disease (see Chapter 1).

HIV/AIDS is a pandemic and has had a severe impact on certain portions of the globe, especially in developing countries where access to treatment is limited. Once again, disparity exists related to this STD because of socioeconomic status, culture, and governmental support of prevention efforts. This disease is an example of the emerging diseases affecting the United States and world as a whole.

Prevention of Sexually Transmitted Diseases

STDs bring additional challenges to prevention efforts. The mode of transmission involves a human behavior that is tied to cultural mores. Changing risky behaviors in general can be difficult, but addressing a behavior that few wish to discuss in public settings and that may be tied to feelings of shame or powerlessness can present barriers to the nurse wishing to intervene. The Syphilis Elimination Project demonstrates that these barriers can be overcome, especially if a population approach is taken that includes consideration of the culture of the target population and that includes that population in the design, implementation, and evaluation of the intervention.

Communicable Diseases and Communicability

Not all diseases caused by an infection are communicable. Understanding the difference between an agent that infects humans and causes disease and the communicability of the agent is based on the transmission of the infection from one person to another. A person may become infected with a disease but no public health response is required to prevent further transmission of the agent to other persons, because the agent is not actually communicable. The following case illustrates the point at which an infection is deemed communicable and may require a public health response and when it does not.

▶ SOLVING THE MYSTERY
The Case of the Flesh-Eating Bug
Public Health Science Topics Covered:
- Epidemiology
- Surveillance

On June 20, 2006, David Walton, a leading economist in the United Kingdom, was admitted to Cheltenham General Hospital complaining of fever and stomach pain. Within 24 hours, he was dead. According to one physician, the infection "seemed to spread before our eyes, down the thigh, growing towards the shoulder and chest."[44]

In another case, a 3-year-old girl, Isabel Maude, was brought to the emergency room with high fever, nausea, and vomiting. Her parents explained that their daughter had recently come down with chickenpox. The physician reviewed the care of chickenpox with the parents and sent the child home. The symptoms worsened and the child was readmitted to the pediatric intensive care unit because of organ failure. The first physician had missed the diagnosis based on the recent history of chickenpox. The child actually had a much more serious infectious disease. She eventually recovered after a 2-month stay at the hospital.[45] The case would have turned out differently if the health-care provider who first saw the little girl asked the question "Whodunit?" The health-care providers failed to solve the mystery when they first saw the girl. They did not go beyond the obvious clinical conclusion that this was chickenpox and ask what else might be going on.

A third case related to this same infectious disease occurred in Lanarkshire, England. Between December 24, 2008, and January 3, 2008, two injecting drug users died of the flesh-eating bug. There was one other confirmed case and one suspected case. These deaths prompted a public health announcement from the public health authorities in Lanarkshire.[46,47] The other two cases did not result in a public health alert. This case in England was different from some of the other infectious disease investigations reviewed in this chapter. In the Case of the Halloween Cider and in the syphilis epidemic in Baltimore City among Hispanics, the infection occurred within a population. The hypothetical *E. coli* outbreak took place at a fair and anyone who attended that fair and drank the unpasteurized cider was at risk for becoming infected. In Baltimore City, an increase in the incidence rate for an STD occurred within a specific ethnic population with less access to care and less awareness about their risk for infection. In both cases, interventions were aimed at reducing the incidence rates within a population. The cases also differed on the CFR. In the first case, though the CFR is low for many *E. coli* outbreaks, many of those deaths are in children and older adults and occur soon after infection. In the second case, the period between infection and death in untreated cases can be as long as 20 years. Therefore, the urgency related to an *E. coli* outbreak is fueled not only by the need to decrease illness but also by the importance of decreasing the risk of mortality, especially in children. Though the virulence of the disease is extreme, as in the case of the flesh-eating bug, in this situation the disease was not spreading to the general public.

One of the issues in communicable diseases is separating the agent from the disease or diseases caused by the agent. In the case of the "flesh-eating bug," the agent can cause rapid death in some cases and no illness at all in other cases. In addition, the disease is linked to more than one agent.[48] This is where the cycle of transmission gets interesting. Though the specific agent may differ, the portal of entry is the same; bacteria are introduced through an opening in the skin. In some cases, the bacteria that are introduced are those that are often found on the skin or in the throat. This was not the case with the drug users. Therefore, though the disease was the same and the portal of entry was the same, the reservoir differed. This then has implications for the decision of whether or not to proceed with a public health alert. In relation to *E. coli* 0157:H7, the primary concern was to deal with an outbreak. In the case of the flesh-eating bug, only one of the scenarios given above resulted in a public health initiative similar that in *E. coli* outbreaks.

To answer the question about whether a public health alert is needed, it helps to go back to the lessons learned in the Case of the Halloween Cider. In that case, the team conducted an assessment to determine whether this was a common source of outbreak. Based on the agent, the team members rightly suspected that this was a foodborne outbreak. In the three scenarios presented related to the flesh-eating bug, the first two cases represented an isolated incident. No new cases were admitted to the hospital. Knowing the usual portal of entry of an agent that causes this disease lowered the public health concern that others were at risk. However, in the third case there were three more

cases in rapid succession. The one thing the patients had in common was IV heroin drug use. This raised the potential threat to the public's health but the focus was IV drug users of heroin, not the public in general.

One reason for the public health response was the virulence of the flesh-eating bug. When it enters the body through a wound, the agents associated with the flesh-eating bug have a very high level of virulence; that is, the severity of the disease produced by the agent and the CFR were high. In the United States, the CFR for this disease ranges from 20 to 30 per 100 cases.[48] However, not all persons exposed to agents that cause this disease become ill. Bacteria that cause this disease include *S. aureus, Clostridium perfringens, Bacteroides fragilis, Aeromonas hydrophila,* and others. Again, the presence of the agent is not what is important, but rather it is the portal of entry. The agent itself can be present on skin or in the throat and cause no disease or mild disease with a very low CFR. However, when introduced to the host through a wound, the disease agent causes changes. The formal name for this infectious disease is necrotizing fasciitis (NF). One of the known agents responsible for this disease is group A β-hemolytic streptococci (GABHS). In the throat, GABHS can cause mild illness, but when introduced into the human body through a break in the skin, NF can result.

This leads us back to the issue of the infectivity of the agent. From one perspective, the infectivity is low because there must be an opening in the skin for the agent to enter and cause disease. Therefore, the CDC does not recommend antibiotic prophylaxis in all persons exposed to the patient, unless there are certain other risk factors present. However, from another perspective, the infectivity of the agent is a key issue. Once the agent has entered the host through a break in the skin it can rapidly multiply in the host, resulting in what is reflected in the quote that the infection "seemed to spread before our eyes, down the thigh, growing towards the shoulder and chest."[44]

For the first two cases, no public health alerts were made, but in the third case there was reason to believe that it was actually a common source outbreak. All of the cases were heroin IV drug users. Though there were only four cases and two deaths, the virulence of the agent prompted action. In addition, a similar outbreak a few years earlier in the United Kingdom had resulted in 43 deaths.[47] What the public health officials discovered was each of the cases had injected heroin that had been contaminated with the causative agent that was in spore form. They had a common source outbreak. This discovery led to a selective prevention effort that targeted those at risk, heroin IV drug users (see Chapter 4). Their efforts included alerting emergency departments. This part of their alert focused on case finding and early treatment.

The three examples of NF provided here illustrate that not all communicable diseases require an immediate public health response and that various issues come into play when making these decisions. Key issues include the virulence of the agent or agents causing the disease, whether or not there is a common source for the outbreak, and whether the public health alert will reduce the occurrence of more cases as well as promote early detection and treatment. Of interest in the second case, the disease resulted in the parents of the child developing an organization, Isabel Healthcare, that provides a diagnosis system that prompts health-care providers to reach a timely diagnosis, thus preventing the delay in treatment experienced by their daughter.[45]

Controlling Communicable Diseases

In all the cases presented here, the main issue is to control the spread of disease. There are three main approaches: (1) changing the environment; (2) inactivating the agent; and (3) increasing host resistance. Changing the environment can involve altering or eliminating the reservoir, controlling the vector, applying personal measures of hygiene, and using aseptic technique. Nurses engage in these measures regularly in patient care settings through their own use of proper hygiene and aseptic technique. In this way, they help to reduce the occurrence of hospital-acquired infections. Public health officials actively engage in these measures on a regular basis through general community-level sanitation measures related to water, food, and sewerage. They also actively participate in vector control. Communities at risk for mosquito-borne diseases have mosquito control programs aimed at eliminating the breeding grounds of the insects. This may include the use of insecticides or the draining of swampy areas.

Inactivating the agent includes the use of physical and chemical agents. Pasteurization of cider uses heat to inactivate infectious agents such as *E. coli* 0157:H7. One of the main issues with transmission of *E. coli* 0157:H7 through beef products is the failure to properly cook the beef at a high enough temperature to inactivate the agent. Cold is also used to inactivate agents in food products. The advent of refrigeration greatly reduced the spread of foodborne diseases. There are specific guidelines related

to adequate refrigeration of foods to prevent the growth of bacteria that can cause disease. Chemical methods involve the use of chemicals to control agents such as the chlorination of water or the use of disinfects to clean potentially infected areas or items.

Finally, breaking the cycle of transmission can be accomplished through increasing host resistance. As mentioned above, resistance can be active or passive. Eradication of smallpox was accomplished through the use of vaccines. This was a global campaign launched in 1967. At that time, smallpox had a case fatality rate of 24% and left most of the survivors either scarred or blind. Once a person had the disease, there was no known treatment. However, since the late 1700s it was known that inoculation with cowpox protected against the disease. The global effort to increase host resistance was successful and in 1977 the last documented case occurred.[28]

The use of vaccines to increase host resistance has dramatically changed the impact of communicable diseases on populations, especially children. **Vaccine** refers to the immunizing agent that is used to increase the host's resistance to viral, rickettsial, and bacterial diseases.[49] They can be killed, modified, or changed into a variant form of the agent. In the United States, children routinely receive a series of vaccines that protect against measles, mumps, diphtheria, poliomyelitis, and rubella. Recently, there has been controversy over the potential risk of autism related to childhood vaccinations despite the lack of scientific evidence to support the link. The CDC has put together a guide for parents on the use of vaccines. The use of vaccines is a good example of evidence-based practice, because all vaccines go through a vigorous process to establish safety and effectiveness prior to being used.[50]

■ EVIDENCE-BASED PRACTICE
Vaccination Recommendations During Childhood
Practice Statement: Vaccination is recommended by the CDC for all children as outlined on the CDC's Web site for parents related to vaccination.[51]
Targeted Outcome: Decrease in incidence of vaccine preventable diseases in children.
Evidence to Support: Childhood vaccinations have been part of pediatric care for more than 60 years with a significant reduction of childhood communicable diseases.
Recommended Approaches: Vaccines are held to the highest standard of safety. The United States currently

has the safest, most effective vaccine supply in history. Years of testing are required by law before a vaccine can be licensed. Once in use, vaccines are continually monitored for safety and efficacy. Immunizations, like any medication, can cause adverse events. However, a decision not to immunize a child also involves risk. It is a decision to put the child and others who come into contact with him or her at risk of contracting a disease that could be dangerous or deadly. Consider measles. One out of 30 children with measles develops pneumonia. For every 1,000 children who get the disease, one or two will die of it. Thanks to vaccines, we have few cases of measles in the United States today. However, the disease is extremely contagious, and each year dozens of cases are imported from abroad into the United States, threatening the health of people who have not been vaccinated and those for whom the vaccine was not effective. Between January 1st and June 27th of 2014 there were 539 cases.[52] The CDC and the Food and Drug Administration continually work to make already safe vaccines even safer. In the rare event that a child is injured by a vaccine, he or she may be compensated through the National Vaccine Injury Compensation Program (VICP).[53]

Vaccines are used to increase host resistance to other diseases. These include influenza, pneumonia, and tetanus. Health-care workers are immunized for hepatitis B. In some countries, a tuberculosis vaccination program is in effect for all members of the population. Several factors influence the decisions of public health agencies to make vaccines mandatory and how much protection will be provided by vaccines. First, vaccines are given when the risk to the population is high. For example, hepatitis B is not given to the general public because the risk is low. Health-care providers are at higher risk from their exposure to blood and bodily fluids; thus, health-care workers providing direct care to patients are required to be vaccinated for hepatitis B. For most of the childhood diseases, the risk is high for all children, so vaccination is often required prior to enrollment in schools and health departments have active outreach programs for all the children in the population.

The vaccine for TB is not used universally in all countries. In a country such as India, where the prevalence of TB is high, the vaccine is used to prevent childhood TB. However, in the United States it is not recommended because of the low risk of infection related to receiving the vaccine and the variability of effectiveness of the vaccine against adult pulmonary TB.[54]

Vaccines continue to be a major prevention tool in public health. Science continues to work at developing new vaccines such as a possible vaccine against HIV. In addition to the development and testing of vaccines, continued efforts are needed to implement effective vaccination programs. Not all persons at risk for increased morbidity and mortality related to influenza and pneumonia get vaccinated. There continues to be negative press related to the side effects of vaccines. However, without vaccines smallpox eradication would not have happened. Altering the environment, inactivating the agent, and increasing the resistance of the host are all powerful tools that nurses can use to decrease the incidence of communicable diseases.

■ Summary Points

- Communicable diseases are a significant health issues that place populations at risk for increased morbidity and mortality.
- Preventing the transmission of disease requires an understanding of the cycle of transmission.
- Specific actions taken by nurses and other health-care providers at the population level include:
  - Participating in an outbreak investigation
  - Instituting appropriate isolation within an acute care setting
  - Screening patients or aggregates for an infectious disease
  - Developing and implementing a community outreach program to educate the public on a specific disease
- Vaccination is an important public health intervention aimed at reduction of the transmission of infectious agents.

▲ CASE STUDY
The Measles Epidemic
Learning Outcomes

By the end of this case study, the student will be able to:

- Gain understanding of the investigation of an epidemic.
- Describe appropriate prevention measures.
- Apply the cycle of transmission to individual infectious agents.

In 2008, from January 1 to April 25 there were 64 confirmed cases of measles reported to the CDC. The

CDC initiated a multistate investigation. Based on these findings, the CDC made recommendations related to isolation procedures and vaccination of health-care workers.

Access the *Morbidity and Mortality Weekly Report* article related to the investigation[55] and then answer the following questions:

1. Is this an example of an epidemic? Why or why not?
2. What is the mode of transmission for the agent?
3. In relation to this specific outbreak, was the key issue(s) the agent, the environment, or the host?
4. The CDC made specific recommendations for prevention in hospital settings. What were they and did they all interrupt the cycle of transmission at the same point?

REFERENCES

1. Centers for Disease Control and Prevention. (2012). *2012 West Nile update as of August 28.* Retrieved from http://www.cdc.gov/ncidod/dvbid/westnile/index.htm.
2. Centers for Disease Control and Prevention. (2012). *Multistate outbreak of Salmonella Typhimurium and* Salmonella *Newport infections linked to cantaloupe (final update).* Retrieved from http://www.cdc.gov/salmonella/typhimurium-cantaloupe-08-12/index.html.
3. Centers for Disease Control and Prevention. (2012). *August 2012 Yosemite National Park outbreak notice.* Retrieved from http://www.cdc.gov/hantavirus/outbreaks/yosemite-national-park-2012.html.
4. World Health Organization. (2015). *Ebola virus disease fact sheet N 103.* Retrieved from http://www.who.int/mediacentre/factsheets/fs103/en/.
5. Centers for Disease Control and Prevention. (2012). *Press release August 16, 2012.* Retrieved from http://www.cdc.gov/nchhstp/newsroom/2012/HCV-Testing-Recs-PressRelease.html.
6. World Health Organization. (2012). *Smallpox: Historical significance [Fact sheet].* Retrieved from http://www.who.int/mediacentre/factsheets/smallpox/en/.
7. *Healthy People 2020.* (2012). *Immunization and communicable diseases.* Retrieved from http://www.healthypeople.gov/2020/topicsobjectives2020/overview.aspx?topicid=23.
8. World Health Organization. (2011). *The top ten causes of death.* Retrieved from http://www.who.int/mediacentre/factsheets/fs310/en/index.html.
9. Martin, P.M.V., & Martin-Granel, E. (2006). 2,500-year evolution of the term *epidemic. Emerging Infectious Diseases, 12*(6), 976-980.
10. Centers for Disease Control and Prevention. (2012). *2011–2012 flu season draws to a close.* Retrieved from http://www.cdc.gov/flu/spotlights/2011-2012-flu-season-wrapup.htm.
11. Mali, S., Tan, K.R., & Arguin, P.M. (2011). Malaria surveillance—United States, 2009. *Morbidity and Mortality Weekly Report Surveillance Summaries, 60*(3), 1-15.
12. World Health Organization. (2012). *Malaria.* Retrieved from http://www.who.int/mediacentre/factsheets/fs094/en/.
13. Centers for Disease Control and Prevention. (2012). *Malaria.* Retrieved from http://www.cdc.gov/malaria/malaria_worldwide/impact.html.
14. World Health Organization. (2012). *HIV.* Retrieved from http://www.who.int/mediacentre/factsheets/fs360/en/index.html.
15. Centers for Disease Control and Prevention. (2012). *HIV in the United States: At a glance.* Retrieved from http://www.cdc.gov/hiv/resources/factsheets/PDF/HIV_at_a_glance.pdf.
16. Centers for Disease Control and Prevention. (2010). *Eliminate disparities in HIV and AIDS.* Retrieved from http://www.cdc.gov/omhd/amh/factsheets/hiv.htm.
17. New York State Department AIDS Institute. (2009). *HIV/AIDS in the United States: Disease burden and resource allocation.* Retrieved from http://www.health.ny.gov/diseases/aids/reports/hiv_aids_in_the_us/2009-07_statistical_brief.pdf.
18. Brooks, J.T., Buchacz, K., Gebo, K.A., & Mermin, J. (2012). HIV infection and older Americans: The public health perspective. *American Journal of Public Health, 102*(8), 1516-1526.
19. U.S. Department of Health and Human Services. (2012). *Healthy People 2020 topics and objectives—HIV.* Retrieved from http://www.healthypeople.gov/2020/topicsobjectives2020/overview.aspx?topicId=22.
20. World Health Organization. (2015). *Diarrhoea.* Retrieved from http://www.who.int/topics/diarrhoea/en/.
21. Centers for Disease Control and Prevention. (2015). *Diarrheal disease in less developed countries.* Retrieved from http://www.cdc.gov/healthywater/hygiene/ldc/diarrheal_diseases.html.
22. Centers for Disease Control and Prevention. (2014). *Rotavirus.* Retrieved from http://www.cdc.gov/rotavirus/index.html.
23. World Health Organization. (2015). *Emerging disease.* Retrieved from http://www.who.int/topics/emerging_diseases/en/.
24. National Center for Emerging and Zoonotic Infectious Diseases. (2015). *About the National Center for Emerging and Zoonotic Infectious Diseases.* Retrieved from http://www.cdc.gov/ncezid/.
25. Centers for Disease Control and Prevention. (2014). Trends in tuberculosis—United Stated 2013. *Morbidity and Mortality Weekly Report, 63*(11), 229-233.
26. Centers for Disease Control and Prevention. (1991). Tuberculosis outbreak among HIV-infected persons. *JAMA, 266*(15), 2058, 2061.
27. World Health Organization. (2014). *Global tuberculosis report 2014.* Geneva, Switzerland: Author.

28. Tipple, M.A., Heirendt, W., Metchock, B., Ijaz, K, & McElroy, P.D. (2004). Tuberculosis outbreak in a community hospital—District of Columbia, 2002. *Morbidity and Mortality Weekly Report, 53*(10), 214–216.

29. Centers for Disease Control and Prevention. (n.d.). *Life cycle of the hookworm.* Retrieved from http://www.dpd.cdc.gov/dpdx/HTML/Hookworm.htm.

30. Centers for Disease Control and Prevention. (n.d.). *Escherichia coli.* Retrieved from http://www.cdc.gov/ecoli/general/index.html.

31. Centers for Disease Control and Prevention. (2009). Recommendations for diagnosis of Shiga toxin-producing *Escherichia coli* infections by clinical laboratories. *Morbidity and Mortality Weekly Report, 58*(RR-12).

32. Centers for Disease Control and Prevention. (1997). Case definition for communicable diseases under public health surveillance. *Morbidity and Mortality Weekly Report, 46*(RR10), 1–55.

33. Rangel, J.M., Sparling, P.H., Crowe, C., Griffin, P.M., & Swerdlow, D.L. (2005). Epidemiology of *Escherichia coli* 0157:H7 outbreaks 1982–2002. *Emerging Infectious Disease, 11*(4), 603–609.

34. Centers for Disease Control and Prevention. (2007). *Multistate outbreak of E. coli 0157 infections linked to Topp's brand ground beef patties.* Retrieved from http://www.cdc.gov/ecoli/2007/october/100207.html.

35. Centers for Disease Control and Prevention. (2006). Ongoing multistate outbreak of *Escherichia coli* serotype 0157:H7 infections associated with consumption of fresh spinach—United Sates, September 2006. *Morbidity and Mortality Weekly Report, 55*(Dispatch), 1–2.

36. Centers for Disease Control and Prevention. (2012). *Reports of selected E. coli outbreaks.* Retrieved from http://www.cdc.gov/ecoli/outbreaks.html.

37. U.S. Department of Health and Human Services. (2015). *Healthy People 2020. Topic—sexually transmitted diseases.* Retrieved from http://www.healthypeople.gov/2020/topicsobjectives2020/overview.aspx?topicid=37.

38. Centers for Disease Control and Prevention. (2011). *Sexually transmitted disease surveillance 2010.* Atlanta, GA: US Department of Health and Human Services. Retrieved from http://www.cdc.gov/std/stats10/surv2010.pdf.

39. Centers for Disease control and Prevention. (2014). *Sexually transmitted disease CDC fact sheet—syphilis.* Retrieved from http://www.cdc.gov/std/syphilis/syphilis-factsheet-July-2014.pdf.

40. Endyke-Doran, C., Gonzalez, R.M., Trujillo, M., Solera, A., Vigilacnd, P.N., Edwards, L.A., et al. (2006). The Syphilis Elimination Project: Targeting the Hispanic community of Baltimore City. *Public Health Nursing, 24*(1), 40–47.

41. Martin P.M.V., & Martin-Granel, E. (2006). 2,500-year evolution of the term *epidemic. Emerging Infectious Diseases, 12*(6), 976–980.

42. Green, M.S., Swartz, T., Mayshar, E., Lev, E.B., Leventhal, A. Slater, P.E., et al. (2002). When is an epidemic an epidemic? *Israel Medical Association Journal, 4,* 3–6.

43. Centers for Disease Control and Prevention. (2012). Monitoring selected national HIV prevention and care objectives by using HIV surveillance data—United States and 6 U.S. dependent areas—2010. *HIV Surveillance Supplemental Report, 17*(3, part A).

44. Koster, O. (2007). Flesh-eating bug killed top economist in 24 hours. *Mail Online.* Retrieved from http://www.dailymail.co.uk/news/article-428234/Flesh-eating-bug-killed-economist-24hours.html.

45. Isabel: The Diagnosis Checklist. (n.d.). *Isabel's story.* Retrieved from http://www.isabelhealthcare.com/home/story.

46. Skin deep. (2008). *The Guardian.* Retrieved from http://www.guardian.co.uk/lifeandstyle/2008/feb/03/healthandwellbeing.features.

47. Scottish Drug Forum. (2009). *Toxic bacterial skin infection claims two lives.* Retrieved from http://www.sdf.org.uk/sdf/2788.html.

48. Wisconsin Division of Public Health: Department of Health and Family Services. (2004). *Necrotizing fasciitis.* Retrieved from http://dhs.wisconsin.gov/communicable/FactSheets/PDFfactsheets/NecrotizingFasciitis_42074_0504.pdf.

49. U.S. Department of Health and Human Services, Vaccines.gov. (n.d.). *Glossary of terms.* Retrieved from http://www.vaccines.gov/more_info/glossary/index.html.

50. Centers for Disease Control and Prevention. (2011). *Vaccine safety information for parents.* Retrieved from http://www.cdc.gov/vaccinesafety/populations/parents.html.

51. Centers for Disease Control and Prevention. (2013) *For Parents: Vaccines for your children.* Retrieved from http://www.cdc.gov/vaccines/parents/index.html.

52. Centers for Disease Control and Prevention (2014). Measles (rubeola). Retrieved from http://www.cdc.gov/measles/.

53. Health Resources and Services Administration. (2014). *National Vaccine Injury Compensation Program.* Retrieved from http://www.hrsa.gov/vaccinecompensation/index.html.

54. Centers for Disease Control and Prevention. (n.d.). *Fact sheet: BCG vaccine.* Retrieved from http://www.cdc.gov/tb/pubs/tbfactsheets/BCG.htm.

55. Redd, S.B., Kutty, P.K., Parker, A.A., LeBaron, C.W., Barskey, A.E., Seward, J.F., et al. (2008). Measles, United States, January 1–April 15, 2008. *Morbidity and Mortality Weekly Report, 57,* 1-4.

Chapter 9

Noncommunicable Diseases

LEARNING OUTCOMES

After reading this chapter, the student will be able to:

1. Describe the impact of noncommunicable diseases on the health of a population.
2. Define the burden of noncommunicable diseases using current epidemiological frameworks.
3. Describe the risk factor at the individual and population levels related to development of a noncommunicable disease.

4. Apply current evidence-based population interventions to the prevention of noncommunicable diseases.

KEY TERMS

Burden of disease
Chronic disease
Chronic disease self-management
Cultural shift
Disability-adjusted life years (DALY)

Health-adjusted life expectancy (HALE)
Health-related quality of life (HRQoL)
Human genome epidemiology
Human genomics

Life expectancy
Monogenetic
Noncommunicable disease (NCD)
Polygenetic
Premature death

Standardized incidence rates (SIRs)
Years of productive life lost (YPLL)

▪ Introduction

In contrast with communicable diseases, a **noncommunicable disease (NCD)** is a disease that is not passed from one person to the next through direct or indirect means and is not associated with an infectious agent. The broader term, **chronic disease,** refers to either communicable diseases such as AIDS or NCDs such as diabetes that have a long duration and usually slow progression, require medical attention over time, and/or limit the ability to perform activities of daily living (ADLs).[1] This chapter focuses only on NCDs that are chronic in nature.

The news and talk shows constantly reference our risk for NCDs and provide chilling facts related to injury. Oprah Winfrey publically struggles with her weight and the negative consequences associated with being overweight. Television doctors such as Sanjay Gupta and Mehmet Oz focus on telling us how to change our lifestyles so we can be healthier and prevent developing a chronic disease. We are told to eat healthfully, engage in regular exercise, and avoid unhealthful behaviors such as tobacco use and risky use of alcohol. For those of us who are currently healthy, it is easy to assume that it does not affect us directly. The truth is that the burden of disease associated with NCDs affects us all. NCDs contribute to the increasing cost of health care and decrease our community's ability to reach optimal productivity and health. If we solely focus on combating NCD on the individual level after disease has occurred, we are doomed to failure in the long run. Many risk factors that contribute to the development of NCD such as exposure to secondary smoke in public places are beyond the ability of an individual to control or modify. True change requires a public health population approach that encompasses population-level as well as individual-level interventions. Nurses in all settings play an important role in prevention of NCD across the continuum of prevention through the use of primary-, secondary-, and tertiary-level interventions.

Noncommunicable Chronic Diseases

The majority of NCDs cannot be prevented or cured through vaccination or medication; rather, they require long-term management. Globally, there is an increase in NCDs, with cardiovascular disease, diabetes, cancers, and chronic respiratory disease the chief causes of death globally.[2–4] In the United States, preventing NCDs is a major priority as reflected in many of the *Healthy People 2020 (HP 2020)* objectives.[5] The World Health Organization (WHO) reported that 63% of all deaths globally were due to NCDs.[4] The majority of NCDs could be prevented through a reduction in behavioral risk, especially a decrease in tobacco use, sedentary lifestyle, and harmful alcohol use, and an increase in healthful eating.[4]

Health-care providers, including nurses, typically care for those with NCDs on an individual basis, often during an acute phase of the disease or at the end stages of disease. More recently, especially with the implementation of the Affordable Care Act, the care of NCDs is moving away from an acute care model to a chronic care model in which the disease is managed over time and the focus is decreasing morbidity and mortality associated with NCDs through an integrated care delivery model (Fig. 9-1).[6,7] This new model requires health-care providers to reframe the care provided from the treatment of acute phases of an NCD within an acute care setting to long-term management in the community. Care of existing an NCD should be provided within a secondary and tertiary prevention framework that focuses on early detection and treatment and a long-term plan of care aimed at reducing morbidity and mortality (see Chapter 2). To accomplish this, nurses must use not only their knowledge of the pathophysiology of an NCD, but an understanding of the public health issues associated with the disease. All nurses have a role to play in reducing the burden of disease related to NCDs in populations they serve. Nurses across settings and specialties become part of national and global efforts aimed at reducing the toll that chronic diseases take on the health of not only individuals but also of populations.

Burden of Disease

NCDs add significantly to the overall burden of disease for a population. The **burden of disease** is defined by the WHO as "the overall impact of diseases and injuries at the individual level, at the societal level, or to the economic costs of diseases."[8] Why is it important to know about the burden of disease associated with a specific disease? First, it takes into account what impact the disease has on the population or community as a whole. Estimating the burden of a particular disease can help a community to prioritize health promotion and prevention efforts by targeting those diseases that account for the greatest burden to the community. Determining the burden of disease takes into account not only the cost of

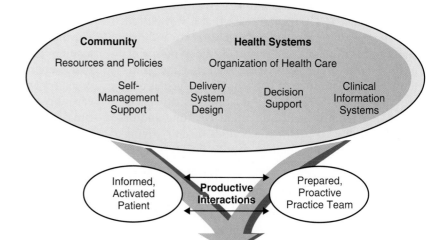

Figure 9-1 The Chronic Care Model.
*(Developed by the MacColl Institute,
°American College of Physicians-ASIM
Journals and Books.)*

treatment but also the social and economic impacts. Analysis of the burden of a particular disease allows for the assessment of the comparative importance of a disease, injury, or risk factor. This assessment takes into account how much the disease, injury, or risk factor contributes to the overall disability and premature death in the population.

For example, if in Berryton, a hypothetical U.S. town of 8,000 adults, the prevalence of type 2 diabetes rose from 160 (2%) to 800 (10%) cases, the impact on the town would involve more than the cost to treat the individuals with the disease. Let's add another aspect to this town. It is a rural farming community recently hit with a downturn in the market price for the farmers' main crop, strawberries. The new cases are occurring for the most part in 35- to 45-year-old males and the closest medical center is 100 miles from the town. With a depressed economy, rural setting, and reduced access to care, the potential for adverse consequences and premature death associated with diabetes is increased. This could result in a decrease in the number of able-bodied people to work on the farms, further depressing the economy. Thus, the impact of an NCD extends beyond individuals and their families. For this community, the disease contributes to reduced productivity and adversely affects the economic viability of the town.

Life Expectancy

Estimating the health of a population is calculated based on a number of measures. First, mortality rates are used to estimate the life expectancy of a group of people. **Life expectancy** is defined as the number of years a person could be expected to live based on the current mortality rates in a specific setting, usually a country. There is great variability across countries in life expectancy, especially between developed and developing countries. For example, the estimated life expectancy in the United States for 2014 was 79.6 years and in Afghanistan it was 50.6 years.[9]

Life expectancy is a valuable tool, but it fails to capture the burden of ill health caused by NCDs.[4,9] To help adjust for these factors, public health officials use the healthy life expectancy measure. **Health-adjusted life expectancy (HALE)** reflects the average number of years that a person can expect to live in good health by adjusting for disease and/or injury. The WHO uses HALEs to measure the average level of health in countries and regions by taking into account population-specific prevalence of disease and injury as well as severity distribution of health states.[10] As a result of problems with comparable health state prevalence data, the WHO uses a four-stage strategy to compute HALE (Box 9-1). This allows

the WHO to estimate HALE for countries across the globe. Epidemiologist compute the HALE for a chronic disease using data related to age, the number of survivors, and the number of years lived.

Premature Death

NCDs often lead to **premature death,** that is, a death that occurs earlier than the standard life expectancy. For those who die prior to reaching the age they would be expected to live, their death is defined as premature. Therefore, premature death reflects the number of potential life years lost. Premature death is usually expressed as the **years of potential life lost (YPLL).** YPLL is calculated by subtracting the age at which a person dies from life expectancy.[10] For example, if a man died of a heart attack in the United States in 2011 at the age of 42, the YPLL would be 36 because the life expectancy in the United States was 78 years that year.[11] In contrast, the YPLL for a man who died in a motor vehicle crash at the age of 21 would be 57.

From a population perspective, premature death is calculated based on the number of potential life years lost prior to the life expectancy of the population per 100,000 persons—in other words, how many total years of useful life were not available to the population because of early death. If you calculated the YPPL for a 50-year-old man

---

| BOX 9–1 | **Application: Health-Adjusted Life Expectancy (HALE): Methods of Estimation** |

The World Health Organization uses death registration data that are reported annually to estimate HALE. This information is part of the WHO Global Burden of Disease (GBD) study. Other sources of data include the WHO Multi-Country Survey Study (MCSS) and World Health Survey (WHS). Information use includes estimates for the incidence, prevalence, duration, and years lived with disability for 135 major causes. However, comparable health state prevalence data are not available for all countries, so a four-stage strategy is used:

- Data from the WHOGBD study are used to estimate severity-adjusted prevalence by age and sex for all countries.
- Data from the WHOMCSS and WHS are used to make independent estimates of severity-adjusted prevalence by age and sex for survey countries.
- Prevalence for all countries is calculated based on GBD, MCSS, and WHS estimates.
- Life tables constructed by WHO are used to compute HALE for countries.

Source: See reference 10.

who died of a heart attack in Afghanistan in 2011, the YPPL would be 0 because the life expectancy for males was 49.

Disability-Adjusted Life Years (DALY)

In addition to premature death, most NCDs lead to disability that can affect an individual's quality of life and productivity. For that reason, YPLL does not adequately capture the full burden of disease. A method for quantifying the burden of disease that takes into account both premature death and disability is called the **disability-adjusted life year (DALY).** This is defined as measurement of the gap that exists between the ideal health status of a disease- and disability-free population that lives to an advanced age.[12] It is calculated using population-level data. One DALY represents 1 lost year of life. It is calculated as a sum of the years of life lost (YLL) related to premature death in the population plus the years lost to disability (YLD) related to the disease.

To calculate the DALY, you start with the YLL. The YLL is the number of deaths multiplied by the standard life expectancy at the age at which death occurs. For this you need the number of deaths attributed to the disease or risk factor and the expectancy at age of death in years. YLL measures lost years of life due to deaths using an incidence perspective (number of new cases or deaths), this perspective is also taken to calculate the YLD. The estimation of the YLD for a particular cause in a particular time period you take the incidence (number of new cases) during that time period and multiply it by the average duration of the disease. To account for the variability of the severity of the disease, a weight factor is included that reflects the severity of the disease on a scale from 0 (perfect health) to 1 (dead). The basic formula for YLD requires multiplying the incidence times the disability weight times the average duration of the disease until remission or death (Box 9-2).[12]

Noncommunicable Diseases in the United States

NCD is the number one cause of death and disability in the United States. The four common risk factors that account for much of the NCD in our country are the same as the risk at the global level and are modifiable. These include (1) nutrition, (2) physical activity, (3) tobacco use, and (4) alcohol use. One-fourth of all persons living in the United States with an NCD have one or more limitations in their daily activities.[3] The overarching goal of *HP 2020* is to "attain high quality, longer lives free of preventable disease, disability, injury, and premature

---

BOX 9–2	**Application: Disability-Adjusted Life Year (DALY) calculation**

DALY = YLL (Years of Life Lost) + YLD (Years of Life Disabled)

The basic formula for YLL is:

$$YLL = N \times L$$

where:
- N = number of deaths
- L = standard life expectancy at age of death in years

The basic formula for YLD is the following (again, without applying social preferences):

$$YLD = I \times DW \times L$$

where:
- I = number of incident cases
- DW = disability weight
- L = average duration of the case until remission or death (years)

Source: See reference 12.

---

death."[5] This requires not only increasing life expectancy but also helping individuals of all ages improve their quality of life.

■ HEALTHY PEOPLE 2020
Noncommunicable Disease

Diabetes

Goal: Reduce the disease and economic burden of diabetes mellitus (DM) and improve the quality of life for all persons who have, or are at risk for, DM.

Overview: DM occurs when the body cannot produce or respond appropriately to insulin. Insulin is a hormone that the body needs to absorb and use glucose (sugar) as fuel for the body's cells. Without a properly functioning insulin-signaling system, blood glucose levels become elevated and other metabolic abnormalities occur, leading to the development of serious, disabling complications. Many forms of diabetes exist. The three common types of DM are:

1. Type 2 diabetes, which results from a combination of resistance to the action of insulin and insufficient insulin production
2. Type 1 diabetes, which results when the body loses its ability to produce insulin
3. Gestational diabetes, a common complication of pregnancy. Gestational diabetes can lead to perinatal

complications in mother and child and substantially increases the likelihood of cesarean section. Gestational diabetes is also a risk factor for subsequent development of type 2 diabetes after pregnancy.[13]

Heart Disease and Stroke

Goal: Improve cardiovascular health and quality of life through prevention, detection, and treatment of risk factors for heart attack and stroke; early identification and treatment of heart attacks and strokes; and prevention of repeat cardiovascular events.

Overview: Heart disease is the leading cause of death in the United States. Stroke is the third leading cause of death in the United States. Together, heart disease and stroke are among the most widespread and costly health problems facing the United States today, accounting for more than $500 billion in health-care expenditures and related expenses in 2010 alone. Fortunately, they are also among the most preventable. The leading modifiable (controllable) risk factors for heart disease and stroke are:

- High blood pressure
- High cholesterol
- Cigarette smoking
- Diabetes
- Poor diet and physical inactivity
- Overweight and obesity[14]

Leading Causes of Death and Disability

According to the Centers for Disease Control and Prevention (CDC), noncommunicable chronic conditions are not only costly but are common and preventable causes of death and disability. Seven of the top ten leading causes of death in the United States are noncomunicable diseases including heart disease; cancer; chronic lower respiratory diseases; stroke (cerebrovascular disease); Alzheimer's disease; diabetes; nephritis; nephrotic syndrome; and nephrosis (Box 9-3).[14–16] Understanding the diseases from a public health perspective is required because treating one person at a time once the person becomes ill with the disease is similar to putting a thumb in one hole in a dike with many holes. The public health perspective allows us to step back and examine the context of these diseases and the causal factors linked to the occurrence of disease.

Heart Disease and Stroke

According to the CDC, cardiovascular disease (CVD) and stroke are the first and fourth leading causes of death in the United States.[17] They are costly and widespread.

BOX 9–3	Top 10 Leading Causes of Death, CDC 2010

- Heart disease: 597,689
- Cancer: 574,743
- Chronic lower respiratory diseases: 138,080
- Stroke (cerebrovascular diseases): 129,476
- Accidents (unintentional injuries): 120,859
- Alzheimer's disease: 83,494
- Diabetes: 69,071
- Nephritis, nephrotic syndrome, and nephrosis: 50,476
- Influenza and pneumonia: 50,097
- Intentional self-harm: 38,364

Source: See reference 16.

Together they account for close to one-third of all deaths in the United States. [17] Though rates for coronary heart disease and stroke dropped from 20.8% in 1999 to 24.4% in 2009 serious issues remain.[17] Over a third of adults have two or more risk factors for heart disease and stroke such as high blood pressure, obesity, or current smoking. Heart disease and stroke account for more than 30% of mortality and are leading causes of disability.[18-20]

Understanding the risk factors for CVD has come from public health science. Before World War II, hypertension was accepted as a part of the normal aging process and little was understood about how to treat it, never mind how to prevent it. As life expectancy improved, the prevalence of CVD grew. Because of this increase in prevalence, the National Heart Institute (now known as the National Heart, Lung, and Blood Institute) initiated a longitudinal cohort study in 1948 (defined in Chapter 3) in Framingham, Massachusetts, which is still going on today.[21] From the data collected over the past six decades, we now know a great deal about the risk factors for CVD and stroke. Based on the findings from this study both individual and population level interventions have been developed aimed at reducing risk and subsequently reducing the prevalence of CVD.[21]

Cancer

While great strides have been made in the prevention and treatment of cancer, it is the second leading cause of death in the United States[16] and is projected to be the leading cause of death worldwide.[22] In the United States, public health efforts to increase screening for breast and colorectal cancer have resulted in a decrease in deaths because of early detection and screening, and the length of cancer survival has increased. However, the United States is losing ground in other areas that increase the risk for cancer such as indoor tanning, secondary smoke exposure, and unexplained cancer-related health disparities among subpopulations such as African Americans and those with low socioeconomic status (Box 9-4).[22] Lung cancer is the leading cause of cancer death in both men and women, with 80% of all lung cancers resulting from smoking or exposure to secondhand smoke.[22]

| BOX 9–4 | **United States Losing Ground in Important Areas That Require Attention: The 2011/2012 Update** |

- Death rates for the most common cancers (prostate, female breast, lung, and colorectal) continued to decline.
- Incidence rates of some cancers continued to rise, including melanoma of the skin, non-Hodgkin lymphoma, childhood cancer, cancers of the kidney and renal pelvis, leukemia, thyroid, pancreas, liver and intrahepatic bile duct, testis, and esophagus.
- Lung cancer incidence rates in women continued to rise, but not as rapidly as before.
- Death rates for cancer of the pancreas, esophagus, thyroid, and liver were increasing.
- Although the percent of smokers attempt to quit smoking continued to rise (50%) there has only been a slight increase in successful quitting rates which continue to be low.
- Although progress was made in all segments of the population, subgroups including children living in homes with smokers, young adults, subgroups of non-smoking workers (for example, blue collar occupations and the hospitality industry), and non-Hispanic blacks have higher rates of exposure to secondhand smoke.
- Dentists were half as likely as physicians to advise their patients to quit smoking.
- More people were overweight and obese, and leisure-time physical activity is not increasing.
- Alcohol consumption rose slightly since the mid-1990s. Fruit and vegetable intake was not increasing. Red meat and fat consumption was not decreasing.
- Adult indoor tanning increased slightly.
- Cancer-treatment spending continued to rise along with total health-care spending.
- Unexplained cancer-related health disparities remained among population subgroups. For example, blacks had the highest rates of both new cancers and cancer deaths.
- Pap test use fell. Rates were 74 percent in 2010. Mammography rates stabilized at 67%; screening for colorectal cancer was lower than Pap testing and mammography, despite its proven effectiveness. However, use of colorectal cancer tests was increasing.

Source: See reference 22.

Risk for cancer is a combination of behavioral, genetic, and environmental factors. For example, in breast cancer all three levels of risk apply. Diet, exercise, and alcohol use have all been associated with increased risk for breast cancer.[23,24] An example of genetic risk is the harmful mutation of *BRCA1* or *BRCA2,* tumor suppressor genes. Women who test positive for this gene mutation have an increased lifetime risk for developing breast and ovarian cancers.[25] There is also emerging evidence that exposure to organic solvents and other chemicals increases the risk for breast cancer.[24]

Chronic Lower Respiratory Diseases

Chronic obstructive pulmonary disease (COPD) includes emphysema and chronic bronchitis. Persons with COPD experience airflow limitation that is not fully reversible. The limitation is usually progressive. The NHLBI and the WHO published a Global Initiative for COPD based on a COPD workshop.[26] The major risk factor for COPD is smoking, and the causative link between the two is the abnormal inflammatory response of the lungs to the noxious particles or gases present in tobacco smoke. Other risk factors include exposure to air pollutants, chemical fumes, and dust from the environment or workplace.

Diabetes

Despite the great improvements that have occurred in the management of diabetes and the reduction in complications such as blindness and diabetes-related end-stage renal disease, the prevalence of diabetes is growing. According to the Centers for Disease Control and Prevention, if current trends continue, 1 in 3 Americans will develop diabetes by 2050.[27] This trend is occurring across the globe with the WHO projecting that by 2030 diabetes will be the 7th leading cause of death.[28] In 2012 a little over 9% of the U.S. population had diabetes. In addition, 25% of those over 65 had diabetes (diagnosed and undiagnosed).[29] The majority of this increase is in type 2 diabetes linked to changes in lifestyle, especially exercising and diet.

Again, public health efforts are in full force in attempting to turn this trend around. The main focus has been on behavioral change, thus reducing individual risk. The American Diabetes Association states that prevention or delay of the onset of type 2 diabetes can happen through a healthy lifestyle that includes making healthful changes to diet, increasing the level of physical activity, and maintaining a healthy weight.[30] These recommendations are based on solid epidemiological data related to risk, that is, persons who exercise regularly, eat healthy, and maintain a normal body mass index (BMI) are at a much lower risk for type 2 diabetes. Type 1 diabetes is another story. Less than 10% of persons with diabetes have type 1. It is usually diagnosed in childhood and is associated with genetic risk rather than behavior risk.

Risk Factors

It is clear that risk for NCD is complex and related to numerous factors, individual behaviors, genetics, and environmental exposure as well as the larger socioeconomic context in which people live.[31] To prevent NCDs, the epidemiologist explores factors that increase the risk of disease occurring. As explained in Chapter 3, two studies are often conducted to help determine what leads to development of disease: a case control study and a cohort study. Based on these studies, we can determine the relative risk or the odds ratio of disease that can occur based on exposure to a risk factor. In chronic diseases, there are two major categories of risk that have received a great deal of attention nationally, lifestyle or behavioral risk factors and socioeconomic risk factors.

▶ SOLVING THE MYSTERY
The Case of the Ill Town
Public Health Science Topics Covered:
- Surveillance
- Assessment

Alice, a nurse working in the oncology unit of the regional health center, noticed a number of recent admissions to the unit from one town. She approached her unit manager with her concern. The manager had just come from a hospital meeting related to increasing collaboration with community organizations in the promotion of health. The manager saw an opportunity for collaboration with the public health department and asked Alice to represent the hospital in the pursuit of this issue. Alice began with the hospital discharge data to determine whether an increase indeed existed and if so, for what types of cancers.

Alice contacted the medical records department and asked them to obtain the discharge data for the past 15 years for her unit by ZIP code and diagnosis. She entered the data into an Excel file that listed the total number of admissions for the oncology unit by year and by the ZIP code of the town of interest to see whether the number of cases increased for the town, and whether the percentage of admissions for the town increased. She found that there was indeed a recent increase in

cases for the town. To help understand the data better, she looked at the admissions for the town based on diagnosis and found that there was a wide range of cancers, but noticed that the number of lung cancer admissions increased in that ZIP code, but not for other ZIP codes and that there were two cases of mesothelioma, a relatively rare cancer of the thin membranes that line the chest and abdomen. Armed with these results, she went back to her manager, who contacted the county public health department and made an arrangement for Alice to meet with them and go over the data. The public health department meanwhile reviewed the cancer registry for the state to look at trends in types of cancers across the state. Based on Alice's report, the public health department formed a team to investigate the matter that included the state cancer registry. They asked Alice to serve on the team as well.

The public health nurse (PHN) on the team began by conducting a cohort study that was retrospective (see Chapter 3). Residents of the town with and without cancer were then surveyed in relation to demographics, smoking history, occupation, family history of cancer, source of their drinking water, and residential history. For persons who had died, family members were asked to give the information. In addition to the hospital discharge data, the team collected data from the cancer registry and mortality statistics to calculate a cancer incidence rate for town residents.

A case was defined as a diagnosis of primary cancer confirmed by the state cancer registry. Because of the potential latency period of 20 to 30 years for cancers related to environmental carcinogens such as asbestos, the survey asked residents for information related to possible exposures for the past 30 years, including duration of residence in the town and place of employment. Data on cases and controls were only available for current residents.

Based on the data, **standardized incidence rates (SIRs)** were calculated for total cancers and for cancer groupings including respiratory cancers and gastrointestinal. A SIR reflects the observed number of cases in the study population divided by the expected number of cases. The expected number of cases is based on the incidence rate of a larger population that is designated as normal or average. They found that the SIR was significantly higher for residents of the town compared to the reference population.

The next step in the investigation was to examine the possible common exposure shared by the residents of the town. At one time, there had been a cement factory in town that was now closed. It had begun operation in the late 1920s and shut down in the early 1970s. The team reexamined the residents who had developed cancer in relation to their work history and the proximity of their residence to the plant. They were able to establish a higher incidence rate of respiratory cancers among workers at the cement plant even after controlling for tobacco use. In addition, they found that residents who lived closer to the plant had a slightly higher incidence rate than did those who lived farther away.

Based on this information, the state and local health departments and the hospital partnered to develop health interventions for exposed workers and residents. The first step was to conduct medical examinations and for those who had respiratory symptoms or screened positive for disease, hospital physicians and nurses provided treatment. In addition, the public health department in conjunction with the cancer registry initiated a case-finding process to locate those who had been exposed but no longer resided in the community. Based on the added risk of respiratory cancers in smokers exposed to asbestos, the public health department again partnered with the hospital to provide a smoking-cessation program for residents of the town at risk for asbestos exposure who were also smokers. Through their efforts, the teams was able to improve chances of survival among those exposed to the carcinogen.

Environmental Risk Factors for Noncommunicable Disease

The Case of the Ill Town illustrates the role that environment plays in the development of NCD (see Chapter 6). Pollutants in the environment increase the risk for asthma, cardiovascular health problems, and cancer.[32,33] These pollutants include those found in the air, the home, the water supply, and the ground. Since 1950, the United States has experienced drastic changes in the food supply, the built environment, increased population, and proliferation of environmental chemicals. The built environment includes the structures that exist in our towns and cities including the buildings, roads, sewage systems, parks, and recreation facilities (see Chapter 6). In 1800, only 3% of the world's population lived in an urban setting. In 2008, 50% of the population was urban and it is projected that by 2050, 70% of the world's population will be urban.[34] The growth of cities reflects a growth in commerce, economic opportunities, and opportunities

for building social capital. However, it also increases issues related to environmental pollutants. For example, most of us are aware of the potential pollutants in the air. Local news stations report on the air quality and alert residents when the air quality places a person at risk for health consequences (see Chapter 6). The environment plays a key role in understanding the risk for NCD and is best understood through the application of public health science methodologies.

Behavioral Risk Factors

The WHO posed a question: "Why treat people's illnesses without changing what made them sick in the first place?"[35] We must strive to understand what contributes to the occurrence of NCDs. In addition to environment, much attention has been given to the role of individual behaviors. In particular, the current focus is on healthy nutrition, adequate exercise, and avoidance of substance misuse, especially tobacco and alcohol (see Chapter 11). The evaluation of risk factors has been the dominant paradigm of the late 20th century and through the first decade of the 21st century. Understanding risk factors requires an understanding of public health science, especially epidemiology. Most of the studies that have established the link between a risk factor and a disease are based on case control and cohort studies (see Chapter 3). Often, the exploration of risk factors begins with a basic community/population assessment (see Chapter 4).

Nutrition, Exercise, and Obesity

In 2009–2010, more than a third of U.S. adults (35.7%) were obese (had a BMI greater than or equal to 30) and 16.7% of children and adolescents were obese.[36] It is well known that obesity and overweight increase the risk for NCDs, especially heart disease, type 2 diabetes, certain cancers, and stroke.

The main risk factors associated with obesity are poor nutrition and lack of exercise, which reflect individual behaviors that are thought to be modifiable; that is, they can be changed with intervention. However, using the web of causation (see Chapter 2), these two risk factors are linked to numerous other factors at the population level, including changes in population behaviors, environmental factors, and socioeconomic factors. The risk factor model often fails to establish the complex link between individual behaviors, population-level factors, and the development of NCD. A good place to start when faced with a growing health problem such as obesity is to do a population-level focused assessment that allows for assessment of both the macro- and micro-level perspective (see Chapter 4). This type of assessment can help to identify who is at greatest risk for obesity as well as the population-level factors that contribute to obesity. For example, the prevalence rate for obesity is higher in the South,[36] which may reflect cultural approaches to nutrition and a higher poverty rate. A more thorough population-level assessment can help the PHN develop an intervention that is culturally relevant and takes into consideration barriers faced by the population.

● APPLYING PUBLIC HEALTH SCIENCE

The Case of the Growing Children

Public Health Science Topics Covered:

- Assessment
- Program planning

In Marksville County, a hypothetical county located in the state of Florida close to the Everglades, there was a growing concern among the citizens about the prevalence of obesity and overweight among the children as well as county adults. The issue arose at a city council meeting in Yonston, the only major city in the county. The mayor and city council charged the health officer with heading up a task force to address this issue and asked the task force members to concentrate on childhood obesity. The most obvious step in addressing the issue was first to conduct an assessment. The county had a population of 10,576. The ethnic profile of the county was 5% Seminole Indians, 11% African American, 17%, Hispanic, 65% Caucasian, and 2% other races. Seventeen percent of the population was under the age of 18. The health officer knew that the first step would be to mobilize a broad band of stakeholders and community residents. Before doing so, the health officer decided to seek a commitment from a smaller group, the steering committee.

After thinking about this in consultation with other people, the health officer chose the following people for the steering committee: the principal of the local high school, a university professor from the local nursing school, the county political representative, CEO of the local hospital, two businesspeople, and the director of the Head Start program. The CEO talked with the nurse manager of the pediatric unit and asked her to represent him on the committee. Orientation meetings were held and goals and objectives of the initiative were set. The overall goal was to conduct a community assessment focused on determining the

extent of obesity and overweight in Marksville County, to examine trends of the epidemic, to identify resources for addressing the issue, and to develop an action plan for the future.

An assessment related to a particular health issue helps bring about a greater understanding of the factors influencing that health issue for that particular population. This committee conducted a focused assessment (see Chapter 4) related to obesity in children and adolescents. Overweight and obesity, which are determined by using weight and height to calculate a BMI, are growing public health problems for adults and children.[36] An adult who has a BMI that ranges between 25.0 and 29.9 is considered overweight. If the BMI is 30 or higher, then the person is considered obese. For children and adolescents, overweight is often defined as at or above the 95 percentile of the sex-specific BMI for age growth chart. Ranges above a normal weight have different labels: at risk for overweight and overweight.[37]

After establishing the steering committee, a larger coalition was formed to build the structure needed to conduct the assessment. Invitations were sent out to a broader constituency to develop a coalition to address the issue. Initially, the public was invited to a town hall meeting. The goal was to increase awareness about obesity and overweight within the community and to gain a commitment to get involved. They provided the community with the data on obesity in their county based on data from the Florida Department of Health.

The committee then presented the community with the facts about why childhood obesity is an important public health issue for their county. They explained that obesity occurs when more calories are consumed than are expended. They further explained that they were tackling this problem because childhood obesity has both immediate and long-term health impacts. If the community did not take action, they would be faced with sicker children as well as the long-term cost of caring for more adults with chronic diseases occurring at an earlier age. According to the CDC, 70% of obese youth have at least one risk factor for cardiovascular disease, such as high cholesterol or hypertension. Obese children and adolescents are at greater risk for bone and joint problems. They also suffer from psychological problems owing to social stigma and low self-esteem. As adults, they are at higher risk for CVD, type 2 diabetes, stroke, cancer, and osteoarthritis.[37]

They were able to grab the community's attention when they gave the facts about type 2 diabetes among the children of the county. Based on hospital discharge data from the county hospitals, 50 of their children were already being treated for type 2 diabetes with an overall prevalence rate of 2.8 per 1,000 children and adolescents, higher than the national prevalence of 1.7 per 1,000. The sub-population most affected in their community was the Seminole Indians, with 14 Seminole children in their county diagnosed with type 2 diabetes, a prevalence rate of 4.9 per 1,000 children under the age of 18. Thus, 28% of the children diagnosed with type 2 diabetes in their county were Seminole Indians.

With the support of the community, the committee added key members suggested by the community to help them complete a more in-depth assessment. They began by reviewing national statistics related to the prevalence of obesity/overweight in children and adolescents and comparing those rates with their own rates. They were able to find national reports on the extent of the problem as well as a national-level concern related to the problem. One of the objectives of *HP 2020* is concerned with reducing the proportion of children and adolescents who are obese.[38]

■ HEALTHY PEOPLE 2020
Nutrition and Weight Status

Objective: Nutrition and weight status (NWS)—children and adolescents

NWS-10: Reduce the proportion of children and adolescents who are considered obese

NWS-10.1	Children aged 2 to 5 years
NWS-10.2	Children aged 6 to 11 years
NWS-10.3	Adolescents aged 12 to 19 years
NWS-10.4	Children and adolescents aged 2 to 19 years

Source: See reference 38.

The team reviewed the National Center for Health Statistics Data Brief and found that the prevalence of obesity among children remained high.[39] After further review they also discovered that on the national level, obesity begins early for Native American children.[40] Another source of secondary data came from the Youth Risk Behavioral Surveillance System (YRBSS), which is a state-based health survey that annually collects information on health conditions, behaviors, preventive practices, and access to health care.[41] It is used to monitor health problems in youth as well as healthy and unhealthy behaviors, including the prevalence of obesity among youth and

BOX 9–5	**Results From the 2009 YRBSS: What Is the Problem?**

The 2009 Florida Youth Risk Behavior Survey indicates that among high school students:
- 10% were obese
  During the 7 days before the survey:
- 78% ate fruits and vegetables fewer than five times per day.
- 19% did not participate in at least 60 minutes of physical activity on any day
- 75% were physically active at least 60 minutes per day on fewer than 7 days
- 56% did not attend physical education (PE) classes in an average week when they were in school
- 73% did not attend PE classes daily when they were in school.
- 38% watched television 3 or more hours per day on an average school day
- 31% used computers 3 or more hours per day on an average school day.

Source: See reference 41.

young adults. They located a summary of the results for Florida from the 2009 YRBSS (Box 9-5).

Based on their review of the YRBSS, they noticed that not only were the health behaviors of individual students assessed, but that environmental factors were included as well. The nurse manager of the pediatric unit at the community hospital remembered a discussion in a recent nursing practice committee meeting about the problem of only focusing on individual risk factors when examining a health problem. She went back to the literature and examined new developments in public health science and again reviewed the web of causation (see Chapter 2). She brought back to the committee her concerns about focusing on behavioral risk factors alone. She argued that the risk factor paradigm targets individual change only and ignores the difference between individual risk factors and population risk factors and encouraged the committee to take a macro-look at risk factors as well.[42] The committee agreed to do this.

Taking this broader view of risk related to healthy diet and exercise in children and adolescents, the committee found literature related to the school environment with a focus on health education, healthy food availability, and physical education (PE). On the CDC's Web site they found information on all these areas at the state level (Box 9-6). They found that as a whole, the state is not consistently promoting healthy behaviors using these three standard school based approaches.

- 21% required students to take two or more health education courses.
- 76% taught 14 key nutrition and dietary behavior topics in a required course.
- 79% taught 12 key physical activity topics in a required course.
- 55% taught a required physical education (PE) course in all grades in the school.
- 15% did not allow students to be exempted from taking a required PE course for certain reasons.
- 64% offered opportunities for all students to participate in intramural activities or physical activity clubs.
- 23% did not sell less nutritious foods and beverages anywhere outside the school food service program.
- 19% always offered fruits or nonfried vegetables in vending machines and school stores, canteens, or snack bars, and during celebrations when foods and beverages are offered.
- 37% prohibited all forms of advertising and promotion of candy, fast food restaurants, or soft drinks in all locations.

Source: See reference 43.

The committee now had some important data using secondary data sources from the national, state, and county level. However, they decided they were missing key information, especially the information found in the YRBSS, because their county data were hampered by a small numbers problem; that is, there were not enough respondents to make any conclusions. They decided to do their own survey of school-age children in the county as well as collect institution-level data on the schools in the county to determine what was being offered related to health education, PE, and nutrition. In addition, they collected data from the Head Start and the Women, Infants, and Children (WIC) programs.

In looking at the data, a growing trend in the community was noted from the 2011 program year and the 2012 program year. During the 2011 program year, 22% of children in Head Start and 18% of children in Early Head Start were identified as overweight. In 2012 the percent for Early Head Start stayed the same but for Head Start it increased to 24%. In the two WIC programs in the county, 18% of children were identified as overweight. These percentages were higher than the population of those under the age of 18 as a whole. These data on the under-5 age group illustrated the need to develop a program that extended beyond

school-age children. Also, based on their earlier data, the population at greatest risk for adverse consequences related to obesity was the Seminole Indian children.

They also examined the school data and found that the county schools performed similarly to the rest of the state on the CDC indicators. Healthy nutrient and dietary behavior habits were taught at both the elementary and high school levels, but they did not include key physical activity topics in these courses. Because of recent budgetary problems, PE was no longer offered in the schools, though they had an intramural sports program at the high school and middle school levels. The vending machines in the school did not sell healthy foods and soft drinks were advertised in the school. Notably, the new school football scoreboard was donated by the Pepsi Cola Company. They also found that the school cafeteria prepared foods using a deep-fat fryer.

Based on these findings, the committee began to put together action steps to address the issues specific to their community. They wanted to develop a broad program that would include children aged 5 and below as well as children and adolescents attending school. They also felt it was important to engage the Seminole Indian community in the planning to make sure that any intervention developed was culturally relevant. They started with the 10 recommendations found on the CDC Web site.[43] They also found visual resources at the CDC that could be used to help build awareness in the community (Fig. 9-2). In this way, the schools became leaders in the fight against childhood obesity and in the promotion of a healthier lifestyle in their community.

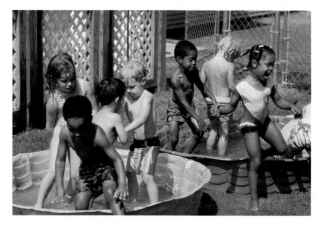

Figure 9-2 Encouraging children to play outdoors along with limiting TV and maintaining a healthy diet. *(From the Centers for Disease Control and Prevention. Photography Jim Gathany, 1990s.)*

Tobacco Use

In addition to nutrition and exercise, tobacco use is a major behavioral risk factor for chronic disease (see Chapter 11). The use of tobacco is strongly associated with increased risk for adverse health outcomes including cancer, pulmonary disease, and cardiovascular disease. According to the CDC, approximately 90% of all lung cancer deaths in men and close to 80% of lung cancer deaths in women are directly related to tobacco smoking.[44] The single most preventable cause of morbidity and mortality in the United States is the use of tobacco. An estimated 443,000 people die each year prematurely of diseases related to smoking or exposure to secondhand smoke, and another 8.6 million experience a serious illness caused by smoking.[45] To address this major health issue, in 2000 *Healthy People 2010* set an objective of reducing tobacco use to 12% of adults aged 18 or older. This goal was met in only two states. The percentage of current smokers in the United States in 2011 by state ranged from 9.3 % in Utah to more than 26.5% in West Virginia, with the highest regional prevalence of smoking in the Huntington–Ashland, West Virginia–Kentucky–Ohio region, where more than a third (34.4%) of the residents were current smokers.[46]

There is strong evidence to support the benefit of smoking cessation in that people who quit smoking have a lower risk of lung cancer than had they continued to smoke.[47] The challenge is that the use of tobacco is more than an individual issue and requires interventions at the population and community level. Both the WHO and the U.S. Department of Health and Human Services have presented population-level strategies aimed at reducing tobacco use. From a global perspective, the WHO initiated an international tobacco treaty in 2005.[48] At the national level, the new *HP 2020* objectives include community- and population-focused objectives to increase the number of sustainable and comprehensive evidence-based tobacco control programs and increase the number of tobacco-free environments.[49]

Alcohol Use

Alcohol use accounts for 4% of the global burden of disease and in the United States is the third leading cause of preventable death.[50, 51] Alcohol consumption, beginning with risky use, is a major avoidable risk factor for disease and injury,[52-55] and in high-income countries cost associated with alcohol accounts for more than 1% of the gross national product.[55] Reduction in the burden of disease associated with alcohol use requires a health-care workforce capable of implementing evidence-based interventions across the continuum of alcohol use and the

life span. If health-care providers understand the continuum of alcohol use across the life span, including adverse alcohol-related health consequences for both the drinker and nondrinker, the scope of prevention and intervention efforts is greatly expanded. Though alcohol consumption is a socially acceptable and normative practice in the United States, it has the potential to adversely affect health across the life span, including but not limited to injury, breast cancer, hypertension, stroke, liver disease, and brain damage.[56- 62] Alcohol use is associated with over 200 diseases and injury.[54]

Genomics and Risk for Noncommunicable Disease

Understanding risk for NCD includes the genetic risk each person or group of genetically related persons has for disease. **Human genomics** is the study of the genetic structure or genome of a living human. Through genomics, evidence clearly demonstrates that there is a genetic role in the major NCD including cancer, diabetes, health disease, and asthma.[63,64] Genetic risk predisposes a person to disease independent of environmental and behavioral risks. Understanding genetic risks and identifying genetic mutations offer hope for both prevention and treatment of chronic disease. An example of genetic risk is the *BRCA1* and *BRCA2* gene mutations, known as tumor suppressors, which increase the risk for breast cancer.[65,66] Persons who screen positive for *BRCA1* and *BRCA2* mutations can choose either to undergo prophylactic surgery (removal of both breasts) or to avoid known risk factors associated with the development of breast cancer.[66] In relation to treatment, genomic research related to diabetes has the potential to result in restoration of insulin production through gene therapy.[67] The WHO has a human genetics research project that is critically evaluating genetic research related to the four NCDs, cancer, asthma, diabetes, and cardiovascular diseases, in the hopes of identifying strategies to control or prevent these diseases.[63]

The CDC has a dedicated site on human genomics and public health. The organization states that the study of the relationship between genes, environment, and behaviors will help us to understand why some people get sick and others do not.[64] The role of family history in the development of disease is not a new concept, but the mapping of the human genome has allowed scientists to identify the actual genes linked to the development of disease and thus increase the ability of researchers to develop and evaluate genetic screening and other interventions that can improve health and prevent disease.

Despite the promise of genomics to help control NCDs, there are potential problems with reliance on genomics to help solve the problem of these diseases. Most chronic disease are not **monogenetic**; that is, the disease is linked to a single gene mutation such as cystic fibrosis. Only 2% of total diseases are monogenetic. All other diseases result from multifactorial causes and are **polygenetic**, meaning multiple genes act together to cause the disease. Many diseases are experienced in the later years of life rather than early in life when genetic interventions are more apt to be beneficial. To further complicate the understanding of the role of genetics in the development of disease, Strohman pointed out in the early 1990s that slower genetic change fails to compensate for rapid environmental change. He explained that "genes are regulated by cellular responses to the external world and that diseases are initiated by those responses."[68] In other words, our genetic makeup is not static and as we age will adapt to the environment we are exposed to. Thus, genetic risk is not a linear source of complex chronic disease but is rather a dynamic process based on interaction between the gene and the environment. The question Strohman raised was whether genomic research should focus on genetic engineering that would fit the individual human organism to a hostile environment or on environmental engineering that would refit the environment to be consistent with the evolving human genome.[68]

Building on the complexity of the interaction between genetics and the environment described in detail by Strohman[68] a new field is emerging, **human genome epidemiology**. This field provides the scientific basis for the study of the distribution of gene variants, gene-disease associations, and gene-environment and gene-gene interactions within and across populations. This allows public health scientists to estimate the absolute, relative, and attributable risks for disease based on genomic factors[66] (see Chapter 3). Thus, the growing understanding of the human genome from a population perspective offers new essential information on the occurrence of chronic disease based on population-level as well as individual risk.

Socioeconomic Risk for Noncommunicable Disease

As demonstrated previously, the development of an NCD is multifactorial. In addition to the physical environment, behavior, and genetic risk, socioeconomic factors play a role in determining who is at greater risk for developing an NCD. Health is remarkably sensitive to the social environment, and those who are less well-off are at greater risk for experiencing ill health.[69] The term often used to describe these factors are the social determinants of health (see Chapter 7). According to the WHO, there are 10 broad socioeconomic categories that contribute to development of disease that also carry policy implications (Box 9-7).[1,69] The premise is that it does not make sense to treat people for disease without addressing the things that make them sick in the first place. Interventions aimed at reducing risk must take into account the social determinants of health and the barriers that exist within a socioeconomic context that reduce the ability of individuals, families, and communities to experience a healthy lifestyle.

Disparity and Noncommunicable Disease

NCD is a major contributor to the disparity in life expectancy.[3] As defined in Chapters 7 and Chapter 23, disparity is a difference or inequality in some aspect of health such as a disparity in the infant mortality rate between two groups. Disparity in morbidity and mortality statistics for NCD persists (see Chapter 7). Age-adjusted stroke and heart disease deaths are higher for African Americans than for whites. African Americans are more

---

BOX 9–7 Social Determinants of Health

- **The Social Gradient:** The further down the social ladder a person is, the more disease will occur and the shorter the life expectancy will be.
- **Stress:** The experience of stressful circumstances when people are worried, anxious, and unable to cope can lead to premature death.
- **Early Life:** Healthy early life and education improve health over the life span.
- **Social Exclusion:** Poverty, social exclusion, and discrimination cost lives.
- **Work:** Stress in the workplace impacts health. People with more control in the workplace have healthier lives.
- **Unemployment:** Higher rates of unemployment are linked to increased disease and premature death.
- **Social Support:** Health is improved through friendship, good social relations, and strong supportive networks.
- **Addiction:** The use of alcohol, drugs, and tobacco leads to poorer health. Such use is influenced by the wider social environment.
- **Food:** Global markets control food supply, so access to healthy food is a political issue.
- **Transport:** Healthy transport reflects less reliance on cars and more walking, biking, and use of public transport.

Source: See reference 1, 69

likely to die of cancer than are any other racial or ethnic group.[70] With diabetes, the groups at greatest risk are American Indians and Alaska Natives who are twice as likely as whites to have diabetes.[71] Much of the disparity in NCDs is associated with economic inequality, specifically the differences between the very wealthy and the very poor, accounting for the higher prevalence of NCDs in those below the poverty level (Chapter 7).[69]

Disparity in NCD rates between different populations is also linked to socioeconomic and geographical factors (see Chapter 7).[18,20] For example, regional disparity exists in the United States related to prevalence rates of NCDs such as diabetes (Fig. 9-3). In 2009, the premature death rate was lowest in New England; four out of the top five states for low YPLL were in New England. In contrast, all but one of the states with the highest YPLL were located in the South.[20] These regional disparities reflect differences in socioeconomic factors and cultural lifestyle. Within states, disparity exists between counties and is often correlated with socioeconomic status, as exemplified by the difference in tobacco use.[46]

The relationship between socioeconomic status and prevalence of NCD presents an ethical dilemma for providers of health care (Box 9-8). A central risk factor for increased morbidity and mortality related to NCD is access to health care including preventive screening, early and ongoing treatment, and resources needed to manage care. In the United States, care is delivered for

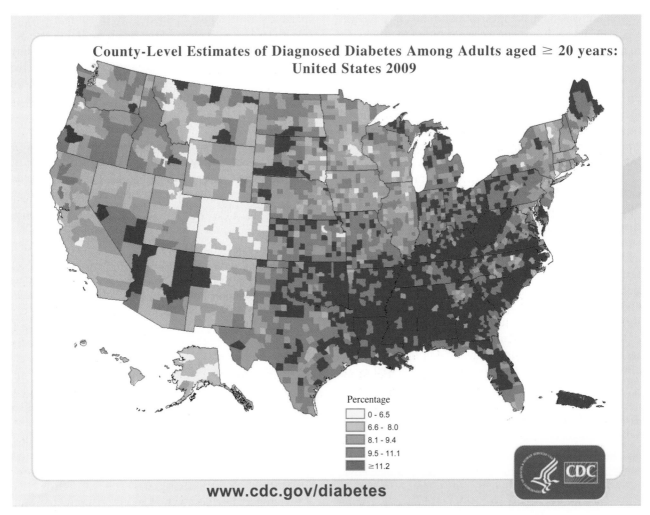

Figure 9-3 County level estimates of adults aged 20 years or older diagnosed with diabetes by state, 2009. *(From the Centers for Disease Control and Prevention. Retrieved from http://apps.nccd.cdc.gov/DDT_STRS2/NationalDiabetesPrevalenceEstimates. aspx?mode=DB.)*

Ethics and Disparity Related to Chronic Diseases

Critical ethical questions related to chronic disease health care include the following:

- Is health care for the management of chronic diseases a right or a privilege?
- Should government pay for medically necessary services when an individual cannot afford those services?
  - If yes, does this approach truly serve the greater good for the greater number?
  - If no, who should be responsible for paying for these services?
- How does failure to provide services to those in need impact the community in general?

the most part based on a fee-for-service basis and health-care providers need to be reimbursed for the care they provide. However, for those who are unable to obtain adequate insurance or do not have adequate transportation to services, care is often delayed until the disease has become advanced. For example, an insulin-dependent diabetic single man who is currently homeless faces daily challenges, which may include maintaining an adequate diet when he is dependent on soup kitchens; checking his blood sugar when he does not have his own glucometer; obtaining insulin and insulin supplies; and storing those supplies in a safe place. In contrast, an insulin-dependent diabetic married man currently employed and domiciled has the financial means and the social support needed to meet those challenges. For both men, diabetic care needs will continue for the rest of their lives. Prevention of morbidity and mortality related to their diagnosis requires careful self-management over time including monitoring of blood sugar, diet and exercise, foot care, adherence to medication regimens, and regular checkups with their health-care provider. Is it ethical for those who have the financial means to have the resources needed to meet their ongoing daily health-care needs necessary for survival while those who do not have the financial means do not? The Affordable Care Act of 2010 attempts to address these issues in part, while still retaining a fee-for-service framework for the delivery of care (Chapter 1).

Gender and Health

Disparity in rates of disease also exists between women and men.[72] These disparities are not just based on physiological differences, but on socioeconomic factors as well. Across the globe, women represent a vulnerable population because of child-rearing responsibilities, lower status, and fewer economic resources (Chapter 7). U.S. men are more likely to report that they have been told they have coronary heart disease and are more likely to report hearing loss than are women. In contrast, women are more likely to have been told they had asthma, hay fever, sinusitis, or chronic bronchitis than are men. In the 2012 national health survey women were more likely to report pain, especially from migraines, neck pain, lower back pain, or face or jaw pain and report feeling sad. Overall, 16% of women reported at least one physical difficulty compared with 12% of men.[73]

Prevention Strategies for Noncommunicable Diseases

Prevention and management of NCDs are global priorities.[1] Prevention strategies extend across the continuum from primary to tertiary prevention (see Chapter 2). Prevention of NCD across all three levels occurs across many settings (see Chapters 14 to 21). Prevention efforts are often focused on reducing the individual risk factors mentioned above, but often the success of prevention efforts require multifaceted interventions at the individual, family, community, and policy levels. For the nurse, these efforts can seem overwhelming. Luckily, national efforts can guide the implementation of evidence-based approaches for prevention. A good example of recommendations made at the policy level related to primary prevention is the 2008 updated *Public Health Action Plan to Prevent Heart Disease and Stroke.*[74] The action plan is intended to help guide both public health and individual health-care providers interested in developing primary programs aimed at preventing cardiovascular disease. There is growing evidence that policy interventions can be effective in the prevention of NCDs, such as the evidence that anti–public smoking laws reduce myocardial infarction (Chapter 22).[75, 76]

At the individual and family levels, primary prevention focuses on behavioral change with a strong emphasis on healthy eating and exercise. There is evidence that interventions aimed at changing behavior can result in healthier lifestyles using various methods such as the Web-based program eHealth Behavior.[77] These approaches not only provide information as to what constitutes a healthy lifestyle, but also provide participants with strategies for making improvements in nutrition and physical activity and accessing the resources needed. The difficulty is that the populations at greatest risk for NCDs are those with limited access to the resources needed to maintain a healthy lifestyle. Thus, population-level primary prevention programs help to change barriers to a healthy lifestyle. For example, obtaining an adequate level of exercise in an urban setting requires safe streets for walking and/or access to recreational activities. This requires action at the community and policy levels. Nurses, especially those working in a public health role, can help facilitate community engagement in improving the safety of streets and improving access to healthy foods at reasonable prices.

Secondary prevention efforts are also associated with reduced morbidity and mortality related to NCD, especially screening (Chapter 2). Examples of screening programs recommended by the CDC for the prevention of NCDs include mammograms and screening for colorectal cancer (CDC, 2009). Such programs result in the early detection of disease and thus in early treatment.

Often the nurse is providing care related to tertiary prevention efforts aimed at reducing the adverse consequences experienced by a person who has already been diagnosed with a disease. The goal is to reduce the morbidity and disability associated with the disease and to prevent premature death. During the course of the disease, there can be periods of acute illness that are usually shorter and often require admission to an acute care facility for care. Chapter 15 provides in-depth coverage of the role of public health science in the nursing care of patients during an acute phase of an NCD. Primary care settings provide care to help patients manage a chronic disease as well as care for milder acute phases of the disease (see Chapter 16). Two concepts used in both of these settings that are grounded in public health prevention models are health-related quality of life and chronic disease self-management.

Health-Related Quality of Life

Health-related quality of life is central to the overarching goals for *HP 2020*. The goal is to attain and promote "a high quality of life for all people, across all life stages."[10] **Health-related quality of life (HRQoL)** is a multidimensional construct related to the desired physical and psychological health outcomes for most of the interventions that nurses provide to individuals and families. HRQoL is defined here as the self-perceived impact of physical and emotional health on quality of life, including the effects on general health, physical functioning, physical health and role, bodily pain, vitality, social functioning, emotional health and role, and mental health.[78,79] The CDC has a whole Web site

dedicated to HRQoL.[79] Included on the Web page is the four-questions measure it uses for HRQoL that can easily be used in any health-care setting and the evidence supports it as a reliable and valid measure of HRQoL. This healthy data measure not only can help in measuring an individual's HRQoL, but according to the CDC, it is also being used at the national and state levels to identify health disparities (see Chapter 7), to track population trends, and to build broad coalitions around a measure of population health. This measure is compatible with the WHO's definition of health (see Chapter 1).[80] The CDC uses the Healthy Days measure in the Behavioral Risk Factor Surveillance system.[78] Based on the CDC's findings, those with NCD experience more unhealthy days than those without. It has also found regional differences.[81]

■ EVIDENCE-BASED PRACTICE
Measuring Health-Related Quality of Life (HRQoL)
Screening for HRQoL

Practice Statement: The use of the HRQoL screening tool can help health-care providers identify persons whose health is negatively impacting their quality of life and can provide a means to measure key health indicators for public health assessments.

Targeted Outcome: Identify those in need of interventions aimed at improving their quality of life and identifying vulnerable populations.

Evidence to Support: The CDC's 14-item HRQoL tool includes the standard four-item set of Healthy Days core questions and the Standard Activity Limitation and Healthy Days Symptoms modules. When used together, these measures make up the full CDC HRQoL-14 Measure. Public health departments have used the tool to identify vulnerable groups when conducting community assessments. The screening tool not only provides a method for assessing an individual's HRQoL, but also provides PHNs with a useful indicator of health at the population level.[74] This measure has been used nationally since the 1990s and has established validity and adequate reliability (Cronbach's alpha 0.57 to 0.75).[81-83]

Recommended Approaches: The CDC HRQoL screening tool is used in community assessments and surveillance. A guide published in the late 1990s described the use of HRQoL as one of the main indictors for monitoring health in populations and evaluating outcomes and is still recommended by the CDC.[79] According to the CDC, "In many cultures, a quality-of-life focus could offer a unifying theme for diverse health and social service programs as well as economic programs which aim to improve population well-being."[79] The CDC uses the tool to compare respondents on HRQoL-based demographic variables (Table 9-1).[78, 83] The tool can also be used to better understand the factors that influence HRQoL.

Sources

Andresen, E.M., Catlin, T.K., Wyrwich, K.W., & Jackson-Thompson, J. (2003). Retest reliability of surveillance questions on health-related quality of life. *Journal of Epidemiology Community Health,* 57(5), 339-343.

Barile, J.P. (2012). Health-related quality of life among older adults with and without functional limitations. *American Journal of Public Health,* 102(3), 496-502. doi:10.2105/AJPH.2011.300500.

Centers for Disease Control and Prevention. (2011). Health-related quality of life methods and measures. Retrieved from http://www.cdc.gov/hrqol/methods.htm.

Hennessy, C.H., Moriarty, D.G., Zack, M.M., Scherr, P.A., & Brackbill, R. (1994). Measuring health-related quality of life for public health surveillance. *Public Health Reports,* 109, 665-672.

Institute of Medicine. (2012). *For the public's health: Investing in a healthier future.* Washington, DC: National Academies Press.

National Research Council. (1997). *Improving health in the community: A role for performance monitoring.* Washington, DC: National Academies Press.

Nelson, D.E., Holtzman, D., Bolen, J. Stanwyck, C.A., & Mack, K.A. (2001). Reliability and validity of measures from the Behavioral Risk Factor Surveillance System (BRFSS). *Sozial- und Praventiv Medizin,* 1(Suppl. 46), S3-S42.

Ware, J.J., Kosinski, M., & Keller, S.D. (1996). A 12-item short-form health survey: Construction of scales and preliminary tests of reliability and validity. *Medical Care,* 34(3), 220-233.

TABLE 9–1 Percentage of Adults Reporting Fair or Poor Self-Rated Health by Demographic Characteristics for Adults ≥ 18 Years of Age: The results below are from the 2009 Behavioral Risk Factor Survey System question, "Would you say that in general your health is excellent, very good, good, fair or poor?"

Variable category	Number of respondents	Percent
Overall Gender	422,199	15.9
Men	160,244	14.8
Women	261,955	14.8
Race		
White non-Hispanic	336,768	13.4
Black non-Hispanic	32,687	20.8
Asian	6,974	9.3
Pacific Islander	689	12.2
American Indian/Alaskan Native	5,900	24.3
Other non-Hispanic	9,170	20.7
Hispanic	25,420	24.7
Annual Household Income Level		
< $15,000	40,578	39.6
$15,000–$24,999	64,396	27.3
$25,000–$34,999	44,409	20.2
$35,000–$49,999	56,660	13.4
> $50,000	159,624	6.2
Unknown/refused	56,532	18.6

Source of data: Centers for Disease Control and Prevention. http://www.cdc.gov/hrqol/data/tables/table1a.htm.

Chronic Disease Self-Management

An evidence-based approach to improving HRQoL for persons with NCD is **chronic disease self-management (CDSM).** It is defined as an ongoing process by which individuals with a chronic illness or condition engages in self-management of medications, symptoms, and promotion of their own health and can be applied to both noncommunicable and communicable chronic disease.[84,85] CDSM requires implementation of health-promotion and health protection strategies, which are fundamental concepts for nursing practice (Chapter 2). Extensive research exists related to the efficacy of patient education programs for specific chronic diseases such as asthma and diabetes.[86,87] Evidence is accumulating that heterogeneous CDSM programs that include persons with different chronic diseases are efficacious, reduce emergency department usage and health distress, and transcend ethnic boundaries[88,89] as well as having applicability to underserved populations who do not have regular health-care providers.[90,91] It has great potential for improving self-efficacy in management of disease, health behaviors, health-care utilization, and health status.

NCD prevention and reduction of risk factors that lead to NCDs drive many of the objectives in *HP 2020.*[11] It is an issue across all health-care settings. Strategies for specific NCDs are discussed across the chapters in this text. The key is to remember that prevention efforts require interventions at all levels with the goal of not only reducing the prevalence of NCD, but also of improving the overall HRQoL for individuals, families, and populations.

Culture and Noncommunicable Diseases

As evidenced by the case study on a hypertension-screening program discussed in Chapter 23, culture plays a big part in the prevention and treatment of NCDs. For the most part, when culture is mentioned in conjunction with prevention of NCDs, the focus is on the role of culture in relation to individual risk behaviors such as food, nutrition, and exercise. Culture is also important in the development of education materials. These issues are well covered in Chapters 2, 7, and 23. However, one issue in relation to culture and NCDs has to do with the cultural shifts that have occurred at the national level in relation to prevention.

Cultural shifts occur over time because no culture is static. In the past 50 years, there have been cultural shifts in the United States in relation to risk behaviors associated with NCDs. A **cultural shift** is defined as a change in society's dominant views, morals, and behaviors. When applied to health, it represents a shift in how society views that issue and the risk factors associated with development of disease. For example, there has been a cultural shift in how society perceives drinking alcohol and driving; once this was viewed as a normal behavior and now it is one that is not tolerated and results in criminal consequences. Another example is the shift in how we view the foods we eat, with the passing of laws in some states prohibiting the sale of large, sugary drinks or the use of deep-fat fryers in schools. A cultural shift changes the way organizations are structured, the environment we live in, and the activities we participate in.

Let's examine a major cultural shift in the United States. In the 1950s, no one questioned a person's right to smoke in public. Smoking occurred in all public places, including banks, hospitals, and restaurants. As the evidence grew that secondhand smoke affected the health of the nonsmoker, public health policy initiatives were begun to reduce smoking in public places. In the beginning, science was driving the change. Based on the evidence, public health policies were put in place that required restaurants to designate no smoking sections and employers constructed separate places for their workers to smoke, often referred to as "butt huts." However, what began as evidence-based public health policy shifted to a social reality. As fewer people smoked, tolerance of smoking declined and the culture shifted from viewing tobacco use in a positive manner to seeing it as a negative and unpleasant behavior. In the 1930s and 1940s, movie stars smoked on screen, and in the 1950s, cigarette ads depicted the smoker as rugged and manly, as in the Marlboro Man. Today, most public spaces are smoke free. It is hard to determine which comes first, the policy or the cultural shift. Often, one reflects the other. However, public polices, to be effective, need the support of the community. When the culture matches the policy, the policy is more apt to actually bring about change. The end result of this cultural shift has been a reduction in morbidity and mortality associated with tobacco use as evidenced by the reduction in admissions for myocardial infarctions following implementation of bans on public smoking of tobacco.[75,76]

Thus, not only does the culture of groups play a role in individual behavior, but also the cultural norms of a population shift over time and can have a significant impact on health. Sometimes there are opposing cultural values in relation to a risk factor such as the use of public policy to restrict the ingredients that restaurants put in foods. Understanding that cultural shifts occur over time related to reducing NCD is important for the nurse who wishes to actively engage in prevention efforts. Nursing can actually play a role in helping the cultural shift along. As the largest segment of the health-care workforce, when nursing is on the forefront of positive cultural shifts related to prevention, the shift can happen at a more rapid pace and populations will get healthier. A world with reduced morbidity and mortality related to NCDs and improved HRQoL can happen and nurses are a major driver of the shift to healthier living as part of our culture.

■ Summary Points

- NCDs contribute significantly to the overall burden of disease.
- The five leading causes of death in the United States are NCDs.
- Risk for NCD is a combination of individual behaviors, the environment, and socioeconomic factors.
- Prevention occurs across the continuum, starting with primary prevention during the perinatal period through tertiary prevention measures such as chronic disease self-management programs.

▲ CASE STUDY
A Journal Club Imitative

The journal club on a medical-surgical unit in a hospital that serves an Appalachian community has decided to tackle the problem of diabetes. One of the nurses has come across an article on the increased prevalence of diabetes in distressed Appalachian counties.[90] She tells the club the article is available online and asks everyone in the club to read it. When the group comes back to discuss the findings in the article, they begin to talk about the patients who are coming into the hospital with diabetes and the problem of readmission rates. The journal club members decide that their next step is to look for evidence-based approaches to prevention across the continuum that would work in the community they serve, but they encounter difficulties finding interventions tailored to Appalachian communities.

1. Choose a county mentioned in the article and map out the demographic information available at the U.S. Census Bureau Web site.
2. Choose a target population based on age and level of intervention (primary secondary and tertiary).

3. Access the county Web site and see what can be learned about:
   a. Cultural considerations
   b. Possible partners for the intervention
   c. Possible barriers
4. Review the literature again for evidence-based interventions relevant to your chosen population and prevention level.
5. Using Chapter 5 as a guide, draft a possible prevention intervention the nurses in the journal club could help initiate.

REFERENCES

1. World Health Organization. (2014). *Chronic diseases.* Retrieved from http://www.who.int/topics/chronic_diseases/en/.
2. Anderson, G., & Howath, J. (2004). The growing burden of chronic disease in America. *Public Health Reports, 119,* 263-270.
3. World Health Organization. (2008). *Noncommunicable diseases now biggest killers.* Retrieved from http://www.who.int/mediacentre/news/releases/2008/pr14/en/index.html.
4. World Health Organization. (2003). *The World Health Report 2003—shaping the future.* Retrieved from http://www.who.int/whr/2003/chapter1/en/print.html.
5. U.S. Department of Health and Human Services. (2014). *Healthy People 2020.* Retrieved from http://healthypeople.gov/HP2020/.
6. World Health Organization. (2003). *Surveillance of noncommunicable disease risk factor.* Retrieved from http://www.who.int/mediacentre/factsheets/fs273/en/print.html.
7. World Health Organization. (2010). *Health systems: Concepts, design & performance.* Retrieved from http://www.emro.who.int/mei/mep/Healthsystems-glossary.htm.
8. World Health Organization. (2014). *Trade, foreign policy, diplomacy and health: Global burden of disease.* Retrieved from http://www.who.int/trade/glossary/story036/en/.
9. Central Intelligence Agency. (2014). *The world fact book: Country comparison life expectancy at birth.* Retrieved from https://www.cia.gov/library/publications/the-world-factbook/rankorder/2102rank.html.
10. World Health Organization. (2014). *Health statistics: Mortality; Health adjusted life expectancy (HALE) at birth (years).* Retrieved from http://www.who.int/healthinfo/statistics/indhale/en/.
11. U.S. Department of Health and Human Services. (2014). *Healthy People 2020*: General health status. Retrieved from http://www.healthypeople.gov/2020/about/genhealthabout.aspx#years.
12. World Health Organization. (2010). *Metrics: Disability adjusted life year (DALY).* Retrieved from http://

www.who.int/healthinfo/global_burden_disease/
metrics_daly/en/print.html.

13. U.S. Department of Health and Human Services.
(2014). *Healthy People 2020*: *Topic—diabetes.*
Retrieved from http://www.healthypeople.gov/2020/
topicsobjectives2020/overview.aspx?topicid=8.

14. U.S. Department of Health and Human Services.
(2014). *Healthy People 2020*: Topic—heart disease and
stroke. Retrieved from http://www.healthypeople.gov/
2020/topicsobjectives2020/overview.aspx?topicid=21.

15. Centers for Disease Control and Prevention. (2014).
Chronic diseases and health promotion. Retrieved
from http://www.cdc.gov/chronicdisease/overview/
index.htm.

16. Centers for Disease Control and Prevention. (2014).
Fast Stats: Top ten leading causes of death. Retrieved
from http://www.cdc.gov/nchs/fastats/leading-causes-
of-death.htm http://www.cdc.gov/nchs/fastats/lcod.htm.

17. Centers for Disease Control and Prevention. (2013).
*Vital signs: Preventable deaths from heart disease &
stroke.* Retrieved from http://www.cdc.gov/VitalSigns/
HeartDisease-Stroke/.

18. National Center for Chronic Disease Prevention.
(2009). *The power of prevention: Chronic disease the
public health challenge of the 21st century.* Retrieved
from http://www.cdc.gov/chronicdisease/pdf/2009-
Power-of-Prevention.pdf.

19. Centers for Disease Control and Prevention. (2010).
*Heart disease and stroke prevention: Addressing the
nation's leading killers at a glance 2010.* Retrieved
from http://www.cdc.gov/chronicdisease/resources/
publications/aag/dhdsp.htm.

20. Centers for Disease Control and Prevention. (2010).
Disparities in premature deaths form from heart disease—50 states and the District of Columbia. *Morbidity and Mortality Weekly Report, 53*(06), 121-126.

21. *Framingham Heart Study.* (2014). Retrieved from
http://www.framinghamheartstudy.org/.

22. National Cancer Institute. (2012). *Cancer trends
progress report 2011/2012 update.* Retrieved from
http://progressreport.cancer.gov/highlights.asp.

23. McTiernan, A. (2003). Behavioral risk factors in breast
cancer: Can risk be modified? *The Oncologist, 8,*
326-334.

24. Brody, J.G., Rudel, R.A., Michels, K.B., Moysich, K.B,
Bernstein, L., Attfield, K.R., & Gray, S. (2007). Environmental pollutants, diet, physical activity, body size
and breast cancer. *Cancer, 109*(12), 2627-2634.

25. National Cancer Institute. (2009). *BRCA1* and *BRCA2:
Cancer risk and genetic testing.* Retrieved from http://
www.cancer.gov/cancertopics/factsheet/Risk/BRCA.

26. Pauwels, R.A., Buist, A.S., Calverley, P.M.A., Jenkins,
C.R., & Hurd, S.S. (2001). Global strategy for the diagnosis, management and prevention of chronic obstructive pulmonary disease. *American Journal of
Respiratory Critical Care, 163,* 1256-1276.

27. Centers for Disease Control and Prevention. (2011).
*Successes and opportunities for population-based
prevention and control at a glance, 2011.* Retrieved
from http://www.cdc.gov/chronicdisease/resources/
publications/AAG/ddt.htm.

28. World Health Organization. (2011). *Global status
report on noncommunicable diseases.* Geneva,
Switzerland: Author.

29. American Diabetes Association. (2014). *Diabetes
statistics.* Retrieved from http://www.diabetes.org/
diabetes-basics/diabetes-statistics/.

30. American Diabetes Association. (2014). *Prevention.*
Retrieved from http://www.diabetes.org/diabetes-
basics/prevention/.

31. Freudenberg, N., & Olden, K. (2011). Getting serious
about the prevention of chronic diseases. *Prevention of
Chronic Disease, 8*(4), A90. Retrieved from http://
www.cdc.gov/pcd/issues/2011/jul/10_0243.htm.

32. Centers for Disease Control and Prevention. (2014).
Air pollutants and respiratory health. Retrieved from
http://www.cdc.gov/nceh/airpollution/.

33. Environmental Protection Agency. (2013). *Air pollution and cardiovascular disease.* Retrieved from http://
www.epa.gov/research/airscience/air-cardiovascular.
htm.

34. Population Reference Bureau. (2013). *Human population: Urbanization.* Retrieved from http://www.prb.
org/Publications/Lesson-Plans/HumanPopulation/
Urbanization.aspx.

35. World Health Organization. (2010). *Social determinants of health posters.* Retrieved from http://www.
who.int/social_determinants/tools/multimedia/
posters/en/index.html.

36. Centers for Disease Control and Prevention. (2012).
Overweight and obesity. Retrieved from http://www.
cdc.gov/obesity/index.html.

37. Centers for Disease Control and Prevention. (2014).
*Basics about childhood obesity: How is childhood
overweight and obesity measured?* Retrieved from
http://www.cdc.gov/obesity/childhood/basics.html.

38. U.S. Department of Health and Human Services.
(2014). *Healthy People 2020 topics and objectives:
Nutrition and weight status.* Retrieved from
http://www.healthypeople.gov/2020/topicsobjec-
tives2020/objectiveslist.aspx?topicId=29.

39. Ogden, C., & Carroll, M., Flegal, Katherine M. (2014).
Prevalence of childhood and adult obesity in the
United States, 2011–2012. *JAMA, 311*(8), 806-814.
doi:10.1001/jama.2014.732.

40. Ogden, C., & Carroll, M. (2010). *Prevalence of obesity
among children and adolescents: United States, trends
1963–1965 through 2007–2008.* National Center for
Health Statistics. Retrieved from http://www.cdc.gov/
nchs/data/hestat/obesity_child_07_08/obesity_child_
07_08.pdf.

41. Centers for Disease Control and Prevention. (2014).
Youth Risk Behavior Surveillance System. Retrieved
from http://www.cdc.gov/HealthyYouth/yrbs/index.
htm.

42. MacDonald, M.A. (2004). From miasma to fractals:
The epidemiology revolution and public health
nursing. *Public Health Nursing, 21*(4), 380-381.

43. Centers for Disease Control and Prevention. (2004).
The role of schools in preventing childhood obesity.
Retrieved from http://www.cdc.gov/HealthyYouth/
physicalactivity/pdf/roleofschools_obesity.pdf.

44. Centers for Disease Control and Prevention. (2013). *Lung cancer: What are the risk factors?* Retrieved from http://www.cdc.gov/cancer/lung/basic_info/risk_factors.htm.

45. Centers for Disease Control and Prevention. (2011). *Tobacco use: Targeting the nation's leading killer.* Retrieved from http://www.cdc.gov/chronicdisease/resources/publications/aag/osh.htm.

46. Davis, S., Malarcher, A., Thorne, S., Maurice, E., Trosclair, A., & Mowery, P. (2009). State-specific prevalence and trends in adult cigarette smoking—United States, 1998–2007. *Morbidity and Mortality Weekly Report, 58*(09), 221-226. Retrieved from http://www.cdc.gov/mmwr/preview/mmwrhtml/mm5809a1.htm.

47. Apelberg, B.J, Onicescu, G., Avila-Tang, E., & Samet, J.M. (2010). Estimating the risks and benefits of nicotine replacement therapy for smoking cessation in the United States. *American Journal of Public Health, 100*(2), 341-347.

48. World Health Organization. (2005). *Global tobacco treaty enters into force with 57 countries already committed.* Retrieved from http://www.who.int/mediacentre/news/releases/2005/pr09/en/print.html.

49. U.S. Department of Health and Human Services. (2014). *Healthy People 2020: Topic tobacco use.* Retrieved from http://www.healthypeople.gov/2020/topicsobjectives2020/overview.aspx?topicid=41.

50. Gulbinat, W. (2008). Alcohol and the burden of disease. *Addiction Research & Theory, 16*, 541-552.

51. Rehm, J., Room, R., Monteiro, M., Gmel, G., Graham, K., Rehn, N. Sempos, C.T., et al. (2003). Alcohol as a risk factor for global burden of disease. *European Addiction Research, 9*(4), 157-164.

52. Mokdad, A.H., Marks, J.S. Stroup D.F., & Gerberding, J.L. (2004). Actual causes of death in the United States, 2000. *JAMA, 291*(10), 1238-1245.

53. Centers for Disease Control and Prevention. (2004). Indicators of chronic disease surveillance. *Morbidity and Mortality Weekly Report, 53*(RR11), 1-6.

54. World Health Organization. (2014). *Global status report on alcohol and health.* Geneva, Switzerland: Author.

55. Rehm, J., Mathers, C., Popova, S., Thavorncharoensap, M., Terrawattananon, Y., & Patra, J. (2009). Global burden of disease and injury and economic costs attributable to alcohol use and alcohol use disorders. *Lancet, 373*, 2223-2233.

56. Caetano, R., Ramisetty-Miker, S., Floyd, L., & McGrath, C. (2006). The epidemiology of drinking among women of childbearing age. *Alcoholism, Clinical and Experimental Research, 30*(6), 1023-1030.

57. National Institute on Alcohol Abuse and Alcoholism. (2006). Underage drinking. *Alcohol Alert, 67.*

58. National Institute on Alcohol Abuse and Alcoholism. (2000). Overall impact. *Alcohol Research and Health, 24,* 3-11.

59. National Highway Traffic Safety Authority. (2007). *Traffic safety facts 2006: Alcohol-impaired driving.* Washington, DC: U.S. Department of Transportation.

60. Wechsler, H., & Nelson, T.F. (2008). What have we learned from the Harvard School of Public Health College Alcohol Study: Focusing attention on college student alcohol consumption and the environmental conditions that promote it. *Journal of Studies on Alcohol and Drugs, 69*(4), 481-490.

61. Ferraroni, M. (2009). Alcohol consumption and risk of breast cancer: A multicentre Italian case–control study. *European Journal of Cancer, 2009, 34*(9), 1403-1409.

62. National Institute on Alcohol Abuse and Alcoholism. (2004). Alcohol: An important women's health issue. *Alcohol Alert, 62.* Retrieved from http://pubs.niaaa.nih.gov/publications/aa62/aa62.htm.

63. World Health Organization. (2014). *Genetics and common diseases.* Retrieved from http://www.who.int/genomics/about/commondiseases/en/index.html.

64. Centers for Disease Control and Prevention. (2014). *Public health genomics.* Retrieved from http://www.cdc.gov/genomics/.

65. Quante, A.S., Whittemore, A.S., Shriver, T., Strauch, K., & Terry, M.B. (2012). Breast cancer risk assessment across the continuum: Genetic and nongenetic risk factors contributing to differential model performance. *Breast Cancer Research, 14*(R144). doi:10.1186/bcr3352.

66. National Cancer Institute. (2009). *BRACA1 and BRACA2: Cancer risk and genetic testing.* Retrieved from http://www.cancer.gov/cancertopics/factsheet/Risk/BRCA.

67. Sanlioglu, A.D., Altunbas, H.A., Balci, M.K., Griffith, T.S., & Sanlioglu, S. (2012). Insulin gene therapy from design to beta cell generation. *Expert Reviews in Molecular Medicine, 14*(e18). doi:10.1017/term.2012.12.

68. Strohman, R.C. (1993). Ancient genomes, wise bodies, unhealthy people: Limits of a genetic paradigm in biology and medicine. *Perspectives in Biology and Medicine, 37*(1), 112-145.

69. Wilkenson, R., & Marmot, M. (2003). *Social determinants of health: The solid facts* (2nd ed.). Copenhagen, Denmark: World Health Organization.

70. U.S. Department of Health and Human Services, Office of Minority Health. (2014). *Stroke and African Americans.* Retrieved from http://minorityhealth.hhs.gov/templates/content.aspx?ID=3022.

71. U.S. Department of Health and Human Services, Office of Minority Health. (2014). *Diabetes and American Indians/Alaska Natives.* Retrieved from http://minorityhealth.hhs.gov/templates/content.aspx?lvl=3&lvlID=5&ID=3024.

72. Centers for Disease Control and Prevention. (2012). *Summary health statistic for U.S. adults: National Health Interview Survey, 2011.* Retrieved from http://www.cdc.gov/nchs/data/series/sr_10/sr10_256.pdf.

73. Centers for Disease Control and Prevention. (2013). *Summary of health statistics for U.S. adults: National Health Interview Survey, 2012.* Retrieved from http://www.cdc.gov/nchs/data/series/sr_10/sr10_260.pdf.

74. Centers for Disease Control and Prevention. (2008). *Update to an action plan to prevent heart disease and stroke.* Retrieved from http://www.cdc.gov/DHDSP/library/action_plan/2008_update/pdfs/2008_Action_Plan_Update.pdf.

75. Sargent, R.P., Shepard, R.M., & Glantz, S.A. (2004). Reduced incidence of admission for myocardial infarction

associated with public smoking ban: Before and after study. *British Medical Journal, 828*(24), 977-983.

76. Herman, P.M., & Walsh, M.E. (2011). Hospital admission for acute myocardial infarction, angina, stroke and asthma after implementation of Arizona's comprehensive statewide smoking ban. *American Journal of Public Health*, 101(3), 491-496. doi: 10.2105/AJPH.2009.179572.

77. Bensley, R.J., Mercer, N., Brusk, J.J., Underhile, R., Rivas, J., Anderson, J., et al. (2004). The eHealth behavior management model: A stage-based approach to behavior change and management. *Prevention Preventing Chronic Disease: Public Health Research Practice and Policy, 1*(4), 1-13.

78. Centers for Disease Control and Prevention. (2011). *Health-related quality of life methods and measures.* Retrieved from http://www.cdc.gov/hrqol/methods.htm.

79. Centers for Disease Control and Prevention. (2012). *Health-related quality of life.* Retrieved from http://www.cdc.gov/hrqol/index.htm.

80. World Health Organization. (2003). *WHO definition of health.* Retrieved from http://www.who.int/about/definition/en/print.html.

81. Centers for Disease Control and Prevention. (2011). *Health-related quality of life: Findings.* Retrieved from http://www.cdc.gov/hrqol/key_findings.htm.

82. Ware, J.J., Kosinski, M., & Keller, S.D. (1996). A 12-item short-form health survey: Construction of scales and preliminary tests of reliability and validity. *Medical Care, 34*(3), 220-233.

83. Barile, J.P. (2012). Health-related quality of life among older adults with and without functional limitations. *American Journal of Public Health, 102*(3), 496-502. doi:10.2105/AJPH.2011.300500.

84. Lorig K.R., Ritter, P., Stewart, A.L., Sobel, D.S., William Brown, B., Bandura, A., et al. (2001). Chronic disease self-management program: 2-year health status and health care utilization outcomes. *Medical Care, 39,* 1217-1223.

85. Lorig K.R., & Holman, H.R. (2003). Self-management education: History, definition, outcomes and mechanisms. *Annals of Behavioral Medicine, 26,* 1-7.

86. Bodenheimer T., Lorig, K., Holman, H., & Grumbach, K. (2002). Patient self-management of chronic disease in primary care. *JAMA, 288,* 2469-2475

87. Marks, R., Allegrante, J.P., & Lorig, K. (2005). A review of the synthesis of research evidence for self-efficacy-enhancing interventions for reducing chronic disability: Implications for health education practice (part II). *Health Promotion Practice, 6,* 37-43.

88. Farrell, K., Wicks, M.N., & Martin, J.C. (2004). Chronic disease self-management improved with enhanced self-efficacy. *Clinical Nursing Research, 13,* 289-308.

89. Lorig, K., Ritter, P.L., & Gonzalez, V.M. (2003). Hispanic chronic disease self-management: A randomized community-based outcome trial. *Nursing Research, 52,* 361-369.

90. Thompson, W.W., Zack, M.M., Krahn, G.L., Andresen, E.M., & Barile, J.P. (2012). Health-related quality of life among older adults with and without functional limitation. *American Journal of Public Health, 102*(3), 496-502.

91. Barker, L. Crespo, R., Shrewsberry, M., Gerzoff, R.B., Cornelius-Averhart, D., & Denham, S. (2010). Residence in a distressed county in Appalachia as a risk factor for diabetes, behavioral risk factor surveillance system, 2006–2007. *Preventing Chronic Disease: Public Health Research Practice and Policy, 7*(5), 1-9.

Chapter 10

Mental Health

LEARNING OUTCOMES

After reading this chapter, the student will be able to:

1. Define the burden of disease related to mental disorders using current epidemiological frameworks.
2. Apply the Institute of Medicine (IOM) framework related to prevention of mental health disorders.
3. Define the difference between behavioral, biological, environmental, and socioeconomic risk factors related to mental health disorders.

4. Apply current evidence-based population-level interventions to the prevention of mental disorders and the promotion of optimal mental health for communities and populations.
5. Describe systems approaches to the promotion of mental health and the prevention and treatment of mental health disorders.

KEY TERMS

Behavioral health
Burden of disease
Deinstitutionalization
Emotional health
Health-related quality
of life (HRQoL)

Indicated prevention
Intersectoral strategies
Major depressive disorder
(MDD)
Mental disorder
Mental health

Mental illness
Protective factors
Resilience
Selective prevention
Serious mental illness
(SMI)

Stigma
Transinsitutionalization
Universal prevention

▮ Introduction

Achieving optimal behavioral health is an essential component of programs aimed at improving the health of populations. The Substance Abuse and Mental Health Services Administration (SAMHSA) defines **behavioral health** as the promotion of emotional health; the prevention of mental illnesses and substance use disorders; and the treatments and services for substance abuse, addiction, substance use disorders, mental illness, and/or mental disorders. Behavioral health is viewed as being essential to health overall.[1,2] In 2005, the Institute of Medicine (IOM) reported that mental or substance use problems and illnesses are the leading cause of combined disability and death for women and the second highest for men.[3] Of the 10 leading health indicator topics of *Healthy People 2020 (HP 2020)*, four topics relate directly to behavioral health, mental health, substance abuse, tobacco, and injury/violence.[4] These four topics come under the umbrella of the term *behavioral health*. Each of these interrelated issues has an impact on the health of individuals, families, and communities. Often mental illness and

substance abuse and/or intentional injury and violence co-occur. Thus, there is a logical and empirical connection between these health issues. Taken together, they make up the most serious and prevalent public health problems of our times. So that each aspect of behavioral health can be covered in depth, these four leading health indicator topics of health are covered in three separate chapters. Chapter 10 covers mental health and mental health disorders; Chapter 11 covers substance use including alcohol, tobacco, and other drugs; and Chapter 12 covers injury and violence.

This chapter focuses on promotion of **mental health**, which is best defined by *HP 2020* as "a state of successful performance of mental function, resulting in productive activities, fulfilling relationships with other people, and the ability to adapt to change and to cope with challenges."[4] The term **emotional health** is used interchangeably with *mental health* and is defined the same way. *HP 2020* includes under the topic of mental health two other terms, *mental disorders* and *mental illness*. *Mental health* reflects a positive state of health, whereas *mental disorders* refers to the diagnosable disorders that negatively affect the mental health of individuals and affect an individual's ability to cope with everyday life. *Mental illness* is a term that refers to all mental disorders collectively. The terms **mental disorder** and **mental illness** are often used interchangeably and are defined as "clusters of symptoms and signs associated with distress and disability (i.e., impairment of functioning), yet whose pathology and etiology are unknown."[1,4] Mental illnesses are disorders, not diseases. A *disease* is a term used when the pathology is known or can be detected, which is not the case with a mental health disorder. Diagnoses that come under the category of mental disorders include depression, anxiety disorders, bipolar disorder, and schizophrenia. Not all mental health disorders have the same etiology (cause) or require the same population-level interventions.

Mental disorders can vary in severity from mild to severe. The term **serious mental illness (SMI)** is used to refer to a diagnosable mental disorder that severely disrupts a person's ability to function socially, to obtain and maintain employment, to have adequate financial resources, and to access appropriate and adequate support or maintain family supports. SMI does not refer to any particular diagnosis; rather, it implies eligibility for specific kinds of support services. The mental disorders that can lead to SMI include major depression, schizophrenia, bipolar disorder, obsessive-compulsive disorder (OCD), panic disorder, post-traumatic stress disorder (PTSD), and borderline personality disorder.

In contrast with mental disorders, mental health represents a state of emotional well-being. Persons who are emotionally healthy are those who are able to meet the demands and stresses of everyday life and function in society. Mental health does not merely represent the absence of a mental disorder, but rather the cognitive and emotional ability to deal with the ups and downs of life while contributing to society through work and play. Viewed from a population perspective, the health of a population reflects not only the physical well-being of the members of the population or community, but also their social and emotional well-being. Because of their overall importance to health, mental health and mental disorders are included in the *HP 2020* list of topics.

■ HEALTHY PEOPLE 2020
Mental Health
Goal: Improve mental health through prevention and by ensuring access to appropriate, quality mental health services.
Overview: *Mental health* is a state of successful performance of mental function, resulting in productive

activities, fulfilling relationships with other people, and the ability to adapt to change and to cope with challenges. Mental health is essential to personal well-being, family and interpersonal relationships, and the ability to contribute to community or society.

Mental disorders are health conditions that are characterized by alterations in thinking, mood, and/or behavior that are associated with distress and/or impaired functioning. Mental disorders contribute to a host of problems that may include disability, pain, or death. *Mental illness* is the term that refers collectively to all diagnosable mental disorders.[4]

Optimal mental health is an essential component of healthy communities. The promotion of mental health involves interventions at the individual and community levels. At the individual level, promotion of optimal mental health requires not only the delivery of interventions focused on behavioral change, but also the provision of adequate systems for care of those with mental health disorders. The mental health of communities depends on the provision of an environment that encourages a strong social network and a safe place to work and live.[5] Because of the importance of mental health in 2012, the World Health Organization issued a resolution on mental health that aims to reduce the global burden of mental disorders and improve the overall mental health of countries. This resolution includes a recognition of "the need for a comprehensive, coordinated response to addressing mental disorders from health and social sectors at the country level. The delegates recognized this includes approaches such as programmes to reduce stigma and discrimination, reintegration of patients into workplace and society, support for care providers and families, and investment in mental health from the health budget."[6]

Epidemiology of Mental Disorders

According to the World Health Organization (WHO), nearly 450 million people worldwide suffer from a mental health disorder.[7] In the United States in 2010, an estimated 25% of adults reported having mental disorders in the previous year, with an estimated economic cost of $317 billion related to SMI.[8] The estimated cost does not take into account costs associated with homelessness, incarceration, or early mortality, all issues associated with SMI.[9] As reviewed in Chapter 9, the **burden of disease** is measured in years of life lost related to ill health and reflects the difference between total life expectancy and disability-adjusted life expectancy. Examining the burden of disease related to mental disorders allows us to take into account what impact mental disorders have on the population or community as a whole. The best place to start is to examine the prevalence of mental disorders across the life span from both a global and international perspective.

Surveillance of Mental Health Disorders

Estimating the prevalence of mental disorders is challenging because there is no current, centralized method for conducting surveillance of mental health disorders in the United States or globally. Recently, the Centers for Disease Control and Prevention (CDC) conducted a compilation of data from numerous surveillance systems to identify gaps in surveillance and make recommendations for an improved method for collecting needed data on mental health disorders. The CDC used eight national surveys and surveillance systems to collect data on mental health in adults. None of these surveys or systems focused specifically on mental health. Through this process of examining data from all data sources, they were not only able to provide some estimates of prevalence of different mental disorders, but also to help make recommendations about how to address the gaps in mental illness surveillance. The data sources included the Pregnancy Risk Assessment Monitoring System (PRAMS), National Nursing Home Survey, National Health Interview Survey, National Hospital Discharge Survey, National Health and Nutrition Examination Survey, National Ambulatory Medical Care Survey, National Hospital Ambulatory

Medical Care Survey, and Behavioral Risk Factor Surveillance System.[8] At the global level, the WHO has developed the World Mental Health Survey to help determine estimates of human capital costs and prevalence of mental disorders in a wide range of countries.[10]

Prevalence of Mental Health Disorders

Mental health is an important part of overall health across the entire life span. Differences exist between age groups in relation to specific disorders. To understand the importance of the issue and evaluate the effectiveness of interventions from a population perspective requires knowledge of the prevalence of mental disorders within and across communities and populations.

The 12-month prevalence is a measure that estimates the occurrence of a disorder within 1 year prior to assessment. In 2012 the 12-month prevalence of all mental disorders not including substance use disorders was 18.6% and was most prevalent in those aged 26 to 49.[11] A little over 4% of the adult population had serious mental illness in 2012.[12]

There are gender, ethnic, and age differences in the prevalence of serious mental illness (Fig. 10-1).[12] In 2012 the 12-month prevalence of any mental disorder was higher in females than in males.[11] American Indian/Alaska Natives are at increased risk for mental health disorders and have a higher rate of lifetime PTSD than others in the national U.S population.[13,14] The lower prevalence of mental disorders in African Americans and Hispanics does not take into account that racial/ethnic minority groups are

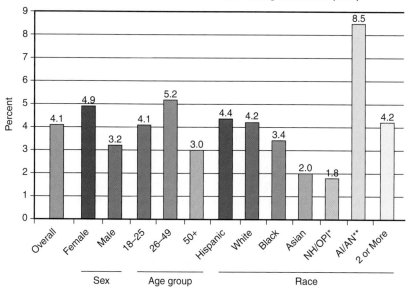

Prevalence of Serious Mental Illness among U.S. Adults (2012)

*NH/OPI = Native Hawaiian/Other Pacific Islander

**AI/AN = American Indian/Alaska Native

Data courtesy of SAMMSA

Figure 10-1 Prevalence of serious mental illness among U.S. adults, 2012. *(See reference 12.)*

disproportionately represented in the homeless and incarcerated populations.[9] These differences persist when examining the prevalence of SMI (see Fig. 10-1).[11] Children also experience mental disorders; about 8% of teens are diagnosed with an anxiety disorder between the ages of 13 and 18 years. However, the symptoms usually begin to emerge around age 6.[15] About 11% of teens are diagnosed with a depressive disorder by the age of 18 years and 25% experience at least mild symptoms of depression.[15]

Under the umbrella of SMI are specific diagnostic categories that have been the focus of population level prevention efforts, especially **major depressive disorder (MDD),** which is a mood disorder that is diagnosed based on the occurrence of one or more major depressive episodes in the absence of a manic or hypomanic episode. About 6.7% of the U.S. population is affected by a MDD within a given year. It is the leading cause of disability for those aged 15 to 44 years and is more prevalent in women than in men.[16] Because of the high prevalence and the impact on health, *HP 2020* includes the reduction of the number of persons who experience an MDD as one of the mental health objectives.

■ HEALTHY PEOPLE 2020

Objectives: Reduce the proportion of persons who experience major depressive episode (MDE)
MHMD-4.1: Adolescents aged 12 to 17 years
Baseline: 8.3% of adolescents aged 12 to 17 years experienced an MDR in 2008.
Target: 7.4%
Target-Setting Method: 10% improvement
Data Source: National Survey on Drug and Health, SAMHSA

Source: See reference 4.

During the past decade, the morbidity and mortality rate associated with SMI has increased, showing that persons diagnosed with an SMI die 25 years earlier than the general population. Part of this is attributed to suicide and injury. The other contributing factor is the strong association between SMI, chronic disease, and substance use.[17–19] Based on these findings, the National Association of State Mental Health Program Directors made specific recommendations aimed at reducing SMI-related morbidity and mortality (Box 10-1): "Understanding how inseparable mental and physical health really are, and how their influence on each other is complex and profound, . . . mental health—neglected for far too long—is crucial to the overall well-being of individuals, societies and countries and must be universally regarded in a new light."[20]

BOX 10–1	**Recommendations of the National Association of State Mental Health Program Directors**

- It should be designated as a priority health disparities population.
- Morbidity and mortality rates of physical conditions should be tracked and monitored.
- Standards of care for prevention, screening, assessment, and treatment of physical conditions ought to be established and implemented.
- Access to integrated physical and mental health-care services must be improved.

Source: See reference 20.

Behavioral, Biological, Environmental, and Socioeconomic Risk Factors

Numerous factors contribute to the development of mental disorders at both the individual and community levels and must be taken into account when attempting to understand the etiology of mental disorders. There is interplay between the individual, the family, and the community environment. From a public health perspective, improving the mental health of a population requires taking all of these factors into account when developing interventions.

Individual-Level Risk Factors for Mental Disorders

At the individual level, both nature and nurture play roles; that is, genetics as well as family environment and individual behavior are associated with the risk of developing a mental disorder, along with socioeconomic factors and community environment. Therefore, it is difficult to define the exact etiology of most mental disorders because the precise cause of mental disorders is poorly understood. There are, however, specific factors that have been associated with the development of mental disorders (Box 10-2). Recent work has helped to demonstrate the link between genotype and mental illness through an environmental pathway. For example, as explained by Schmidt, 30% to 50% of persons with a certain genotype who are exposed to most types of trauma will develop PTSD; however, when the trauma is severe, the prevalence rate increases to close to 100%.[21]

Another issue related to the development of a mental disorder is the relationship between physiology and mental health. Conditions that affect brain chemistry; hormonal imbalances; or exposure in utero to viruses, toxins, or poor nutrition can increase the risk for

BOX 10–2	Risk Factors for Mental Illness

- Family history of mental disorders or history of being diagnosed with a mental disorder in the past
- Traumatic events: military combat, assault, or witness to a violent crime
- In utero exposure to viruses and toxins; poor nutrition
- Cerebral injury: experiencing brain damage as a result of a serious injury such as a violent blow to the head, traumatic brain injury
- Stressful life situations: financial problems, the death of a loved one, or marital problems and/or divorce
- Social isolation: having few friends or few healthy relationships
- Developmental delays
- Substance use: illicit drugs, alcohol, medication side effects, and drug interactions
- Poor health: living with a chronic medical condition such as cancer
- History of being abused or neglected as a child
- Low self-esteem, social isolation, poor social skills
- Gay/Lesbian/Bisexual/Transgender (GLBT) adolescents and anxiety, depression, suicidal tendencies
- Poverty and socioeconomic level
- Rural versus urban populations
- Lower education level
- Dangerous communities, high crime rates

development of a mental disorder.[22,23] Physical trauma such as traumatic brain injury is also associated with an increased risk of developing a mental disorder. Individuals with developmental delays and low IQ are also at higher risk for development of a mental disorder.[24] Another issue is the role of medication side effects and drug interactions in mental disorders.[25] Persons with general poor health and/or a chronic medical condition such as cancer are also at increased risk.[22,26,27] Conversely, there is evidence that mental disorders are themselves independent risk factors for cardiovascular disease, type 2 diabetes, and injuries.[28]

Instability of the family is a factor in the development of mental disorders, with a higher incidence rate in individuals raised in situations of abuse or neglect, including sexual abuse, or for those who have experienced exposure to traumatic events including serious loss.[22,25,26] In addition, children of parents with mental disorders are at increased risk for developing mental disorders themselves because of the negative impact a mental disorder has on parenting skills. The home environment in itself can have an impact on family members including safety of the home, and issues such as ready access to guns, a risk factor for suicide.[27] Exposure to family stress

owing to poor financial situations, death, divorce, or unemployment is also associated with mental disorders.[22] Along with family environment, individual characteristics can increase the risk for development of a mental disorder. For example, individuals with low self-esteem, who are lonely, isolated, and/or have poor social skills, and those who have unhealthy thinking patterns are at higher risk. Some behavioral choices also increase the risk of mental disorders, such as substance use (Chapter 11).[22,25,26]

An emerging issue is the increased incidence of mental disorders in Gay/Lesbian/ Bisexual/Transgender adolescents. They are more likely to be depressed and anxious, and attempt and/or commit suicide because of insecurity and difficulty in negotiating their coming out, family disapproval, rejection, victimization, and chronic stress from stigmatization.[23] Thus, the development of a mental disorder is a complex combination of genetics, other physical disorders, and family environment.

Community-Level Risk Factors for Mental Disorders

The determinants of health also play a role in the development of mental disorders because the community environment plays a pivotal role. There is a clear inverse relationship between poverty and prevalence of mental disorders, with a greater prevalence of mental disorders in populations and communities that are experiencing social and economic disadvantages.[27,29,30] Differences also exist between rural and urban populations. Those living in rural areas with a high poverty rate are different from the mainstream population and have a higher prevalence rate of mental disorders. Part of this risk is associated with a lower level of education and fewer job opportunities and decreased access to mental health services.[29] Living in dangerous communities (Chapter 12), especially those with high crime rates, is another risk factor.

Protective Factors: Building Resilience

Although a risk-based approach is one strategy for addressing the prevention of mental disorders, an examination of protective factors is equally important. Understanding why some individuals are able to overcome adversity is a key component in the development of intervention programs focused on prevention of mental disorders. **Protective factors** are processes within individuals, families, or communities that exist, can be strengthened, or can be incorporated into interventions for purposes of building resilience. They are the supports and opportunities that buffer adversity.[31] **Resilience** is an individual's ability to access protective factors that exist at different levels to withstand chronic stress or recover from traumatic life events (Box 10-3).[32] Protective factors can reduce risk for mental health disorders and promote optimal mental health. Understanding what factors help individuals, families, and communities reach optimal health, then, is as important as understanding the factors that increase the risk for developing a mental disorder. Both prevention and treatment interventions can build on these protective factors to help promote optimal mental health.

Research on individual protective factors provides the foundation for supporting protective factors in prevention interventions. Werner and Smith followed 700 high-risk children into adulthood and found that only one out of six adults had poor health and social outcomes in adulthood.[33] These findings provide evidence of the resilience of people despite adverse childhoods and suggest the need to identify characteristics that are protective. Similar findings have been reported in studies conducted with those seeking treatment for an alcohol use disorder. For example, in one study protective resources such as building self-efficacy or bonding with family, friends, and coworkers predicted remission.[34] According to Bernard, successful outcomes and positive development are dependent on the quality of relationships, expectations, and opportunities for participation, three characteristics that work synergistically in a dynamic process to promote mental health and resilience.[31]

A decade ago, the report from the President's New Freedom Commission on Mental Health was published, emphasizing that the transformation of the mental health delivery system depends on a focus on coping with challenges in life and building resilience.[35,36] Resilience is recognized by strengths such as social competence, problem-solving ability, autonomy, and a sense of purpose.[31] Interventions to promote resilience focus on building these strengths. Because these strengths are

inherent psychological needs, humans are compelled to meet them throughout their lifetime, and the factors determining whether they do meet them are often dependent on the wider systems in which an individual interacts, including families, schools, and communities.[31]

A community can also be viewed as resilient.[32] Similar to how resilience in an individual is defined, a resilient community is characterized by social competence, problem-solving, a sense of identity, and hope for the future. The availability of resources important for human development is evidence of a resilient community. These resources include health care, childcare, housing, education, job training, employment, and recreation.[31] A recent study examined community differences in the quality of childcare and the mental health of children attending the childcare centers in British Columbia, Canada.[37] Based on socioeconomic criteria, the communities were classified as better off or worse off. There were fewer mental health problems, and childcare quality was higher in the resilient community compared with the other communities. When children grow up in a poor community, it is easy to see how the erosion of resilience can occur.

A community's resilience contributes to an individual's capacity to develop resilience and whether a MHD is present or not. The community develops and nurtures resilience by valuing and providing the means of connectedness, by supporting and nurturing commitment and shared values where everyone participates in meaningful structure and role responsibilities, and by engaging in critical reflection and skill building that feeds back into the community.[38] The ability of a community to build resilience is called *community capacity*.[31]

An example of community-level resilience is that of community members and organizations working in partnership with youths, families, and schools. A sense of connectedness can result when schools work in partnership with students, families, and community groups. An example of this connectedness is a program called Elev8 in Baltimore, Maryland, which is focused on improving educational and social outcomes for middle grade adolescents and their families in East Baltimore. "Each Elev8 Baltimore school is assigned a site manager and a family advocate responsible for collaborating with the principal and staff; building relationships with students and families; responding to the needs of students, parents and school staff; promoting the integration of learning, health and family support strategy; and developing a family engagement plan to facilitate connections among families, the school and the broader community."[39]

BOX 10–3	**Protective Factors and Resilience**

- Environmental capital: structural factors and features of the natural and built environments
- Environment that enhance community capacity for well-being
- Social capital: norms, networks and distribution of resources that enhance community trust, cohesion, influence, and cooperation for mutual benefit
- Emotional and cognitive capital as resources that buffer stress and/or determine outcomes and contribute to individual resilience and capability

Source: See reference 32.

School connectedness is an example of building community resilience. Such programs demonstrate that building resilience at the community level not only can improve the mental health of children and youth but also can have a positive impact on the behavioral and academic outcomes of children.[40,38] The importance of interdisciplinary programs working together to build community resilience is also increasingly recognized as an approach to address social determinants of health, inequities in education, and the urban environment overall.[32,41] Some programs operate at the intersection of public health, education, and urban planning. Examples include the Obama administration's Neighborhood Revitalization Initiative, which focuses on standardized test scores and educational inequities, and the Choice Neighborhoods program, which is based on Hope VI, that targets severely distressed public housing developments.[42,43] A focus in these programs is to develop community health centers and full-service community schools, and to pursue community development for purposes of revitalizing neighborhoods.[38]

Culture, Stigma, and Mental Health Disorders

Culture has tremendous influence on the meaning of mental illness for individuals, families, and communities. A culture's deeply rooted beliefs and attitudes exert considerable influence on how mental illness is viewed by society, the individual with the illness, his family, and the community. It may be viewed as real or imagined, adaptive or maladaptive, or as valued distinction or intentional deviance from the norm. Beliefs and attitudes determine how likely support will be available and whether a person with a mental health disorder will seek help or accept treatment.[44–47] Some Latinos and African Americans, for example, tend to voice resistance toward mental health care, tend to downplay and normalize mental illness, and offer alternative explanations for problems other than a biomedical perspective.[46]

Stigma is one of the barriers to the treatment of mental health problems.[45] Goffman's classic definition views stigma as a combination of personal attributes and societal stereotypes related to human characteristics viewed as unacceptable.[48–50] Stigma refers to a trait or attribute of a person that results in the discrediting of that person. Stigma occurs when the person rather than the trait or condition is held responsible for the inability to perform an action.[50] Cultural belief systems can produce stigma, the form of social disapproval that pervades the attitudes

and actions of the community, the family, and even the individual.

Stigma acts as a barrier to achieving health and well-being and can greatly undermine a community's efforts to capitalize on strengths. There is a growing awareness of disparities in access and utilization of mental health services among ethnic and racial minority populations. Treatment disparities among African Americans, for example, are related to a lack of insurance coverage, a tendency not to receive an antidepressant or selective serotonin reuptake inhibitors, and nonresponsiveness to traditional pharmacological interventions for depression.[47] The many pathways possibly explaining these disparities include variations in expression of symptoms, bias or prejudice among providers, experiences of mistreatment, difficulties in accessing treatment, and stigma among various populations.[46] Stigma can cause individuals with mental illness to adopt a number of behaviors that serve to protect them from stigma but may result in failure to seek treatment (Box 10-4).[51]

The National Alliance for Mental Health has developed strategies to address issues related to culture and stigma. These strategies address challenges related to the complexity of the issue, including illness progression, family history and cultural influences, impenetrable isolation reinforced by stigma, and multiple system failures. An example is the organization's recommendations for providing culturally competent care for Korean Americans diagnosed with a mental disorder (see Box 10-5).[52–54]

The importance of culture and stigma is best exemplified by the incident that occurred on April 16, 2007. Seunghui Cho, aged 23 years and a senior at Virginia Polytechnic Institute and State University, wounded 25 people and killed 32 and then himself in a shooting rampage that lasted several hours. Cho was only 8 years old when his family arrived in the United States from South Korea. He was a shy child and apparently was bullied. His childhood years had been troubled, and in middle school, he was diagnosed with selective mutism, a severe anxiety disorder, and a major depressive disorder. He began to receive treatment

BOX 10–4	**Reaction to Stigma**

- Pretend nothing is wrong
- Refuse to seek treatment
- Be rejected by family and friends
- Experience difficulty finding housing and employment
- Be subjected to physical violence or harassment
- Have inadequate health insurance coverage for mental illness

Source: See reference 51.

BOX 10–5	National Alliance for Mental Health Key Cultural Concepts for the Korean American Community

- Mental health providers need to understand cultural and stigmatizing barriers and to be willing to take advantage of opportunities to intervene and treat using programs that are specifically tailored to the ethnicity of the population.
- Public health practitioners should be aware of cultural concepts.
- Three central cultural concepts are:
  Haan—Suppressed anger, unexpressed grievance, resentment
  Jeong—Strong feeling of kinship/interpersonal trust, emotional bonding
  Noon-chi—Capacity to quickly evaluate another person or social situation
  Cultivating *jeong* in the consumer-provider relationship, practicing *noon-chi*, and acknowledging the presence of *haan* is a good beginning for clinicians who wish to develop a trusting and beneficial relationship with Korean American patients.
- Korean Americans are very responsive to family and group psychoeducational interventions, which have been shown to increase coping skills, decrease stigma, and lessen symptom severity.
- Korean Americans, and other Asian Americans can experience more debilitating side effects from psychiatric medications because their bodies respond differently than other ethnic groups to medications because of a noted gene mutation. Providers need to work closely with the family to maximize the benefits of pharmacological treatment

Sources: See references 52–54.

and therapy, which continued through his sophomore year in high school. During college, he was hospitalized for mental illness symptoms and offered treatment, which he declined.[55,56]

The tragic incident led campus police and state government officials to investigate and make recommendations. Due to this incident and others, colleges and universities across the nation have evaluated and revised safety and security plans and strengthened campus mental health services.[56] This case illustrates that a traumatic experience of this nature has a widespread impact on a community, with lasting psychological distress. Violent acts such as this one, the Columbine High School shootings, the movie theater shootings in Aurora, Colorado, and the shootings in Newtown, Connecticut, that left 20 first-grade students dead are linked with mental disorders and social-identity threats.[56,57]

The high-profile case at Virginia Polytech is an example of the impact that culture has on understanding the expressions and presentation of mental disorders. Korean Americans make up 10% of the Asian population in America and make up to 4% of the total American population. Approximately 40% of the Korean population have arrived in the United States since 1990, and are therefore considered recent immigrants.[58,59] Jang and colleagues reported that South Korean individuals are unlikely to present to a health-care provider and complain of mental problems. Rather, their concerns are focused on schooling and vocational or employment-related problems. Families are likely to insist that a family member suffering with mental problems should keep her or his problems hidden because of the shame it can bring on the family. By the time help is sought, the problems have often become severe.[60]

Prevention of Mental Disorders and Promotion of Mental Health

Because mental health is not simply the absence of a mental disorder, prevention of mental disorders and promotion of mental health are key components of efforts to optimize the mental health of individuals and communities. Promotion focuses on building communities with living conditions and environments that support mental health.[5] Prevention focuses on implementing strategies that prevent mental disorders and providing early intervention and adequate treatment for those with mental disorders.

Measure of Mental Health: Health-Related Quality of Life

One way to assess mental health is to measure **health-related quality of life (HRQoL).** It is a marker not only of physical health, but also of mental health. As noted in Chapter 9, HRQoL is central to the overarching goals for *HP 2020*. HRQoL as defined in Chapter 9 is the self-perceived impact of physical and emotional health on quality of life, including the effects on general health, physical functioning, physical health and role, bodily pain, vitality, social functioning, emotional health and role, and mental health.[61,62] The HRQoL measure used by the CDC includes items specifically aimed at measuring emotional and mental health. It is a useful tool for the nurse who wishes to assess the level of mental health in a patient as well as a tool for assessing the overall mental health in a population. The tool is available on the CDC Web site and can be easily downloaded.

Institute of Medicine Model of Prevention

In 1997, the IOM reported that the primary, secondary, and tertiary continuum of prevention was confusing when applied to mental disorders and developed a new model that more clearly separates prevention from treatment.[63] This framework, presented in Chapter 2 and again in Chapter 11, divides the prevention category into three levels that were developed specifically for behavioral health issues: (1) universal, (2) selective (also referred to as selected), and (3) indicated, with possible interventions at each level. **Universal prevention** refers to prevention interventions provided to the entire population, not just those who may be at risk. The interventions include but are not limited to public service announcements provided to the public at large through billboards, media messages (print and electronic), or general health education programs. **Selective prevention** includes interventions provided to specific subgroups that are known to be at high risk for mental disorders owing to biological, psychological, social, or environmental factors but that have not yet been diagnosed with mental disorders. High-risk subgroups include but are not limited to those with a family history of mental disorders, history of adverse childhood events, or victims of violence. An example is counseling delivered to students at a school where violence has occurred such as the extensive counseling required following the Newtown, Connecticut, shootings. Selective interventions include opportunities for learning strategies to prevent the development of a mental disorder as well as early warning signs to help individuals and families seek help early. **Indicated prevention** addresses specific subgroups at highest risk for development of a mental disorder, or that are showing early signs of a mental disorder. The purpose of indicated techniques is to delay or reduce the severity of a mental disorder. At this level, there is less concern about community prevention and more emphasis on individuals who demonstrate early signs of mental disorders.[63]

Promotion of Mental Health and Policy

The WHO strongly supports the implementation of strategies that will create healthful living conditions and environments that result in optimal mental health. The organization stated that mental health promotion depends on **intersectoral strategies.** These are defined as strategies that engage more than one sector of society with a shared interest such as governmental agencies, grass roots citizen groups, nonprofit groups, and/or businesses. Some of the strategies proposed by the WHO include those that address needs of specific age groups, vulnerable populations, and women. Other strategies focus on the environment such as the workplace, schools, housing, and community development. They recommend that governments mainstream mental health promotion across policies and programs.[5] The WHO warns against focusing only on mental disorder treatment and stresses that an upstream approach (see Chapter 2) is vital to the health of communities.

To support its efforts related to mental health improvement, the WHO developed a model to guide its activities called the Mental Health Improvements for Nations' Development (MIND) (Fig. 10-2). It includes four components: (1) Action in Countries, (2) Mental Health Policy, Planning & Service, (3) Mental Health, Human Rights & Legislation, and (4) Mental Health, Poverty & Development. This model demonstrates not only the need for intersectoral strategies, but also for interrelationships between multiple factors that contribute to mental health.[64]

Secondary Prevention: Screening for Mental Disorders

The focus of the IOM report *Improving the Quality of Health Care for Mental and Substance-Use Conditions: Quality Chasm Series* is the need for appropriate behavioral health treatment.[65] The report has a strong emphasis on early identification and treatment. The model for secondary intervention in mental health is screening, brief intervention, and referral for treatment (SBIRT), an approach also used in secondary prevention programs related to at-risk alcohol use (Chapter 11). The Substance Abuse and Mental Health Service Administration (SAMSHA) issued a report on the use of screening for behavioral health that includes screening for depression and trauma/anxiety disorders. Though SAMSHA concludes that no evidence exists to support a comprehensive SBIRT program for these disorders, there is evidence that screening is effective.[66]

A number of reliable screening tools exist that have validity across the life span and across health-care settings. Tools differ based on the specific mental disorder being screened. The screening tools most often used in primary care are for depression and anxiety disorders. Tools to screen for depression include the Patient Health Questionnaire 2 and the Center for Epidemiological Studies Depression Scale. Screening tools for anxiety disorders include the Brief Symptom Checklist-18 of the My Mood Monitor.[66] The challenge is not only to screen but also to provide care to those who screen positive. Thus, universal screening for depression is only recommended in situations in which accurate diagnosis and treatment are available.[66]

One approach related to screening and engagement into treatment for disorders is to integrate care for

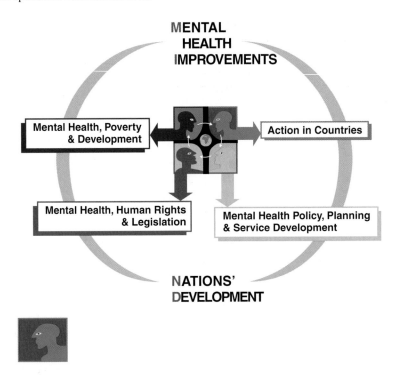

- Action in countries: nations at work
  Supporting countries to improve the lives of people with mental disorders.

- Mental health policy, planning & service development: integration for better services
  Mental health policy and action plans are essential because they coordinate, through a common vision, all programs and services related to mental health.

- Mental health, human rights & legislation: denied citizens including the excluded
  Too many people with mental disability are exposed to a wide range of human rights violations both within psychiatric institutions and in the community.

Figure 10-2 WHO Mental Health Improvements for Nations' Development (MIND). *(From World Health Organization. [2012]. Mental Health, MIND—mental health in development. Retrieved from http://www.who.int/mental_health/policy/en/index.html.)*

- Mental health, poverty, & development: mental health core to development
  Mental health is integral to achieving many development priorities. However people with mental and psychosocial disabilities are not only missed by development programs, but can be actively excluded from these programs.

mental disorders within primary care settings. Because most people who are identified with mental disorders are seen in a primary care setting, integrating care within this setting is a logical approach. Without an integrated system, those who screen positive may not receive the care they need.

● APPLYING PUBLIC HEALTH SCIENCE

The Case of the Baby Blues

Peg, a recent graduate nurse, began working in a labor and delivery unit in an urban hospital and was rapidly learning what she needed to know to function on the unit. In her second month on the unit, she was involved in the care of Abigail, who delivered her first baby after a long labor. During Abigail's labor, Peg learned a lot about Abigail and her husband, Frank, and was impressed by their story. Frank came from Albania and owned and operated a restaurant in Florida. Abigail had grown up in the Northeast and graduated from a culinary academy. They met the day Abigail applied for the pastry chef job at Frank's restaurant and thus began what appeared to be a wonderful love story.

A year after Abigail's son was born, Peg learned that Frank and Abigail's story had taken a tragic turn. Abigail committed suicide after suffering for months with severe postpartum depression (PPD). Abigail had a history of depression and severe premenstrual syndrome symptoms, which may increase a woman's risk for PPD. Peg wondered whether they had screened Abigail on admission for depression and realized that she had not picked up on any warning signs during Abigail's labor. She decided she needed to know more about PPD.

Peg discovered that PPD is not well understood and that it is different from "postpartum blues." According to what she read, there is an underlying biological basis for PPD because it is in part triggered by the massive drop in hormones that occurs after delivery.[67] She remembered learning about this in school, but what she did not realize was that severe PPD, if it occurs, occurs soon after delivery. But Abigail had been discharged within 24 hours of her son's birth. Was there anything that they as nurses could do to prevent this from happening again? She read more and found that PPD can intensify to include delusions, and that nearly 5% of women with postpartum psychosis commit suicide. A very small proportion (4%) of these women will kill their babies.[67]

Peg read that, in another study, the CDC found in three states that about 12% of women reported being moderately depressed and 6% being very depressed after delivery.[68] The study was based on the PRAMS survey conducted by the CDC. PRAMS is a surveillance system of the CDC and state departments that monitors mothers' experiences and attitudes before, during, and after pregnancy. It provides nurses with important data that are broken down by state.[68] An analysis of data from 2004 to 2008 reveals that 14.5% of PRAMS respondents reported symptoms of PPD evidenced by answering "always" or "often" to two questions: (1) Since your new baby was born, how often have you felt down, depressed, or hopeless? and (2) Since your new baby was born, how often have you had little interest in doing things? The prevalence varies by age, with a greater prevalence among those women aged 19 years or younger (23.3%) and among non-Hispanic black women (21.5%).[69]

She brought this information to her nurse manager and wondered whether it would be a good idea to conduct a quality improvement project on how they were screening for PPD on their unit. The manager agreed, and Peg began to review their current process for screening and the current recommendations for screening. Peg was amazed to find that there was no clear evidence on what screening tool to use, whom to screen, and when the best time to screen was.[70–72] She also found that her unit had no clear guidelines.

Following a more thorough search, she found guidelines that had been instituted at the University of Louisville, Kentucky, and submitted them for consideration on her unit. They were modeled after the program in Louisville. On admission to labor and delivery, all new mothers will be assessed for PPD. Those who screen positive will be referred to the attending obstetrician. The evening prior to discharge, all mothers will fill out a questionnaire using a valid and reliable screening tool specific to PPD and appropriate persons will be notified (social worker, physician, and the discharge nurse). The nurse will review the results of the screening with the mother and her support person and inform them of the symptoms of depression, should there be any. The nurse will also provide the mother with a list of available resources in the community (Evidence-Based Practice).

■ EVIDENCE-BASED PRACTICE
Screening for Postpartum Depression

Practice Statement: All women should be screened for postpartum depression using a validated and reliable screening tool during the prenatal period.

Targeted Outcome: Identification of those at risk, initiation of prevention strategies, and, when indicated, referral to treatment

Evidence to Support: The evidence for the effectiveness of screening for PPD is under current scrutiny. The Affordable Care Act of 2010 under Section 2952 includes a requirement that the Department of Health and Human Services conduct a study on the benefits of screening for postpartum depression. A current validated and reliable tool is the Edinburgh Postnatal Depression Scale (EPDS). It has also appropriate reliability across cultures. Though there are valid and reliable tools available to screen for PPD, there is no clear evidence that screening results in improved outcomes or engagement in care.

Sources:

Berger, E., Wu, A., Smulian, E.A., Quinoes, J.N., Curet, S., . . . Smulian, J.C. (2014). Universal versus risk factor-targeted early inpatient postpartum depression screening. *Journal of Maternal, Fetal and Neonatal Medicine*, 1-6. Advance online publication. doi:10.3109/14767058.2014.932764.

Bergink V., Kooistra L., Lambregtse-van den Berg M.P., Wijnen H., Bunevicius R., . . . Pop V. (2011). Validation of the Edinburgh Depression Scale during pregnancy. *Journal of Psychosomatic Research*, 70(4), 385-389. doi:10.1016/j.jpsychores.2010.07.008.

Kheirabadi, G.R., Maracy, M.R., Akbaripour, S., & Masaeli, N. (2014). Psychometric properties and diagnostic accuracy of the Edinburgh postnatal depression scale in a sample of Iranian women. *Iran Journal of Medical Science*, 37(1), 32-38.

Stewart, R.C., Umar, E., Tomenson, B., & Creed, F. (2013). Validation of screening tools for antenatal depression in Malawi—a comparison of the Edinburgh Postnatal Depression Scale and Self Reporting Questionnaire. *Journal of Affective Disorders*, 150(3), 1041-1047. doi:10.1016/j.jad.2013.05.036.

Tertiary Prevention: Treatment for Mental Disorders

At the individual level, a person diagnosed with a mental disorder has to meet the clinical criteria for the diagnosis. Because there are no definitive diagnostic laboratory tests or scans that are useful for diagnosing mental disorders, experts in the field developed a manual, the *Diagnostic and Statistical Manual of Mental Disorders* (DSM), to guide diagnostic decision making and provide consistency and accuracy in diagnoses among clinicians. The new revision of the manual, DSM-5, is organized so the chapters are based on underlying vulnerabilities as well as symptom characteristics. The goal is to facilitate a more comprehensive approach to diagnosis and treatment and the DSM-5 represents a major change from earlier versions of the manual.[73] Thus, at the individual level experts have recently reexamined diagnostic criteria based on the best evidence. Treatment of mental health usually focuses on the individual and can include many different treatment modalities. At the population level, tertiary treatment and policy are closely related with access to treatment as the central issue.

Mental Health Policy Related to Treatment

Access to treatment and the type of treatment available have been central issues since the end of World War II. Prevention at the population level related to treatment entails reduction of disparity in access to treatment, whereas promotion of mental health requires policies that will strengthen the mental health of populations.[74] Historically, government policy focused on treatment of mental disorders and was influenced by underlying attitudes concerning mental disorders. Most recently, policy changes were put in place that led to deinstitutionalization in the latter half of the 20th century. Other events that influenced policy related to treatment included pharmacological advances, for example, the introduction of drugs such as Thorazine, as well as a cultural change from focusing on treatment of those with mental disorders to improving mental health for all.

Supreme Court judgments also affected policy, for example, the "least restrictive alternative" principle in the ruling in *Shelton v. Tucker* (1960), which allowed involuntary admission to a psychiatric facility only if there were no another alternative that would allow more freedom, and the ruling in *O'Connor v. Donaldson* (1975), which stated that mental patients who were not dangerous and who were involuntarily institutionalized had the right to be treated or discharged.[75] These landmark decisions resulted in **deinstitutionalization** of those diagnosed with mental disorders from psychiatric hospitals to independent living arrangements, thus shifting the burden of treatment to the community. President John F. Kennedy signed the Community Mental Health Centers Act in 1963, which opened the way for a network of community mental health centers to provide comprehensive services and continuity of care.[76]

Unfortunately, community facilities did not develop at the same pace as deinstitutionalization. In addition, the lack of planning for alternative facilities and services (medical and psychiatric care, social services, housing and nutrition, income and employment, and vocational and social rehabilitation) resulted in thousands of vulnerable and severely ill persons left behind to become imprisoned by poverty, neglect, victimization, substance abuse, and homelessness, all conditions that exacerbate psychiatric disorders.[77] The term **transinstitutionaliza-tion** began to appear in the literature in the 1980s and refers to the growing numbers of mentally ill persons ending up on the streets, in jails and prisons, in nursing homes, boarding houses, and homeless shelters, and not in places of their own or in the hospital. Today, it is estimated that between 30% and 50% of persons in the United States who are homeless are also mentally ill.[75]

The Mental Health Parity Act represents a step forward as the United States grapples with accepting treatment of mental illness as integral to promoting and ensuring a healthy public. The Paul Wellstone and Pete Domenici Mental Health Parity and Addiction Equity Act of 2008 was signed into law October 3, 2008, and mandates that group health plans of 50 or more persons, which cover mental health and substance use disorders, must provide benefits equivalent to (or better than) those benefits provided for medical or surgical benefits. The Affordable Care Act of 2010 helps to fill in some of the gaps by requiring Medicaid and plans purchased by small businesses to include mental health and substance abuse coverage starting in 2014. Further work is needed to transform the delivery of health care to those with mental disorders. In particular, attention is needed not only on parity but also on the ethics of providing treatment for mental disorders in parity with treatment for physical disorders (Box 10-5).

Summary Points

1. Behavioral health is essential to health overall.
2. Behavioral health disorders will surpass all physical diseases as a major cause of disability worldwide.
3. Mental health, substance abuse, and violence are interconnected.
4. Mental health is the vehicle for developing meaningful relationships, sound thinking, skills for learning and communication, emotional maturity, resilience, and self-esteem.
5. Resilience is an individual's ability to access protective factors.
6. Risk factors and protective factors related to mental health outcomes occur at several levels: individual, family, social, and community.
7. Interventions occur at all levels, but societal interventions in particular are critical to transforming the mental health system.

▲ CASE STUDY
Promoting Mental Health in Adolescents
Learning Outcomes

At the end of this case study, the student will be able to:

- Apply demographic methods to determine the severity of a problem at the population level.
- Examine the role that members of the community play in addressing a population level health issue.
- Discuss policy approaches to a population-level health problem.
- Examine the evidence to support a population-based intervention.

The nurses working for the Indian Health Services at a reservation health clinic were concerned about the increase in suicides among adolescents living on the reservation. One of the nurses brought in an article written by Senator Byron L. Dorgan.[70] They found the opening story about Jami Rose Jetty, who committed suicide at that age of 14, especially disturbing because, according to the article, the health-care providers had told Jami's mom that Jami was just a typical teenager. The nurses decided to investigate what steps they might be able to take to address this type of situation in their own family clinic. One of the nurses stated they could not proceed without including members of the community. How should they begin?

To complete this case study, do the following:

1. Starting with Dorgan's article, review the national statistics on teen suicide among Native Americans.
2. Determine which stakeholders should be involved in helping to design a community-level intervention.
3. Critique proposed policy initiatives in relation to their utility in reducing suicide in Native Americans—are there any?
4. Critique the evidence for programs aimed at preventing teen suicide and evaluate whether they have been tested with Native American populations.
5. Complete a draft plan.

REFERENCES

1. Substance Abuse and Mental Health Services Administration. (2010). *Leading change: A plan for SAMHSA's roles and actions 2011–2014.* Retrieved from http://www.samhsa.gov/about/sidocs/SAMHSA_SI_paper.pdf.
2. World Health Organization. (2001). *Strengthening mental health promotion.* Geneva, Switzerland: Author.
3. Institute of Medicine. (n.d.). *Improving the quality of health care for mental and substance-use conditions: Quality chasm series.* Retrieved from http://www.iom.edu/Reports/2005/Improving-the-Quality-of-Health-Care-for-Mental-and-Substance-Use-Conditions-Quality-Chasm-Series.aspx.
4. *Healthy People 2020.* (n.d.). Retrieved from http://www.healthypeople.gov/2020/topicsobjectives2020/default.aspx.
5. Centers for Disease Control and Prevention. (2011). *Designing and building healthy places.* Accessed from http://www.cdc.gov/healthyplaces/.
6. World Health Organization. (2012). *The 65th World Health Assembly closes with new global health measures.* Retrieved from http://www.who.int/mediacentre/news/releases/2012/wha65_closes_20120526/en/index.html.
7. World Health Organization. (2010). *Mental health: Strengthening our response* (Fact sheet N220). Retrieved from, http://www.who.int/mediacentre/factsheets/fs220/en/.
8. Centers for Disease Control and Prevention. (2011). Mental illness surveillance among adults in the United States. *Morbidity and Mortality Weekly Report, 60*(3), 1-32.
9. Insel, T.R. (2008). Assessing the economic costs of serious mental illness. *American Journal of Psychiatry, 165*(6), 663-665.
10. Harvard School of Medicine. (2005). *The world mental health survey initiative.* Retrieved from http://www.hcp.med.harvard.edu/wmh/.
11. Substance Abuse and Mental Health Services Administration. (2015). *Behavioral Health Barometer: United States, 2014.* HHS Publication No. SMA-15-4895. Rockville, MD: Substance Abuse and Mental Health Services Administration.
12. National Institute on Mental Health. (2013). *Serious mental illness (SMI) among adults.* Retrieved from http://www.nimh.nih.gov/statistics/SMI_AASR.shtml.
13. Broome, B., & Broome, R. (2007). Native Americans: Traditional healing. *Urologic Nursing, 27*(2), 161-173.
14. Beals, J., Novins, D.K., Whitesell, N.R., Spicer, P., Mitchell, C.M., & Manson, S.M. (2005). Prevalence of mental disorders and utilization of mental health services in two American Indian reservation populations: Mental health disparities in a national context. *American Journal of Psychiatry, 162*(9), 1723-1732.
15. National Institute for Health Care Management. (2010). Improving early identification and treatment of adolescent depression: Considerations and strategies for health plans. Retrieved from: http://nihcm.org/pdf/Adol_MH_Issue_Brief_FINAL.pdf.
16. National Institute of Mental Health. (2012). *The numbers count: Mental disorders in America.* Retrieved from http://www.lb7.uscourts.gov/documents/12-cv-1072url2.pdf
17. Centers for Disease Control and Prevention. (n.d.). *Burden of mental illness.* Retrieved from http://www.cdc.gov/mentalhealth/basics/burden.htm.
18. Kessler, R.C., Chiu, W.T., Demler, O., & Walters, E.E. (2005). Prevalence, severity, and comorbidity of 12-month DSM-IV disorders in the National Comorbidity Survey Replication. *Archives of General Psychiatry, 62,* 617-627. Retrieved from http://archpsyc.ama-assn.org/cgi/content/full/62/6/617.
19. Gadermann, A.M., Alonso, J., Vilagut, G., Zaslavsky, A.M., & Kessler, R.C. (2012). Comorbidity and disease burden in the National Comorbidity Survey Replication (NCS-R). *Depression and Anxiety, 9,* 797-806. doi:10.1002/da.21924.
20. Parks, J., Svendsen, D., Singer, P., Foti, M. E., & Mauer, B. (2006). *Morbidity and mortality in people with serious mental illness National Association of State Mental Health Program Directors, Medical Directors Council.* Retrieved from http://www.nasmhpd.org/docs/publications/MDCdocs/Mortality%20and%20Morbidity%20Final%20Report%208.18.08.pdf.
21. Schmidt, C.W. (2007). Environmental connections: A deeper look into mental illness. *Environmental Health Perspective, 115*(8), A404-A410.
22. Centers for Disease Control and Prevention. (2012). *Genomics and health.* Retrieved from http://www.cdc.gov/genomics/resources/diseases/mental.htm
23. Mayo Clinic. (2015). *Mental illness. Risk factors.* Retrieved from http://www.mayoclinic.org/diseases-conditions/mental-illness/basics/risk-factors/CON-20033813
24. Bostwick, W. (2007). *National Alliance on Mental Illness. Mental health risk factors among GLBT youth.* Retrieved from http://www.nami.org/Content/ContentGroups/Multicultural_Support1/Fact_Sheets1/MH_Risk_Factors_among_GLBT_Youth_07.pdf.
25. Goodman, A., Fleitlich-Bilyk, B., Pate,l V., & Goodman, R. (2007). Child, family, school and community risk factors for poor mental health in Brazilian schoolchildren. *Journal of the American Academy of Child and Adolescent Psychiatry, 46*(4), 448-456.
26. Moore, C., Mink, M., Probst, J., Tompkins, M., Johnson, A., & Hughley, S. (2005). *Mental health risk factors, unmet needs, and provider availability for rural children.* Retrieved from http://rhr.sph.sc.edu/report/(41)%20Mental%20Health%20Risk%20Factors.pdf.
27. Smith, M., Segal, R., & Segal, J. (2012). *Improving emotional health.* Retrieved from http://www.helpguide.org/mental/mental_emotional_health.htm.
28. World Health Organization. (2015). *Risk factors of ill health among older people.* Retrieved from http://www.euro.who.int/en/health-topics/Life-stages/healthy-ageing/data-and-statistics/risk-factors-of-ill-health-among-older-people.
29. Baxter, A., Charlson, F., Somerville, A., & Whiteford, H. (2011). Mental disorders as risk factors: Assessing

the evidence for the global burden of disease study. *BMC Medicine, 9*, 134. doi:10.1186/1741-7015-9-134.

30. Kessler, R. (2012). *Risk factor: World Health Organization world mental health survey.* Retrieved from http://www.hcp.med.harvard.edu/research/projects/kessler_WMH.

31. Bernard, B. (2010). Individual, family, and community resilience. In L. Cohen, V. Chavez, & S. Chehimi (Eds.), *Prevention is primary.* San Francisco, CA: Jossey-Bass.

32. World Health Organization. (2009). *Mental health resilience and inequalities.* Retrieved from http://www.euro.who.int/__data/assets/pdf_file/0012/100821/E92227.pdf.

33. Werner, E.E., & Smith, R.S. (2001). *Journeys from childhood to the midlife: Risk, resilience, and recovery.* Ithaca, NY: Cornell University Press.

34. Moos, R.H., & Moos, B.S. (2007). Protective resources and long-term recovery from alcohol use disorders. *Drug and Alcohol Dependence, 86,* 46-54.

35. Shapiro, V.B., & LeBuffe, P.A. (2006). Using protective factors in practice: Lessons learned about resilience from a study of children aged five to thirteen. *Annuals of the New York Academy of Science, 1094,* 350-353.

36. New Freedom Commission on Mental Health. (2003). *Achieving the promise: Transforming mental health care in America, Final Report.* (DHHS Publication No. SMA-03-3832). Rockville, MD: U.S. Department of Health and Human Services.

37. Maggi, S., Roberts, W., MacLennan, D., & D'Angiulli, A. (2011). Community resilience, quality childcare, and preschoolers' mental health: A three-city comparison. *Social Science & Medicine, 73,* 1080-1087.

38. Kelly, S.E. (2010). *Personal and community resilience: Building it and sustaining it.* (PowerPoint slides; ppt. #24). Bureau for Behavioral Health and Health Facilities, West Virginia Department of Health and Human Resources. Retrieved from http://www.wvdhhr.org/healthprep/common/resiliency.ppt.

39. *Elev8 Baltimore.* (n.d.). Retrieved from http://www.elev8kids.org/local-initiatives/content/baltimore.

40. World Health Organization (2015). Child and adolescent mental health. Retrieved from http://www.who.int/mental_health/maternal-child/child_adolescent/en/.

41. Monahan, K.C., Oesterle, S., & Hawkins, J.D. (2010). Predictors and consequences of school connectedness: The case of prevention. *The Prevention Researcher, 17*(3), 3-6.

42. Wegmann, K.M., & Bowen, G.L. (2010). Strengthening connections between schools and diverse families: A cultural capital perspective. *The Prevention Researcher, 17*(3), 7-10.

43. Thompson, J.W. (1994). Trends in the development of psychiatric services, 1844–1994. *Hospital and Community Psychiatry, 45*(10), 987-992.

44. Vega, W.A., Rodriguez, M.A., & Ang, A. (2010). Addressing stigma of depression in Latino care patents. *General Hospital Psychiatry, 32,* 182-191.

45. Alvidrez, J., Snowden, L.R., & Patel, S. G. (2010). The relationship between stigma and other treatment concerns and subsequent treatment engagement among black mental health clients. *Issues in Mental Health Nursing, 31,* 257-264.

46. Carpenter-Song, E., Chu, E., Drake, R.E., Ritsema, M., Smith, B., & Alverson, H. (2010). Ethno-cultural variations in the experience and meaning of mental illness and treatment: Implications for access and utilization. *Transcultural Psychiatry, 47,* 224-251.

47. Bailey, R.K., Blackman, H.L., & Stevens, F.L. (2009). Major depressive disorder in the African American population: Meeting the challenges of stigma, misdiagnosis, and treatment disparities. *Journal of the National Medical Association, 101*(11), 1084-1089.

48. Goffman, E. (1963). *Notes on the management of spoiled identity.* Englewood Cliffs, NJ: Prentice-Hall.

49. Horsfall, J., Cleary, M., & Hunt, G.E. (2010). Stigma in mental health: Clients and professionals. *Issues in Mental Health Nursing, 31,* 450-455.

50. Centers for Disease Control and Prevention. (2013). Stigma and illness. Retrieved from http://www.cdc.gov/mentalhealth/about_us/stigma-illness.htm.

51. Mayo Clinic.com. (n.d.). *Mental illness: Mental health; Overcoming the stigma of mental illness.* Retrieved from http://www.mayoclinic.com/health/mental-health/MH00076.

52. NAMI: National Alliance on Mental Illness. (n.d.) *Korean American community mental health fact sheet.* Retrieved from http://www.nami.org/Template.cfm?Section=Fact_Sheets1&Template=/ContentManagement/ContentDisplay.cfm&ContentID=46216.

53. Jang, Y., Chiriboga, D.A., & Okazakib, S. (2009). Attitudes toward mental health services: Age-group differences in Korean American adults. *Aging and Mental Health, 13*(1), 127-134.

54. Kim, I.J., Kim, L.I.C., & Kelly, J.G. (2006). Developing cultural competence in working with Korean immigrant families. *Journal of Community Psychology, 34*(2), 149-165.

55. Seung-Hui-Cho. (n.d.). *Biography.* Retrieved from http://www.biography.com/articles/Seung-Hui-Cho-235991.

56. *CHO's mental health history.* (n.d.). Retrieved from http://www.vtreviewpanel.org/report/report/11_CHAPTER_IV.pdf.

57. Brown, R.P., Osterman, L.L., & Barnes, C.D. (2009). School violence and the culture of honor. *Psychological Science, 20*(11), 1400-1405.

58. Vicary, A.M., & Fraley, R.C. (2010). Student reactions to the shootings at Virginia Tech and Northern Illinois University: Does sharing grief and support over the Internet affect recovery? *Personality and Social Psychology Bulletin, 36*(11), 155-163.

59. Number Of.net. (2010). *Number of Koreans in America.* Retrieved from http://www.numberof.net/number-of-koreans-in-america/.

60. Jang, Y., Chiriboga, D.A., & Okazakib, S. (2009). Attitudes toward mental health services: Age-group differences in Korean American adults. *Aging and Mental Health, 13*(1), 127-134.

61. Centers for Disease Control and Prevention. (2015). *Health-related quality of life.* Retrieved from http://www.cdc.gov/hrqol/.

62. Gandek, B., Sinclair, S.J., Kosinski, M., & Ware, J.E., Jr. (2004). Psychometric evaluation of the SF-36 health survey in Medicare managed care. *Health Care Finance Review, 25*(4), 5-25.

63. Substance Abuse and Mental Health Services Administration. (n.d.). *Levels of risk and levels of intervention.* Retrieved from http://captus.samhsa.gov/prevention-practice/prevention-and-behavioral-health/levels-risk-levels-intervention/2.

64. World Health Organization. (2015). *Mental Health, MIND—mental health in development.* Retrieved from http://www.who.int/mental_health/policy/en/index.html.

65. Institute of Medicine. (2005). *Improving the quality of health care for mental and substance-use conditions: Quality Chasm Series.* Retrieved from http://www.iom.edu/Reports/2005/Improving-the-Quality-of-Health-Care-for-Mental-and-Substance-Use-Conditions-Quality-Chasm-Series.aspx.

66. Substance Abuse and Mental Health Services Administration. (2011). *Screening, brief intervention and referral to treatment (SBIRT) in behavioral healthcare.* Retrieved from http://www.samhsa.gov/prevention/sbirt/SBIRT whitepaper.pdf.

67. Olds, D.L., Kitzman, H.J., Cole, R.E., Hanks, C.A., Arcoleo, K.J., Anson, E.A., et al. (2010). Enduring effects of prenatal and infancy home visiting by nurses on maternal life course and government spending: Follow-up of a randomized trial among children at age 12 years, *Archives of Pediatrics and Adolescent Medicine, 164*(5), 419-424.

68. Centers for Disease Control and Prevention. (2004, June). *Pregnancy Risk Assessment Monitoring System (PRAMS): PRAMS and postpartum depression.* Retrieved from http://www.cdc.gov/prams/ppd.htm.

69. Centers for Disease Control and Prevention. (2011). *Mental illness surveillance among adults in the United States.* Retrieved from http://www.cdc.gov/mmwr/preview/mmwrhtml/su6003a1.htm.

70. Agency for Healthcare Research and Quality. (2012). *Efficacy and screening for postpartum depression.* Retrieved from http://effectivehealthcare.ahrq.gov/index.cfm/search-for-guides-reviews-and-reports/?pageaction=displayproduct&productid=997#4918.

71. Logsdon, M.C. (2012). Identification of mothers at risk for postpartum depression by hospital-based perinatal nurses. *American Journal of Maternal Child Nursing, 37*(4), 218-225.

72. Hewitt, C., Gilbody, S., Brealey, S., Paulden, M., Palmer, S., Mann, R., et al. (2009). Methods to identify postnatal depression in primary care: An integrated evidence synthesis and value of information analysis. *Health Technology Assessment, 13*(36), 1-145, 147-230.

73. American Psychiatric Association (2013). Diagnostic and Statistical Manual of Mental Disorders (5th ed.). Arlington, VA; American Psychiatric Association.

74. Thompson, J.W. (1994). Trends in the development of psychiatric services, 1844–1994. *Hospital and Community Psychiatry, 45*(10), 987-992.

75. Krieg, R.G. (2001). An interdisciplinary look at the deinstitutionalization of the mentally ill. *The Social Science Journal.* Retrieved from http://www.accessmylibrary.com/article-1G1-78901856/interdisciplinary-look-deinstitutionalization-mentally.html.

76. Talbott, J.A. (1982). Twentieth-century developments in American psychiatry. *Psychiatric Quarterly, 54*(4), 207-219.

77. Reddi, V. (2005). *Dorthea Lynde Dix (1802–1887).* Center for Nursing Advocacy. Retrieved from http://www.nursingadvocacy.org/press/pioneers/dix.html.

Chapter 11

Substance Use and the Health of Communities

LEARNING OUTCOMES

After reading this chapter, the student will be able to:

1. Describe the impact of substance use on the health of a population.
2. Define the burden of disease-related substance use using current epidemiological frameworks.
3. Apply current evidence-based population interventions to the prevention of substance use disorders.
4. Describe population-level approaches to the prevention and treatment of substance use disorders.
5. Apply current frameworks related to prevention of substance use disorders.

KEY TERMS

Abstinence
Addiction
Alcohol Use Disorder
At-risk use
Binge drinking
Blood alcohol concentration (BAC)
Duration

Environmental tobacco smoke (ETS)
Frequency
Harmful use
Heavy drinking
Heavy episodic drinking
Low risk use

Moderate use
Pattern
Physiological dependence
Psychoactive substances (drugs)
Psychological dependence
Quantity
Risky use

Screening and brief intervention (SBI)
Secondhand smoke exposure
Stigma
Substance use
Substance use disorder

■ Introduction

Across the globe, use of alcohol, tobacco, and other drugs is linked to adverse health consequences for individuals, families, and communities. From a public health perspective the consequences go beyond the negative impact on the health of the individual using the substance. Substance use increases the risk for injury, crime, adverse health issues, and the environment—not just for those who use the substances, but also for the community as a whole. For example, psychoactive drug use is linked to increased crime in a neighborhood, driving under the influence is linked to an increased risk for motor vehicle crashes that affect drinkers and nondrinkers alike, and tobacco use pollutes the environment. Substance use is a major public health issue affecting all ages, populations, and countries.

Substance Use and the Global Burden of Disease

Substance use is a term used across the globe in reference to the use of **psychoactive substances (drugs)** (Box 11-1). These are chemical substances that have a pharmacological effect on the brain and the central nervous system (CNS). The effects of these substances on an individual include altered mood, perception, and level of consciousness.[1] The classes of psychoactive substances include stimulants, depressants, inhalants, dissociative anesthetics, narcotics, hallucinogens, and cannabis (Table 11-1).[2,3] Some are legal, such as alcohol; some are illegal (or illicit), such as heroin; and some are legal with a prescription, such as narcotics prescribed for pain or, in a growing number of states, marijuana (cannabis). In addition, in 2014 marijuana became legal for recreation use in two states (Washington and Colorado).

BOX 11–1	Psychoactive Substances

Depressants:

Alcohol, sedatives

Stimulants:

Amphetamine, cocaine, nicotine, methamphetamine

Hallucinogens:

LSD, cannabis, PCP

Inhalants:

Nitrous oxide, hydrocarbons

Narcotics/Opioids:

Heroin, codeine

Source: See reference 2.

All of these substances have the potential to result in a substance use disorder. A **substance use disorder** is defined as "a maladaptive pattern of substance use leading to clinically significant impairment or distress" and can be diagnosed as moderate or severe.[4] The broader term used to refer to substance use disorders is **addiction**, defined as meeting the criteria for a substance use disorder. In recent years, the professional literature has moved away from that term as well as the term dependence in an effort to view the full continuum of risk rather than

dichotomize the problem into categorizing a person as addicted or not addicted, thus negating the full continuum of harm associated with substance use. The gold standard used by health-care providers to diagnose a substance use disorder is the *Diagnostic and Statistical Manual of Mental Disorders* (DSM). In the 2013 DSM-5 (the fifth edition of the manual), the criteria for diagnosis of dependence are located under the Substance Use and Addictive Disorders section. The new criteria are a radical change from the approach used in the DSM-IV, which included two diagnoses, substance abuse and substance dependence. With the DSM-5, a substance use disorder is presented as a continuum that uses severity, evidence of physiological dependence, and course of treatment to classify the disorder (Box 11-2). The disorder can be established with or without physiological dependence. **Physiological dependence** is defined as evidence of tolerance or withdrawal.[4] Globally, the ICD-10 coding system is used to code for a substance use disorder.

For years, much of the focus was on the treatment of those who met the criteria for a substance use disorder, in other words, a downstream approach (Chapter 2) with a simultaneous policy approach that focused on criminalization of illegal substance use and control of access to legal psychoactive substances such as alcohol and

TABLE 11–1	Classes of Psychoactive Drugs		
Category	Description: The drugs in this category:		Examples
Stimulants	Overstimulate the CNS, resulting in accelerated heart rate, blood pressure and other symptoms related to stimulation of the CNS		Cocaine, amphetamines, methylphenidate, nicotine, methamphetamine, Ritalin, caffeine, and Methadrine
Narcotics	Relieve pain, and can result in a state of euphoria and other mood changes		Vicodin and OxyContin, opium, morphine, heroin, codeine, hydromorphone, meperidine, methadone, Darvon
Dissociative anesthetics	Inhibit the body's ability to perceive pain		PCP
Depressants	Depress the CNS, thus slowing down the brain and the body		Alcohol, barbiturates, and anti-anxiety tranquilizers (e.g., Valium, Librium, Xanax, Prozac, and Thorazine)
Inhalants	Come from a wide range of chemicals that are inhaled producing mind-altering effects		Butyl nitrite, amyl nitrite gas used in some aerosol cans, gasoline and toluene vapors from correction fluid, glue, marking pens
Hallucinogens	Result in altered perception of reality		PCP, LSD, mescaline, peyote, psilocybin, ecstasy, PCE, and methamphetamine, and *Cannabis*
Cannabis	Result in a feeling of euphoria, and can include distorted perceptions, memory impairment, as well as difficulty thinking and solving problems		Cannabinoids including, marijuana, tetrahydrocannabinol or THC, hashish, hashish oil and synthetics like Dronabinol.

Sources: See references 2 and 3.

<table>
</table>

BOX 11–2	Diagnosis of Substance Use and Addictive Disorders

Severity specifiers:
Moderate: Two to three criteria positive
Severe: Four or more criteria positive
Specify if:
With Physiological Dependence: evidence of tolerance or withdrawal (i.e., either Item 4 or 5 is present)
Without Physiological Dependence: no evidence of tolerance or withdrawal (i.e., neither item 4 nor 5 is present)
Course specifiers (see reference 4 for definitions):
Early Full Remission
Early Partial Remission
Sustained Full Remission
Sustained Partial Remission
On Agonist Therapy
In a Controlled Environment

Source: See reference 4.

tobacco. Over the past few decades, the global focus has shifted to include a broader upstream approach aimed at reducing harm at the population level through prevention of harmful substance use and early treatment of substance use disorders, decriminalization of substance use, and broader policy initiatives.[5-7]

Substance use is linked to a wide spectrum of adverse health consequences at the individual, family, and community levels (Table 11-2). Worldwide, tobacco and alcohol are among the top 10 risk factors for mortality, with tobacco being the number 1 risk factor in high-income countries.[8] Alcohol use is the most prevalent substance use worldwide, with more than 50% of adults reporting current use of alcohol. When broken down by gender, 65% of males and 45% of women report current alcohol use.[5] In the United States, the statistics are similar, with a little over 50% of adults reporting current alcohol use. This is followed by tobacco use, with 19% of adults in the United States reporting current tobacco use.[9,10] The World Health Organization (WHO) reported that in 2008, 155 to 250 million people, or 3.5% to 5.7% of the global population, used psychoactive substances other than alcohol and tobacco. The most commonly used substance after alcohol and tobacco was marijuana (cannabis).[11] The percentage of adults aged 12 or older in the United States who report current drug use is higher at 8.9% of the population age 12.[9]

Measurement and Surveillance

Before developing interventions to help reduce the harm related to substance use, it is important to understand how surveillance of substance use and associated adverse health outcomes (see Chapter 3) is conducted in the United States and across the globe in relation to the prevalence of substance use and adverse health consequences associated with use. The first step in conducting surveillance is important to defining how substance use is measured. Across all substances, there is a classification of use that reflects the level of risk associated with use (Fig. 11-1). As multiple terms are sometimes used, clarity is needed. The first term is **abstinence,** which is defined as no use of the substance. For alcohol, it is usually measured as two or fewer drinks in the past 12 months. **Low-risk use** or **moderate use** is use of the substance that places the user at little or no risk. For example, if a person drinks at or below the recommended limits for alcohol

TABLE 11–2	Adverse Consequences Related to Substance Use			
Level	Injury	Environment	Physical Health	Psychosocial Health
Individual	Increased risk for unintentional injury and suicide		Increased risk for adverse health outcomes	Negative impact on: • Mental health • Employment • Social networks
Family	Increased risk for intentional and unintentional injury	Adverse effect on home environment, e.g., secondhand smoke in the home	Increased risk for adverse health outcomes secondary to impaired family member	Negative impact on: • Mental health • Employment • Social networks
Community	Increased risk for intentional and unintentional injury	• Secondhand smoke • Increased crime • Decreased property values	Increased burden for cost of health care	Negative impact on: • Community Social networks

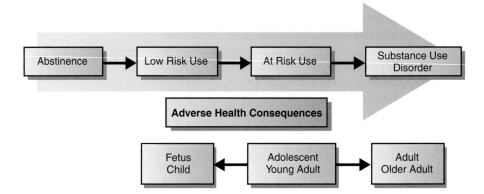

Figure 11-1 Substance use across the continuum of use and the life span.

consumption of no more than two drinks in one day for adult men (one drink for adult women) and no more than 14 drinks (7 drinks for women) in a week, that person is considered to be at low risk.[12] A number of terms are used to describe the next level of use, including risky use, at-risk use, binge drinking, heavy episodic drinking, harmful use, and nondependent heavy use. **Risky use** or **at-risk use** refers to any use of alcohol that places the person at risk for physical, psychological, or social harm who does not meet the criteria for a substance use disorder at risk for adverse consequences. This includes **binge drinking** and **heavy episodic drinking**, which is defined as consuming five or more drinks for a man or four or more drinks for a woman at a single occasion. For the purpose of this chapter, we will use the term *at-risk use*. At-risk use for alcohol includes **heavy drinking,** defined as drinking more than the recommended limits, and episodic heavy (binge) drinking, defined as five or more drinks (four or more for women) consumed on a single drinking occasion. At-risk use of substances also includes **harmful use,** defined as use that is associated with harm to the individual, family, and/or community.[5,12,13]

For substances other than alcohol, the distinction between low-risk use and risky use is less clearly defined. In general, any use of tobacco and illicit substances is considered at-risk use. Use of psychoactive substances that are available by prescription is termed risky use when the use is not in alignment with the prescription. At the end of the spectrum, is substance use dependence described above. For some substances or some situations, all use is seen as at risk. For example, there is no level of low (moderate) use of substances during pregnancy including tobacco, alcohol, and psychoactive drugs.

Another aspect of measuring substance use is to determine the quantity, frequency, pattern, and duration of use. These are measures of use, while the terms reviewed in the previous paragraph rank the level of risk related to use. When collecting individual substance use data, it is important to measure these four aspects of consumption of use. For example, in measurement of alcohol use, **quantity** reflects the amount (dose) consumed and for some substances there is a standard measure. For example alcohol is measured as a standard drink so that the intake reflects the amount of alcohol consumed rather than the amount of the beverage consumed. For some substances, especially street drugs such as heroin, quantity is hard to determine because there is no standard. **Frequency** refers to how often the substance is used, such as how many times a week. **Duration** refers to how long over the lifetime the substance has been used, and **pattern** refers to whether the use is constant or varies. These terms are important not only when asking an individual about substance use, but also when measuring use at the population level. Surveillance related to substance use is conducted on a regular basis to help measure the prevalence of substance use. How use is measured in these surveys helps public health officials determine the level of risk at the population level. Eleven different national surveillance surveys are listed on the Centers for Disease Control and Prevention (CDC) Web site that involve the collection of data on substance use, including the Behavioral Risk Factor Surveillance System, the National Survey on Drug Use and Health, and the National Epidemiologic Survey on Alcohol and Related Conditions. This surveillance process provides information on the distribution of substance use and substance use disorders as well as information on health-related consequences (Fig.11-2). Understanding the terms helps in the interpretation of the findings. For example, the report on binge drinking in the United States released by the CDC requires an understanding of what binge drinking is and is not.[14]

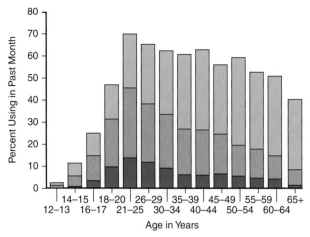

Figure 11-2 Current, binge, and heavy alcohol use among persons aged 12 years or older, by age, 2009. *(From the National Survey on Drug Use and Health: Vol. 1. Summary of national findings. U.S. Department of Health and Human Services, Substance Abuse and Mental Health Services Administration, Office of Applied Studies. Retrieved from http://www.samhsa.gov/ data/NSDUH/2k9NSDUH/2k9Results.htm#2.2.)*

Models for Prevention and Treatment of Substance Use Disorders

Prevention efforts related to substance use and adverse health consequences have shifted during the past 20 years from a narrow focus on the end of the continuum of use, substance use disorders, to a broader focus that includes the continuum of use across the life span. There are two models used across the globe that guide prevention efforts, the harm reduction model and the Institute of Medicine's prevention model presented in Chapter 2.

Institute of Medicine Prevention Model

Prevention is aimed at promoting resilience. In 1997, the Institute of Medicine identified the primary-secondary and tertiary continuum of prevention as confusing and developed a new, simpler model that more clearly separates prevention from treatment.[15] As explained in Chapter 2, this framework divides the prevention category into three levels—universal, selective, and indicated—and includes possible interventions at each level that can be applied easily to behavioral health issues.

Universal Level of Prevention

The universal level of prevention addresses identified populations regardless of identified risk. In the case of substance abuse prevention, older adults, pregnant women, and teenagers can be offered skills to allow the postponement of use of substances of abuse. Universal prevention techniques include education regarding the effects of alcohol, tobacco, and other drugs on one's own health, on the health of children, and the danger of fetal alcohol syndrome/effects and risk factors; the danger of using substances of abuse when using prescribed medication; and special education for older adults in an age-appropriate manner. It includes appropriated decision making and social skills to empower the participants to make good decisions.

Selective Level of Prevention

With substance abuse, the selective level of prevention addresses specific subgroups that are known to be at risk for substance abuse by virtue of biological, psychological, social, or environmental factors. Whether or not individual members of the specific subgroups are using alcohol, tobacco, or other drugs is not taken into consideration when applying selective interventions. What is important here is that the subgroups are at higher risk for substance abuse than the general population. The selective interventions are tailored to specific characteristics of the subgroups such as age, gender, reproductive status, availability of drugs in the communities in which the members live, community attitudes toward substance abuse, substance abuse by peers, family history of substance abuse, family attitudes, social problems, history of sexual abuse, and marginal or poor academic achievement in school. Selective interventions include opportunities for learning social skills that might delay initial use of alcohol, tobacco, and other drugs. Interventions such as after-school activities, community centers, job interview skills acquisition, drug and alcohol education, role-playing, self-esteem–building exercises and opportunities are examples of selective interventions.

Indicated Level of Prevention

The indicated level of prevention addresses specific subgroups at highest risk for development of a substance use disorder, or that are showing early signs of substance use disorder. These groups may appear to be experimenting with substances of abuse and, while this may be the case, without aggressive preventive action, some members of the group will develop full-fledged substance use disorder. In addition to delaying initial substance use, the purpose of indicated techniques includes delaying or reducing the severity of a substance use disorder. At this level, there is less concern about community prevention and more emphasis on those demonstrating early substance use disorder. Indicated techniques might include continued alcohol and drug education with specific attention paid to the consequences of continued use, and self-tests to determine the level of substance use disorder a person might be experiencing, providing an opportunity for the early user to identify his or her risk factors and any signs or symptoms of substance use disorder that might be present.

Harm Reduction Model

Another model used in the prevention of adverse consequences associated with alcohol and drug use is the harm reduction model. Harm reduction refers to any program, policy, and/or intervention that seeks to reduce the harm related to alcohol and drug use or other high-risk behavior, rather than focusing solely on attainment of abstinence of the risky behavior at the individual level.[16] Thus, it includes a wide spectrum of interventions from safer use (needle exchange programs) to abstinence. Those engaged in risky use of substances who are not willing or able to engage in treatment that leads to abstinence are provided with options to minimize the harm associated with substance use. From a public health perspective, harm reduction is used to minimize the physical, emotional, social, and economic harm associated with substance use, not only in relation to the individual but also to the larger population and the community. The guiding principles of harm reduction are based on the assumption that interventions aimed at reduction of the adverse consequences associated with substance use should be free of judgment or blame. The Canadian Center for Substance Abuse proposed guiding principles for harm reduction (Box 11-3).[17] The reduction of the harm associated with substance abuse is a goal of *Healthy People 2020 (HP 2020)*.[18]

■ HEALTHY PEOPLE 2020
Substance Use

Goal: Reduce substance abuse to protect the health, safety, and quality of life for all, especially children

Overview: In 2005, an estimated 22 million Americans struggled with a drug or alcohol problem. Almost 95% of people with substance use problems are considered unaware of their problem. Of those who recognize their problem, 273,000 have made an unsuccessful effort to obtain treatment. These estimates highlight the importance of increasing prevention efforts and improving access to treatment for substance abuse and comorbid disorders

Source: See *HP 2020* for background, objectives, interventions, and resources. See reference 18.

Alcohol Use

Alcohol consumption is a socially acceptable and normative practice in the United States. As noted above, more than half of the U.S. population aged 12 years or older reported current use of alcohol. In the United States in 2010, nearly a quarter (23.1%) of Americans aged 12 years and older reported heavy episodic alcohol use (five or more drinks on the same occasion at least once in the past 30 days) and 6.8% reported heavy alcohol use (five or more drinks on the same occasion on at least 5 different days in the past 30 days) (see Fig. 11-2).[9,19]

BOX 11–3	Guiding Principles on Harm Reduction

- Clients are responsive to culturally competent, nonjudgmental services, delivered in a manner that demonstrates respect for individual dignity, personal strength, and self-determination.
- Service providers are responsible to the wider community for delivering interventions that attempt to reduce the economic, social, and physical consequences of drug- and alcohol-related harm and harms associated with other behaviors or practices that put individuals at risk.
- Because those engaged in unsafe health practices are often difficult to reach through traditional service venues, the service continuum must seek creative opportunities and develop new strategies to engage, motivate, and intervene with potential clients.

- Comprehensive treatments need to include strategies that reduce harm for those clients who are unable or unwilling to modify their unsafe behavior.
- Relapse or periods of return to unsafe health practices should not be equated with or conceptualized as "failure of treatment."
- Each program within a system of comprehensive services can be strengthened by working collaboratively with other programs in the system.
- People change in incremental ways and must be offered a range of treatment outcomes in a continuum of care, from reducing unsafe practices to abstaining from dangerous behavior.

Sources: See references 16 and 17.

According to the WHO, harmful alcohol use is the third leading risk factor for poor health, with approximately 2.5 million deaths each year associated with the harmful use of alcohol. Worldwide, heavy episodic drinking is highest in middle to high per capita consumption countries and is higher for males than it is for females (Table 11-3).[5]

Though much of the current focus in health care is on the person with an **alcohol use disorder** (AUD), an AUD takes time to develop, whereas one episode of heavy/at-risk alcohol use can lead to serious adverse health consequences such as motor vehicle crashes, drowning, and alcohol poisoning. Health issues related to at-risk alcohol use occur across the life span beginning with fetal exposure to alcohol, and can affect the nondrinker as well. In 2009, for example, 14% of all motor vehicle crashes that resulted in the death of a child were the result of alcohol-impaired driving. In addition, close to one-third (32%) of all motor vehicle crashes were alcohol related.[20] At-risk alcohol use also increases the risk for other adverse consequences not normally associated with alcohol. For example, a recent study demonstrated a link between alcohol use and the increased risk of breast cancer.[21]

Prevention of adverse alcohol-related health consequences is a major public health issue across the life span. Since its inception, *Healthy People* has included prevention of adverse alcohol-related consequences related to at-risk/heavy alcohol use including reduction in motor vehicle crash deaths and injuries, alcohol-related hospital emergency department visits, alcohol-related violence, lost productivity related to alcohol use, and deaths of adolescents riding with a driver who has been using alcohol.[18] In total, there are 21 objectives listed under the substance abuse topic, 10 of which are specific to alcohol. The objectives include primary, secondary, and tertiary prevention. The objectives are grouped under three headings: Policy and Prevention, Screening and Treatment, and Epidemiology and Surveillance. An example of an objective listed under Prevention and Policy is aimed at reducing the number of adolescents who ride with an intoxicated driver.

■ HEALTHY PEOPLE 2020
Substance Abuse
HP topic relevant to alcohol use reduction
Targeted Topic: Substance use
Specific Objectives: Alcohol use reduction objective SA1 (substance abuse 1)
Objective: Reduce the proportion of adolescents who report that they rode, during the previous 30 days, with a driver who had been drinking alcohol
Baseline: 28.3 percent of students in grades 9 through 12 reported that they rode, during the previous 30 days, with a driver who had been drinking alcohol in 2009
Target: 25.5%
Source: Youth Risk Behavior Surveillance System (YRBSS), CDC, National Center for Chronic Disease Prevention and Health Promotion/CDC (NCCDPHP/CDC)[18]

Thus, timely prevention and early treatment are key to saving lives, and the professional health-care workforce is the key to meeting national and global objectives related to reducing alcohol-related morbidity and mortality and increasing the age and proportion of adolescents who remain alcohol free.

Consequences of Alcohol Use

Alcohol is a causal factor in over 200 types of diseases and injuries[5, 22–34] and accounts for almost 5.1% of the global burden of disease.[5] Alcohol has the ability to cause multiorgan toxicity, and toxicity in one organ system affects other systems.[22] Damages occur not only in the liver and brain but also in the gastrointestinal (intestinal mucosa), endocrine (pancreas), and other organ systems. Acetaldehyde, the primary metabolic product of ethanol,

TABLE 11–3	Ranking of Selected Risk Factors: Ten Leading Risk Factor Causes of Death by Income Group, 2004			
Substance	World	Low-Income Countries	Middle-Income Countries	High-Income Countries
Tobacco	Ranked #2	Ranked #7	Ranked #2	Ranked #1
	5.1 million deaths	1 million deaths	2.6 million deaths	1.5 million deaths
Alcohol use	Ranked #8	Not in top 10	#5	#9
	2.3 million deaths		1.6 million deaths	0.1 million deaths

Source of data: See reference 8.

is thought to be the instrumental toxin in developing alcohol-related disease.[22,23]

In addition to physical problems, there are many psychosocial consequences associated with alcohol use for individuals and their families.[35] These can include legal problems such as traffic violations, driving while intoxicated, and public intoxication. Early employment problems can include lateness, frequent absences, an inability to concentrate on the job, and decreased competency, which can eventually lead to on-the-job accidents and injury or loss of employment that leads to chronic unemployment. It does not take a great deal of exposure to problem drinking for the family also to manifest dysfunction. Family conflict, erratic child discipline, neglect of responsibilities, and social isolation can progress to divorce, spousal abuse, and child abuse or neglect.

Other problems associated with at-risk alcohol use include injury (Chapter 12) and psychiatric illness. In 2001, the CDC reported that there were 40,933 injury-related deaths in the United States associated with excessive alcohol use.[36] In addition, alcohol use is associated with unintentional injury in adolescents.[37] Comorbidity of psychiatric illness and alcohol use is also common, with evidence that alcohol is a causal factor for depression.[38]

Vulnerable Populations Across the Life Span

The effects of alcohol use can be viewed across the life span, with a particular focus on vulnerable populations interacting with their environment at key points over time (see Fig. 11-1). Adverse pregnancy outcomes, for example, referred to as *fetal alcohol spectrum disorders,* are often characterized by prenatal or postnatal growth deficiency, certain facial features, and CNS structure or function changes.[39] Alcohol is the leading teratogen and it is estimated that the percentage of children born with fetal alcohol syndrome, the most severe of the disorders, ranges from 0.5 to 2 per 1,000 live births and are found in all racial and ethnic groups.[40]

The vulnerable time periods following pregnancy are those of childhood and early adolescence, followed by early adulthood. Adolescence is a time often marked by willingness to take risks and to experiment with alcohol, a period that can extend into early adulthood.[37] In 2010, among young adults aged 18 to 25 the rate of binge drinking was 40.6% compared with 23% for all persons aged 12 and older.[9] This underlines the need to begin primary prevention with children prior to the age of 12. The significance of focusing on children is twofold. First, children who initiate drinking before the age of 15 are five times more likely to report a diagnosis of an

AUD than are persons who first used alcohol after the age of 20.[41] In addition, the brain is developing during adolescence, indicating that the lack of executive functioning may inhibit good decision making as well as the fact that unique characteristics in the brain may increase the reaction to the rewarding sensations of alcohol use.[42,43]

Older adults are another group that may be at particular risk of detrimental consequences of alcohol use (Chapter 20). For older adults who continue to drink heavily throughout their life, the cumulative effect of alcohol exposure may result in damage to cells, tissues, and organs.[44] In addition, there is the possibility that even low-risk alcohol use may place the older adult at risk because of the potential for falls, the problem of comorbid health conditions that may impact the ability to metabolize alcohol, and the interaction of alcohol with prescription drugs for comorbid conditions.[45]

Screening Brief Intervention and Referral for Treatment

From a public health perspective, screening for at-risk alcohol use is an essential component in the fight to prevent the harm related to alcohol use.[5] In the past, screening tools were developed to help identify those who may be alcohol dependent, but screening tools now in use also help the health-care provider to identify persons at risk for adverse consequences related to alcohol use across the continuum of use (see Fig. 11-1).[46] More recently, acute care settings are adopting a universal approach to screening for alcohol use.[47,48]

● APPLYING PUBLIC HEALTH SCIENCE

The Case of the Drinking Trauma Patients

Public Health Science Topics Covered:
- Setting assessment
  - Secondary data analysis
- Screening

John and Kelly worked at a Level II trauma unit located in regional hospital in the Midwest. Their manager had reported at a staff meeting that there was a new requirement instituted by the American College of Surgeons that all Level I and II trauma centers must implement the use of alcohol screening and brief interventions (SBI) for unhealthy [at-risk] alcohol use.[47] The unit would be put this plan into place and the manager wanted volunteers to work on developing, implementing, and evaluating the plan. They had no idea where to begin but had cared for so many patients with life-threatening injuries, incurred especially after drinking and driving, that they agreed to be co-chairs of the committee.

Their first step was to look for information on the Internet. They discovered that the use of **screening and brief interventions (SBI)** is an evidence-based approach that focuses on engaging people who are not seeking help for alcohol problems but who are engaged in at-risk drinking in adopting strategies that can help them reduce at-risk alcohol use.[46] The first step in SBI is to screen for at-risk alcohol use. For those who screen positive for at-risk drinking, the second step is to assess for an alcohol use disorder. The third step is to advise and assist, using brief interventions that consist of raising the subject of alcohol use, providing feedback, enhancing motivation to change drinking behaviors, and negotiating and advising. Brief interventions are designed to take about 10 to 15 minutes and can be delivered in one to four sessions. There are different approaches to brief intervention for those at-risk compared with those with a possible AUD.[46–50]

Next, they located a step-by-step SBI implementation guide for trauma centers.[51] They could not believe their luck. At first glance, it appeared that this was going to be easy. All the information they needed seemed to be right at their fingertips. But John remembered that in his undergraduate program, the professor teaching the public health course had stressed that the first step in planning a health program was to conduct an assessment (Chapter 4). Kelly thought that was a good idea but questioned whether they would need more people on their task force to help them. So, following the guidelines for implementing SBI in trauma centers,[51] they identified a few other team members and called for a meeting. The initial team examined the guide and identified others who should be on the team, resulting in a final team that represented key disciplines working on the trauma unit including nursing, medicine, pharmacy, social work, and clergy.

John and Kelly then explained to the full team the idea of doing an assessment. John reviewed his public health textbook from nursing school to determine what type of population-level assessment was appropriate for their issue. He concluded that they could conduct a setting-specific assessment that focused on one health issue—unhealthy alcohol use (Chapter 4). Some of the members of the team asked John and Kelly why it was necessary to do this first step. They explained that this would provide them with additional data needed not to only design the SBI program, but also to establish baseline data. They further explained that baseline data would be essential in evaluating the effectiveness of the program. John and Kelly agreed to take primary responsibility for doing the initial assessment.

First, Kelly and John decided to determine the prevalence of alcohol-related trauma at their institution during the past 6 months. They examined the number of patients admitted to their unit with a possible alcohol-related injury. They classified the injury as alcohol related if there was documentation in the chart by a health-care provider that the patient was intoxicated or had a **blood alcohol concentration** (BAC) above the legal limit (for their state, that was 0.08% or greater). BAC is defined as the amount of alcohol contained in a person's blood and is measured as weight per unit of volume. The measurement is converted to a percentage that reflects what percentage of a person's blood is alcohol. Thus, a BAC of 0.1% indicates that one-tenth of one percent of a person's blood is alcohol. They then checked the medical record to see how many of the patients with alcohol-related injuries had screened positive for an AUD. They found that 42% of the visits were alcohol related, a little higher than national rates.[52] They also found that on their unit, only 10% of patients positive for an alcohol-related visit screened positive using the screening tool currently in use on the unit, the CAGE questionnaire, a four-question screening test, to determine whether the patient might have an AUD,[53,54] and fewer than a quarter of the charts had documentation that a brief intervention had been done.

They then examined the current system used to assess for alcohol use on their trauma unit. The nursing assessment form included an item that asked the patient whether they consumed alcohol (yes or no). The assessment form then directed the nurse to administer the CAGE. Based on their earlier findings, they concluded that their current system of screening using the CAGE did not help them identify patients who would most benefit from SBI and did not use an evidence-based approach to screen for at-risk use; rather, the CAGE alone would identify only those who *probably* had an AUD.

Upon further reading, John and Kelly found clear evidence that the use of SBI in trauma patients with at-risk drinking could result in a change in drinking habits and that the SBI was designed for use with those who did not yet meet the criteria for an AUD. They then undertook a review of current screening instruments. One of the most popular instruments to screen for alcohol use is the Alcohol Use Disorders Identification Test (AUDIT), a 10-item screening test developed by the WHO to enhance cultural and linguistic generalizability. The AUDIT screens for at-risk use as well as AUDs.[51,55,56] They also found the new publication on alcohol screening with adolescents put out by the National Institute on Alcohol Abuse and Alcoholism (NIAAA).[57]

Kelly and John put together samples of the tools (Box 11-4) and a table that compared the utility of each of the screening tools available and presented them to the team (Table 11-4). These tools included the Consumption + CAGE, the AUDIT, the single-question binge drinking screen, and the CRAFFT. They also presented the team with the NIAAA guide for clinicians to help guide the decision on what screening tool to use on their unit. The team decided to use a universal approach and administer the single-question screening tool for initial screening of risk for all patients aged 12 and older coming on to the unit. They then decided to obtain a BAC for all those suspected of an alcohol-related injury to help validate recent alcohol consumption. For adults who screened positive

BOX 11–4 Tools for Assessing Substance Abuse

Consumption + CAGE

Consumption
1. On average, how many days per week do you have a drink containing alcohol?
2. On a typical day when you drink alcohol, how many drinks do you have?
3. How many times in the past year have you had x (x = 5 for men; x = 4 or more for women) or more drinks in a day?

CAGE
4. **C**ut Down—Have you ever felt you should cut down on your drinking?
5. **A**nnoyed—Have people annoyed you by criticizing your drinking?
6. **G**uilty—Have you ever felt bad or guilty about your drinking?
7. **E**ye opener—Have you ever had a drink first thing in the morning to steady your nerves or to get rid of a hangover?[53]

AUDIT

The Alcohol Use Disorders Identification Test (AUDIT) can detect alcohol problems experienced in the past year. A score of 8+ on the AUDIT generally indicates harmful or hazardous drinking. Questions 1–8 = 0, 1, 2, 3, or 4 points. Questions 9 and 10 are scored 0, 2, or 4 only.[56]

Some items below ask questions about how many drinks you have had. For the purpose of this screening test, a drink is defined as follows: (1) a single small (8 ounces; half pint) glass of beer, (2) a single

shot/measure of liquor/spirits, (3) a single glass of wine.

1. How often do you have a drink containing alcohol?
   a. Never
   b. Monthly or less
   c. Two to four times/month
   d. Two to three times/week
   e. Four or more times/week
2. How many drinks containing alcohol do you have on a typical day when drinking? (make sure you understand how each drink is defined—see Drink Definitions, above)
   a. 1 or 2
   b. 3 or 4
   c. 5 or 6
   d. 7, 8, or 9
   e. 10 or more
3. How often do you have 6 drinks or more drinks on one occasion?
   a. Never
   b. Less than monthly
   c. Monthly
   d. Weekly
4. How often during the past year have you found that you were not able to stop drinking once you had started?
   a. Never
   b. Less than monthly
   c. Monthly
   d. Weekly
   e. Daily or almost daily

BOX 11-4 Tools for Assessing Substance Abuse—cont'd

5. How often during the last year have you failed to do what was normally expected from you because of drinking?
   a. Never
   b. Less than monthly
   c. Monthly
   d. Weekly
   e. Daily or almost daily
6. How often during the last year have you needed a first drink in the morning to get yourself going after a heavy drinking session?
   a. Never
   b. Less than monthly
   c. Monthly
   d. Weekly
   e. Daily or almost daily
7. How often during the past year have you had a feeling of guilt or remorse after drinking?
   a. Never
   b. Less than monthly
   c. Monthly
   d. Weekly
   e. Daily or almost daily
8. How often during the past year have you been unable to remember what happened the night before because you had been drinking?
   a. Never
   b. Less than monthly
   c. Monthly
   d. Weekly
   e. Daily or almost daily
9. Have you or someone else been injured as a result of your drinking?
   a. No
   b. Yes, but not in the past year
   c. Yes, during the past year
10. Has a relative or friend or doctor or other health worker been concerned about your drinking or suggested you cut down?
   a. No
   b. Yes, but not in the past year
   c. Yes, during the past year[57]

Single Question Screening Tool

When was the last time you had more than x (x = 5 for men; x = 4 or more for women) drinks in one day?[46]

CRAFFT (for Adolescents)

1. Have you ever ridden in a **C**ar driven by someone (including yourself) who was high or had been using alcohol or drugs?
2. Do you ever use alcohol or drugs to **R**elax, feel better about yourself, or fit in?
3. Do you ever use alcohol or drugs by yourself **A**lone?
4. Do you ever **F**orget things you did while using alcohol or drugs?
5. Do your **F**amily or **F**riends ever tell you that you should cut down on your drinking or drug use?
6. Have you ever gotten into **T**rouble while you were using alcohol or drugs?

A score of 2 or more (each yes counts as one) is correlated with a substance abuse–related diagnosis or the need for treatment.[57]

TABLE 11-4 Alcohol-Screening Tools

	Blood Alcohol Level (BAC)	Single Screening Question	AUDIT	Consumption + CAGE	CRAFFT
+ or − screen	X	X	X	X	X
Evaluates problems			X		X
Likely dependence			X	X	
# or questions		1	10	7	6

Sources: See references 46, 50, and 57.

with the BAC and/or the single screening question, a second round of screening would be done to assess for an AUD. All those who reported at-risk alcohol use would receive a brief intervention. Those who might have an AUD would receive further assessment from the health-care providers on staff with expertise in addictions for possible referral for treatment.

Based on John's and Kelly's assessment, the program planning team was able to address the directive to implement an SBI program on their trauma unit that not only met the requirements of the American College of Surgeons, but also met the specific needs of their patients. This program also had the potential to reduce alcohol-related injuries in the population they served. To further help the team plan the program, they began to use other aspects of the assessment to answer key questions:

- Who will administer the screening tools?
- Who will administer the brief intervention?
- Who will be responsible for referring patients for treatment if they may have an AUD?
- How will they know that SBI worked with their patients?

John and Kelly's leadership resulted in the implementation of an evidence-based SBI program on the trauma unit that was based not only on national guidelines, but also on data from their own population. The program planning included all the key stakeholders and provided the baseline data needed to evaluate the effectiveness of the program over time.

Policy-Level Interventions to Reduce Alcohol-Related Harm

The interest in developing and disseminating both evidence-based practices and policies to minimize the harms associated with alcohol misuse is widespread.[5,58] From a policy perspective, the WHO has brought together member states to come up with policy strategies. They have outlined 10 areas for national action and four at the global level (Box 11-5).[5] In the United States, alcohol policies focus on five main areas. The first is the regulation of the physical availability of alcohol (e.g., minimum age; restrictions on sites). Next is altering the drinking context (e.g., not serving intoxicated clients). A third policy approach is limiting alcohol promotion, such as the ban on advertising hard liquor on television. A fourth policy is deterrence though sanctions on drunk driving. The fifth approach is developing policies related

---

BOX 11–5 World Health Organization Global Strategy to Reduce Harmful Alcohol Use

The ten areas for national action are:
1. leadership, awareness and commitment;
2. health services' response;
3. community action;
4. drink-driving policies and countermeasures;
5. availability of alcohol;
6. marketing of alcoholic beverages;
7. pricing policies;
8. reducing the negative consequences of drinking and alcohol intoxication;
9. reducing the public health impact of illicit alcohol and informally produced alcohol;
10. monitoring and surveillance.

The four priority areas for global action are:
1. public health advocacy and partnership;
2. technical support and capacity building;
3. production and dissemination of knowledge;
4. resource mobilization.

Source: See reference 5.

---

to treatment and early intervention as evidenced by the policy on including SBI on Level I and Level II trauma units. These policies can be enacted at the national, state, and local levels, or may be instituted outside of the government.

Another approach to policy is driven by health-care groups that determine best practices. An example is the National Quality Forum (NQF), which uses a consensus process to evaluate the evidence and how to translate that evidence into clinical practice through the development of practice guidelines and best practices. The NQF and others have published information on best practices in the treatment of substance use disorders.[59-61] The NRQ report is based on a rigorous evaluation of the evidence and sets a standard of care for clinical practice. Other examples of evidence-based practice related to alcohol can be found online at the National Registry of Evidence-Based Programs and Practices, an online registry of mental health and substance abuse interventions reviewed by independent reviewers.[62]

■ EVIDENCE-BASED PRACTICE
Brief Alcohol Screening and Intervention for College Students (BASICS): A Harm Reduction Approach

Practice Statement: BASICS is designed to help students make better alcohol use decisions and reduce their alcohol use to decrease the negative consequences of drinking.

Targeted Outcome: Frequency of alcohol use, quantity of alcohol use, negative consequences of alcohol use

Evidence to Support: The program has been implemented in 1,100 sites and has reached 20,000 individuals. Six studies have been conducted.

Recommended Approaches: The intervention is conducted over two 1-hour interviews and with an online assessment survey that gathers data about alcohol consumption, beliefs about alcohol, and drinking history. A customized feedback profile is developed for the second interview, which compares personal alcohol use with alcohol use norms. Motivational interviewing is used to reveal the discrepancy between the risky drinking behavior and the student's goals and values. It is designed to help students make changes to decrease alcohol consumption or abstain altogether from alcohol.

Sources

Amaro, H., Reed, E., Rowe, E., Picci, J., Mantella, P., & Prado, G. (2010). Brief screening and intervention for alcohol and drug use in a college student health clinic: Feasibility, implementation, and outcomes. *Journal of American College Health, 58*(4), 357–364.

Dimeff, L.A., Baer, J.S., Kivlahan, D.R., & Marlatt, G.A. (1999). *Brief Alcohol Screening and Intervention for College Students (BASICS): A harm reduction approach.* New York, NY: Guilford Press.

Grossbard, J.R., Mastroleo, N.R., Kilmer, J.R., Lee, C.M., Turrisi, R., Larimer, M.E., & Ray, A. (2010). Substance use patterns among first-year college students: Secondary effects of a combined alcohol intervention. *Journal of Substance Abuse Treatment, 39*(4), 384–390. doi:10.1016/j.jsat.2010.07.001.

Turrisi, R., Larimer, M.E., Mallett, K.A., Kilmer, J.R., Ray, A.E., Mastroleo, N.R., et al. (2009). A randomized clinical trial evaluating a combined alcohol intervention for high-risk college students. *Journal of Studies on Alcohol and Drugs, 70*(4), 555–567.

Source: See reference 63.

Tobacco Use

Tobacco is the number one cause of preventable death in the United States, causing approximately 443,000 premature deaths each year attributable to smoking and accounts for one out of every five deaths.[64,65] It is the only legal product that causes the death of half of its regular users.

More than a billion people use tobacco products worldwide.[66] For more than 50 years, the U.S. Surgeon General's reports on smoking and health indicate that there is enough evidence to infer a causal relationship between cigarette smoking and a number of diseases and conditions, many of which were not, initially, seen as smoking-attributable diseases or conditions.[67,68] The devastating effects were documented in the 2010 Surgeon General's report, which explains how tobacco causes disease.[69]

Smokers are directly exposed through three routes: (1) smoking cigarettes, pipes, or cigars; (2) chewing smokeless tobacco; and (3) inhaling snuff. Tobacco use through any of these routes is a major public health issue for smokers and nonsmokers alike. **Secondhand smoke exposure** occurs when nonsmokers are exposed to a mixture of the smoke produced from the end of the cigarette, cigar, or pipe as well as the smoke exhaled by the smoker. Because exposure to secondhand smoke is an environmental issue, it is also referred to as **environmental tobacco smoke** (ETS) as well as involuntary or passive smoking. According to the U.S. Environmental Protection Agency, ETS contains more than 4,000 substances, including substances known to cause cancer in humans.[69]

Tobacco use in the United States is on the decline. In 2010, a little less than a fifth of adults (19.3%) were current smokers, down from 20.9% in 2005 and 25.5% in 1990. Youth cigarette use declined sharply from 1997 to 2003. In 2009, 17.2% of high school students were current smokers, compared with 19.8% in 2006.[9] Tobacco use varies by state and region, from 17.5% in Utah to more than 28% in Kentucky. The region with the highest reported tobacco use is the Ashland, Kentucky / Huntington, West Virginia, region, where a third of adults (34.2%) use tobacco.[70]

Alcohol, tobacco, and/or psychoactive drugs are often used together, increasing the risk for adverse health consequences. Two-thirds (66.2%) of smokers reported past month alcohol use compared with 44.7% of nonsmokers, and almost a quarter (22.6%) reported past month illicit drug use compared with 4.9% of nonsmokers. Alcohol and tobacco co-use occurs more often in men than in women.[9,71] Thus, prevention of tobacco use has the potential to have a subsequent reduction in the at-risk use of alcohol and psychoactive drugs. *HP 2020* addresses this important health issue under the topic of Tobacco Use.

■ HEALTHY PEOPLE 2020
Topic Relevant to Tobacco

Targeted Topic: Tobacco use

Goal: Reduce illness, disability, and death related to tobacco use and secondhand smoke exposure

Overview: Scientific knowledge about the health effects of tobacco use has increased greatly since the first Surgeon General's report on tobacco was released in 1964.
Source: See *HP 2020* for background, objectives, interventions, and resources.[18]

Consequences of Tobacco Use

The adverse health consequences experienced by tobacco users include cardiovascular disease; cancer; chronic obstructive pulmonary disorders; adverse effects on the oral cavity and teeth; and adverse maternal and neonatal outcomes (Box 11-6).[72–75] For nonsmokers exposed to ETS, the adverse effects are similar but also include other serious health risks, especially in children, including increased risk for asthma, sudden infant death syndrome (SIDS), middle ear infections, and lower respiratory tract infections.[72]

Vulnerable Populations Across the Life Span

Risk factors for cigarette smoking include being male (23.5%), living in poverty (31.1%), and for those adults aged 25 years or greater, having less than a high school education (28.5%). Based on national data, populations with higher prevalence of tobacco use include adolescents, males, and those with a comorbid mental disorder.[9,76] In 2010, tobacco use was 8.9 times higher in youths who used illicit drugs in the past month, with more than half (52.9%) of youths aged 12 to 17 years who smoked reporting illicit drug use compared with 6.2% of

---

BOX 11–6	**Risk for Adverse Health Consequences for Users of Tobacco**

Compared with nonsmokers, smoking is estimated to increase the risk of:
- Coronary heart disease by 2 to 4 times
- Stroke by 2 to 4 times
- Men developing lung cancer by 23 times
- Women developing lung cancer by 13 times
- Dying from chronic obstructive lung diseases (such as chronic bronchitis and emphysema) by 12 to 13 times

Smokeless tobacco is associated with:
- Oral cancer
- Recession of the gums, gum disease, and tooth decay

Tobacco use and reproductive health:
- All forms of tobacco use are associated with adverse maternal and neonatal outcomes including preeclampsia, premature birth, and low birth weight

Sources: See references 70 and 71.

---

nonsmoking youth.[9] For some mental disorders, the prevalence of tobacco use is high. Up to 90% of persons with schizophrenia smoke, almost half (45% to 50%) of persons with major depression smoke, and more than half (50% to 70%) of persons with a bipolar disorder smoke.[76] Differences exist in the prevalence of current tobacco use across ethnic groups, with American Indians/Alaska Natives having the highest prevalence (35.8%) followed by non-Hispanic whites (29.5%), African Americans (27.3%), Hispanics (21.9%), and Asian/Pacific Islanders (12.5%).[9]

Differences in the prevalence of tobacco use also exist between countries. Though tobacco use is declining in the United States, it is increasing globally, especially in low-income countries. According to the WHO, "The tobacco epidemic is one of the biggest public health threats the world has ever faced."[77] Almost 80% of smokers live in middle- or low-income countries.

Finally, those who are most vulnerable to the adverse effects of tobacco use are, in many cases, children of smokers. From conception, children of smokers are at higher risk. Mothers who smoke during pregnancy are more apt to have children who are small for gestational age. In addition, fetal exposure to tobacco increases the risk for SIDS. Children exposed to ETS in their home have higher rates of asthma and upper respiratory infections.[78] This fact has resulted in a public service announcement campaign from the CDC to inform the public of the risk (Fig. 11-3).

Another concern is that youth are the most vulnerable population for initiation of tobacco use. According to the National Cancer Institute, initiation of tobacco use begins for most smokers prior to the age of 18.[79] Based on this, of the six objectives in *HP 2020* related to tobacco, three are focused on adolescents. The tobacco use objective aimed at the reduction of the initiation of tobacco use among children, adolescents, and young adults has eight targets. However, after graduation from high school, 25% of those who report that they were not current users prior to graduation began tobacco use after graduation, with those who do not attend college being at higher risk for becoming tobacco users after graduation. Thus, efforts to prevent tobacco use now include both adolescents and young adults.

Screening and Treatment for Tobacco Use

Screening for tobacco use is less complex than screening for at-risk alcohol or drug use, and focuses on quantity and type of tobacco use. Most users of tobacco are daily users, thus the standard screening question asks the

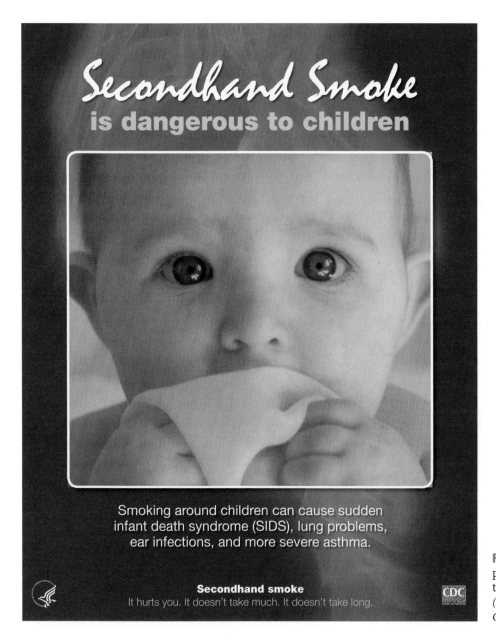

Figure 11-3 CDC campaign poster on prevention of tobacco-associated SIDS. *(From Centers for Disease Control and Prevention, 2006.)*

person whether they use tobacco products, and if so, how much on average per day. The key is how the question is framed. The question should be, "Do you now use tobacco?" rather than, "Do you smoke cigarettes?" because tobacco use includes smokeless tobacco, cigars, pipes, and other forms of inhaling tobacco. If the person is a current tobacco user, the next step in the screening process is to determine whether the person is ready to quit. If the person is not a current tobacco user, it is important to determine whether he or she is a former user of tobacco and whether the person is at risk for relapse (Fig. 11-4).[80]

The targeted levels set by *HP 2020* are reduction of cigarette use to 12% of the population and smokeless tobacco to 0.3% of the population.[81] Implementation of evidence-based tobacco use cessation programs are needed to achieve these objectives. One approach is included in the clinician's guide that incorporates both screening and interventions (Box 11-7).[80] The guide acknowledges the challenges of treatment for tobacco dependence but provides an excellent overview of interventions that can be instituted at the individual level, including both prescription and over-the-counter pharmacological approaches

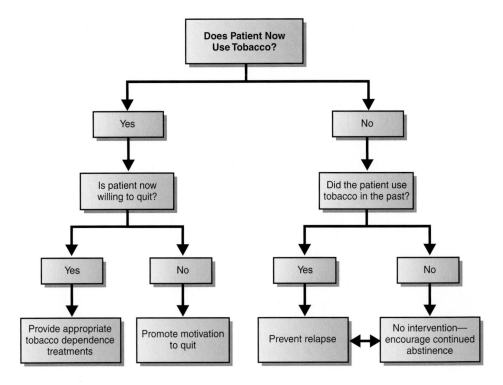

Figure 11-4 Screen for tobacco use status.

BOX 11-7 | **Smoking Cessation Strategies**

• ASK about tobacco use on every visit.
• ADVISE all tobacco users to quit.
• ASSESS readiness to quit.
• ASSIST tobacco users with a quit plan.
• ARRANGE follow-up visits.

Source: See reference 80.

as well as the use of self-help groups. During the past two decades, clinical trials have resulted in treatment advances that demonstrate the effectiveness of multiple methods in assisting an individual to successfully cease tobacco use.[80,82]

Policy-Level Intervention to Reduce Tobacco-Related Harm

There are a number of events in our history that have coincided with changes in the smoking behavior of the American public, many of them associated with policy. Tobacco use in the United States rose steadily from the Great Depression through World War II, and then peaked during the 1960s and 1970s (Fig. 11-5). The period from 1934 to the end of World War II (1945) saw a consistent, almost 300% increase in the number of cigarettes consumed. Consumption dropped off again in the

mid-1950s, when the first evidence of the association of cancer and cigarette smoking was found. Both of those periods of reduced cigarette consumption were followed by a rebound to levels higher than they had been previously. In 1964, this phenomenon ceased.[69,83]

With the release of the first Surgeon General's report on smoking and health, a period began of reduced cigarette consumption that has continued over the past three decades. In addition, the Federal Communication Commission applied the Fair Trade Act of 1949 to tobacco advertising. The point of this was to offer an opportunity, at no cost, to present health information that was directed toward smoking cessation. The application of the Fair Trade Act would have given the same amount of time to the anti-smoking initiatives (at no cost) as was purchased by the cigarette industry for advertising. Application of the Fair Trade Act seems associated with a marked decrease in number of cigarettes smoked. Shortly following the ban on television advertising, and the resulting elimination of free antismoking advertising, and coupled with the smoker's rights movement, cigarette smoking frequency increased, but the Great American Smokeout of 1977 appears to have been the beginning of a fairly consistent decline in cigarette consumption. In the 1980s, nonsmokers' rights movements began with eventual changes in policies related to smoking in public places, advertising restrictions, and increased taxes.[83]

FIGURE 1. Annual adult per capita cigarette consumption and major smoking and health events — United States, 1900–1998

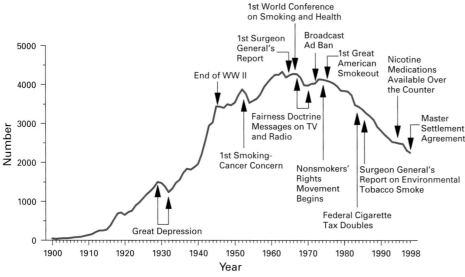

Sources: United States Department of Agriculture; 1986 Surgeon General's Report.

Figure 11-5 Annual adult per capita cigarette consumption and major smoking and health events—United States, 1900–1998. *(From U.S. Department of Agriculture; 1986 Surgeon General's Report. Retrieved from http://www.cdc.gov/mmwr/PDF/wk/mm4843.pdf.)*

Currently global and national public health efforts focus on population-level strategies with the objective of reducing tobacco use. In 2005, the WHO initiated an international tobacco treaty. Though the United States signed the treaty, as of 2011 it had not ratified it; however, 68 countries have done so.[84] Despite the failure to ratify the treaty, in June 2009, the president signed into law the Smoking Prevention and Tobacco Control Act. This act grants the Food and Drug Administration the authority to regulate the advertising and labeling of tobacco products, to preempt state regulation, to control the development of a "safer" cigarette, to set performance standards, and to collect user fees and taxes.[85,86] The prevalence of tobacco use continues to decline, which may be reflective of the effectiveness of these policies.

Illicit and Licit Drug Use

In 2010, it was estimated that 22.8 million (8.6%) Americans reported psychoactive drug use during the previous 30 days.[9] The most prevalent psychoactive drug used was marijuana (6.9%), followed by nonmedical use of psychotherapeutics (sedatives, painkillers, stimulants) (2.7%), cocaine (0.6%), and hallucinogens (0.6%). Males were more apt to report current illicit drug use (Fig. 11-6). Illicit drug use varies across age groups with those 18 to 20 reporting the highest current use (23.1%). There was an overall decline in illicit drug use among those aged 12

to 17 years from a high of 11.6% in 2002 to 10.1% in 2010. Rates declined across age groups with those 65 or older reported the lowest use at 1.1%. However, current illicit drug use is higher among adults aged 50 to 59 with an increase from 2.7% in 2002 to 6.2% in 2009.[9] This may be owing to the aging of the baby boom cohort, which has a higher illicit drug use rate than previous cohorts.[87]

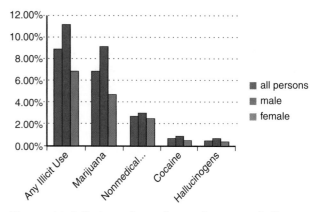

Figure 11-6 Estimated prevalence of past month illicit drug use in those 12 years of age or older. *(From Substance Abuse and Mental Health Services Administration. [2011]. Results from the 2010 National Survey on Drug Use and Health: Summary of National Findings, NSDUH Series H-41 [HHS Publication No. SMA 11-458]. Rockville, MD: Author. Retrieved from http://www.oas.samhsa.gov/NSDUH/2k10NSDUH/2k10Results.pdf.)*

▶ SOLVING THE MYSTERY

The Case of Increasing Emergency Room Visits and the Explosion at Motel LaBelle

Public Health Science Topics Covered:

- Epidemiology
- Surveillance

Up to this point, we have largely been talking about substance abuse disorders in relation to individuals or populations. The fact is, however, that substance use is a community-wide problem, affecting not just individuals but also society. In one case, health-care providers sought to answer these questions: (1) Why was there an increase in the number of admissions to the local emergency room during the past 6 months? (2) What was the cause of the explosion at the local motel that resulted in two admissions to a local hospital and a referral to the regional hospital for severe burns?

Taylor Hospital is a small community hospital in a rural farming community in a midwestern state and serves the local community of approximately 2,500 people. During the past 6 months, there was a 20% increase in the number of visits to the emergency room. The majority of the complaints were typical for the area, with the exception of an increase in minor burns as well as child injuries that resulted in child neglect reports to child services for the county. In addition, a few of the patients presented with euphoria and hallucinations as well as extreme fevers that were noteworthy.

Another exceptional event occurred in the local motel in Grant County. In the past week, there had been a report of an explosion at Motel Labelle. Local fire and ambulance personnel rushed to the scene to find that the explosion had resulted in the evacuation of 30 people from the motel and the admission of two people to the local hospital for burns, one of whom was referred to the regional hospital for severe burns. An examination of the damage revealed that the door in the room where the explosion occurred had been blown off its hinges, the bathtub had been ripped from the wall, and the windows were shattered.

What is happening in this county? What could explain the increase in emergency room visits and an increased number of child service reports for child neglect? Is the explosion at the local hotel the result of faulty pipes, as initially explained in the newspaper?

With further investigation into the explosion, the investigative team actually discovered the remnants of pseudoephedrine products in the motel room. What is the meaning of this event?

The investigators found that the culprit was methamphetamine. Few substances of abuse pose as extensive a threat to a community as does methamphetamine production and use. Methamphetamine (meth), also known as crank, crystal, glass, ice, rock, is a CNS-stimulant drug providing the user with a sense of euphoria that is similar to the effects of cocaine. The effect of meth lasts longer than that of cocaine, making it more attractive than cocaine to many stimulant users. However, the "crash" that is experienced when the effect of meth is over is much more pronounced than with other stimulants. This often leads the user to repeated use of increasing dosages, tolerance, and dependence on the drug.

Persons who use meth present in a number of ways. They can appear euphoric, tremulous, anorexic, with dilated pupils, and with diaphoresis. Continued use results in weight loss, strong body odor, dry mouth, and tactile hallucinations that often take the form of imagined insects under the skin. These tactile hallucinations can result in infections and lesions on the skin where the user scratches or tries to remove the insects. In an attempt to relieve dry mouth, the user often drinks copious amounts of sugary beverages, which results in decayed and missing teeth. Long-term use can result in cachexia, alopecia, corneal ulcerations, repetitive behavior patterns, and severe mental illness symptoms. Harm done to the family is predictably similar to the harm done by the use of other substances. Meth is less expensive than cocaine or heroin, so it appeals to those in lower socioeconomic groups, that is, those that can least afford it financially.[88]

Meth is easily manufactured, particularly so in states lacking laws regulating the sale of the key components for manufacture. Interestingly, the early centers of manufacture were the farming communities of the midwestern and western United States. The ease with which meth is manufactured and its increasing popularity facilitated the spread of meth "labs" throughout the United States and Mexico. These labs can be located in homes, apartments, trailers, campers, caves, or any place of shelter.[89]

Some of the chemical components of meth are quite caustic in their own right, and include pool acid/muratic acid, lye, acetone, brake fluid, brake cleaner, iodine crystals, lithium metal/lithium batteries, lighter fluid, drain cleaners, cold medicine containing pseudoephedrine or ephedrine, ethyl ether (in engine-starting fluid), anhydrous ammonia (stored in propane tanks or coolers), sodium metal, and red phosphorous. Often, manufacturers of meth are either careless or lack knowledge regarding the proper handling of the nature of the components, which often leads to fires and explosions.[90]

It has been reported that some "superlabs" can manufacture up to 100 pounds of meth per day. For every pound of meth produced, there are 5 to 6 pounds of toxic waste produced as well. This is an environmental disaster in the making. The manufacturers of meth dispose of the waste in a number of ways: flushing down the toilet, pouring into drains, burying, and pouring on the ground.[90]

Thus, unlike other psychoactive drugs, pollution of the environment with a hazardous chemical is a major issue. The threat to the water supply, health of the soil, and people in the surrounding areas is clear. Toxic waste by-products from meth production can be in suspension in the air and settle on furniture, carpeting, floors, tables, food, and toys, creating a serious threat to those who reside where the labs are located, especially children. Children in such environments not only suffer from neglect but also are exposed to hazardous materials. When a meth lab is seized by law enforcement officials, assuming welfare of the children and treatment and/or incarceration for the users/manufacturers is only a beginning. For first responders, there are occupational health hazards that need to be addressed. HAZMAT teams must be summoned to decontaminate and clean up the area where the lab was located. This process usually costs thousands of dollars or more, depending on the size of the lab.[90,91]

The impact of methamphetamine and the demand to work from a regional perspective is illustrated by another case example.[89] In the early 1990s, a methamphetamine lab was established in a rural Iowa farming community. The lab was run by five men aged 22 to 26 years, who were seeking to increase their income by selling meth to anyone interested in its purchase. Their efforts were successful in that they sold meth to individuals in the same rural area in which they lived, and to individuals in a low-income area of Davenport, Iowa. They also found that they could earn money by selling the recipe they used for the meth manufacture. In the late 1990s, there were an estimated 161 labs in Iowa, Nebraska, Kansas, and Missouri. Many labs were identified after explosions or fires occurred as a consequence of improper handling of the components. Some labs were discovered when social

service workers investigated cases of child neglect or when police investigated reports of strange behavior and odor associated with a nearby residence. Despite arrests and referrals for treatment, the industry grew, as did the problems it caused. By 2000, it was estimated that there were more than 175 meth labs and 2,500 meth users in Iowa, Nebraska, Kansas, and Missouri.[89]

In response the governments of the four states joined together to eradicate methamphetamine production and use in their states. Budgets for this enterprise were increased significantly; law enforcement, fire, social services, and health-care providers underwent training specific to managing methamphetamine manufacture and use. Funding for treatment of meth addicts was increased, as was the number of HAZMAT teams. By 2005, the problem was reduced to barely noticeable levels. This was determined by the absence of fires and explosions from meth production, and the significant reduction in the number of individuals arriving at hospitals and emergency departments with signs and symptoms of methamphetamine use. What does this case illustrate to you about the need for collaboration in public health care?

Consequences of Psychoactive Drug Use

The consequences of psychoactive drug use for individuals vary based on the pharmacokinetics of the drug used. For example, cocaine is a stimulant; thus, while under the effect of the drug, the individual experiences a stimulation of the CNS. These effects include an increase in energy and mental alertness, and a decreased need for sleep. It also has a stimulant effect on the cardiovascular system including constriction of the blood vessels, dilated pupils, and increased heart rate and blood pressure. Once the drug has left the system, the person experiences a rebound effect, an understimulation of the CNS that can result in depression and decreased energy.[92] Persons who use drugs are at increased risk for comorbid mental disorders, sexually transmitted infections (STIs), and other adverse effects on health secondary to the use of the specific drug.[93]

Vulnerable Populations Across the Life Span

As with alcohol and tobacco, the most vulnerable populations are the fetus, the adolescent, and the young adult. Use of drugs has been associated with adverse maternal and infant outcomes. The variation of the adverse effects again relates to the pharmacokinetics of the drug used. Adverse effects include prematurity, being small for gestational age, neonatal withdrawal, and birth defects. In addition, women who use drugs during pregnancy are at higher risk for poor nutrition, are more apt to engage in prenatal care later, and are at greater risk for STIs.[94]

For youths and young adults, the focus is on prevention of use. In 2010, 10.1% of adolescents aged 12 to 17 reported current use of an illicit drug. In young adults, the rate increased to a little over one-fifth (21.5%) of those aged 18 to 25 reporting current illicit drug use. Three of the objectives in *HP 2020* related to substance abuse focus on the adolescent, specifically increasing the proportion who report never using substances, who disapprove of substance use, and who perceive great risk associated with substance use.[18]

Screening and Treatment for Psychoactive Drug Use

A number of screening instruments are available to screen for drug use. One widely used is the Drug Abuse Screening Test (DAST-10). It screens for drug use excluding alcoholic beverages. The DAST-10 has been shown to be reliable and valid with English-speaking and Spanish-speaking populations, and with those individuals seeking treatment for attention deficit-hyperactivity disorder.[95] Another tool is the National Institute on Drug Abuse (NIDA) ASSIST tool. It is available online and covers the different types of drugs of abuse.[95]

As with alcohol and tobacco, there is a clinician's guide that incorporates both screening, brief interventions and referral to treatment.[96] The guide provides the health-care provider with an excellent overview of interventions that can be instituted at the individual level, including pharmacological approaches, the use of self-help groups, and behavioral therapies.

Policy-Level Intervention to Reduce Psychoactive Drug Use–Related Harm

Policy related to drug use has been a hot topic for decades. The majority of policy has focused on controlling drug use through prosecution and jail time. From the U.S. standpoint, drug policy has come under the title of a "war on drugs," complete with a federal-level drug "czar," whose official title is director of the Office of National Drug Control Policy (ONDCP). In 2012, the drug czar was Richard Gil Kerlikowske.[97] Under President Obama, the focus of the ONDCP has shifted from prosecution to increasing access to treatment.[97]

This reflects shifting from a downstream approach to a broader focus on prevention (upstream) and early intervention with those engaged in risky use of psychoactive drugs or nonmedical use of prescription drugs. A specific focus on decriminalizing drug use has been marijuana

on two fronts: the use of marijuana for medical purposes and the reduction of criminal penalties for those who are not engaged in criminal activity related to the production, transportation, or distribution of marijuana. As of 2012, 18 states have adopted laws that permit medical use of marijuana with a prescription. In 2014, two states, Colorado and Washington, have legalized recreational marijuana use. Reduction in legal consequences includes imposing civil fines, requiring drug education, or instigating treatment. Some states have specified that various marijuana offenses are the lowest priority of law enforcement. This shift in laws related to marijuana reflects the wider shift in focus to upstream and midstream approaches.

Culture, Substance Use, and Stigma

Substance use has a long history of being viewed from a moral standpoint. Moral views of substance use vary based on ethnic culture, social practices, the specific substance in question, and the gender of the substance user. Often, the person who engages in risky substance use suffers stigma. **Stigma** is defined as a mark of disgrace or reproach. The person who is suffering from stigma often experiences shame, which, in turn, affects engagement in treatment.[98]

Stigma is a continuing concern for persons who engage in risky use, especially if it becomes a barrier to treatment. Stigma is pervasive in the general and medical community. Examples of stigma in the nursing literature can be found, such as in articles about pregnant women who are engaged in psychoactive drug use.[99] Stigma arises from the perception that risky substance use is a personal choice and the consequences are self-inflicted. The ONDCP support of midstream interventions reflects a growing emphasis on educating the national population on the benefits of treatment and the potential cost of continuing to treat substance use from a legal war on drugs approach.

Stigma has not always been experienced with substance use if the use is seen as a social norm. For example, tobacco use was a culturally acceptable practice for men in the United States, especially during the early- to mid-20th century. However, prior to World War II it was not socially acceptable for women to smoke. Many of the early tobacco ads aimed at getting women to smoke suggested that women should defy this moral standard and smoke. By the 1960s and early 1970s, some tobacco companies took this one step further and created a specific brand for women such as Virginia Slims and created ads that linked cigarette use to the feminist movement. By the 1990s, the pendulum had swung the other way and cigarette smoking shifted from an acceptable social practice to a culturally reprehensible practice. The scientific evidence that ETS results in adverse effects for the non-smoker, coupled with a growing intolerance of the odor of tobacco smoke in public places, resulted in bans against public smoking with a subsequent benefit to the population as a whole. But has this shift also resulted in a moral shunning of the tobacco user?

The stigma related to alcohol use has for the most part focused on risky and dependent use. One exception is the temperance movement in the late 1800s and early 1900s that resulted in the passing of the 18th Amendment in 1919, which effectively turned alcohol into an illicit drug. It was repealed in 1933, and alcohol once again became a socially acceptable and normative practice. However, the judgment that a person who has an alcohol use disorder is morally reprehensible did not change. The stigma associated with being an "alcoholic" resulted in the creation of 12-step programs that hold confidentiality as a core principle.

An example of a cultural shift related to alcohol use is the banning of drinking and driving. In the 1950s, the phrase "one for the road" was actually socially accepted. Though law enforcement attempted to deal with drunk driving, it was hard to determine what constituted drunkenness. A number of events contributed to a cultural shift in our view of driving under the influence (DUI). These include the advent of the Mothers Against Drunk Driving (MADD) movement, technological advances in measuring BAC, and evidence related to what constitutes impaired driving. The MADD movement was the beginning of a cultural shift that began in relation to public tolerance of the person driving under the influence. Another example of addressing stigma is the change in how we reference the person who has a substance use disorder. Instead of labeling the person with a title such as *addict, alcoholic*, or *druggie*, professional literature uses the phrase *person living with (recovering from) a substance use disorder* or *a person engaged in risky use of substances*.[100] As nurses we can combat stigma and help individuals, families, and communities reduce the harm associated with use without prejudice against the persons struggling with at-risk use.

Summary Points

- At-risk substance use affects the overall health of the individual, family, and the community.
- Substance use varies across the life span with increased vulnerability for adolescents, young adults, and pregnant women.

- Evidence-based practices exist in relation to prevention programs, screening, brief intervention, and treatment.
- Substance use, especially use of tobacco and alcohol, are serious public health issues and policy initiatives exist at the global, national, state, and local levels aimed at reducing the harm associated with at-risk substance use.
- Cultural context for substance use has shifted over time, but stigma continues to be a barrier for entrance into treatment for the person with at-risk use or a substance use disorder.

▲ CASE STUDY
Screening and Brief Intervention for Alcohol Use
Learning Outcomes
At the end of this case study, the student will be able to:

- Apply program planning to the development and implementation of a health prevention program.
- Examine current standards of care related to substance use.
- Identify strategies for training health-care providers in the use of screening tools relevant to substance use.

There has been an increased emphasis on using SBI for at-risk alcohol use in acute care medical settings. You have been assigned the task to develop an SBI program for a medical-surgical unit in a large urban hospital. Begin with the current American College of Surgeons guide for implementing SBI on a trauma unit and adapt it to the medical-surgical unit. Based on your review of the guide and building on what you learned about program planning in Chapters 4 and 5, develop an SBI program for the medical-surgical unit. Be sure you include the following:

- Current alcohol SBI recommendations from The Joint Commission on Hospital Accreditation
- A plan to train health-care personnel on the use of alcohol SBI:
  - Training methods
  - Cultural and stigma considerations
  - What other strategies could you use?
- An evaluation plan

REFERENCES

1. World Health Organization. (2012). *Management of substance abuse.* Retrieved from http://www.who.int/substance_abuse/en/.
2. The International Drug Evaluation and Classification program. (n.d.). *The 7 drug categories.* Retrieved from http://www.decp.org/experts/7categories.htm.
3. The National Institute on Drug Abuse. (2010). *Marijuana.* Retrieved from http://www.nida.nih.gov/DrugPages/Marijuana.html.
4. American Psychiatric Association. (2013). *Diagnostic and statistical manual of mental disorders* (5th ed.). Washington, DC: American Psychiatric Publishing.
5. World Health Organization. (2014). *Global status report on alcohol and health 2014.* Retrieved from http://www.who.int/substance_abuse/publications/global_alcohol_report/en/.
6. United Nations. (2011). *World drug report.* Retrieved from http://www.unodc.org/documents/data-and-analysis/WDR2011/World_Drug_Report_2011_ebook.pdf.
7. Global Commission on Drug Policy. (2011). *War on drugs: Report of the Global Commission on Drug Policy.* Retrieved from http://online.wsj.com/public/resources/documents/GlobalCommissionReport0601.pdf.
8. World Health Organization. (2009). *Global health risks. Mortality and burden of disease attributable to selected major risks.* Retrieved from http://www.who.int/healthinfo/global_burden_disease/GlobalHealthRisks_report_part2.pdf.
9. Substance Abuse and Mental Health Services Administration. (2011). *Results from the 2010 National Survey on Drug Use and Health: Summary of National Findings, NSDUH Series H-41* (HHS Publication No. SMA-11-458). Rockville, MD: Author. Retrieved from http://www.oas.samhsa.gov/NSDUH/2k10NSDUH/2k10Results.pdf.
10. U.S. Department of Health and Human Services. (2012). *Summary health statistics for US adults: National health interview survey.* Retrieved from http://www.cdc.gov/nchs/data/series/sr_10/sr10_252.pdf.
11. World Health Organization. (2012). *Management of substance abuse: Other psychoactive substances.* Retrieved from http://www.who.int/substance_abuse/facts/psychoactives/en/index.html.
12. Centers for Disease Control and Prevention. (2011). *Alcohol and public health: Frequently asked questions.* Retrieved from http://www.cdc.gov/alcohol/faqs.htm#moderateDrinking.
13. Centers for Disease Control and Prevention. (2011). *Fact sheets: Alcohol and health.* Retrieved from http://www.cdc.gov/alcohol/fact-sheets/alcohol-use.htm.
14. Centers for Disease Control and Prevention. (2010). Vital signs: Binge drinking among high school students and adults—United States, 2010. *Morbidity and Mortality Weekly Report, 59*(39), 1274-1279. Retrieved from http://www.cdc.gov/mmwr/preview/mmwrhtml/mm5939a4.htm?s_cid=mm5939a4_w.
15. Institute of Medicine (IOM) Prevention Model. (1997). *Drug abuse prevention: What works* (pp 10-15). Rockville, MD: National Institute of Drug Abuse.
16. San Francisco Department of Public Health. (n.d.). *Community behavioral services, harm reduction policy.* Retrieved from http://www.sfdph.org/dph/comupg/oservices/mentalHlth/SubstanceAbuse/HarmReduction/default.asp.
17. Beirness, D.J., Jesseman, R., Notaradrea, R., & Perron, M. (2008). *Harm reduction, what's in a name. Canadian Center on Substance Abuse.* Retrieved from http://www.ccsa.ca/2008%20CCSA%20Documents2/ccsa0115302008e.pdf.
18. U.S. Department of Health and Human Services. (2012). *Healthy People 2020 topics and objectives: Substance abuse.* Retrieved from http://www.healthypeople.gov/2020/topicsobjectives2020/overview.aspx?topicid=40.
19. U.S. Department of Health and Human Services. (2012). *Summary health statistics for US adults: National health interview survey.* Retrieved from http://www.cdc.gov/nchs/data/series/sr_10/sr10_252.pdf.
20. Centers for Disease Control and Prevention. (2011). *Impaired driving: Get the facts.* Retrieved from http://www.cdc.gov/MotorVehicleSafety/Impaired_Driving/impaired-drv_factsheet.html.
21. Zhang, S.M., Lee, I.M., Manson, J.E., Cook, N.R., Willett, W.C., & Buring, J.E. (2007). Alcohol consumption and breast cancer risk in the Women's Health Study. *American Journal of Epidemiology, 165*(6), 667-676.
22. Gunzerath, L., Hewitt, B.G., Li, T.-K., & Warren, K.R. (2011). Alcohol research: Past, present, and future. *Annals of the New York Academy of Sciences, 1216,* 1-23. doi:10.1111/j.1749-6632.2010.05832.x.
23. Guo, R., & Ren, J. (2010). Alcohol and acetaldehyde in public health: From marvel to menace. *International Journal on Environmental Research and Public Health, 4,* 1285-1301.
24. Ceccanti, M., Attili, A., Balducci, G., Attilia, F., Giacomelli, S., Rotondo, C., et al. (2006). Acute alcoholic hepatitis. *Journal of Clinical Gastroenterology, 40*(9), 833-841.
25. Apte, M., McCarroll, J., Pirola, R., & Wilson, J. (2007). Pancreatic MAP kinase pathways and acetaldehyde. *Novartis Foundation Symposium, 285,* 200.
26. Zhang, X., Li, S., Brown, R., & Ren, J. (2004). Ethanol and acetaldehyde in alcoholic cardiomyopathy: From bad to ugly en route to oxidative stress. *Alcohol, 32,* 175-186.
27. Bujanda, L. (2000). The effects of alcohol consumption upon the gastrointestinal tract. *American Journal of Gastroenterology, 95*(12), 3374-3382.
28. Gurvits, G.E. (2010). Black esophagus: Acute esophageal necrosis syndrome. *World Journal of Gastroenterology, 16*(26), 3219-3225.
29. Dodi, F., Centanaro, M., Campolucci, A., Valente, U., & Pagano, G. (2010). Pneumocystis jiroveci and cytomegalovirus pneumonia in patients with alcoholic hepatic cirrhosis. *Le Infezioni in Medicina, 18*(2), 120-123.

30. Harper, C. (2009). The neuropathology of alcohol-related brain damage. *Alcohol and Alcoholism, 44*(2), 136-140. doi:10.1093/alcalc/agn102.

31. Blume, S.B., & Russell, M. (2001). Alcohol and substance abuse in obstetrics and gynecology practice. In N.L. Stotland (Ed.), *Psychological aspects of women's health care: The interface between psychiatry and obstetrics and gynecology* (2nd ed). Washington, DC: American Psychological Press.

32. Nolen-Hoeksema, S. (2004). Gender differences in risk factors and consequences for alcohol use and problems. *Clinical Psychology Review, 24*(8), 981-1010. doi:10.1016/j.cpr.2004.08.003.

33. Poschl, G., & Seitz, H.K. (2004). Alcohol and cancer. *Alcohol & Alcoholism, 39*(3), 155.

34. Boffera, P., & Hashibei, M. (2006). Alcohol and cancer. *Lancet, 7*, 149-156.

35. Benishek, L., Kirby, K., & Dugosh, K. (2011). Prevalence and frequency of problems of concerned family members with a substance-using loved one. *The American Journal of Drug and Alcohol Abuse, 37*(2), 82-88. doi:10.3109/00952990.2010.540276.

36. Centers for Disease Control and Prevention. (2004). Alcohol-attributable deaths and years of potential life lost. United States 2001. *Morbidity and Mortality Weekly Report, 53*, 866-870.

37. Sleet, D.A., Ballesteros, M.F., & Borse, N.N. (2010). A review of unintentional injuries in adolescents. *Annual Review of Public Health, 31*,195-212.

38. Jane-Llopis, E., & Matytsina, I. (2006). Mental health and alcohol, drugs and tobacco: A review of the comorbidity between mental disorders and the use of alcohol, tobacco and illicit drugs. *Drug Alcohol Review, 25*(6), 515-536.

39. Manning, M.A., & Hoyme, H.E. (2007). Fetal alcohol spectrums: A practical clinical approach to diagnosis. *Neuroscience & Biobehavioral Reviews, 31*(2), 230-238.

40. May, P.A., & Gossage, J.P. (2001). Estimating the prevalence of fetal alcohol syndrome, summary. *Alcohol, Research & Health, 25*, 159-167.

41. Substance Abuse and Mental Health Services Administration. (2004). *The National Survey on Drug Use and Health Report: Alcohol dependence or abuse and age of first use.* Retrieved from http://www.oas.samhsa.gov/2k4/agedependence/agedependence.htm.

42. National Institute on Alcohol Abuse and Alcoholism. (2012). *Facts about alcohol and adolescent health.* Retrieved from http://www.niaaa.nih.gov/About NIAAA/NIAAASponsoredPrograms/Pages/Alcohol AdolescentHealth.aspx.

43. Bava, S., & Tapert, S. (2010). Adolescent brain development and the risk for alcohol and other drug problems. *Neuropsychological Review, 20*, 398-413.

44. Duru, O.K., Xu, H., Tseng, C.H., Mirkin, M., Ang, A., Tallen, L., et al. (2010). Correlates of alcohol-related discussions between older adults and their physicians. *Journal of American Geriatric Society. 58*(12), 2369-2374. doi:10.1111/j.1532–5415.2010.03176.x.

45. Savage, C.L. (2008). Screening for alcohol use in older adults. *Directions in Addiction Treatment and Prevention, 12*(2), 17-26.

46. National Institute on Alcohol Abuse and Alcoholism. (2005). *Helping patients who drink too much: A clinician's guide.* Rockville MD: Author.

47. American College of Surgeons Committee on Trauma. (n.d.). *Alcohol screening and brief intervention for trauma patients.* Retrieved from http://www.facs.org/trauma/publications/sbirtguide.pdf.

48. Madras, B.K., Compton, W.M., Avula, D., Stegbauer, T., Stein, J.B., & Clark, J.W. (2009). Screening, brief interventions, referral to treatment (SBIRT) for illicit drug and alcohol use at multiple healthcare sites: Comparison at intake and six months. *Drug and Alcohol Dependence, 99*(1–3), 280-295.

49. ATTC Addiction Messenger. (n.d.). *SBIRT Part 2. Breaking the model down.* Retrieved from http://www.nattc.org/find/news/attcnews/epubs/addmsg/aug2010article.asp.

50. Barbor, T.F., McRee, B.G., Kassebaum, P.A., Grimaldi, P.L., Ahmed, K., & Bray, J. (2007). Screening, Brief Intervention, and Referral to Treatment (SBIRT): Toward a public health approach to the management of substance abuse. *Substance Abuse, 28*(3), 7-30.

51. Higgins-Biddle, J., Hungerford, D., & Cates-Wessel, K. (2009). *Screening and Brief Interventions (SBI) for unhealthy alcohol use: A step-by-step implementation guide for trauma centers.* Atlanta, GA: Centers for Disease Control and Prevention, National Center for Injury Prevention and Control.

52. Macleaod, J.B., & Hungerford, D.W. (2011). Alcohol-related injury visits: Do we know the true prevalence in the U.S. trauma centers? *Injury, 42*(9), 922-926.

53. Ewing, J.A. (1984). Detecting alcoholism: The CAGE questionnaire. *Journal of the American Medical Association, 252*(14), 1905–1907.

54. Dhalla, S., & Kopec, J.A. (2007). The CAGE questionnaire for alcohol misuse: A review of reliability and validity studies. *Clinical and Investigative Medicine, 30*(1), 33-41.

55. Vitesnikova, J., Dinh, M., Leonard, E., Boufous, S., Conigrave, K. Use of AUDIT-C as a tool to identify hazardous alcohol consumption in admitted trauma patients. *Injury. 45*(9), 1440-1444.

56. Daeppen, J.B., Yersin, B., Landry, U., Pecoud, A., & Decrey, H. (2000). Reliability and validity of the Alcohol Use Disorders Identification Test (AUDIT) imbedded with a general health risk screening questionnaire: Results of a survey in 332 primary care patients. *Alcoholism: Clinical and Experimental Research, 24*(5), 659-665.

57. National Institute on Alcohol Abuse and Alcoholism. (2011). *Alcohol screening and brief intervention for youth: A practitioner's guide.* Bethesda, MD: Author.

58. Lam, T.H., & Chim, D. (2010). Controlling alcohol-related global health problems. *Asia Pacific Journal of Public Health, 22* (Suppl. 3), 203S-208S.

59. National Quality Forum. (2007). Steering committee member. *National Voluntary Consensus Standards for the Treatment of Substance Use Conditions: Evidence-Based treatment practices.* Washington DC: Author.

60. Savage, C.L. (2008). Clinical reviews: National Quality Forum's consensus on evidence-based treatment of substance use illnesses; A report. *Journal of Addictions Nursing, 19*(4).

61. Glasner-Edwards, S., & Rawson, R. (2010). Evidence-based practices in addiction treatment: Review and recommendations for public policy. *Health Policy.* doi:10.1016/j.healthpol.2010.05.013.

62. Substance Abuse and Mental Health Services Administration. (2012). *The National Registry of Evidence-based Programs and Practices.* Retrieved from http://www.nrepp.samhsa.gov/AboutNREPP.aspx.

63. Substance Abuse and Mental Health Services Administration. (2008). *The National Registry of Evidence-Based Programs and Practices: Brief alcohol screening and intervention for college students.* Retrieved from http://www.nrepp.samhsa.gov/ViewIntervention. aspx?id=124.

64. Centers for Disease Control and Prevention. (2011). *Tobacco-related mortality.* Retrieved from http://www.cdc.gov/tobacco/data_statistics/fact_sheets/health_effects/tobacco_related_mortality/.

65. Mokdad, A.H., Marks, J.S., Stroup, D.F., & Gerberding, J.L. (2004). Actual causes of death in the United States, 2000. *JAMA, 291*(10), 1238-1245.

66. World Health Organization. (2011). *Tobacco fact sheet.* Retrieved from http://www.who.int/mediacentre/factsheets/fs339/en/index.html.

67. U.S. Department of Health, Education, and Welfare. (1964). *Smoking and health: Report of the Advisory Committee to the Surgeon General of the Public Health Service* (PHS Publication No. 1103). Washington, DC: U.S. Department of Health, Education, and Welfare, Public Health Service, Centers for Disease Control.

68. U.S. Department of Health and Human Services. (1988). *The health consequences of smoking: Nicotine addiction. A Report of the Surgeon General* (DHHS Publication No. [CDC] 88-8406). Atlanta, GA: U.S. Department of Health and Human Services, Public Health Service, Centers for Disease Control, National Center for Chronic Disease Prevention and Health Promotion, Office on Smoking and Health.

69. Centers for Disease Control and Prevention. (2012). *2010 Surgeon General's report—How tobacco smoke causes disease: The biology and behavioral basis for smoking-attributable disease.* Retrieved from http://www.cdc.gov/tobacco/data_statistics/sgr/2010/index.htm.

70. Centers for Disease Control and Prevention. (2010). Surveillance of certain health behaviors and conditions among states and selected local areas—Behavioral Risk Factor Surveillance System, United States, 2007. *Morbidity and Mortality Weekly Report, 59*(SS01),1-220. Retrieved from http://www.cdc.gov/mmwr/preview/mmwrhtml/ss5901a1.htm#tab28.

71. Dube, S.R., McClave, A., James, C., Caraballo, R., Kaufmann, R., & Pechacek, T. (2010). Vital signs: Current cigarette smoking among adults aged > 18 years—United States, 2009. *Morbidity and Mortality Weekly Report, 59*(35), 1135-1140.

72. U.S. Environmental Protection Agency. (2011). *Health effects of exposure to second hand smoke.* Retrieved from http://www.epa.gov/smokefree/healtheffects.html.

73. Centers for Disease Control and Prevention. (2012). *Smoking and tobacco use: Health effects of smoking.* Retrieved from http://www.cdc.gov/tobacco/data_statistics/fact_sheets/health_effects/effects_cig_smoking/.

74. Centers for Disease Control and Prevention. (2011). *Smoking and tobacco use: Smokeless tobacco facts.* Retrieved from http://www.cdc.gov/tobacco/data_statistics/fact_sheets/smokeless/smokeless_facts/.

75. Centers for Disease Control and Prevention. (2011). *Smoking and tobacco use: Frequently asked questions.* Retrieved from http://apps.nccd.cdc.gov/osh_faq/topic.aspx?TopicID=16.

76. Grant, B.F., Hasin D.S., Chou, P.S., Stinson, F.S., & Dawson, D.A. (2004). Nicotine dependence and psychiatric disorders in the United States: Results from the National Epidemiologic Survey on Alcohol and Related Conditions. *Archives of General Psychiatry, 61*(11), 1107-1115.

77. World Health Organization. (2011). *Tobacco fact sheet.* Retrieved from http://www.who.int/mediacentre/factsheets/fs339/en/index.html.

78. Centers for Disease Control and Prevention. (2012). *Health effects of secondhand smoke.* Retrieved from http://www.cdc.gov/tobacco/data_statistics/fact_sheets/secondhand_smoke/health_effects/index.htm.

79. National Cancer Institute. (2010). *Cancer trends progress report—2009/2010 update.* Bethesda, MD: National Cancer Institute, NIH, DHHS. Retrieved from http://progressreport.cancer.gov.

80. Fiore, M.C., Bailey, W.C., Cohen, S.J., Bailey, W.C., Benowitz, N.L., Curry, S.J., Dorfman, S.F., et al. (2000, October). *Treating tobacco use and dependence: Quick reference guide for clinicians.* Rockville, MD: U.S. Department of Health and Human Services. Public Health Service. Retrieved from http://www.surgeongeneral.gov/tobacco/tobaqrg.html#Identification.

81. U.S. Department of Health and Human Services. (2010). *2020 topics and objectives: Tobacco use.* Retrieved from http://www.healthypeople.gov/2020/topicsobjectives2020/objectiveslist.aspx?topicId=41.

82. Centers for Disease Control and Prevention. (2011). *Smoking and tobacco use: Smoking cessation.* Retrieved from http://www.cdc.gov/tobacco/data_statistics/fact_sheets/cessation/quitting/index.htm.

83. Centers for Disease Control and Prevention. (1999). Achievements in public health, 1900-1999: Tobacco use—United States, 1900–1999. *Morbidity and Mortality Weekly Report, 48*(43), 986–993.

84. The World Health Organization. (2011). Tobacco-free initiative. Retrieved from http://www.who.int/tobacco/framework/countrylist/en/index.html.

85. Gostin, L.O. (2009). FDA regulation of tobacco: Politics law and the public's health. *JAMA, 3*(13), 1459-1460.

86. Bayer, R., & Kelly, M. (2010). Tobacco control and free speech—an American dilemma. *New England Journal of Medicine, 362*(4), 281-283.

87. Han, B., Gfroerer, J.C., & Colliver, J.D. (2009, August). An examination of the trends in illicit drug use among adults aged 50–59 in the United States. *OAS Data Review.* Retrieved from http://www.oas.samhsa.gov/2k9/OlderAdults/OAS_data_review_OlderAdults.pdf.

88. Society for Public Health Education, Agency for Toxic Substances and Disease Registry: The American College of Medical Toxicology. (2007). *Helping communities combat clandestine methamphetamine laboratories: Meth tool kit.* Retrieved from http://www.sophe.org/sophe/pdf/Meth%20Toolkit_final_.pdf.

89. NIDA. (n.d.). Methamphetamine abuse and addiction. How is methamphetamine abused? *NIDA News—Research Report Series.* Retrieved from http://www.nida.nih.gov/researchreports/methamph/methamph3.html.

90. U.S. Environmental Protection Agency. (2008). RCRA hazardous waste identification of methamphetamine production process byproducts. *Report to Congress Under the USA Patriot Improvement and Reauthorization Act of 2005.* Retrieved from http://www.epa.gov/wastes/hazard/wastetypes/wasteid/downloads/rtc-meth.pdf.

91. McFadden, D., Fitzgerald, S., Kub, J., & Lamar. E. (2006). Occupational health hazards to first responders. *Journal of Addictions Nursing, 1*(3), 169-174.

92. National Institute on Drug Abuse. (2011). *Info facts: Cocaine.* Retrieved from http://www.drugabuse.gov/publications/infofacts/cocaine.

93. National Institute on Drug Abuse. (2012). *Info facts.* Retrieved from http://www.drugabuse.gov/publications/term/160/InfoFacts.

94. March of Dimes. (2008). *Smoking, alcohol and drugs.* Retrieved from http://www.marchofdimes.com/pregnancy/alcohol_illicitdrug.html.

95. McCann, B.S., Simpson, T.L., & Ries, P.R. (2000). Reliability and validity of screening instruments for drug and alcohol abuse in adults seeking evaluation for attention-deficit/hyperactivity disorder. *American Journal on Addictions, 9*(1), 1-9. doi:10.1080/10550490050172173.

96. National Institute on Drug Abuse. (2012). *NIDA quick screen.* Retrieved from http://www.drugabuse.gov/nmassist/.

97. National Institute on Drug Abuse. (2009). *Screening for drug use in medical settings.* Retrieved from http://www.drugabuse.gov/publications/resource-guide .

98. Office of National Drug Abuse Policy. (n.d.). *National drug control strategy.* Retrieved from http://www.whitehouse.gov/ondcp/2011-national-drug-control-strategy.

99. Fortney, J., Mukherjee, S., Curran, G., Fortney, S., Han, X., & Both, B.M. (2004). Factors associated with perceived stigma for alcohol use and treatment among at-risk drinkers. *Journal of Behavioral Health Services Research, 31*(4), 418-429.

100. Savage, C.L. (2009). Clinical reviews: A proposed framework related to the care of addicted mothers *Journal of Addictions Nursing, 19*(3), 158-160.

101. Broyles, L.M., Binswanger, I.A., Jenkins, J.A., Finnell D.S., Faseru, B. Gordon, A.J. et al. (2014). Confronting inadvertent Stigma and Pejorative Language in Addiction Scholarship: A Recognition and Response. *Substance Abuse,* doi:10.1080/08897077.2014.930372. Retrieved from http://www.tandfonline.com/doi/pdf/10.1080/08897077.2014.930372.

Chapter 12

Injury and Violence

OBJECTIVES

After reading this chapter, the student will be able to:

1. Describe the impact of injury and violence on the health of a population.
2. Define the burden of disease related to injury and violence using current epidemiological frameworks.
3. Use appropriate frameworks in the assessment of injury and violence.
4. Understand the role of policy in injury and violence prevention.
5. Apply current evidence-based population interventions to the prevention of injury and violence.

KEY TERMS

Acquaintance violence
Alcohol-impaired driving
Child maltreatment
Collective violence
Community violence
Emotional abuse
Emotional neglect
Family violence
Fire-related injury

Haddon Matrix
Injury
Intentional injury
Interpersonal violence
Intimate partner violence
Motor vehicle crashes (MVCs)
Physical abuse
Physical neglect

Physical violence
Poisoning
Post-traumatic stress disorder (PTSD)
Psychological/emotional violence
Road traffic injury (RTI)
Self-inflicted violence
Sexual abuse

Sexual violence
Stranger violence
Suicide
Threat of physical/sexual violence
Unintentional injury
Violence
War

■ Introduction

Overview of Injury

Injury is a serious public health issue that kills more than 5 million people globally and causes harm to many more. Injury occurs as the result of a wide variety of events, including motor vehicle crashes (MVCs), drowning, poisoning, falls, burns, assault, self-inflicted violence, or acts of war. According to the World Health Organization (WHO), 9% of global mortality is attributable to injury.[1] Injury disproportionately affects the young and the impoverished and in the United States is the number one cause of death for those aged 1 to 44.[1,2] Injury not only affects the person who is injured, but also can have an effect on family members, friends, coworkers, employers, and communities.[2] Thus, injury is a serious public health issue, not only because of mortality, but also in relation to disability, health-care costs, and the need for emergency care.

Types of Injuries

An **injury** is defined as damage or harm done to or suffered by a person or thing. There are two types of injury, unintentional and intentional. An **unintentional injury** is defined as an injury to a person for which there is no predetermined intent to injure another or oneself. Unintentional injuries include MVCs, drowning, falls, poisoning, burns, and other injuries. Although the media use the term *accident* when referring to unintentional injuries, these injuries are often predictable and preventable and not the result of random unavoidable accidental events.[3]

In the United States, unintentional injuries account for more than 120,000 deaths and more than 27 million emergency department (ED) visits. The highest number of deaths is related to MVCs, followed by falls and poisonings (Box 12-1).[4] The population most at risk is males under the age of 45. Of special concern are

BOX 12–1	**Top 10 Causes of Injury-Related Mortality, 2009**

1. Unintentional motor vehicle crashes
2. Unintentional poisonings
3. Unintentional falls
4. Suicide/firearm
5. Homicide/firearm
6. Suicide/suffocation
7. Suicide/poisoning
8. Unintentional suffocation
9. Unintentional, unspecified
10. Unintentional drowning

Source: See reference 3.

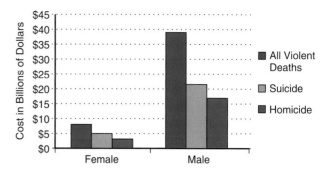

Total deaths: 10,491 females and 40,682 males

Figure 12-1 Total combined medical and work loss costs of violent deaths, by sex and intent in the United States, 2005. *(Data from Centers for Disease Control and Prevention. [2012]. Injury prevention and control: Injury center; Cost of violent deaths in the U.S., 2005.)*

infants less than 1 year and children aged 1 to 19 years. More than a third (37%) of all deaths for children aged 1 to 19 are related to injury, making it the leading cause of death in this age group. For infants under the age of 1 year and newborns, it is the fifth leading cause of death.[2,4] Unintentional injuries not only contribute to premature death, but nonfatal injuries also have consequences that range from temporary pain to long-term disability, chronic pain, and a diminished health-related quality of life. Twenty-six million emergency visits per year are for unintentional injury.[5] Following an injury, a person often requires hospitalization and/or rehabilitation services.

Overview of Violence

Intentional injuries are defined as injuries that occur because of a deliberate act that causes harm either to the self or others. **Violence** is a broader term used in conjunction with intentional injury in the public health literature and refers to physical force used to violate, damage, or abuse others or oneself. According to the WHO, violence is among the leading causes of death for those aged 15 to 44 years.[6] Violence is equally threatening to a community and often occurs along with mental illness and/or substance use (Chapters 10 and 11). Annually in the United States, more than 51,000 deaths are attributable to violence. A recent cost estimate of violence in the United States was $47.2 billion, including direct health-care costs and costs related to work loss. This translates to a per capita cost of $160 (Fig. 12-1).[7]

Types of Violence

The WHO presented a topology of violence that separates violence into two contexts, family violence and community violence, and three categories, self-inflicted

violence, interpersonal violence, and collective violence. **Self-inflicted violence** is violence in which the perpetrator and the victim are one and the same, and includes suicide and self-inflicted injury. **Interpersonal violence** occurs between individuals and includes two different contexts in which the violence occurs. The first is **family violence,** which includes intimate partner violence, child abuse/maltreatment, and elder abuse. The second is **community violence,** which occurs in the context of the community and includes **acquaintance violence,** violence between individuals who know each other, and **stranger violence,** violence that occurs between individuals who do not know each other. **Collective violence** occurs when a large group of people engage in violent behavior and covers various types of violent acts such as conflicts between nations and groups, terrorism instigated by groups or states, rape as a weapon of war, and gang warfare.

Violent acts are broken out into four types of violence: (1) neglect, (2) psychological violence, (3) physical violence, and (4) sexual assault. The topology proposed by the WHO helps to demonstrate the context in which violence occurs and the four types of violence that can occur (Fig. 12-2).[6]

Injury and violence are of major concern worldwide and in the United States *Healthy People 2020 (HP 2020)* health topics include prevention of unintentional injury and violence. This topic area was included because of the mortality and disability associated with injury. Under this topic, there is a total of 43 objectives: 28 related to unintentional injury and 15 related to violence.

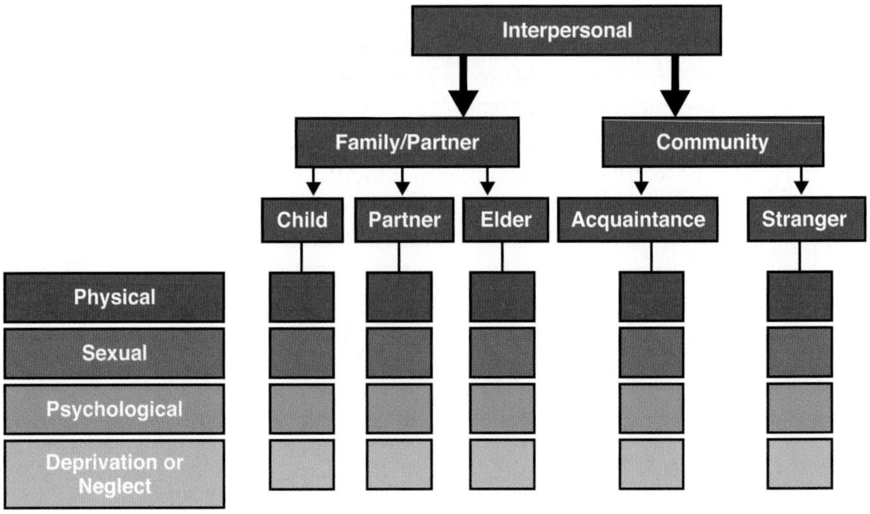

Figure 12-2 The topology of violence. *(From the World Health Organization. [2002]. World report on violence and health. Geneva, Switzerland: Author.)*

■ HEALTHY PEOPLE 2020
Injury and Violence Prevention

Goal: Prevent unintentional injuries and violence, and reduce their consequences

Overview: Injuries and violence are widespread in society. Both unintentional injuries and those caused by acts of violence are among the top 15 killers for Americans of all ages.[1] Many people accept them as accidents, acts of fate, or as part of life. However, most events resulting in injury, disability, or death are predictable and preventable. The Injury and Violence Prevention Objectives for 2020 represent a broad range of issues which, if adequately addressed, will improve the health of the Nation.[8]

Surveillance of Injury and Violence

Injury surveillance is conducted via various reporting mechanisms at the local, state, and national levels. In relation to unintentional injury, various tracking methods exist. For example, MVCs are tracked through the department of motor vehicles, department of transportation, and, for fatal MVCs, through vital statistics. Some categories of injury such as poisoning are tracked through the department of public health. Some injuries are not routinely tracked at the governmental level, such as injury due to falls, but are tracked by institutions for patient-related falls and through public health departments and child protective services for child-related falls.

Tracking of intentional injury became more centralized in 2002 when the Centers for Disease Control and Prevention (CDC) received funding to establish the National

Violent Death Reporting System. This system pools data on violent deaths from various state-level databases to create an anonymous database that could help states develop programs and monitor outcomes. Sources of data include death certificates, police reports, medical examiner reports, and other available data. Thus, multiple sources of data can be used to examine the impact of injury at the population level.[9]

Determining Risk for Injury or Violence

Tracking the incidence of injury is only one part of the puzzle. A key step in prevention of injury it to determine who is at greater risk for incurring an injury. The risk factors for injury vary based on the type of injury but come under the same main categories as chronic disease, behavioral, environmental, and socioeconomic risk factors. For example, in an MVC several factors come into play. The behavioral level includes such issues as wearing seat belts, texting while driving, or driving under the influence of alcohol. In addition, environmental factors such as weather conditions and traffic control may play a role. Socioeconomic factors also play a role; for example, those with fewer economic resources may have older cars that may not be adequately maintained, and poorer countries, states, or municipalities may not be able to maintain safe roads. Analysis of risk for a particular injury requires a complex evaluation of a number of factors.

The Haddon Matrix

A common method used to determine injury risk is the **Haddon Matrix.** This matrix was developed based on the epidemiological triangle (see Chapter 3) and incorporates the three constructs in the triangle: (1) agent, (2) host, and (3) environment. It was designed by William Haddon, Jr., the first head of what is now the National Highway Traffic Safety Administration. The original purpose was to examine the problem of traffic safety.[10]

The Haddon Matrix has a minimum of 12 empty boxes to be filled in. The rows reflect the time around the event—"pre-event," "event," and "post-event"—and the columns are related to the host, agent, and environment (Fig. 12-3). Filling in the boxes provides a method of viewing the factors that contribute to the event and help in the planning of injury interventions and prevention strategies. The matrix can also help set up the process for data collection. The process helps to identify interventions that could occur at multiple points by prevention of the injury (pre-event) or mitigating the impact of the event (event or post-event).

Phases	Host/Human	Agent Vehicle/Equipment	Physical Environment	Social Environment
Pre-Event				
Event				
Post-Event				

Partially Filled-In Haddon Matrix: Analysis of a Motor Vehicle Crash

Complete the matrix by filling in possible factors for agent and environment based on the time phases.

Assess the contributing factors or characteristics from the perspective of:

1. *Host/Human:* What were the Host or Human Factors that contributed to the event?
2. *Agent Vehicle/Equipment:* What was the crash worthiness of the vehicle?
3. *Physical Environment:* What was the status of the roadway design or safety features?
4. *Social Environment:* For example, passage and enforcement of seat belt laws.

Combine with time phases:

1. *Pre-Event:* What factors affect the host before the event occurs?
2. *Event:* What are factors related to the crash phase?
3. *Post-Event:* What are the factors related to the post-event crash phase?

Phases	Host/Human	Agent Vehicle/Equipment	Physical Environment	Social Environment
Pre-Event	Poor vision Texting/Cell phone Reaction time Alcohol Risk taking Driving experience	Failed brakes Missing lights	Narrow shoulders Rain storm	
Event	Failure to wear seat belt	Malfunctioning seat belts		
Post-Event	High susceptibility Alcohol			

Figure 12-3 Twelve boxes of the Haddon Matrix.

Although this matrix was originally developed for the evaluation of MVCs, it can be used for any category of injury. Because it uses a classic epidemiological framework, it has applicability across settings. For example, it could be useful in an acute care setting to evaluate patient falls. It also provides needed information to develop primary prevention strategies (prevention of the event) and mitigation of the impact of the event, both during the event and following the event (secondary and tertiary prevention).

Figure 12-3 includes a blank Haddon Matrix and then a partially filled-out matrix related to MVCs that can be used with your own county or city data. If you begin filling out the partially filled-out form you can begin to identify areas where interventions could be developed at all three levels: pre-crash, crash, and following the crash. The first part of the matrix provides vital information on what contributes to the injury and the consequences of the injury and the second dimension provides vital information to help planners compare possible interventions on a variety of dimensions. The matrix becomes three dimensional by adding decision criteria for each level and includes consideration of the effectiveness, cost, feasibility, and other identified criteria used to decide what would be the best intervention.[10] This can help planners choose from a variety of possible interventions.

Prevention of Injury and Violence

Prevention of injury and violence is a major public health initiative. The CDC has a national center dedicated to injury prevention.[2] The home page for this center illustrates the vast array of serious injury issues for the country, including poisoning (especially in children), traumatic brain injury, falls, MVCs, and drowning. The top unintentional injury prevention priorities are MVCs and falls in the older adult. The injury center not only collects surveillance data on injury; it also provides leadership and funds research aimed at reducing injury.

Nursing Role in Prevention

Nurses play a key role in addressing the issue of injury and violence through the care they provide, the interventions they develop, and their active role in policy making. There is constant national attention from the media on injury issues that help raise awareness and in many cases result in policy-level interventions. For example, the issue of violence against women has received international attention, especially after a number of cases of rape occurred on public transportation in India and South America. Nurses directly helped shape policy here in the United Sates to help prevent violence against women. For example, public health nurse researchers, such as Dr. Jacquelyn Campbell, and nursing organizations, especially the ANA, were actively involved in the passing of the 2013 Violence Against Women Act. Nurses also play a role on the front lines every day providing care for persons following injury, especially in trauma centers.

The importance of the role of nurses is evidenced by the involvement of nurses on the national and local levels. The Society of Trauma Nurses (STN) includes injury prevention and education in its mission statement. It has an active committee dedicated to injury prevention. In line with the STN priorities, an injury prevention program was initiated by trauma nurses at Cincinnati Children's Hospital Medical Center (CCHMC). The nurses developed and implemented a child passenger safety program. The program was offered to low-income families and was conducted at 46 "fitting" stations located in the community, including fire stations and health departments, so that parents could receive help on car seat installation, that is "fitting" the seats into their cars. Other programs initiated by these nurses included a bike safety program, community health fairs, and leadership with the Safe Kids Coalition.

Because injury prevention is an essential component of what nurses provide to their communities, how would you begin? A good place to start is to examine the injury data related to the setting in which you work and the population for whom you care. If you work in the emergency department (ED), you are most likely confronted with injury on a daily basis. As almost all injury is preventable, it is important to take an upstream approach while tending to the victims downstream, as did the nurses at CCHMC. To review from Chapter 2, the upstream metaphor in public health refers to the following: People are drowning in a river and rescue workers keep pulling them out, trying to save them from drowning. Pretty soon, the rescuers realize that no matter how hard they work at pulling people out, more keep floating downstream. They decide to walk upstream to find out why people are falling in the river in the first place. Effort is then put into fixing the problem upstream that is causing people to fall into the river.

The problem for the individual nurse is that it feels as though there is no time to walk upstream. There are just too many patients coming for nursing care who have already fallen into the water. Luckily, the upstream approach is done as a collaborative effort across disciplines and entities. Take, for example, the child safety initiative at CCHMC. The programs were offered in community settings and included nurses at the hospital, the public health department, the fire department, and the police department. The key is to have someone ask the question, "What is happening upstream?" and then have a team not only ready to find out, but also committed to fixing the issues upstream.

Policy Aimed at Prevention of Injury and Violence

Many examples of policies exist at the state and local levels aimed at preventing injury. For example, most local municipalities require that a fence be in place around a swimming pool to prevent accidental drowning. Pedestrian laws and signs at crosswalks are in place to prevent injury to pedestrians. The list is long and demonstrates that policy efforts are effective in reducing injury. Seat belt laws alone have resulted in reduction in fatal MVCs. Policy aimed at reducing violence often comes through the judicial system. However, other approaches are also effective, such as creating neighborhood watch groups, increasing lighting on streets at night, and reducing density of alcohol outlets. Policy initiatives often arise from the grassroots and often effectiveness is contingent on neighborhood buy-in (Chapters 4 and 22).

Epidemiology of Unintentional Injury: Motor Vehicle Crashes

Motor vehicle crashes (MVCs) are a major public health concern worldwide, particularly for the young. An MVC is defined as the collision of a motor vehicle with another vehicle, a stationary object, or a person that results in injury or death. The term *crash* has been substituted for the term *accident* because most MVCs are not random accidental events, but are related to preventable causes. To help encompass the broader issue of road-related injury, the WHO uses the term **road traffic injury (RTI)**. The WHO's definition of an RTI is similar to the definition of an MVC, but includes the term *public road*. Thus, its definition is an injury that occurs as the result of a collision on a public road with involvement of at least one vehicle.[11]

In the United States, for children from infancy to 19 years old, MVCs are the leading cause of unintentional injury deaths. For those aged 5 to 19, MVCs account for 67% of all unintentional injury deaths in this age group.[12] There has been a decline over time in MVC-related injury, which may reflect an increase in the use of seatbelts, car seats, and booster seats. Factors associated with a decline in MVCs include a decrease in driving while alcohol impaired, vehicle design, changes in driver's license requirements, and improved road environments.[13,14]

Estimates of the economic burden of MVCs are difficult to determine. In an attempt to understand the impact, the National Safety Council used available national data to estimate costs that reflect the dollars spent and income not received because of fatal and nonfatal injury. They calculated the average economic cost per death from an injury or crash. The costs included wage and productivity losses, medical expenses, damage to the motor vehicle, and employers' uninsured costs. The average economic cost per death was $1,300,000. For a nonfatal disabling injury, the cost was $63,500.[15] Using these estimates can be helpful in determining the economic burden experienced at the state level. For example, you can access information on state Web sites on the number of MVCs in a year. If in one state there were 158 MVC-related fatalities it would mean a total economic cost of $205,400,000!

Risk Factors for Motor Vehicle Crashes

As noted above, when considering MVCs, a number of factors come into play. The behavioral level includes such issues as wearing seat belts, texting while driving, or driving under the influence of alcohol. In addition, environmental factors may play a role, for example, weather conditions and traffic control. Socioeconomic factors also play a role; for example, those with fewer economic resources may have older cars that may not be adequately maintained, and poorer countries, states, or municipalities may not be able to maintain safe roads.

The study of risk factors for MVCs is complex, as evidenced by the study by Ramano, Peck, and Voas in which they examined the role of impaired driving and other driver characteristics such as age, gender, and environmental factors.[16] Driving while under the influence of alcohol is a major risk factor for MVCs. **Alcohol-impaired driving** is driving with a blood alcohol level at 0.08 or above, and laws have been enacted that make it illegal to drive impaired. An emerging issue related to MVCs is understanding the role of driver distraction. Evidence has emerged that texting, eating, using handheld devices, and drowsiness when driving can result in driver impairment that is, at times, equal to or greater than alcohol impairment.

Speed is a major contributing factor to the severity of the injury associated with MVCs. According to Elvick, speed contributes more than any other factor because of its impact on reaction time, the amount of kinetic energy created, and ability to control the vehicle.[17] Other contributing factors include weather, road conditions, and vehicle safety features.[11] Once again, behavioral and environmental factors and socioeconomic status play roles.

Other injury issues exist when the broader context of all RTIs is taken into account. Other vehicles such as all-terrain vehicles, motorcycles, and bicycles as well as pedestrian injuries are major public health issues, especially owing to the high mortality rates associated with these types of injuries. The same risk factors apply across all RTIs.

Prevention of Motor Vehicle Crashes

Reduction in MVC-associated injury has in part occurred owing to changes at the policy level. Laws related to seat belt use, car seats, booster seats, and use of handheld phones have had a positive effect on the reduction in injury and mortality. A case in point is the issue of texting while driving. Under the Haddon Matrix, this risk factor would come under the Host/Human column as a pre-crash factor (see Fig. 12-3). This risk factor came to the forefront of media attention in 2009 based on data that indicated that an increasing number of motorists were texting while driving prior to a MVC. The CDC now includes texting as one of the examples of distracted driving that is often equated with driving while intoxicated. Response to this risk factor has been reflected in laws enacted against texting while driving, making it illegal.

Much of the prevention efforts at the primary level in the United States have focused on reducing risky behaviors such as alcohol-impaired driving and public education aimed at increasing awareness of the importance of using proper safety measures. Back in the late 1970s, hospitals put into effect a policy that all parents must have a car seat in place prior to taking their newborns home from the hospital. Another approach has been to put in place a graduated driver licensing system aimed at reducing teen MVCs. In Connecticut, this policy resulted in a significant reduction in MVCs among teen drivers, with a 40% decreased MCV rate in 16-year-olds and a 30% decreased rate for 17-year-olds.[13]

Other prevention efforts are aimed at the environment, improving roads, and installing traffic lights and pedestrian walkway signs. These types of prevention approaches are more difficult to put in place in Low-and-Middle-Income Countries (LMIC) that lack the resources and that have not placed a strong emphasis on injury prevention.[11] The WHO has adopted a global plan for road safety for the decade 2011–2020. The plan has five pillars or categories of prevention efforts. These include: "1) building road safety management capacity; 2) improving the safety of road infrastructure and broader transport networks; 3) further developing the safety of vehicles; 4) enhancing the behavior of road users; and 5) improving post-crash care."[11] The CDC has become a part of this effort to put the focus on road safety here in the United States.[18]

In the United States, there have been dramatic improvements in post-crash care, resulting in a reduction in MVC-associated mortality and morbidity. Much of this is due to the development of Level I trauma units, use of flight teams to bring helicopters to the crash site and transport victims directly to a trauma center, and the development of interventions aimed at decreasing the time from the initial trauma to the initiation of treatment. Such efforts to improve post-crash care help to reduce the long-term disability and the survival rate of injury associated with MVCs.

■ HEALTHY PEOPLE 2020
Injury and Violence (IVP)

Objective: IVP-13
IVP-13.1: Reduce MVC-related deaths: deaths per 100,000 population
Baseline: 13.8 deaths per 100,000 population were caused by motor vehicle crashes in 2007 (age adjusted to the year 2000 standard population)
Target: 12.4 deaths per 100,000 population
Target-Setting Method: 10% improvement
Source: See reference 8.

Epidemiology of Unintentional Injury: Fire-Related Injuries

Fire-related injuries include burns, smoke inhalation, or any other injury sustained as the result of a fire such as falls or lacerations. These injuries are the fourth most common type of trauma worldwide, making it a major public health issue. Fire-related injuries account globally for 300,000 deaths annually and 10 million disability-adjusted life years lost.[19] More than 90% of the fatal fire-related burns occur in LMICs, with over half occurring in Southeast Asia. For those burns requiring medical care, the incidence is 20 times higher in Asia. Burns are among the most devastating of all injuries and are almost always preventable.[20] Burns are difficult to treat in very high-income countries, and with limited resources even more difficult to treat in LMICs.

In the United States, 450,000 people receive treatment for burns annually. Fires and burns account for 3,500 deaths, 3,000 in residential fires. The other 500 die due to electrical and chemical fires and fires in motor vehicle and airplane crashes. Of those burned, 45,000 are hospitalized with 25,000 hospitalized in burn centers.[21] Most burns occur in the home, with an increased incidence in women, children, and older adults. For children, 80% of the fire-related injuries occur while they are unsupervised.[20] However, in LMICs the epidemiology is different from what it is in high-income countries. In LMICs, a greater proportion of the population live as joint families, resulting in more supervision of children and older adults and thus reducing the incidence of burns in these two age groups.[22]

Risk Factors for Burn Injuries

Using the epidemiological data, the associated risk factors for burn injuries are influenced by behavioral, social, cultural, and economic factors. Women and children in LMICs are at greatest risk because they spend more time at home using open fires to cook food and heat water. In LMICs in colder climates, there is exposure to heaters and stoves to keep homes warm.[21,22] Thus, the risk for fire-related injury is more strongly associated with socioeconomic status than with culture or education.[22] Behavioral risk factors include alcohol use, tobacco use, history of seizures, and history of a psychiatric disorder. According to Atiyeh, Costagliola, and Hayek, the major risk factors are poverty, education, and type of residence.[22] Environmental risk factors include the safety of the built environment, population density, the work environment, and the natural environment. For example, some areas of the United States are more prone to large forest fires that pose a risk to populations based on the natural flora (e.g., dry tinder) and weather.

Prevention of Burn Injuries

Prevention is an essential component in any burn management program, especially with the high incidence in LMICs.[22] As in all injury, the main focus is on reduction of risk. For burns, primary prevention focuses on environmental measures in the home and behavioral changes (Box 12-2). In the United States, many of the public health interventions focus on children and measures that can be taken to reduce risk (Box 12-3).[23] In LMICs the challenge for prevention is greater, where there is less governmental emphasis on prevention of injury as well as limited resources.[22]

In the United States, policy has played a large role in reduction in fire-related morbidity and mortality. In 1911, a devastating fire in the Triangle Shirtwaist factory in New York City took the lives of 146 garment workers, most of them women. Based on that event, laws were put in place to improve safety of the workplace. Another fire, the Coconut Grove fire that occurred in Boston in 1942, resulted in the deaths of 462 people, the deadliest nightclub fire in U.S. history. The club was decorated in a South Pacific motif using decorations made of flammable materials that covered exit signs. The fire spread rapidly,

| BOX 12–2 | **Primary Prevention of Burns** |

There are several measures you can take to prevent burns and fires in the U.S., as follows:
- Do not smoke in bed.
- Keep water heater at 120°F or lower.
- Store cleaning solutions and other flammable material in ventilated area.
- Keep trash cleaned up in attics, basements, and garages.
- Use proper fuses and do not overload electrical outlets.
- Avoid fireworks at home.
- Take action to avoid being struck by lightning.

With children there are additional measures:
- Keep matches out of the hands of children and keep children away from open flames.
- Keep children away from stoves and always turn pot handles away from a child's reach.
- Never smoke or have hot liquids near or when holding a child.
- Do not heat baby bottles in a microwave.
- Cover outlets and do not let children play or chew on electrical cords.
- Keep chemicals and cleaning solutions that can burn children out of their reach.

Sources: See references 23 and 24.

| BOX 12–3 | **Secondary Prevention for Burns** |

- Have working smoke alarms.
- Have a fire escape plan for the home.
- Have a fire extinguisher.
- As soon as children can understand, teach them to Stop, Drop, and Roll if their clothes are on fire; if they are in a burning building, they need to drop below the smoke and crawl to safety.

Source: See reference 23.

engulfing the club within 5 minutes of the first flame. The main entrance was a single revolving door that quickly became jammed as panicked customers tried to escape. This fire resulted in the institution of fire code regulations that are in place today, such as restriction on the use of flammable materials as decorations and requirements for clearly marked exit signs. It also resulted in the mandate that all revolving doors be flanked by two regular doors equipped with panic bars. So the next time you go through a revolving door, you will notice that this safety measure is always in place.

Secondary prevention focuses on what to do in the event of a fire. Stop, Drop, and Roll is an example of a successful campaign to teach children, workers, and others what to do if their clothes or hair are on fire (Fig. 12-4).

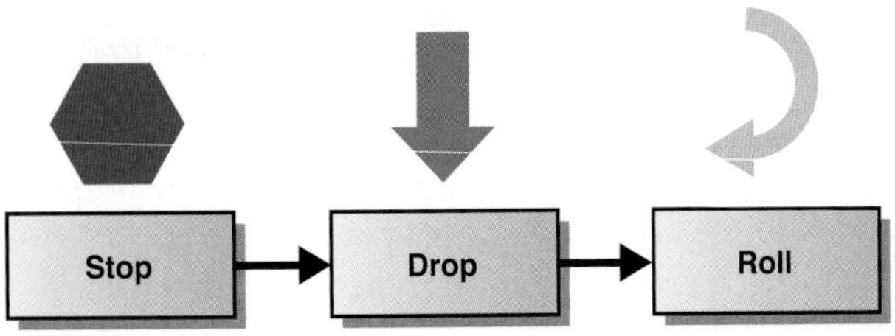

Figure 12-4 Stop, Drop, and Roll.

The purpose is to mitigate the extent of the burns by using a technique that is effective in extinguishing the flames. Strides have also occurred in the management of burns, resulting in a worldwide decline in fire-related mortality.[22] Care of a fire-related injury must also take into account the issues of disability, disfigurement, emotional impact, and pain.

▶ SOLVING THE MYSTERY
The Case of the Exploding Barrel
Public Health Science Topics Covered:

- Assessment
- Epidemiology
- Health planning

In May, Ben Smith, RN, moved from a large metropolitan area in to a rural region of the country. He took a job working in the ED in a regional medical center serving six counties. After working there for 2 months, he became concerned about the number of injuries from firecrackers that he saw, especially injuries to teenagers. His concern grew when two teenagers who had sustained eventually fatal injuries after placing a 50-gallon metal barrel over a sparkler bomb were admitted to the ED. After this event, Ben approached his supervisor about his concerns and the supervisor commented that this was something they saw every summer, especially in July. Ben wanted to know whether the number of injuries was up this year and whether their ED had been involved in any prevention efforts. His supervisor thought that was a good question and suggested that Ben look into the issue.

Ben applied basic public health principles that he had learned in his undergraduate community health courses to begin investigating the problem. He began by reviewing their records for the number of fireworks-related injuries treated in the ED during the past 5 years, including age of the patient, month the injury occurred, and the severity of the injury based on triage level. This first phase of his investigation required a basic understanding

of epidemiology (see Chapter 3), specifically how to calculate incidence rates, track the rates over time, and compare them with national rates. It also required basic community assessment skills. In this case, he did a focused assessment (see Chapter 4), that is, he started with a specific focus of fireworks-related injury. He found that the CDC had a portion of its Web site dedicated to this issue. This helped guide his investigation because the site provided information on the most common risk factors, current laws and regulations, and possible solutions.[24]

Using 5 years of data, he found that the two deaths he had encountered in the ED were the only deaths in the past 5 years, but that various fireworks-related injuries had been treated during the past 5 years that were similar to national data; most of the injuries had occurred to the fingers, hands, and eyes and the majority were burns. He calculated incidence rates for the entire population living in the region served by the medical center, using population estimates for each of the 5 years (Box 12-4).[25] He then looked at the frequency of injuries based on separate age groups including children under the age of 5, children aged 6 to 12, youths aged 13 to 18, and adults over the age of 18, and for each county. Based on the information, he determined that the overall incidence rate for the five-county region was higher than the national rate. He also found that the injury rate had decreased in children under the age of 6, but had increased in those aged 6 to 18. Starting in 2010, the majority of cases were between the ages of 13 and 18.

BOX 12–4	**Estimating Injury Rates**

The populations of the following five counties are considered here when estimating injury rates:

County Q	44,516
County R	42,316
County X	40,383
County Y	17,934
County Z	28,093

- The total population for the preceding counties in 2012 = 173,242.
- The total number of ED visits for fireworks injuries = 25.
- Rate of fireworks-related injury for the region = 12.9 per 100,000.
- The 2012 population for the United States as a whole = 313,780,968.
- The estimated number of ED visits in the United States for fireworks-related injury in 2012 = 9,300.
- Rate of fireworks-related injury in the United States = 2.9 per 100,000.

Ben then looked into community information that might help explain the decreased incidence rate in one age group and the increased rate in the other age group. After talking with his colleagues in the pediatric units, he discovered that the community had initiated a fireworks safety initiative with new parents in 2011. The health departments in all five counties had developed a brochure that was handed out at all the well-baby clinics and had been provided to the pediatricians as well. For children less than 5 years of age, the prevention program from the public health departments appeared to have been effective. But why was the rate going up in the older children, especially among teenagers?

Ben did some further research on the laws surrounding the sale of fireworks. He found that there was a wide variance in the state laws. The state in which he was working had strict laws that went beyond the Federal Hazardous Substances Act, which prohibits the sale of highly dangerous fireworks and the components that are used to make them. However, the region his hospital served was close to the border of another state that had more lax laws and allowed the sale of fireworks that were just under the legal limit of no more than 50 milligrams of explosive powder and no more than 130 milligrams of flash powder. In 2013, two new fireworks stores had opened right across the state border. This increased availability was a possible factor in the increased incidence.

He then applied the Haddon Matrix to the problem. He started with the incident that had resulted in the death of the two teenagers and filled out the Haddon Matrix using factors related to the two boys pre-event, event, and post-event. He accessed local news reports, police reports, and fire department reports on fireworks-related injuries and filled in the matrix. He found that the social environment pre-event played a big role, with a growing peer-related interest in using more dramatic fireworks. He also found that most of the injuries were clustered in the counties closest to the state border.

The Haddon Matrix assisted Ben in his assessment in another way. It helped him to examine whether there were factors during the event or post-event that also influenced the outcome of the injury. The two counties that were closest to the state border were also farthest from the regional medical center and were quite rural. For some of the events, the time for emergency personnel to arrive on the scene was 20 minutes or more. Transportation to the regional medical center averaged 25 minutes from the time the emergency personnel arrived on the scene and the time the victim arrived at the medical center.

Following his assessment, Ben was able to recommend possible action that could be taken by the hospital in conjunction with the public health departments, the schools, the emergency providers, and other stakeholders to reduce the number of these incidents. He made a recommendation that suggested prevention at the three levels of pre-event, event, and post-event. In some cases, his information opened the door for a discussion on injury prevention in the region at a higher level. Ben felt that the post-event issue related to emergency response time was bigger than just the fireworks injury issue. Ben's approach to a problem led to the development of a comprehensive fireworks prevention program spearheaded by the regional hospital that built on the work done with the preschool children. Ben now had baseline data to track the effectiveness of the intervention. Based on his work, the community put in place an injury prevention committee.

Epidemiology of Unintentional Injury: Drowning

Drowning is the leading cause globally of unintentional injury death in children aged 0 to 4 based on WHO data, with an average total global mortality rate of 7.4 per 100,000. It is highest in China, and is the number one cause of death in children 15 years and younger in that country. In the United States, in children aged 1 to 14 it is the second leading cause of all unintentional injuries and death.[26,27] It is a major social and economic burden, and in the United States, the economic loss is more than $5.7 billion annually.[26] Every day in the United States, 10 people unintentionally drown. This adds up to 3,443 fatal drownings a year, one-fifth of them children. Those who receive emergency care for nonfatal submersion frequently require a high level of hospitalization, and if they suffer potential brain damage, they can become a heavy burden to society.[27]

Risk Factors for Drowning

We know that globally age is a risk factor for drowning. Age plays a role for the older adult as their swimming ability declines. For young children, risk is tied to multiple issues. Their inquisitiveness and their lack of coordination make them susceptible to falls into bodies of water such as swimming pools, lakes, ponds, ditches of water, bathtubs, and buckets. Children aged 1 to 4 have the highest drowning rate. In the United States, young males are 10 times more likely to drown than young females, with 80% of all drowning victims being male.[27] In the United States, the most common sites for drowning are bathtubs and 5-gallon buckets for infants; for children aged 1 to 4 the greatest risk is swimming pools; and for older children, the most common sites are pools, lakes, and rivers. Drowning rates for all rural residents are three times higher than for urban residents and drowning usually occurs in open water such as ponds, rivers, irrigation canals, and lakes. Children usually die of drowning in sites where they are without adequate supervision.[26] Another risk factor is hair or body entrapment in drains of pools or spas. Children and adults are at greater risk of drowning while swimming in open bodies of water without lifeguard supervision, or while boating, especially when alcohol is being consumed by the driver of the boat or other occupants in the boat.

Not having the ability to swim is a significant risk factor and is more common in females than males and more common in African Americans than whites. On August 3, 2010, six teens from two African American families died in the Red River near Shreveport, Louisiana. One unknowingly stepped off the shallow edge and slipped into the deep river and six more teens went in to rescue him. Only one made it back. None of them knew how to swim and neither did their parents, watching from the shore. In the United States, African Americans, American Indians, and Alaska Natives all have a drowning rate among adolescents more than double the national average. According to national statistics, approximately 60% of African American and Hispanic/Latino children are unable to swim, while only 30% of white/Caucasian children do not know how to swim.[28] Thus, the fact that no one in a family knows how to swim increases the risk, because family members often are the only ones supervising children when they swim. Similar risk is found in LMICs, which also have very low rate of citizens who know how to swim across all ages, with especially low rates in females. In addition, mothers in LMICs often have more children and are the sole caretakers of the children, making it more difficult to provide good supervision.[26]

Prevention of Drowning

Prevention requires a concerted effort on the part of health-care providers, public health officials, and family members. The American Academy of Pediatrics (APA) issued a policy statement aimed at increasing the role that pediatricians can play in preventing drowning in children. It can also serve as a guide to nurses. The policy statement focuses on prevention interventions aimed at both primary and secondary levels of prevention. The scope is broad and includes supervising, learning to swim

(both caretakers and children), and making changes to the environment such as fences and drain covers.[29] The CDC breaks down primary prevention into the following categories: barriers, supervision, learning to swim, life jacket use, and alcohol use.[27] From a secondary prevention viewpoint, both the APA and CDC recommend learning cardiopulmonary resuscitation (CPR). The CDC also includes recommendations to help prevent drowning in natural bodies of water. There is a clear consensus on the actions that can be taken to prevent drowning and in the event of a drowning, to provide early and effective treatment to prevent mortality (Box 12-5).

BOX 12–5	**Primary Prevention for Drowning in the United States**

- Pool fencing on all four sides at a 4-foot height would reduce drowning by 83%.
- Clear the pool and the deck of the pool so children are not tempted to return to the pool area.
- Provide one-on-one supervision for small children whenever they are in or near water including bathtubs. With preschool children, the adult should be close enough to touch them and not engage in any other activity.
- Be aware of the weather in natural bodies of water. Be knowledgeable about riptides.
- A child should always swim with a buddy.
- Children should swim under the supervision of a lifeguard.
- All children need to learn to swim and receive water safety instructions. Participation in formal swimming lessons can reduce the risk of drowning by 88% among children aged 1 to 4 years.
- Learn CPR. CPR performed by bystanders has been shown to improve outcomes in drowning victims. The more quickly intervention occurs, the more likely will be the chance of improved outcomes.
- Do not use alcohol while boating, during other water recreation, or when supervising children in or near the water.
- Provide continuous supervision of small children if there is a pool on the property. Most young children who drowned in pools were last seen in the home, had been out of sight less than 5 minutes, and were in the care of one or both parents at the time.
- Wear a life jacket when boating (in boating accidents, 90% of drowning victims were not wearing life jackets).
- The most common accidental death of people with seizure disorders is accidental death by drowning (in the bathtub; safer to use a shower).
- Do not use personal flotation devices, as they are not designed to keep people safe.

Sources: See references 26–30.

Epidemiology of Unintentional Injury: Falls in Children

The two populations at greatest risk for fall-related injuries are children and older adults. Falls in older adults are covered in Chapter 20; here we discuss falls in children. Falls are the seventh leading cause of unintentional injury deaths in children less than 19 years of age,[12] and the leading cause of injury for children aged 14 years and younger.[30] Each year there are 2.3 million nonfatal falls in children with almost half occurring in children under the age of 5.[30] The mortality rate has remained steady at 0.2 per 100,000 among persons aged 0 to 19 years.[12]

Risk Factors for Falls in Children

The majority of falls in children occur on the playground, from windows, from beds or other furniture, or with baby walkers/riders that allow an infant to independently move from place to place, including ride-on toys and circular walkers.[30,31] Age, socioeconomic status, and gender play roles as well. The population at greatest risk is made up of those under the age of 11. Males are more likely to be victims of a fall.[30] The type of fall changes based on the age and stage of development. Fall risk increases once an infant becomes mobile, and in early infancy is most apt to involve a fall from furniture or on stairs. Preschool and school-age children are at risk for playground-related falls. As children enter middle school and engage in athletics, sports-related falls predominate. Window-related falls are perhaps the most dramatic, as underscored in Eric Clapton's song "Tears in Heaven." In 1991, his 4-year-old son Conor fell from a 53rd floor apartment window in New York City. Window falls occur most often in urban, low-income, and multidwelling settings.

Prevention of Falls in Children

Prevention efforts begin with home safety interventions. Parents are encouraged to put in place stair and window guards to prevent falls and, as with drowning prevention, maintaining supervision of children in the home and on the playground. Product regulation has also played a role in increasing the safety of baby walkers and playground equipment. The U.S. Consumer Product Safety Commission has a playground equipment safety guideline publication that clearly outlines how to prevent playground-related injury.[32] Both window guards and baby walkers must meet product safety requirements.

■ EVIDENCE-BASED PRACTICE
Use of Window Guards

Practice Statement: Window guards should be placed on all windows in multidwelling buildings.
Targeted Outcome: Reduction in incidence of window-related falls in children
Evidence to Support: The majority of the evidence is linked to surveillance data tracking the incidence of window-related falls in children before and afer the enactment of window guard laws. In New York City, the incidence dropped 35% in the 2 years following the enactment of the requirement for window guards.
Recommended Approaches: Legislative approaches that require landlords and owners of multidwelling buildings to install window guards, access to window guards for those who may not be able to purchase them, and provision of public information on prevention of the window-related falls in children (Box 12-6).
Sources: See references 33 and 34.

BOX 12–6 New York City Window Guard Program

In 1976, the New York City Board of Health enacted legislation known as *Health Code Section 131.15*, the window guard law. It requires owners of multiple dwellings (buildings of three or more apartments) to provide and properly install approved window guards on all windows, including first floor bathroom and windows leading onto a balcony or terrace in an apartment where a child (or children) 10 years of age or younger reside and in each hallway window, if any, in such buildings.

The exceptions to this law are:
• Windows that open onto fire escapes
• A window on the first floor that is a required secondary exit in a building in which there are fire escapes on the second floor and up

If tenants or occupants want window guards for any reason, even if there are no resident children in the covered age category, they should request them in writing and they may not be refused. Examples:
• Grandparents who have visiting children
• Parents who share intermittent custody
• Occupants who provide childcare

If required or requested window guards have not been installed or if they appear to be insecure or improperly installed, or if there is more than 4.5 inches of open, unguarded space in the window opening, a complaint should be made immediately to 311.

For more information on Window Guards, call 311.

Source: See reference 34.

Epidemiology of Unintentional Injury: Poisonings

According to the CDC, in the United States, 31,758 died from unintentional poisoning.[35] Unintentional poisoning is responsible for the deaths of 87 people and 2,277 ED visits each day, and accounts for 7% of all mortality in children.[35,36] In 2010, unintentional poisoning caused about 831,295 ED visits and 25% of these resulted in hospitalization or transfer to another facility.[35,37] **Poisoning,** defined as the ingestion, inhalation, injection, or absorption of a harmful substance into the body, is a significant problem, costing our country $33.4 billion in medical and productivity costs each year.[38] A means of monitoring poisonings is the National Poison Data System, an electronic surveillance system documenting all calls made to poison centers across the United States. The system was initiated in 1985 and receives more than 50 million calls per year, with 80% of them related to children.[39]

Risk Factors for Unintentional Poisonings

As noted above, there are differences in unintentional poisoning mortality rates based on demographic characteristics such as age, gender, and ethnicity. Men are twice as likely to die as women and the highest mortality is for people aged 45 to 49 years old. Rates also seem to vary based on ethnic group. American Indians/Alaska Natives have the highest death rates, followed by whites and then African Americans.[35]

Although poisonings can be intentional or unintentional, most poisonings in the United States (76%) are unintentional and caused by the excessive use of drugs or chemicals for nonmedical purposes. Those aged 25 to 64 years are most at risk, and in 2009 poisonings actually caused more deaths for this age group than did MVCs.[35] This is especially apparent among youths aged 19 to 25, a group in which there has been an increase in poisoning deaths, some of which is attributable to the increase in prescription drug misuse (see Chapter 11).[40] The class of drugs known as prescription painkillers (methadone, hydrocodone, and oxycodone) are the drugs most commonly involved in an overdose, followed by cocaine and heroin (see Chapter 11). From 2000 to 2009, the poisoning death rate among teens aged 15 to 19 doubled (1.7 to 3.3/100,000) and is also associated with an increase in prescription drug overdose.[40,41]

An area of concern is the rate of unintentional poisoning in children. Children 5 years of age and younger are more likely to be taken to the ED for unintentional poisonings than are older children, and male children are more likely to experience unintentional poisoning than are female children.[41] For the most part, the unintentional poisoning in children is related to ingestion of household products or medicines, with household products accounting for 60% of all childhood poisoning.[41] Poison-related death and injury in children account for almost $22 billion in costs annually.[38]

A major issue related to children and poisoning is the home environment. Most childhood poisonings occur in the home.[42] Children who live in older homes are at greater risk for lead poisoning as a result of the presence of lead-based paint, or carbon monoxide poisoning from older heating systems. The other issue is ingestion of poisonous substances found in the home. In a study of children aged 5 years and younger, researchers examined pediatric medication poisonings from 2001 to 2008 for children who were evaluated in a health-care facility. They found that the greatest morbidity was related to self-ingestion of prescription products, especially opioids, sedative-hypnotics, and cardiovascular agents.[43] Other risk factors associated with poisoning in children are socioeconomic status and lower education level of the mother.[41] Poisoning in children is also a global issue. In some countries that rely on kerosene and petrol for cooking fires and heat, these chemicals are often stored in old soda bottles or juice containers, increasing the risk that children will ingest these products.

Prevention of Unintentional Poisoning

With the predominant problem of overdose related to prescription medications, the most obvious approach to prevention is a focus on proper use and labeling of medications, not sharing medications, proper storage of medications, and proper disposal of drugs. In order to raise awareness of child injury in particular, the National Action Plan for Child Injury Prevention was recently developed by the CDC and more than 60 stakeholders. It has six action steps that have relevance to preventing unintentional injury in children and adolescents (Table 12-1).[42]

Epidemiology of Self-Directed Violence: Suicide

Self-directed violence (SDV), both fatal and nonfatal, is a serious public health issue and includes behavior that results in injury or the potential of injury. It includes both **suicide** and nonsuicidal acts.[44] In an effort to improve surveillance, the National Center for Injury Prevention and Control published definitions related to SDV (Box 12-7).[44]

TABLE 12–1	Six Goals and Select Strategies of National Action Plan for Child Injury Prevention (NAP)
Goal	Select Strategies
Data and surveillance	Improve data systems such as prescription drug–monitoring programs.
	Identify inappropriate prescribing of controlled prescription drugs.
Research	Conduct research on the fate of prescription drugs dispensed to adolescents.
	Estimate the impact of current medication disposal programs on the prevalence of unused drugs of abuse in the home that teens could divert to nonmedical use.
Communication	Encourage widespread use of public information campaigns such as the CDC's partnership with the Up and Away initiative. (This educational program reminds families of the importance of safe medication storage.)
Education and training	Educate health-care providers on the appropriate prescribing of controlled prescription drugs to minors to include proper dosages, quantities, and conditions for which these drugs' benefits outweigh their risks.
	Educate health-care providers on how to identify and address drug misuse and abuse in adolescents.
Health systems and health care	Create guidelines for prescribing controlled prescription drugs to children that can be implemented by health-care systems and insurers.
	Leverage insurer and pharmacy benefit manager mechanisms to reduce the amount of unused medications available for diversion, abuse, and overdose.
Policy	Improve access of law enforcement agencies to data from state prescription drug–monitoring programs to help identify "pill mills," which flood communities that are prone to abuse with prescription drugs.
	Better enforce Food and Drug Administration regulations prohibiting the marketing to providers of off-label uses of psychotherapeutic drugs, e.g., sleep aids, in children.

Source: See reference 42.

BOX 12–7	Definitions of Self-Directed Violence

Self-Directed Violence: Behavior that is self-directed and deliberately results in injury or the potential for injury to oneself. This does not include behaviors such as parachuting, gambling, substance abuse, tobacco use, or other risk-taking activities, such as excessive speeding in motor vehicles. These are complex behaviors, some of which are risk factors for SDV but are defined as behavior that while likely to be life threatening is not recognized by the individual as behavior intended to destroy or injure the self. (Farberow, N.L. [Ed.]. [1980]. *The many faces of suicide.* New York, NY: McGraw-Hill.) These behaviors may have a high probability of injury or death as an outcome but the injury or death is usually considered unintentional. (Hanzlick, R., Hunsaker, J.C., & Davis, G.J. [n.d.]. *Guide for manner of death classification.* National Association of Medical Examiners. Retrieved from http://www.charlydmiller.com/LIB03/2002NAMEmannerofdeath.pdf.)

Nonsuicidal Self-Directed Violence: Behavior that is self-directed and deliberately results in injury or potential for injury to oneself. There is no evidence, whether implicit or explicit, of suicidal intent.

Suicidal Self-Directed Violence: Behavior that is self-directed and deliberately results in injury or the potential for injury to oneself. There is evidence, whether implicit or explicit, of suicidal intent.

Undetermined Self-Directed Violence: Behavior that is self-directed and deliberately results in injury or the potential for injury to oneself. Suicidal intent is unclear based on the available evidence.

Suicide Attempt: A nonfatal self-directed potentially injurious behavior with any intent to die as a result of the behavior. A suicide attempt may or may not result in injury.

Interrupted Self-Directed Violence—by Other or by Self:

By other—A person takes steps to injure self but is stopped by another person prior to fatal injury. The interruption can occur at any point during the act, such as after the initial thought or after onset of behavior.

By self (in other documents may be termed "aborted" suicidal behavior)—A person takes steps to injure self but is stopped by self prior to fatal injury.

Source: See reference 44.

There is a growing concern about the fact that annually there are more than 1.5 million suicides worldwide.[45] In the United States, there were 38,364 suicide deaths in 2010, with suicide ranking as the tenth leading cause of death.[46] It is the fourth leading cause of death for adults aged 18 to 65, with a significant increase in suicide rates from 1999 to 2010 for those aged 35 to 64 years.[47,48] Although suicide has typically been seen in older adults, the most recent data show that suicide rates are highest among persons aged 40 to 54 years in the United States for non-Hispanic whites, a trend that has been seen since 2006. In addition, rates overall are higher among males than females, and among American Indians/Alaska Natives and non-Hispanic whites compared with non-Hispanic blacks. Asian/Pacific Islanders have the highest rate for suicide among those 65 years and older.[49]

There are many more suicide attempts than actual suicides. It is estimated that there are 11 attempted suicides for every suicide death and that women and young people are more likely to attempt suicide than are men and older adults.[50] It is critical to realize that suicide attempts are expressions of distress, not just attention-seeking behavior, warranting immediate mental health treatment.[48]

Risk Factors for Suicide

Although in the United States suicide has been viewed as a moral problem or a sign of personal weakness by some, in reality it often reflects an underlying mental health disorder (see Chapter 10), and therefore should be treated as a part of the larger public health issue of mental health.[51] Based on the finding of research studies, greater than 90% of persons who die by suicide are suffering with a diagnosable mental health disorder at the time of death, most often with depression and less often with bipolar disorder, anxiety, and/or alcohol or substance abuse disorders. Yet only 33.8% were being treated for a mental health disorder.[52] Mood disorders, previous suicide attempts, experience of a crisis in the preceding 2 weeks, intimate partner problems (family violence), and physical health problems are significant risk factors for suicide.[44] Other risk factors include age, sex, marital status, family history of mental illness or substance abuse, incarceration, or exposure to suicidal behaviors of others.[53,54] The presence of co-occurring substance abuse disorders is also significant, with alcohol use associated in one-third of suicides.[44] The availability of a lethal method such as firearms is another important factor, because the three most common methods of suicide are firearms, suffocation, and poisonings.[54]

Prevention of Suicide

A recent systematic review of studies published between 1966 and 2005 examined interventions in several domains: education and awareness of the general public and for professionals, the use of screening tools, treatment of psychiatric disorders, restricting access to the means of committing suicide, and the role of the media. The two methods that were effective at preventing suicide were the education of physicians and restricting the access to lethal means.[51] The education of the primary care provider is important, because some studies have found that education improves detection and increased treatment of depression. This is significant because most individuals who commit suicide have had contact with a provider within a month of death.[53] Another important strategy is the education of gatekeepers in the community, including clergy; first responders; pharmacists; caregivers; personnel staff; and those employed in school, prisons, and other institutions.[51]

Some work has been done to develop interventions that are specific to ethnic populations. It is critical to design programs that are culturally appropriate because it is recognized that culturally sensitive interventions can improve access to services.[54, 55] For example, American Indians/Alaska Natives are twice as likely to experience suicide in comparison with other groups.[56] The Indian Health Service and the Substance Abuse and Mental Health Services Administration have established a Web site that provides AI/AN tribes with the information to adapt evidence-based mainstream programs to their own cultural context.[57] This is an excellent example of developing public health interventions that take into account the cultural context of the population.

Epidemiology of Family Violence

As mentioned earlier, family violence includes violence between intimate partners, maltreatment of children, and elder abuse. The context of the violence is the family and occurs between individuals.[6] The victims and the perpetrators have an established family-based relationship. Because violence against the older adult is covered in Chapter 20, the focus of this section is on child maltreatment and intimate partner violence.

Child Maltreatment

Child maltreatment is defined by the federal Keeping Children and Families Safe Act of 2003 P.L. 108-36 as "any recent act or failure to act on the part of a parent or caretaker which results in death, serious physical or emotional harm, sexual abuse or exploitation" or "an act or failure to act which presents imminent risk or serious harm."[58]

Child maltreatment includes child physical abuse, child emotional abuse, child neglect, and child sexual abuse. In 2011, there were more than 681,000 children who experienced child neglect or some form of child abuse in the United States. The highest rate of victimization occurs for children from birth to age 1. The majority of children experienced neglect (79%), then physical abuse (18%), sexual abuse (9%), and other abuse (10%)[59] Of these, 1,570 died due to the abuse.[59]

Child neglect is the most prevalent form of child maltreatment and includes both physical neglect and emotional neglect. **Physical neglect** includes the withholding of food, shelter, clothing, and/or medical or dental care, whereas **emotional neglect** involves the omission of caring, nurturing, and acceptance. **Emotional abuse** is defined as extreme debasement of feelings whereas **physical abuse** is nonaccidental physical harm such as bruising, bites, thermal burns, or cigarette burns, severe fractures, and even death.[59-61] **Sexual abuse** defined by the federal Child Abuse Prevention and Treatment Act,[42] as amended by the Keeping Children and Families Safe Act of 2003 is "the employment, use, persuasion, inducement, enticement, or coercion of any child to engage in, or assist any other person to engage in, any sexually explicit conduct or simulation of such conduct for the purpose of producing a visual depiction of such conduct; or the rape, and in cases of caretaker or interfamilial relationships, statutory rape, molestation, prostitution, or other form of sexual exploitation of children, or incest with children."[58]

The National Child Abuse and Neglect Data System is the surveillance system that monitors trends of child maltreatment by collecting Child Protective Service reports from 49 states, Puerto Rico, and the District of Columbia.[61] A recent analysis of ethnic differences using these data (2011) demonstrated that African Americans have the highest rate of victimization at 14.3 per 1,000 children in the same ethnic population followed by American Indians (11.4) and multiple race (10.1).[62] These data are dependent on the actual reporting of cases.

The consequences of childhood maltreatment are long lasting, not only affecting the initial development of the child but also influencing adult health. A recent meta-analysis of 16 epidemiological studies found that childhood maltreatment is associated with clinically relevant measures of depression.[64] Emotional abuse, for example, often results in feelings of inadequacy and feeling uncared for and worthless.[59] Children experiencing child maltreatment are at increased risk of poor physical health into adulthood, and for those experiencing child sexual abuse there is a risk of medical, psychological, behavioral, and sexual disorders.[63,64] Based on the estimated lifetime cost per person, the total economic burden of fatal and nonfatal child maltreatment in the United States is $124 billion.[65]

Risk Factors for Child Maltreatment

Risk factors for childhood maltreatment focus on problematic family contexts as well as community-level factors.[60, 64,] Maternal socioeconomic factors play a role, for example, the level of mother's education and poverty, and parental behavioral issues such as mental health disorders or substance use place a child at higher risk.[60] For some, a parent's history of child abuse in the family of origin is significant, whereas for other families current substance abuse and/or mental health issues including depression in the family are predictors of child maltreatment. Other risk factors include parents' lack of understanding of children's needs, child development, and parenting skills, or parental thoughts and emotions that tend to support or justify maltreatment behaviors.[643,66] The presence of a nonbiological, transient caregiver in the home is another risk factor for sexual abuse in particular (e.g., mother's male partner).[60] In a nationally representative sample of 2,017 children aged 2 to 9 years, alcohol or drug problems and residential instability were related to child neglect.[60] Community-level risk factors include low socioeconomic status and living in an impoverished community.[64] A history of childhood maltreatment can lead to lifelong health issues in adults.[67,68]

Prevention of Child Maltreatment

The focus of childhood maltreatment prevention programs is often on parental education, support, and /or public awareness campaigns.[69] Tertiary prevention is also important to prevent recurrence of abuse or to decrease impairment. One study, for example, found a dose-response relationship between the number of chronic reports of maltreatment over the course of childhood and negative outcomes (suicide attempts, mental health treatment, substance abuse, sexually transmitted infections [STIs]) into adolescence, whereas another found that chronicity of maltreatment is related to the initiation of early substance use in adolescence.[70, 71]

Home visitation in particular has been implemented for the prevention of child maltreatment. Focusing on selective protective factors is the focus of many of these programs. Protective factors for child maltreatment include nurturing parenting skills; promoting stable family relationships; promoting household rules and child monitoring; and assisting with parental employment, adequate housing, or access to health care and social services.[72] Home visitation programs include the Nurse Family Partnership Model, which has undergone rigorous evaluations and shows promise for the prevention of child maltreatment.[73] Other programs include the Triple P program, Sure Start, Family Connections, and Together for Kids.[74-78] The actual translation of evidence-based practice into real practice settings is a challenge for a number of reasons, including training, resources, and specificity to the populations. A tailored or tiered-level approach can be used to include basic services such as employment services or outreach to more intense curriculum-based strategies.[79]

Epidemiology of Intimate Partner Violence

Intimate partner violence is violence that occurs between two people in an intimate relationship. It includes physical violence, sexual violence, and psychological/emotional violence as well as threats of physical/sexual violence.[80] **Physical violence** is the intentional use of physical force with the potential for causing death, disability, injury, or harm. Physical violence includes, but is not limited to, scratching; pushing; shoving; throwing; grabbing; biting; choking; shaking; slapping; punching; burning; use of a weapon; and use of restraints or one's body, size, or strength against another person. **Sexual violence** is divided into three categories: (1) use of physical force to compel a person to engage in a sexual act against his or her will, whether or not the act is completed; (2) attempted or completed sexual act involving a person who is unable to understand the nature or condition of the act, to decline participation, or to communicate unwillingness to engage in the sexual act (e.g., because of illness, disability, or the influence of alcohol or other drugs, or because of intimidation or pressure); and (3) abusive sexual contact. **Threat of physical or sexual violence** is the use of words, gestures, or weapons to communicate the intent to cause death, disability, injury, or physical harm. **Psychological/emotional violence** involves trauma to the victim caused by acts, threats of acts, or coercive tactics. Psychological/emotional abuse can include, but is not limited to, humiliating the victim, controlling what the victim can and cannot do, withholding information from the victim, deliberately doing something to make the victim feel diminished or embarrassed, isolating the victim from friends and family, and denying the victim access to money or other basic resources.[80]

About 1 in 4 American women experiences some type of abuse in her lifetime.[81] Surveillance of intimate partner violence occurs through various databases (Box 12-8).[82] This abuse can start early in dating relationships. Among sexually experienced adolescent girls, for example, 1 in 5 girls reported being physically hurt by a date in the previous year.[83] In another study in Chicago, the prevalence of physical victimization was reported by approximately one-third of tenth- and eleventh-grade, inner-city female adolescents. In this same study, Hispanic adolescents were more likely to report psychological violence victimization, whereas African American adolescents reported greater physical violence perpetration.[84]

Although intimate partner violence victimization is usually focused on heterosexual females, males also experience some form of lifetime intimate partner violence, at a ratio of 1 in 7 men.[85-87] Lesbian, gay, bisexual, and transgender persons (LGBT) also experience abuse.[88] A survey in Massachusetts found that the lifetime physical abuse rate among transgender respondents was 34.6%, and for gay or lesbian individuals it was 14%.[89]

Intimate partner violence has significant negative effects on health.[82] A recent study examined medical records and self-reports of past year experiences with intimate partner violence. Among 3,568 women randomly sampled from a U.S. health insurance plan, women who had experienced violence in the past year had significantly higher relative risks for psychosocial/mental diagnoses, musculoskeletal disorders, female reproductive disorders; a threefold increased risk of being diagnosed with an STI (3.15); a twofold increased risk of lacerations (2.17); and increased risks of acute respiratory tract infections, gastroesophageal reflux disease, chest pain, abdominal pain, urinary tract infections, headaches, and contusions/abrasions.[90] Abused women are also more likely to use medical services including outpatient primary care, EDs, and mental and substance abuse services.[91]

BOX 12–8	**Resources for Information on Intimate Partner Violence**

Behavioral Risk Factor Surveillance System (BRFSS)
National Violence Against Women Survey
National Violent Death Reporting System
The National Survey of Family Growth
Pregnancy Risk Assessment Monitoring System
CDC's Youth Risk Behavior Surveillance System
Federal Bureau of Investigation (FBI)
National Crime Victimization Survey

Source: See reference 82.

The negative effects of intimate partner violence are more widespread than affecting just the individual. It also affects the family, community, and society. Within the family, children exposed to the violence are at increased risk of emotional, physical, and sexual abuse as well as other emotional and behavioral problems.[92,93] At the community level, homicide, which is unfortunately not uncommon, is the most extreme negative outcome. In a national surveillance system tracking violent deaths in 16 states, there were 612 intimate partner deaths in 2007, with the majority being females.[94] Pregnancy is a particular time when women are at more risk of being killed. A study of the analysis of pregnancy-associated homicides between 1993 and 2008 in Maryland examined police and medical examiner reports, linked birth and death certificates, and evaluated news publications. Close to two-thirds of the 110 homicides were committed by an intimate partner.[95] At the societal level, the acceptance of intimate partner violence can become a part of the culture and social norms. A recent qualitative study in Tanzania, for example, found that a prevailing norm was the acceptance of women's subordination, which was used to justify male violence toward women.[96]

Risk Factors for Intimate Partner Violence

Risk for intimate partner violence occurs at many levels. At the individual level, risk factors include female gender, young age, being unmarried, being uninsured or on medical assistance, low income, and a history of child maltreatment.[91] In addition, at-risk alcohol use by either the woman, man, or both is associated with intimate partner violence perpetration.[97] Other risk factors include low self-esteem, mental health problems, unemployment, or desire for power and control in relationships.[98] At the family level, exposure as an adolescent to severe intimate partner violence between caregivers increases the risk for relationship violence in early adulthood.[99] At the community level, residence in an area characterized by poverty and social disadvantage as well as by an increased density of alcohol outlets is an example of a factor associated with intimate partner violence–related ED visits.[100]

Prevention of Intimate Partner Violence

The CDC's prevention work targeted toward intimate partner violence is focused on four categories: (1) tracking the problem, (2) developing and evaluating prevention strategies, (3) supporting and enhancing prevention programs, and (4) providing prevention resources. According to the CDC, reducing risk requires promoting change at all the levels of social ecology (individual, relationship,

community, and society).[101] Safe Dates is an example of an effective prevention program focused on adolescents. It is a 10-session curriculum targeted toward eighth and ninth graders. The theoretical basis of the curriculum is that of changing norms and addressing conflict management as a means of preventing violence.[102,103]

Screening and referral for treatment are two key steps for prevention of intimate partner violence at the secondary prevention level and have been tested over time.[104–106] An example of a screening with high sensitivity for pregnant women is the Abuse Assessment Screen.[106] For nonpregnant women, routine screening is also recommended by many major medical organizations.[107–110] Disclosure of intimate partner violence requires action by the provider, further assessment, appropriate referrals, and discussion of a safety plan.[108] To help practitioners, the Massachusetts Medical Society developed a guide with the acronym RADAR as its title (Box 12-9). The purpose is to provide easy steps for conducting screening with all women.[112] Though a number of screening instruments have been developed, none have been tested against intimate partner violence outcomes, and further research is needed to determine best practices in this area.[110–112]

Although these clinical recommendations guide providers, there is actually a dearth of studies examining evidence-based approaches to intimate partner violence, both for the victim and for interventions focused on perpetrators.[104,110,113] The majority of tested interventions focus on changing practices of healthcare providers, including assessment protocol, which requires changing practice at the organization and systems levels.[114,115] Intimate partner violence is a global health priority. To help move prevention efforts forward, the WHO released a new tool, *Preventing Intimate Partner and Sexual Violence Against Women: Taking Action and Generating Evidence,* with the goal of engaging policy makers and program planners in establishing evidence-based approaches to primary and secondary prevention.[116]

BOX 12–9 **Clinician's Guide to Intimate Partner Violence Screening and Referral (RADAR)**

R: Perform routine screening
A: Ask direct questions
D: Document findings
A: Assess patient (and children) safety
R: Review patient options and provide referrals

Source: See reference 112.

Epidemiology of Community Violence

Community violence is defined as an event that includes crime, weapons use, and violence or potential violence and is perpetrated in a local neighborhood.[117] The violence that receives the most media attention at the community level is homicide, a significant crime indicator affecting public health. In 2007, homicide was the second leading cause of death for 10- to 24-year-olds.[118] Although the trends in crime overall are on a decline, in 2010 there were 12,996 murder victims in the United States, of which most were male (77%) and most involved the use of a firearm.[119] In cases for which the relationships of murder victims and offenders were known, more than half of the victims (53%) were killed by someone they knew (acquaintance, neighbor, friend, boyfriend), whereas 24.8% were slain by family members. The actual percentage of murders shows that most victims were African American (53.1%), whereas 44.6% were white.[119] Other forms of violence within a community include assault, which is the most prevalent form of violent crimes (62.5%), followed by robbery (29.5%) and forcible rape (6.8%).[120]

The impact of violence on a community is widespread. Exposure to the constant stress of living within an unsafe community takes its toll on all of its citizens. It can lead to a sense of isolation for older adults who limit their activity outside their home because of violence. It can lead to a lack of physical activity in children and families because parents are concerned about the safety of their children. It can lead to psychiatric sequelae because of the feelings of fear and stress.

Community violence can also occur in towns and neighborhoods where violence is not the norm, such as the killing of 20 children and 6 adults at Sandy Hook Elementary School in Newtown, Connecticut. This event sent a shock wave through the nation and brought calls for stricter gun control laws. Another example of seemingly random violence that impacts a community was the Aurora, Colorado, movie theater massacre that resulted in the death of 12 and the injury of 70 others. Both of these events highlighted the relationship between mental illness and violence, with both perpetrators having a long-standing history of mental illness. In other cases, such as the Boston Marathon bombing, the violence that occurred was linked to terrorism rather than mental illness. All three events brought their communities together to help the victims as well as work to implement polices to help reduce the risk of further violence.

Thus, violence in a community can occur in different ways. For some, it is an unexpected event that takes a community unaware, and in others, the violence is part of everyday life. In the case of war, one expects to be exposed to death, trauma, and stress. Unfortunately, certain neighborhoods in our cities have often been compared to war zones where it is not uncommon to be exposed to severe violence. An example of how exposure to violence in the community can affect a person is explained here through Carl's experience (hypothetical person). He is a 25-year-old homeless unemployed African American male who has been living on the streets of Baltimore for the past 7 years. He has a difficult family history marked by physical abuse, a mother who was incarcerated both for assault and battery of a male partner and for dealing drugs. Carl has a history of abusing alcohol beginning at age 10 and has been injecting heroin for the past 2 years, although he has been clean for the past 3 months. Violence and drug use are often associated and Carl's history reveals a number of incarcerations related to violence. Carl spent the past month in jail because of assault and was released only 5 days ago. Without a home, he tends to wander to shelters but occasionally goes to boarded-up homes, a common sight in Baltimore, and slips through the broken edges of the boards to find a place to sleep. This night was not unlike any other except that he was shocked to find a dead body when he entered the boarded-up home.

Cases like this are not uncommon. In fact, a recent epidemiological study assessing the prevalence of exposure to dead bodies among drug users in Baltimore found that in a sample of 951 respondents enrolled in a human immunodeficiency virus (HIV) prevention project, 17% reported that they had found a dead body in their lifetime. These deaths were related to violence (37%), natural causes (22.2%), drug overdose (21.6%), accidental death (3.1%), and suicide (2.5%).[121]

Although finding a dead body seems like an extreme example, the fact is that exposure to some form of violence is common, especially in our cities. A recent study of 3,614 adolescents from a U.S. national household probability sample found that 38% witnessed community violence.[122] This exposure to community violence (i.e., seeing someone be shot; someone being stabbed, molested, raped, mugged, threatened with a knife, gun or weapon; or someone being beaten up or hurt) is often associated with psychiatric sequelae including post-traumatic stress disorder (PTSD).[117,123,124] **Post-traumatic stress disorder (PTSD)** is a type of anxiety disorder in children and adults who witness horrific events within their community. PTSD can develop in response to a variety of traumatic events such as witnessing a violent act or crime, experiencing a natural or unnatural disaster, and experiencing physical or sexual abuse.[123] Other comorbid psychiatric symptoms include anxiety and major depressive episode. Substance use and behavior problems are also seen in children who are exposed to violence.[125]

Risk Factors for Community Violence

Young people perpetrate violent acts at a higher rate than any other age group. The risk factors for youth violence include low socioeconomic status, poor parental supervision, delinquent peers, and harsh parenting.[126] Individual risks associated with community violence exposure vary as a function of age (older youths are more vulnerable), being a person of color, living within a city, or living in a single-parent home.[127]

In addition to individual risk factors, certain characteristics of neighborhoods are also associated with self-reported involvement with the justice system. A recent study developed a tool to examine characteristics of the built and social environments potentially related to increasing the risk of violence, alcohol, and other drug exposure. It consists of six domains (physical layout, structures on the block, dwelling type, youth and adult activity, physical order and disorder, social order and disorder) and was used to examine 242 residential neighborhoods in Baltimore, Maryland (Table 12-2).[128] The tool was further tested by combining data from a previous study of urban substance users with the characteristics of the neighborhoods. This study found that living in a neighborhood with moderate or high levels of disorder and drinking alcohol every day or nearly every day was associated with an incarceration history.[125] Other studies have found that neighborhood deficits in social cohesion, institutional resources, collective efficacy, and informal social control are other factors associated with violence.[123]

Protective Factors for Community Violence

Promoting youth development is one strategy used to decrease youth violence within the community. This is based on the fact that social connectedness is a protective factor inversely associated with rates of crime at the community level.[130,131] Resilience is the ability to successfully adapt and function despite exposure to chronic stress and adversity.[132,127] Resilience is achieved through support from a family, school, or peer groups.[127] In addition, the importance of strengthening the community overall is another strategy that is used to promote the positive development of youths. One example of a community-level approach is the Ivanhoe Neighborhood Council Youth Project, which is located within an inner-city, predominately African American community in Kansas City, Missouri. A group of 85 residents and community partners created a vision for the neighborhood called Thriving Neighborhoods in Harmony, and developed a strategic plan focused on crime, safety, and youth development.[131]

Other strategies to prevent youth violence and promote positive youth development include the implementation of evidence-based practices in the community and mobilizing communities for these changes (Box 12-10).[134–135] Effective and promising programs include Blueprints for Violence Prevention, Substance Abuse and Mental Health Services Administration Model Program, and STRYVE (Striving to Reduce Youth Violence Everywhere), a national initiative led by the CDC to prevent youth violence, developed by the University of Boulder in Colorado in response to a series of school shootings that occurred in the 1990s.[135] (See Chapter 18 on School-Based Approaches.) The CDC is also developing a national public

TABLE 12–2	Domain and Sample Items of the Neighborhood Inventory for Environmental Typology
Domain	Sample Items
Physical layout of the block face	Length and width of the block; presence of alleys; presence of medians
Types of structures	Number and type of residential and commercial properties; number of churches
Adult activity	Number of adults on the street; adults supervising young people; adults exercising
Youth activity	Number of children on the street; young people riding bicycles; young people doing drugs
Physical disorder and order	Number of broken windows; abandoned houses; vacant lots; presence of trash; evidence of vandalism; number of potholes, number of abandoned vehicles; evidence of landscaping
Social disorder and order	Presence of homeless people; people yelling, fighting, loitering; intoxicated persons; evidence of prostitution; positive adult interaction
Violence, alcohol and other drug indicators	Shell casings; police tape/outlines; memorials on the block; number of people smoking tobacco, consuming alcohol, using or selling drugs

Source: See reference 128.

BOX 12–10 | **Centers for Disease Control and Prevention Framework for Action; Strengthen the Personal Capacity of Youth to Resist Violence**

Strengthen the Personal Capacity of Youth to Resist Violence

• **Social, emotional, and behavioral skill-building strategies** that help young people develop healthy, peaceful relationships; enhance positive connections to home, school, and community; and establish or strengthen nonviolent beliefs and attitudes
• **Youth engagement, development, and leadership strategies** that promote youth involvement in safe and structured opportunities that enable them to build their talents and interests, self-confidence, social relationships, and leadership potential
• **Human service strategies** that ensure that young people exposed to violence and trauma have opportunities to heal; and that young people with social, emotional, behavioral, mental health, and substance abuse problems receive appropriate early intervention and treatment services

Build and Support Positive Relationships Between Youth and Adults

• **Family and school-based strategies** that promote good communication skills and safe, stable, and nurturing connections between young people and their parents, other caregivers, teachers, and school personnel, which are established at birth and continued through young adulthood

• **Mentoring strategies** that provide young people with caring, supportive role models who can provide guidance and advocacy when needed and create strong bonds between young people and adults in communities

Promote Thriving, Safe, and Connected Communities

• **Economic, vocational, and educational strategies** that make available and link young people with opportunities; that ensure young people who have been or are at risk of suspension or expulsion from school are directed to alternative programs and activities; and that help young people graduate from high school
• **Community-oriented safety strategies** that protect and provide for the safety of all people in the community. Examples include crisis intervention, improved police–community relations, and violence prevention through environmental design

Create a Society That Promotes Safety and Health

• **Collaborative strategies** that engage multisector, multidisciplinary, national, state, and local entities in developing, investing in, and implementing comprehensive, coordinated youth-violence prevention strategies
• **Evidence-informed policy strategies** that address disparities in wealth, educational and occupational opportunities, and access to services

Source: See reference 134-135.

---

health strategy to prevent youth violence. This includes strengthening the personal capacity of youths to resist violence; building and supporting positive relationships between youths and adults; promoting thriving, safer, and more connected communities; and creating a safer and healthier society.[136]

Epidemiology of War: An Example of Collective Violence

War as defined in the *Stanford Encyclopedia of Philosophy* is the "actual, intentional and widespread armed conflict between political communities."[137] This excludes individuals or families fighting, gangs fighting, and other smaller community entities. Traditional war is thought of as the fighting between two political states or countries, but just as common is the fighting between two groups within a state (civil war) that are aspiring to become the political entity for the state. War is a violent way of determining who will govern. War and its violence create serious social

consequences that affect all the political communities involved.[137] These consequences can be a result of a prolonged conflict, extreme aggression, excessive mortality and morbidity, and/or high financial cost, all of which reduce resources for social needs.

In their book on *War and Public Health,* Levy and Sidel write:

War accounts for more death and disability than many major diseases combined. It destroys families, communities, and sometimes whole cultures. It directs scarce resources away from protection and promotion of health, medical care, and other human services. It destroys the infrastructure that supports health. It limits human rights and contributes to social injustice. It leads many people to think that violence is the only way to resolve conflicts—a mindset that contributes to domestic violence, street crime, and other kinds of violence. And it contributes to the destruction of the environment and overuse of nonrenewable resources. In sum, war threatens much of the fabric of our civilization (p. 3, 138).

War affects more than the combatants. In the 20th century, it is estimated that 136.5 to 148.5 million people died in war and conflict. However, many feel the largest death toll comes not from the direct conflict but from the residual effects of the war such as disease and malnutrition.[139]

Worldwide, there are still many ongoing wars including ones in Afghanistan, Iraq, Somalia, Sudan, Congo, and those in the Middle East. However, the good news is that there are now actually fewer wars than in the past. More than 40 wars (both between nations and civil wars) began in the 1990s compared with fewer than 10 in the first decade of this century. There also were fewer deaths caused directly by war-related violence from 2000 to 2010 than in any decade in the past 100 years. One contributing factor to lower mortality is that the nature of war has changed. There are no longer huge armies in battle with massive human destruction. However, more countries have access to weapons of mass destruction and the number of countries with active nuclear warheads has grown from two in the 1940s to nine by 2013.

With the use of social media, there has also been more reporting of wars and the atrocities of war. The reporting occurs almost at the moment they occur. It makes the violence seem greater, because of the immediacy with which it is being reported. There is some indication that with this increased awareness, the societal tolerance for this type of violence is lessening.[140] In addition, when traditional reporting by journalists is impeded, as occurred in the Syrian conflict, social media provided an alternative source of news for those inside and outside the country.

Even with fewer wars and numbers of deaths, the war-related effects of current conflicts are enormous. There is an obvious breakdown in public health systems with the displacement of resources to war and away from health services including prevention services, increase in disease transmission, and other changes in the social systems that had previously kept the population healthy. The results of war are many and can devastate a country (Box 12-11).[139, 141]

There are many other examples of the destructiveness of war: the use of child soldiers, resulting in severe physical and emotional abuse of the children and making it very difficult for them to reintegrate in civil society; the forced movements of refugees and displaced persons from their own homes to areas with decreased health and safety; and the increased acceptability of violence in solving problems.

Role of the Nurse in War

One of the roles of the nurse in war and the consequences of war is prevention. Starting with primary

BOX 12–11	**The Impact of War**

- Psychologically impaired individuals, both combatant and noncombatant
- Individuals chronically disabled as a result of war injuries
- Increased rape and other gender-based violence
- Brutality, ethnic cleansing, and genocide against opponent forces
- Increase in substance abuse
- Malnutrition and starvation
- Environmental degradation
- Fragmentation of communities
- Disruption in policy decisions, policy making, and policy implementation

Sources: See references 1, 5, and 6.

prevention, the nurse can support actions to prevent war. If war ensues, the nurse may try to minimize the effects of the war as part of secondary prevention. After the war is over, the nurse at the tertiary level may help to treat the victims of the war and minimize the political, economic, social, and environmental destruction. Nurses can help in surveillance and documentation of what happens during the war and report it to the appropriate agencies; advocate for the use of nonviolence and, during wars, advocate to minimize the results of war; and work with the refugees and displaced persons from the war either in the United States or in other countries to improve their health and their social reintegration into society. With additional training, nurses can provide the emergency relief that is frequently needed during and immediately at the end of the war. Nurses can also help document and understand the most appropriate interventions for refugees and displaced persons, which are frequently specific to the affected population. Using this additional information, the reintegration of individuals into the postwar social systems can be facilitated.[138]

Summary Points

- Injury is a major public issue that includes both intentional and unintentional injury, most of which is preventable.
- Risk factors associated with injury and violence are complex and include a combination of individual behaviors, environment, socioeconomic status, and culture.
- Violence can occur at the family or community level, with the most vulnerable being children, women, and the older adults.

▲ CASE STUDY
All Children Learn to Swim

Learning Outcomes

At the end of this case study, students will be able to:

- Describe the components of developing a public health injury prevention program.
- Compare the effectiveness of different approaches to prevention.
- Explain the role of stakeholders in prevention program planning.
- Discuss the benefits of incorporating cultural components into a health program.

The nurses in a large metropolitan children's hospital emergency room were concerned about the increase in drowning among African American and Hispanic children in their area. One of the nurses brought in a report about how the U.S. Consumer Product Safety Commission was launching a campaign to advocate for increased swimming education for blacks and Hispanics. One of the nurses discussed a recent incident in which four children drowned while their parents looked on because the parents also couldn't swim. The nurses wondered whether they could partner with other members of the community to address the issue the same way the Cincinnati Children's Hospital Medical Center nurses did to address use of car seats and booster seats. One of the nurses wondered what approaches they should take: Should they focus on teaching children to swim, teaching parents to swim, or improving water rescue and resuscitation skills during a drowning incident? To complete this case study, do the following:

1. Review national initiatives and, using the Institute of Medicine's prevention model (Chapters 10 and 11), choose an example of a universal, a selected, and a targeted prevention approach.
2. Critique proposed policy initiatives in relation to their utility in reducing drowning in African American and Hispanic communities.
3. Determine what stakeholders should be at the table to help design a community-level intervention.
4. Come to a conclusion on how the nurses can develop a learn-to-swim program in their community and include:
   a. A draft plan
   b. Cultural concerns
   c. Establishment of objectives that align with *HP 2020* (Injury and Violence Prevention objective #25)

REFERENCES

1. World Health Organization. (2012). *Health topics: Injury.* Retrieved from http://www.who.int/topics/injuries/en/.
2. Centers for Disease Control and Prevention. (2012). *Injury prevention and control.* Retrieved from http://www.cdc.gov/injury/overview/.
3. Centers for Disease Control and Prevention. (2012). *Injury prevention and control: Injury center.* Retrieved from http://www.cdc.gov/ncipc/about/about.htm.
4. Centers for Disease Control and Prevention. (2012). *10 Leading causes of injury death by age group highlighting unintentional injury death, United States 2009.* Retrieved from http://www.cdc.gov/Injury/wisqars/pdf/Leading_Causes_injury_Deaths_Age_GRoup_Highlighting_Unintentional_Injury%20Deaths_US_2009-a.pdf.
5. Centers for Disease Control and Prevention. (2010). *Fast Stats: Unintentional injury.* Retrieved from http://www.cdc.gov/nchs/fastats/acc-inj.htm.
6. World Health Organization. (2002). *World report on violence and health.* Geneva, Switzerland; Author.
7. Centers for Disease Control and Prevention. (2014). *Injury prevention and control: Injury center; Cost of violent deaths in the U.S., 2005.* Retrieved from http://www.cdc.gov/violenceprevention/violentdeaths/.
8. U.S. Department of Health and Human Services. (2014). *Healthy People 2020: Health topics and objectives; injury and violence prevention. Data from National Vital Statistics System–Mortality (NVSS–M), CDC, NCHS.* Retrieved from http://www.healthypeople.gov/2020/topicsobjectives2020/overview.aspx?topicid=24.
9. Centers for Disease Control and Prevention. (2011). *National Violent Death Reporting System.* Retrieved from http://www.cdc.gov/ViolencePrevention/NVDRS/.
10. Haddon, W., Jr. (1999). The changing approach to the epidemiology, prevention, and amelioration of trauma: The transition to approaches etiologically rather than descriptively based. *Injury Prevention, 5*(3), 161-162.
11. World Health Organization. (2013). *Global Plan for the Decade of Action for Road Safety 2011–2020.* Retrieved from http://www.who.int/roadsafety/decade_of_action/plan/en/index.html.
12. Centers for Disease Control and Prevention. (2012). Vital signs: Unintentional injury deaths among persons aged 0–19 years—United States, 2000–2009. *Morbidity and Mortality Weekly Report, 61*(15), 270-276.
13. Rogers, S.C., Bentley, G.C., Campbell, B., Borrup, K., Saleheed, H., Wang, Z., & Lapidus, G. (2011). Impact of Connecticut's graduated driver licensing system on teenage motor vehicle crash rates. *The Journal of Trauma, Injury, Infection and Critical Care, 71*(5), S527-S530.
14. Centers for Disease Control and Prevention. (2012). *Winnable battles: Motor vehicle injuries.* Retrieved from http://www.cdc.gov/WinnableBattles/MotorVehicleInjury/.

15. National Safety Council. (2010). *Estimating the cost of unintentional injuries.* Retrieved from http://www.nsc.org/news_resources/injury_and_death_statistics/Pages/EstimatingtheCostsofUnintentionalInjuries.aspx.

16. Romano, E.O., Peck, R.C., & Voas, R.B. (2012). Traffic environment and demographic factors affecting impaired driving and crashes. *Journal of Safety Research, 43,* 75-82. doi:10.1016/j.jsr.2011.12.001.

17. Elvik, R. (2012). Speed limits, enforcement, and health consequence. *Annual Review Public Health, 33,* 225-238.

18. Centers for Disease Control and Prevention. (2011). *Motor vehicle safety.* Retrieved from http://www.cdc.gov/motorvehiclesafety/.

19. McKibben, J.B., Ekselius, L., Girasek, D.C., Gould, N.F., Holzer, C., Rosenberg, M., et al. (2009). Epidemiology of burn injuries II: Psychiatric and behavioral perspectives. *International Review of Psychiatry, 21*(6), 512-521.

20. Peck, M. (2010). *Epidemiology of burn injuries globally.* Retrieved from http://www.uptodate.com/contents/epidemiology-of-burn-injuries-globally.

21. American Burn Association. (2011). *American Burn Association National Burn Repository.* Retrieved from http://www.ameriburn.org/resources_factsheet.php.

22. Atiyeh, B.S., Costagliola, M., & Hayek, S.N. (2009). Burn prevention mechanisms and outcomes: Pitfalls, failures and successes. *Burns, 35,* 181-193. doi:10.1016/j.burns.2008.06.002.

23. Mayo Clinic. (2012). *Infant and toddler health: Burn safety: Protect your child from burns.* Retrieved from http://www.mayoclinic.com/health/child-safety/CC00044/NSECTIONGROUP=2.

24. Centers for Disease Control and Prevention. (2010). *Fireworks-related injury.* Retrieved from http://www.cdc.gov/homeandrecreationalsafety/fireworks/index.html.

25. National Safety Council. (2010). *Estimating the cost of unintentional injuries.* Retrieved from http://www.nsc.org/news_resources/injury_and_death_statistics/Pages/EstimatingtheCostsofUnintentionalInjuries.aspx.

26. Hyder, A., Borse, B., Blum, L., Khan, R., El Arifeen, S., & Baqui, A. (2008). Childhood drowning in low- and middle-income countries: Urgent need for intervention trials. *Journal of Paediatrics and Child Health, 44,* 221-228. doi:10.1111/j.1440-1754.2007.01273.x.

27. Centers for Disease Control and Prevention. (2014). *Injury prevention and control: Home and recreational safety. Unintentional drowning: Fact sheet.* Retrieved from http://www.cdc.gov/HomeandRecreationalSafety/Water-Safety/waterinjuries-factsheet.html.

28. USA Swimming. (2010). *Make a splash.* Retrieved from http://www.usaswimming.org/DesktopDefault.aspx?TabId=1699.

29. Committee on Injury, Violence and Poison Prevention, America Academy of Pediatrics. (2010). Policy statement: Prevention of drowning. *Pediatrics, 126.* Retrieved from http://pediatrics.aappublications.org/content/early/2010/05/24/peds.2010-1264.full.pdf+html. doi:10.1542/peds.2010-1264.

30. Wang, D., Zhao, W., Wheeler, K., Yang, G., & Xiang, H. (2012). Unintentional fall injuries among U.S. children: A study based on the National ED sample. *International Journal of Injury Control and Safety Promotion.* doi:10.1080/17457300.2012.656316.

31. Safe Kids USA. (2011). *Safety from falls.* Retrieved from http://www.safekids.org/assets/docs/ourwork/research/2011-falls.pdf.

32. The U.S. Consumer Product Safety Commission. (2010). *Public playground safety handbook.* Retrieved from http://www.cpsc.gov/cpscpub/pubs/325.pdf.

33. McClure, R., Nixon, J., Spinks, A., & Turner, C. (2005). Community-based programmes to prevent falls in children: A systematic review. *Journal of Paediatrics and Child Health, 41,* 465-470.

34. New York City Department of Health and Mental Hygiene. (2012). *Windows fall prevention program: Understanding the basics.* Retrieved from http://www.nyc.gov/html/doh/html/win/winbas2.shtml.

35. Centers for Disease Control. (2012). *Poisoning in the United States: Fact sheet.* http://www.cdc.gov/HomeandRecreationalSafety/Poisoning/poisoning-factsheet.htm.

36. National SAFE KIDS Campaign. (2004). *Poisoning fact sheet.* Washington, DC: Author.

37. Centers for Disease Control. (2012). *Prevent unintentional poisoning.* Retrieved from http://www.cdc.gov/Features/PoisonPrevention/.

38. Gilchrist, J., Ballesteros, M.F., & Parker, E. (2012). Vital signs: Unintentional injury deaths among persons. Aged 0–19 years—United States, 2000–2009. *Morbidity and Mortality Weekly Report, 61*(15), 270-276.

39. Finkelstein, E., Corso, P., & Miller, T. (2006). *The incidence and economic costs of injury in the United States.* New York, NY: Oxford University Press.

40. Centers for Disease Control and Prevention. (2011). *Prescription painkiller overdoses in the U.S. Vital signs.* Atlanta, GA: U.S. Department of Health and Human Services, Centers for Disease Control and Prevention.

41. American Association of Poison Control Centers. (n.d.). *Poison data.* Retrieved from http://www.aapcc.org/dnn/NPDSPoisonData.aspx.

42. Centers for Disease Control and Prevention. (2013). *A national action plan for child injury prevention. Reducing poisoning injuries in children.* Retrieved from http://www.cdc.gov/safechild/nap/overviews/poison.html.

43. Bond, G.R., Woodward, R.W., & Ho, M. (2012). The growing impact of pediatric pharmaceutical poisoning. *Journal of Pediatrics, 160,* 265-270.

44. Crosby, A.E., Ortega, L., & Melanson, C. (2011). *Self-directed violence: Uniform definition and recommended data elements.* Atlanta, GA: Centers for Disease Control and Prevention, National Center for Injury Prevention and Control.

45. Hoven, C.W., Mandell, D.J., & Bertolote, J.M. (2010). Prevention of mental ill-health and suicide: Public health perspectives. *European Psychiatry, 25,* 252-256.

46. Centers for Disease Control and Prevention. (2013). *Fast Stats: Suicide and self-inflicted injury.* Retrieved from http://www.cdc.gov/nchs/fastats/suicide.htm.

47. American Foundation for Suicide Prevention. (2012). *Facts and figures.* Retrieved from http://www.

afsp.org/index.cfm?fuseaction=home.viewPage&page_id=050FEA9F-B064-4092-B1135C3A70DE1FDA.

48. Centers for Disease Control and Prevention. (2013). Suicide among adults aged 35–64 years—United States, 1999–2010. *Morbidity and Mortality Weekly Report, 62*(17), 321-322.

49. Crosby, A., Ortega, L., & Stevens, M.R. (2011). Suicides—United States, 1999–2007. *Morbidity and Mortality Weekly Report, 60*(1), 56-59.

50. Nation Institute of Mental Health. (n.d) *Suicide in the U.S.: Statistics and prevention* (NIH Publication No. 06-4594). Retrieved from http://www.nimh.nih.gov/health/publications/suicide-in-the-us-statistics-and-prevention/index.shtml.

51. Silverman, M.M., Frankel, M.J., & Miller, A.C. (2001). *Office of the Surgeon General National Strategy for Suicide Prevention: National Council For Suicide Prevention: Goal 1.* Retrieved from http://www.ncbi.nlm.nih.gov/bookshelf/br.fcgi?book=suicide&part=A4682.

52. National Institute of Mental Health. (2010). *The numbers count: Mental disorders in America.* Retrieved from http://www.nimh.nih.gov/health/publications/the-numbers-count-mental-disorders-in-america/index.shtml.

53. Mann, J.J., Apter, A., Bertolote, J., Beautrais, A., Currier, D., Haas, A., et al. (2005). Suicide prevention strategies. *JAMA, 294*(16), 2064-2074.

54. National Institute of Mental Health. (2010). *Suicide in the United States: Statistics and prevention.* Retrieved from http://www.nimh.nih.gov/health/publications/suicide-in-the-us-statistics-and-prevention/index.shtml#factors.

55. Schulberg, H.C., Bruce, M.L., Lee, P.W., Williams, J.W., & Dietrich, A.J. (2004). Preventing suicide in primary care patients: The primary care physician's role. *General Hospital Psychiatry, 26,* 337-345.

56. Walker, R.D., Loudon, L., Walker, P.S., & Frizzell, L. (2006). *A guide to suicide prevention for American Indian and Alaska Native communities.* Retrieved from http://www.oneskycenter.org/pp/documents/AGuidetoSuicidePreventionFINAL.pdf.

57. Indian Health Service. (n.d.). *American and Alaska Native suicide prevention.* Retrieved from http://www.ihs.gov/nonmedicalprograms/nspn/.

58. US Department of Health and Human Services, Administration for children and Families. (n.d.). *Keeping Children Safe Act.* Retrieved from https://www.childwelfare.gov/systemwide/laws_policies/federal/index.cfm?event=federalLegislation.viewLegis&id=45.

59. Centers for Disease Control and Prevention. (2013). *Child maltreatment: Facts at a glance.* Retrieved from http://www.cdc.gov/violenceprevention/pdf/cm-data-sheet—2013.pdf.

60. Turner, H.A, Finkelhor, D., Ormrod, R., Hamby, S., Leeb, R.T., Mercy, J.A., et al. (2012). Family context, victimization, and child trauma symptoms: Variations in safe, stable, and nurturing relationships during early and middle childhood. *American Journal of Orthopsychiatry, 82*(2), 209-219. doi:10.1111/j.1939-0025.2012.01147.x.

61. Centers for Disease Control and Prevention. (2014). *Child maltreatment: Risk and protective factors.* Retrieved from http://www.cdc.gov/violenceprevention/childmaltreatment/riskprotectivefactors.html.

62. US Department of Health and Human Services, Children's Bureau. (n.d.). *Reporting systems.* Retrieved from http://www.acf.hhs.gov/programs/cb/research-data-technology/reporting-systems.

63. U.S. Department of Health and Human Services. (2011). *Child maltreatment 2011.* Retrieved from http://www.acf.hhs.gov/sites/default/files/cb/cm11.pdf.

64. Dakil, S.R., Cox, M., Hua, L., & Flores, G. (2011). Racial and ethnic disparities in physical abuse reporting and child protective services interventions in the United States. *Journal of the National Medical Association, 103* (9/10), 926-931.

65. Fang, X., Brown, D.S., Florence, C., Mercy, J.A. (2012). The economic burden of child maltreatment in the United States and implications for prevention. *Child Abuse and Neglect, 36*(2), 156-165.

66. Wegman, H.L., & Stetler, C. (2009). A meta-analytic review of the effects of childhood abuse on medical outcomes in adulthood. *Psychosomatic Medicine, 71,* 805-812.

67. Maniglio, R. (2009). The impact of child sexual abuse on health: A systematic review of reviews. *Clinical Psychology Review, 29,* 647-657.

68. Nanni, V., Uher, R., & Danese, A. (2012). Childhood maltreatment predicts unfavorable course of illness and treatment outcome in depression: A meta-analysis. *American Journal of Psychiatry, 169* (2), 141-151.

69. Gonzalez, A., & MacMillan, H.L. (2008). Preventing child maltreatment: An evidence-based update. *Journal of Postgraduate Medicine, 54*(4), 280-286.

70. Johnson-Reid, M., Kohl, P.L, & Drake, B. (2012). Child and adult outcomes of chronic child maltreatment. *Pediatrics, 129*(5), 839-845.

71. Dube, S.R., Miller, J.W., Brown, D.W., Giles, W.H., Felitti, V.J., Dong, M, & Anda, R.F. (2006). Adverse childhood experiences and the association with ever using alcohol and initiating alcohol use during adolescence. *Journal of Adolescent Health, 38*(4), 1-10.

72. Berger, L.R., Wallace, L.J.D., & Bill, N.M. (2009). Injuries and injury prevention among indigenous children and young people. *Pediatric Clinics in North America, 56,* 1519-1537.

73. Olds, D.L. (2002). Prenatal and infancy home visiting by nurses: From randomized trials to community replication. *Preventive Science, 3,* 153-172.

74. Sanders, M.R., Cann, W., & Markie-Dadds, C. (2003). The Triple P-Positive Parenting Programme: A universal population-level approach to the prevention of child abuse. *Child Abuse Review, 12,* 155-171.

75. Carpenter, J., Brown, S., & Griffin, M. (2007). Prevention in integrated children's services: The impact of Sure Start on referrals to social services and child protection registrations. *Child Abuse Review, 16,* 17-31.

76. Onyskiw, J.E., Harrison, M.J., Spady, D., & McConnan, L. (1999). Formative evaluation of a collaborative community-based child abuse prevention project. *Child Abuse and Neglect, 23,* 1069-1081.

77. DePanfilis, D., & Dubowitz, H. (2005). Family Connections: A program for preventing child neglect. *Child Maltreatment, 10*, 108-123.

78. Krugman, S.D., Lane, W.G., & Walsh, C.M. (2007). Update on child abuse prevention. *Current Opinions Pediatrics, 19*, 11-18.

79. Toth, S.L., & Manly, J.T. (2011). Bridging research and practice: Challenges and successes in implementing evidence-based preventive intervention strategies for child maltreatment. *Child Abuse and Neglect, 35*(8), 633-636.

80. Saltzman, L.E., Fanslow, J.L., McMahon, P.M., & Shelley, G.A. (2002). *Intimate partner violence surveillance: Uniform definitions and recommended data elements* (Version 1.0). Atlanta, GA: Centers for Disease Control and Prevention, National Center for Injury Prevention and Control.

81. Zolotor, A.J., Denham, A., & Weil, A. (2009). Intimate partner violence. *Primary Care Clinic Office Practice, 36*, 167-179.

82. Centers for Disease Control and Prevention. (2010). *Intimate partner violence: Data sources.* Retrieved from http://www.cdc.gov/ViolencePrevention/intimatepartnerviolence/datasources.html.

83. Silverman, J.G., Raj, A., & Clements, K. (2004). Dating violence and associated sexual risk and pregnancy among adolescent girls in the United States. *Pediatrics, 114*(2), e220-e225.

84. Alleyne-Green, B., Coleman-Cowger, V.H., & Henry, D.B. (2012). Dating violence perpetration and/or victimization and associated sexual risk behaviors among a sample of inner-city African American and Hispanic adolescent females. *Journal of Interpersonal Violence, 27*, 1457-1473.

85. Cho, H. (2012). Examining gender differences in the nature and context of intimate partner violence. *Journal of Interpersonal Violence, 27*(13), 2665-2684. doi:10.1177/0886260512436391.

86. O'Leary, K.D, & Slep, A.M. (2011). Prevention of partner violence by focusing on behaviors of both young males and females. *Preventive Science, 13*(4), 329-339. doi:10.1007/s11121-011-0237-2.

87. Breiding, M.J., Black, M.C., & Ryan, G.W. (2008). Prevalence and risk factors of intimate partner violence in eighteen U.S. states/territories, 2005. *American Journal of Preventive Medicine, 34*(2), 112-118.

88. Kimberg, L.S. (2008). Addressing intimate partner violence with patients: A review and introduction of pilot guidelines. *Journal of General Internal Medicine, 23*(12), 2071-2078.

89. Massachusetts Department of Health. (2009). *The health of lesbian, gay, bisexual, and transgender.* Retrieved from http://www.mass.gov/eohhs/docs/dph/commissioner/lgbt-health-report.pdf.

90. Bonomi A.E., Anderson, M.L., Reid, R.J., Rivara, F.P., Carrell, D., & Thompson, R.S. (2009). Medical and psychosocial diagnoses in women with a history of intimate partner violence. *Archives Internal Medicine, 169*(18), 1692-1697.

91. Gottlieb, A.S. (2008). Intimate partner violence: A clinical review of screening and intervention. *Women's Health, 4*(5), 529-539.

92. Holt, S., Buckley, H., & Whelan, S. (2008). The impact of exposure to domestic violence on children and young people: A review of the literature. *Child Abuse and Neglect, 32*, 797-810.

93. Wolfe, D.A., Crooks, C.V., Lee, V., McIntyre-Smith, A., & Jaffe, P.G. (2003). The effects of children's exposure to domestic violence: A meta-analysis and critique. *Clinical Child and Family Psychology Review, 6*(3), 171-187.

94. Karch, D.L., Dahlberg, L.L., & Patel, N. (2010, May 14). Surveillance for violent deaths—national violent death reporting system, 16 states, 2007. Division of Violence Prevention, National Center for Injury Prevention and Control, CDC. *Morbidity and Mortality Weekly Report (MMWR) Surveillance Summaries, 59*(SS04), 1-50. Retrieved from http://www.cdc.gov/mmwr/preview/mmwrhtml/ss5904a1.htm.

95. Cheng, D., & Horon, I.L. (2010). Intimate-partner homicide among pregnant and postpartum women. *Obstetrics Gynecology, 115*(6), 1181-1186.

96. Laisser, R.M., Nystrom, L., Lugina, H.I., & Emmelin, M. (2011). Community perceptions of intimate partner violence—a qualitative study from urban Tanzania. *BMC Women's Health, 11*, 13.

97. Testa, M., Kubiak, A., Quigley, B.M., Houston, R.J., Derrick, J.L., Levitt, A., et al. (2012). Husband and wife alcohol use as independent or interactive predictors of intimate partner violence. *Journal of Studies on Alcohol and Drugs, 73*, 268-276.

98. Centers for Disease Control and Prevention. (2010). *Intimate partner violence: Risk and protective factors.* Retrieved from http://www.cdc.gov/ViolencePrevention/intimatepartnerviolence/riskprotectivefactors.html.

99. Smith, C.A., Ireland, T.O., Park, A., Elwyn, L., & Thornberry, T.P. (2011). Intergenerational continuities and discontinuities in intimate partner violence: A two-generational prospective study. *Journal of Interpersonal Violence, 26*(18), 3720-3752.

100. Cunradi, C.B., Mair, C., Ponicki, W., & Remer, L. (2012). Alcohol outlet density and intimate partner violence-related emergency room visits. *Alcoholism: Clinical and Experimental Research, 36*(5), 847-853.

101. Centers for Disease Control and Prevention. (n.d.). *Preventing intimate partner and sexual violence.* Retrieved from http://www.cdc.gov/violenceprevention/pdf/IPV-SV_Program_Activities_Guide-a.pdf.

102. Centers for Disease Control and Prevention. (2010). *Intimate partner violence: Prevention strategies.* Retrieved from http://www.cdc.gov/ViolencePrevention/intimatepartnerviolence/prevention.html.

103. Foshee V.A., Linder, G.F., Bauman, K.E., Langwick, S.A., Arriaga, X.B., Heath, J.L., et al. (1996). The Safe Dates Project: Theoretical basis, evaluation design, and selected baseline findings. *American Journal of Preventive Medicine, 12*(Suppl. 5), 39-47.

104. Foshee, V.A., Bauman, K.E., Ennett, S.T., Suchindran, C., Benefield, T., & Linder, G.F (2005). Assessing the effects of the dating violence prevention program "Safe Dates" using random coefficient regression modeling. *Preventive Science, 6*(3), 245-258.

105. Wathen, C.N., & MacMillan, H.L. (2003). Interventions for violence against women. *JAMA, 289*(5), 589-600.

106. McFarlane & Parker, (2002). An intervention to increase safety behaviors of abused women: Results of a randomized clinical trial. *Nursing Research, 51*(60), 347-354.

107. Chambliss, L.R. (2008). Intimate partner violence and its implication for pregnancy. *Clinical Obstetrics and Gynecology, 51*(2), 385-397.

108. O'Campo, P., Kirst, M., Tsamis, C., Chambers, C., & Ahmad, F. (2010). Implementing successful intimate partner violence screening programs in health care settings: Evidence generated from a realist-informed systematic review. *Social Science & Medicine, 72*(6), 855-866.

109. Hawley, D.A., & Barker, A.C. (2012). Survivors of intimate partner violence: Implications for nursing care. *Critical Care Nursing Clinics of North America, 24,* 27-39.

110. Fulton, D. (2000). Recognition and documentation of domestic violence in the clinical setting. *Critical Care Nurse, 23*(2), 26-34.

111. Todahl, J., & Walters, E. (2011). Universal screening for intimate partner violence: A systematic review. *Journal of Marital & Family Therapy, 37*(3), 355-369.

112. Massachusetts Medical Society. (2010). *Intimate Partner Violence: A clinician's guide.* (5th ed.). Retrieved from http://www.ahrq.gov/downloads/pub/prevent/pdfser/famviolser.pdf.

113. Krug, E.G., Dahlberg, L.L., Mercy, J.A., Zwi, A.B., & Lozano, R. (Eds.). (2002). *World report on violence and health.* Geneva, Switzerland: World Health Organization. Retrieved from http://whqlibdoc.who.int/publications/2002/9241545615_eng.pdf.

114. Smith-Stover, C., Meadows, A.L., & Kaufman, J. (2009). Interventions for intimate partner violence: Review and implications for evidence-based practice. *Professional Psychology Research and Practice, 40*(3), 223-233.

115. Chibber, K.S., & Krishnan, S. (2011). Confronting intimate partner violence: A global health priority. *Mount Sinai Journal of Medicine, 78,* 449-457.

116. World Health Organization. (2012). *Violence and injury prevention: Prevention of intimate partner violence and sexual violence.* Retrieved from http://www.who.int/violence_injury_prevention/violence/activities/intimate/en/index.html.

117. Bell, C., & Jenkins, E.J. (1993). Community violence and children on Chicago's Southside. *Psychiatry: Interpersonal and Biological Processes, 56,* 46-54.

118. Centers for Disease Control and Prevention. (2012). *Injuries and violence are leading causes of death: Key data and statistics.* Retrieved from http://www.cdc.gov/injury/overview/data.html.

119. Federal Bureau of Investigation. (n.d.). *Crime in the United States.* Retrieved from http://www.fbi.gov/about-us/cjis/ucr/crime-in-the-u.s/2010/crime-in-the-u.s.-2010/offenses-known-to-law-enforcement/expanded/expandhomicidemain.

120. Federal Bureau of Investigation. (n.d.). *Crime in the United States.* Retrieved from http://www.fbi.gov/about-us/cjis/ucr/crime-in-the-u.s/2010/crime-in-the-u.s.-2010/violent-crime/violent-crime.

121. Latkin, C., Yang, C., Ehrhardt, B., & Hulbert, A. (2013). The epidemiology of finding a dead body: Reports from inner-city Baltimore, Maryland U.S. *Community Mental Health Journal. 49*(1), 106-109. doi:10.1007/s10597-012-9492-3.

122. Zinzow, H.M., Ruggiero, K.J., Resnick, H., Hanson, R., Smith, D., Saunders, B., & Kilpatrick, D. (2009). Prevalence and mental health correlates of witnessed parental and community violence in a national sample of adolescents. *Journal of Child Psychology and Psychiatry, 50*(4), 441-450.

123. Blizzard, S.J., Kemppainen, J., & Taylor, J. (2009). Posttraumatic stress disorder and community violence: An update for nurse practitioners. *Journal of the American Academy of Nurse Practitioners, 21,* 535-541.

124. Bell, C.C., & Jenkins, E.J. (1991). Traumatic stress and children. *Journal of Health Care for the Poor and Underserved, 2*(1), 175-185.

125. Horowitz, K., McKay, M., & Marshall, R. (2005). Community violence and urban families: Experiences, effects, and directions for intervention. *American Journal of Orthopsychiatry, 75*(3), 356-368.

126. Hahn, R., Fuquia-Whitley, D., Wethington, H., Lowry, J., Crosby, A., Fullilove, M., et al. (2007). Effectiveness of universal school-based programs to prevent violence and aggressive behavior. *American Journal of Preventive Medicine, 33*(Suppl. 2), S114-S129.

127. Aisenberg, E., & Herrenkohl, T. (2008). Community violence in context: Risk and resilience in children and families. *Journal of Interpersonal Violence, 23,* 296-315.

128. Furr-Holden, C.D.M., Smart, M.J., Pokorni, J.L, Ialongo, N.S., Leaf, P.J., Holder, H.D., & Anthony, J.C. (2008). The NifETy method for environmental assessment of neighborhood-level indicators of violence, alcohol, and other drug exposure. *Preventive Science, 9,* 245-255.

129. Whitaker, D., Graham, C., Furr-Holden, D., Milam, A., & Latimer, W. (2011). Neighborhood disorder and incarceration history among urban substance users. *Journal of Correctional Health Care, 17*(4), 309-318. doi:10.1177/1078345811413092.

130. Kawachi, I., Kennedy, B.P., & Wilkinson, R.G. (1999). Crime, social disorganization and relative deprivation. *Social Science Medicine, 48,* 719-731.

131. Watson-Thompson, J., Fawcett, S.B., & Schultz, J.A. (2008). A framework for community mobilization to promote healthy youth development. *American Journal of Preventive Medicine, 34*(Suppl. 3), S72-S81.

132. Garmezy, N. (1981). Children under stress: Perspectives on antecedents and correlates of vulnerability and resistance to psychopathology. In I.A. Rabin, J. Arnoff, A.M. Barclay, & R.A. Zucker (Eds.), *Further explorations in personality* (pp 196-269). New York, NY: John Wiley.

133. Allison, K.W., Edmonds, T., Wilson, K., Pope, M., & Farrell, A.D. (2011). Connecting youth violence prevention, positive youth development, and community mobilization. *American Journal of Community Psychology, 48*(1-2), 8-20.

134. Backer, T.E., & Guerra, N.G (2011). Mobilizing communities to implement evidence-based practices in youth violence prevention: The state of the art. *American Journal of Community Psychology, 48*(1-2), 31-42.

135. Centers for Disease Control and Prevention. (2011). *Youth violence: Prevention strategies.* Retrieved from http://www.cdc.gov/ViolencePrevention/ youthviolence/prevention.html.

136. Centers for Disease Control and Prevention. (2009). *Framework for action.* Retrieved from http:// www.cdc.gov/violenceprevention/pdf/ PreventYouthViolence-a.pdf.

137. Orend, B. (2008). War. In E.N. Zalta (Ed.), *The Stanford encyclopedia of philosophy.* Retrieved from http://plato.stanford.edu/archives/fall2008/entries/war/.

138. Levy, B., & Sidel, V. (Eds.). (2007). *War and public health* (2nd ed.). Oxford, England: Oxford University Press.

139. Leitenberg, M. (2006). *Deaths in wars and conflicts in the 20th century.* Retrieved from http://www. cissm.umd.edu/papers/files/deathswarsconflicts june52006.pdf.

140. Goldstein, J. (2011, September-October). Think again: War. *Foreign Policy.* Retrieved from http://www.foreignpolicy.com/articles/2011/08/15/ think_again_war?page=full.

141. Benjamin, D. (2007). War and public health. *Health Generations, 7*(3), 1-3.

Chapter 13

Nursing and Global Health

LEARNING OUTCOMES

After reading this chapter, the student will be able to:

1. Define the concept of global health and its importance to nursing.
2. Explain the term *primary health care* in the context of the global community, and differentiate it from *primary care*.
3. Identify collaborating national and international agencies in global health.
4. Discuss the importance of the eight Millennium Development Goals in achieving better health for all.
5. Identify the current major global health problems and the future trends.
6. Discuss the importance of the neglected and emerging diseases.
7. Identify the new emerging roles of nurses in the framework of global health.

KEY TERMS

Bilateral organizations
Burden of disease
Disability-adjusted life year (DALY)
Environmental sustainability
Food security
Global health
High-income countries
Life expectancy
Low-income countries
Maternal mortality
Middle-income countries
Millennium Development Goals (MDGs)
Multilateral organizations
Nongovernmental organization
Primary care
Primary health care
Select agent
Sustainable Development Goals (SDGs)

■ Introduction

Health, one of the foundations of the global civil society, promotes social and cultural growth, political stability, and economic sustainability. Yet health is an area in which large portions of the world are losing ground. Several countries are seeing health measures such as life expectancy decline, despite the tremendous medical advances that have been made over the last few decades. **Global health** reflects "health issues that transcend national boundaries and governments and call for actions on the global forces that determine the health of people."[1] Using a more dynamic approach, Beaglehole and Bonita defined global health as "the collaborative trans-national research and action for promoting health for all."[2] Global health stands for a new approach to the concept of international health.

One of the most popular and quoted definitions of global health was written in 2009 by the Consortium of Universities for Global Health: "Global health is an area for study, research, and practice that places a priority on improving health and achieving equity in health for all people worldwide. Global health emphasizes transnational health issues, determinants, and solutions; involves many disciplines within and beyond the health sciences and promotes interdisciplinary collaboration; and is a synthesis of population based prevention with individual-level clinical care."[3] Health in the context of global health is defined broadly and supports the World Health Organization (WHO) classic definition of health: "a state of complete physical, mental and social wellbeing and not merely the absence of disease or infirmity."[4] The constitution of the WHO further recognized "the enjoyment of the highest attainable standard of health . . . as one of the fundamental rights of every human being."[5]

One of the variables associated with differences between countries is their economic well-being. The terms most often used to differentiate countries based on country-level income data are **high-income countries (HICs)**, middle-income countries (MICs), and **low-income countries (LICs)**. The World Bank classifies countries into these categories based on current economic ranges of the per capita gross national income (GNI). For example, in 2012 an LIC was a country with a GNI equal to or less than US$1,035, an MIC's GNI ranged from US$1,036 to $12,615 and an HIC's GNI was equal to or greater than US$12,616. To further assist in classifying countries, MICs represent two groups: low-middle-income countries (GNI range US$1,036 to $4,085) and high-middle-income countries (GNI range US$4,086 to $12,615).[6] These terms replace the earlier terms of *developed* and *developing* countries. From a global health perspective, a major concern is the growing disparity between LICs and both HICs and MICs. Previously, international health-care workers in low- and middle-income countries looked for solutions to health care within the country or developed collaboration with one other country. The key conceptual change in global health is the emphasis on the interdependence of countries; the interdependence of the health of people in all countries; and the interdependence of the policies, economics, and values that arise related to health.[1]

The ultimate goal of any global health endeavor is to promote optimal health for all and eliminate the disparity in health status between countries. According to the WHO, "In the 21st century, health is a shared responsibility, involving equitable access to essential care and collective defence against transnational threats."[4] Thus, a global health perspective envisions health in a way that encompasses all nations and peoples. Nursing plays an important part across the world, providing care, developing population-level interventions, and conducting needed research on how best to improve health for vulnerable populations.

Measuring Global Health

Life Expectancy

One way to measure the health of populations and to compare them from a global perspective is through life expectancy. **Life expectancy** is the average number of years a person born in a given country would live if mortality rates at each age were to remain constant in the future.[7] Based on 2013 estimates worldwide, there is a wide range (49.07 years to 89.63 years) among countries in relation to the average life expectancy at birth.[7] One of the reasons for lower life expectancy in MICs and LICs is that they experience more difficulty with control and eradication of communicable diseases and the illnesses that are associated with maternal, child, and women's health. These differences between LICs and MICs

demonstrate the health benefits of stable economies with advanced industrial and technological development. It also reflects the greater financial emphasis placed on the health-care needs of people in HICs, especially in relation to providing universal health care. The United States, which enacted the Affordable Care Act in 2014, was the last HIC to have some form of universal health care. Despite the availability of state of the art health care, in 2013 the United States ranked 51 out of 223 countries in relation to life expectancy. For example, the average life expectancy in the United States was 78.62 years compared with 89.63 years in Monaco.[7]

In the past 100 years, great strides in improving life expectancy have occurred in HICs. For example, a person born in the United States in 1910 could hope to live to be 48 years old if male and 52 years old if female.[7] Overall life expectancy in the United States in 2013 was 78.62. Thus, since 1910 the average life span has increased by 30 years, whereas infant mortality decreased by 93%. Of this increase in life span, 25 years of the 30-year increase are attributed to the advances in public health practices.[8] These improvements include vaccinations, motor vehicle safety, safer workplaces, control of communicable disease by specifically having clean water and sanitation, decline in coronary disease and stroke, safer and healthier foods, healthier mothers and babies, family planning, recognition of the dangers of tobacco, and fluoridation of the water.[8]

Worldwide in 2012, 6.6 million children under 5 died, a decrease of 47% from 1990 when the total number of deaths was 12.4 million.[9] Most of these deaths are preventable and are a result of such things as respiratory infection and diarrhea that result from a lack of clean water and good sanitation.[9] With the world population already at 6.1 billion, rapid population growth in several countries has stressed economies and put enormous strain on country resources, including the need for more housing, more food, and more schools. At the same time, approximately 800 women a day die from complications of pregnancy and childbirth each year, with 99% of maternal deaths occurring in LICs.[10] These global health issues not only affect those living in the developing world, but also directly have an impact on Americans. As the U.S. Agency for International Development (USAID) pointed out:[11]

- Healthy citizens are essential for global economic growth
- Stable populations reduce the risk of humanitarian crises
- Good communicable disease programs reduce the threats of epidemics and pandemics

- New technologies developed through research in the developing world can also be applied in the U.S. health-care system

Importance to the United States

According to a statement by Institute of Medicine (IOM) made at the end of the 20th century, "The failure to engage in the fight to anticipate, prevent, and ameliorate global health problems would diminish America's stature in the realm of health and jeopardize our own health, economy, and national security."[12] Americans can gain a new awareness of their own health by looking at the health of the world. *Global* refers to the scope of the problem and not to its location. One way is to study different facets of health-care delivery throughout the world, the outcome of these health services, the impact health has on all government and private institutions, especially on economic development, and how intertwined all of these components are with the people of the United States. Outbreak of disease in one country can decrease animal and plant crops for export. Malaria can reduce production of goods over significantly large areas, limiting economic development.[13] Droughts can have devastating effects on food supplies, producing starvation and malnutrition in some areas and economic and political destabilization in others.[14] Communicable diseases are spread without difficulty in our global community with rapid and easily accessed transport. New forms of rapid communication can also affect transfers of culture, goods, and disease. In addition, harmful lifestyles, pollution, toxic substances, and unsafe goods and products are easily transported, moving quickly across borders.

Importance to Nursing

Nursing in the era of globalization has many opportunities and several challenges. Globalization is an irreversible process that is both complex and diverse and places considerable emphasis on areas other than health such as economics, social relationships, politics, and culture. The urbanization of the world and economic growth creates both positive and negative changes, sometimes too many changes too fast. Nurses respond in several ways to these changes. Nurses can be prepared to practice in environments with emerging and reemerging communicable diseases, providing care to increasingly diverse populations, and focus on evidence-based practice (EBP) and research that includes the global community. Nurses the world over need to remember that innovation and knowledge are not restricted to the HICs, and they can all learn from one another. Nurses will want to understand not only their local community but also

their national and global communities. In developing countries, nurses can develop leadership skills to insert themselves within the health-care system in a way that will guarantee that they can have an impact on health care and the roles of nurses in the future.[15,16] The new IOM Report, *The Future of Nursing: Leading Change, Advancing Health*, encourages all U.S. nurses to take collective action to amplify nursing's voice in transforming their healthcare system.[17] In doing this, nurses can also have a voice in global health and be on the forefront of any potential changes. In support of this approach, Sigma Theta Tau International, the nursing honor society, has a mission to improve nursing care worldwide as a means of improving health at the global level.[18]

● APPLYING PUBLIC HEALTH SCIENCE
The Case of Nurse Gladys
Public Health Science Topics Covered:

- Environmental health
- Resource allocation
- Building capacity

Nurses in low-income countries (LICs) have the potential to demonstrate leadership in global health initiatives. Nurses form the biggest health-care force the world over, and they spend more time with the patients and clients in the health-care system than any other health-care provider. However, nurses in LICs such as Uganda face grand challenges that affect their work and affect their contribution to the global health initiatives. Some of the challenges include a serious nurse shortage, low status as nurses with low salaries, a large family to care for, a national health-care system that is inadequately budgeted, and the heavy impact of communicable diseases, specifically malaria, HIV/AIDS, and pneumonia.

Uganda is a small, landlocked country in East Africa that borders Lake Victoria and has for neighbors Kenya, Tanzania, Sudan, Democratic Republic of Congo, and Rwanda. It is 87% rural with only a few major cities. Agriculture is the major occupation of the rural residents. Communication has been made easier with universal cell phone usage, but currently consistent Internet service is not readily available and there is very limited reception in the rural areas.

Nurses in Uganda train at various levels. There are a few baccalaureate registered nurses, but the majority are registered comprehensive nurses (diploma nurses) and enrolled comprehensive nurses (licensed practical nurses). The majority of these nurses at all levels are also registered midwives. Many new nurses graduate from their respective institutions every year, but there has not been any change in the nurse-to-population ratio. This is in part because of the high population growth of 3.3% annually, but more important, the nurses who graduate from the various nursing schools cannot find work because the Ministry of Health, the biggest employer, does not have the money to fill hundreds of empty positions. As a result, nurses who are lucky to be employed are severely overworked.

The National Health Care system in Uganda, which provides free care and medication to Ugandans, comprises two National Referral and Teaching Hospitals: Butabika for mental and psychiatric illnesses and Mulago for all other health conditions. There are regional referral hospitals, district hospitals, and health centers, but most are significantly under resourced with very limited stocks of pharmaceuticals, working equipment, laboratory testing, or other essentials necessary in primary health care. There are private not-for-profit hospitals—mainly faith-based nongovernment organizations (NGOs)—and some private-for-profit hospitals and clinics. These nonpublic institutions charge patient fees, so only a few Ugandans can afford to use them, and the number of nursing positions is limited.

The nurses working in the major government hospitals are overworked because of the overwhelming numbers of patients and are frustrated by a lack of resources. In addition to the preceding, those in the community clinics work without supervision. To be able to contribute positively to the global health initiative, nurses must have current information; however, most nurses in Uganda have no access to current information. For some, there is a lack of physical access with no journals, no books, and no computer or Internet access where the nurses work. The nurses may also not know how to get information, or they may not have the time and money required to access the information.

Consider the typical life of Ugandan registered nurse Gladys Namusisi (fictional name). Gladys was trained at the diploma level, lives in a rural community, and works in her district hospital. Gladys's training prepared her with knowledge and skills to perform her duties in a hospital setting. Owing to the nurse shortage, she is frequently responsible for 40 inpatients whose diagnoses include severe malaria (frequently cerebral malaria), pneumonia, tuberculosis (TB),

HIV/AIDS, trauma, diabetes, and other emerging noncommunicable diseases. She is thankful that each patient has a family member staying with the patient to provide the basic hygiene care, assist with feeding the patient, and also help Gladys with some of the clinical procedures. However, the family members can also add to her stress with their demands and need for constant reassurance.

Today there is no running water in the hospital, so she has asked one of the staff to get water for her. There is also sporadic electricity but this is not a serious problem during sunlight because she has no electrical equipment. She is frustrated today because she has once again run out of the second-line malaria drugs that she must have for three of her patients. She also gave her only blood pressure cuff to the obstetrical nurse who has two women with preeclampsia and no way to measure their blood pressure. She has no machines, no one to help monitor the IV setups, and no one to monitor patient status. At the end of her shift she is exhausted, but her colleague Patricia does not turn up owing to family problems and Gladys has to stay for one more shift.

Nurse Gladys does her routine work of monitoring and evaluating her patients, giving the medication, starting IVs, and completing the ordered procedures. She does some occasional patient ward teaching but has no time to spend teaching individual patients. She continues to do her work as she was taught because there are no resources such as the Internet, journals, or books to look for new information. Therefore, Gladys's work continues the same way, year in and year out.

There are many factors contributing to Gladys not being able to improve her skills. She is very tired with the heavy hospital workload and the extended hospital hours, and she works in a private clinic on her day off to supplement her meager salary. She cannot afford to pay for Internet services in an Internet cafe just next to the hospital where she works because her salary is too low. Gladys has many personal financial demands, and paying for Internet access is not a priority. The only free Internet access in the hospital is in the hospital director's office, which only the hospital physicians can use. The hospital director is even frustrated because the Internet reception is intermittent, and when it is on, it is very slow. Even if Gladys had the access to the Internet, she is not computer literate and has no skills to search for literature. Therefore, Gladys continues to work diligently as she was taught in nursing school, unaware that health care is dynamic and continually changing.

The other limitation for Gladys is that the only opportunity for her to have continuing nursing education is through training workshops that are organized by the hospital or nurse managers and are not guaranteed on a regular basis. Besides, when these do take place, the issues discussed in the workshops are determined by the leaders and frequently they are not of interest to Gladys.

In the Ugandan culture, Gladys has significant family responsibilities. Like many of her colleagues, Gladys has responsibility for her immediate and her large extended-family members. She is one of only a few in her large extended family that is employed with a salary. Also, she is a nurse and she is expected to give medical support to her whole family. This is because getting medical care if you are poor in Uganda is difficult; without insurance or income, you must use the government system. Gladys's family considers themselves very lucky because they have a nurse to help address their medical problems. Typical families are very large given Uganda's high fertility rate. Even though Gladys has only four biological children, she has many children to care for as the nephews and nieces are also considered her children. She must also help her aged parents because there is no safety net such as Social Security. Two of the nieces and one nephew are orphans as a result of the HIV/AIDS epidemic, and two others need support because their mother (Gladys's sister) died in childbirth. Gladys is totally responsible for these five additional children. Some of Gladys's nine siblings have no income because they are uneducated and have never gone to school because of family financial constraints, and cannot help her out. Gladys is obliged to care for these children because if she does not educate them now and help them be independent, her own children will suffer the consequences in the future. That is, they will have to provide economic support for their cousins who never went to school.

However, although Gladys has good intentions, she cannot afford to give quality education to all. Therefore, most of the nieces and nephews and even Gladys's biological children will be forced to drop out of school at the end of the primary level or will have to stop their study at secondary level because university education is too expensive. Even if free universal primary education has been in place for some years now in Uganda and universal secondary education was introduced recently, the uniforms and scholastic

materials are not affordable for poor parents and they, like Gladys, cannot keep their children in school. This means that Gladys's children may end up not having enough education for a good job with adequate pay. The vicious circle of poverty continues.

The AIDs epidemic has worsened the situation for Gladys. The epidemic affects Gladys in two ways, at the workplace and the family levels. At the workplace, there is an increased overload of patients who are very ill and there is the additional fear of getting infected with occupational exposure. There are limited protective devices and even gloves are not always easily available. On the family side, AIDS has increased Gladys's social/family responsibility with many additional people for whom she is responsible.

In talking with people in her village, the community leader suggested she might want to seek out two NGOs in the neighborhood. These organizations tell her about the new initiatives funded to help Uganda meet the Millennium Development Goals (MDGs), eight global health goals with a target date of 2015 aimed at improving health for all (see below). She finds that there are resources from these groups to help pay school fees to ensure that all of her children get a full primary education and can even continue in secondary education if they have good grades. There are also potential referrals to a new free clinic in the neighboring community that can provide more holistic care for the two nieces who were born with HIV. She feels some relief for now and is glad that she is a nurse and can care for so many of her fellow Ugandans. She hopes that not too far in the future the burden of disease for her family and for her community will decrease. She is also hopeful that her children will grow up in a better world.

Primary Health Care

Nurses such as Gladys working in LICs in acute care settings face challenges in the delivery of care. These challenges have prompted the effort to increase the number of nurses as providers of primary health care outside the acute care setting to help communities stay well. The term *primary health care* from a global perspective is quite different from the term *primary care* used in the United States. **Primary health care** refers to the essential care needed to have healthy individuals and a healthy community. In contrast, the term **primary care,** as often used in the United States, refers to personal health services. It is usually the first point of consultation for all patients who are typically seen by a family physician or a nurse practitioner. The primary care providers usually see the patient on a continuing basis and include primary, secondary, and tertiary prevention in their care. Primary care can be thought of as one of the components of the broader term *primary health care.*

The concept of primary health care originated at the 1978 WHO Alma-Ata conference, which brought together 134 nations in Kazakhstan. These nations committed themselves to the goal of "Health for All" by the year 2000. The conference participants felt that, if the new approach of primary health care was initiated in the communities and if individual governments met their obligation to fund primary health-care services, this goal could be reached in the next 20 years. The essential components of primary health care, as defined at Alma-Ata, were broad and encompassed eight components that contribute to health, in addition to direct care service:[19]

- Education concerning prevailing health problems and the methods of preventing and controlling them
- Promotion of food supply and proper nutrition
- Adequate supply of safe water and basic sanitation
- Maternal and child health care, including family planning
- Immunization against the major communicable diseases
- Prevention and control of locally endemic diseases
- Appropriate treatment of common diseases and injuries
- Provision of essential drugs

Countries have added onto these basic components to include:

- Principles of equity
- Affordable and accessible care
- Availability of resources
- Use of a multi-sectored approach
- Appropriate technology
- Emphasis on primary and secondary prevention

Globally, there are many examples of public health nurses (PHNs) working in LICs providing primary health care in local villages, which includes activities that seem at first to be outside the normal services provided by nurses. Nurses have introduced activities such as construction of dish-drying racks made from everyday local resources to decrease contamination, assisted in construction of pit latrines, demonstrated how to use banana fiber to cover the latrine openings, and helped in removing brush near the homes to decrease mosquito breeding grounds for malaria.

Since its inception in the late 1970s, primary health care remains a focus of the WHO's commitment to achieving optimal health for all (Box 13-1). Since 1978, significant improvement in health has occurred, with many countries adopting a primary health-care model, with efforts continuing to bring primary health care to more countries.[20]

Global Initiatives: Millennium Development Goals

The **Millennium Development Goals (MDGs)** are the world's time-bound and quantified targets for addressing extreme poverty in its many dimensions—income poverty, hunger, disease, lack of adequate shelter, and exclusion—while promoting gender equality, education, and environmental sustainability. They are also basic human rights, that is, the rights of each person on the planet to health, education, shelter, and security.[20] In September 2000 at the United Nations (UN) headquarters in New York City, 147 world leaders, the largest gathering of world leaders at that time, met for the Millennium Summit. After 3 days of discussion, on September 8, the leaders ratified the UN Millennium Declaration. In total, 189 member states adopted the declaration. It advocates for improving people's lives through the development of international partners to work together to create peace, reduce poverty, decrease ill health, improve education, protect the environment, promote clean water and sanitation, decrease gender inequality, and implement development goals to guarantee that economic development reaches all, including LICs. The broad concepts of health were threaded throughout. The result was eight international development goals

BOX 13–1	The WHO Primary Health-Care Key Elements

The ultimate goal of primary health care is better health for all. The WHO has identified five key elements to achieving that goal:
1. Reducing exclusion and social disparities in health (universal coverage reforms)
2. Organizing health services around people's needs and expectations (service delivery reforms)
3. Integrating health into all sectors (public policy reforms)
4. Pursuing collaborative models of policy dialogue (leadership reforms)
5. Increasing stakeholder participation

Source: See reference 20.

following the adoption of the UN Millennium Declaration (Fig. 13-1). The International Council of Nurses backs the UN's MDGs to relieve poor health conditions around the world and to establish positive steps to improve living conditions. The WHO projected that if these goals are reached by 2015, world poverty will be cut by half, tens of millions of lives saved, and billions will benefit from the world economy.[20]

Global Health Organizations

Central to the adoption of a global approach to health as evident in the development of the MDGs is collaboration between and within countries and across organizations, both public and private. As global health becomes a reality, more national and international agencies are building partnerships to improve the health of countries, regions, and the world. Organizations are usually classified as a multilateral, bilateral, or NGO.

Goal 1: Eradicate extreme poverty and hunger

Goal 2: Achieve universal primary education

Goal 3: Promote gender equality and empower women

Goal 4: Reduce child mortality

Goal 5: Improve maternal health

Goal 6: Combat HIV/AIDS, malaria, and other diseases

Goal 7: Ensure environmental sustainability

Goal 8: Develop a Global Partnership of Development Source (88)

Figure 13-1 The Millennium Developmental Goals. *(From the World Health Organization,[20]*

Multilateral Organizations

The term **multilateral organizations** means that the collaborative work and funding come from multiple governments, as well as from nongovernmental sources, and is distributed to many different countries. Examples of multilateral organizations include the WHO, the World Bank, the UN Children Fund (UNICEF), and the UN Development Programme.[21]

World Health Organization

All of the major multilateral health organizations are part of the UN. The WHO is the directing and coordinating authority for health within the UN's system. The organization was created in 1946, and has as its creed, "Health for All." As a representative body of the 193 member states, the WHO, through its constitution, is mandated to provide leadership in matters of global health, provide norms and standards established on EBP, monitor trends of health and disease, set the research agenda, and provide technical support to countries. It is also especially concerned with protecting the health of vulnerable and poor communities and countries.[3,22] The WHO has a six-point agenda as a response to the rapidly changing global community and the changing areas of public health.[23]

1. **Promoting development:** These activities give priority to health outcomes in poor, disadvantaged, or vulnerable groups. This objective coincides with the MDGs (see below), and addresses health development with particular concerns about preventing and treating noncommunicable diseases and the neglected tropical diseases.
2. **Fostering health security:** The focus is on preventing and controlling outbreaks of emerging and epidemic-prone diseases. These outbreaks are more common with increased and rapid urbanization, poor environmental controls, poor or inappropriate food distribution, and the misuse of antibiotics.
3. **Strengthening health systems:** The goal is to guarantee the provision of health care to the underserved and those living in poverty. This is done by increasing the number of trained health-care providers, encouraging adequate financing, providing available technology and pharmaceuticals, and collecting vital statistics.
4. **Harnessing research, information, and evidence:** The WHO gathers data to set norms and standards, articulates evidence-based policy options, and monitors the evolving global heath situation.
5. **Enhancing partnerships:** The WHO works with many partners, both governmental and nongovernmental,

and encourages these partners to align with the WHO agenda and the individual country priorities using the best technical guidelines and published EBP.

6. **Improving performance:** The agencies continue to do quality assurance to make sure the staff are motivated and rewarded by their work and meet the performance criteria at local and international levels.

The WHO is a large organization with a budget for 2006–2007 of US$3.3 billion. Of this amount, just over one-quarter comes from regular dues from the WHO's member states, whereas more than 70% is money that countries, agencies, and other partners give to the WHO voluntarily. The primary publication from the WHO is the *World Health Report,* which is useful in understanding current global health, in referencing current statistics, and in helping to make policy and funding decisions.[24] Other publications include *World Health Statistics,* the *International Classification of Disease,* and its journal *Bulletin of the World Health Organization.*

The Pan American Health Organization

The Pan American Health Organization, started more than 100 years ago, is an international public health agency working to improve health and living standards of the countries of the Americas. It joined with the WHO when the WHO was created in 1946 and is now part of the UN system. There are 36 member states from the Americas. Accomplishments include the eradication of small pox in 1973 and of polio in the Americas in 1994. Their current work focuses on decreasing infant mortality, fighting against the use of tobacco, and raising concern about prevention of the noncommunicable diseases.[25]

World Bank

The World Bank is a source of financial and technical assistance to developing countries around the world. It is not a bank in the traditional sense. It is made up of two institutions, the International Bank for Reconstruction and Development and the International Development Association, both owned by the 187 member countries. The money is loaned to poor countries on positive terms not available in commercial markets. In 2010, the World Bank's focus was on helping countries achieve the MDGs. The World Bank notes that its mission is to help people help themselves by providing resources, sharing knowledge, and building capacity. World Bank goals are to build capacity, create infrastructure, develop financial systems, and combat corruption. In 2009, it provided $46.9 billion for 303 diverse projects all over the world.[26]

Bilateral Organizations

Bilateral organizations in general represent a single government that gives aid to developing countries. Examples of this type of organization in the United States include USAID and Centers for Disease Control and Prevention (CDC). Each of the major industrialized countries has similar organizations within their government structure. Their efforts are usually directed toward developing countries, and for political and historical reasons some of the governments concentrate their aid in specific countries or regions.[20]

U.S. Agency for International Development

The U.S. government, through the USAID, is committed to global health and is determined to prevent suffering, save lives, and help families in the developing world. USAID provides resources to improve the quality, availability, and use of essential health services. It provides resources for field programs in child and maternal health, reproductive health, and in communicable diseases such as HIV/AIDS, malaria, and TB. It also encourages research and innovations to develop and transfer new technology to the field. The requested budget for 2014 was $20.4 billion.[27]

Top priorities have long included: (1) child immunizations—more than 100 million children receive a basic set each year; (2) nutrition—malnutrition has been reduced by 15%; and (3) prenatal care and safe motherhood. Over the past 20 years, the United States has committed more than $6 billion in support through USAID's global child survival efforts. For example, almost a billion episodes of child diarrhea are treated with lifesaving oral rehydration therapy each year, reducing child deaths from diarrheal disease by more than 50%.[27]

Centers for Disease Control and Prevention

The overall mission of the CDC is to collaborate to create the expertise, information, and tools that people and communities need to protect their health through health promotion, prevention of disease, injury and disability, and preparedness for new health threats. The CDC has established global health goals (Box 13-2) and provides information relevant to global health on its Web site. It has become a leader in promoting public health, protecting the United States, and supporting the *Healthy People* goal of "healthy people in a healthy world." The CDC focuses on preventing and controlling communicable and noncommunicable diseases; responds to international disasters; and builds global health capacity by training epidemiologists, laboratory scientists, and public health managers.[27]

BOX 13–2	Centers for Disease Control and Prevention (CDC) Global Health Goals

CDC leverages its core strengths to advance four overarching global health goals:
1. Improving the health and well-being of people around the world
2. Improving capabilities for preparing for and responding to infectious diseases and emerging health threats
3. Building country public health capacity
4. Maximizing organizational capacity

Source: See reference 29.

Global Health Center

The *Global Health Initiative* is a new initiative in the Global Health Center introduced by President Obama in 2009. The total U.S. investment for 2009 to 2015 was $63 billion, a 33% increase in spending, to help partner countries improve health outcomes through strengthened health systems.[28] The focus is on the most vulnerable, including women and girls, and gender equality along with six other core principles (Box 13-3). The programs include efforts to protect communities against communicable disease, saving the lives of mothers and children, and creating an AIDS-free generation. The outcome measures specifically target reductions in death and disease. There is a fundamental emphasis on the principles that reflect an effort to assist countries in meeting the MDGs by 2015.[29]

Nongovernmental Organizations

Nongovernmental organizations (NGOs) are voluntary groups organized at the local, national, or international level to provide service and humanitarian relief, advocacy, development, and sustainable programs, and to monitor policies and provide information. NGOs provide at least 20% of all aid to developing countries that includes, among other activities, direct health services in the country. There are more than 40,000 operating international NGOs, many very small and often affiliated with a religious organization. Some examples of the larger NGOs include CARE, Project Hope, Catholic Relief Society, International Committee of the Red Cross, Médecins Sans Frontières (Doctors Without Borders), and International Red Cross and Red Crescent Movement.[21] Several NGOs have put health in their mission and developed objectives to promote health as part of their work.

CARE

One of the largest and leading humanitarian organizations, CARE fights global poverty and supports primary

BOX 13–3	The U.S. Global Health Initiative (GHI)

Focusing on Women, Girls, and Gender Equity

This principle aims to address gender imbalances related to health, promote the empowerment of women and girls, and improve health outcomes for individuals, families, and communities.

Country Ownership

Country ownership challenges the U.S. government, recipient nations, and donor countries alike to work tirelessly to create sustainable health systems that are eventually owned, managed, and operated by the host government and its people.

Health Systems Strengthening

Weak health systems are often identified as the binding, or rate-limiting, constraint to further progress.

Promoting Global Health Partnership

Partnership relationships can be an integral part of reaching objectives since not one donor, organization, or partner country can address all health needs.

Integration

The integration of health sector activities with activities in other sectors—such as water and sanitation, education, food security, agriculture, economic growth, microfinance, and democracy and governance—can achieve high-yield gains for health.

Research and Innovation

Achievement of the GHI goals requires innovative translation of investments in health research into real and measurable population-level health outcomes. GHI encourages innovation along the scientific continuum, reflected in the full range of U.S. government-funded research.

Improve Metrics, Monitoring, and Evaluation

Monitoring and evaluation should be incorporated throughout the program process, beginning with the assessment of needs and program planning through routine monitoring of implementation with a robust evaluation agenda.

Source: See reference 28.

health care. Founded in 1945 to provide relief to European survivors of World War II, CARE is trusted for its compassion and generosity to millions. It has evolved over the last half century to meet the changing needs of the world. Much of the focus of its current programs is on women. Its reasoning is that if its can help the women, the women will help both their families and the community. The core of the programs promotes basic education, prevents the spread of HIV, improves water and sanitation, expands economic opportunities, and protects the environment. CARE also provides humanitarian relief to populations that have experienced wars and natural disasters.[30]

CARE has supported more than 800 poverty-fighting projects in 72 countries and has reached more than 59 million people. It not only deals with the obvious problems but also looks for the root causes so people can solve these problems and become self-sufficient. The agency advocates for global responsibility.[30]

Catholic Relief Service

Catholic Relief Services, like CARE, was founded at the end of World War II to provide relief to European survivors. These services have also evolved and now the organization provides services to more than 100 million people in more than 100 countries. The organization was founded by Catholic bishops in the United States and is a religiously affiliated NGO. Although its service is based on the social teachings of the Catholic Church, it serves all people based only on need and not on religion or race or ethnicity. Its key areas of service globally are hunger prevention, emergency aid, education, health promotion, and peace.[31] For example, in one of the many countries in Africa in which Catholic Relief Service works, it provides a wide array of services including HIV/AIDS services, agriculture, microfinancing, water and sanitation, partnership building, and emergency preparedness.[32]

Achieving the Millennium Development Goals

The UN has continued to review the global process to help evaluate the progress toward attaining each of the eight MDGs, with a target date of 2015.[20] Under each goal, there are targets and indicators such as the target under MDG 5 of reducing maternal mortality ratio by 75% (Table 13-1).[33] These outcomes are globally aggregated and do not serve as a measure of progress in individual countries, with progress toward reaching the

TABLE 13–1	Millennium Goals With MDG Targets and Selected Examples of Indicators
Millennium Development Goals (MDGs) *Goals and Targets (from the Millennium Declaration)*	*Indicators for Monitoring Progress*
Goal 1: Eradicate extreme poverty and hunger	
Target 1.A: Halve, between 1990 and 2015, the proportion of people whose income is less than one dollar a day	1.1 Proportion of population below $1 (PPP) per day 1.2 Poverty gap ratio
Target 1.B: Achieve full and productive employment and decent work for all, including women and young people	1.3 Proportion of employed people living below $1 (PPP) per day
Target 1.C: Halve, between 1990 and 2015, the proportion of people who suffer from hunger	1.4 Prevalence of underweight children under 5 years of age 1.5 Proportion of population below minimum level of dietary energy consumption
Goal 2: Achieve universal primary education	
Target 2.A: Ensure that, by 2015, children everywhere, boys and girls alike, will be able to complete a full course of primary schooling	2.1 Net enrolment ratio in primary education 2.2 Proportion of pupils starting grade 1 who reach last grade of primary
Goal 3: Promote gender equality and empower women	
Target 3.A: Eliminate gender disparity in primary and secondary education, preferably by 2005, and in all levels of education no later than 2015	3.1 Ratios of girls to boys in primary, secondary and tertiary education
Goal 4: Reduce child mortality	
Target 4.A: Reduce by two-thirds, between 1990 and 2015, the under-5 mortality rate	4.1 Under-5 mortality rate 4.2 Infant mortality rate
Goal 5: Improve maternal health	
Target 5.A: Reduce by three-quarters, between 1990 and 2015, the maternal mortality ratio	5.1 Maternal mortality ratio 5.2 Proportion of births attended by skilled health personnel
Target 5.B: Achieve, by 2015, universal access to reproductive health	5.3 Contraceptive prevalence rate 5.4 Adolescent birth rate

Continued

TABLE 13–1	Millennium Goals With MDG Targets and Selected Examples of Indicators—cont'd

Millennium Development Goals (MDGs) *Goals and Targets (from the Millennium Declaration)*	*Indicators for Monitoring Progress*
Goal 6: Combat HIV/AIDS, malaria, and other diseases	
Target 6.A: Have halted by 2015 and begun to reverse the spread of HIV/AIDS	6.1 HIV prevalence among population aged 15 to 24 years 6.2 Proportion of population aged 15 to 24 years with comprehensive correct knowledge of HIV/AIDS
Target 6.B: Achieve, by 2010, universal access to treatment for HIV/AIDS for all those who need it	6.3 Proportion of population with advanced HIV infection with access to antiretroviral drugs
Target 6.C: Have halted by 2015 and begun to reverse the incidence of malaria and other major diseases	6.4 Incidence and death rates associated with malaria 6.5 Incidence, prevalence and death rates associated with tuberculosis
Goal 7: Ensure environmental sustainability	
Target 7.A: Integrate the principles of sustainable development into country policies and programmes and reverse the loss of environmental resources **Target 7.B:** Reduce biodiversity loss, achieving, by 2010, a significant reduction in the rate of loss	7.1 Proportion of land area covered by forest 7.2 CO_2 emissions, total, per capita and per $1 GDP (PPP) 7.3 Proportion of terrestrial and marine areas protected 7.4 Proportion of species threatened with extinction
Target 7.C: Halve, by 2015, the proportion of people without sustainable access to safe drinking water and basic sanitation	7.5 Proportion of population using an improved drinking water source 7.6 Proportion of population using an improved sanitation facility
Target 7.D: By 2020, to have achieved a significant improvement in the lives of at least 100 million slum dwellers	7.7 Proportion of urban population living in slums*
Goal 8: Develop a global partnership for development	
Target 8.A: Develop further an open, rule-based, predictable, nondiscriminatory trading and financial system. Includes a commitment to good governance, development and poverty reduction—both nationally and internationally	*Some of the indicators listed below are monitored separately for the least developed countries (LDCs), Africa, landlocked developing countries and small island developing States.* **Official Development Assistance (ODA)**
Target 8.B: Address the special needs of the least developed countries. Includes tariff and quota free access for the least developed countries' exports; enhanced programme of debt relief for heavily indebted poor countries (HIPC) and cancellation of official bilateral debt; and more generous ODA for countries committed to poverty reduction **Target 8.C:** Address the special needs of landlocked developing countries and small island developing States (through the Programme of Action for the Sustainable Development of Small Island Developing States and the outcome of the twenty-second special session of the General Assembly) **Target 8.D:** Deal comprehensively with the debt problems of developing countries through national and international measures in order to make debt sustainable in the long term	8.1 Net ODA, total and to the least developed countries, as percentage of ORGANISATION FOR ECONOMIC CO-OPERATION AND DEVELOPMENT/ Development Assistance Committee (OECD/DAC) donors' gross national income 8.2 Proportion of total bilateral, sector-allocable ODA of OECD/DAC donors to basic social services (basic education, primary health care, nutrition, safe water and sanitation) 8.3 ODA received in small island developing States as a proportion of their gross national incomes **Market access** 8.4 Proportion of total developed country imports (by value and excluding arms) from developing countries and least developed countries, admitted free of duty **Debt sustainability** 8.5 Total number of countries that have reached their HIPC decision points and number that have reached their HIPC completion points (cumulative) 8.6 Debt relief committed under HIPC and MDRI Initiatives 8.7 Debt service as a percentage of exports of goods and services

TABLE 13–1	Millennium Goals With MDG Targets and Selected Examples of Indicators—cont'd

Millennium Development Goals (MDGs)

Goals and Targets (from the Millennium Declaration)	Indicators for Monitoring Progress
Target 8.E: In cooperation with pharmaceutical companies, provide access to affordable essential drugs in developing countries	8.8 Proportion of population with access to affordable essential drugs on a sustainable basis
Target 8.F: In cooperation with the private sector, make available the benefits of new technologies, especially information and communications	8.9 Fixed telephone lines per 100 inhabitants 8.10 Mobile cellular subscriptions per 100 inhabitants 8.11 Internet users per 100 inhabitants

Source: See reference 35.

*For monitoring country poverty trends, indicators based on national poverty lines should be used, where available. The actual proportion of people living in slums is measured by a proxy, represented by the urban population living in households with at least one of the four characteristics: (1) lack of access to improved water supply; (2) lack of access to improved sanitation; (3) overcrowding (three or more persons per room); and (4) dwellings made of nondurable material.

goals varying by region and country.[34] The goals are all interdependent and each goal speaks directly to a health issue, such as reducing child mortality, or relies on a healthy population to be able to reach the goal, such as achieving universal primary education. These goals are for the entire international community, but there is also an allowance for specific country objectives to be included and tailored to meet the country's development needs, such as the addition of a ninth goal of national security added to the Afghanistan MDGs.[34]

Progress toward reaching the goals was uneven, as of 2013. Some countries achieved many of the goals, whereas others were not on track to realize any.[34,35] The Inter-agency and Expert Group on MDG Indicators (IAEG) regularly reviews and discusses countries' needs in building capacity for the production and analysis of MDGs and development indicators, work with national statistical offices to identify priorities in capacity building and to facilitate the coordination of technical assistance activities, and provides periodic reports. Data are analyzed at the global and country levels.[33]

In the 2013 report on the MDGs, the UN provided evidence that significant progress had been made in improving health and reducing mortality, with several MDG targets met or were close to being met, but in some areas it recommended that "accelerated progress and bolder action" was needed to achieve the MDGs by 2015.[35] Despite the achievements at the global level in meeting the MDGs, variation occurred between countries based on a number of issues including resource availability, conflict, and the structure used to support the implementation of evidence-based interventions.[34–36]

It is clear that there is a synergism and interrelatedness of the goals. Countries working with all the goals at the same time have produced better results than the

countries emphasizing one goal at a time. It is also clear that different regions of the world have different outcomes and different successes. Those areas that have recently been in conflict or are now in conflict, 40% in sub-Saharan Africa, in general have less political and social structure and aren't performing as well with the MDGs.[34] Several external issues have affected the achievement of the MDGs. High food prices and the international/economic crisis had an impact on Goal 1, to eradicate extreme poverty and hunger. Climate changes have also affected food production. In addition, rapid urbanization in the developing world stresses the social infrastructure.[37] In the 2013 MDG report, specific progress was evident in meeting a number of the goals. For example, the mortality rate for malaria had dropped 25% and it was projected that the tuberculosis infection rate would be halved by 2015. It was also projected that the goal of halving the hunger rate was within reach. In addition, the mortality rate for children under the age of 5 had dropped by 41% and the HIV infection rate had declined.[35] Thus, it is apparent that this global commitment to improving health has had an impact. The WHO provided a summary of the key facts related to the MDGs in 2013 (Box 13-4).

Goal 1: Eradicate Extreme Poverty and Hunger

For MDG 1, achievements by 2013 included halving the poverty rates, yet the global recession widened the global job gap. In addition, although there has been progress in combating hunger, 1 in 8 persons still goes to bed hungry.[35] **Food security** is defined as continuous access to sufficient, safe, and nutritious food, and is essential to meet the second target.[38] The commitment to improving food security remains an issue for the global community.

BOX 13–4	**Millennium Development Goals: Key Facts, 2013**

- Globally, the number of deaths of children under 5 years of age fell from 12.6 million in 1990 to 6.6 million in 2012.
- In developing countries, the percentage of underweight children under 5 years old dropped from 28% in 1990 to 17% in 2012.
- Whereas the proportion of births attended by a skilled health worker has increased globally, fewer than 50% of births are attended in the WHO African Region.
- Globally, new HIV infections declined by 33% between 2001 and 2012.
- Existing cases of tuberculosis are declining, along with deaths among HIV-negative tuberculosis cases.
- In 2010, the world met the United Nations Millennium Development Goals target on access to safe drinking water, as measured by the proxy indicator of access to improved drinking-water sources, but more needs to be done to achieve the sanitation target.

Source: See reference 51.

■ EVIDENCE-BASED PRACTICE
Improving Nutrition of Children

Practice Statement: Interventions are needed at the population level that will reduce malnutrition and stunting in children.

Targeted Outcome: Millennium Developmental Goal to reduce by half the proportion of people who suffer from hunger

Evidence to Support: In a study in six central states in Mexico, families participating in a large-scale, incentive-based welfare program were randomly surveyed. The program provided participating families with:

- Fortified nutrition supplements for the children and pregnant and lactating women
- Nutrition education, health care, and cash transfers, of which one part was associated with school attendance of the children

The low-income rural infants and children participating in the program who received the nutritional intervention had better growth and lower rates of anemia. The information was used to improve this large-scale program to provide the intervention to 4.5 million families in Mexico.

Source: Rivera, J., Sotres-Alvarez, D., Habicht, J., Shamah, T., & Villalpando, S. (2004). Impact of the Mexican Program for education, health, and nutrition (Progresa) on rates of growth and anemia in infants and young children: A randomized effectiveness study. *JAMA, 291*(21), 2563-2570.

Goal 2: Achieve Universal Primary Education

The UN reported that progress has been made in reaching this goal, with the number of children out of school declining by almost half (from 102 million to 57 million) (Fig. 13-2). Despite this accomplishment, the UN noted that barriers to education continue to exist, with some countries denying children their right to education.[35] This denial was highlighted by the young girl Malala from Afghanistan, who at the age of 15 was shot because of her outspoken support for educating girls. She began to promote education for girls and to detail her life under the Taliban through a BBC-supported blog. On October 9, 2012, as she boarded her school bus, a gunman asked for Malala and then shot her. She survived the attack and has gone on to write a book and continues to promote education for women and girls.[37]

Goal 3: Promote Gender Equality and Empower Women

By 2013, progress had been made in achieving gender equality, but further progress was needed. For example, one of the indicators for achieving this goal is primary education of girls, yet out of 130 countries only two countries had achieved the targeted levels of education. Other indicators for this goal included increasing wage-earning jobs for women and increasing women's representation in governments. The UN reported that in 2013,

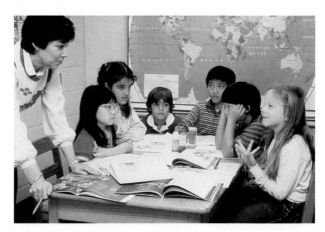

Figure 13-2 School-age children. *(Rudd, K., & Kocisko, D. [2014]. Pediatric nursing: The critical components of nursing care. F.A. Davis Company, Philadelphia.)*

women held 40 out of every 100 nonagricultural jobs and only 20% of seats in parliaments were held by women (Fig. 13-3).[35]

Goal 4: Reduce Child Mortality

In MICs and LICs, children under 5 years of age generally die from preventable conditions and most die from one of six causes: diarrhea, HIV/AIDS, malaria, measles, neonatal causes, and/or pneumonia. Malnutrition increases the risk of the child dying from any one of the above conditions. About 40% of the deaths occur in the first month of life because of a preterm delivery, sepsis, and birth asphyxia. Pneumonia (19%), diarrhea (18%), and malaria (8%) are the areas that need the most intervention for the older children younger than 5 years of age.[38] Despite gains made in reaching this goal, further action is needed. Although the mortality rate for children under 5 dropped by 41% between 1990 and 2011, this fell short of the target for 2015 of a reduction in the rate by two-thirds. The majority of the deaths occur in LICs during the first month of life[35] (see Chapter 18 for more in-depth discussion of maternal and infant health).

Goal 5: Improve Maternal Health

Maternal mortality is a measure of the death of women during pregnancy, childbirth, or the 6 weeks after delivery (see Chapter 18). As with child mortality, progress had occurred by 2013, with the maternal mortality ratio dropping by 47% since 1990. This fell short of the 2015 target of reducing the ratio by three-quarters.[35]

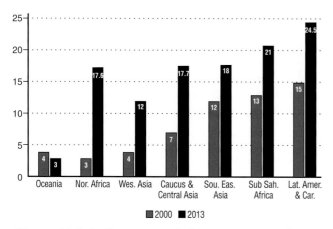

Figure 13-3 Millennium Goal Three: Proportion of seats held by women in single or lower houses of national parliaments, 2000 and 2013 (percentage). *(From the United Nations Development Programme. [2013]. The Millennium Developmental Goals report 2013 [p. 22]. New York, NY: United Nations. Retrieved from www.un.org/en/development/desa/publications/mdgs-report-2013.html.)*

The causes of mortality are preventable, especially if there is no delay in seeking care. One of the ways to understand the lack of seeking treatment is the "three delays." Developed in the early 1990s, the framework has helped explain some of the decision-making process. The three delays are points at which access to care is delayed, and that lack of care leads to maternal death:[38–40] (1) deciding to seek care, (2) arriving at the health center, and (3) receiving adequate care once at the health center.[41–43] The cost of the transport, the cost of the health care, and the quality of the care can influence seeking care.

1. **Delay Deciding to Seek Care.** Women with limited resources will hesitate to seek care if they know they cannot afford it. One woman said that for her to seek care she would have to sell her goat, the only family investment, and the other children would then suffer. She died in childbirth.[38] Pregnant women who do not know the danger signs of pregnancy may delay seeking care, thinking the problem is not serious enough. Teaching the community the danger signs of pregnancy and helping them organize an evacuation plan when there is a problem can assist in decreasing the first two delays.[38]

2. **Delay Arriving at the Health Center.** Significant delays in arriving at the health center can occur when the woman must walk or be carried 5 to 10 miles to the local health center on narrow paths, down mountains, across rivers without bridges, and along poorly constructed roads. Cell phones have helped with communication to the health center even in very rural communities. This can decrease the second delay if transport can be sent to meet the woman on the passable roads, and can decrease the third delay because the doctors and nurses will be expecting her.[38]

3. **Delay Receiving Adequate Care at the Health Center.** Once the woman has arrived at the hospital, if she cannot pay for care she probably will not be seen. One woman arrived at a hospital hemorrhaging with part of a retained placenta. Without NGO monetary intervention, she would have died. The NGO arranged for a blood transfusion to be brought to the site, provided money for the gasoline to run the generator to power the surgical suite, and paid for the surgical supplies necessary to save her life.[38]

Goal 6: Combat HIV/AIDS, Malaria, and Other Diseases

In 2013, there was a reported decline in new cases of HIV infections. In addition, access to antiretroviral therapy was approaching the 2015 target. However, knowledge related to prevention of HIV transmission remained low. From 1995 to 2011, treatment for TB has saved 20 million lives, and in several areas of the globe the death rate was projected to be halved by 2015. Gains were made in reducing morbidity associated with malaria when 1.1 million deaths from malaria were averted, representing a 25% reduction in malaria deaths between 2000 and 2010.[35]

Goal 7: Ensure Environmental Sustainability

Environmental sustainability based on the MDG 7 refers to access to potable water, reduction in slum dwelling, and reversal of the loss of environmental resources.[35] Access to water sources, sanitation facilities, durable housing, and adequate living space improved for 200 million slum dwellers, exceeding the target of 100 million. Despite these gains, environmental sustainability continued to be a problem. Specific concerns included acceleration in carbon dioxide (CO_2) emissions, deforestation, and diminished yields in marine fishing due to diminishing stocks. On the positive side, more land and marine areas were under protection, but the extinction rate for animals has increased.[35]

Of particular concern globally is the issue of access to potable water. Fresh water is a finite resource and is essential for life, not only for drinking, but also for agriculture, for animals, and for hygiene. Infant mortality drops precipitously when there is a clean supply of water. The waterborne diseases such as cholera, typhoid, hepatitis, and diarrhea diminish as the clean water supply increases. Purifying water has been shown to decrease general mortality, not just waterborne diseases but also pneumonia, heart disease, and TB.[44–46] The health dividends of safe water are enormous.

Water is a difficult resource for many people to access. Often, safe drinking water must be carried a long distance, on average 1 to 3 miles in India and Africa, where supplies are limited. Children and women walk to get the water in the developing world. For example, in the African country of Burkina Faso women carry 40 pounds of water on their heads, walking 1 to 2 and a half hours daily, 300 days a year. Individuals in hot climates require a minimum of 7.5 liters per day (± 8 quarts/2 gallons) for ingestion (cooking and drinking).[44] Placing a water standpipe in a village can reduce time needed to get water from 2 hours to 30 minutes.[45]

Another concern is improved sanitation. Despite the gains in access to sanitation facilities, continued improvement is needed to help promote health. Without proper sewerage, disposal infections such as schistosomiasis, trachoma, viral hepatitis, cholera, and those caused by nematodes are easily spread.[46] Even if the MDG is reached for sanitation, 25% of the world's population will still have no basic sanitation. One of the biggest challenges is to provide adequate sanitation to the very rapidly growing megacities in the developing world. With much of the growth occurring in the slums and squatter areas of these cities, there is limited or no sanitation and limited waste removal.[46]

Another environmental issue in the LICs is the increased environmental pollution from burning biomass fuels for cooking in enclosed or unventilated space. More than half of the world's population cooks over open fires, or they use traditional stoves that also emit high levels of pollutants. These pollutants have the biggest impact on children younger than age 5 years whose airways are still developing, causing acute lower respiratory pneumonia. It was found to be responsible for more than a quarter of all deaths in children aged 1 to 4 years in India. The time that the child spent indoors and the proximity to the fire increased the risk, making girls more susceptible.[47] Currently, improved stoves have been developed to burn fuel more efficiently and they have incorporated a chimney or flue for ventilation. In Honduras, women using the improved stove reported fewer respiratory symptoms, but the actual health impact was more difficult to measure.[48] In Africa, they also found that better stove ventilation was a significant means for decreasing lower respiratory infections in younger children.[49] A study done in Bangladesh suggests that if cleaner fuel cannot be afforded, then fuel-efficient stoves should be used, the kitchen should be located peripheral to the house, the kitchen should be made of permeable materials to allow for ventilation, and a chimney tall enough to allow smoke dispersion over a large area should be selected. Another suggestion was that women in the same household should rotate the cooking role to decrease exposure.[50]

Goal 8: Develop a Global Partnership for Development

NGOs, the private sector, and a number of developing countries are becoming increasingly significant sources of development assistance. However, bilateral aid and contributions to multilateral development institutions will need to increase to meet the MDGs by 2015. Progress did occur with the debt service to revenue ratio of all LICs at 3.1% in 2011. Other achievements included an improvement in duty-free market access, with a positive impact on LIC exports. However, in 2012 less aid money was available, negatively affecting LICs.[35]

Another issue related to development is access to medications. Pharmaceuticals are one of the leading resource limitations in many of the clinical facilities in the LICs. According to the WHO, in 2010 in 44 LICs the public sector had only 44% and the private sector 66% of the generic medicine on the essential medicine list. Without the medicine, the patient is forced to do without or to purchase in the private sector at 630% more than the international reference price.[51]

Post-2015 Developmental Framework

By 2012, the UN began to focus on a post-2015 developmental framework (Box 13-5). The challenge was to build on the original MDG framework within the context of a changing world.[52] Challenges that emerged include sustainability, inequalities, inter- and intranational conflict, food security, and political structures.[50,53] The idea presented by the UN was to establish **Sustainable Development Goals (SDGs)** that preserve the benefits of the MDG framework and merge with the post-2015 agenda. The SDGs grew out of the 2012 Rio+20 sustainable development conference that took place in Rio de Janeiro, Brazil. According to the UN, it was the largest UN conference ever held.[52] The result was a document titled *The Future We Want*. To develop the SDGs, the UN put together a 30-member open working group of the General Assembly in the beginning of 2013. The open working group was tasked with preparing a proposal on the SDGs. Post-2015, the WHO will begin the process of implementing the SDGs and tracking progress in meeting goals using methods similar to what was done with the MDGs.[54]

Global Health Challenges

Global health at the beginning of the 21st century is faced with numerous challenges. Providing optimal health to the world's population is impeded by various issues including human rights and differing governmental priorities and resources. Organizations such as the WHO seek to provide guidance from a global perspective that helps to foster collaboration between countries and provide a united front to protect human rights.

Human Rights

The *Universal Declaration of Human Rights,* specifically article 25, adopted by the General Assembly of the UN in 1948, provides the framework for global human rights and equity in health (see Chapter 7 for a more thorough discussion). The Alma-Ata Declaration, as suggested in the discussion of primary health care in this chapter, also supports the idea that health care is a human right of all people in the world.[19] However, as has been pointed out in this chapter and in Chapter 7, there are still vast differences in the amount of health care received and health outcomes achieved among LICs, MICs, and HICs.

Globalization has had a direct impact on country health systems and social determinants of health by increasing the inequity of health. Currently, globalization is benefiting the more developed countries with increased concentration of wealth. There is a growing gap between the best and the worst off countries. There are several disadvantages for the poorest countries in the global market with increase in poverty in these countries. These include growing inequality between skilled and unskilled workers, gender inequality in the workforce, and marginalization of women. Another major health issue facing the world today is lack of access to safe water because it is treated as a commodity, one that the very poor cannot afford. Nutrition is a concern not only in LICs but in MICs and HICs. Changes in diet have occurred worldwide with the proliferation of Western-style fast food and the move to urban areas. This has contributed to a higher prevalence of obesity and chronic noncommunicable diseases such as hypertension and diabetes. In addition, changes in tariffs and public revenue have decreased the government money available for health, education, water, and sanitation.[55]

BOX 13–5   Sustainable Development Goals: What We Want

The document calls for a wide range of actions, among many other points, including:
- Launching a process to establish sustainable development goals
- Detailing how the green economy can be used as a tool to achieve sustainable development
- Strengthening the UN Environment Programme and establishing a new forum for sustainable development
- Promoting corporate sustainability reporting measures
- Taking steps to go beyond GDP to assess the well-being of a country
- Developing a strategy for sustainable development financing
- Adopting a framework for tackling sustainable consumption and production
- Focusing on improving gender equality
- Stressing the need to engage civil society and incorporate science into policy
- Recognizing the importance of voluntary commitments on sustainable development

Source: See reference 54.

The human right to health means that everyone has the right to the highest attainable standard of physical and mental health, which includes access to all medical services, sanitation, adequate food, decent housing, healthy working conditions, and a clean environment.[55] The human right to health care means that hospitals, clinics, medicines, and doctors' services must be accessible, available, acceptable, and of good quality for everyone, on an equitable basis, where and when needed. Health care must be affordable and comprehensive for everyone, and physically accessible where and when needed. The ability of each nation to meet its obligation to the health of its population is shrinking as globalization grows. The policies, practices, and operation of many of the large international organizations can produce more power than that of a national government, limiting the government in its ability to protect and promote human rights of its citizens.[52]

Paul Farmer, a physician who has worked extensively in LICs such as Haiti, Peru, and Rwanda, explains that the lack of health care in LICs with heavy disease burdens poses an ethical and moral dilemma. In alignment with MDG 6, he reasons that reliable and reasonable treatments for the three major killers—tuberculosis, malaria, and HIV/AIDS—should be made available to everyone, regardless of where they live. The challenge for health-care providers in countries with limited access to treatment resources is in reconciling diagnosing individuals with these health problems with not being able to provide treatment, often restricting the availability of options to palliative care despite the existence of treatments that can result in a reduction in mortality and morbidity.[56]

Availability of Health-Care Providers

Another challenge is the availability of an adequate health-care provider workforce. Many LICs have a poor infrastructure for health services and have limited numbers of skilled doctors and nurses. In sub-Saharan Africa in 2010, WHO, with support from the President's Emergency Plan for AIDS Relief (PEPFAR) and other U.S. agencies, provided grants to African higher education institutions to dramatically increase the numbers of physicians educated to better meet needs of individual African countries. PEPFAR continues to work at the global level with the ultimate goal of creating an AIDS-free generation.[57] For those countries that do act to provide education aimed at increasing their number of health-care providers, they are met with the challenge of keeping them at home. There is evidence of a significant brain drain among these doctors and nurses to other countries

where the workplace and income are better, leaving a situation where it is incredibly difficult to increase capacity. With skilled nurses leaving, there is even more limited primary health care, fewer vaccines given, and less-skilled deliveries and care for newborns.[58]

The movement of health personnel is occurring internally within Africa with nurses and physicians moving from rural areas to urban settings. There is also a loss of health-care providers who emigrate to HICs such as the United Kingdom and United States, where the aging population is creating an increased demand for nurses.

There have been several suggestions on how to stop brain drain. For example, if the nursing education programs provided relevant nursing education that taught the local endemic diseases, provided opportunities for the nurses to gain experience as students in the rural areas, taught the students best practices with limited resources, and recruited students from rural areas who would return home to work, LICs might be able to retain more nurses.[58]

Communicable Diseases, Noncommunicable Diseases, Injury, and Violence

Globally, the issue of communicable disease has come to the forefront (see Chapter 8). As noted above under achievements in MDG 6 (Combat HIV/AIDS, Malaria, and Other Diseases), communicable diseases continue to be an issue, especially for sub-Saharan Africa.[35] Communicable diseases produce a heavy global toll, with 35.3 million people living with HIV/AIDS in 2012,[59] and 8.6 million people newly infected with tuberculosis.[60] In addition, there were an estimated 660,000 malaria deaths in 2010 and an estimated 219 million cases.[61] These communicable diseases are also concentrated in the tropical climate zones, mainly in sub-Saharan Africa, South and Central America, and Southeast Asia.

In contrast, the noncommunicable diseases such as stroke, cancer, heart disease, diabetes, and chronic respiratory diseases are the actual leading causes of mortality in the world. Of the 35 million people who die each year of a noncommunicable disease, it is surprising that 80% of these deaths occur in LICs and MICs. These are the same countries that experience the heavy toll of communicable disease. This epidemic of noncommunicable diseases is less visible, but has a profound impact on the economies of these MICs and LICs, with significant impact on premature death and disability and decreased economic output.[62]

As a result of the decrease in maternal and child mortality, the distribution of deaths by age group in LICs and MICs is shifting from younger populations to older adults.[60,61] In many sub-Saharan countries in Africa, half the population was under 16 years and the percentage older than 60 was very small. With a continuing major decline anticipated in the mortality and disability from communicable, maternal, perinatal, and nutritional disorders, the population pyramids will shift toward having proportionately fewer in the younger age groups and a higher percentage in the middle and older age group (see Chapter 20). As the proportion of populations in older age groups increases, there will be a transition from communicable diseases to noncommunicable diseases. Other factors that are associated with the increase in noncommunicable diseases in MICs and LICs include the increase in tobacco use, an increased consumption of high-fat foods, a decrease in exercise, and an increase in obesity.[62]

Other patterns of change in health and disease include the increasing levels of injury as countries industrialize as well as experience increased morbidity and mortality related to violence, especially in regions in conflict (see Chapter 12). All of this provides a continuing challenge to public health professionals including PHNs. The cause of death disparity between the poorest and the richest in the world shows that the poorest are still experiencing considerably higher rates of morbidity and mortality associated with communicable disease[62–64] and the shift to provide the limited resources for noncommunicable disease should be done thoughtfully to avoid creating increased inequity among the very poor.[64]

Global Burden of Disease

As is apparent from the MDGs, the health of individuals and families affects all aspects of a country's development. For example, if a member of a family in sub-Saharan Africa becomes infected with malaria, the family must provide sick care, money for diagnoses and treatment, and may lose wages as a result of work time lost by the caregiver and/or the sick individual. As discussed in detail in Chapter 9, public health science provides methods for measuring this impact of a health problem on a population using indicators such as monetary cost, mortality, and morbidity, and refers to this as the burden of disease. As recalled, the **burden of disease** is defined by the WHO as "the total significance of disease for society beyond the immediate cost of treatment. It is measured in years of life lost to ill health as the difference between total life expectancy and disability-adjusted life expectancy."[63] To help measure the burden of disease,

statisticians calculate the **disability-adjusted life years (DALY)** that takes into account not only mortality but also the morbidity and the disability associated with a disease or risk factor. DALY is defined as a measurement of the gap that exists between those with the disease and the ideal population that lives to an advanced age free of disability and disease. It is an important measure of population health. Calculation of DALYs allows for the comparison of disease burden across countries and helps to predict the impact of an intervention aimed at preventing the disease.[66] In the 1990s, the WHO began the Global Burden of Disease Project that has helped to evaluate the burden of disease from a global perspective.[67] These data help evaluate the impact of interventions and identify areas for action (see Chapter 9 for additional information and how to calculate DALY).

Neglected Diseases

The neglected tropical diseases such as dengue fever, cholera, and shigellosis receive less attention in the global health arena, but they are still deadly. These "neglected diseases" sicken and kill more than a billion each year worldwide. Certain diseases that could be prevented receive less media attention than other diseases. In response, the Bill and Melinda Gates Foundation has a specific strategy related to neglected diseases with the stated goal: "to reduce the burden of neglected infectious diseases on the world's poorest people through targeted and effective control, elimination, and eradication efforts."[68] One example of a neglected disease is lymphatic filariasis, also known as elephantiasis. In 2012, more than 120 million people were infected with lymphatic filariasis.[69] Cholera is a neglected disease that got media attention during the Haiti earthquake. There are an estimated 3 to 5 million cases of cholera cases and as many as 120,000 deaths annually.[70] As another example, in 2012, there were more than 182,000 cases of leprosy.[71]

Pharmaceutical companies are not financially motivated to help combat these diseases through development of new drugs that are safe, effective, and affordable because the populations with the diseases are poor and have little ability to purchase these drugs. HICs that have substantial government research dollars do not have citizens with these diseases and the diseases remain low on pharmaceutical companies' research priority list. To help address the gap in resources needed and improve access to prevention and treatment, in 2013 the WHO adopted a resolution to address all 17 neglected tropical diseases.[72]

Leishmaniasis

Leishmaniasis is a parasitic disease caused by a single-celled protozoan called *Leishmania*. The disease is spread by infected sand flies. There are two common forms, cutaneous and visceral. Cutaneous leishmaniasis leads to severe, disfiguring skin lesions; the visceral form, also known as kala-azar or black fever, affects internal organs, especially the liver, spleen, and bone marrow.[73]

Leishmaniasis is prevalent in many countries but the biggest percentage occurs in Bangladesh, Brazil, India, Nepal, and Sudan. Many cases of the disease have been reported in the United States among troops returning from Iraq and Afghanistan. Leishmaniasis occurs in tropical rural areas and in poor urban areas where sand flies thrive in cracked walls and earthen floors, and breed in garbage piles. The disease frequently coexists with HIV/AIDS.[73]

Cutaneous leishmaniasis is diagnosed by the presenting symptoms. The disease starts as an initial solid red lump at the site of the sand fly bite, and slowly forms ulcers as the infection spreads. The infection can spread over large parts of the skin, especially in immune-suppressed people. Visceral leishmaniasis symptoms include high fever, loss of appetite, and severe weight loss. The disease can infect the bone marrow in advanced stages, leading to anemia, an enlarged spleen, and skin changes. Definitive diagnosis may require invasive procedures where tissue biopsies are done on affected organs.[73]

The first-line drugs for treatment of leishmaniasis are toxic as they contain metal antimony, and the second-line drugs are also dangerous. The drugs are administered intramuscularly or intravenously, which is problematic in resource-limited settings.

To improve treatment, there is need for non-invasive diagnostic tests suitable for use in resource-limited settings to ensure early detection of disease, fewer toxic drugs for treatment and prophylaxis, a vaccine to prevent the spread of disease, and environmental measures to control the sand fly.[73]

Chagas Disease

Chagas disease, also known as American trypanosomiasis, is a parasitic infection caused by *Trypanosoma cruzi*. The disease can be transmitted through feces of an infected triatomine bug, through blood transfusions, with organ transplant, and from a pregnant mother to the fetus. This communicable disease can cause destruction of the heart and digestive tract, and is the leading cause of chronic heart disease in the areas where it is most common.[73]

Although the triatone bugs are found in the Americas, the disease transmission rate and occurrence of Chagas disease is much higher in Central and South America and in Mexico because the bugs live in lower-quality housing in poor rural areas. Chagas disease affects 9 million people of all ages, both sexes, and state of health (healthy and unhealthy). However, there is increased risk in people whose immune systems are compromised, for example, HIV/AIDS or other noncommunicable diseases. With far-ranging travel and migration of people from endemic areas in the Americas, it is becoming necessary worldwide to prepare blood banks to screen blood donors for Chagas, perform donor and recipient screening for organ transplantation, screen women of child-bearing age who are at risk of having been infected and infecting their children, organize outpatient clinics to care for these patients, and train personnel to diagnose and treat Chagas disease. In the United States, Chagas disease is transmitted through blood transfusion, which has led to the screening of all donated blood for Chagas disease. There are approximately 390,000 infected people living in countries with no natural vector but the disease can spread through contaminated blood.[74]

During the acute phase of the disease, there may be swelling around the site of infection, and in infants it may cause severe illness and death. While many people remain asymptomatic throughout their lives, more than one-third of those infected develop debilitating fatal disease of the heart and intestinal tract. Diagnosis is possible in the acute phase with blood microscopy, but in the early phase there are few or no symptoms. In the chronic phase, the disease is difficult to diagnose because accurate diagnosis requires complicated blood tests.[74]

Treatment of Chagas disease is by two antiparasitic medications taken for several months. These medications can cause serious side effects and they are contraindicated for pregnant women and patients with liver or kidney disease. Because of the complications of the treatment, medical interventions focus on addressing the complications of Chagas disease such as cardiac arrhythmias or congestive heart failure.[74]

To improve treatment, there is a need to develop a vaccine to prevent infection, drugs with fewer side effects, drugs suitable for pregnant women, and drugs that can treat the chronic stage of the disease; improve screening of blood supplies and donated organs; and control the triatomine bugs by indoor spraying, use of bed nets, and improved housing.[74]

Dengue

Dengue, also known as "breaking bone fever," is a disease caused by one of four related viruses spread to humans through the bite of an infected *Aedes* mosquito. Infection with one version of the virus gives lifelong protection to the infected person from the particular virus but not from the other three. Dengue hemorrhagic fever is the most common serious complication of dengue, with a fatality rate of 20%, and is one of the leading causes of hospitalization and death among children in India. Dengue is endemic in more than 100 countries and it is estimated by the WHO that more than one-third of the world's population is at risk. The range of dengue disease has expanded because of climate change and increased international travel and trade. Cases of dengue in the United States have been attributed to travel in endemic areas. However, there have been isolated cases in the U.S. South. Dengue can infect anyone, once that person has been bitten by an infected *Aedes* mosquito, and evidence has shown that multiple infections increase a person's chance of development of dengue hemorrhagic fevcer.[75,76]

Diagnosis of dengue is made through its symptoms, including rapid development of high fever, joint pain, a rash, and intense headache. Death is rare if the disease does not develop to dengue hemorrhagic fever. There is no current treatment for dengue disease. There is need for faster specific diagnostic tests in locations where dengue hemorrhagic fever is suspected, development of a vaccine against the disease, and improved vector control strategies.[75]

Emerging and Reemerging Diseases

Emerging diseases such as H7N9, H1N1, SARS, HIV/AIDS, avian influenza ("bird flu"), and reemerging disease such as Ebola can be potentially deadly, especially when preventive measures, early detection, and treatment are not readily available. As globalization increases, the impact of these diseases on the economy, politics, health, and travel in the world takes on more meaning. Many of these diseases mutate from animals and become transmissible in humans, creating potentially dangerous situations; others that were once on the decline in humans have reemerged.[76-79]

Reasons for the emergence or reemergence of these diseases include the expansion of the growing human population into new areas, climate change, and globalization of trade. The increasing movement of animal species, civil wars, microbial evolution, and ecological disruption also increase the potential for new emerging diseases at an accelerated rate. Some of these diseases mutate as they spread around the world, rendering vaccines less effective. About 75% of the emerging diseases that affected humans since 1995 originated from animals (Table 13-2). Developing primary and secondary prevention for these diseases

TABLE 13–2	**Examples of Emerging Diseases Since 1973**		
Year	Microbe	Disease	Original Host
1977	Ebola virus	Ebola hemorrhagic fever	Bats
1977	*Legionella pneumophila*	Legionnaires' disease	Unknown
1977	Hantaan virus	Hemorrhagic fever with renal syndrome	Field rodents
1982	*Borrelia burgdorferi*	Lyme disease	Rodents
1983	Human immunodeficiency virus (HIV-1)	AIDS	Primates
1986	HIV-2	AIDS	Primates
1989	Hepatitis C	Parenterally transmitted non-A, non-B hepatitis	Primates
1997	Avian influenza virus (H5N1)	Highly pathological influenza	Chickens
1999	West Nile–like virus	Encephalitis	Birds
2003	Influenza A virus (H5N1)	Influenza	Birds
2003	SARS coronavirus	Severe acute respiratory syndrome (SARS)	Palm civets
2008	Influenza A virus (H1N1)	Influenza	Pigs
2013	Influenza A virus (H7N9)	Influenza	Birds

Sources: See references 76 and 77.

can be quite difficult and generally complex.[77,78] Because the emergence of new diseases is not predictable, it is very important that nurses and other health-care providers carefully monitor disease and focus on surveillance, including new animal diseases that could eventually spread to humans. In surveillance, there should be no delay in sharing information and coordination at the local, national, and international levels.

Severe Acute Respiratory Syndrome

Severe acute respiratory syndrome (SARS) is a classic example of an emerging disease that spread quickly across borders. It was a disease that had no vaccine, no treatment, and no cure. There was also significant delay in reporting the new disease. SARS started in the markets of Guangdong, China, and was identified as a coronavirus that is 99% similar to an animal virus found in Guangdong's meat markets, and was finally isolated in the palm civet, a small mammal that is a member of the viverridae family and a native of Asia.[78]

The first person to be diagnosed with SARS was a farmer in the Guangdong providence on November 16, 2002. Several health providers who were caring for the farmer before he died contracted the disease and also died. There seems to have been no outside communication about the outbreak. The second outbreak occurred again in China on February 1, 2003, at the time of the New Year celebration, and within 2 weeks, 45 people had contracted the disease. That likewise was not reported. The third outbreak occurred when, unknowingly, on February 22 a doctor who had treated patients in the second outbreak carried the virus to a hotel in Hong Kong. Eight travellers were infected and they then carried it to Vietnam, Canada, and Singapore. It was also transported to Bangkok, New York, Germany, and Ireland.[79]

Health-care providers in Hong Kong were not prepared to contain the disease, and it continued to spread. A global alert finally went out on March 12 when health-care providers were concerned that the illness might be avian influenza, and within 3 days an alert of a similar disease came from Vietnam, Canada, and Singapore. Travel advisories with screenings were implemented, and the WHO established lab networks and information sharing among more than 100 experts in 17 countries. It took until June 30 to contain the outbreak, and the last known infection occurred on July 5, 2003. SARS had rapidly reached 37 countries and infected 8,437 people, with a case fatality rate of 9.6% (813 people). Quarantine was used in several countries and strictly enforced to stop the spread.[79]

Since the outbreak, global health agencies have continued to track SARS and since 2004 there have been no new cases reported.[80] Because of the continued threat of another outbreak in 2012, SARS was labeled as a select agent by the National Select Agent Registry Program. A **select agent** is defined as a bacterium, virus, or toxin that could potentially pose a severe threat to both public health and safety.[80]

Influenza

Seasonal flu is a serious public health issue that has resulted in a strong public health effort to vaccinate entire populations.[81,82] In many hospitals, it is now mandatory for all employees to receive the flu vaccine in the early fall. Globally, there has been a concern about emerging flu strains such as the H1N1 outbreak in 2009 and avian influenza. Avian influenza is the disease that occurs when a person becomes infected by one of the avian bird influenza type A viruses.[83] Other influenza viruses of global concern include swine flu virus. These viruses do not normally infect humans, but there have been cases of variant swine flu viruses that have infected humans.[82]

HINI

An influenza pandemic occurred in 2009 caused by the H1N1 virus. It began in March 2009 in children in California and other cases in Mexico. By April 25, 2009, as the numbers of cases increased, the director general of WHO declared H1N1 an emergency of national concern; 2 days later he raised the concern to a pandemic alert; and on April 29, he raised it to phase 5, a pandemic imminent. The outbreaks in April spread rapidly. Travel to Mexico was initially curtailed to help prevent the spread. Scientists immediately began preparing a new vaccine for the H1N1. The United States also bolstered its laboratories to provide better testing. The largest age groups infected were between 5 and 24 years, and the older children and young adults were the ones most likely hospitalized. Those over 65, who are usually the sickest with the influenza virus, had few cases and rarely were hospitalized.[84]

On June 11, the fourth month into the outbreak, a pandemic was declared. Seventy-four counties had cases of the virus. By that time, every U.S. state had a percentage of the population that had been infected. The virus showed new seasonal pattern differences with multiple cases in the summer months, and most of the deaths occurring in young, otherwise healthy people, pregnant women, and young children.[84]

In July 2009, H1N1 started to take on the pattern of seasonal flu in the southern hemisphere. In October and

November, H1N1 took on the seasonal pattern of influenza in the United States. By the end of September, there were more than 400,000 cases and nearly 5,000 deaths. In October, after careful preparation for how best to administer the vaccine, it was ready for use. It was used in targeted groups until enough was manufactured for complete vaccine coverage. By late December, the number of cases had dramatically decreased, and there was enough vaccine available for everyone.[84]

It was not until August 10, 2010, that the director general of the WHO declared the pandemic outbreak over. She noted that the world was lucky with this new virus because it had not mutated into a more lethal form, it did not become resistant to the viral drugs, and the vaccine was very effective.[85]

Avian Influenza (H5N1 and H7N9).

Avian influenza has raised concerns globally of another emerging disease that originated in animals. There has been more than one strain of the virus, with H5N1 and H7N9 causing the most concern. The first human case of avian influenza, H5N1, occurred in 1997, and as of October 2010, there had been 505 confirmed cases and 300 deaths. Most cases of avian influenza infection in humans resulted from contact with infected poultry (e.g., domesticated chicken, ducks, and turkeys) or surfaces contaminated with secretion/excretions from the infected birds. The more virulent form of the virus is highly contagious in poultry and can produce 90% to 100% mortality in the birds in just 48 hours. Most of the infected humans were previously healthy children or young adults who had contact with infected birds. H5N1 does not spread easily from birds to humans, and the spread of avian influenza viruses from human to human is extremely rare. There have probably been only two such incidences, one in Thailand, in which a mother contracted it from her sick child, and another in Indonesia, in which one family member may have infected several other members. In neither case did it spread further.[85]

Symptoms of avian influenza in humans have ranged from typical human influenza–like symptoms (e.g., fever, cough, sore throat, and muscle aches) to eye infections, pneumonia, severe respiratory diseases (such as acute respiratory distress), and other severe and life-threatening complications. The case fatality rate is very high.[85]

Because the virus does not spread from person to person, it is not currently a major risk to humans. However, as all influenza viruses mutate, there is the very real danger that someday the virus will spread more easily among humans. Because no one has immune protection, it is predicted that it will spread rapidly from person to person, producing a pandemic. This is of grave concern, considering the very high mortality rate. Experts from around the world are watching the H5N1 situation in Asia and Europe very closely and are preparing for the possibility that the virus may begin to spread more easily and widely from person to person.[85]

Another avian flu virus, H7N9, emerged in humans in 2013 in China. Most of the reported cases of human infection resulted in severe respiratory illness. In the month following the report of the first case, more than 100 people had been infected, an unusually high rate for a new infection; a fifth of those patients had died, a fifth had recovered, and the rest remained critically ill. Research regarding background and transmission is ongoing. It has been established that many of the human cases of H7N9 appear to have a link to live bird markets. Currently, no vaccine exists, but the use of influenza antiviral drugs known as neuraminidase inhibitors in cases of early infection may be effective. The CDC is following this situation closely[86] (Fig. 13-4).

Ebola

Ebola is an example of a remerging disease with the 2014 outbreak. It is a severe, often fatal, disease in humans first identified in 1976. The Ebola virus is transmitted through contact with the bodily fluids of an infected person or corpse. The case fatality rate ranges from 25 percent to 90 percent.[87] Due to the high case fatality rate and the absence of a vaccine, the world took notice when, on March 21, 2014, a confirmed identification of a case of Ebola was made in Guinea, West Africa. Ebola rapidly became an epidemic not only in Guinea but in the neighboring countries of Liberia and Sierra Leone.

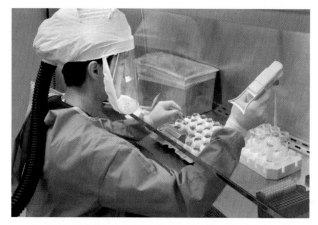

Figure 13-4 CDC scientist harvests H7N9 virus. *(From the CDC, courtesy of Douglas E. Jordan. Photographer James Gathany, 2013.)*

Health-care providers were soon overwhelmed by the rapid geographical dispersion of the disease, the complexity of trying to contain transmission, and the magnitude of operational needs to provide care.[88] This region of Africa had not experienced an outbreak of this disease and the population had no idea what to expect. Past outbreaks in equatorial Africa occurred in rural areas and spread of the disease was swiftly controlled within affected villages. In contrast, the 2014–2015 outbreak occurred in urban settings. The difficulty of containing the outbreak in these areas was compounded by weak public health infrastructure in all three countries and porous borders with a very mobile population. Poor roads, transportation systems, and limited telecommunication also contributed to difficulty with distribution of health services.

In July 2014, Ebola spread to Nigeria for the first time via air travel, and then to the United States and Lagos.[88] In these three countries, the disease was quickly contained. The United States had two imported cases, two locally acquired cases (both nurses caring for one of the patients), and one death. The highest risk of transmission of the disease was to health-care providers and to friends and family members of the infected individual. By March 2015, 839 health-care providers had been infected and 491 had died.[88]

In August 2014, the WHO had declared the Ebola epidemic an international public health emergency. WHO noted, "This has demonstrated the lack of international capacity to respond to a severe, sustained, and geographically dispersed public health crisis."[89] By the end of 2014, many international, national, and government organizations were working together to stop the spread and to provide good, supportive clinical care. Lessons learned from this epidemic include the importance of investing in strong and equitable health systems in all countries, knowing that preparedness works, no single intervention works but rather a coordination of activities, and the importance of community engagement.[88]

As of March 6, 2015, the last case in Liberia was discharged and there were no new cases reported for the week in that country. Between March 2014 and March 2015, 23,948 cases and 9,855 deaths were officially reported, a case fatality rate of 41 percent . These numbers may not reflect the full picture due to possible underreporting of cases.[90] The consequences of the epidemic went beyond the number of cases. For example, it was estimated that there were at least 30,000 children now orphaned, as well as the loss of economic productivity. Despite the apparent end of the epidemic in Liberia, in March 2015, Guinea and Sierra Leone were still reporting new cases.[90]

Health Delivery Systems From a Global Perspective

Each country has its own unique health-care system dependent on such things as history, resources, form of government, the priority given to health, national policies, and how decisions are made in the country. Many of the differences in health-care systems have to do with how health care is financed and who is eligible to use the care. In many countries, the tax system or other fiscal components of the government finance a universal health-care system and all citizens can access the care without charge. In other countries, there is a private health-care system that can be nonprofit or for profit, and individuals accessing the system must pay out of pocket or through an insurance program for the care. In general, most countries have a mixture of both government and privately funded health care that can make the systems quite complex. In some health systems, the traditional birth attendant, the herbalist, traditional healers, and the pharmacist play a large role in primary care, especially when Western medicine is not easily accessible, affordable, or acceptable. In some countries in which there is internal and/or external military conflict, the health-care systems may no longer be functioning, and in other countries with poorly functioning systems, the majority of the care could be provided by external NGOs.

Successful health-care systems usually share common attributes. They:

- Provide universal equitable coverage and quality care
- Emphasize primary prevention
- Are acceptable, affordable, and accessible to the individual
- Are efficient
- Have adequate human and material resources including pharmaceuticals
- Have a good documentation system and an appropriate referral system for more specialized care as needed

It is clear that "Health for All" as defined at Alma-Ata was not achieved in 2000 and it is clear that many countries, especially the LICs in sub-Saharan Africa, found it difficult to reach the MDGs. It is also clear that most of the LICs and MICs need to put more emphasis on the evolving noncommunicable diseases as the life expectancy in those countries rises.

Primary health care is an important component of a successful health-care delivery system. There are several potential reasons it has not been as effective a tool globally as it could be. Governments have not put health as a top priority, even with the knowledge that economic development is closely linked to a healthy population. There has not always been good oversight of the health-care delivery system, including both assessments and evaluations. There has been rapid population growth in some of the developing countries, placing a strain on the system and having an impact on an already poorly resourced health structure that lacks both human and material resources, especially at the primary health-care sites. There has also been a lack of essential pharmaceuticals at all levels of care. Walley, colleagues, and members of the Lancet Alma-Ata Working Group have suggested several changes to the primary health-care system to improve outcomes:

- A continuum of care for maternal and child care
- Integrated evidence-based and country-specific packages of preventive and curative care
- Community partnerships, with their participation in the primary health care of sanitation, water, and nutrition
- Attention to the noncommunicable diseases, including mental health

They caution that progress should be measured and accountability assured.[91]

Culture

Another essential component of global health is sensitivity and understanding of how culture has a direct impact on health care and how health care is delivered (see Chapter 23). Culture is not to be confused with poverty, inequality, and lack of knowledge about health at the community level. As Paul Farmer states in his book *AIDS and Accusations*, HIV/AIDS is about poverty and not about voodoo and superstition.[92] However, culture does affect how patients seek care, how they perceive birth and death, and how they maintain their traditions. The following case study illustrates how culture can have an impact on nursing care.

● APPLYING PUBLIC HEALTH SCIENCE

The Case of Student Nurse Kelly in Africa

Public Health Science Topics Covered:

- Cultural humility
- Cultural assessment

Culture has a major impact on how nursing care is delivered in all parts of the world. This became apparent when Kelly, a student nurse from the United States, was providing nursing care in a large hospital in a country in Africa as part of an exchange clinical experience. Kelly was working on a pediatric ward with two wings, each with more than 30 beds. All the beds were full, and there was some overflow that caused there to be two infants per bed. There was little space to move, and to add to the confusion and crowding there was at least one family member with each of the children to provide basic care 24 hours a day. These family members would sleep on the floor near the child at night.

Most of the children had malaria, pneumonia, meningitis, or other communicable diseases. Kelly had been assigned to monitor a very small infant, a little more than 5 weeks old and less than 5 pounds. The child had just arrived at the referral hospital with an undiagnosed heart condition, had not responded to any previous therapy, and was not taking breast milk well. The mother and baby were from a rural area, a bus ride of several hours away. The mother came alone without other family members because the family could not afford more than one bus ticket. The mother had never been to an urban area before, and had no experience with a large hospital.

Kelly was asked to assist with an emergency; when she returned to her new patient, the child did not appear to be breathing. Kelly and Lillian, a student nurse from the local university, started resuscitation and eventually were assisted by a medical student, the only doctor on the unit at the time. Without any emergency medicine, the baby did not respond and died. Kelly was very upset and found it difficult to communicate with the mother, who spoke very little English. Kelly did what she had been taught in the United States. She removed the resuscitation equipment, washed the baby's face, wrapped the baby well in a blanket, and gave the baby to the mother to hold. The mother, who had intuitively understood what happened, began to scream and pushed the baby away. She started to cry quite loudly and Kelly realized she definitely did not want to hold the baby. Kelly then offered to take her to a quiet place where she could grieve. The mother's yelling and crying had brought all the others mothers to see what had happened.

Lillian, who was of the same culture as the mother, offered her cultural interpretation and wisdom to Kelly. She pointed out that in their culture, if a young woman were to hold a dead baby, doing so would bring bad luck to her next pregnancy and cause that baby also to die. Lillian also reported that women grieve very openly and really want support from other women. The other women in the ward were always willing to help a mother deal with the death of her child. Removing the mother from the comfort of these women, although she didn't know them, would be very stressful. Kelly asked Lillian to share some of the other cultural practices so she could be more sensitive the next time.

Different Nursing Roles for Global Health

Nurses are no longer being educated to work in one local, specialized setting. Nurses are mobile and their work is always changing. The global health approach allows nurses to consider things from multiple angles and to work collaboratively in a world that is becoming more and more complex. Nurses are beginning to view health from a global perspective as the interconnectedness of health-care provision across the globe becomes more apparent. Global nursing provides a new worldview that is full of contradictions, has increasing diversity, and places considerable value on the larger population and communities. It also opens up many opportunities for nursing to make a difference (Box 13-6).

There are technical solutions to many of the major global health problems, but it will take nurses in countries

BOX 13–6	**Actions Nurses Can Take at the National and Global Level**

- Advocate with policy makers, especially government policy makers, for more research funding to help specifically with the prevention, treatment, and control of communicable and chronic diseases worldwide.
- Build cultural competency (see Chapter 23) to the needs of individuals who have come to live in the United States from other countries.
- Asses those born outside the United States for past health history, possible exposure to communicable diseases, and possible exposure to violence.
- Be a good consumer of current knowledge about globalization and progress toward achieving global-level goals such as the SDGs.
- Get to know the nurses you work with who have emigrated from other countries.
- Choose to volunteer or work globally. There are many volunteer opportunities to work with some of them, such as Project Hope (see Web Resources).

of all levels (HICs, MICs, and LICs) to help move these solutions into reality. It will take political, financial, and policy changes to close the gap and guarantee health for all. Nurses, indeed, all health-care providers, need to increase partnerships to enhance better health outcomes. As health-care providers, nurses can build on the belief that health is a valuable economic resource, enhance the development of countries and regions, and increase the resources available to continue to positively change the health of the population. Nurses can also affirm that health is a right of all people whether they live in the United States, Kenya, Sweden, or Indonesia.

A central key role for nurses in community settings across the globe is to provide health education. Health literacy is an important aspect of improving health (see Chapter 2). For example, if the population does not understand germ theory or that malaria is transmitted by the mosquito, the distribution of mosquito nets may not be effective. Nurses working with the context of primary health care should assess the population for health literacy on the major health issues prior to implementing an intervention aimed at preventing disease (see Chapter 4) and often need to build a health education component into the development, implementation, and evaluation of health programs in populations with low levels of health literacy (see Chapter 4).

■ Summary Points

- Global health emphasizes the interdependence of policies, economics, and values that arise related to health. The focus of global health is on transnational issues, determinants, and solutions and the promotion of interdisciplinary collaboration.
- Primary health care is a broad concept that includes the provision of all the components that contribute to health (e.g., food, water and sanitation, medicines) in addition to direct services.
- There are many partners in global health and they include multilateral and bilateral organizations and NGOs that work to improve the health of countries and regions as well as worldwide.
- Significant progress was made in reaching the Millennium Development Goals at the global level, which helped to frame the post-2015 Sustainable Development Goals.
- Though health care is seen as a human right at the global level, there is still considerable inequity in who receives that care and how much care they receive.
- LICs bear the greatest global burden of disease.

- In LICs, there continues to be a heavy burden of communicable disease, especially tuberculosis, malaria, and HIV/AIDS. However, there are also a growing number of individuals with noncommunicable diseases that include cardiovascular disease, cancer, diabetes, and chronic respiratory disease.
- Neglected diseases and emerging diseases are also having an impact on the morbidity and mortality of the world.
- Global nursing provides a new worldview of nursing and health care. Nurses have an important role in improving the health of populations from the local level to the global level as advocates, health planners, health educators, and deliverers of care, especially to those who are most vulnerable.

▲ CASE STUDY
Chronic Disease in the Village
Learning Outcomes

At the end of this case study, the student will be able to:

- Identify the impact of noncommunicable disease in LICs.
- Explore the process for designing health education programs appropriate for populations in an LIC.
- Discuss the process for implementing and evaluating a health education program with limited resources.

In an LIC's local health center, one of the district nurses, Edith, has been providing nursing care at a community clinic for the past 5 years. The clinic sees between 200 and 300 patients daily. Three weeks ago, some nursing faculty from the local university visited the clinic. They had been told that the prevalence of malaria and childhood pneumonia had dropped significantly since Edith had been the charge nurse at the clinic. The nursing visitors wanted to explore how this decrease in disease had happened.

Edith was glad to share information but she wanted something in return. Edith had heard the doctor talking with some visitors from the Ministry of Health, and they were discussing the increase in heart disease and diabetes in the district. Edith wanted to do something about the increase in noncommunicable disease in her community, but had no idea where to begin. She also mentioned that her colleagues in the district also had no idea how to attack this problem.

The visiting members of the nursing faculty suggested that Edith develop community health education classes in conjunction with a communicable disease management program tailored to the clinic population.

Answer the following questions to help Edith and her colleagues attack the problem of noncommunicable disease:

1. What topic(s) should be included in the health education program?
2. When should the classes be given? How long should the program last? Who should give the educational information?
3. How should the classes be taught? Should there be clinical practice in the class?
4. What should the chronic disease management program look like in Edith's clinic?
5. How would Edith assess community needs when designing this program?
6. What could she do with her limited available time to really make a difference?
7. How could she involve her community workers?

Sources

1. Kearney, P., Whelton, M., Reynolds, K., Muntner, P., Whelton, K., & He, J. (2005). Global burden of hypertension: Analysis of worldwide data. *Lancet, 365,* 217-223.
2. Good, L. (2010). Hypertension highlights; Blood pressure targets, global risk factors, and diabetes—the latest data are not encouraging. *Medscape Today.* Retrieved from www.medscape.com/viewarticle/715584.
3. World Health Organization. (2010). Implementation of the global strategy on diet, physical activity and health. Retrieved from www.who.int/dietphysicalactivity/implementation/en/.

REFERENCES

1. Kickbush, I. (2006). The need for a European strategy on global health. *Scandinavian Journal of Public Health, 34,* 561-565.
2. Beaglehole, R., & Bonita, R. (2010). What is global health? *Global Health Action, 3.* doi:10.3402/gha.v3i0.5142.
3. Koplan, J., Bond, C., Merson, M., Rodriquez, M., Sewankambo, N., & Wasserheit, J. (2009). Toward a common definition of global health. *Lancet, 373,* 1993-1995.
4. World Health Organization. (2013). *About the WHO.* Retrieved from www.who.int/about/en/.
5. World Health Organization. (2013). *Governance: WHO constitution.* Retrieved from www.who.int/governance/eb/constitution/en/.

6. World Bank. (2013). *How we classify countries.* Retrieved from data.worldbank.org/about/country-classifications.

7. U.S. Central Intelligence Agency. (2013). *World fact book.* Retrieved from www.cia.gov/library/publications/the-world-factbook/rankorder/2102rank.html.

8. Centers for Disease Control and Prevention. (1999). Ten great public health achievements—United States, 1900-1999. *Mortality and Morbidity Weekly Report, 48*(12), 241-243. Retrieved from www.cdc.gov/mmwr/preview/mmwrhtml/00056796.htm.

9. World Health Organization. (2013). *Global health observatory: Under five mortality.* Retrieved from www.who.int/gho/child_health/mortality/mortality_under_five/en/index.html.

10. World Health Organization. (2012). *Media center: MATERNAL mortality.* Retrieved from www.who.int/mediacentre/factsheets/fs348/en/.

11. U.S. Aid for International Development. (2013). *Global health.* Retrieved from www.usaid.gov/global-health.

12. Institute of Medicine. (1997). *America's vital interest in global health.* Washington, DC: National Academies Press.

13. World Health Organization. (2013). *Malaria: Data and statistics.* Retrieved from www.who.int/malaria/data/en/.

14. World Health Organization. (2013). *Drought technical hazard sheet natural disaster profiles.* Retrieved from www.who.int/hac/techguidance/ems/drought/en/index.html.

15. Hegarty, J., Condon, C., Walsh, E., & Sweeney, J. (2009). The undergraduate education of nurses: Looking to the future. *International Journal of Nursing Education Scholarship, 6*(1), 1-11.

16. da Silva, A. (2008). Nursing in the era of globalization: Challenges for the 21st century. *Revista Latino-Americana de Enfermagem, 16*(4), 787-790.

17. Institute of Medicine. (2010). Report at a glance. *The future of nursing: Leading change, advancing health.* Retrieved from www.iom.edu/Reports/2010/The-Future-of-Nursing-Leading-Change-Advancing-Health/Report-Brief.aspx.

18. Sigma Theta Tau International. (2013). *STTI's global initiatives.* Retrieved from www.nursingsociety.org/GlobalAction/Initiatives/Pages/building_global.aspx.

19. Declaration of Alma-Ata. (1978, September). *International Conference on Primary Health Care, Alma-Ata, USSR.* Retrieved from www.who.int/hpr/NPH/docs/declaration_almaata.pdf.

20. World Health Organization. (2013). *Millennium development goals.* Retrieved from www.who.int/topics/millennium_development_goals/en/index.html.

21. International Medical Volunteer Organization. (n.d.). *The major international health organizations.* Retrieved from www.imva.org/Pages/orgfrm.htm.

22. Yach, D. (1995). *Health and illness: The definition of the World Health Organization. Geneva, World Health Organization.* Retrieved from www.medizin-ethik.ch/publik/health_illness.htm#4.

23. World Health Organization. (2013). *The WHO agenda.* Retrieved from www.who.int/about/agenda/en/index.html.

24. World Health Organization. (2013). *World health report.* Retrieved from www.who.int/whr/en/index.html.

25. Pan American Health Organization. (2010). *About PAHO.* Retrieved from new.paho.org/hq/index.php?option=com_content&task=view&id=91&Itemid=220.

26. World Bank. (2013). *About us.* Retrieved from www.worldbank.org/en/about.

27. U.S. Agency for International Development. (2013). *About USAID.* Retrieved from www.usaid.gov/about_usaid/.

28. *The Global Health Initiative.* (2013). Retrieved from www.ghi.gov/principles/index.html#.U9AfWvwnLIU

29. Centers for Disease Control and Prevention. (2013). *Global health.* Retrieved from www.cdc.gov/globalhealth/index.html.

30. CARE. (2013). *About CARE.* Retrieved from www.care.org/about/index.asp.

31. Catholic Relief Services. (2013). *About Catholic Relief Services.* Retrieved from http://crs.org/about/.

32. Catholic Relief Services. (2010). *Where we serve.* Retrieved from http://crs.org/where/.

33. United Nations Statistics Division. (2013). *Inter-agency and Expert Group on MDG Indicators.* Retrieved from http://mdgs.un.org/unsd/mdg/Host.aspx?Content=IAEG.htm.

34. Hill, P., Mansoor, G., & Claudio, F. (2010). Conflict in least-developed countries: Challenging the Millennium Development Goals. *Bulletin of the World Health Organization, 88*, 562-563.

35. United Nations Development Programme. (2013). *The Millennium Developmental Goals report 2013.* New York, NY: United Nations. Retrieved from www.un.org/en/development/desa/publications/mdgs-report-2013.html.

36. Yousafzai, M. (2013). *I am Malala: The girl who stood up for education and was shot by the Taliban.* London, England: Weidenfeld & Nicolson, Orion Pub.

37. Pucher, P.H., Macdonnell, M., & Arulkumaran, S. (2013). Global lessons on transforming strategy into action to save mother's lives. *International Journal of Gynecology and Obstetrics, 123*, 167-172.

38. Thaddeus, S., & Maine, D. (1994). Too far to walk: Maternal mortality in context. *Social Science & Medicine, 38*(8), 1091-1110.

39. Shaikh, A. (2009). *Maternal mortality—the three delays.* Retrieved from http://humanrights.change.org/blog/view/maternal_mortality_-_the_three_delays.

40. Cham, M., Sundby, J., & Vangen, S. (2005). Maternal mortality in the rural Gambia: A qualitative study on access to emergency obstetric care. *Reproductive Health, 2*(3). doi:10.1186/1742-4755-2-3.

41. World Health Organization. (2013). *Millennium Developmental Goals key facts.* Retrieved from www.who.int/mediacentre/factsheets/fs290/en/index.html.

42. World Health Organization. (2010). *Food security: Trade, foreign policy, diplomacy and health.* Retrieved from www.who.int/trade/glossary/story028/en/.
43. Bryce, J., Boschi-Pinto, C., Shibuya, K., & Black, R. (2005). WHO estimates of the causes of death in children. *Lancet, 365,* 1147-1152.
44. Vidyasagar, D. (2007). Global minute: Water and health—walking for water and water wars. *Journal of Perinatology, 27,* 56-58.
45. Moe, C., & Rheingans, R. (2006). Global challenges in water, sanitation and health. *Journal of Water and Health* (Suppl. 4), 41-57.
46. World Health Organization. (2010). *Health through safe drinking water and basic sanitation.* Retrieved from www.who.int/water_sanitation_health/mdg1/en/index.html.
47. Bassani, D., Jha, P., Dhingra, N., & Kuman, R. (2010). Child mortality from solid-fuel use in India: A nationally-representative case-control study. *BMC Public Health, 10,* 491.
48. Clark, M., Reynolds, S., Burch, J., Conway, S., Bachand, A., & Peel, J. (2010). Indoor air pollution, cookstove quality, and housing characteristics in two Honduran communities. *Environmental Research, 110*(1), 12-18.
49. Rehfuess, E., Tzala, L., Best, N., Briggs, D., & Joffe, M. (2009). Solid fuel use and cooking practices as a major risk factor for ALRI mortality among African children. *Journal of Epidemiology and Community Health, 63,* 887-892.
50. Dasgupta, S., Wheeler, D., Hug, M., & Khaliquzzaman, M. (2009). Improving indoor air quality for poor families: A controlled experiment in Bangladesh. *Indoor Air, 19,* 22-32.
51. World Health Organization. (2010). *Fact sheet: Millennium Goals: Progress toward the health-related Millennium Development Goals.* Retrieved from www.who.int/mediacentre/factsheets/fs290/en/index.html.
52. United Nations Economic and Social Council. (2012). *Post-2015 UN Development Framework.* Retrieved from www.un.org/en/ecosoc/newfunct/pdf/post_2015_un_development_framework_summary.pdf.
53. D'Ambruoso, L. (2013). Global health post-2015: The case for universal health equity. *Global Health Action, 6,* 19661. Retrieved from http://dx.doi.org/10.3402/gha.v610.19661.
54. United Nations. (n.d.). *Sustainable Development Goals.* Retrieved from http://sustainabledevelopment.un.org/index.php?menu=1300.
55. Chapman, A. (2009). Globalization, human rights, and the social determinants of health. *Bioethics, 23*(2), 97-111.
56. Farmer, P., & Campos, N. (2003). Rethinking medical ethics: A view from below. *Developing World Bioethics, 4*(1), 17-41.
57. The President's Emergency Plan for AIDS Relief. (2014). *Strategy.* Retrieved from www.pepfar.gov/about/strategy/index.htm.
58. Hurst, S. (2008). Physician brain drain: Can nothing be done? *Public Health Ethics, 1*(2), 180-192.
59. World Health Organization. (2013). *HIV fact sheet.* Retrieved from www.who.int/mediacentre/factsheets/fs360/en/.
60. World Health Organization. (2013). *Tuberculosis fact sheet.* Retrieved from www.who.int/mediacentre/factsheets/fs104/en/.
61. World Health Organization. (2013). *Malaria fact sheet.* Retrieved from www.who.int/mediacentre/factsheets/fs094/en/.
62. World Health Organization. (2013). *Chronic diseases and health promotion.* Retrieved from www.who.int/chp/en/.
63. Murray, C., & Lopez, A. (1997). Alternative projections of mortality and disability by cause 1990–1920: Global Burden of Disease Study. *The Lancet, 349,* 1498-1504.
64. Heuveline, P., Guillot, M., & Gwatkin, D. (2002). The uneven tides of the health transition. *Social Science and Medicine, 55,* 312-322.
65. World Health Organization. (2013). *Health data and statistics.* Retrieved from www.who.int/healthinfo/statistics/en/.
66. World Health Organization. (2013). *Metrics: Disability-adjusted life year (DALY).* Retrieved from www.who.int/healthinfo/global_burden_disease/metrics_daly/en/.
67. World Health Organization. (2013). *About the Global Burden of Disease Project.* Retrieved from www.who.int/healthinfo/global_burden_disease/about/en/index.html.
68. Bill and Melinda Gates Foundation. (2010). *Neglected disease overview.* Retrieved from www.gatesfoundation.org/topics/Pages/neglected-diseases.aspx.
69. World Health Organization. (2013). *Lymphatic filariasis fact sheet.* Retrieved from www.who.int/mediacentre/factsheets/fs102/en/.
70. World Health Organization. (2013). *Cholera fact sheet.* Retrieved from www.who.int/mediacentre/factsheets/fs107/en/.
71. World Health Organization. (2013). *Leprosy fact sheet.* Retrieved from www.who.int/mediacentre/factsheets/fs101/en/.
72. World Health Organization. (2013). *World Health Assembly adopts resolution on all 17 neglected tropical diseases.* Retrieved from www.who.int/neglected_diseases/WHA_66_seventh_day_resolution_adopted/en/index.html.
73. Centers for Disease Control and Prevention. (2013). *Parasites—leishmaniasis.* Retrieved from www.cdc.gov/parasites/leishmaniasis/.
74. Centers for Disease Control and Prevention. (2013). *Parasites—American trypanosomiasis (also known as Chagas).* Retrieved from www.cdc.gov/parasites/chagas/.
75. World Health Organization. (n.d.). *Dengue.* Retrieved from www.who.int/topics/dengue/en/.
76. Centers for Disease Control and Prevention. (2013). *Dengue.* Retrieved from www.cdc.gov/dengue/.
77. National Institute of Allergy and Infectious Diseases. (2013). *Emerging and re-emerging diseases.* Retrieved from www.niaid.nih.gov/topics/emerging/Pages/introduction.aspx.

78. Wang, M., Yan, M., Xu, H., Liang, W., Kan, B., Zheng, B., et al. SARS-CoV infection in a restaurant from palm civet. *Emerging Infectious Diseases* [serial on the Internet]. Retrieved from http://dx.doi.org/10.3201/eid1112.041293.

79. Xu, R., He, J., Evans, M.R., Peng, G., Field, H.E., Schnur, A., et al. (2004). Epidemiological clues to SARS origin in China. *Emerging Infectious Diseases, 10*(6), 1030-1037.

80. Centers for Disease Control and Prevention. (2013). *Severe acute respiratory syndrome (SARS).* Retrieved from www.cdc.gov/sars/

81. Flu.gov. (n.d.). *Pandemic flu history.* Retrieved from www.flu.gov/pandemic/history/index.html#.

82. Centers for Disease Control and Prevention. (2014). *Seasonal flu.* Retrieved from www.cdc.gov/flu/index.htm.

83. Centers for Disease Control and Prevention. (2014). *Seasonal influenza (flu): Information on avian influenza.* Retrieved from www.cdc.gov/flu/avianflu/.

84. Centers for Disease Control and Prevention. (2010). *H1N1 virus.* Retrieved from www.cdc.gov/h1n1flu/background.htm.

85. World Health Organization. (2010). *Pandemic (H1N1) 2009.* Retrieved from www.who.int/csr/disease/swineflu/en/.

86. Centers for Disease Control and Prevention. (2013). *H7N9.* Retrieved from www.cdc.gov/flu/avianflu/h7n9-virus.htm.

87. World Health Organization (2015). *Ebola virus disease.* Retrieved from www.who.int/mediacentre/factsheets/fs103/en/.

88. World Health Organization (2015) *Global alert and response.* Retrieved from who.int/csr/disease/ebola/one-year-report/response-in-2015/en/.

89. British Broadcasting Company News (2015) *Ebola: Mapping the outbreak.* Retrieved from www.bbc.com/news/world-africa-28755033.

90. World Health Organization (2015). *Ebola situation Report, 4 March 2015.* Retrieved from http://apps.who.int/ebola/current-situation/ebola-situation-report-4-march-2015.

91. Walley, J., Lawn, J., Tinker, A., de Francisco, A., Chopra, M., Rudan, I., et al. (2008). Primary health care: Making Alma-Ata a reality. *Lancet, 372*(9642), 1001-1007. doi:10.1016/S0140-6736(08)61409-9.

92. Farmer, P. (1992). *AIDS and accusations. Haiti and the geography of blame (comparative studies of health systems and medical care).* Berkeley: University of California Press.

Chapter 14

Health Planning for Local Public Health Departments

LEARNING OUTCOMES

After reading this chapter, the student will be able to:

1. Describe the historical development of public health departments (abbreviated in this chapter as PHDs).
2. Describe the structure and services of PHDs.
3. Describe the interdisciplinary workforce in PHDs.
4. Analyze key roles and responsibilities of public health nurses (PHNs) in PHDs.
5. Discuss current issues related to delivery of essential public health services by PHDs.
6. Investigate the role of PHDs in community assessment and planning for health needs of the community.
7. Identify the most frequent activities and services provided by PHDs.
8. Discuss financial and information technology resources needed to support PHDs.
9. Describe the challenges facing PHDs.
10. Discuss accreditation and evaluation of services provided by PHDs.

KEY TERMS

Behavioral Risk Factor Surveillance System (BRFSS)
Categorical funding
Centralized system
Community health assessment
Decentralized system
Directly observed therapy
Federally qualified health centers (FQHCs)
Fetal death
Geographic information system (GIS)
Healthy Start
Medication electronic monitoring system
Public health department (PHD)
Public health informatics
Public health system
Public health systems and services research
Shared or mixed system
Vital statistics
Women, Infants, and Children (WIC)

◼ Introduction

An official governmental body responsible for assuring the health of citizens residing within a county, municipality, township, or territory is called a **public health department (PHD)**. PHDs are seen as trusted conveners that facilitate partnerships and coalitions to assess and address local public health issues.

The basic mandate of the PHD is to protect and improve health in partnership with the community (see Chapter 1). Citizens generally think that the PHD is responsible for providing services related to communicable diseases or immunization services. They may not be aware of the overarching mission of the PHD to promote and protect the health, defined more broadly than communicable diseases, of all people in the community. This mission can only be accomplished through a host of health-care providers and community partners who pool together resources and coordinate services. These partners and their services make up the **public health system.**[1] Although the PHD is not responsible for providing all health services for a population, governmental agencies are responsible for assuring essential community health services.[2]

The purpose of this chapter is threefold. It is important for all nurses to be aware of the role of local health departments in order to access support and appropriate services for the people they are serving, to describe the role of the public health nurse in a PHD, and to discuss the challenges facing PHDs today.

History of Public Health Departments

Local official agencies in the United States developed out of local boards of health in the late 18th century.[3] The first city to form a board of health was Philadelphia (1794), followed by Baltimore (1797), Boston (1799), Washington, DC (1802), New Orleans (1804), and New York City (1805).[4] The concerns at that time were focused on communicable diseases within densely populated cities. With a growing understanding of the connection between proper sanitation and disease, there was an expansion of municipal health departments in the 1880s and early 1900s.[5] Another major growth period occurred with the passage of the Social Security Act in 1935, which provided millions of dollars for maternal and child health services for public health.[4]

The rural experience was slightly different. Prior to the establishment of formalized governmental units in rural areas, district nurses provided much of the work of public health.[5] With time and population growth, county health departments developed in these growing communities and their responsibilities expanded outside the centers to address sanitary needs. Jefferson County in Kentucky is often considered the first PHD to provide public health services. This county department was formed in 1908, and in 1911 two others followed. Guilford County in North Carolina sought school health programs, and Yakima County in Washington State responded to a typhoid epidemic.[6] The first exclusive rural county health department was in Robeson County in North Carolina. By 1921, the county movement had spread to 186 counties in 23 states, often with the help of private foundations.[7] The Rockefeller Foundation developed rural programs between 1910 and 1913 to:[4]

- Educate medical professionals and the public about hookworm disease
- Provide funds to sanitize communities for protection
- Fund the employment of personnel to continue work in the counties

This support from the Rockefeller Foundation and other private foundations allowed the development of county health departments and this support eventually was combined with funding from the Public Health Service (PHS).

Mission of Public Health

The mission of public health had its beginnings in the mid-19th century when physicians, housing reformers, advocates for the poor, and scientists trained in housing and civil engineering came together to fight problems of urbanization, industrialization, and immigration.[8] The focus was largely on housing conditions and communicable diseases. The work of social reformers at Hull House in Chicago or the Henry Street Settlement with Lillian Wald (Chapter 1) are examples of this work.

Beginning in the 1920s, the Committee on Administrative Practice of the American Public Health Association (APHA) sought to define the mission of public health agencies.[3,9] In 1933, the Committee on Administrative Practice of APHA listed two primary goals for local public health agencies:[3]

- Control of communicable diseases
- Promotion of child health

These goals reflected the basic public health needs of the time, recognizing that children suffered the most from communicable diseases. By 1940, another APHA statement produced a clearer listing of the six minimum functions of local health departments:[10]

- Vital statistics
- Environmental sanitation
- Communicable disease control
- Public health laboratories
- Maternal and child health
- Public health education

The mission of public health was revisited with the Institute of Medicine (IOM) report in 1988. At that time, public health was redefined (see Chapter 1) and the mission was defined as fulfilling society's interest in assuring conditions in which people can be healthy.[11] The three core functions of assurance, assessment, and policy formation evolved from this work.

Structure of Public Health Departments

As hospitals have different corporate and organizational structures, so does the infrastructure for public health agencies vary on the state and local levels. Thus the adage, "When you have seen one health department, you have seen one health department,"[1] meaning no two health departments are alike. Knowing how the PHD is organized is of key importance for nurses to understand how public health services are delivered in their state and community. Generally, PHDs are organized by one of three major delivery modes:

- **Centralized system:** PHDs are operated by a state health agency or board of health and the PHD functions under the state agency (6 states).
- **Decentralized system:** PHDs are operated by local government with or without a board of health (27 states).
- **Shared or mixed system:** PHDs are operated under shared or combined authority of the state health agency, board of health, and local government (16 states).[12,13]

Similar to the size of the hospital (number of beds) and nurse-to-patient ratio, the size of the population the PHD serves is a critical factor in local public health service delivery. Figure 14-1 illustrates the percentage of small, medium, and large PHDs and the percentage of the U.S. population served by these PHDs. It is interesting to note that 49% of the population is served by only 5% of PHDs, whereas 63% of PHDs cover 11% of the population.[12]

Another organizational factor is the type of jurisdiction or territory the PHD serves. The majority of PHDs (68%) are county based, 4% serve a combined city/county (e.g., Miami-Dade in Florida), whereas 21% serve a city or town[12] (Fig. 14-2). Multicounty or regional jurisdictions make up 8% of PHDs and are proposed as a method for strengthening public health services in rural areas.[12,13]

PHDs located in rural areas are challenged by pronounced problems in infrastructure related to limited

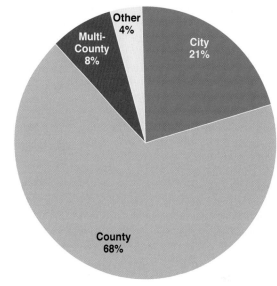

N=2,565
Note: Due to rounding, percentages do not add to 100%.

Figure 14-2 Percentage distribution of PHDs by type of geographical jurisdiction. *(From the National Association of County and City Health Officers. [2011]. The 2010 national profile of local health departments, Washington, DC: Author. Retrieved from http://www.naccho.org/topics/infrastructure/profile/resources/2010report/upload/2010_Profile_main_report-web.pdf.)*

resources and isolation.[14] And yet, they are often called upon to address health outcomes that are different and sometimes worse than those in urban areas. For example, rural areas have higher morbidity and mortality rates and environmental health challenges related to agriculture pollution and unsafe mining and logging practices.

Public Health Workforce

The PHD workforce is interdisciplinary and the majority of PHDs have fewer than than 100 employees. The types of occupations typically found in PHDs include physicians, environmental health specialists, nutritionists, social workers, pharmacists, epidemiologists, information technology specialists, health educators, public information specialists, and nurses. Of these, nurses made up 17% of the public health workforce in the 2010 National Association of City and County Health Officials (NACCHO) survey, down from 24% in 2005 (Fig. 14-3).[12] Depending on the jurisdiction, some PHDs may have mental health service providers as part of their workforce. Staffing patterns vary depending on the size and services provided by the PHD.

Historically, the cultural diversity of the public health workforce is less likely to represent the diversity of the

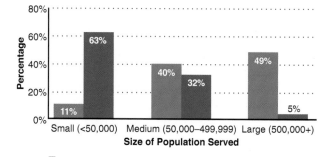

Percentage of U.S. Population Served
Percentage of All LHDs
N=2,565

Figure 14-1 Percentage of PHDs and percentage of U.S. population served, by size of population served. *(From the National Association of County and City Health Officers. [2011]. The 2010 national profile of local health departments, Washington, DC: Author. Retrieved from http://www.naccho.org/topics/infrastructure/profile/resources/2010report/upload/2010_Profile_main_report-web.pdf.)*

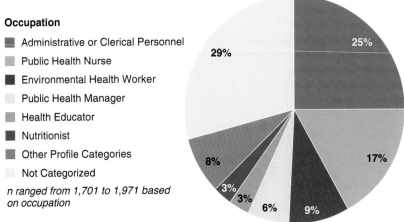

Occupation

■ Administrative or Clerical Personnel
▨ Public Health Nurse
■ Environmental Health Worker
▫ Public Health Manager
▨ Health Educator
■ Nutritionist
▨ Other Profile Categories
▫ Not Categorized

n ranged from 1,701 to 1,971 based on occupation

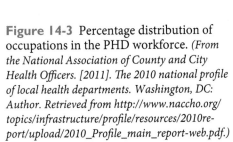

Figure 14-3 Percentage distribution of occupations in the PHD workforce. *(From the National Association of County and City Health Officers. [2011]. The 2010 national profile of local health departments. Washington, DC: Author. Retrieved from http://www.naccho.org/topics/infrastructure/profile/resources/2010report/upload/2010_Profile_main_report-web.pdf.)*

communities they serve. A PHD workforce study found the average PHD racial and ethnic staff representation to be 57% white, nonhispanic; 31% race other than white; and 12% Hispanic, nonblack.[12] Larger PHDs typically have a more diverse workforce than do smaller PHDs. However, PHD workforce diversity still remains less than the population served.

Role of Public Health Nurses in Public Health Departments

Nurses who work within a PHD are usually considered public health nurses (PHNs). Public health nurses make up one of largest professional groups within the health department. Not all PHNs work within an official agency.

The relevance of nursing to public health was recognized in the early 1920s when C.E Winslow's definition of public health highlighted the role of nursing services:[15]

> Public health is the science and art of preventing disease, prolonging life, and promoting physical, and mental health and well-being through organized community effort for the sanitation of the environment, the control of communicable infections, the organization of medical and nursing services for the early diagnosis and prevention of disease, the education of the individual in personal health, and the development of social machinery to assure everyone a standard of living adequate for the maintenance or improvement of health.

In addition, APHA's 1933 and 1940 statements of the mission of public health emphasized the role of public health nursing in several functions of the health department, especially communicable disease and maternal-child health.[3]

Core Functions

Today, PHNs who work in PHDs promote and protect the health of the entire population in a community through the three core public health functions:[11]

- Population assessment
- Assurance of a well coordinated system of health promotion and health-care services
- Policy development to support health of the community

These functions and their related essential services[16] were introduced in Chapter 1 (see Box 1-1) and their relevance for guiding local health departments is further explored in this chapter.

We can apply these core functions to public health nursing within a PHD setting using immunization as an example of an intervention to promote the health of a population/community. Assessment is illustrated when PHNs working in PHDs gather epidemiological data to determine the rate of children fully immunized against specific communicable diseases (e.g., measles, H1N1 influenza). A high immunization rate (> 70%) is needed to provide a community level of immunity (herd immunity) to protect the population (see Chapter 8).[17] Another example of the application of core functions by PHNs in PHDs is their involvement in writing and implementing policies that require immunizations for entry into day care, schools, and colleges to help ensure that herd immunity level is obtained for the protection of students, staff, and families. If the rate is lower, PHNs assure immunization services are provided by mobilizing community partners to target specific groups that have low immunization rates and by providing easily accessible immunizations in pediatric clinics and schools.

This example demonstrates the role of PHD PHNs in assessment, assurance, and policy development to decrease the risk of communicable disease transmission in their community. Underlying these three functions is the assumption that the PHD PHN will provide ethical and moral leadership in providing public health services as outlined by the Public Health Leadership Society[18] (Box 14-1).

BOX 14–1	**Principles of the Ethical Practice of Public Health**

- Public health should address principally the fundamental causes of disease and requirements for health, aiming to prevent adverse health outcomes.
- Public health should achieve community health in a way that respects the rights of individuals in the community.
- Public health policies, programs, and priorities should be developed and evaluated through processes that ensure an opportunity for input from community members.
- Public health should advocate and work for the empowerment of disenfranchised community members, aiming to ensure that the basic resources and conditions necessary for health are accessible to all.
- Public health should seek the information needed to implement effective policies and programs that protect and promote health.
- Public health institutions should provide communities with the information they have that is needed for decisions on policies or programs and should obtain the community's consent for their implementation.
- Public health institutions should act in a timely manner on the information they have within the resources and the mandate given to them by the public.
- Public health programs and policies should incorporate a variety of approaches that anticipate and respect diverse values, beliefs, and cultures in the community.
- Public health programs and policies should be implemented in a manner that most enhances the physical and social environment.
- Public health institutions should protect the confidentiality of information that can bring harm to an individual or community if made public. Exceptions must be justified on the basis of the high likelihood of significant harm to the individual or others.
- Public health institutions should ensure the professional competence of their employees.
- Public health institutions and their employees should engage in collaborations and affiliations in ways that build the public's trust and the institution's effectiveness.

Source: See reference 18.

Essential Services

The core functions are further delineated in the 10 essential public health services that illustrate to legislators and the general public what public health does (see Chapter 1) (Fig. 14-4). For example, the assurance function is further defined in one of the essential public health services, that of linking people to needed personal health services and assuring the provision of health care when otherwise unavailable.[16] Continuing with the immunization example, PHD PHNs refer college students to their primary care provider, college health center, or local health department to obtain needed immunizations.

Public Health Interventions

A useful conceptual framework for understanding how a health department provides population-based care is the Intervention Wheel, which was introduced in Chapter 2.[19] The Intervention Wheel depicts 17 PHN interventions that are provided on the individual, community, or systems level to affect the health of individuals and families that make up the community.

PHD PHNs usually provide several types of interventions to address a single issue and these interventions

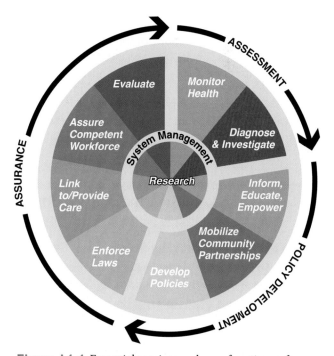

Figure 14-4 Essential services and core functions of public health. *(From the Public Health Functions Steering Committee, 1995. Retrieved from http://www.health.gov/phfunctions/public.htm.)*

may be directed at different levels of care. The Intervention Wheel model depicts three levels of care: (1) individual, (2) community, and (3) systems.[19] For example, interventions for reducing tobacco use can be provided for all three levels of care. On the individual level, a PHD PHN may counsel a pregnant woman on how to stop smoking. A community-level intervention may be used to have an impact on more smokers through group education. The PHD PHN may teach tobacco cessation classes that target teens. Nurses working in PHDs also direct interventions at a systems level, which affects the health of the populations and may have the greatest potential for improving health-care outcomes. For example, in considering a population, the most effective tobacco cessation program may not be counseling individuals but, instead, intervening on the systems and policy levels to levy tobacco taxes[20] (see Chapter 11).

What does intervening at a systems level mean? For at least the past 10 years, the Tobacco Control Research Branch of the National Cancer Institute has been studying a transdisciplinary initiative to explore systems thinking approaches and methods in tobacco prevention and control, resulting in 2007 in a monograph titled *Greater Than the Sum: Systems Thinking in Tobacco Control*.[21] The complexity involved in systems thinking was recently discussed, for example, by presenting a framework for investigating the social ecology of tobacco use. The multiple factors at play include actions of the tobacco industry, regulatory systems (smoke-free laws, taxation levels), and the tobacco use control subsystem (quit lines, social marketing, multilevel networks).[22, 23] One can address any of these factors from a systems perspective.

Ideally, PHD PHNs and community partners work together to implement the core functions, essential services, and public health nursing interventions to ultimately meet the *Healthy People 2020 (HP 2020)* vision of a "society in which all people live long, healthy lives."[24] To help illustrate how this is done, the next section describes how a PHD implements core functions, essentials services, and interventions to address high infant mortality rates in their community (Fig. 14-5).

▶ SOLVING THE MYSTERY
The Case of the Dying Babies

Public Health Science Topics Covered:
- Assessment
- Epidemiology
  - Surveillance
  - Rates

Health problems are identified in a variety of ways, often simultaneously. In hypothetical Beach County, the death of a 5-month-old infant of a 14-year-old mother was highly publicized in the local media and community members were outraged that this occurred in their "backyard." A nurse leader at the PHD was asked to convene a community work group to assess the issues, especially because this was not viewed as an isolated case, and make recommendations for addressing infant mortality in her community.

The nurse leader decided to begin by conducting an assessment on the population level. **Community health assessments** (see Chapter 4) are ongoing activities by PHDs, and formal community health assessments are usually conducted every 3 to 5 years.[25] There are several frameworks for conducting a community health assessment, including the Community Health Assessment aNd Group Evaluation tool (CHANGE) (see Chapters 4 and 5). Beach Health Department selected the Mobilizing for Action Through Planning and Partnerships (MAPP) because of its emphasis on a community-driven process facilitated by the PHD.[25] This framework, which consists of four different types of assessments, allows communities to apply strategic thinking to prioritize public health issues and identify resources to address them (see Chapters 4 and 5). In this case, the PHD was very concerned about the infant mortality issue and decided to focus its assessment on a specific population: mothers and babies. Because a comprehensive assessment was due in approximately 2 years, this phase was viewed as a narrower perspective for identifying the issues surrounding the infant mortality problem.

There were several steps involved in the assessment, all exhibiting evidence of the essential services. The nurse leader contacted the state department of health and arranged for training on MAPP, thus assuring a competent workforce, the eighth essential public health service. A MAPP committee was formed to guide the health planning process, with broad representation of the community and local public health system including community members, nurses, and health-care providers from the local hospital, schools, and private practices. Elected officials were asked to join as well as a pregnant woman and teen mothers. This committee is an example of the fourth essential public health service: mobilizing community partnerships to identify and solve health problems. The assessment was initiated by the PHD in this case, bringing not only a public health perspective to the issue but also a governmental legitimacy and sense of urgency.

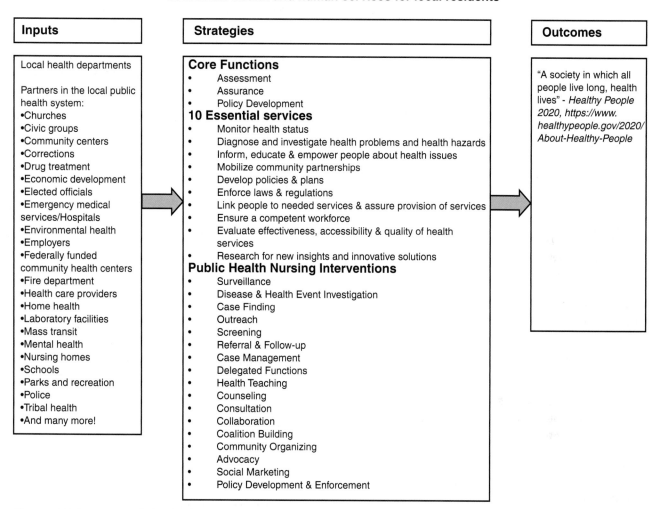

Vision: A healthy and safe community where individuals can thrive and prosper
Mission: Collaborate with community partners to promote and assure high quality, accessible health and human services for local residents

Inputs	Strategies	Outcomes
Local health departments Partners in the local public health system: •Churches •Civic groups •Community centers •Corrections •Drug treatment •Economic development •Elected officials •Emergency medical services/Hospitals •Environmental health •Employers •Federally funded community health centers •Fire department •Health care providers •Home health •Laboratory facilities •Mass transit •Mental health •Nursing homes •Schools •Parks and recreation •Police •Tribal health •And many more!	**Core Functions** • Assessment • Assurance • Policy Development **10 Essential services** • Monitor health status • Diagnose and investigate health problems and health hazards • Inform, educate & empower people about health issues • Mobilize community partnerships • Develop policies & plans • Enforce laws & regulations • Link people to needed services & assure provision of services • Ensure a competent workforce • Evaluate effectiveness, accessibility & quality of health services • Research for new insights and innovative solutions **Public Health Nursing Interventions** • Surveillance • Disease & Health Event Investigation • Case Finding • Outreach • Screening • Referral & Follow-up • Case Management • Delegated Functions • Health Teaching • Counseling • Consultation • Collaboration • Coalition Building • Community Organizing • Advocacy • Social Marketing • Policy Development & Enforcement	"A society in which all people live long, health lives" - *Healthy People 2020, https://www. healthypeople.gov/2020/ About-Healthy-People*

Figure 14-5 Framework for the delivery of population-focused health services on the local level. *(Created by B. Little and S. Bulecza, 2013.)*

The committee began with a brainstorming activity to formulate a shared community vision and values statements to guide the community-driven planning process. A time line was established and a preliminary plan was written that identified the work to be done. As explained in Chapter 4, MAPP is divided into four assessments:[25]

1. The **Community Themes and Strengths Assessment** provides a deep understanding of the issues that residents feel are important by answering the open-ended questions about what is important to the community. In this case, it might involve some key informant interviews or focus groups assessing the strengths and problems surrounding the care of mothers in the community.

2. The **Local Public Health System Assessment** focuses on all of the organizations and entities that contribute to the public's health. In this case, it would be important to assess the organizations providing services to mothers and babies.

3. The **Community Health Status Assessment** identifies priority community health and quality of life issues. It includes identifying the indicators focused on maternal-child health and gathering

secondary and primary data related to these indicators.

4. The **Forces of Change Assessment** focuses on identifying forces such as legislation, technology, and other impending changes that affect the context in which the community and its public health system operate. In this case, a key question was focused on the impending changes regarding funding for maternal child services in the county.

The members of the core steering committee divided themselves according to interest or expertise into one of four groups. The nurse and the PHD epidemiologist provided support to each of the subcommittees. This assessment illustrates how the PHD implements the essential services of monitoring health status to identify, diagnose, and investigate health problems and health hazards in the community.

During the next several months, subcommittees met on a regular basis and periodically reported on progress and findings to each other. For example, the Forces of Change subcommittee reported on a newly funded grant for the development of a federally funded health center to be located in a neighborhood with a high infant mortality rate. The Community Health Status subcommittee asked the PHD epidemiologist for additional vital statistics and geographic information systems (GIS) data, described later in this chapter, and assistance with analyzing the rate of infant mortality and teen births by ZIP code, race, and age. The committee also gathered secondary data from the state and county **Behavioral Risk Factor Surveillance System (BRFSS)** survey data about high-risk behaviors as well as county data about neonatal mortality, infant mortality, percentage low birth weight, percentage very low birth weight, percentage of prenatal care initiated in the first trimester, percentage of mothers who smoke, and the prevalence of sudden infant death syndrome (SIDS). BRFSS is a behavioral and noncommunicable disease surveillance system sponsored by the Centers for Disease Control and Prevention (CDC).[26] The surveys are conducted via land line telephones and recently expanded to include cell phones. The Community Themes and Strengths Assessment group decided to focus on a series of listening or focus groups with minority residents and youth, whereas the Local Public Health System Assessment group focused on identifying resources within the community addressing the health concerns. They conducted an Inventory of Resources (see Chapter 4).

After the subcommittees completed their assessments, the nurse leader compiled the results and prepared a presentation and agenda for the next MAPP committee meeting. The report consisted of county-specific data, health status compared with state objectives, trends, disparities, assets, and summary conclusions. The results showed that the infant mortality rate was 9.6 deaths per 1,000 live births compared with 7.1 for the state, and there were racial differences with a rate of 12.7 deaths per 1,000 live births for African Americans and a rate of 6.2 for the white population. Only 68.4% of the African American population received prenatal care in the first trimester compared with 80% for the total population. Fifteen percent of the pregnant women smoked in Beach County compared with 12% in the state as a whole. The percentage of low birth weight was much higher for the minority population (12%) compared with that of the white population (7.8%). Low birth weight was similar to the state findings. The teen birth rate was 71 per 1,000 live births compared with 67 per 1,000 live births only 2 years earlier.

The core committee met to review the data. Community issues were discussed and a list of four issues were identified and arranged by priority. In Beach County, some of the issues directly related to infant mortality were delayed prenatal care, increased low birth weight, high birth rates among teens, and tobacco use during pregnancy. Each issue was further researched for best practices, and goals and strategies were developed. In addition, the committee established a community goal for reducing infant mortality to 6 per 1,000 live births within 3 years.

This MAPP example illustrates the PHD role in conducting community assessments, facilitating health planning, and collaborating with partners to target high-priority issues. During the next year, the MAPP committee entered the action cycle and sought funding from public and private donors to establish a Nurse-Family Partnership[27, 28] community health program with nurse home visitors for low-income, first-time mothers. Through administration of the home visitation program, the PHD addressed the essential service of linking people to needed personal health services and assuring the provision of health care when otherwise unavailable.

■ EVIDENCE-BASED PRACTICE

The Nurse-Family Partnership Model for Providing Home-Visiting for Low-Income, First-Time Mothers and Their Children

Practice Statement: Nurses provide prenatal and child health education, care coordination, and life coaching during home visits that begin during pregnancy and continue through the child's second birthday.

Targeted Outcome: Improved prenatal health, fewer childhood injuries, fewer subsequent pregnancies, increased intervals between births, increased maternal employment, improved school readiness

Evidence to Support: Randomized controlled trials and economic analysis suggest improved long-term outcomes for mothers and children in the nurse-family partnership home visitation program. Nurse-family partnership programs are available in 43 states and participate in a Web-based data collection and evaluation system that allows programs to measure progress toward meeting nurse-family partnership benchmarks for maternal and child health outcomes.

Recommended Approaches: The nurse-family relationship is the cornerstone of the home-visiting program that is based on a client-centered, strengths-based approach to support personal and family functioning. Nurses are equipped with tools, education, and resources to improve family outcomes. The nurse-family partnership agency provides the infrastructure to ensure high quality implementation and ongoing program evaluation in local communities.

Sources

1. Nurse-Family Partnership. (2010a). *Overview*. Retrieved from http://www.nursefamilypartnership. org/assets/PDF/Fact-sheets/NFP_Overview.
2. Nurse-Family Partnership. (2010b). *Research trials and outcomes*. Retrieved from http://www. nursefamilypartnership.org/assets/PDF/Fact-sheets/ NFP_Research_Outcomes.
3. Nurse-Family Partnership. (2011). *Nurses and mothers*. Retrieved from http://www.nursefamilypartnership.org/ assets/PDF/Fact-sheets/NFP_Nurses-Mothers.

Local Health Department Activities

In 2010, PHDs were surveyed by NACCHO to identify not only structure but also function and capacities of local PHDs. The roles of PHDs have changed during the past century and have been shaped by historical events. The events of September 11, 2001, brought to the forefront an awareness of the role of PHDs in disasters. More recently, threats such as Superstorm Sandy emphasized this even more.

The following section describes a contemporary view of the activities of PHDs and recognizes that separating out activities solely performed by local health departments is indeed difficult. The 2010 NACCHO survey asked PHDs to report those activities performed only by the PHD, those done in concert with the state, and those done by contracting out to other members of the public health system. The 10 most frequent activities and services provided by PHDs directly are found in Table 14-1.[12] It is clear that more than three-fourths of PHDs provide these services. Other services are provided through contractual relationships with other organizations such as lab services, by other governmental agencies (animal control), or through nongovernmental organizations (NGOs). The contractual agreements are one way for PHDs to assure that needed health services are available to its citizens.[29]

There are five categories used to summarize the major activities of PHDs:[30]

1. Environmental health services
2. Data collection and analysis: health and vital statistics

TABLE 14-1	Percentage of Public Health Department Jurisdictions With 10 Most Frequent Activities and Services

Available Through PHDs Directly

Activity or Service	Percentage of Jurisdictions
Adult Immunization Provision	92%
Communicable/Infectious Disease Surveillance	92%
Child Immunizations Provision	92%
Tuberculosis Screening	85%
Food Service Establishment Inspection	78%
Environmental Health Surveillance	78%
Food Safety Education	76%
Tuberculosis Treatment	75%
Schools/Day Care Center Inspection	74%
Population-Based Nutrition Services	71%

Source: See reference 12.

3. Individual and community health
4. Disease control, epidemiology, and surveillance
5. Regulation, licensing, and inspection

Environmental Health Services

Environmental health services are focused around activities ensuring that communities have safe water and food and sanitary environments. For example, local health departments located near beaches are responsible for conducting periodic water sampling to ensure that the water does not contain high levels of contaminants or bacteria. If bacteria or contaminants are found at levels out of normal range that pose a risk to persons swimming at the beach, then local health departments have the authority to close the beach until levels return to an acceptable range.

Environmental services are the backbone of public health infrastructure in developed countries and have eliminated such problems as cholera and diarrheal disease. In fact, in 1940 environmental sanitation was viewed as a minimum function of local health departments to address proper public and private water supply systems and sewage disposal, restaurant inspections, insect and rodent control, housing inspections, and environmental complaints.[3] The development of solid waste management is interesting. At the time of the infectious epidemics in the 1800s, funding was not available for a regional approach to solid waste management, which resulted in municipal approaches to dealing with the problems.[30] Today, solid waste management is largely handled by municipalities and operated by private companies.

Environmental concerns today are often seen as responsibilities of both local and state agencies as well as other local governmental agencies or NGOs. In the most recent NACCHO 2010 survey, food safety education and vector control activities were most often connected with the PHD as the resource. State health departments were most often listed as resources for many other activities such as indoor air quality, groundwater protection, noise pollution, hazardous waste disposal, air pollution, and radiation control.[12] With any of these activities, there is a great deal of variability, with many agencies often assuming some level of responsibility. In another study examining the combined roles of state and local health departments, the PHD was typically found to oversee private water supplies and septic systems.[32] A list of typical environmental concerns is found in Box 14-2 (see Chapter 6).

Data Collection and Analysis: Health and Vital Statistics

Most data collection and analysis activities are state-level functions, although the process of collecting statistics

begins at the local level. **Vital statistics** are data collected regarding births, deaths, marriages, and divorces. Data are forwarded to the state, where they are compiled and sent to the CDC National Vital Statistics System.[33] This is the oldest process for sharing public health data across governmental agencies. It requires that these agencies share standards and procedures so that the National Center for Health Statistics can monitor, store, and disseminate the nation's official vital statistics.

When a baby is born, the hospital completes a birth form that is submitted to the PHD. The PHD then issues the official birth certificate to the child's parents. The birth record includes data that can be found on the official birth certificate such as the birth date, place of birth, and parents' names. It also includes a wealth of other information not listed on the official birth certificate. These data include neonatal outcomes, risk factors related to adverse outcomes, and protective factors related to positive outcomes.[34] Information is included on parental demographic and behavioral variables such as age; level of education; race; and maternal use of alcohol, tobacco, and other drugs during pregnancy. Information is also collected related to the pregnancy and the delivery such as the number of prenatal visits, when the trimester prenatal care began, and the type of delivery. Finally, data are collected on the newborn. In addition to weight, head circumference, and length, data are collected on information related to the neonate's weeks of gestation and congenital defects. Data are obtained from the medical record, the health provider of record, and from family members. These data provide important information needed to understand population-level trends related to birth and allows evaluation of how well *HP 2020* objectives are being met.

Likewise, PHDs collect mortality data based on the information collected on death records. The first part of the document includes basic demographic information on the deceased and is completed by the funeral director or other person in charge of internment. This same person is also responsible for filing the certificate with the registrar where the death occurred. The medical examiner or coroner certifying the death completes the second section of the document that includes information related to the cause of death. The certificate includes essential demographic data as well as date and time of death, where the death occurred, and the primary cause of death. Like the birth record, the death record includes more data than what is included in the death certificate. These include a record of conditions that contributed to the death, history of tobacco use, race, and other variables.[34] These data are used to evaluate mortality trends at the population level. If the death was due to an injury, information related to the injury is also collected. Cause of death data are compiled from death certificates and used to determine specific disease, injury, or mode of death rates within communities and for the state. For example, death data are used to determine the number of cancer deaths in a community and help during community assessments and health system planning. For infants aged less than 1 year, linked birth and death certificate files provide even more information to help determine risk factors related to fetal mortality.

Another required vital record is fetal death. **Fetal death** is a spontaneous intrauterine death of a fetus at any time during pregnancy. Again, the record includes a section to complete the basic information related to parental demographic data, time and date of delivery, and gender of the fetus. The second section relates to the cause and conditions contributing to the fetal death. Again, the data not only provide an official record of the death, but also provide additional information to help with population-level assessments and program planning. Most states report fetal deaths of 20 weeks of gestation or more and/or birth weight of 350 grams or more.

Although states are responsible for the analysis of most data, reportable diseases is one category wherein

the PHD is often responsible for the collection and analysis of data.[12] In addition, in some states with local boards of health, morbidity data are sometimes collected at the local level.

There are many uses for vital statistics. Birth and death certificates are used to legally establish citizenship and to obtain drivers licenses and Social Security cards, and are required in the probating of a will. Vital statistics help genealogists conduct family research and establish ties between individuals. Most important, vital statistics from a global perspective are vital to understanding the health of populations, determining life expectancy, and helping to guide interventions aimed at improving health.

Individual and Community Health

For some PHDs, assuring the health of populations sometimes involves providing direct individual care as well as providing care at the community level. Direct individual care provided by PHDs can include a variety of services such as prenatal and well-baby clinics, clinics for communicable diseases (e.g., tuberculosis [TB], sexually transmitted infections [STIs]), primary care clinics, school health services, and vaccination clinics. Comparing PHDs, there is probably no area within the local public health system with as much diversity in programs for the provision of direct individual care. Some health departments provide no direct care at all, whereas others provide a wide variety of care. The City of Cincinnati Health Department, for example, includes home-care services, pharmacy, school nursing, and multiple clinics.[35] Other PHDs contract out services or the services are available only through NGOs.

At one time, the provision of primary care services (see Chapter 16), particularly to underserved and economically disadvantaged citizens (and areas), were part of the mainstream of public health activities. There has been a national effort to have governmental public health services return their attention to more population-based public health services.[36] Consequently, a transfer of services has taken place and this has been done in many different formats. PHDs have contracted or networked with their local hospital system to fund primary care services as an alternative to emergency room visits for the same service. In some cases, the most recent 2010 NACCHO survey found that certain activities were exclusively provided through contracts:[12]

- Laboratory services, 21%
- HIV/AIDS treatment, 12%
- Cancer screening, 11%
- STI screening, 9%

- Tobacco prevention, 9%
- Oral health, 9%
- Tuberculosis treatment, 9%
- STI treatment 9%
- Child immunization, 9%

Another process for PHDs to obtain funding for providing care is through federally qualified health centers. **Federally qualified health centers (FQHC)** are funded through the Health Resources and Service Administration (HRSA) under section 330 of the Public Health Service Act. There are multiple benefits for having a FQHC, including enhanced reimbursement from Medicare and Medicaid. Federally qualified health centers must serve an underserved area or population, offer a sliding fee scale, and provide comprehensive services.[37] They must also have an ongoing quality assurance program with a governing board of directors.

Maternal and Child Health

Maternal-child services have traditionally been a key component of any PHD (See Chapter 18). This goes back to the early 20th century as evidenced in the APHA mission statements.[9,10] The overall goal of maternal-child services has been to improve the health of mothers and children through the delivery of preventive interventions. Although these efforts have changed overtime, they are still an important aspect of PHD services. PHDs either provide these services directly or help to link their constituents with available services. For maternal-child health services overall, the 2010 NACCHO survey shows that the current services provided most often in PHDs are MCH home visits (61%), **Women, Infants, and Children (WIC)** services (64%), and family planning (55%).[12] In addition, the importance of these programs was underscored by HRSA in 2010 when they provided $90 million in the Affordable Care Act (ACA) Funding for Maternal, Infant, and Childhood Home Visiting Program grants.[38]

One example of a comprehensive maternal-child health program is **Healthy Start,** which focuses on reducing infant mortality and low birth weight. The Healthy Start initiative was signed into law in 1991 and is funded through HRSA.[39] In this program, nurses working at PHDs engage in multiple services from group-level activities, such as health education to expectant and new mothers to individual care in prenatal and well-baby clinics or home visiting. It addresses multiple issues such as providing adequate prenatal care, meeting basic health needs, reducing barriers to access, and empowering clients. There is growing evidence that these programs have been successful in lowering preterm births and low birth weight.[40]

In addition to maternity care programs, PHDs provide nutritional support for pregnant women and children through the federally funded WIC programs. WIC was established as a pilot program in 1972, made permanent in 1974, and is administered at the federal level by the Food and Nutrition Service of the U.S. Department of Agriculture. In April 2008, there were 9.5 million women, infants, and children enrolled in the WIC program and two-thirds of them were at or below the poverty line.[41] Nurses and nutritionists work collaboratively to provide nutrition counseling and breastfeeding support.

Family planning programs are a third example of maternal-child health care in PHDs. Family planning programs began in the 1960s and 1970s as a result of the need to meet the reproductive needs of populations at some level. Family planning grew out of federal legislation, originally the Office of Economic Opportunity in 1965 and then the enactment of Family Planning Services and Population Research Act of 1970, or Title X.[42] Family planning programs did not share a universal acceptance upon their inception. These programs coincided with the approval of oral contraceptives and were temporally associated with the changing societal mores regarding sexual activity. Many communities initially resisted the provision of these services. Over the years, levels of acceptance of these programs have risen and fallen, with most of the controversy focusing on whether there should be public financing of family planning. This demonstrates the role that public opinion plays in public health policy. Core family planning services have centered on individual counseling on method selection, annual physicals, and follow-up services.

An example of comprehensive family planning services can be found at the New York State Department of Health Web site: http://www.health.state.ny.us/health_care/medicaid/program/longterm/familyplanbenprog.htm. The purpose of the program is to ". . . increase access to family planning services and to enable individuals of childbearing age to prevent or reduce the incidence of unintentional pregnancies."[43]

School Health

School health is concerned with assuring the health of the entire school population, students, and staff (Chapter 19). As the health-care expert in the school setting, school nurses take a leadership role in developing policies and providing clinical care that promote health and assure safe health-care practices in a nonmedical setting including medication administration, immunizations, and emergency response to medical crises or disasters.

School-based screening programs for vision, hearing, and obesity identify children with potential health problems that may be a barrier to academic achievement or indicate an underlying medical condition necessitating the nurse to make referrals to other providers and conduct follow-up to assure access to care and adherence to treatment (see Chapter 19).[44] By delivering case management services, school nurses coordinate care and help families locate resources for medical, social, and mental health services. School-based wellness programs are designed to address common childhood issues such as obesity; dental caries; asthma; and health education needs related to growth and development, communicable diseases, and sexuality. Funding and staffing patterns for school nurses employed by PHDs and school districts vary between states and counties. Not every school has a school nurse, which is unfortunate as 9% of children do not have health insurance and the school nurse may be their only access to care.[45]

Immunization and Health Protection Programs

Providing immunizations to protect a population from communicable diseases is an essential component of public health. Vaccinations are mandated by school districts and in some cases employers, especially in health-care settings. If an outbreak of disease occurs, the PHD is often the entity responsible for mass immunization, as occurred in the H1N1 influenza outbreak in 2009.

Immunization practices have been in place for centuries. For example, variolation (the exposure of well persons to material from an infected person such as pus or scabs) was used to prevent smallpox. Though variolation resulted in death for some, the overall death rate fell. In the late 1700s, Edward Jenner, a physician, discovered that milkmaids exposed to cowpox, a less deadly disease, developed immunity to smallpox. The term *vaccine* comes from the word *vaca,* which means "cow" in Latin. He exposed a small boy to pus from a milkmaid with cowpox and then exposed him to smallpox. The boy did not contract the disease. Though it took a while for vaccinations to enter into mainstream practice, by 1800 they were being used across Europe and other parts of the globe.[46] Today, owing to a global campaign, smallpox has been eradicated worldwide.

Immunizations are a major responsibility of PHDs. PHDs manage the programmatic requirements associated with administration and utilization of vaccines for preventable diseases. Immunization administration may be integrated into the PHD clinical service program. Immunization program components include ordering and tracking vaccines, ensuring that individual immunizations

are recorded into registries if used in that jurisdiction, and coordinating special immunization clinics. In addition, immunization programs coordinate the Vaccine for Children program. This program helps to get supplies of vaccine to health-care providers who provide services to children to make sure they have adequate supplies to vaccinate the children in their care. This helps to ensure that all children, regardless of ability to pay, have access to immunizations for vaccine-preventable diseases.

In addition to childhood vaccination programs, PHD immunization programs provide services to other populations at risk. This includes international travel vaccination. They also provide the rabies postexposure prophylaxis vaccine. PHDs often work with community partners to provide clinics where anyone can come for immunizations for diseases such as influenza. These types of clinics help increase a community's level of immunity from these diseases. PHNs often coordinate the planning and implementation of these open clinics. Schools have often been a place where immunizations and other child-focused services are provided. Through these activities, not only does the PHD protect individuals who receive the vaccine, but also the programs are instrumental in reducing the overall prevalence of communicable diseases, thus reducing the opportunity for the spread of disease and providing herd immunity (see Chapter 8).

Role of Nurses in Providing Individual Care

Nurses are often employed by PHDs to provide the direct individual care at the clinics. The nursing care provided often includes one-on-one clinical interventions such as vaccinations, prenatal care, and dispensing of medications for STIs or TB. In addition, PHNs often provide home visiting and a focus on high-risk families as part of these services.[47] Establishing working relationships with these families has been a strength of public health nursing and the value of these home visitations has been proved.[48,49] A recent qualitative study illustrates that PHNs are especially good at recognizing the sociohistorical factors that influence families, focusing on strengths and chaotic lives simultaneously, and working flexibly.[47]

Community Health Primary Prevention Efforts

As described in Chapter 2, primary prevention occurs before illness or injury has occurred in an effort to prevent it from happening. In addition to services focused on individuals, PHDs provide a wide array of primary prevention services aimed at health promotion and protection at the community level. Health promotion includes activities that focus on improving the ability of individuals and populations to practice healthy living. Health protection interventions focus on protecting the individuals or populations from disease by improving the immune system through vaccination for individuals or providing protective barriers such as the use of personal protective equipment by health-care providers.

Health promotion efforts at the community level include educating about healthy lifestyles. Examples of health education include HIV prevention education for teens or Back to Sleep campaigns for reducing SIDS. The Back to Sleep campaigns began in 1994 and focused on educating parents, caregivers, and health-care providers about ways to reduce the risk of SIDS. Since the campaign started, there has been a 50% reduction in SIDS deaths, and the percentage of babies being placed on their backs to sleep has increased significantly.[50]

Communication is a key component to the provision of primary prevention programs for PHDs. In today's world, there are multiple methods for communicating important health data and health promotion information. For example, during the H1N1 influenza outbreak in 2009, PHDs used multiple methods to communicate to their communities where to get immunizations and which groups had priority. They used TV, radio, and print media to get the message out as well as sending information home with schoolchildren. Social media such as YouTube, Twitter, and Facebook are being used with increasing frequency by PHDs as effective avenues for providing health information.

A Healthy Community: Sarasota, Florida: An example of a community-wide health promotion initiative is the Community Health Improvement Partnership in Sarasota, Florida.[51] The Sarasota PHD led this partnership and brought together many stakeholders from the community. Partners included community organizations, individual citizens, and health-care professionals. Together, they identified evidence-based strategies and chose those that had the most applicability to their community. These strategies were multipronged; that is, they used different venues and methods to engage the community in a healthier lifestyle. They developed Healthy Living kiosks throughout the community. These kiosks provided information about health insurance options, health-care resources, and consumer tips. Users were able to access a county health scorecard that provided data on health status, and linkage to a community pharmacy where those who were uninsured or underinsured could have access to needed medications. The development of this required that PHD nurses understand the basics of public health science so that they could develop an intervention based on the community priority health needs and service gaps

within the community. It also required understanding implementation and evaluation strategies to determine whether the kiosk was an effective intervention. PHDs provide essential leadership and skills in the promotion of the health of the community they serve.

Disease Control, Epidemiology, and Surveillance

Disease Control

Because communicable disease is a primary concern of PHDs, their ability to provide necessary training and services surrounding communicable diseases is important. This will vary depending on the size of the public health system. Many small health departments gather private physician case reports and provide the information to a regional or central office for analysis and compilation. Larger PHDs may have internal units devoted to the communicable disease program, including core epidemiological services and supporting the biostatistical analysis of the determinants of diseases in animals and man.

Tuberculosis Management: TB management is one of public health's oldest communicable disease programs for one of the oldest diseases noted in history. With the advent of effective therapies, elimination of TB was considered a possibility. However, this remarkable organism continues to be a major threat to public health both globally and in the United States. A resurgence of the disease is sometimes now accompanied by a rise in multidrug resistant TB (MDR-TB), which is defined as TB that is resistant to the two most effective first-line therapeutic drugs, isoniazid and rifampin. The CDC established a task force to develop a plan of action to address the issue of drug-resistant TB.[52] Tuberculosis is a complex interaction of medical, societal, behavioral, and economic factors.

● APPLYING PUBLIC HEALTH SCIENCE

The Case of the Tuberculosis Neighborhood Investigation

Public Health Science Topics Covered:

- Surveillance
- Disease investigation
- Prevention

Sara Johnson, communicable disease nurse at Creek County Health Department, received a call from the infection control nurse at Providence Hospital reporting a newly diagnosed case of TB in a hospitalized patient. The patient was a 40-year-old male (Mr. H.) who worked for the grounds maintenance unit of the local college. Sara advised the infection control nurse that she would come to the hospital that day to review the chart and interview the patient. She remembered that there had been another university employee from the same unit diagnosed a year ago and all of the employees had received appropriate TB testing. No other cases had been identified during that case follow-up, so she was somewhat concerned about the appearance of this case.

Sara learned the following from her chart review and patient interview:

- The patient had only been employed with the university for 4 months.
- He lived with his girlfriend and her two daughters.
- He presented with classic TB symptoms—night sweats, weight loss, no appetite, and persistent cough. His sputum was acid-fact bacillus (AFB) positive and his chest x-ray was indicative of pulmonary TB. Pharmacological therapy was consistent with the CDC's TB treatment protocols. He would be hospitalized in isolation until three consecutive AFB sputum smears were negative.
- Names of coworkers, family, and friends were obtained.
- He wasn't sure whether he had been around anybody with TB. One of his neighbors had been sick a few months ago with similar symptoms, but the patient didn't know what the neighbor had.

Based on the above information, Sara ruled out that he had been exposed from the previous case and began to prioritize the contact list for follow-up. What criteria should Sara use to prioritize the contacts? To answer this question and the rest of the questions related to this case, see Box 14-3.[53–55]

Sara contacted the patient's girlfriend and arranged for her and her daughters to come to the health department for evaluation and tuberculin skin testing because they had closest contact with the patient. Then, she contacted the patient's supervisor to advise him of the situation and the need to interview coworkers. To minimize disruption to the workers, Sara agreed to bring a small interview team to the site to conduct evaluations and provide tuberculin skin testing. She agreed to go back to the site to read the tests 72 hours later so the workers would not have to miss work.

After about a week, Sara received notification from the hospital that the patient was ready for discharge

BOX 14-3 Questions Related to the Neighborhood Investigation of Tuberculosis

1. How is the infectious period for TB defined?
2. What is the difference between active and latent TB infection?
3. What factors had an impact on the decision to initiate a contact investigation? What are the goals of a contact investigation?
4. What groups are most at risk for TB infection? How should the nurse prioritize contact for follow-up?
5. What factors would require a contact be placed on chemoprophylaxis?
6. Directly observed treatment is a resource-intensive intervention. How should the nurse prioritize contacts for it?
7. If the neighborhood had been different, what other interventions could have been used to reach the neighbors?
8. Discuss challenges with and solutions for providing directly observed therapy with someone who is homeless.
9. This investigation may attract the attention of the media. What strategies should the nurse use for communicating with the media?

The following are recommended sources for answering the preceding questions:
1. Centers for Disease Control and Prevention. (2005). Guidelines for the investigation of contacts of persons with infectious tuberculosis. *Morbidity and Mortality Weekly Report, 54*(RR15), 1-37. Retrieved from http://www.cdc.gov/mmwr/preview/mmwrhtml/rr5415a1.htm.
2. CDC TB Web site: http://www.cdc.gov/tb/.

and he would need to be on **directly observed therapy** for several months to ensure adherence to the medication regimen. It was decided that Sara would meet the patient at his home the next day after he was discharged. During this meeting, Sara reviewed activity restrictions and the medication plan, explained the process of directly observed therapy, and told him that she would be coming to his home each day to watch him take the medications.

Two key issues in the treatment of TB are the length of treatment and the emergence of MDR-TB. For the most part, MDR-TB occurred because of nonadherence to recommended treatment. That is, those with an active infection did not complete the required drug regimen and the bacterium became resistant to the drug. Today, the World Health Organization (WHO) recommends treatment to continue for

6 months or longer.[56] In the United States, the populations most at risk for active TB are often those hardest to reach (e.g., foreign-born persons from countries with a high TB prevalence, those exposed to persons with active TB, those who are immune-compromised, persons with alcohol or substance abuse, and persons with latent TB infections [they are infected but do not have active disease]).[55] To assist with this, nurses working in PHDs often function as case managers to help ensure that patients with TB follow through with the required treatment. Nurses apply their holistic approach to care and are able to appreciate and mitigate factors that exist in the patient's life.

A key function of TB case management is ensuring adherence to the medication regimen. As noted earlier, one of the oldest ways of ensuring that is through the use of directly observed therapy, in which the patient takes the required daily medication in the presence of a public health-care provider, often a nurse. Either the patient goes directly to the PHD, or the public health-care provider comes to the patient's home. As with other areas of health care, technology has been developed that enhances the ability to monitor medication adherence. One example is a **medication electronic monitoring system,** which tracks adherence to a medication regimen through a chip placed in the medication bottle cap that uploads the date and time the cap is opened.[57] Other examples include use of text messaging, phone call reminders, and e-mail reminders.

With case management under way in the case of Mr. H., it was critical to continue to investigate for additional exposures. In trying to determine how he may have been exposed, Sara began reviewing previous cases. She found that the case from the prior year lived on the same street as the patient and that there had been several contacts who could not be found. She also determined that there had been another, earlier case on the same street. Based on this information, should Sara expand the contact investigation? Sara determined that there needed to be outreach to all the neighbors to ensure there were not any additional undiagnosed cases. She decided to learn more about the neighborhood by conducting a windshield survey of the street. Her findings were the following: (1) The street was isolated and not connected to a larger neighborhood; (2) there were about 15 houses; (3) there appeared to be children of all ages living on the street; and (4) there were several open, grassy areas on the street.

Sara decided that a community information fair and testing clinic would be the best way to provide outreach

services to the neighbors without compromising the patient's privacy. She developed the plan and presented it to the health department administrator for approval. After the plan was approved, she identified a Saturday for the event, recruited health department staff to assist, and solicited other health department programs to participate or provide information or give-away items. The event was very successful, with many of the neighbors receiving testing and information. Fortunately, no new cases were identified but several people with latent TB infection were placed on prophylaxis therapy.

Because of the communicability of TB, PHDs and PHNs take a leading role in both the prevention and treatment of TB. One approach by state and PHDs is to provide TB clinics that include screening assessment, diagnosis, and treatment components. Efforts at the local, state, and national levels have resulted overall in a reduced incidence of TB.[54] It is possible that TB could be eliminated in the United States. It will take continued efforts on the part of PHDs to continue to screen those at risk, assess persons with positive screens, and treat those with active disease.

Sexually Transmitted Infections: Communities also rely on PHDs to provide surveillance, prevention, and treatment of STIs. Most STIs are reportable diseases and the PHD reports each case to the state department of health, which then reports to the CDC. PHDs also combine clinical care for the diagnosis and treatment of the disease with a strong field investigative component needed to identify and notify contacts. Many PHDs conduct primary prevention programs, especially with teens, aimed at preventing STIs with outreach to schools, correctional facilities, gay bathhouses, and other community settings.

There is an enormous burden of STIs in the United States with more than 1.4 million cases of chlamydia infections, 321,849 cases of gonorrhea, and 49,273 new cases of HIV infection in 2011.[58,] With a disease burden of this magnitude in addition to the costs for society, the investigative role of PHDs is critical. The investigation of STIs includes three steps:

1. Screening for possible infection. Persons with suspected STIs are screened using appropriate tests. Depending on the STI, a positive screen may require further laboratory confirmation.
2. Treatment.
3. Screening all known sexual contacts of the person with the confirmed STI and treat if necessary.

Public health nurses often conduct the follow-up investigations for persons diagnosed with an STI such as syphilis. The PHN follows up with the patient to ensure he has adhered to the prescribed medications and obtain contact information for any sexual contacts before he was treated.

In 2010, NACCHO published a policy statement about the prevention and control of STIs.[59] PHDs have traditionally provided a critical role in this arena but there is a current threat to this coverage because of dwindling funds. In the first half of 2010, more than 53% of PHDs had to make cuts in their core programs, which in some cases resulted in an elimination of programs and services.[60]

Epidemiology and Surveillance

● APPLYING PUBLIC HEALTH SCIENCE
The Case of the Mysterious Illness

Public Health Science Topics Covered:

- Case finding
- Disease investigation

When Hannah Miles, a school nurse, arrived at the elementary school early one morning, she found Alexis, a sickly looking second grade student, waiting for her. Ms. Miles had seen Alexis just last week when she enrolled in the school after moving into the nearby homeless family shelter. Alexis has asthma and Ms. Miles referred the mother to the county health department for assistance with Medicaid eligibility and a primary care provider. The school nurse's assessment of Alexis found a temperature of 101.5°F, a dry cough, wheezing, inflamed throat, and runny nose. Alexis also complained of diarrhea and aching all over.

Earlier that week, the county epidemiologist sent all the school nurses an e-mail with an update on the novel influenza A (H1N1) flu outbreak. The WHO raised the pandemic flu alert to 5 and the CDC issued daily updates on the status of the outbreak, which involved 30 countries, 47 states, 4,298 confirmed and probable cases, and 3 deaths. After reviewing influenza signs and symptoms, the school nurse decided to refer the child for a medical evaluation. She called the mother at the shelter and explained that the child needed to be seen by a medical provider that day. Alexis was given a mask to wear and quarantined in the health room until the homeless shelter arranged for transportation to take her and her mother to the county health department because they did not have a primary care provider.

The school nurse also called the county health department to report the influenza-like illness case to the communicable disease/epidemiology staff and advise them of the child's imminent arrival at the clinic. She told them of the child's living situation so that the county health department could alert the shelter management of the need for vigilance in cleaning and hygiene and to be on the lookout for other residents with symptoms. The epidemiologist asked Ms. Miles to conduct active surveillance by checking with Alexis's teacher about other children with the same symptoms and by reviewing the absentee list to determine whether an abnormal number of students were absent from that class. In addition, students with symptoms of influenza-like illness seen in the health rooms were to be reported by fax to the communicable disease/epidemiology office.

Meanwhile, the county health department administrative team called a meeting of the medical director, nursing director, epidemiologist, communicable disease director, planning staff, and public information officer to review and implement their pandemic flu response plan in collaboration with county emergency operations, emergency response (law enforcement, fire service, and emergency medical services), local hospitals, and the school district. Staff provided the following updates:

- The clinic nursing supervisor reported that three suspect cases had been tested in the clinic, resulting in questions on disease containment in the waiting rooms and the need for a follow-up disease investigation.
- The local airport called and was seeking guidance on how to handle passengers in the terminal. Pilots have jurisdiction of passengers while they are on board but it was unclear who determined how to handle sick passengers within the terminal prior to boarding.
- The media were awaiting information on the suspect cases and was anxious to get the word out to the public.

A primary role of the PHD is to provide a central collection point for data on communicable diseases, emerging infections, illness, and disease in the community. Although new pharmaceutical products and vaccines have been developed to address communicable diseases, the dual threats of antibiotic resistance and the emergence of new pathogens have focused more attention on communicable disease epidemiology.

States, working in cooperation with the CDC, have a list of reportable diseases that private health-care systems are required to report. As described in Chapter 8, surveillance of communicable diseases on a regular basis works as an early warning system of a possible outbreak. If the reported cases of a communicable disease exceed the normal incidence, the PHD can begin a timely investigation into the outbreak.

The size of the PHD may hamper the ability of the department to collect the individual case report data. Although small departments may need the assistance, the emergence of an outbreak in the community will trigger an investigation, either independently or with assistance from state or federal (CDC) officials.

Emerging or Reemerging Infections: As we move ahead into the 21st century, PHDs will face two significant challenges: increased mobility due to globalization and emergence of new human pathogens. Joshua Lederberg coined the term *emerging infections* for the IOM in 2000. Emerging infections are diseases whose incidence in humans has increased within the past 2 decades or threatens to increase in the near future.[61] Reemerging communicable diseases include cholera and plague, whose geographical ranges are expanding.[62]

Our global society and rapid transit around the globe can result in the rapid dissemination of pathogens throughout the world. A case example is that of H1N1 influenza, a viral infection unheard of not too long ago as well as the 2003 severe acute respiratory syndrome (SARS) epidemic. SARS originated in China and was rapidly spread across the globe as infected persons traveled by airplane from China to other countries. As noted in Chapter 13, SARS infected 8,437 people with a case fatality rate of 9.6% (813 people).[63] Other recent examples of rapid global dissemination of a communicable disease are that of H1N1 and H7N9 (see Chapter 13). For H1N1, the Mexican government disseminated a wide array of pamphlets and posters to alert their population about mitigating the impact of H1N1 by slowing the transmission and lowering mortality.[64]

Besides globalization, the second factor most frequently underlined in the emergence of communicable diseases is that of demographic growth in urban settings.[62] The results are the growth of shantytowns, slums, and *barrios* where people live in less than healthy conditions, and the effects of urban poverty are evident in outbreaks of global pandemics such as dengue fever; trench fever *(Bartonella quintana)*; cholera; and the three major threats of AIDS, TB, and malaria.

Zoonotic Diseases: Another challenge in the modern world is the growth of cities and suburbia, which encroaches on the natural habitats of wild animals. Across the United States, deer, fox, and other wild animals are now living in suburbia and even in urban settings, increasing the likelihood of the transmission of zoonotic disease. Zoonotic diseases are diseases transmitted from animals to humans in the community through direct contact, as with rabies, or indirect contact through a vector such as Lyme disease[65] (see Chapter 8). PHDs are called on to conduct surveillance of zoonotic disease and institute prevention programs.

Rabies is a preventable viral disease of mammals that is usually transmitted through the bite of a rabid animal such as a dog or a raccoon. Owing to efforts from public health departments, both local and state levels, the incidence of rabies in the United States has dramatically decreased during the past 100 years.[66] Through public health campaigns to vaccinate domestic animals, 90% of all cases reported to the CDC are now in bats and wild carnivores. Human deaths due to rabies rarely occur because of effective and early intervention with post-bite exposure prophylaxis. The PHD provides education to health-care providers, tracks and reports to the state department of health all known cases, both animal and human, and works in partnership with animal control programs and veterinarians

Disaster Preparedness: An increasingly prominent role of PHDs, especially PHNs, is public health preparedness for responding to emergencies and disasters. Prior to the events of 2001, the preparedness functions were dictated by the regularity of events that affected the population and the health-care systems. Southeastern coastal states regularly face hurricanes. Midwestern states continually experience tornados. West Coast states are constantly threatened by earthquakes and fires. All have created robust emergency response systems. However, the realities of the 21st century have placed an additional responsibility on these systems because of threats caused by humans. Disaster planning programs evolved into "all hazards" planning. For example, a biological event, whether it is an anthrax attack or a widely distributed *Escherichia coli* contamination calls for a concerted response action. Preparedness has four major requirements PHDs need to address (see Chapter 25):

- Preparedness
- Mitigation
- Response
- Recovery

In 2002, the *Bioterrorism and Emergency Readiness Competencies for All Public Health Workers* was developed and has become the standard for ensuring the public health workforce is prepared and ready to respond to emergencies and disasters.[67]

Preparedness functions and planning rely heavily on the use of partners and data sets to achieve success. Each community is different in the resources it can bring to bear on dealing with an emergency or disaster. Consistently, the PHD is looked to as the community lead in collaboration with local emergency management for health and medical response activities in an emergency or disaster. Public health nurses have key roles to play in disaster planning and preparedness efforts. A key preparedness function uses a basic public health nursing skill, community assessment. By knowing the aspects of the community, plans can be written to meet the unique needs of that community during an emergency or disaster. During the disaster, the PHN's role may center on staffing emergency shelters for persons with special health and medical needs. During the recovery phase of a disaster, the PHN may be assigned to go into the community to assess the current and long-term needs of the area. Identification of these needs is essential to ensure the delivery of services to the community so that normal functioning may return.

Regulation, Licensing, and Inspection

Regulatory, licensing, and inspection activities are common roles for a PHD. The 2010 NACCHO survey of PHDs revealed that the areas of particular focus in PHD were food service, swimming pools, septic systems, and private drinking water.[12] Other areas included schools or day-care centers, camps, campgrounds, and, in some cases, housing.

Public Health Department Challenges for the Future

HP 2020 Objectives

As one thinks about the future, the objectives for *HP 2020* provide some insight into the issues of importance to the functioning of local health departments. *HP 2020*'s goal is to increase public health infrastructure. An example of an objective is "to increase the proportion of Tribal and State public health agencies that provide or assure comprehensive laboratory services to support essential public health services."[68] Other objectives relate to assuring the workers' competencies, monitoring performance, and assuring practice that is guided by standards. In an effort to highlight the need to strengthen the public health workforce, increased workforce diversity and reducing the shortage are critical and are reflected in the objectives

added to *HP 2020* that target public health education and competencies.

■ HEALTHY PEOPLE 2020
Healthy People 2020 Objectives Relevant to Public Health Department Infrastructure

Selected Objectives:

PHI HP2020–1: Increase the proportion of Tribal and State public health agencies that provide or assure comprehensive laboratory services to support essential public health services.

PHI HP2020–2: Increase the proportion of Tribal, State, and local public health agencies that provide or assure comprehensive epidemiology services to support essential public health services.

PHI HP2020–6: Increase the proportion of Federal, Tribal, State, and local public health agencies that incorporate core competencies for public health professionals into job descriptions and performance evaluations.

PHI HP2020–7: Increase the proportion of Council on Education for Public Health (CEPH) accredited schools of public health, CEPH accredited academic programs, and schools of nursing (with a public health or community health component) that integrate core competencies in public health into curricula.

PHI HP2020–8: (Developmental) Increase the proportion of Tribal, State, and local public health personnel who receive continuing education consistent with the core competencies for public health professionals.

PHI HP2020-9: Increase the proportion of State and local public health jurisdictions that conduct performance assessment and improvement activities in the public health system using national standards.

PHI HP 2020-10: Increase the proportion of Tribal, State, and local public health agencies that have implemented a health improvement plan and increase the proportion of local health jurisdictions that have implemented a health improvement plan linked with their State plan.

PHI HP2020-17: Increase the proportion of Tribal, State, and local public health agencies that are accredited.

PHI HP2020-18: Increase the proportion of Tribal, State, and local public health agencies that have implemented an agency wide quality improvement process.

PHI HP2020-19 Increase the proportion of public health laboratory systems (including State, Tribal, and local) that perform at a high level of quality in support of the 10 Essential Public Health Services.

Other challenges of PHDs include issues of relevance to the public health workforce, information technology, quality improvement and PHD accreditation, and PHD financing, especially as it relates to the economic recession.

Public Health Workforce

Currently, there is a shortage of public health workers and this shortage is projected to increase in the coming years. In 2010, the Association of State and Territorial Health Officials conducted a survey of state agencies. It found there were more than 12,500 vacant public health workforce positions, an average of 11% per state health agency. There are a number of factors contributing to this shortage, including budget reductions and hiring freezes, a rapidly aging workforce whose average age was 47 years in state agencies, and 24% of the workforce eligible to retire by 2014.[69] All of these issues raise concern for PHDs as well.

The U.S. public health workforce has been of sufficient interest to policy makers during the past four decades to lead to regular efforts to enumerate it. In 1980, there was a ratio of public health workers to the general population of 220/100,000, and in 2000 that had dropped to 158/100,000.[70] Although there is an overall shortage, the critical shortage of PHNs is a threat to the public's health and of great concern because they make up a large sector of the public health workforce.[71,72] Executive leadership for PHDs is also a major concern, especially in light of the aging public health workforce and projected shortages.[73]

Core competencies for various public health workers or in specific functions have been developed to enhance the public health workforce capacity. These include the *Public Health Nursing: Scope and Standards of Practice*,[74] *Bioterrorism and Emergency Preparedness Core Competencies for Public Health Workers*,[75] *Council on Linkages: Core Competencies for Public Health Professionals*,[76] and *Competencies for Public Health Informaticions Competencies*.[77]

Because the public health workforce comprises a broad range of educational backgrounds and training, these competencies provide a common framework for measuring and improving public health workforce skills and abilities[78] (Box 14-4). In addition, there has been some discussion about credentialing public health workers.[78]

Sustainment of the public health workforce is a major concern and is influenced by several factors. First, many of the health-care professions have experienced shortages in available workers, thus many health-care facilities are competing for the same candidates. Second, many PHD jurisdictions are located in rural or remote areas, making

recruitment of qualified personnel difficult. Third, limited financial resources may make it difficult for PHDs to provide compensation that is competitive with private-sector entities. Finally, there are faculty shortages within the academic setting that limit the ability of colleges and universities to graduate large numbers of qualified individuals.[78] Currently, there are critical PHN nursing faculty shortages that have significantly limited the exposure to and specialization in public health nursing.[80]

Information Technology

Information technology (IT) is a key infrastructure component within a PHD, from clinical records management to supporting a PHD Web site. IT is used in every aspect of operations. All persons working in a PHD use IT at varying degrees. The level of use and knowledge required is position dependent. For example, an administrative assistant would require just basic knowledge and skills to use IT for general office functions, whereas an epidemiologist will need more advanced knowledge and skills for data collection and analysis. IT is much more than just using computer equipment and programs. The field of **public health informatics** focuses on the use of information technology by public health professionals. There are several definitions for public health informatics, all of which essentially define it as public health information systems and infrastructure that are population based and used for surveillance, program outcome evaluation, quality assurance, systems analysis, and evidence-based disease management.[81]

In 2002, the CDC created a work group of subject matter experts to define overarching public health informatics competencies for all persons working in public health. These competencies focused on three areas: (1) information for public health practice, (2) use of IT by the public health professional to enhance personal performance, and (3) utilization of IT projects to improve PHD effectiveness.[77] These competencies provide the framework to ensure that PHDs have the capacity to adequately perform in today's technologically demanding environment.

Although PHDs use IT to support general business operations, new regulations and technology create new demands on PHDs to enhance IT use. Two key examples of this are **geographic information system (GIS)** application and electronic health records. Both of these activities have required PHDs to expand staff knowledge and hardware capacity in order to effectively integrate these applications into daily operations.[82] The use of GIS has transformed a number of functions within PHDs. It can be used to visualize data geographically within a designated area. For example, in a disease outbreak, the case data can be entered into a GIS program and maps can then be created to show various characteristics of the cases. An epidemiology nurse can easily identify where cases may be clustering geographically or identify density of cases through a color-coding system. Likewise, the PHN can use GIS to identify potential exposure risk from environmental hazards by applying layers of demographic data to environmental data layers. GIS technology is a very effective tool for understanding the dynamics between health status, health system access, and physical environment.

New regulations and requirements to move health records from paper-based systems to electronic systems have resulted in a paradigm shift for medical record management. PHDs have faced unique challenges in implementing these systems because public health practitioners' health focus is much broader than that in clinical care. Public health electronic systems need to (1) integrate clinical data from all providers for public health use such as disease surveillance and investigation, and (2) include expanded capacity for psychosocial, behavioral, and environmental client data collected by PHDs.[83] The impact of electronic health record implementation affects public health systems in two ways: (1) There is a need to implement an electronic system for individual patient care; and (2) PHDs need to maintain the ability to conduct population-based core functions such as assessment, policy development, and assurance through interfaced integration of electronic data from providers. This will require public and private providers to come together to ensure electronic health record systems include a public health orientation. By effectively integrating this focus, reporting duplication can be reduced and community decision making can be enhanced through more comprehensive data availability.[84]

Quality Improvement and Public Health Department Accreditation

The emerging areas of PHD accreditation and **public health systems and services research** expand our knowledge about the relationship between characteristics of PHDs, local public health system performance, and public health outcomes. Continuous quality improvement initiatives are led by multidisciplinary teams to systematically apply evidence-based practice, improve service delivery, and achieve the best outcomes. In the NACCHO 2010 survey of PHDs, 84% of PHDs reported conducting some type of quality improvement activities.[12] The Public Health Accreditation Board is developing a national voluntary accreditation program for state and PHDs to formalize and advance quality and performance of PHDs and improve population health outcomes.[85,86]

Studies show that the strongest predictor of PHD performance is the size of the jurisdiction population.[1,73,87] In general, PHDs serving larger populations with greater numbers of staff and higher funding per capita perform better than PHDs serving populations of less than 50,000.[2] PHD leadership structure also influences staffing models and service focus. Bekemeier and Jones[87] found there were distinct differences between programmatic service delivery and the core functions of assessment and planning in PHDs led by nurse executives and non-nurse executives. PHDs under nurse executive leadership had stronger prevention programs such as unintended pregnancy, obesity, and injury prevention, immunization, and maternal-child health than nonnurse-led PHDs.[88] However, assessment and planning functions were performed less by nurse executives than by medical or nonclinical senior executives, indicating the need for additional training in these areas.

Public Health Department Financing

Public health systems have historically been designed as a function of local (county or city) government operations. The structure of PHDs previously described has an impact on PHD financing. The vast majority of states have county-operated systems, usually governed by local boards of health, but large metropolitan areas, such as Los Angeles or New York City, may have city structures as well. Some states (e.g., Florida) have a state-centered program with contractual agreements with counties for provision of public health services. The financing of PHD operations can become very complex, related to disparities in county size, needs, and local community capabilities to provide services.

The three primary funding streams for PHDs are federal, state, and local. There is not an overriding formula for any of these financing layers. However, there are guidelines developed to assure that allocations are used appropriately and may be designated for specific programs or services. These funds, often called **categorical funds,** are usually federal funds ether directly disbursed to PHDs from the federal government through grants, or received by the states and reallocated to the PHDs. Either way, budgets must show the expenditures by category (personnel, expenses, fixed capital) and require annual reporting back to the federal government.[89] An example of this might be a PHN position that performs family planning, STI, and school-based health services. The PHN will then need to record her time spent in each service area to ensure her time is allocated to the appropriate funding source. This is a common occurrence in PHDs; therefore, tracking systems and reporting procedures have been developed to manage the funding reporting requirements.

In January/February 2010, NACCHO conducted a survey of PHDs and found that in the last 6 months of 2009, nearly half of the PHDs (46%) lost skilled people because there were 8,000 jobs lost, resulting in a cumulative 23,000 jobs lost from 2008 to 2009.[89] The economic recession had a significant impact on jobs, budgets, and programs. Many of the PHDs reported that the cuts are most often in local and state funding, and that the dramatic cuts threaten the general use funds that enable PHDs to respond to urgent community needs not covered by specific disease grants.

One way the PHDs have survived these changes has been through one-time funding for diseases, for example, as happened in the H1N1 influenza outbreak. What is needed, however, is stable, long-term funding. The key to funding the PHD in the future will be the ability to clearly articulate its mission. Policy makers will need to support PHDs by ensuring an adequate investment in public health by assuring that prevention dollars do go to PHDs to help build their capacities. It is anticipated that the Patient Protection and Affordable Care Act will benefit PHDs and public health. This is critical, considering the important role that PHDs play in keeping communities safe. "[PHDS] have been described as the country's 'best kept secret.' As one PHD official states, 'Unless there is an outbreak, no one even knows that we exist. We operate diligently and quietly in the background, keeping our community healthy and safe.'"[89]

Additional Challenges

Keeping the community healthy and safe is key. Although there is a growing emphasis on emerging or reemerging communicable disease or on disaster preparedness, in reality a major threat to the health of populations is noncommunicable disease. PHDs often lack structure as well as money to address noncommunicable disease. This challenge raises issues of what strategies to use in addressing multiple health issues as well as how to finance new

initiatives. Some health departments provide an exemplar of what can be done. From 2002 to 2007, for example, the New York City Health Department, with a long history of innovation, implemented both policy-based initiatives as well as health-care initiatives.[90] Some of these policy initiatives included taxation; a smoke-free air law; mass-media campaigns; a phase-out of the use of trans-fats in restaurants; required calorie labeling in restaurants; and citywide health standards for food in day care, schools, prisons, homeless shelters, and other city agencies. The factors associated with their success include strong technology systems, skillful epidemiology, expertise in communications using modern media, policy-making authority, and, most important, political support.[90]

PHDs in California provide some insight into how to build the infrastructure and programs in difficult times. In many cases, target risk factors are brought together—tobacco, physical activity, nutrition, injury, and violence in ongoing partnering.[91] The PHDs built their capacity by relying on categorical funding supplemented by flexible funding and sometimes the use of state revenue.

■ Summary Points

- The basic mandate of the PHD is to protect and improve health in partnership with the community.
- PHDs are organized by three major delivery modes: centralized system, decentralized system, and shared or mixed system.
- The PHD workforce is interdisciplinary, with nurses making up 17% of it.
- The 10 most frequent activities and services available through the direct services of the PHD are: adult immunization provision, communicable disease surveillance, child immunization provision, tuberculosis screening, food service establishment inspection, environmental surveillance, food safety education, TB treatment, schools/day-care center inspections, and population-based nutrition services.
- PHDs also work in collaboration with the state or contract with other partners in order to fulfill the core functions of public health.
- The major responsibilities of PHDs lie with environmental health services, data collection and analysis (which includes the collection of vital statistics), assurance of individual and community health, communicable diseases, epidemiology and surveillance, and licensing.
- Nurses' roles within health departments include providing primary prevention efforts, making health policy, designing health programs, and providing

care at the individual and community levels. The role of the nurse in a public health department varies depending on the services being provided and the level of expertise needed.

- Challenges for PHDs include the shortage of public health workers, using IT to enhance care, quality improvement, and financing efforts in the future.
- PHD accreditation is being proposed as a voluntary program to advance quality and performance of PHDs.
- The mission of public health is to assure conditions in which people can be healthy. Although there are emerging and reemerging infections from a global concern that affects population health, noncommunicable diseases, which are additional challenge for PHDs, are the major threats to the health of populations.

▲ CASE STUDY
Collaborating With Community Partners

Learning Outcomes

At the end of this case study, the student will be able to:

- Investigate the role of PHDs in community assessment and planning for health needs of the community.
- Describe the structure and services of your PHD.
- Identify the major partners involved in community health planning.

You have been asked by your hospital to be the representative on a community needs assessment. This will involve measuring and evaluating health status and developing collaborative programs that will address the health needs of your community. You realize that you need to learn more about your local health department and the population that it serves. Research your local health department and answer the following questions:

1. What type of public health system is used in your state (centralized, decentralized, mixed, shared)?
2. What type of jurisdiction does your PHD serve (city, town, county, multiple county, district, region)?
3. Is there a local board of health and, if so, what is its role and function?
4. What types of assessment and planning are under way? Who are the main community partners?
5. Where is the PHD located? Are there branch offices?
6. What types of services are provided? What services exist that (a) ensure a safe environment; (b) provide preventive and/or primary health care; (c) monitor, detect, and investigate disease outbreaks; (d) track and record health data about the community; (e) promote healthy behaviors; and (f) prepare the health department to support communities during times of disasters or emergency?
7. What roles and services do nurses perform? How many nurses are employed? What are the educational and certification requirements?

REFERENCES

1. Scutchfield, F.D., Knight, E.A., Kelly, A.V., Bhandarie, M.W., & Vasilescu, I.P. (2004). Local public health agency capacity and its relationship to public health system performance. *Journal of Public Health Management Practice, 10*(3), 204-215.
2. Erwin, P.C. (2008). The performance of local health departments: A review of the literature. *Journal of Public Health Management and Practice, 14*(2), E9-E18.
3. Jekel, J.F. (1991). Health departments in the U.S. 1920–1988: Statements of mission with special reference to the role of C.E.A Winslow. *The Yale Journal of Biology and Medicine, 64,* 467-479.
4. Fee, E., & Brown, T. (2007). The unidentified promise of public health: Déjà vu all over again. *Health Affairs, 26*(6), 31.
5. Meit, M., & Knudson, A. (2009). Why is rural public health important? A look to the future. *Journal of Public Health Management and Practice, 15*(3), 185-190.
6. U.S. Public Health Service. (1936). *Health of county health organizations in the United States: 1908–1933.* Washington, DC: US Government Printing Office.
7. Hiscock, I. (1937). [Review of the book *History of county health organizations in the United States, 1908–1933,* by the U.S. Public Health Service]. *American Journal of Public Health Nations Health, 27,* 90.
8. Fairchild, A.L., Rosner, D., Colgrave, J., Bayer, R., & Fried, L.P. (2010). The exodus of public health. *American Journal of Public Health, 100*(1), 54-63.
9. Vaughan, H.F. (1972). Local health services in the United States: The story of the CAP. *American Public Health Association, 62,* 95-111.
10. APHA. (1940, September). An official declaration of attitude of the American Public Health Association on desirable minimum functions and suitable organization of health activities. *American Journal of Public Health,* 1099-1106.
11. Institute of Medicine. (1988). *The future of public health.* Washington, DC: National Academies Press.
12. National Association of County and City Health Officers. (2011). *2010 national profile of local health departments.* Washington, DC: Author. Retrieved from http://www.naccho.org/topics/infrastructure/profile/resources/2010report/upload/2010_Profile_main_report-web.pdf.
13. Association of State and Territorial Health Officers. (2007). *Understanding state public health.* Retrieved

from http://www.astho.org/Display/AssetDisplay.aspx?id=2884.

14. Kansas Health Institute. (2006). *Local public health at the crossroads: The structure of health departments in rural areas.* Topeka, KS: Author. Retrieved from http://media.khi.org/news/documents/2009/09/02/40-0601HealthDeptStructureHRSABrief.pdf.

15. Winslow, C.E. A. (1920). The untilled fields of public health. *Science, 51,* 23-33.

16. Centers for Disease Control and Prevention. (n.d.). *Ten essential public health services.* Retrieved from http://www.cdc.gov/od/ocphp/nphpsp/essentialphservices.htm.

17. Fris, R.H., & Sellers, T.A. (2009). *Epidemiology for public health practice.* Sudbury, MA: Jones & Bartlett.

18. Public Health Leadership Society. (2002). *Principles of the ethical practice of public health, version 2.2.* Retrieved from http://www.phls.org/home/section/3-26/.

19. Keller, L., Strohschein, S., Lia-Hoagberg, C., & Schaffer, M. (2004). Population-based interventions: Innovations in practice, teaching and management. Part II. *Public Health Nursing, 21*(5), 469-487.

20. Levy, D., Chaloupka, F., & Gitchell, J. (2004). The effects of tobacco control policies in smoking cessation rates: A tobacco control scorecard. *Journal of Public Health Management Practice, 10*(4), 338-353.

21. National Cancer Institute. (2007). *Greater than the sum: Systems thinking in tobacco control.* Retrieved from http://cancercontrol.cancer.gov/Brp/tcrb/monographs/18/monograph18.html.

22. Marcus, S.E., Leischow, S.J., Mabry, P.L., & Clark, P.J. (2010). Lessons learned from the application of systems science to tobacco control at the National Cancer Institute. *American Journal of Public Health, 100*(7), 1163-1165.

23. Borland, R., Young, D., Coghill, K., & Zhang, J.Y. (2010). The tobacco use management system: Analyzing tobacco control from a systems perspective. *American Journal of Public Health, 100*(7), 1229-1236.

24. U.S. Department of Health and Human Services. (n.d.). *Healthy People 2020.* Retrieved from http://www.healthypeople.gov/hp2020/objectives/framework.aspx.

25. National Association of County and City Health Officers. (n.d.). *Mobilizing for action through planning and partnerships.* Retrieved from http://www.naccho.org/topics/infrastructure/mapp/index.cfm.

26. Centers for Disease Control and Prevention. (n.d.). *Behavioral Risk Factor Surveillance System.* Retrieved from http://www.cdc.gov/brfss/about/index.htm.

27. Nurse-Family Partnership. (2010a). *Overview.* Retrieved from http://www.nursefamilypartnership.org/assets/PDF/Fact-sheets/NFP_Overview.

28. Nurse-Family Partnership. (2010b). *Research trials and outcomes.* Retrieved from http://www.nursefamilypartnership.org/assets/PDF/Fact-sheets/NFP_Research_Outcomes.

29. Nurse-Family Partnership. (2011). *Nurses and mothers.* Retrieved from http://www.nursefamilypartnership.org/assets/PDF/Fact-sheets/NFP_Nurses-Mothers.

30. Bazzoli, G.J., Stein, R., Alexander, J.A., Conrad, D.A., Sofaer, S., & Shortell, S.M. (1997). Public-private collaboration in health and human service delivery: Evidence from community partnerships. *The Milbank Quarterly, 75*(4), 533-561.

31. Beitsch, L.M., Grigg, M., Menachemini, N., & Brooks, R.G. (2006). Roles of local public health agencies within the state public health system. *Journal of Public Health Management and Practice, 12*(3), 232-241.

32. Louis, G.E. (2004). A historical context of municipal solid waste management in the United States. *Waste Management & Research, 22,* 306-322.

33. Centers for Disease Control and Prevention. (n.d.). *National Vital Statistics System.* Retrieved from http://www.cdc.gov/nchs/nvss.htm.

34. Centers for Disease Control and Prevention. (2003). *Revisions of the U.S. Standard Certificates of Live Birth and Death and the Fetal Death Report.* Retrieved from http://www.cdc.gov/nchs/nvss/vital_certificate_revisions.htm.

35. City of Cincinnati Health Department. (2014.). *Health department: Working for Cincinnati's health & wellness.* Retrieved from http://www.cincinnati-oh.gov/health/.

36. Institute of Medicine. (2003). *The future of the public's health in the 21st century.* Washington, DC: National Academies Press.

37. Rural Assistance Center. (2009). *What is a federally qualified health center and what are the benefits?* Retrieved from http://www.raconline.org/info_guides/clinics/fqhcfaq.php#whatis.

38. Maternal and Child Health Bureau. (n.d.). *Maternal and child health home.* Retrieved from http://mchb.hrsa.gov/index.html.

39. National Healthy Start Program. (n.d.). *The Healthy Start Program.* Retrieved from http://www.healthystartassoc.org/hswpp6.html.

40. Promising Practices Network. (2008). *On children, families and communities.* Retrieved from http://www.promisingpractices.net/program.asp?programid=118.

41. U.S. Department of Agriculture, Food and Nutrition Service, Office of Research and Analysis. (n.d.). *WIC participant and program characteristics 2008* (WIC-08-PC). Washington, DC: Author.

42. Office of Population Affairs. (n.d.). *Family planning.* Retrieved from http://www.hhs.gov/opa/familyplanning/index.html.

43. New York State Department of Health. (n.d.). *Family Planning Benefit Program.* Retrieved from http://www.health.state.ny.us/health_care/medicaid/program/longterm/familyplanbenprog.htm.

44. National Association of School Nurses. (2002). *The role of the school nurse.* Silver Spring, MD: Author. Retrieved from http://www.nasn.org/Default.aspx?tabid=279.

45. Data Resource Center for Child and Adolescent Health. (2007). *National survey of children's health.* Retrieved from http://nschdata.org/DataQuery/SurveyQuestions.aspx?yid=2&tid=44&geoid=0.

46. Riedel, S. (2005). Edward Jenner and the history of smallpox and vaccination. *BUMC Proceedings, 18,* 21-25.

47. Browne, H., Reimer, J., MacLead, M., & McLellan, E. (2010). Public health nursing practice with "high priority" families: The significance of contextualizing "risk." *Nursing Inquiry, 17,* 27-38.

48. Heaman, M., Chalmers, K., Woodgate, R., & Brown, J. (2006). Early childhood home visiting programme: Factors contributing to success. *Journal of Advanced Nursing, 55,* 291-300.

49. Olds, D., Robinson, J., O'Brien, R., Luckey, D., Pettitt, L., Henderson, C., et al. (2002). Home visiting by paraprofessionals and by nurses: A randomized, controlled trial. *Pediatrics, 110,* 486-496

50. National Institute of Child Health and Human Development. (n.d.). *Back to Sleep campaign.* Retrieved from http://www.nichd.nih.gov/sids/.

51. Sarasota County Health Department. (n.d.). *Community health improvement partnership.* Retrieved from http://www.chip4health.org/whatwedo/index.htm.

52. LoBue, P., Sizemore, C., & Castro, K.G. (2009). Plan to combat extensively drug-resistant tuberculosis: Recommendations of the federal Tuberculosis Task Force. *Morbidity and Mortality Weekly Report, 5*(RR03), 1-43. Retrieved from http://www.cdc.gov/mmwr/preview/mmwrhtml/rr5803a1.htm?s_cid=rr5803a1_e.

53. Centers for Disease Control and Prevention. (2005). Guidelines for the investigation of contacts of persons with infectious tuberculosis. *Morbidity and Mortality Weekly Report, 54*(RR15), 1-37.

54. Centers for Disease Control and Prevention. (2005). Controlling tuberculosis in the United States. *Morbidity and Mortality Weekly Report, 54*(RR12), 1-81. Retrieved from http://www.who.int/tb/features_archive/new_treatment_guidelines_may2010/en/index.html.

55. Centers for Disease Control and Prevention. (2010). *Tuberculosis.* Retrieved from http://www.cdc.gov/tb/.

56. World Health Organization. (2009). *Treatment of tuberculosis guidelines.* Retrieved from http://whqlibdoc.who.int/publications/2010/9789241547833_eng.pdf.

57. Ailinger, R.L., Black, P.L., & Lima-Garcia, N. (2008). Use of electronic monitoring in clinical nursing research. *Clinical Nursing Research, 17*(2), 89-97.

58. Centers for Disease Control and Prevention. (2012). *Sexually transmitted disease surveillance, 2011.* Atlanta, GA: U.S. Department of Health and Human Services.

59. National Association of County and City Health Officials. (2010). *Statement of policy prevention and control of sexually transmitted infections.* Retrieved from http://www.naccho.org/advocacy/positions/upload/09-10-Prevention-and-Control-of-STI.pdf.

60. National Association of County and City Health Officials. (2010). *Survey of local health department job losses and program cuts.* Washington, DC: Author.

61. Davis, J.R., & Lederberg, J. (Eds.). (2000). *Public health systems and emerging infections: Assessing the capabilities of the public and private sectors.* Washington, DC: National Academies Press.

62. Snowden, F.M. (2008). Emerging and reemerging diseases: A historical perspective. *Immunological Reviews, 225,* 9-26.

63. World Health Organization. (2003). *Summary of probable SARS cases with onset of illness from 1 November 2002 to 31 July 2003.* Retrieved from http://www.who.int/csr/sars/country/table2004_04_21/en/index.html.

64. Stern, A.M., & Markel, H. (2009). What Mexico taught the world about pandemic influenza preparedness and community mitigation strategies. *JAMA, 302*(11), 1221-1222.

65. Centers for Disease Control and Prevention. (2008). *Animals.* Retrieved from http://www.cdc.gov/ncidod/dpd/animals.htm.

66. Centers for Disease Control and Prevention. (2010). *Rabies.* Retrieved from http://www.cdc.gov/rabies/.

67. Centers for Disease Control and Prevention. (2002) *Bioterrorism & Emergency Preparedness Core Council on linkages between academia and public health practice.* Retrieved from http://training.fema.gov/emiweb/downloads/BioTerrorism%20and%20Emergency%20Readiness.pdf.

68. Department of Health and Human Services. (2014). *About Healthy People 2020.* Retrieved from http://healthypeople.gov/2020/about/default.aspx.

69. Association of State and Territorial Health Officials. (2011). *Profile of state public health* (Vol. 2). Retrieved from http://www.astho.org/uploadedFiles/_Publications/Files/Survey_Research/ASTHO_State_Profiles_Single%5B1%5D%20lo%20res.pdf.

70. Merrill, J., Btoush, R., Gupta, M., & Gebbie, K. (2003). A history of public health workforce enumeration. *Journal of Public Health Management, 9*(6), 459-470.

71. Bekemeier, B., & Jones, M. (2010). Relationship between local public health agency functions and agency leadership and staffing: A look at nurses. *Journal of Public Health Management and Practice, 16*(2), E8-E16.

72. Quad Council of Public Health Nursing Organizations. (2007). *The public health nursing shortage: A threat to the public's health.* Retrieved from http://www.resourcenter.net/images/ACHNE/Files/QCShortagePaperFinal2-07.pdf.

73. Bhandari, M., Scutchfield, F.D., Charnigo, R., Riddel, M., & Mays, G.P. (2010). New data, same story? Revising studies on the relationship of local public health systems characteristics to public health performance. *Journal of Public Health Management and Practice, 16*(2), 110-117.

74. American Nurses Association. (2013). *Public health nursing: Scope and standards of practice* (2nd ed.). Silver Spring, MD: Author.

75. Columbia University School of Nursing Center for Health Policy. (2002). *Bioterrorism and emergency preparedness competencies for all public health workers.* Retrieved from http://www.nursing.columbia.edu/chp/pdfArchive/btcomps.pdf.

76. Public Health Foundation. (n.d.). *Council on Linkages: Core competencies for public health professionals.* Retrieved from http://www.phf.org/link/corecompetencies.htm.

77. U.S. Department of Health and Human Services. (2009). *Competencies for public health informaticians.* Retrieved from http://www.cphi.washington.edu/resources/PHICompetencies.pdf.

78. Gebbie, K.M., & Turnock, B.J. (2006). The public health workforce, 2006: New challenges. *Health Affairs, 25*(4), 923-933.

79. National Association of County and City Health Officers. (2007). *The local health department workforce: Findings from the 2005 National Profile of Local Health Departments study.* Washington, DC: Author.

80. Collier, J., Davidson, G., Allen, C.B., Dieckmann, J., Hoke, M.M., & Sawaya, M.A. (2010). Academic faculty qualification for community/public health nursing: An association of community health nursing educators position paper. *Public Health Nursing, 27*(1), 89-93.

81. Araujo, J., Pepper, C., Richards, J., Choi, M., Xing, J., & Li, W. (2009). The profession of public health informatics: Still emerging? *International Journal of Medical Informatics, 78,* 375-385.

82. Centers for Disease Control and Prevention. (2006). *Geographic information systems at CDC.* Retrieved from http://www.cdc.gov/gis/.

83. Kukafka, R., Ancker, J.S., Chan, C., Chelico, J., Khan, S., Mortoti, S., et al. (2007). Redesigning electronic health record systems to support public health. *Journal of Biomedical Informatics, 40,* 398-409.

84. Beitsch, L.M., Leep, C., Shah, G., Brooks, R.G., & Pestronk, R.M. (2010). Quality improvements in local health departments: Results of the NACCHO 2008 survey. *Journal of Public Health Management Practice, 16*(1), 49-54.

85. Bender, K., & Halverson, P.K., (2010) Quality improvement and accreditation: What might it look like? *Journal of Public Health Management and Practice, 16*(1), 79-82.

86. Mays, G.P., McHugh, M.C., Shim, K., Perry, N., Lenaway, D., Halverson, P.K., & Moonesinghe, R. (2006). Institutional and economic determinants of public health system performance. *American Journal of Public Health, 96*(3), 523-531.

87. Bekemeier, B., & Jones, M. (2010). Relationship between local public health agency functions and agency leadership and staffing: A look at nurses. *Journal of Public Health Management and Practice, 16*(2), E8-E16.

88. Buehler, J.W., & Holtgrave, D.R. (2007). Who gets how much: Funding formulas in federal public health programs. *Journal of Public Health Management Practice, 13*(2), 151-155.

89. National Association of County and City Health Officials. (2010). *Research brief: Local health department job losses and program cuts.* Retrieved from http://www.naccho.org/topics/infrastructure/lhdbudget/upload/Job-Losses-and-Program-Cuts-5-10.pdf.

90. Frieden, T.R., Bassett, M.T., Thorpe, L.E., & Farley, T.A. (2008). Public health in New York City, 2002–2007: Confronting epidemics of the modern era. *International Journal of Epidemiology, 37,* 966-977.

91. Prentice, B., & Flores, G. (2007). Local health departments and the challenge of chronic disease: Lessons from California. *Preventing Chronic Disease, 4*(1), 1-6.

Health Planning for Acute Care Settings

LEARNING OUTCOMES

After reading this chapter, the student will be able to:

1. Describe the relationship between acute care and population health.
2. Identify the role of population-level data in the development of the discipline of critical care.
3. Discuss the relevance of cohort studies to the delivery of tertiary care.

4. Explain the application of health planning in an acute care setting.
5. Recognize the basic steps in the quality improvement process.
6. Identify key infection control issues related to the acute care setting.

KEY TERMS

Acute care
Acute coronary syndrome
Acute myocardial ischemia
Cardiopulmonary resuscitation (CPR)
Critical care nursing
Critically ill/injured patients
Door to balloon time

Electronic medical record (EMR)
Epidemiology
Healthcare-associated infections (HAIs)
Hospital discharge rate
Hospital recidivism
Institutional review board

International Classification of Diseases, 9th Revision (ICD9)
Major diagnostic category (MDC)
Multiple drug-resistant organisms
PSDA cycle

Patient populations
Polio
Performance improvement
Quality improvement
Sepsis
ST-elevated myocardial infarction
Survival rate

◾ Introduction

Sixty percent of the nursing workforce works in an acute care setting.[1] **Acute care** is defined as care that is provided during a severe episode of illness, following surgery, or following a traumatic injury. Acute care usually occurs in a hospital setting and requires skilled care provided by health-care providers. Acute care is provided for a short time during the severe episode and may be followed by chronic care in the home or other long-term care facility.[2]

Acute care occurs mostly at the tertiary prevention level (see Chapter 2), where care is provided to patients who have been diagnosed with a clinical disease or have already experienced an injury. The focus of the care is to prevent further morbidity and reduce disability related to the disease or injury. The majority of the care is clinical rather than environmental or even behavioral. Though an effort is made during the hospital stay to provide education on

behavioral changes that will increase the chances of return to a more healthy state and reduce the chances of death or disability, the primary focus of the hospital stay is provision of direct clinical interventions.

Hospitals provide care to persons who are acutely ill, many of them critically ill. Adults who seek care in a hospital setting require highly skilled nurses competent to provide care to the individual and aimed at addressing the acute episode of illness or aftermath of an injury. It would seem at first glance that the public health sciences have little to contribute to the acute care setting. However, the high level of care now available to patients experiencing an acute episode of illness or injury is based on a clear understanding of the natural history of disease that evolved out of cohort and case control studies (see Chapter 3). Our knowledge of the effectiveness of interventions is based on the findings from rigorous clinical trials (see Chapter 3). These research designs have their basis in epidemiology.

Nurses have a long history of applying population-level research and an understanding of determinants of health to their delivery of care at both the macro (population) level and the micro (individual) level. As hospitals strive to meet criteria for accreditation and recognition of excellence, the role of the staff nurse in improving patient outcomes encompasses nurses actively applying public health science to the evaluation and improvement of the care they provide.

The Acute Care Setting and Population Health

Often, the distinction between the community/public health nurse (PHN) and the nurse working in a hospital is based on the concept of direct and indirect care as presented in the new *Essentials of Doctorate Education for Advanced Nursing Practice*.[3] However, that distinction gets blurred because many nurses who define themselves as PHNs provide care to individuals, for example, administering flu vaccines, whereas hospital-based nurses frequently tackle problems from a public health perspective, for example, reducing the rate of healthcare infections (HAIs) or improving targeted patient outcomes for a particular population.

If, instead of a dichotomous concept of direct and indirect care, nursing practice is viewed across the continuum of care from micro/individual health to macro/population health, it is easier to demonstrate the application of public health science to nursing practice in acute care settings. Nurses in acute care settings are continuously involved in efforts to improve care for the populations they serve, not just for each individual. If nurses on a unit are working on a performance improvement project, they have moved along the continuum to look at an issue at the group level, the group they serve. To develop an understanding of the patient data they collect for the project requires the application of epidemiology such as computing discharge rates, establishing odds ratios (see Chapter 3), or looking at HAI rates. In most hospitals, the performance improvement committee provides frequent updates on care issues within the hospital and evidence to demonstrate whether efforts to address specific problems have resulted in improved patient outcomes.

The challenge is differentiating the term *population* used in public health and the term *population* used in a hospital setting. In Chapter 1, the term was defined as a mass of people that make up a definable unit to which measurements pertain. Chapter 1 explains that population health occurs within the context of the social, economic, cultural, and environmental influences on populations and, thus, on individuals. This implies that from a public health perspective, population includes persons who share a similar social setting, culture, and/or geographical community over a period of time. In a hospital setting, populations are instead grouped based on a particular health issue or a hospital unit with individuals rapidly entering and exiting the population. For example, within the hospital the concern may be the diabetic population being treated at the hospital, or it may be the **patient population** on a specific unit. Thus, the term *population* within a hospital context does not usually refer to a group of persons who share other attributes other than being admitted to the hospital on a certain unit and/or having a specific diagnosis.

▶ SOLVING THE MYSTERY
The Case of the Nurse Who Wanted to Know "Who, Why, What, Where, and When?"

Public Health Science Topics Covered:

- Assessment
- Epidemiology
  - Computing rates
  - Comparing rates with national rates
- Health planning
  - Conducting a setting specific assessment
  - Population-level conclusions: Identifying priorities

A large midwestern teaching hospital contracted with a college of nursing to have a faculty member with research experience provide mentorship to the staff engaged in nursing practice research. A nurse researcher who was also a PHN, Cheryl, was assigned to the project. She found that the hospital had a history of nurses on the units initiating small nursing-practice studies or review of the literature to examine the evidence related to a particular nursing intervention. These projects were conducted by individual nurses and typically culminated in a brief report on their findings from the literature. The projects did not necessarily result in change in practice. There was no information on the effect any of these activities had on patient outcomes. The newly appointed chief nursing officer (CNO), Janet, stated that she wanted to change the process so there was evidence that demonstrated whether these studies or projects resulted in a change in how nursing care was delivered and if there was a positive impact on patient outcomes. Janet asked Cheryl how to change the process so that it was clear what patient outcomes should be targeted, how to plan change, and how to evaluate the impact of the change.

Cheryl explained to Janet that a good starting point was to take a public health perspective. When Janet asked her to explain, Cheryl replied that a health-planning model was the best approach (Chapters 4 and 5) that included an assessment phase and health program phase. Cheryl said the best place to begin was to answer the questions related to who, why, what, where, and when. That is, to find out who was being admitted to their hospital, why were they being admitted (diagnosis), what were their outcomes, where were they coming from, and whether there was a variation in these variables over the months and years.

As explained in Chapter 4, there are different types of community/population assessments. Cheryl proposed to Janet that the nursing department conduct a setting-focused assessment. In addition, Cheryl explained that this assessment would be conducted using an epidemiological model. That is, the assessment would focus on quantifying hospital-based data using existing data sources and would then compare these data with national data such as the data available from the Healthcare Cost and Utilization Project (HCUP).[4] The purpose of the assessment would be to determine what patient issues were priorities for nursing practice research in the hospital. The choice of priorities would be based on the discharge diagnostic category with the highest volume, longest mean length of stay, and highest mean charges as well as trends over time.

The CNO liked this approach and together with Cheryl assembled a small team of graduate student nurses and nurses familiar with the nursing units. They were able to use a de-identified database (no patient names or other means of identification) that included all hospital discharges during a 5-year period. For each discharge, they had information on gender, diagnoses (including primary diagnosis and all other diagnoses applied during the hospital stay), procedures, length of stay, hospital charges, zip code, and payer source. They used the HCUP Web site[4] to access national-level data to compare these parameters with national statistics.

The team first calculated hospital discharge rates for each diagnostic category. A **hospital discharge rate** is defined as the rate of a particular discharge diagnosis divided by the total number of discharges times a constant and is computed in the same way other rates are computed (see Chapter 2). Thus, a hospital discharge

rate represents the number of discharges for that diagnosis in comparison with all other discharges for that time period. It is calculated using the number of discharges for the diagnostic category or group divided by all discharges times a constant, usually per 100 discharges (Box 15-1).

While doing the assessment, one of the students asked Cheryl to explain the difference between *International Classification of Diseases, 9th Revision (ICD9)* codes and the Major Diagnostic Categories (MDC) used by HCUP. Cheryl explained that the **major diagnostic category (MDC)** is a taxonomy that groups the principal diagnosis of patients into similar diagnosis-related groups. There are 25 categories based on systems that are designed to be mutually exclusive.[4] Conversely, although *ICD9* is also a taxonomy, it was developed to code very specific diagnoses related to the discharge rather than categories of diagnoses, although the codes can be collapsed into broader categories based on systems such the circulatory system or disease group such as neoplasms. A person with diabetes who may have heart failure also referred to as congestive heart failure (CHF) as a result of the diabetes may be admitted primarily to treat the an acute episode of CHF. Therefore, the primary diagnosis coded using an *ICD9* code would be specific to CHF. They may have subsequent secondary and tertiary *ICD9* codes entered related to the circulatory system, and would have an *ICD9* code for diabetes listed as the fourth or fifth diagnosis. *ICD9* allows the hospital to code for billing a very specific diagnosis under the broader *ICD9* category that indicates exactly what particular diagnoses were related to this admission. To help illustrate this for the student, Cheryl took the data for one admission from the database and demonstrated what *ICD9* categories were entered for

---

BOX 15-1   Calculating a Discharge Rate

The total number of discharges in 2010 assigned the MDC Cardiovascular System was 4,179 and the total number of discharges was 29,585.

The discharge rate per 1,000 discharges is as follows:

$$4,179/25,585 \times 100$$

and is read as

14.1 per 100 discharges in 2009

Note: This reflects discharges, not patients.

that patient including the primary diagnosis and all other diagnoses related to the admission (Table 15-1). She then pointed out that only one MDC category was applied to that specific admission. In this case, the MDC was used to identify the principal diagnosis for admission and was a broader category, whereas the *ICD9* code identified for what specific diseases the patient was being treated during the admission (Table 15-1).

The team ran frequencies on the discharge data to determine the top five MDCs, which MDC had the highest mean length of stay, and which had the highest mean charges. They also calculated hospital discharge rates for each MDC. The MDC with the highest discharge rate was the circulatory system. They constructed a table that displayed the top ten MDC discharge rate bases on gender and age (Table 15-2). They then compared these data with the available national

data related to hospital discharges. They found that although their discharge rate was higher, when compared with the national data, the hospital had a lower mean length of stay and mean charges for that MDC. Despite the evidence that they were better than the national norms on these two indicators, they concluded that owing to the high discharge rate the patients admitted with an MDC related to the circulatory system would be a focus area for development of health programs aimed at improving outcomes.

The team had now answered the "why" question. They went on to answer the rest of the questions. They used gender, payer source, and place of residence to answer the "who" and "where" questions. They completed the analysis for each of the 5 years of data and trending discharge rates during the 5 years and by month. They then used the discharge status variable to

TABLE 15–1	Comparison of Major Diagnostic Category Listing and *ICD9* Codes for a Discharge				
MDC	Major Diagnostic Category	*ICD9* Primary Diagnostic Category	*ICD9* Secondary Diagnostic Category	*ICD9* Primary Diagnostic Code	*ICD9* Secondary Diagnostic Code
Discharge	6	2	7	197.6	401.9
Diagnoses	Diseases of the digestive system	Neoplasms	Diseases of the circulatory system	Malignant neoplasms	Hypertensive disease

TABLE 15–2	Top 10 Major Diagnostic Categories for Nonmaternal Nonneonatal Hospitalizations				
Major Diagnostic Category	Rank Males Aged 0–85+	Rank Females Aged 0–85+	Rank All Genders Aged 18–44	Rank All Genders Aged 45–64	Rank All Genders Aged 65+
Diseases of the circulatory system	1	1	4	1	1
Disease of the respiratory system	2	2	6	4	2
Diseases of the digestive system	3	4	2	3	4
Disease of the musculoskeletal system and connective tissue	4	3	3	2	3
Disease of the nervous system	5	5	5	5	5
Diseases of the kidney and urinary tract	6	6	10	6	6
Mental disorders	7	7	1	8	12
Infectious and parasitic diseases	8	8	14	9	7
Disease of the hepatobiliary system	9	11	7	7	9
Endocrine, nutritional, and metabolic systems	10	9	8	10	8
Diseases of the female reproductive system		10	9	12	15

examine outcomes. This was an extensive project, but provided answers to their questions and, most important, provided a clear picture of the patients they served and the subpopulations most at risk for poorer outcomes. They also identified other information that they wished to add to the assessment such as **hospital recidivism,** that is, readmission to the hospital within 30 days of discharge.

The assessment project not only helped the nursing department establish these priorities, but also provided baseline data from the past 5 years. In this way, the nursing department could track discharge rates and other quality indicators such as length of stay and charges over the next 5 years to help determine whether institution or revision of nursing interventions resulted in any changes in patient outcomes. At this hospital, the nursing department moved from focusing on the evaluation of effectiveness of nursing interventions on individual patient outcomes to an inclusion of the population-level perspective and the evaluation of the outcomes for both levels.

Culture and Acute Care Settings

As discussed in Chapter 23, culture is an important aspect of nursing care within an acute care setting. Nurses understand the need for culturally relevant care for individuals and families, but it also helps if nurses working in an acute care setting are aware of the different cultures represented in their community. An excellent hypothetical example based on an actual story is the issue of the Burundian refugees who settled in a midwestern city. In this example a total of 106 Burundian refugees came to the city with support from the Catholic Archdiocese of the city. They were able to find housing in one of the poorer sections of the city and faced multiple challenges, including obtaining health care. They had lived in refugee camps since the 1970s and were unable to speak English, with low literacy in their own language.

To address the challenges faced by these refugees, the parish nurse employed by a large urban hospital as part of their community outreach project began to work with the Burundians to help establish a means for them to access care and communicate with health-care providers. This required that she learn their culture and normative health-care practices. The parish nurse located an interpreter and began meeting with the women in the community on a regular basis. Together they learned from one another: The Burundians learned the culture of their new country and the parish nurse learned the culture of the Burundians. She was able to use this cultural knowledge to provide the

hospital with key cultural insights into Burundian culture, especially in relation to health beliefs, so that the physicians and nurses providing care would understand health from a Burundian perspective. Without the work of the parish nurse, the hospital would have had difficulty not only in understanding the Burundians when they came for care but also in understanding their cultural perspective on the care received.

The Epidemiology of Populations Treated in Acute Care Settings in the United States

As defined in Chapter 3, **epidemiology** is the study and quantification of illness and disease within human and animal populations. From an acute care perspective, epidemiology provides the framework for the study of the frequency, distribution, cause, and control of diseases or injury in persons who receive care in an acute care setting. Thus, epidemiology revolves around several factors, including patients with noncommunicable, communicable diseases, violence, abuse, and injury. Its purpose is to assist public health officials as well as the registered nurse (RN) to understand the causes of disease as well as the distribution and impact of disease and the groups at risk so that prevention efforts along the continuum from primary to tertiary levels can be developed. Hospital morbidity and mortality rates are published each year by the Centers of Disease Control and Prevention (CDC) and the Agency for Healthcare Research and Quality (AHRQ). Public health nurses as well as nurses working in the acute care setting may access any of these databases to determine specific health risk factors based on age group, gender, and residence. This information may then be used to target interventions to improve the health of those they care for in acute care settings.

According to the CDC, in 2013 the top two leading causes of death in the United States were heart disease and cancer for both males and females. There were differences between genders; the third leading cause of death for males was unintentional injuries, and for females, it was stroke (Table 15-3). Following cancer and stroke were chronic respiratory diseases, accidents, Alzheimer's disease, diabetes, influenza and pneumonia, nephritis, and septicemia (see Box 10-4, Chapter 10).[5] In 2010, the CDC published "National Hospital Discharge Summary Data for 2007," which provided estimates about the number of patients discharged from U.S. hospitals as well as the associated diseases resulting in an inpatient hospitalization.[6] During 2007, there were an estimated 34 million hospital discharges in the United States, not including newborns. The AHRQ reported the average length of stay (ALOS) in a hospital was 4.6 days, a decrease from the ALOS of 5.7 days in 1993.[7]

TABLE 15–3	2007 Differences in Top 10 Leading Causes of Death by Gender		
Leading Causes of Death Males	Percentage	Leading Causes of Death Females	Percentage
1. Heart disease	25.7	1. Heart disease	25.1
2. Cancer	24.3	2. Cancer	22.1
3. Unintentional injuries	6.6	3. Stroke	6.7
4. Chronic lower respiratory diseases	5.1	4. Chronic lower respiratory diseases	5.5
5. Stroke	4.5	5. Alzheimer's disease	4.3
6. Diabetes	2.9	6. Unintentional injuries	3.6
7. Suicide	2.3	7. Diabetes	2.9
8. Influenza and pneumonia	2.0	8. Influenza and pneumonia	2.3
9. Kidney disease	1.9	9. Kidney disease	2.0
10. Alzheimer's disease	1.8	10. Septicemia	1.6

In 2008, circulatory-related conditions such as heart attack and stroke accounted for almost 6 million hospital admissions (15%), followed by pneumonia and CHF. Females accounted for more of the overall hospital stays of 18.6 million versus the 16.5 million for males, excluding pregnancy or childbirth stays. Osteoarthritis discharges increased by threefold for persons aged 45 to 64 years and by 73% for persons aged 65 to 84.[7] The most common procedures performed at hospitals included blood transfusions, episiotomies, caesarean sections, percutaneous transluminal coronary angioplasty, respiratory intubation and ventilation, and coronary artery bypass grafts. When the data are reviewed for these procedures, it appears that they coincide with the major causes of deaths in the United States, specifically heart attack and chronic respiratory illnesses.[7]

Age and Gender Statistics

Reporting of hospital patient data is done based on gender and age. Chapter 18 covers data related to maternal child populations. In this chapter, the focus is the adult 18 years and older who seeks care at a hospital setting. The main source of data is the HCUP used in Solving the Mystery.[4] As explained in Chapter 2 and demonstrated in Solving the Mystery, understanding the "who" is an essential piece of information, in this case, who is seeking care in U.S. hospitals.

During 2011, approximately 42% of all nonmaternal, nonneonatal hospital admissions were male patients. The top 10 major diagnostic categories varied by age and gender (Table 15-2). For all nonmaternal, nonneonatal discharges, there was not much difference in the top 10 diagnoses between males and females. However, for those aged 18 to 44, mental disorder was the top discharge diagnosis but dropped to eighth place for those aged 45 to 64, and for those older than age 64, it fell to 12th place. Across all adult age groups, diseases of the cardiovascular system, digestive system, musculoskeletal system, and nervous system were in the top five.[7]

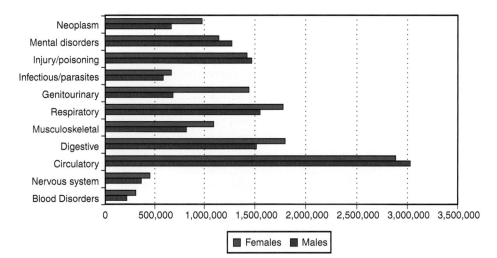

Figure 15-1 Hospital discharge data by first listed diagnosis males versus females, 2007. *(U.S. Department of Health and Human Services. [2011]. Understanding the Health Care Reform Act.)*

Discharge Status of Hospitalized Patients

The goal on discharge is to return the patient to his optimal state of health and, if possible, to independent living. Return to independent living is attainable for 72% of all hospitalized adults in the United States. Ten percent of patients are able to return to their home environment with home health-care services. Thirteen percent of patients were transferred to an extended care facility for both short-term and long-term stays. The remaining 5% of patients may have been discharged to another hospital, expired, or left against medical advice (Fig. 15-2).[7] Assessing patients at the time of admission and developing individual discharge plans will make the postdischarge transition easier for all of those involved. Tracking discharge status is another indicator of patient outcomes and could easily be added to an ongoing hospital population assessment such as the one conducted by Janet and Cheryl.

Inpatient Populations

Understanding public health science and its daily role in the hospital setting is an essential competency for all nurses working across various units including critical care, emergency departments (EDs), and medical-surgical units. They participate through their daily activities in the improvement of health for the patients for whom they care, the patients' families, and the communities to which those patients return. Understanding the patients they care for within the broader context of the community served by the hospital can be a challenge, but as the nation takes its slow march toward health promotion and disease prevention, as evidenced in the Affordable Care Act of 2010,[8] the need for more activities on the population end of the continuum of health care will increase and nurses working in acute care settings will have an important role to play.

Within hospitals, there are numerous settings that are usually referred to as units. These units vary based on the type of services required (e.g., surgery, medical, emergency care) and the severity of the patients' condition (e.g., intensive care, trauma, step-down units). Hospitals also vary in relation to the level of care they provide, the communities they serve, and whether or not they are teaching hospitals. Also, some services, such as infection control, are provided across all units of the hospital. Community hospitals that are located in suburban or rural areas are less apt to provide care to high-level-of-acuity patients such as those requiring complex surgical procedures or trauma one–level care. In contrast, a large urban medical center, especially one affiliated with a large university, has a wide array of units with many providing complex or specialized services.

Critical Care

An excellent example of the relationship between public health science and acute care settings is the role that public health science has played in the development of critical care as a specialty in the acute care setting. **Critical care nursing** requires specialized skills related to human responses to life-threatening health problems,[9] and is usually provided within an area in the hospital designed to provide care to the most critically ill or injured patients. **Critically ill** or **injured patients** can be defined as patients who are at high risk for actual or potential life-threatening health-care problems.[9] Critical illness can result from a progressive disease such as chronic obstructive pulmonary disease or may occur in an acute situation such as myocardial infarction (MI). Acute illness can involve a rapid change in condition for the worse or a condition that arises quickly, such as an exacerbation of fluid overload in the patient with heart failure. Patients in the critical care arena have varied disease etiologies, background demographics, socioeconomic status, and

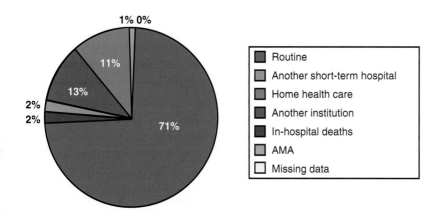

Figure 15-2 Hospital discharge status, 2008. *(From Wier, L.M., Levit, K., Stranges, E., Ryan, K., Pfuntner, A., Vandivort, R., et al. [2010]. HCUP facts and figures: Statistics on hospital based care in the U.S., 2008. Agency for Healthcare Research and Quality.)*

complexities. Also, a patient may be in critical condition from blood loss due to an acute injury sustained in motor vehicle crash. The more critically ill the patient is, the more vulnerable for instability and threat to life, requiring intense and highly skilled nursing care.

The care of the critically ill patient takes place in several different arenas within the hospital setting. This patient population can be found in areas that include intensive care units (ICUs), step-down or transitional care units, EDs, postanesthesia care units (PACU), cardiac catheter laboratories (cardiac cath), and cardiac care units. The focus of the critical care nurse is not only on the patient's responses to illness and optimal care, but also on the family's response. Nurses who care for patients in the critical care area account for an estimated 37% of the total number of nurses working in the hospital setting. There are more than half a million nurses in the United States who are caring for the critically ill and injured. Of these, 229,914 spend at least half their time in an ICU; 92,826 spend at least half their time in step-down or transitional care units; 117,637 spend at least half their time in EDs; and 62,747 spend at least half their time in the PACU.[10] Critical care nurses rely on a vast body of knowledge, skill, and experience so that they can provide care to the patient and the patient's family while performing as a patient advocate and liaison. Included in the body of knowledge is public health science.

Though nurses working in critical care settings spend the majority of their time providing individual care to patients and families, hospital-based, population-level data are needed to evaluate the effectiveness of that care. Nurses use well-established epidemiological models to guide their health prevention activities, mostly at the tertiary prevention level. These activities include health education and careful discharge planning to promote recovery and reduce the risk of disability and mortality. In addition, over time critical care nurses actively engage in population-level care through performance improvement activities and participation in research studies aimed at gathering evidence to demonstrate the effectiveness of interventions for improving the outcomes of the patient populations they serve.

Evolution of Critical Care: Population Driven

Over the past few decades, critical care nursing has been recognized as a distinct and essential specialty, providing care to those who are the most severely ill or injured.[9] The origin and development of the critical care field occurred in response to several different factors, each of which was population driven. The initiating factors first occurred in response to wartime injury. The progression of critical care can be attributed to the advancement in technology and the utilization of an improvement process shaped by evidence-based practice.

War: Critical care, in part, was developed using knowledge and skill obtained during wartime efforts. The true origin has been difficult to establish, but Florence Nightingale[11] is considered to be the first to have used an ICU approach to help focus care on those who were in the need of the highest level of nursing care. She served with the British during the Crimean War from 1854 to 1856. In her book *Notes on Hospitals*, she wrote about the advantages of establishing a separate area of the hospital for the sickest or most severely injured soldiers. She maintained this area close to her nursing station where she could keep a close watch on their condition and provide quick help when needed. The next report of a similar effort was in 1929, when Dr. Walter Dandy of Johns Hopkins Hospital in Baltimore developed a specialized postoperative unit containing three beds for neurosurgical patients.[12]

Advancements in caring for the critically ill also occurred as a consequence of wartime injuries. During World War I, the importance of recognizing shock and treating it with the intravascular volume replacement using saline and colloid solutions was demonstrated. Early in World War I, before the United States entered into the war, blood transfusion was first introduced by Bruce Robertson. He was a Canadian physician who, while training in the United States, became convinced that whole blood was superior to saline infusions. The blood was collected from soldiers on the battlefield who were willing and ready to donate. It was not until World War II that the technique of blood transfusion was widely used. This war provided the stimulus for organized blood collection; as the war progressed, a national blood program was established, which provided massive quantities of blood for overseas use.[13]

Also during World War II, advances in surgical techniques led to survival of injuries that were previously considered lethal. These injured soldiers subsequently needed prolonged supportive care for recovery. Shock wards were developed to resuscitate and care for the soldiers injured in battle or undergoing surgery, and postoperative patients were admitted to recovery rooms to facilitate nursing care.[14]

With each subsequent war, advances have been made in the care of the critically ill and injured. In the Iraq and Afghanistan wars, significant advances were made in the treatment of traumatic brain injuries that resulted from roadside bomb explosions. These have translated into advances in caring for civilian injuries both unintentional, such as motor vehicle accidents (MVAs) and football injuries, and intentional, such as the gunshot to the head sustained by U.S. Representative Gabrielle Giffords in 2011. These advances occurred because of the focus on the care of a population, in this case soldiers, and the particular type of injuries they were experiencing. This has resulted in a steady improvement in the mortality rate of soldiers in U.S. conflicts.[15,16] During the American Civil War, the chance of dying was about one in four (250 per 1,000). Only a fraction actually died during battle because much of the deaths were attributable to disease and infections of wounds sustained during battle.[17] By the time of the war in Vietnam, the death rate dropped to 21.8 per 1,000, which was five times higher than the death rate in the Iraq war.[18] Some of these advancements were a result of innovations not that dissimilar to what Florence Nightingale did in the Crimean War. For example, in Iraq medical teams were deployed closer to combat areas and evacuation times were greatly improved.[18]

All of these innovations in care were driven by population-level data. In particular, these changes were made to improve the health outcomes of soldiers sustaining life-threatening injuries or disease on the battlefield. The practices continued to be refined and used because population-level data demonstrated that survival rates improved. **Survival rate** is defined as the number of persons who survive an event divided by the total number of persons who experience an event. Thus, these innovative clinicians, including Florence Nightingale (see Chapter 1), effectively used public health science to improve the health of the critically ill.

Polio and Intensive Care: Critical care has evolved not only through the care of those injured during war but also through advances related to communicable diseases (see Chapter 8) and noncommunicable chronic diseases (see Chapter 9). Innovations in the delivery of care to those who are critically ill have occurred in response to communicable disease outbreaks. In other cases, public health science findings resulted in changes in how we care for chronic diseases.

A good example of how a communicable disease outbreak changed practices in critical care is the poliomyelitis (polio) epidemic that started in the late 1940s. **Polio,** one of the most dreaded diseases of childhood during the 21st century, is caused by the poliovirus, a human enterovirus member of the family Picornaviridae. It is transmitted from person to person via the fecal-oral route. Until the 20th century, the virus was readily transmitted via water, and most exposures to the virus occurred during infancy. At this young age, when most

have at least partial protection via maternal antibodies, the resulting infection was subclinical. This asymptomatic infection in turn gave lifelong immunity. Only a few suffered from paralysis, which was labeled *infantile paralysis.* As advancements in water treatment took place, the early childhood exposure to the poliovirus decreased. As a consequence of better hygiene, the first exposure to the virus was more apt to occur during late childhood or young adulthood. In this older age group, the infection caused more severe sequelae: a paralysis syndrome. At the peak of the epidemic in 1952, there were more than 21,000 cases. With the introduction of the Salk vaccine, the incidence rapidly decreased. By 1965, there were only 61 cases and the last known case caused by wild poliovirus was in 1993.[19]

Prior to the introduction of the vaccine, the epidemic in the late 1940s and early 1950s resulted in an increased demand on the health-care system. Although more than 90% of poliovirus infections are asymptomatic, the most severe effect of the virus is paralysis. The paralytic syndromes range from paralysis of one or more limbs to respiratory muscle paralysis. The mortality rate from respiratory polio was greater than 90%. Boston Children's Hospital was the first to use a mechanical respiratory machine called the *iron lung* to prevent likely death (Fig. 15-3). Use of this respiratory therapy resulted in a significant reduction of mortality, but was found to

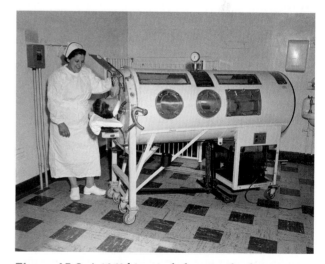

Figure 15-3 A 1960 historical photograph of a nurse caring for a victim of a Rhode Island polio epidemic, who was inside an Emerson respirator, also sometimes referred to as an "iron lung" machine. *(From Centers for Disease Control and Prevention, Public Health Image Library No. 12009. Retrieved from http://phil.cdc.gov/phil/details.asp.)*

be cumbersome and expensive, and made it difficult to provide nursing care. As years passed, improvements were made to this mechanical respiratory unit and it was broadly used throughout North America and Europe during severe polio outbreaks.

In 1952, during a large polio outbreak in Denmark, Bjorn Ibsen, an anesthetist in Blegdam Hospital, used the positive pressure ventilation concept used in the operating room for the respiratory support for the polio victims. Dr. Bjorn had his medical students hand-ventilate dozens of patients through tracheostomy tubes until the worst of the paralytic phase had passed. For efficiency and convenience, the patients who needed the respiratory support were placed in a single location within the hospital. This is often cited as the world's first intensive care unit (ICU), "a ward where physicians and nurses observe and treat 'desperately ill' patients 24 hours a day."[12,20] The introduction of a defined area of the hospital that is used for the support of patients in respiratory failure was the origin of today's ICU. Again, improved outcomes and decreased mortality for this particular hospital-based population drove the development of these interventions.

Despite the innovative use of an iron lung and an ICU concept, the polio pandemic spurred public health research aimed at primary prevention. Based on the epidemiological triangle reviewed in Chapter 8, clinicians had the choice to eradicate the virus, change the environment, or protect the host (humans). There was a major public health public program using public service announcements that warned parents about the risk of polio with a focus on public swimming areas. Polio outbreaks often occurred during the summer months as a result of children swimming in contaminated water. Thus, initial efforts were to alter the chance of exposure. However, public health research concentrated on protecting the host through the development of a vaccine that would boost human resistance to the virus. It was the introduction of the Salk vaccine in 1952 and the Sabin vaccine in 1962 that dramatically reduced the incidence of polio to less than one per 100,000 persons annually in the early 1960s. Thus, public health science can often help bring solutions to health issues, which can result in the need for critical care. Since the initiation of the ICU concept during the polio pandemic, ICUs have been instituted to provide care for many different kinds of patients from the neonate to adults with specific intensive care needs (Box 15-2).

Technology and Acute Care: Cardiopulmonary Resuscitation): Advances in technology have also resulted in changes in the delivery of critical care. The use of these

BOX 15–2 **Specialized Types of Intensive Care Units**

- Neonatal intensive care unit (NICU)
- Special care nursery (SCN)
- Pediatric intensive care unit (PICU)
- Psychiatric intensive care unit (PICU)
- Coronary care unit (CCU)
- Cardiac surgery intensive care unit (CSICU)
- Cardiovascular intensive care unit (CVICU)
- Medical intensive care unit (MICU)
- Medical surgical intensive care unit (MSICU)
- Surgical intensive care unit (SICU)
- Overnight intensive recovery (OIR)
- Neurotrauma intensive care unit (NICU)
- Neurointensive care unit (NICU)
- Burn wound intensive care unit (BWICU)
- Trauma intensive care unit (TICU)
- Surgical trauma intensive care unit (STICU)
- Trauma-neuro critical care (TNCC)
- Respiratory intensive care unit (RICU)
- Geriatric intensive care unit (GICU)
- Mobile intensive care unit (MICU)

technologies demonstrates a combination of population data, advances in the understanding of human physiology, and technological advances. As in the field of pharmacy, the randomized clinical trial (Chapter 3) is the gold standard for determining the effectiveness and efficacy of technological interventions in critical care. These advances often began with bench science but in the end translate into how care is provided owing to positive changes in the outcomes of the patient populations involved. One of the most dramatic examples is the whole issue of **cardiopulmonary resuscitation (CPR)**, an emergency procedure that includes the use of external cardiac massage and artificial respiration for persons who experience sudden cardiac arrest. The technique was developed within the acute care setting and adopted for use by the general public. Overall, CPR has dramatically reduced mortality that is attributed to a variety of events that result in cessation of breathing, heartbeat, or both.

Peter J. Safar, the "father" of CPR, converted the method of CPR used in the hospital for use by the general public. He promoted the development of life-supporting first aid, which is known as basic life support. In 1957, he publicized the "A" (airway), "B" (breathing), and "C" (circulation system). Safar was a public health advocate who gave the first step to the general public to aid others in an emergency. He worked hard to popularize the procedure around the world and collaborated with a Norwegian company to create "Resusci Anne," the first CPR

CHAPTER 15 • Health Planning for Acute Care Settings *359*

training manikin. His contribution to life-saving medical technique has earned him a reputation as one of the pioneers of critical care medicine and has saved uncountable numbers of lives.[21]

In 1960, the American Heart Association (AHA) started a program to acquaint physicians with closed-chest cardiac resuscitation and became the forerunner of CPR training for the general public. Although only 40 communities in the United States regularly measure and report survival rates, these population-level data have proved invaluable in the evaluation of the success of CPR and the development of changes aimed at improvement of survival rates. Initially, it was recommended that laypersons administering CPR first clear the airway (A), then administer breaths (B), and then initiate chest compressions (C). In 2010, dramatic revisions were made to the CPR guidelines. The recommendations are for the three steps of CPR to be rearranged: the new first step is now chest compressions instead of first establishing the airway, and then administering breaths. Newborns are an exception to the change. Thus, A-B-C has become C-A-B for compressions, airway, and breathing (Fig. 15-4). For laypersons, the AHA states that the most effective approach is to immediately deliver chest compressions at a rate of greater than 100 compressions per minute "the same rhythm as the beat of the Bee Gees' song, 'Stayin' Alive.'"[22] Although it is difficult to determine the exact survival rate, the American Public Health Association examines the factors that are associated with long-term survival rate and uses this information to guide the administration of CPR and the development of supportive programs such as public access defibrillation programs aimed at improving survival rates.[23,24]

Role of Cohort Studies in the Delivery of Acute Care

Population data have not only been gathered from within the hospital to help improve patient outcomes, but have also been gathered from general populations. A longitudinal cohort study (see Chapter 3) provides valuable evidence on who will potentially develop disease based on different risk factors. At baseline, information is collected about the health of the individuals in the cohort and then these individuals are tracked over time to determine who develops disease and who does not. A cohort study can be focused on a particular disease, for example, the Framingham Health Study (FHS)[25] or a particular population such as the Nurses' Health Study.[26]

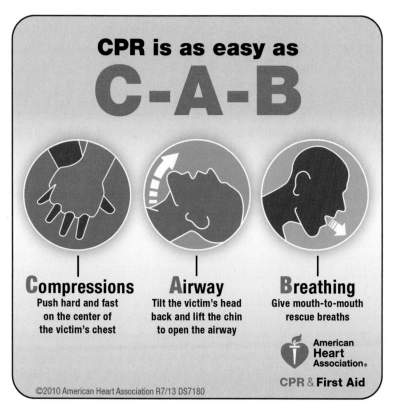

Figure 15-4 C-A-B for cardiopulmonary resuscitation. *(See reference 24. Used with permission.)*

The Framingham Heart Study and Cardiovascular Disease

As reported in Chapter 9, the leading cause of death in the United States is cardiovascular disease (CVD). Nearly 2,300 Americans die of CVD each day, an average of one death every 38 seconds. CVD claims more lives each year than cancer, chronic lower respiratory diseases, and accidents combined. There are an estimated 81,100,000 American adults (more than one in three) with CVD. Of these, 38,100,000 are estimated to be age 60 or older.[26] As staggering as these numbers appear, a recent study examining deaths from CVD in the United States from 1980 to 2000 found that there was about a 47% decrease.[27] This was attributable to evidence-based medical therapies and changes in risk factors. The FHS is directly responsible for the remarkable advances made in the prevention of heart disease in the United States and throughout the world.

In 1948, the town of Framingham, Massachusetts, was selected by the U.S. Public Health Service as the study site, and 5,209 healthy residents between 30 and 60 years of age, both men and women, were enrolled as the first cohort of participants. It was the first major cardiovascular study to recruit women participants. At the time, little was known about the general causes of heart disease and stroke, but the death rates for CVD had been increasing steadily since the beginning of the 20th century and had become an American epidemic. The FHS became a joint project of the National Heart, Lung, & Blood Institute (NHLBI) and Boston University.[25]

The objective of the FHS was to identify the common risk factors that contribute to CVD by following its development over a long period of time in a large group of participants who had not yet developed overt symptoms of CVD or suffered a heart attack or stroke. Since 1948, the subjects have continued to return to the study every 2 years for a detailed medical history, physical examination, and laboratory tests. In 1971, the study enrolled a second generation, 5,124 of the original participants' adult children and their spouses, to participate in similar examinations. In 1994, the need to establish a new study including a more diverse community of Framingham was recognized, and the first Omni cohort of the FHS was enrolled. In April 2002, the study entered a new phase, the enrollment of a third generation of participants, the grandchildren of the original cohort. In 2003, a second group of Omni participants was enrolled.[25]

The FHS continues to make important scientific contributions by enhancing its research capabilities and capitalizing on its inherent resources. Some of the more recent data from the FHS show from the original and offspring cohorts (1980–2003) that the average annual rate of first major cardiovascular events is on the rise. Events have gone from 3 per 1,000 in men at ages 35 to 44, to 74 per 1,000 at ages 85 to 94. For women, comparable rates occur 10 years later in life, and the gap narrows with advancing age. Before age 75, a higher proportion of CVD events due to coronary heart disease (CHD) occur in men than in women, and a higher proportion of events due to stroke occur in women than in men. From 1996 to 2006, death rates from CVD declined 29.2%. Data from the FHS indicate that the lifetime risk for CVD is two in three for men and more than one in two for women at age 40.[25] Over time, the impact of the study on heart health is substantial (Box 15-3).[28,29]

Woman and Cardiovascular Disease

Earlier, CVD was perceived by many health-care providers as a predominately male disease linked to stress and lifestyle. It was thought that women had a low risk for developing CVD and were protected by female sex hormones. The assumption that CVD was primarily a male disease had a profound effect on the underdiagnosing, underinvestigating, and undertreating of the female population with CVD.[30]

As mentioned above, the FHS is one of the few long-term prospective studies of CVD that has included both men and women. Women participated from the very beginning and investigators recognized that CVD occurs later in life and with lower frequency in females. With follow-up of 5,209 original study participants (2,873 women and 2,336 men), researchers have documented information about the incidence of CVD the in FHS women and risk factors that are unique to women.[30]

There are specific physiological, pathophysiological, clinical, and socioeconomic issues that differentiate women and men with CVD. Because of these differences, symptoms of an MI are different between genders. Women are more likely to experience atypical chest pain, abdominal pain, dyspnea, nausea, and fatigue during a cardiovascular event. Because these symptoms are different from the "elephant sitting on the chest" type of pain that males often experience, the atypical presentation may be missed or be attributed to another etiology. If the suspicion of CVD has not been raised by symptoms, underinvestigation and undertreatment may occur. Women typically wait longer to seek medical assistance and this may be due to the atypical presentation of symptoms.[31,32] Delay of treatment has a devastating

BOX 15–3	Framingham Heart Study Milestones

1960	Cigarette smoking found to increase the risk of heart disease.
1961	Cholesterol level, blood pressure, and electrocardiogram abnormalities found to increase the risk of heart disease.
1967	Physical activity found to reduce the risk of heart disease and obesity to increase the risk of heart disease.
1970	High blood pressure found to increase the risk of stroke.
1976	Menopause found to increase the risk of heart disease.
1978	Psychosocial factors found to affect heart disease.
1988	High levels of high-density lipoprotein cholesterol found to reduce risk of death.
1994	Enlarged left ventricle (one of two lower chambers of the heart) shown to increase the risk of stroke.
1996	Progression from hypertension to heart failure described.
1998	Development of simple coronary disease prediction algorithm involving risk factor categories to allow physicians to predict multivariate CHD risk in patients without overt CHD.
1999	Lifetime risk at age 40 years of developing CHD is one in two for men and one in three for women.
2001	High-normal blood pressure is associated with an increased risk of CVD, emphasizing the need to determine whether lowering high-normal blood pressure can reduce the risk of CVD.
2002	Lifetime risk of developing high blood pressure in middle-aged adults is 9 in 10.
2002	Obesity is a risk factor for heart failure.
2004	Serum aldosterone levels predict future risk of hypertension in nonhypertensive individuals.
2005	Lifetime risk of becoming overweight exceeds 70%; that for obesity approximates one in two.
2006	The NHLBI of the National Institutes of Health announced a new genomewide association study at the FHS in collaboration with Boston University School of Medicine to be known as the SHARe project (SNP Health Association Resource).
2007	Based on evaluation of a densely interconnected social network of 12,067 people assessed as part of the FHS, network phenomena appear to be relevant to the biological and behavioral trait of obesity, and obesity appears to spread through social ties.
2008	Based on analysis of a social network of 12,067 people participating in the FHS, researchers discover that social networks exert key influences on decision to quit smoking.
2008	Discovery by FHS and publication of four risk factors that raise probability of developing precursor of heart failure; new 30-year risk estimates developed for serious cardiac events.
2009	FHS cited by the AHA as among the top 10 cardiovascular research achievements of 2009, "Genome-wide Association Study of Blood Pressure and Hypertension: Genome-wide Association Study Identifies Eight Loci Associated With Blood Pressure."
2009	A new genetic variant associated with increased susceptibility for atrial fibrillation, a prominent risk factor for stroke and heart failure, is reported in two studies based on data from the FHS.
2009	FHS researchers find parental dementia may lead to poor memory in middle-aged adults.

Source: See reference 29.

effect on the outcome of a cardiovascular event, which certainly may be seen in the mortality rate for a woman following an MI (Box 15-4). The risk of CVD increases with age. In 2005, more than 36 million American women were aged 55 or older; as noted in Chapter 20, as the baby boomers age, this number will grow. Owing to this increasing number, it is important to raise awareness of this major public health issue for older women. Within 1 year after a heart attack, women are more likely to die than men. Within 5 years following a first heart attack at the age of 70 or older, 56% of white women and 62% of black woman will die.[31] As life expectancy continues to increase, the burden of CVD for woman will also continue to increase.[27,32]

●APPLYING PUBLIC HEALTH SCIENCE

The Case of the Waiting Women

Public Health Science Topics Covered:

- Health planning
  - Conducting a setting-specific assessment
  - Population-level conclusions: Identifying priorities

Two nurses, Susan and Maria, work together in a cardiac catheterization laboratory (cath lab) in a large urban tertiary center. The cath lab is a very busy area within this medical center. This specialized area holds

| BOX 15–4 | Facts About Woman and Cardiovascular Disease |

- CVD, particularly coronary heart disease (CHD) and stroke, remain the leading causes of death of women in America and most developed countries, with nearly 37% of all female deaths in the United States occurring from CVD.
- CVD is a particularly important problem among minority women. The death rate due to CVD is higher in black women than in white women.
- One in 2.7 females who die, die of heart disease, stroke, and other CVD compared with one in 30 who die of breast cancer.
- In 2005, CVD claimed the lives of 454,613 females—cancer, 268,890.
- CHD claims the lives of 213,572 females annually compared with 41,116 lives from breast cancer and 69,105 from lung cancer.
- At age 40 and older, 23% of women compared with 18% of men will die within 1 year after a heart attack.

Source: See reference 30.

diagnostic imaging equipment used to support diagnostic and interventional procedures. The cath lab is staffed by a multidisciplinary team including physicians (interventional cardiologists, vascular surgeons, or radiologists), nurses, and radiology technicians.

A diagnostic procedure called a cardiac catheterization is performed in the cath lab to determine the extent of disease present in the vascular system. Left heart catheterization (arterial) is performed to determine blockages in the coronary vascular system. Right heart catheterization (venous) is performed to determine how well the heart valves are functioning and how effectively the heart is pumping blood to the lungs. The method involves threading a catheter through a femoral artery or vein or the radial artery and then threading it into the heart. During cardiac cath, a radio-opaque dye is injected through the catheter to highlight the coronary arteries. This test is called a coronary angiogram or coronary arteriogram.

Depending on what is found during the coronary angiogram, different interventions may occur during the cardiac cath. For example, an angioplasty that uses a balloon on the end of the catheter is able to open narrowed coronary arteries. Stents, which are small, meshlike devices made of metal that act as supports, or scaffolds, inside of a vessel, may be placed at the time of angioplasty.

During one particularly busy shift in the cath lab, Susan relieved Maria for lunch and received a report on a patient who was coming from the ED with a diagnosis of a suspected MI. The patient was a 60-year-old woman with no known history of CVD, who arrived in the ED about an hour before with vague complaints of fatigue, shortness of breath, and chest pressure. After a detailed history and physical, this patient was found to have an **ST-elevation myocardial infarction (STEMI)**, a heart attack caused by a prolonged period of blocked blood supply.[33] While Susan was with this patient in the cath lab, the coronary angiogram showed a severely occluded left main coronary artery, a surprising discovery given her atypical complaints. Knowing that this type of obstructive disease holds an increased mortality risk, Susan wanted to know why this patient was in the ED for such a long time before the diagnosis was made. She was also concerned because the door-to-balloon time was just at the 90-minute mark.

Door-to-balloon time is defined as the amount of time between a patient's arrival at the hospital and the time he/she receives percutaneous coronary intervention, such as angioplasty.[33] Because "time is muscle," meaning that delays in treating a MI increase the likelihood and amount of myocardial damage resulting from localized hypoxia, the American College of Cardiologists and the AHA guidelines recommend a door-to-balloon time of no more than 90 minutes. A national Door-to-Balloon Initiative was launched in November 2006 and has become a core quality measure for The Joint Commission.

When Maria returned from her lunch break, she and Susan discussed the circumstances of the patient with the STEMI. Susan voiced her concerns about the severity of the CVD in the presence of atypical complaints and the length of door-to-balloon time despite the success of the intervention. Maria was equally concerned in light of the fact that she had just cared for a postmenopausal patient with a STEMI who also presented with vague complaints earlier in the day that had gone beyond the 90-minute door-to-balloon time. After much discussion and a review of the recorded door-to-balloon times during the past several months, which showed other cases of women with prolonged times, both nurses felt strongly that they needed to take action so that they could make a difference in the care of woman with CVD.

Unsure of what to do next, Susan and Maria decided to consult Karen, the director of nursing research at the hospital. They knew that their short-term goal was to discover the red flags that could be used to alert the

ED personnel to the possibility of CVD in the post-menopausal woman with atypical symptoms. After educating the ED staff, Susan and Maria then wanted take this information and educate women at risk.

Karen encouraged them to learn more about the population at risk. Was the event that Susan witnessed unusual or more the norm in the ED? What was the evidence to support the door-to-balloon time frame? Were women at greater risk than men? Susan and Maria had hunches but no real data on the issue. Karen suggested that they conduct a retrospective chart review to answer these questions. She reminded them that they would have to follow the hospital policies related to chart reviews. The two nurses, with Karen's help, wrote up a proposal for doing the review.

Focused Assessment

The purpose of their review was not only to determine the length of time between arrival in the ED and treatment, but also to determine the length of time between the point at which the women first had symptoms and their arrival at the ED. Thus, the team embarked on a focused assessment (Chapter 4) that allowed them to examine the population of women who arrived in the ED over a specified period of time. They collected data on all adult women who arrived with a nontrauma event and then compared the presenting symptoms for those who actually had STEMI with those who did not. They collected information on time from first symptoms to arrival at the ED and what those first symptoms were. All of these assessment data were needed not only to determine whether indeed the door-to-balloon time standard was or was not being met, but also to describe more accurately the presenting symptoms of the women with a STEMI compared with those without a STEMI. This vital information helped in the development of an intervention for health-care providers and for the educational program they wanted to develop for women at risk for a STEMI. Both centered on how to recognize a possible STEMI and both interventions used a population approach.

Ethics in an Acute Care Setting

One issue faced by Susan and Maria was how to address the privacy of the patient information they obtained during their chart review. Karen showed them how to write a proposal, which they would then send to the institutional review board for approval. Karen explained to them that they could not access patient data without going through this process. In that way, they would design the review so that they would ensure the privacy of the patients and also allow them to disseminate their findings at an aggregate level with no personal identifiers.

Nurses interested in using population-level data to improve patient outcomes must be fully aware of the ethics of utilizing individual patient-level data for purposes other than what they were intended. There are two legal areas that nurses must remember at all times when conducting assessments or doing health program evaluations using patients data. The Health Insurance Portability and Accountability Act (HIPAA) of 1996 was designed to protect the use of electronic patient data. It set national standards for the security of electronic protected health information such as the **electronic medical record (EMR).** An EMR is a digital version of the patient chart that has replaced paper charts in most acute care settings. It is used to store the medical records of patients. It also provided rules on the use of identifiable confidential patient information to analyze patient safety events and improve patient safety.[34]

Though patient information obtained during a hospital stay is protected under HIPAA, there are times when the information can be shared. This represents the conflict between the individual's right to privacy and the public health perspective of protecting the health of the whole. The law has built into it regulations that recognize the need for public health authorities and others mandated to protect the public safety to have access to patient data. Thus, a physician may report information on dog bites or gunshot wounds to those with authority. Agencies with such authority include state and local health departments, the Food and Drug Administration (FDA), the CDC, and the Occupational Safety and Health Administration. Situations in which individual information may be shared to help protect the public include child abuse or neglect, adverse events associated with an FDA-approved activity or product, and reportable communicable diseases. It is important to note that the information may only be released to agencies with recognized authority as stipulated in the law.[34]

The HIPAA law is an important factor for nurses who plan to collect patient data to conduct a study related to their care. For example, in some cases nurses make changes to practice based on existing evidence and do this within the scope of their practice. They do not report the assessment data or the success of their program outside of their hospital because it is not a research study. Susan and Maria remembered covering human subjects' research in their research class, but were not sure how to proceed. Their hospital had a policy that all projects that involved obtaining data from patient records and/or collecting patient data from patients must be reviewed by the institutional review board (IRB) prior to collecting any data. An **institutional review board** is a committee formally charged with reviewing biomedical and behavioral research conducted with human subjects to ensure the protection of research participants. These committees must comply with federal regulations related to conducting research with human subjects. The two nurses worked with the hospital nurse researcher to delineate exactly what their process was and then provided the information as required to their institution's IRB. They clarified that when collecting the data from the medical records, they would include information on the residence of the patient and that they would need to link medical records from two different clinics. Though they were planning to utilize the information for an internal change in practice, they wished also to examine whether there was a difference between those patients who actually had a STEMI and those who did not and then report those findings in a journal article or at a conference. Thus, they wished to generalize the findings of their assessment. They submitted their proposal with specific information on how they would protect the privacy of the patient's medical record. The IRB determined that it did constitute human subjects research but met the requirements for an expedited review because it involved a review of medical records only, with minimal risk to the patients.

Thus, nurses working in the acute care settings are faced with multiple ethical issues. From a public health perspective, the nurse must be aware of the need to protect the health of the public while protecting the right to individual privacy. In addition, as more hospitals encourage nurses working in acute care settings to engage in research, they must become aware of the ethical dilemmas posed in the collection of patient data. Improving patient outcomes requires a constant review of the evidence and health planning to improve practice. During this process, human subjects must always be protected from unnecessary risk.

The Nurses' Health Study

The Nurses' Health Study is similar to the FHS, but focuses on the health of women rather than a particular

disease. It started in 1976, and has expanded to include two more cohorts, one in 1989 and one in 2008. Initially, the primary objective was to study the long-term consequences related to the use of oral contraceptives. However, the findings from the studies are providing insights into a broad array of health issues including breast cancer, diabetes, and CVD in women. The results of the studies confirm that diet, physical activity, and other lifestyle factors significantly promote better health and reduce risk for disease.[26]

Health Planning and Acute Care

The approach instituted at the hospital described in the first case study, Solving the Mystery, used a health planning approach to the delivery of nursing care in a hospital setting. The team completed the first step in heath planning, the assessment (see Chapter 4). The data helped to identify populations at risk for poorer outcomes. Armed with these data, the nursing department could now move to the next step, the development, implementation, and evaluation of a health program aimed at improving patient outcomes (see Chapter 5). For Cheryl who wanted to know the who, what, why, when, and where, the final results of the assessment identified the areas in need of nursing activities related to searching for the evidence to support practice as well as conducting research studies aimed at improving outcomes. For the CNO, the assessment provided her with the outcomes-focused approach and the baseline data she needed to evaluate change over time from an organizational perspective. The results were distributed to the nursing staff as a whole, and nursing units were encouraged to explore opportunities to develop population-level interventions that would improve outcomes for patients admitted with a diagnosis that matched those included in Table 15-2.

Noncommunicable Diseases and Acute Care Settings

Chapter 9 provided an overview of noncommunicable diseases and their contribution to the overall burden of disease. Acute care settings provide care to persons with noncommunicable diseases when they are experiencing an acute stage of the disease. They may come to the hospital when they have first been diagnosed, or the admission may be one of many related to the noncommunicable disease. Providing acute care for a disease process that will not result in a cure leaves the care provider focused on decreasing disease related morbidity and disability and reducing the risk of premature death. Thus, the nurse in the acute care setting caring for a person with a noncommunicable disease is providing tertiary prevention (see Chapter 2). This can be challenging for the nurse because of short hospital stays. The nurse must adapt the plan of care to fit the individual's needs. However, development of a program that addresses population-level barriers to care and improves the ability of patients to self-manage their disease on discharge can make a big difference. This again requires using a population approach and often requires the identification of subpopulations within the patient population who may be experiencing significant barriers to self-management of their diseases.

The first step for the nurse working on a hospital unit who wishes to develop an intervention program is to identify the level of prevention involved in the intervention. For example, if a nurse wanted to develop a program focused on **acute coronary syndrome** (ACS), she would have to begin with an understanding of the disease. ACS is defined by the AHA as any set of clinical symptoms associated with acute myocardial ischemia. **Acute myocardial ischemia** presents as chest pain that is due to an insufficient blood supply to the heart muscle. The underlying cause is CAD. The majority of known risk factors for CAD are modifiable by specific preventive measures. Primary prevention focuses on prevention of disease in those who do not have the disease (see Chapter 2). The AHA goal for primary prevention is to educate all adults about the levels and significance of risk factors related to CAD. The AHA guide to primary prevention of CAD has a risk reduction focus. The major risk factors targeted include smoking, blood pressure control, dietary intake, blood lipid management, physical activity, and weight management. Comprehensive risk factor interventions can prevent disease from occurring. In addition, secondary prevention, early identification of those with subclinical disease, can extend overall survival, improve health-related quality of life, and decrease need for interventional procedures such as angioplasty and bypass grafting and ultimately reduce the incidence of subsequent heart attack (MI). Examples of secondary prevention include identifying and treating people with established disease and those at very high risk of developing CAD. Examples of tertiary prevention include treating and rehabilitating patients who have had a heart attack or to prevent another cardiovascular event. *Healthy People 2020 (HP 2020)* includes heart disease and stroke as one of its topics, and one objective is to reduce hospitalizations.[35] Meeting these objectives requires interventions across the prevention continuum and a population health perspective.

■ HEALTHY PEOPLE 2020
Heart Disease and Stroke (HDS)

HDS Objective 24: Reduce hospitalizations of older adults with heart failure as the principal diagnosis.

HDS-24-1 Adults Aged 65 to 74 Years

Baseline: 9.8 hospitalizations for heart failure per 1,000 population aged 65 to 74 years occurred in 2007
Target: 8.8 hospitalizations per 1,000 population
Target Setting Method: 10% improvement
Data Source: Chronic Conditions Warehouse (CCW), CMS

HDS 24-1 Adults Aged 75 to 84 Years

Baseline: 22.4 hospitalizations for heart failure per 1,000 population aged 75 to 84 occurred in 2007
Target: 20.2 hospitalizations per 1,000 population
Target Setting Method: 10% improvement
Data Source: Chronic Conditions Warehouse (CCW), CMS

HDS 24-3 Adults Aged 85 Years and Older

Baseline: 42.9 hospitalizations for heart failure per 1,000 population aged 75 to 84 occurred in 2007
Target: 38.6 hospitalizations per 1,000 population
Target Setting Method: 10% improvement
Data Source: Chronic Conditions Warehouse (CCW), CMS
Source: See reference 35.

Performance Improvement and Acute Care Settings

One of the most important aspects in the progression of hospital-based health care has been the change in emphasis from the hospital as a location or a place that holds acutely ill patients to a focus on the provision of evidence-based care with documented improved patient outcomes. To achieve this goal, acute care settings use a specific process called quality improvement and/or performance improvement that works to provide safe and consistent care to the acutely ill and injured. This process is population based and provides the appropriate framework for conducting studies that evaluate the effectiveness of actions taken. The type of studies conducted may involve calculation of rates such as infections, determining the impact of risks such as diabetes on MI, and developing interventions such as a walking program to decrease risks of osteoporosis.

According to Margolis, Provost, Schoettker, and Britto, **quality improvement** (QI) in health care may be defined as "systematic data guides activities designed to bring about positive changes in the delivery of healthcare in particular settings."[36] *Public Health Nursing: Scope and Standards of Practice*[37] defines **performance improvement** (PI) as a "process that considers the organizational context, describes desired performance, identifies gaps between desired and actual performance, identifies root causes, selects interventions to close the gaps, and measures changes in performances with the goal of achieving desired results or outcomes."

The terms *quality improvement* and *performance improvement* are often used interchangeably with the difference being that performance improvement takes a more bottom-up approach and acknowledges that improvement is an ongoing rather than a static process. For the purposes of this chapter, the term *PI* is used because it matches the term used in *Public Health Nursing: Scope and Standards of Practice*. Basically, the goal is to improve the care of hospitalized patients through the implementation of evidence-based practices or system changes. No project is generally deemed too small if it improves patient outcomes. For the majority of direct patient care staff, questioning a specific practice by asking, "Why do we do this task this way?" may initiate a PI project.

In order for programs to be successful, data collection must occur within the context of a continuous improvement strategy so that the caregivers in the acute care setting can implement changes that improve the quality of health care.[38] Two examples of PI projects are (1) comparison of hospital antibiotic timing rates among patients who receive required preoperative antibiotics before the start of the operative procedure with data from the Centers for Medicare & Medicaid Services and (2) comparing the rates of postoperative infections against the national rates reported by the CDC.[39]

Why Do We Need PI in Acute Care Settings?

A groundbreaking report published by the Institute of Medicine (IOM) at the start of the 21st century entitled *To Err Is Human: Building a Safer Health Care System* created a stir in the health-care industry.[40] Its findings brought to the forefront the lack of consistent quality programs in hospitals in the United States. The report identified the following deficiencies:

- In 1997, there were more than 33.6 million admissions to U.S. hospitals.

- Approximately 44,000 Americans die each year as a result of medical errors, and other data suggest that the number may be as high as 98,000.
- More people die because of medical errors than MVAs, breast cancer, and AIDS each year.
- Total national costs (including loss of income, disability, and health-care costs) were estimated to be between $37 and $50 billion for adverse events, and for preventable adverse events between $17 and $29 billion.
- In terms of lost lives, patient safety is as important as worker safety. More than 6,000 American workers die each year of workplace injuries as compared with the 1993 reported medication error deaths at 7,000 lives.

As a result of the findings presented in the initial IOM report, the group recommended a fundamental redesign of the entire health-care system. It recommended the following six aims for improving the system around the following core needs of health care:

1. Safe—Avoid injuries to patients.
2. Effective—Care should be evidence and scientifically based.
3. Patient centered—Care should be built upon patient preferences, needs, and values.
4. Timely—Reduce waits and delays.
5. Efficient—Avoid wastes.
6. Equitable—Care should be equal to all person regardless of age, gender, ethnicity, location, and socioeconomic status.[40]

Based on the IOM report and recommendations, the Institute for Healthcare Improvement (IHI) developed a patient safety initiative because it believes that patients deserve safe and effective health care. The IHI exists to close the gap between the health care we have and the health care we should have.[41] Thus, the IHI launched its 100,000 Lives Campaign, the goal of which was to save 100,000 patient lives through quality improvements to six patient safety initiatives based on several core practices. These initiatives include the following; (1) Deploy rapid response teams; (2) deliver reliable and evidence-based care for acute MI patients; (3) prevent adverse drug events through medication reconciliation; (4) prevent central line infections; (5) prevent surgical site infections; and (6) prevent ventilator associated pneumonia.[42] To assist hospitals in implementing these PI projects, the IHI supplies template tools to implement as well as track progress in achieving these goals. The IHI created steps for incorporating these quality improvement initiatives (Box 15-5).

BOX 15–5	Institute for Healthcare Improvement Steps for Incorporating Quality Improvement Initiatives

- Set AIM—Defining the specific population to be studied and what the group wishes to accomplish.
- MEASURE results—Specific rate or number as a benchmark for comparison to determine whether the changes being made lead to improvement (e.g., reduction in bloodstream infections, or reduction in the wait time from ED visit to hospital room).
- TEST changes—This may be accomplished through the Plan (P) Do (D) Study (S) Act (A) cycle (PDSA) (Fig. 15-5).
  - Plan = Plan the change
    - Determine the key personnel
    - Where/when it will take place
    - How it will be tested
    - What data need to be collected
    - Who will collect the data and record the results
  - Do = Test the change/intervention
  - Study = Determine the results—did it work?
  - Act = Was the intervention/change successful?
    - If yes, can it be expanded to more patients?
    - If yes, then implement another PDSA cycle
  - If the intervention/change did not work:
    - Determine why it failed
    - Reassess and develop a new plan and test it again
- IMPLEMENT changes—moving the program on a broader scale. This may include other shifts on the nursing unit, similar nursing units or hospitalwide.

Source: See reference 41.

● APPLYING PUBLIC HEALTH SCIENCE

The Case of the Hospital Partners

Public Health Science Topics Covered:

- Epidemiology and biostatistics
  - Determining rates
- Assessment

In 2003, a group of 10 Cincinnati area hospitals collaborated to reduce HAIs as part of a patient safety initiative. One goal of the project was to reduce catheter-related bloodstream infections (CR-BSI) through the implementation of evidence-based practice (EBP). The hospitals met monthly to discuss their progress and share information about their progress toward meeting their specific goal.[43] A team was formed in Hospital A to work on their institutional-level efforts to meet the regional goals. The group not

only used the IHI model described above, but also applied the four-step Plan-Do-Study-Act (PDSA) cycle to their PI project. The **PDSA cycle** is an interactive process adopted from business, is also known as the Deming Wheel, and has been around since the 1920s (Fig. 15-5). This cycle is based on action-oriented learning; provides shorthand for testing a change; and is accomplished through a cycle of planning the change, trying it, observing the results, and then acting on what is learned.[44]

The first step in the IHI process is to set an aim. For hospital A, they decided their aim statement would be: to reduce CR-BSIs. The second step is the Measurement statement, which would be: a reduction in CR-BSI by 50% over the next 12 months. The reason this was important was based on the evidence that over 200,000 CR-BSIs occur each year in the United States, and have an associated mortality of 4% to 35%.[43] Hospital A determined that to reduce the rates of CR-BSIs, they would first have to develop a tool to measure adherence to treatment with best practices outlined by the CDC (Box 15-6).[43] These best practices included performing hand hygiene before insertion of catheters, applying maximum sterile barriers (gowns, masks, head cover, and sterile gloves) prior to the insertion of central line catheters, covering the patient with a full body drape, and prepping the insertion site with a chlorhexidine-based product.[45]

Once the nursing staff determined what they wanted to measure, they initiated the PDSA cycle

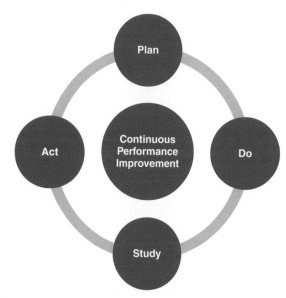

Figure 15-5 Plan (P) Do (D) Study (S) Act (A) cycle.

BOX 15–6 | Central Line Insertion Guidelines

With each central line insertion, the nursing staff collected data on each of the best practices and reported adherence back to all end users on the following:

- Percentage adherence to hand hygiene
- Percentage adherence to maximum barriers (mask, head cover, surgeon gown, and sterile gloves)
- Percentage adherence to full body drapes
- Percentage adherence to chlorhexidine antiseptic for each central line insertion

Source: See reference 43.

(see Fig. 15-5). The **PLAN** identified the key personnel to be included in the central line insertion—the chief medical resident and patient's registered nurse (RN). The line insertion would take place in a patient's room on day shift in the medical intensive care unit (MICU). The data to be collected were outlined on a central line check sheet developed by Hospital A, and the person collecting the information would be the charge RN.

The next step is **DO.** Once it was determined there was a patient who needed a central line, the charge nurse gathered all the supplies including central line insertion tray, surgical attire from the operating room, a large surgical thyroid drape with an opening (fenestration) near the top of the drape, and the chlorhexidine antiseptic swabs. The MICU RN and the chief resident donned the sterile garb. The MICU charge RN applied a mask and remained at the bedside to act as a circulating nurse and also to record the events and to complete the checklist. The medical resident and the MICU RN applied the drape and prepped the patient's insertion site with chlorhexidine. The resident inserted the central line per hospital protocol.

The next step is **STUDY.** During the covering with the sterile drape, several problems were encountered. First, neither the chief medical resident nor the MICU RN had much experience with applying a large surgical drape and had difficulty maintaining sterility. Thus, they went through several drapes during the application process. Using several drapes decreased the volume in the operating room. This resulted in placing an urgent order to the manufacturer. This had an impact on the cost of the procedure. Also, the current central line kit was found to be missing some of the supplies needed to meet the CDC recommendations,[45] so the MICU charge RN had to leave the room several times to find the supplies not included in the current central line trays.

The final step is **ACT.** The group concluded that this first test was not successful and regrouped. They determined there were a number of processes that needed to be corrected before they proceeded on with the next line insertion: requesting the OR staff the MICU nurses/residents with in-service teaching on the proper application of a full body drape; working with the purchasing department to have more drapes stocked in the MICU and the operating room; and reviewing the contents of the current central line kits to determine what supplies would be needed to meet the intent of the CDC recommendations to decrease the number of interruptions during the insertion process. The group asked the purchasing department to schedule meetings with the central line tray manufacturers to revise the trays to include the supplies needed.

The group concluded that employing the PDSA cycle allowed them to test the new protocols before instituting it in all the other ICUs and the hospital. This was a new approach, replacing the usual practice in which a policy was developed and the users were then required to determine how they would adhere to it. They were able to determine what worked on a small scale and what needed to be corrected in order to provide their patients with the best care they deserved. Eventually, the group was able to work with the manufacturers of surgical drapes and central line insertion trays to develop efficient and EBP central line trays and surgical packs.

They collected data by using the check sheets and reported adherence to the best practices back to the end users, and published the rates in their respective units for staff, physicians, and families to review. The nurses were empowered to stop any procedure wherein any of the components on the checklist were not followed. Eventually, through repeated PDSA cycles, the MICU unit reduced their CR-BSI rates by over 50%, and the process was instituted in the rest of the hospital.[39] The checklist was followed throughout Hospital A for all central line insertions. Adherence rates continued to be reported to all users and committees and infection rates were then posted in all ICUs, allowing for immediate action and the continuous use of the PDSA cycle.

Infection Control and Acute Care Settings

The CDC defines a **healthcare-associated infection (HAI)** as a localized or systemic condition resulting from an adverse reaction to the presence of an infectious agent(s) or its toxin(s) that (1) occurs in a patient in a health-care setting (e.g., a hospital or outpatient clinic); (2) was not found to be present or incubating at the time of admission unless the infection was related to a previous admission to the same setting; and (3) if the setting is a hospital, meets the criteria for a specific infection site as defined by the CDC.[46] The major issues include sepsis/bacteremias, pneumonia, and urinary tract infections (UTIs).

■ HEALTHY PEOPLE 2020
Healthcare-Associated Infections
Targeted Topic: Healthcare-Associated Infections
Goal: Prevent, reduce, and ultimately eliminate HAIs.
Overview: HAIs are infections that patients get while receiving treatment for medical or surgical conditions. They are among the leading causes of preventable deaths in the United States and are associated with a substantial increase in health-care costs each year.
Source: See reference 35.

Sepsis

According to the National Center for Health Statistics, sepsis is the 10th leading cause of death in the United States.[47] **Sepsis** is defined as "a systemic inflammatory syndrome in response to infection. When associated with acute organ dysfunction, such as acute renal failure, it is said to be severe."[48] Sepsis is the body's response to the invasion of pathogenic microorganisms in which severe sepsis and septic shock are the end results of the interaction between infecting organisms and the body's host responses. These responses cause inflammation, immunosuppression, abnormal coagulation, and blood flow and circulatory dysfunction, which leads to organ injury and cell death.[49]

Sepsis also includes a robust systemic inflammatory response also known as systemic inflammatory response syndrome (SIRS). The SIRS syndrome may include fever or hypothermia, tachycardia, tachypnea, leukocytosis or leukopenia, or the presence of immature neutrophils. The patient's temperature may be greater than 38°C or less than 36°C, heart rate greater than 90 beats per minute, respiratory rate greater than 20 breaths per minute, white blood cell count (WBC) greater than 12,000 or less than 4000.[47,50]

When sepsis causes dysfunction in one organ, it is diagnosed as severe sepsis. Signs and symptoms of sepsis include fever; chills; inflammatory responses such as increased WBC and increased serum concentrations of C-reactive protein; hemodynamic symptoms of increased heart rate; increased cardiac output; low oxygen saturation rate; metabolic responses such as increased insulin requirements; tissue perfusion changes such as altered skin perfusion and decreases in urinary output; and organ dysfunction such as increases in urea and creatinine levels, decreases in platelets, and coagulation abnormalities.[50] If sepsis results in induced hypotension that does not respond to increased fluid challenges, then the diagnosis of septic shock is made. In some situations, the rapid implementation of antibiotics therapy is critical for survival. In other cases, débridement of infected tissues, such as those associated with necrotizing fasciitis, is urgently required for survival.[51]

Initial antibiotic therapies are based on the likely source of the infection and the most common pathogens. For instance, urosepsis treatment is based on the most likely source of UTIs such as *Escherichia coli* and enterococcal species. Antibiotic therapies should begin as soon as possible and always within the first hours of recognized sepsis and septic shock.[52] Blood, urine, and sputum cultures should be sent to the laboratory before antibiotics are given for proper identification of the incriminating organism. Once the organism is identified, antibiotic treatments should be reassessed to decrease the risk of antibiotic resistance.[53]

Ventilatory and volume support are also crucial for patient survival to combat hypotension and respiratory insufficiency. Hemodynamic support includes fluid replacement, crystalloids, or colloids. Vasopressor support includes dopamine and norepinephrine; inotropic therapy may include dobutamine. Steroids may be used when hypotension responds poorly to fluids and vasopressors. Other supportive measures may include blood products, glucose control, and renal replacement therapy (e.g., dialysis and continuous renal replacement therapy, deep venous thrombosis prophylaxis, and stress ulcer prophylaxis).[53]

A patient who survives sepsis can be expected to stay in an ICU for at least 7 to 14 days, most likely on ventilator support. Most patients have an additional hospital stay of 10 to 14 days after leaving the ICU. The overall hospital length of stay ranges from 3 to 5 weeks. The incidence of sepsis occurs more frequently in persons with diabetes, malignancies, chronic immunosuppressive therapy, and HIV. Higher fatality rates are seen in older adults. Sepsis affects most of the major body systems including pulmonary, circulatory, renal, metabolic, coagulation, and gastrointestinal, which originates from a bacterial source and has invaded the bloodstream.[54]

Sepsis in Older Adults

Of particular concern is the risk for sepsis in older adults (see Chapter 20). Each year in the United States, over 2,500 cases per 100,000 persons of sepsis occur in persons older than 85 years. Older adults (persons over the age of 65) are more likely to develop sepsis than younger adults, especially due to gram-negative organisms, specifically, *E. coli* and methicillin-resistant *Staphylococcus aureus* (MRSA). These incidences of sepsis in the older population are frequently associated with UTIs in over 50% of the bacteremia episodes in persons older than 89 years. Risk factors leading to sepsis in the older population include urinary catheters and pressure ulcers.[55]

Because of their increased age and variance of presenting symptoms, older adults frequently do not develop fever. Thus, initial treatment is geared toward antibiotic therapy, after urine, sputum, blood, or wound cultures have been analyzed. The initial antibiotics are geared toward a broader spectrum of suspected pathogens such as *E. coli* and MRSA. In addition to antibiotic therapy, fluid resuscitation as well as invasive monitoring for blood pressure, urinary catheters for renal output, and oxygen therapy must be considered and used as needed. Older adult patients do respond well to treatment protocols, but health-care providers need to have a high level of suspicion for sepsis in older adults so that treatment may begin in a timely manner.[55]

Cerebral Spinal Infections

Meningitis is defined as an inflammation of the meninges, the membrane that covers the brain and spinal cord. Meningitis is frequently caused by *Streptococcus pneumoniae* and *Neisseria meningitidis*. *N. meningitidis* is a gram-negative diplococcus, which is transmitted from respiratory droplets from the nose and throat of an infected person. The incubation period is generally 3 to 4 days.[56]

Signs and symptoms of meningitis include fever, stiff neck, changes in mental status, and headache. A classic petechial rash is common, which appears on the trunk and lower extremities and correlates to the thrombocytopenia.[57] If the infection is not diagnosed early and antibiotics are not initiated promptly, especially in cases caused by *N. meningitidis*, patients may develop sepsis (meningococcemia), which results in hypotension and bilateral adrenal hemorrhage. Case fatality rates may be as high as 25% and occur rapidly. Thus, IV antibiotics

must be initiated promptly.[58] Antibiotic therapy may include ceftriaxone or penicillin G (PCN); for those with cephalosporin or PCN allergies, chloramphenicol may be given.[57]

Once a diagnosis of meningitis has been determined, close contacts of patients diagnosed with *N. meningitidis*, such as household members, young children in day care, military persons who shared the same sleeping quarters, and health-care workers who were involved in resuscitation efforts (intubation and mouth-to-mouth resuscitation), should be monitored for signs and symptoms of infection. In addition, upon confirmation of *N. meningitidis,* these persons should be given prophylaxis, which includes ceftriaxone and ciprofloxacin.[56]

Skin and Soft Tissues Infections

Skin and soft tissue infections may first present as cellulitis but later may develop into an abscess, progress to necrotizing fasciitis, and then to sepsis. If sepsis occurs, the patient will require treatment in an ICU setting. Survival is dependent on early diagnosis and treatment as well as surgical intervention such as draining of the abscess or débridement of the tissues. Signs and symptoms of skin and soft tissue infections may first begin with erythema, edema with/without wound drainage. Progression to necrotizing fasciitis includes the presence of vesicular or bullous lesions, skin necrosis, and crepitus in the surrounding tissues, along with systemic symptoms of pain, fever, tachycardia, diaphoresis, and central nervous system changes. In addition, the presence of purple or red bullous lesions, pain on palpitation over unaffected areas, and loss of sensation distal to the affected area with rapid progression denote a deeper, more serious infection.[59]

Other systemic symptoms may include renal failure, hypotension and acidosis, elevated WBC counts over 15, 000, and sodium levels less than 135. Radiology exams (x-rays) may demonstrate gas in the soft tissues and computed tomography / magnetic resonance imaging may reveal abscesses. The organisms frequently associated with these skin and soft tissue infections include streptococcus, staphylococcus, and clostridium. Other organisms implicated include gram-negative strains such as pseudomonas, *Klebsiella*, and *Serratia*. Risk factors for deep and necrotizing fasciitis include patients with recent trauma, recent abdominal surgery, diabetes, alcoholism, and renal diseases.[51]

Treatment of necrotizing fasciitis includes a combination of antibiotics, surgical débridement, and hyperbaric oxygen therapies. Antibiotic therapy is generally a combination of several different classifications. Surgical débridement includes removal of infected tissues until viable tissues may be found, and is sometimes repeated daily for several days. Hyperbaric oxygen therapy is thought to be effective since it delivers oxygen to the ischemic and infected tissues, which improves the tissue viability and increases the body's ability to fight the infection.[59] Recently, the use of vacuum-assisted wound closure therapy has been shown to decrease the time for wound healing, decrease drainage, and improve patient comfort.[60]

Toxic Shock Syndrome (TSS)

Toxic shock syndrome (TSS) is characterized by sudden onset of fever, chills, vomiting, diarrhea, muscle aches, and rash. It can rapidly progress to severe and intractable hypotension and multisystem organ failure.[61] Approximately one to two cases per 100,000 women are infected each year with TSS. It was first described in the late 1970s when an increasing number of menstruating women were seen in EDs with a sudden onset of fever, gastrointestinal symptoms (such as nausea, vomiting, and diarrhea), and a macular skin rash that rapidly progresses to hypotension. The implicating organism was found to be *Staphylococcus aureus.*

Many young women required massive fluid resuscitation, vasopressure support, acute dialysis for renal failure, and ventilator supports for acute respiratory distress syndrome.[62] The initial case fatality rate was as high as 15%. By the 1980s, as many as 1,000 cases were reported to the CDC, which was eventually able to link this new syndrome epidemiologically to high-absorbency tampons. Women who used these high-absorbency tampons were found to leave them in place longer than other less absorbent tampons. Other theories suggested that women may have been colonized with *S. aureus* and using the high absorbency tampons increased the risk for the toxin to be produced and released.[61,62]

Pneumonia

One of the most frequent cases of community-acquired pneumonia (CAP) is *S. pneumoniae*. It is a gram-positive organism and frequently colonizes the nasopharynx.[63] *S. pneumoniae* is also referred to as pneumococcal pneumonia and it estimated to infect at least 100 adults per 100,000 population each year in the United States and Europe. Droplets and direct oral contact are the means of transmission. The incubation period is 1 to 3 days.[56] Predisposing factors include cigarette smoking, chronic lung disease, heart failure, diabetes, malignancy, immunosuppression, alcohol abuse, and cancer.[63] The case fatality rate may be 10% among hospitalized patients,

but may be as high as 20% to 40% among patients with alcoholism and underlying disease.[56]

Signs and symptoms include sudden onset of high fever (102°F to 103°F) accompanied by chills and rigors, diaphoresis, myalgias, headache and malaise, pleural pain, increased respirations (20 to 24 breaths per minute), tachycardia (90 to 110 beats per minute), dyspnea, and productive cough of rust-colored sputum. Older patients may have a slight fever but are more prone to have a higher respiratory rate and signs of confusion or mental status changes. Chest x-rays may show lobar consolidation and pleural effusions; however, only around 10% of patients need a thoracentesis. Most patients have a WBC greater than 12,000.[56,63]

One complication of *S. pneumoniae* includes an empyema, which may occur in about 5% of patients diagnosed with *S. pneumoniae*. It is made evident by persistence of high fever and leukocytosis after appropriate antibiotic therapy.[53] Treatment includes both IV and oral therapy. Outpatient therapy, for patients who do not require hospitalization, includes quinolones, macrolides, penicillins, and doxycycline. Intravenous therapy for hospitalized patients includes penicillin, ampicillin, or ceftriaxone; macrolides may be given to those with PCN and cephalosporin allergies.[56,63]

Prevention includes vaccination with the pneumococcal vaccine, a polysaccharide vaccine, which protects against 23 types of pneumococcal bacteria. Protection against infection develops within 2 to 3 weeks of receiving the vaccine. The CDC recommends it for all persons 65 years or older; children under the age of 2 years; persons with underlying respiratory illnesses, smokers; those with chronic illnesses (heart disease, sickle cell disease, diabetes, alcoholism, cirrhosis); persons with weakened immune systems; and those receiving long-term steroids, chemotherapy, and radiation therapy. Generally, only one dose of vaccine is required. However, in certain populations a second dose may be required in persons over the age of 65 years who received their initial dose before they were 65 years and if it has been more than 5 years from the initial dose. Other populations in whom a second dose is given include those who have a damaged or no spleen; those with sickle cell anemia; those who have HIV or AIDS, cancer, nephritic syndrome, or previous organ transplantation; or those who are receiving long-term steroids or chemotherapy.[64]

Catheter-Acquired Urinary Tract Infections

More than 30 million Foley catheters are inserted each year in the United States and contribute to over 1 million

UTIs. Catheter-associated UTIs (CA-UTIs) are the most frequent type of infections seen in hospital settings, and account for as much as 36% of all HAIs. Risk factors associated with CA-UTIs include presence of a Foley catheter for over 6 days, being female, having diabetes, malnutrition, azotemia, and ureteral stents.[65,66]

Complications of an indwelling Foley catheter include UTI, secondary bacteremias (urosepsis), sepsis, and acute pyelonephritis. Urosepsis is defined when the organism(s) cultured from the urinary tract is the same as what is cultured and identified in the blood. Urosepsis may occur more frequently in patients with preexisting renal disease, patients with urethral stents, and those with history of renal stones. Adverse outcomes include increased hospital stays, increased mortality, and ureteral strictures.[61] The organisms most frequently implicated in CA-UTIs generally originate from the gastrointestinal tract—enterococcus (Fig. 15-6) and *E. coli.*[52,65]

According to the CDC,[64] preventing CA-UTIs includes the following key components:

- Practice hand hygiene before and after catheter insertion and when manipulating the catheter site or device.
- Use aseptic technique when inserting the catheter and obtaining urine samples, and always use sterile equipment.
- Properly secure the catheter to prevent movement and urethral traction.

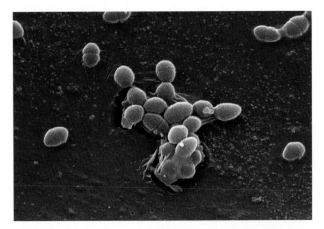

Figure 15-6 Enterococci, leading causes of nosocomial bacteremia, surgical wound infection, and urinary tract infection. *(From Centers for Disease Control and Prevention Public Health Image Library, photograph by Pete Wardell. Retrieved from http://phil.cdc.gov/phil/details.asp.)*

- Consider using portable ultrasound devices to assess the volume of urine in the bladder and to reduce unnecessary catheterization.
- Maintain a closed drainage system and unobstructed flow of urine.

Quality improvement programs have been implemented to promote proper usage of urinary catheters and to reduce the risk of CA-UTIs. Key initiatives include appropriate use of catheters, removing catheters when no longer needed, monitoring adherence to hand hygiene practices and proper care of catheters, developing alert systems or reminders among patients with catheters for early removal, and developing protocols for placement of catheters, for the use of ultrasound devices and for assessing the need for catheters.[64]

Catheter-Related Bloodstream Infections

According to the Association for Professionals in Infection Control and Epidemiology,[65] over 90,000 catheter-associated bloodstream infections (CA-BSIs) occur annually in the United States with associated costs of over $2.3 billion in the United States each year. Over 15 million central line catheters are inserted each year in the United States, and most infections are related to the type of lines that are inserted to provide fluids, medications, and parenteral nutrition; monitor cardiac outputs; and provide temporary hemodialysis to critically ill patients.[67] The associated mortality rate is 12% to 25% among critically ill patients and the associated cost per infection is estimated between $34,508 and $56,000.[65,68] Risk factors for developing CA-BSIs include underlying diseases, neutopenia, prolonged hospitalization, presence of a central line catheter, systemic antibiotics, active infection at another site, mechanical ventilation, and ICU stay.[69]

Signs and symptoms of CR-BSIs include fever, chills, hypotension, increased respirations, and confusion; also, there may be inflammation and purulent drainage at the insertion site.[69] The organisms frequently implicated in CR-BSIs are coagulase-negative staphylococci, *S. aureus, Candida, Enterococcus,* and emerging gram-negative organisms such as *Enterobacter* and *Klebsiella* strains. The pathogenesis of CR-BSIs frequently involves migration of skin organisms at the insertion site into the catheter tract or contamination of the catheter hub; catheters might become hematogenously seeded from another focus of infection (e.g., urinary tract or osteomyelitis).[68] Treatment of a CR-BSI generally depends on the severity of the patient's clinical disease, risk factors for the infection, and the bacteria associated with the infection. Complications may include septic thrombosis and infective endocarditis, which require long-term antibiotic treatment.[67]

■ EVIDENCE-BASED PRACTICE
Prevention of CR-BSI

Practice Statement: Patients in acute care settings are at risk of developing CR-BSIs because of the need for invasive monitoring in critical care medicine. A patient safety goal for ICU patients is to reduce the risks of CR-BSI through the adoption of best practices including: hand hygiene, maximal sterile barriers, full body drapes, and chlorhexidine-based products for insertion site antisepsis.

Targeted Outcome: Reduction in CR-BSI

Evidence to Support: The CDC[69] has always supported the use of maximum sterile barriers and covering the patient with a full sheet during insertion of central lines as a means to reduce CR-BSIs. Pronovost et al.[70] determined the use of these EBPs to reduce CR-BSIs were effective in reducing this type of infection by over 60% in a collaborative cohort study in Michigan among 108 participating hospitals. Render et al.[43] found similar results in their study in which 10 greater Cincinnati hospitals participated in a collaborative project to reduce CR-BSIs and saw a 50% reduction in CR-BSIs when adherence to best practices was at least 95%.

Recommended Approaches and Resources: Insert central line catheters into the subclavian site when possible. Femoral sites have been associated with higher rates of infection.

- Perform hand hygiene before insertion of catheters as well as when manipulating or accessing central line catheters.
- Apply maximum sterile barriers (gowns, masks, head cover and sterile gloves) prior to the insertion of central line catheters.
- Cover the patient with a full body drape.
- Prepare the insertion site using chlorhexidine-based products.
- Cover the insertion site with a sterile occlusive dressing.
- Use aseptic technique when accessing or changing central line dressing.
- Remove catheters when no longer needed.

Sources: See references 68 and 69.

Healthcare-Associated Infections and Multiple Drug-Resistant Organisms

Multiple drug-resistant organisms (MDROs) pose a public health issue for hospitals. An MDRO is defined by the CDC as "microorganisms, predominantly bacteria, that are resistant to one or more classes of antimicrobial agents."[71] One example is the carbapenem-resistant Enterobacteriaceae family of infectious agents. This family of pathogens presents a challenge to health-care workers in acute care settings because these infections are resistant to most front-line antibiotics. Some Enterobacteriaceae are normally present in the human gut and can become carbaepem-resistant through enzymes that break down these antibiotics so that they are no longer effective.[72] Other MDROs include MRSA, *Clostridium difficile,* and vancomycin-resistant enterococci.

The most common mechanism for acquiring a MDRO in a hospital is patient-to-patient via the hands of a health-care worker. Prevention efforts include a wide range of interventions that are conducted at the organizational and individual levels. They require the application of public health principles and an understanding of how communicable diseases are transmitted. The CDC lists the following as components of an MDRO prevention program: education, judicious use of antimicrobials, MDRO surveillance, infection control precautions, and environmental controls aimed at reducing transmission.[71]

■ Summary Points

- A public health perspective applies to the acute care setting.
- Focused assessments related to acute care population–level data provide the necessary information for setting priorities.
- The improvement of health-care delivery and patient outcomes in an acute care setting has occurred because of population-level interventions.
- Differences exist between males and females in relation to health care received in the acute care setting.
- The evolution of critical care has occurred at the population level.
- Health planning occurs in acute care settings using the same process used in community settings.
- Performance improvement within an acute care setting uses public health science and health planning principles throughout the process.
- The prevention of HAIs is a major public health issue and the responsibility of every nurse.

▲ CASE STUDY
Health Planning to Prevent Falls

Learning Outcomes

At the end of this case study, the student will be able to:

- Apply the techniques for a focused assessment.
- Identify risk factors associated with an identified patient safety issue.
- Apply program planning to the development, implementation, and evaluation of a hospital fall prevention program.

The recent safety reports for the medical units in a hospital caught the attention of the nursing department because there had been an increase in falls. The chief nursing officer asked the nurse managers of the medical units to determine what was behind the increased fall incidence rate. After examining the hospital incident report data, they found that three medical units had an increased fall rate and two did not. The nurse mangers formed a committee of nurses across the five units to examine the issues related to falls and develop a fall prevention program.

To complete this case study, answer the following questions:

1. What further information do the nurse managers need for the assessment phase of their investigation (see Chapter 4)?
2. What are the risk factors are associated with falls in an acute care setting from a national perspective?
3. How would you construct a hypothetical case control study for three of the major risk factors (see Chapter 3)?
   a. What sources of data would you use?
   b. Would this require IRB approval?
4. What evidence-based interventions are relevant to fall prevention in an acute care setting?
5. What recommendations would you make for implementing an intervention?
6. What outcome measures would be relevant to evaluating the effectiveness of the intervention?

REFERENCES

1. Bureau of Labor Statistics. (2011). *Occupational outlook handbook 2010–2011 edition: Registered nurses.* Retrieved from http://www.bls.gov/oco/ocos083.htm.
2. Acute care. (2015). *The free dictionary.* Retrieved from http://medical-dictionary.thefreedictionary.com/acute+care.
3. American Association of Colleges of Nursing. (2006). *The essentials of doctorate education for advanced nursing practice.* Washington, DC: Author.
4. U.S. Department of Health and Human Services, Agency for Health Research and Quality. (2011). *Healthcare Cost and Utilization Project (HCUP).* Retrieved from http://hcupnet.ahrq.gov/.
5. Centers for Disease Control and Prevention. (2015). *Leading causes of death.* Retrieved from http://www.cdc.gov/nchs/fastats/leading-causes-of-death.htm.
6. Hall, M.J, DeFrances, C.J., Williams, S.N., Golosinskiy, A., & Schwartzman, A. (2010). National Hospital Discharge Survey: 2007 Summary. *National Health Statistics Reports, 29,* 1-24. Retrieved from http://www.cdc.gov/nchs/data/nhsr/nhsr029.pdf.
7. Agency for Healthcare Research and Quality. (n.d.). *Welcome to HCUP-net.* Retrieved from http://hcupnet.ahrq.gov/HCUPnet.jsp.
8. U.S. Department of Health and Human Services. (2015). *Understanding the Health Care Reform Act.* Retrieved from http://www.healthcare.gov/law/introduction/index.html.
9. American Association of Critical Care Nurses. (n.d.). *About critical care nursing.* Retrieved from http://www.aacn.org/wd/pressroom/content/aboutcritical-carenursing.pcms?pid=1&&menu=.
10. U.S. Department of Health and Human Services. (2008). *The registered nurse population: Findings from the 2008 National Sample Survey of Registered Nurses.* Retrieved from http://bhpr.hrsa.gov/healthworkforce/rnsurvey/2008/.
11. Nightingale, F. (1863). *Notes on hospitals* (3rd ed.). London, England: Longmans, Green.
12. Hall, J.R. (1990). Critical-care medicine and the acute care laboratory. *Clinical Chemistry, 36*(8B), 1552-1556.
13. Hanson, C.W., III, Durbin C.G., Jr., Maccioli, G.A., Maccioli, G.A., Deutschman, C.S., et al. (2001). The anesthesiologist in critical care medicine: Past, present, and future. *Anesthesiology, 95*(3), 781-788.
14. Society of Critical Care Medicine. (n.d.). *History of critical care.* Retrieved from http://www.sccm.org/SCCM/History+of+Critical+Care/.
15. Okie, S. (2005). Retrospective TBI in the war zone. *New England Journal of Medicine, 352,* 2043-2047.
16. Warden, D. (2006). Military TBI during the Iraq and Afghanistan wars. *Journal of Head Trauma Rehabilitation, 21*(5), 398-410.
17. eHistory archive. (2011). *Statistics on the Civil War and medicine.* Retrieved from http://ehistory.osu.edu/uscw/features/medicine/cwsurgeon/statistics.cfm.
18. Preston, S.H., & Buzzell, E. (2006). *Mortality of American troops in Iraq.* Retrieved from http://repository.upenn.edu/cgi/viewcontent.cgi?article=1000&context=psc_working_papers.
19. Centers for Disease Control and Prevention. (2014). *Polio disease—questions and answers.* Retrieved from http://www.cdc.gov/vaccines/vpd-vac/polio/dis-faqs.htm.
20. Berthelsen, P., & Cronqvist, M. (2003). The first intensive care unit in the world: Copenhagen 1953. *Acta anaesthesiology Scandinavia, 47*(10), 1190-1195.

21. Milka, M. (2003). Father of CPR, innovator, teacher, humanist. *Journal of the American Medical Association, 289*(19), 2485-2486.

22. American Health Association. (2010). *2010 AHA guidelines for CPR and ECC.* Retrieved from http://static.heart.org/eccguidelines/reprint-2010-aha-guidelines-for-cpr.html.

23. American Health Association. (2011). *Cardiopulmonary resuscitation statistics.* Retrieved from http://www.americanheart.org/presenter.jhtml?identifier=4483.

24. Travers, A., Rea, T., Bowbrow, B., Edelson, D.P., Berg, R.A., Swor, R.A., et al. (2010). Part 4: CPR Overview: 2010 American Heart Association guidelines for cardiopulmonary resuscitation and emergency cardiovascular care. *Circulation, 122,* S676-S684.

25. The Framingham Heart Study. (2015). *History of the Framingham Heart Study.* Retrieved from http://www.framinghamheartstudy.org/about/history.html.

26. The Nurses' Health Study. (2015). Retrieved from http://www.channing.harvard.edu/nhs/.

27. American Heart Association. (n.d.). *Heart disease and stroke statistics: 2010 update-at-a-glance.* Retrieved from http://www.americanheart.org/downloadable/heart/1265665152970DS-3241%20HeartStroke Update_2010.pdf.

28. Ford, E., Ajani, U., Croft, J., Critchley, J., Labarthe, D., et al. (2007). Explaining the decrease in U.S. deaths from coronary disease, 1980–2000. *New England Journal of Medicine, 356,* 2388-2398.

29. The Framingham Heart Study. (2015). *Milestones.* Retrieved from http://www.framinghamheartstudy.org/about/milestones.htm.

30. American Heart Association. (n.d.). *Woman and heart disease.* Retrieved from http://www.americanheart.org/presenter.jhtml?identifier=2859.

31. Rosenfeld, A., Lindauer, A., & Darney, B. (2005). Understanding treatment-seeking delay in women with acute myocardial infarction: Descriptions of decision making patterns. *American Journal of Critical Care, 14*(4), 285-293.

32. Mosca, L., Benjamin, E.J., Berra, K., Benzanson, J.L., Doal, R.J., et al. (2011). Effectiveness-based guidelines for the prevention of cardiovascular disease in women 2011 update: A guideline From the American Heart Association. *Circulation, 123,* 1243-1262. . doi:10.1161/CIR.0b013e31820faaf8.

33. American College of Cardiology and American Heart Association. (2004). Guidelines for the management of patients with ST-Elevation Myocardial Infarction. *Journal of the American College of Cardiology, 44,* 671-719.

34. U.S. Department of Health and Human Services. (n.d.). *Health information privacy: Public health.* Retrieved from http://www.hhs.gov/ocr/privacy/hipaa/understanding/special/publichealth/index.html.

35. United States Department of Health and Human Services. (2015). *Healthy People 2020 topics: Heart disease and stroke.* Retrieved from http://www.healthypeople.gov/2020/topicsobjectives2020/objectiveslist.aspx?topicid=21.

36. Margolis, P., Provost, L.P., Schoettker, P.J., & Britto, M.T. (2009). Quality improvement, clinical research, and quality improvement research: Opportunities for integration. *Pediatric Clinics of North America, 56,* 831-841.

37. American Nurses Association. (2007). *Public health nursing: Scope and standards of practice.* Silver Spring, MD: Nursesbook.org.

38. U.S. Department of Health and Human Services Health Resources and Services Administration. (2011). *Managing data for performance improvement.* Retrieved from http://www.hrsa.gov/quality/toolbox/508pdfs/managingdataperformanceimprovement.pdf.

39. Lo, B., & Groman, M. (2003). Oversight of quality improvement. *Archives Internal Medicine, 163,* 1481-1486.

40. Kohn, L.T., Corrigan, J.M., & Donaldson, M.S. (2000). *To err is human: Building a safer health care system.* Washington, DC: Institute of Medicine, National Academies Press. Retrieved from http://www/nap/edu/openbook.php?record_id+9728&page-1.

41. Institute for Healthcare Improvement. (2005). *Testing change.* Retrieved from http://www.ihi.org/IHI/Topics/Improvement/ImprovementMethods/HowToImprove/testingchanges.htm.

42. Berwick, D.M., Calkins, D.R., Cannon, C.J., & Hackbarth, A.D. (2006). The 100,000 lives campaign: Setting a goal and a deadline for improving health care quality. *JAMA, 295*(3), 324-327.

43. Render, M., Brungs, S., Kotagal, U., Nicholson, M., Burns, P., Ellis, D., et al. (2006). Evidence-based practices to reduce central line infections. *Joint Commission Journal on Quality and Patient Safety, 32*(5), 253-260.

44. Langley, G.J., Moen, R., Nolan, K.M., Nolan, T.W., Norman, C.L., & Provost, L.P. (2010). *The improvement guide: A practical approach to enhancing organizational performance* (2nd ed.). San Francisco, CA: Jossey-Bass.

45. Centers for Disease Control and Prevention. (2011). Guidelines for the prevention of intravascular catheter related infections. Retrieved from http://www.cdc.gov/hicpac/pdf/guidelines/bsi-guidelines-2011.pdf.

46. McKibben, L., Horan, T., Tolkars, J.I., Folwer, G., Cardo, D.M., Pearson, M.L., Brennan, P.J., & Healthcare Infection Control Practices Advisory Council. (2005). Guidance on public health reporting of healthcare associated infections: Recommendations of the Healthcare Infection Control Practices Advisory Committee. *American Journal of Infection Control, 33*(4), 217-226.

47. Melamed, A., & Sorvillo, F.J. (2008). The burden of sepsis-associated mortality in the United States from 1999–2005: An analysis of multiple-cause-of-death data. *Critical Care, 13*(1), 1-8.

48. Angus, D.C., Linde-Zwirble, W.T., Lidicker, J., Clermont, G., Carcillo, J., & Oinsky, M.R. (2001). Epidemiology of severe sepsis in the United States: Analysis of incidence, outcome and associated costs of care. *Critical Care Medicine, 29*(7), 1303-1310.

49. Nduka, O.O., & Parrillo, J.E. (2009). The pathophysiology of septic shock. *Critical Care Clinics, 25,* 677-702.

50. Dombrovskiy, V.Y., Martin, A.A., Sunderram, J., & Paz, H.L. (2005). Facing the challenge: Decreasing case fatality rates in severe sepsis despite increasing hospitalizations. *Critical Care Medicine, 33*(11), 2555-2562.

51. Dawson, D. (2002). Sepsis recognition—a greater role for nursing? *Intensive and Critical Care Nursing, 18,* 135-137.

52. Nicolasora, N., & Kaul, D.R. (2008). Infectious diseases emergencies. *The Medical Clinics of North America, 92,* 427-441.

53. Cunha, B.A. (2008). Sepsis and septic shock: Selection of empiric antimicrobial therapy. *Critical Care Clinics, 24,* 313-334.

54. Dellinger, R.P., Levy, M.M., Carlet, J.M., Bion, J., Parker, M.M., Jaeschke, R., et al. (2008). Surviving sepsis campaign: International guidelines for management of severe sepsis and septic shock: 2008. *Critical Care Medicine, 36*(1), 296-327.

55. Martin, J.B., & Wheeler, A.P. (2009). Approach to the patient with sepsis. *Clinical Chest Medicine, 30,* 1-16.

56. Girard, T.D., & Ely, E.W. (2007). Bacteremia and sepsis in older adults. *Clinics in Geriatric Medicine, 23,* 677-702.

57. Heymann, D.L. (2004). *Control of communicable diseases manual* (18th ed.). Washington, DC: American Public Health Association.

58. Apicella, M.A. (2004). Neisseria meningitidis. In G.L. Mandell, J.E. Bennett, & R. Dolin (Eds.), *Principles and practices of infectious diseases* (pp 2498-2510). Philadelphia, PA: Elsevier, Churchill, Livingston.

59. Hans, D., Kelly, E., Wilhelmson, K., & Katz, E.D. (2008). Rapidly fatal infections. *Emerging Clinics of North America, 26,* 259-279.

60. Napolitano, L.M. (2009). Severe soft tissue infections. *Infectious Disease Clinics of North America, 23,* 571-591.

61. Younggren, B.N., & Denny, M., (2007). Emergency management of difficult wounds: Part II. *Emergency Medicine Clinics of North America, 25,* 123-134.

62. Centers for Disease Control and Prevention. (2005). *Toxic shock syndrome.* Retrieved from http://www.cdc.gov/ncidod/dbmd/diseaseinfo/toxicshock_t.htm.

63. Light, R.B. (2009). Plaques in the ICU: A brief history of community-acquired epidemic and endemic transmissible infections leading to intensive care admission. *Critical Care Clinics, 25,* 67-81.

64. Musher, D.M. (2004). Streptococcus pneumonia. In G.L. Mandell, J.E. Bennett, & R. Dolin (Eds.), *Principles and practices of infectious diseases* (pp 2392-2407). Philadelphia, PA: Elsevier, Churchill, Livingston.

65. Centers for Disease Control and Prevention. (2015). *Pneumococcal polysaccharide vaccine—Vaccine information sheet.* Retrieved from http://www.cdc.gov/vaccines/hcp/vis/vis-statements/ppv.html.

66. Association for Professionals in Infection Control and Epidemiology. (2009). *Guide to the elimination of catheter related bloodstream infections.* Washington, DC: Author.

67. Lo, E., Nicolle, L., Classen, D., Arias, K.M., Podgorny, K., Anderson, D.J., et al. (2008). Strategies to prevent catheter-associated urinary tract infections in acute care hospital. *Infection Control and Hospital Epidemiology, 29*(1), S41-S50.

68. Mermel, L.A., Farn, B.M., Sheretz, R.J., Reed, I.I., O'Grady, N.O., Harris, J.S., & Craven, D.E. (2001). Guideline for the management of intravascular catheter-related infections. *Clinical Infectious Diseases, 32,* 1249-1272.

69. O'Grady, N.P., Alexander, M., Burns, M.T., Dellinger, E. P., Garland, J., et al. Healthcare Infection Control Practices Advisory Committee (HICPAC). (2011). *Guidelines for the prevention of intravascular catheter related infections. Centers for Disease Control and Prevention.* Retrieved from http://www.cdc.gov/hicpac/pdf/guidelines/bsi-guidelines-2011.pdf.

70. Pronovost, P., Needham, D., Berenholtz, S., Sinopoli, D., Chu, H.C., Cosgrove, S., et al. (2006). An intervention to decrease catheter related bloodstream infections in the ICU. *The New England Journal of Medicine, 355*(26), 2725-2732.

71. Centers for Disease Control and Prevention. (2006). *Management of multiple drug resistant organisms in health care settings.* Retrieved from http://www.cdc.gov/hicpac/mdro/mdro_2.html.

72. Centers for Disease Control and Prevention. (2015). *Health care associated infections, Carbapenem-resistant Enterobacteriaceae (CRE).* Retrieved from http://www.cdc.gov/hai/organisms/cre/ http://www.cdc.gov/hai/organisms/cre/.

Chapter 16

Health Planning for Primary Care Settings

LEARNING OUTCOMES

After reading this chapter, the student will be able to:

1. Describe the evolution of primary care at the national and global levels.
2. Apply the principles of epidemiology to the primary care setting.
3. Discuss the integration of primary, secondary, and tertiary care interventions in the primary care setting.
4. Describe chronic disease management and case management.
5. Discuss current policy issues related to the delivery of primary care.
6. Describe the patient centered medical home (PCMH) component of the Affordable Care Act.

KEY TERMS

Case management

Food desert

Health promotion

Health protection/risk reduction

Patient centered medical home (PCMH)

Primary care

Primary health care

Vaccine

Introduction

"Primary health care now more than ever" was declared by the World Health Organization (WHO) in a 2008 article.[1] Still, barriers remain. The issue at the forefront in the United States is the diminishing primary care workforce. A 2009, *USA Today* headline read, "Shortage of primary care threatens health system."[2] In 2010 the American Medical Association asked the question, "Are primary care physicians an endangered species?"[3] In response to the looming shortage, more states have sought to expand the role of nurse practitioners (NPs) as a way of increasing access to primary care. This effort has placed nursing in the center of the struggle to address the increasing demand for primary care services in the United States. What is behind the focus on primary care and what does primary care have to do with public health?

Populations that have access to health care, especially preventive care on a primary and secondary level, are healthier.[1] Primary health care includes preventive care such as vaccines and immunizations, health education, health promotion, and monitoring of health status. **Primary care** provides to individuals and families vital secondary prevention such as screening and early treatment. These efforts can decrease the overall burden of disease experienced by a population through the prevention of disease and reduction of mortality and morbidity. Primary care is central to the health of the public, and primary health-care providers who apply public health science to their practice become active participants in the promotion of health in the populations they serve. Primary care is delivered across a continuum from the individual to the community as a whole (Fig. 16-1).

Evolution of Primary Care

According to the WHO, globalization is putting the social cohesion of countries under stress and health-care systems are not performing at the level needed to adequately address the health-care needs of their citizens. The WHO argues that primary health care can make a difference in the capability of health-care systems to

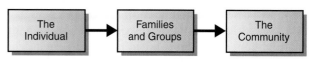

Figure 16-1 The continuum of primary care.

respond better and faster to the need for services (Chapter 13).[1] Despite overall improvement worldwide in health and life expectancy, these improvements are not consistent across countries or populations. In addition, trends in the delivery of health-care services are problematic, especially the following:

- The focus by health-care systems is on curative care.
- The approach to disease control is short term and fragments service delivery.
- A laissez-fare approach to health systems has allowed unregulated commercialization of health care.[1]

United States

Primary care, as we think of it today in the United States, has evolved out of population demand and political changes across time. The definition of primary care is dependent on the services provided to the patient and the provider of that service, and for the most part focuses on the method for delivery of primary health-care services to individuals and families. In the past, the local general practitioner cared for a patient from birth to death. After World War II, that method of care delivery dwindled and specialty care grew. It was not until the late 1960s and early 1970s, because of population demand, that family practice became a new specialty with a launch of family practice medical education programs in 1969.[4] According to the American Academy of Family Physicians (AAFP), to define primary care one must describe the nature of services provided and identify the provider of these services.[5]

The core of primary care is the patient. For primary care to be effective, patients must be partners in their care. Primary care is often referred to as the gatekeeper, the control center for access to care. It is the entryway to the maze known as the health-care system. Though this is true, we should also see the opportunity that primary care brings to fully meet the needs of the patient. The services delivered encompass health promotion, disease prevention, health maintenance, counseling, patient education, diagnosis, and treatment of acute and chronic illness.[5] In addition to providing health care to patients, the primary care provider also acts as a patient advocate. The primary care environment promotes patient-centered care that is cost effective and focused on both accomplishing the goals of individual patients and reducing morbidity and mortality in the population served through prevention, early detection of disease, and engagement in treatment. The importance of increasing access to care is part of the *Healthy People 2020 (HP 2020)* objectives.[6]

Global

In 1978, the international conference held in Alma-Ata resulted in a declaration that urged action from all governments, health-care workers, and the global community to protect and promote the health of all peoples. As noted in Chapter 13, they defined primary health care as follows:

> Primary health care is essential health care based on practical, scientifically sound and socially acceptable methods and technology made universally accessible to individuals and families in the community through their full participation and at a cost that the community and country can afford to maintain at every stage of their development in the spirit of self-reliance and self-determination. It forms an integral part both of the country's health system, of which it is the central function and main focus, and of the overall social and economic development of the community. It is the first level of contact of individuals, the family and community with the national health system bringing health care as close as possible to where people live and work, and constitutes the first element of a continuing health care process.[1]

The goal set at the end of the conference was to achieve an acceptable level of health care for all people of the world by 2000. Although this has not been achieved, a 2008 report by the WHO showed some progress in the building of primary health-care infrastructure; however, it also pointed to the existence of barriers. The WHO makes the argument that the core values of primary health care are equity, solidarity, and the active participation of people in the decisions that affect their health. These values then drive reforms that reflect concrete expectations of citizens within developing and developed societies (Fig. 16-2).[1]

Thus, from a global perspective, the term **primary health care** has a broader meaning. As envisioned at the International Conference on Primary Health Care in

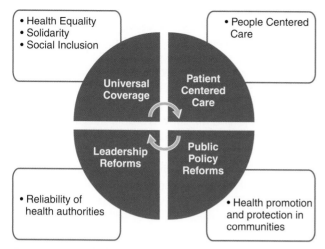

Figure 16-2 Social values that drive primary health care and the corresponding set of reforms. *(Adapted from the World Health Organization.)*

Alma-Ata, USSR, in 1978, primary health care was defined using a population perspective (Chapter 13). In contrast in the United States, the term primary health care is used to describe the level of delivery of care to individuals and families rather than to populations. The difference in the definition of primary care from the global perspective is evident in the central values of the Alma-Ata Declaration that are related to the achievement of health for all. The declaration began a movement that tackled political, social, and economic inequalities in health care. The agenda for the 2008 WHO report was to renew the effort to reform health-care systems across the globe to achieve that equality.[1]

Where the two perspectives of primary care come together is the central commitment to people-centered health care built on the development of a personal relationship between the health-care providers and the seekers of care. Both function under the belief that people are partners in the management of their health. Primary health care as stated by the WHO takes it one step further with the idea that primary care is responsible for the health of the community as a whole across the life span, and that primary care must tackle the determinants of ill health.[1]

This approach has brought criticisms. Some thought the Alma-Ata Declaration primarily supported the creation of one health-care delivery system that had the potential of providing inadequate health care to the poor.[1] In reality, the declaration addressed much larger issues than just providing care to one group. Since 1978, large gaps have been exposed in the ability of current health systems to address the changing health needs of

populations. Many systems are facing increased demands and changing expectations of what the health-care system should deliver. In addition, the issues raised by emerging chronic and communicable diseases are bringing to the forefront the evidence that primary health care not only meets the needs of individuals but also can improve the health of entire communities.

A good example is the country of Sri Lanka. This lower-middle-income country took on the issue of maternal-child health using a primary health-care system approach with excellent success.[7] In 1960, the maternal mortality rate (MMR) in Sri Lanka was almost nine times greater than in the United States for that same year (340 per 100,000 births compared with 37.6). By 2005, the MMR in Sri Lanka fell to 43 per 100,000 live births compared with 11 in the United States There were similar significant drops in the infant mortality rate and the under-5 mortality rate.

What do these changes in the overall health of the population have to do with primary health care? The government of Sri Lanka made a commitment to take action so that health and social services could reach the poor. They expanded their services and targeted the universal provision of health care. They then targeted women and children. Thus, the health issues facing the population as a whole and the social determinants of adverse health outcomes were targeted. In this case, the issues were antenatal care and skilled attendance at births. To this, they added measures to improve the education, employment, and social engagement of women. Thus, the delivery of primary health care to women during pregnancy and birth were provided within the larger context of improving the overall economic and social status of women. Despite these advances, countries such as Sri Lanka continue to face challenges. The ability to achieve optimal health care for all members of the country is impeded by shortages of health-care workers and the high rate of malnutrition owing to food scarcity. To be successful at the population level, a primary health-care system must take into account the social, economic, and political context in which it functions.

Epidemiology and Targeted Prevention Levels in Primary Care

Primary care encompasses all levels of prevention, primary, secondary, and tertiary. Interventions vary based on the level of prevention, gender, and age. Helping our country achieve optimal health requires a comprehensive understanding of the community. Health promotion and protection should be provided to all members of the community despite their disease status. Primary care nurses who apply public health science including assessment and health planning skills will not only have a better chance of providing optimal care to individuals and families, but also are more apt to contribute to the building of a healthier community. Public health nurses (PHNs) who work in primary care settings develop health programs that help to prevent disease and manage noncommunicable disease (NCD). Examples of the programs implemented for populations include case management, health education programs, and community outreach.

A major challenge in the United States and globally is access to primary care services. The Patient Protection and Affordable Care Act (ACA) of 2010 (see Chapter 1) is built on the assumption that increasing access to care will improve the health of the U.S. population. In particular, monies were made available to create and support nurse-managed clinics that would focus on promoting and maintaining optimal health. The primary care setting is central to the reform bill and the interventions provided by nurses working in primary care are built on the application of public health science. This requires that nurses working in primary care settings have knowledge not only of the health of individuals seeking care, but also an understanding of the context in which they live. Thus, nurses working in a primary care setting who are caring for individuals, families, and/or communities and populations must have current information on the prevalence of diseases within the community they serve, information on the current recommendations for primary and secondary prevention relevant to their community, and the ability to engage community partners in development of sustainable and effective interventions.

▶ SOLVING THE MYSTERY
The Case of the Sleeping Mom
Public Health Science Topics Covered:

• Assessment
• Advocacy

Nurses who know the community their clients live and work in have a great advantage in primary care. Sometimes they are able to intervene at a level that goes beyond assessment, diagnosis, and treatment. Consider Terry, a nurse working at a primary care clinic located in one of the poorer neighborhoods in New York City. Brenda, a single African American mother, came in with her 4-month-old baby for a routine well-baby checkup. The mother was seen initially by the primary

care physician working in the clinic. He came out of the examining room and asked Terry to put together a social services referral. The physician told Terry, "This mother has real problems. When I was examining the baby, the mother fell asleep in the chair and I had to keep waking her up to answer questions. She obviously is not capable of caring for this child if she can't stay awake in the middle of the day!" Terry told the physician that she would go in and talk with the mother.

When Terry went into the room, she found the baby safely nestled in the car seat and Brenda asleep in the chair. Terry gently woke up Brenda up and identified herself. She asked Brenda to tell her about her baby. Brenda glowed and said that the baby was wonderful. Terry then told her that she noticed Brenda was asleep when she came in. Was there a reason for this? Brenda hesitated and said that it was nothing. Terry probed gently and Brenda explained that she has been staying up at night because the apartment in which she is living is infested with rats. If she doesn't stay awake, the rats will get into the baby's crib and hurt him. She was pleased that she has been able to keep her baby safe, but worried that she was so tired that she may fall asleep during the night.

Terry asked her whether she had issued a complaint. Brenda said she had complained to the landlord but nothing had happened. Terry assured her that there are steps that can be taken to address the issue and then began the process, not for a social service visit, but to work with the public health department and the housing authority to implement the process for getting the rodents eliminated from the building. In addition, Terry looked through the charts to find other families attending the clinic who lived in the same building and called each one to determine whether the rat problem was being experienced throughout the building. Many of the clients complained of a similar problem and Terry helped the tenants to begin to work together to address the issue as well. Within a short period of time, an effective program was put in place that included action from the public health department, the housing authority, and the newly formed tenants group. The end result was landlord compliance with rodent eradication and elimination of rats from the building. Brenda was at last able to sleep at night.

Terry built on the knowledge she had obtained in her community health course. When she accepted the job, she took the time to learn about the community that the clinic was located in, including identifying key contacts in the public health department. This knowledge had helped her in the past to address prob-lems with immunization of children, distribution of the swine flu vaccine, and now a problem with rodent in-festation. Over time, she not only knew the patients who came to the clinic, but also had a growing under-standing of the environment in which they lived. This knowledge meant that she immediately understood the possibility that there was an alternative explanation for the sleeping mom. Her knowledge of key stakeholders helped her determine who had the power to take ac-tion. In addition, her understanding of how a commu-nity works helped her to include the residents of the building in the problem-solving process.

An important component to all levels of prevention is the education of patients about what they can do to min-imize their own risk factors for disease (see Chapter 2). Understanding the relationship of diet, exercise, and maintaining a healthy weight can be key to disease pre-vention or minimizing complications of disease. The di-abetic who controls his blood sugar will minimize the micro- and macrovascular complications. The smoker will reduce the risk of cardiovascular disease and chronic obstructive pulmonary disease if he enters a smoking ces-sation program. Other important items a nurse can ad-dress with a patient during a primary care visit include use of sunscreen, dental hygiene, and alcohol intake. When these risks occur across a group of patients, the nurse can develop population-level interventions such as education packets or working with the health department to implement the use of public safety announcements specific to their community.

Primary Prevention Within the Primary Care Setting

The first and desired level of intervention is primary pre-vention to keep a person free of disease (see Chapter 2). For individuals free of disease who seek primary care, the major focus for the nurse is to conduct a routine checkup, provide health education (see Chapter 2), support positive health practices, and provide infor-mation and support related to changing unhealthy be-haviors. The challenge for the nurse working in a primary care setting is how to engage in primary pre-vention at the aggregate level as well as the individual and family levels. This requires knowledge of the com-munity, the resources available, leaders within the community, and the other stakeholders in the com-munity who can support efforts to promote and pro-tect the health of the community. Thus, it is important

to know how to conduct a community assessment and make a plan (see Chapters 4 and 5).

Let's consider the example of the nurses working in a primary care setting in Ashland, Kentucky, where a key behavioral issue is the high rate of tobacco use. Accord-ing to the Centers for Disease Control and Prevention (CDC), the highest regional prevalence of smoking is in the Huntington-Ashland, region where more than a third (34.4%) of the population smokes.[8] Furthermore, between 2000 and 2004, Kentucky had the highest rate of tobacco-attributable deaths—370.6 per 100,000 com-pared with 248.5 for the United States.[9] A comprehensive smoking cessation program at the clinic should include not only efforts to help individuals quit, but also primary prevention programs at the community level. If nurses seek further information at the community level, they will identify the resources available to the community. They will also be able to identify cultural issues related to tobacco use that may influence the success of a smoking prevention campaign. Knowledge of the community will also help them engage other potential partners in the community for doing an anti-smoking campaign among the youth of the community.

Primary prevention is the first step in reducing the number of adults who smoke over the next decade. In the example of tobacco use in a Kentucky community, the primary care nurse could collaborate with the school system to develop a culturally grounded antismoking campaign, in the hope that over time they would see fewer patients in their clinic suffering from smoking-related adverse health consequences. Such a campaign could encompass the development of policies that not only reduce youth access to tobacco products, but also reduce exposure to secondary smoke.

To be effective, primary prevention in a primary care setting requires both individual- and community-level interventions. It includes both health promotion and health protection activities. As defined in Chapter 1, **health promotion** at the individual and family levels helps people change their lifestyle to achieve optimal health.[10] As stated in Chapter 2, **health protection/risk reduction** includes primary prevention interventions that protect the individual from disease by reducing risk. Thus, health promotion usually focuses on behavioral change with health education a main tool, whereas health protection involves a clinical intervention such as immu-nization (Table 16-1).

Health Promotion

The majority of health promotion in primary health-care settings is delivered at the individual and family levels.

TABLE 16–1	Levels of Prevention in Primary Care and Recommended Interventions

Primary Prevention—Adult (to prevent illness from occurring)

Primary Prevention Focus	Examples
Health protection: Immunizations	• Flu shot • Pneumococcal vaccination • Tetanus booster (every 10 years) • Human papillomavirus (females aged 9–26) • Chicken pox (VZV) for those born after 1980
Health promotion: Education	• Healthy diet • Exercise • Weight loss • Smoking cessation • Low-risk alcohol use

Secondary Prevention—Adult (to identify disease in a patient with asymptomatic illness)

Men	Age Range	Testing
	19–39	• Blood pressure (BP), body mass index (BMI), health risks • HIV discussion • Depression screening • Diabetes screening • Lipids for men at age 35
	40–49	• BP, BMI, health risks • HIV discussion • Depression screening • Diabetes screening • Lipids every 5 years
	50–70	• BP, BMI, health risks • HIV discussion • Depression screening • Diabetes screening • Colorectal screening (at age 50)
	70 and older	• BP, BMI, health risks • Depression screening • Diabetes screening • Colorectal screening until 75

Women	Age Range	Testing
	19–39	• BP, BMI, health risks • HIV discussion • Depression screening • Diabetes screening • Chlamydia/gonorrhea (sexually active women through age 24 and then as needed) • Cervical cancer (first should be done at age 21 or 3 years after first sexual contact, then every 3 years)
	40–49	• BP, BMI, health risks • HIV discussion • Depression screening • Diabetes screening • Cervical cancer (every 3 years) • Mammography (optional as a baseline every 2 years)

TABLE 16-1	Levels of Prevention in Primary Care and Recommended Interventions—cont'd

Secondary Prevention—Adult (to identify disease in a patient with asymptomatic illness)

Women	Age Range	Testing
	50–70	• BP, BMI, health risks • Depression screening • Diabetes screening • Cervical cancer screening up to age 65 • Colorectal screening (at age 50) • Mammography (every 2 years) • Bone density (age 65 or women at a high risk for fractures per risk factors) • Lipids optional every 5 years until 70 as per risk factors
	71 and over	• BP, BMI, health risks • Depression screening • Diabetes screening • Colorectal screening • Mammography every 1 to 2 years until 74, then optional

Tertiary Prevention—Adult (identifies the disease state the patient may have to minimize complications)

Diabetes		• Tight glycemic control • Lipid management • BP control • Healthy weight • Exercise • Foot care
Cardiovascular		• Lipid management • BP control • Healthy weight • Exercise

For further information on interventions in primary care refer to:

1. Agency for Healthcare Research and Quality (2012). *Guide to clinical prevention services, 2012.* Retrieved from http://www.ahrq.gov/professionals/clinicians-providers/guidelines-recommendations/guide/index.html.
2. Agency for Healthcare Research and Quality National Guideline Clearinghouse at http://www.ahrq.gov/professionals/clinicians-providers/guidelines-recommendations/ngc/index.html.
3. US Preventitive Services Task Force at http://www.uspreventiveservicesraskforce.org/BrowseRec/Index/browse-recommendations.

However, to be effective, these interventions should be developed, implemented, and evaluated from a population level (see Chapter 5). This requires an understanding of the community, including cultural, environmental, socioeconomic aspects of the community, and the resources available in the community.

For example, if you worked in a primary care setting in Arizona with a high percentage of Pima Indians as clients, it would be important to know what diseases this population is most at risk for. Based on data from the CDC, a major concern would be prevention of type 2 diabetes in Pima youth (Table 16-2).[11] This requires a review of population-level information related to risk factors. In the case of the Pima Indians, the risk factors include genetic predisposition and a shift in diet from traditional foods they grew themselves to processed

TABLE 16-2	Prevalence of Type 2 Diabetes in the 0- to 19-Year Age Group

Ethnic Group	Prevalence
Pima Indians	50.9/1,000
All U.S. American Indians	4.5/1,000
All U.S. youth	1.7/1,000

Source: See reference 12.

foods.[12,13] Primary prevention strategies would require buy-in from the community and should begin during the prenatal period rather than when a child develops type 2 diabetes. Partnering with the community would be a key first step prior to initiating evidence-based prevention strategies that have been used in other parts of the country. The Pima Indians have their own unique culture as well as a genetic predisposition that requires modification of any other programs to match the specific needs of the community. Fortunately, much work has been done in partnership with Pima Indians to understand how to improve their health.[12] Again, primary care requires a population perspective not only as the starting point but also for ongoing evaluation of the effectiveness of interventions delivered across the continuum in primary care (see Fig. 16-1).

Immunization and Health Protection

Immunization through the administration of a vaccine is one of the most frequently used health protection efforts conducted in primary care. As explained in Chapter 8, a **vaccine** refers to the immunizing agent that is used to increase the host's resistance to viral, rickettsial, and bacterial diseases. They can be killed, modified, or become a variant form of the agent. In the United States, the CDC provides detailed guidance to the health-care provider related to the recommended vaccination schedule for all age groups. An example is the recommended adult immunization schedule compiled for the health-care provider (Fig. 16-3). The schedule includes immunizations recommended for all adults based on age group, including:

- Tetanus
- Human papillomavirus
- Varicella

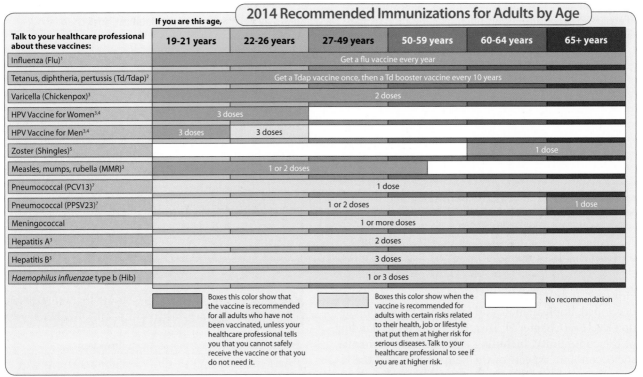

2014 Recommended Immunizations for Adults by Age

If you are this age,

Talk to your healthcare professional about these vaccines:	19-21 years	22-26 years	27-49 years	50-59 years	60-64 years	65+ years
Influenza (Flu)[1]	Get a flu vaccine every year					
Tetanus, diphtheria, pertussis (Td/Tdap)[2]	Get a Tdap vaccine once, then a Td booster vaccine every 10 years					
Varicella (Chickenpox)[3]	2 doses					
HPV Vaccine for Women[3,4]	3 doses					
HPV Vaccine for Men[3,4]	3 doses	3 doses				
Zoster (Shingles)[5]					1 dose	
Measles, mumps, rubella (MMR)[3]	1 or 2 doses					
Pneumococcal (PCV13)[7]	1 dose					
Pneumococcal (PPSV23)[7]	1 or 2 doses					1 dose
Meningococcal	1 or more doses					
Hepatitis A[3]	2 doses					
Hepatitis B[3]	3 doses					
Haemophilus influenzae type b (Hib)	1 or 3 doses					

Boxes this color show that the vaccine is recommended for all adults who have not been vaccinated, unless your healthcare professional tells you that you cannot safely receive the vaccine or that you do not need it.

Boxes this color show when the vaccine is recommended for adults with certain risks related to their health, job or lifestyle that put them at higher risk for serious diseases. Talk to your healthcare professional to see if you are at higher risk.

No recommendation

FOOTNOTES:

1. Influenza vaccine: There are several flu vaccines available—talk to your healthcare professional about which flu vaccine is right for you.
2. Td/Tdap vaccine: Pregnant women are recommended to get Tdap vaccine with each pregnancy in the third trimester to increase protection for infants who are too young for vaccination, but at highest risk for severe illness and death from pertussis (whooping cough). People who have not had Tdap vaccine since age 11 should get a dose of Tdap followed by Td booster doses every 10 years.
3. Varicella, HPV, MMR, Hepatitis A, Hepatitis B vaccine: These vaccines are needed for adults who didn't get these vaccines when they were children.
4. HPV vaccine: There are two HPV vaccines, but only one, HPV (Gardasil®), should be given to men. Gay men or men who have sex with men who are 22 through 26 years old should get HPV vaccine if they haven't already started or completed the series.
5. Zoster vaccine: You should get the zoster vaccine even if you've had shingles before.
6. MMR vaccine: If you were born in 1957 or after, and don't have a record of being vaccinated or having had these infections, talk to your healthcare professional about how many doses you may need.
7. Pneumococcal vaccine: There are two different types of pneumococcal vaccines: PCV13 and PPSV23. Talk with your healthcare professional to find out if one or both pneumococcal vaccines are recommended for you.

If you are traveling outside of the United States, you may need additional vaccines. Ask your healthcare professional which vaccines you may need.
For more information, call toll free 1-800-CDC-INFO (1-800-232-4636) or visit http://www.cdc.gov/vaccines

Figure 16-3 Recommended adult immunization schedule. *(From the Centers for Disease Control and Prevention, http://www. cdc.gov/vaccines/recs/schedules/downloads/adult/2010/adult-schedule-6x4-5-pss.pdf.)*

- Measles, mumps, and rubella
- Influenza

Other vaccines are recommended if some risk factor is present, such as the occupational risk of exposure to hepatitis A and B for health-care providers.[14] The primary care nurse often administers the vaccine. Nurses providing the vaccines use population-level data related to risk, helping them identify persons who would most benefit from the vaccine. Recommendations for vaccination from the CDC are based on age, risk factors, and medical conditions.[15]

Immunizations are central to the patient's risk reduction and health promotion. Every interaction with the health-care team is an opportunity to assist the patient in making choices that will enhance his/her health. Patient education regarding how immunizations can affect health is often the role of the primary care nurse. With every interaction with each patient, the nurse has the opportunity to make the information relate to that patient and his concerns or needs. The young mother who cannot miss work for illness needs to understand that getting the flu vaccine could decrease her risk for illness this year. The farmer working in the soil needs to understand how important his tetanus booster is to keep him working without a problem. The student starting a career in health care needs to see the relationship between getting his/her hepatitis B series and his/her new role. One of many things the primary care nurse does well is to draw this picture: showing patients the relationship between their own needs and how preventive health care can help them meet those needs. The understanding and then availability of immunizations such as the flu vaccine helps the patient adhere to this mandate. Thus, the primary care nurse actively participates in the achievement of the *HP 2020* goal related to immunization.

HP 2020 goals for immunization and communicable diseases are rooted in evidence-based clinical and community activities and services for the prevention and treatment of infectious diseases. Objectives new to *HP 2020* focus on technological advancements and ensuring that states, local public health departments, and nongovernmental organizations are strong partners in the federal attempt to control the spread of communicable diseases. Objectives for 2020 reflect a more mobile society and the fact that diseases do not stop at geopolitical borders. Awareness of disease and completing prevention and treatment courses remain essential components for reducing transmission of communicable disease.[16]

■ HEALTHY PEOPLE 2020
Immunization and Infectious Disease

Goal: Increase immunization rates and reduce preventable infectious diseases.
Targeted Topic: Immunizations and infectious diseases
Overview: The increase in life expectancy during the 20th century is largely due to improvements in child survival; this increase is associated with reductions in infectious disease mortality, due largely to immunization.[1] However, infectious diseases remain a major cause of illness, disability, and death. Immunization recommendations in the United States currently target 17 vaccine-preventable diseases across the life span.
Source: U.S. Department of Health and Human Services (2012). *Healthy People 2020 topics and objectives: Immunizations and infectious diseases.* Retrieved from http://www.healthypeople.gov/2020/topicsobjectives 2020/overview.aspx?topicid=23.

Secondary Prevention Within the Primary Care Setting

Secondary prevention is a major activity in primary care. Secondary prevention focuses on identifying individuals with subclinical disease and initiating early treatment. The activity usually associated with secondary prevention is screening. Most primary care settings follow the current recommendations for screening. Screening in primary care includes a wide range of tests, from taking weight and height done in the office to colonoscopies that require anesthesia. (For more detail on screening, see Chapter 2.) Primary care settings are where most screening occurs; thus, primary care providers are essential to the process of early detection and treatment. However, note again that aggregate-level approaches are also vital to the success of screening. Some screening procedures such as colonoscopy can be expensive and require access to health-care facilities that provide the service. Knowledge about the community and the population served can help improve access to screening services, thus improving the health of the population served.

Screening

Here's an example of how nurses take an active role in screening and health promotion. Access to mammography screening in the rural communities of southeastern Indiana was limited. In response, nurses developed a screening program that has resulted in a regional drive to bring screening to the women living in these communities. This program, funded by the Susan G. Komen Foundation and others, uses the mammography van from a local hospital to go to the women who need the service. With advanced advertisement, women are registered for a screening, clinical breast exam, and education.

This example of a grassroots approach to breast cancer screening has been very successful. Many women have been reached, screened, and referred for follow-up care. A parallel opportunity that came out of this project in southern Indiana was the development of a nurse-run clinic for the uninsured. This free clinic opens twice a month, staffed by nurses, a pharmacist, and a nurse practitioner who offer education, episodic intervention, and referral to primary care providers in the community who will care for patients using an economic sliding scale. These interventions were implemented by nurses living in the area who identified a need and responded to it from a primary care perspective. Nurses in the community applied their understanding of the community to find a way to respond to that need. This included knowledge of the community demographics, the regional and ethnic cultural practices, and community resources such as treatment facilities available for those who screened positive for breast cancer. The focus was secondary prevention with the long-term goal of reducing morbidity and mortality in a population of women at risk.[17]

The CDC is an excellent source for recommendations related to screening in primary care settings. For example, it has a Web page dedicated to HIV screening in primary care with a recommendation that all patients aged 13 to 64 be screened.[18] The CDC also has recommendations on screening for cancer, including breast and colorectal cancers.[19,20]

Screening is basic to care because health-care providers are looking for illness that is asymptomatic. In the primary care population, we screen routinely for blood pressure, cholesterol, and glucose levels. We screen for these because we know through evidence-based practice that people who have these underlying issues are at greatest risk for disease. Hypertension, hyperlipidemia, and diabetes are the root causes for diseases that have the highest incidence of mortality and morbidity. Taking a blood pressure is noninvasive and simple to do, uses minimal equipment, and can identify the patient who is at risk for coronary artery disease. To identify this patient and then offer the education and opportunities to improve their health is foundational to primary care. Screening must be followed up by education that includes information on lifestyle changes such as diet, exercise, weight loss, and medications. Screening without follow-up

leaves the patient without the direction or knowledge to take charge of his health.

Ethics of Screening in Primary Care

Chapter 2 addressed the ethical issues related to screening in detail, but the importance of ethics in screening bears repeating here. A major issue in primary care is conducting screening when treatment is not available. Prior to screening, the primary care nurse must first know what to do if the patient screens positive. Is this something the patient wants to know? Does the family want to know? For example, you may have a woman with two sisters who wants to know whether she carries the gene for breast cancer, but the other sisters do not want to know. This can become an ethical issue for the family. Think about the family in which a member may have a disease for which there is no known cure, such as amyotrophic lateral sclerosis, also known as Lou Gehrig's disease. Do the children want to know whether they are carriers and how does this affect their lives going forward? Does the nurse know what facilities are available to the client to take the next steps—assessment, diagnosis, and treatment? Availability includes geographical availability, the patient's access to transportation to get the facility, and whether the patient has the ability to pay for the treatment. For example, if a surgical intervention is required and the patient is uninsured and has no savings, the only option may be Medicaid. The state Medicaid program may require that the patient sell any assets, such as a home, prior to qualifying for Medicaid. These ethical issues related to screening should be considered prior to conducting routine screening.

Tertiary Prevention Within the Primary Care Setting

Despite our best efforts with primary prevention, people become ill with either a communicable disease (Chapter 8) or an NCD (Chapter 9). Certainly, primary care plays a key role during the acute phase of the illness, but it also is crucial to successful tertiary care. The goal of tertiary prevention is to minimize the complications or sequelae to NCDs. All NCDs carry the risk of lifelong complications.

Nurses are familiar with the macro- and microvascular changes that occur if diabetes is not well controlled. A cerebral vascular accident or myocardial infarction can occur in the patient with uncontrolled hypertension or hyperlipidemia. It is the follow-up, management, and education of the patient with an NCD in primary care that reduce this risk. Reeducation of risk of complication occurs through the careful evaluation of the patient that is done on a set schedule of appointments. However, care recommendations made to a patient are based not only on patient-specific data but also on population-level data. For example, the recommendations that the diabetic patient on insulin should be seen every 3 months and the diabetic patient on oral agents should be seen every 4 to 6 months are based on the epidemiological evidence that these time frames provide adequate coverage. This schedule of care minimizes complication by a careful evaluation on the success of the current plan of care or the opportunity to adjust the interventions.

Management of Noncommunicable Diseases

As reviewed in Chapter 9, management of NCDs is an essential component of care aimed at reducing the associated morbidity and premature death. For example, patients with diabetes require long-term management related to regulation of blood sugar, medications, foot care, diet, and exercise. Though management of diabetes is most frequently delivered to the individual, a population approach is also required. Primary care nurses rely on already developed health education materials to help teach their patients how to self-manage their disease. However, not all materials work across populations because of a lack of cultural relevance (see Chapter 23) or health literacy levels (see Chapter 2). One PHN in Cincinnati conducted a survey of diabetic patients related to diabetic education and concluded that the health education materials currently in use by the area clinics were not at the appropriate reading level and did not address the needs of patients with low literacy levels. This simple approach to collecting population-level data led to the development of educational materials aimed at this subpopulation that addressed their needs.[21] The application of public health science in a primary care setting does not always require time-consuming, sophisticated studies. It can often be accomplished through the use of simple assessment tools.

Case Management

Visits to primary care allow health education to be reinforced and questions to be answered. It is this follow-up that establishes the trust and provides the basis for outcomes that will improve the patient's overall health and well-being. To help guide this effort, nurses in primary care often use a case management approach. According to the Case Management Society of America, **case management** is "a collaborative process of assessment, planning, facilitation and advocacy for options and services to meet an individual's health needs through communication and available resources to promote quality cost-effective outcomes."[22] Case management involves the monitoring and managing of all of a patient's health needs. The role can be designated in different ways. A case manager can be diagnosis-focused (diabetes, heart failure, multiple sclerosis), patient type-focused (homeless, older adult, obese, pediatric), or site-focused (hospital, clinic, shelter).

Nurse case managers actively participate with their clients to identify and facilitate options and services for meeting individuals' health needs to reduce fragmentation and duplication of care.[23] Contemporary case management began in the 1970s as a way to assure both quality outcomes and cost containment.[24,25] The essence of case management is the incorporation of the client, the family, and the community into meeting the needs of the patient. Case management has a positive impact on cost containment and improves patient outcomes.[26-28] This focus on patient outcomes improves the quality of patient care and, therefore, the overall health of the community.

Public Primary Care

Primary care occurs in public settings such as health clinics run by public health departments, federally qualified health centers, and free clinics. Not all public health departments have primary care clinics and most are located in urban areas. Federally qualified health centers provide health care to underserved populations on a sliding scale and have received grants under section 330 of the Public Health Service Act. These clinics qualify for enhanced reimbursement from Medicare and Medicaid. They must also provide comprehensive services.[29] These primary care settings are funded at the federal, state, or local level and aim to improve access to primary care for populations who have limited resources.

Another source of primary care for the underserved population is a free health clinic.

The National Association of Free Health Clinics says the following about free health clinics:

> Free clinics are volunteer-based, safety-net health care organizations that provide a range of medical, dental, pharmacy, and/or behavioral health services to economically disadvantaged individuals who are predominately uninsured. Free clinics are 501(c)(3) tax-exempt organizations, or operate as a program component or affiliate of a 501(c)(3) organization. Entities that otherwise meet the above definition, but charge a nominal fee to patients, may still be considered free clinics provided essential services are delivered regardless of the patient's ability to pay.[30]

These organizations are not directly supported by public funds and depend heavily on a volunteer workforce.

The passing of the ACA in 2010 brought an increased focus on primary care and the need to build the workforce. In 2010, the Department of Health and Human Services announced the availability of $250 million aimed at increasing the number of health-care providers working in primary care, especially in clinics that provide care to underserved populations. One of the major aims of the ACA was to increase access to primary care with the goal of reducing the morbidity and mortality related to untreated disease and lack of preventive care.

Increasing the capacity of public primary care through public health clinics helps to provide care to those with limited access. One of the challenges for these clinics is matching a care to the resources available to promote and protect health. Once again, nurses who restrict themselves to the individual level of care miss opportunities to maximize the ability of a community to support healthy living. In the case of one primary care nurse, the identification of the lack of nutritional resources led to a communitywide effort that far exceeded her initial one-on-one health education with her patients.

● APPLYING PUBLIC HEALTH SCIENCE

The Case of the Nurse Who Thought She Lived in the City— Not the Desert

Public Health Science Topics Covered:

- Assessment
- Collaboration
- Health planning

Katherine, a nurse, lived and worked in the inner city for many years. "I'm a city girl," she would often say, explaining that she could get whatever she needed in the city. However, she heard that there was a problem with hunger in the city. She noticed an article that discussed inner-city nutrition and the article used the term *food desert*. From a public health perspective, a **food desert** is a large, often isolated, geographical area where there is little or no access to the food needed to maintain an affordable and healthy diet.[31] In many major cities, large grocery stores are closing their doors in inner-city neighborhoods, especially poor neighborhoods, thus limiting access to fresh produce, food varieties, and nutritional choices. In the

United States, food deserts tend to be located in urban and rural low-income neighborhoods, where residents are less likely to have access to supermarkets or grocery stores that provide healthy food choices.

Through her review of the literature on food deserts, Katherine discovered that an increasing number of communities had few food retailers or supermarkets that regularly stocked fresh produce, low-fat dairy, whole grains, and other healthy foods.[32,33] This phenomenon has been slowly occurring over time with the movement of people out of the city, the economic downswing, and the loss of jobs. The 2008 Farm Bill directed the U.S. Department of Agriculture (USDA) to study food deserts in the United States, to assess their incidence and prevalence, to identify characteristics and factors causing and influencing food deserts, and to determine the overall effect of food deserts on local populations.[33] Based on this, the USDA was asked to provide recommendations for addressing the causes and effects. The Economic Research Service is the lead agency in this effort and is collaborating with other agencies within the USDA such as the Food and Nutrition Service and the Cooperative State Research, Education, and Extension Service. Legislation also instructed the USDA to work with other organizations, including the Institute of Medicine and the National Research Council.[34] The 2009 report stated that 4.1 million low-income people live more than a mile from a grocery store or supermarket. It concluded that urban areas with decreased access had higher racial segregation and greater income inequality.[33]

Katherine realized that a major supermarket had left the community in which her clinic is located, and she wondered about the impact. With this on her mind, she began to ask the patients in the primary care clinic where she worked a simple question: "Where do you shop for food?" The responses of the patients began to identify this as a real concern. The convenience store or fast-food restaurants were the most common answers. The patients explained lack of transportation as the main reason for shopping at the convenience store even though the prices were higher. Ms. Reid, an older adult patient, related how hard it was for her to get on the bus and carry groceries home. James told Katherine that the convenience store was close by but so expensive that he could not purchase much food. The most disturbing comment came from Mary, the mother of four children, who said, "I know my children need fresh fruits and vegetables but I cannot get that around here." All of the patients, in one way or another, felt the impact of living in a "desert."

Katherine did further reading and found that the economic and nutritional sequelae to this loss of access to supermarkets were far reaching. It is well documented that dietary choice may reverse or lessen the disease burden of many NCDs as well as prevent communicable diseases.[34] When the choice is limited to red meats, fatty foods, added fats, desserts, and sweets, there is a substantially increased risk for obesity, type 2 diabetes, and heart disease.[35,36] The effect goes across the life span, affecting adults, older adults, and the younger population. The growth and development of the child and adolescent are compromised by the lack of quality available foods. The long-term effect for the younger population is twofold: It affects their health, certainly, but it also provides a pattern of eating that will be detrimental for the rest of their life. The goal of adequate nutrition in childhood is to prevent nutritional disorders such as malnutrition and overweight, as well as the increased morbidity and mortality that accompany them.[37] According to the National Restaurant Association, in 2012, 48% of the share in the food dollar was spent at a restaurant, with total sales of $631.8 billion, up from $379 billion in 2000.[38] Snack, convenience, and fast foods and sweets continue to dominate food advertisements viewed by children. The marketing of these items contributes to the fast-food consumption of U.S. children.[39,40] Children spend more time, an average of 44.5 hours per week, in front of a television, computer, and/or game screen than in any other activity except sleeping.[41] They are repeatedly exposed to advertisements and often cannot distinguish between an advertisement and programming.[39]

Katherine and the other nurses at her clinic reviewed *HP 2020* objectives related to nutrition and weight status and found a new objective, NWS-4. It was listed as developmental and the objective was to "...increase the proportion of Americans who have access to a food retail outlet that sells a variety of foods that are encouraged by the Dietary Guidelines for Americans."[42] Based on this, the nurses decided to attack this problem on two fronts. They realized that education must take place to inform and advise the patients on the importance of good nutrition. In addition, since the lack of availability of the food was a serious barrier to healthy eating, the food desert in their community needed to change first. Katherine decided to investigate ways to get a neighborhood farmer's market into the city. She learned that this concept helps bring fresh produce, eggs, and meats to the city as well as helps the small farm owner.[43] It can

also be a method to develop local gardens, new business, employment, and camaraderie in a neighborhood. In 2012, there were 7,864 farmers' markets registered with the USDA's national farmers' market directory, up 9.6% from 2011, and more than double the number registered in 2004.[44] She realized that this was something doable, and contacted a group in New York City, Greenmarket, to find out where to start. Greenmarket began in 1976 with 12 farmers and one farmers' market located in Manhattan. It grew to 54 markets and 230 family farms and fishermen.[45] The registered nurse group that Katherine worked with on this project used what they learned in their undergraduate public health nursing courses to tackle the problem. They knew they had to begin with an assessment, but had little time in their busy clinic schedules to do this. One of the more recent graduates of a local school of nursing suggested that they enlist the help of the students and the nearby school of nursing. They added a member of the nursing faculty from the school to their planning group. The faculty member agreed to have students who were taking their public health nursing practicum help conduct the assessment and contribute to the planning and evaluation stages of the project. The nurses now had a team.

The team began with a geographical assessment of their community and the surrounding area, plotting the location of fast-food restaurants, convenience stores, and the closest supermarkets (see Chapter 4). They then plotted the public transportation routes. To help with the assessment, they asked members of the community to join their team. The community members described the realities of trying to shop for food. With the help of the community members, they conducted a more formal survey of the patients coming to their clinics, asking about their nutritional intake and for information on where they purchased their food. This provided them with baseline data.

Using the data from their community-specific assessment, the team constructed a viable plan to bring farmers' markets into the community, which included measurable objectives, impact, and outcomes (see Chapter 5). The plan included organizing local food cooperatives and farmers' markets to set up sites in the neighborhoods. Once availability of the food was in place, the group of nurses supplemented their nutritional education for patients with added knowledge of what was available in the community. They provided their patients with pamphlets and information about the new offerings. They put up posters in their office.

After 6 months, they reissued their survey and found that the nutritional intake had improved and that patients reported easier access to healthy foods through the farmers' markets. Thus, Katherine's concern as well as application of basic public health assessments and program planning resulted in a change of the health of an entire neighborhood.

Private Primary Care

Primary care is also provided through private practices. Providers include physicians, nurse practitioners, nurses, and other health-care providers. Private practices do not receive direct federal support, but most accept payment through federal programs such as Medicaid and Medicare. The financial structure is based on a fee-for-service model. However, the delivery of care is the same. Again, the nurse must be attuned to the larger context of the community in which the patients of the clinic live. This understanding helps the nurse to identify issues that require intervention at the community level.

▶ SOLVING THE MYSTERY
The Case of the Wobbly Men
Public Health Science Topics Covered:

- Surveillance and case finding
- Epidemiology
- Communication

Madelyn, a nurse who works as the intake nurse at the primary care office in Rivertown, Ohio, began her busy day reviewing the schedule. She noticed that James T., a 45-year-old male, was on the schedule again for a chief complaint of "feeling weak, a wobbly gait, and his wife says he is irritable." Madelyn recalled that James was at the clinic last month with a similar complaint, and that he was not the only one. She wondered why the local men had been visiting the office so often recently. Usually, it is very difficult to get this age bracket of men into the office for risk prevention and routine checks. James was the fifth man this week with a similar complaint.

As she did the initial intake of James T's history, she noticed a listing of symptoms that she had heard recently from the other five middle-aged male patients. The complaints of weakness, unsteady gait, and feeling depressed and irritable were new for these patients. She decided to explore this change in the usual patient population. She realized that these symptoms can be

attributed to many different diagnoses but it was the similarity of the symptoms in a particular group of male patients in the same age group that got her attention.

Madelyn pulled the charts of all five of the men with similar chief complaints and started on a basic public health mission, looking for anything that might link these five men. They did not live on the same street and they worked at different jobs. She then called each of the men and asked them other questions to try and find a link between them. She found one very quickly when she asked whether they knew each other. They reported that they had formed an informal fishing group and fished regularly for relaxation. Because the majority of their wives did not like to clean the fish or cook it, they ate most of the catch the same day on the boat. The rest they cleaned themselves and froze for eating during the week. They regularly caught Rock Bass, Smallmouth Bass, and Yellow Bullhead. They also threw back the smaller fish, even those that met regulations, and sought the bigger fish. When asked how many times a week they ate fish that they had caught, they replied that they ate between three and four meals per week. For Madelyn, the common denominator across this patient population was the ingestion of large quantities of river fish over the past few years. She found no other common denominator. She remembered hearing something about freshwater fish being contaminated with chemicals. She reviewed the men's symptoms again and noticed that the symptoms pointed to mercury poisoning. Madelyn's attention to detail and her understanding of basic epidemiology led her to a possible solution to the puzzle of the wobbly men. She explained her conclusions to the physician and the two nurse practitioners who worked in the clinic with her. She shared her information with the providers in the office, who then followed up on her recommendation to test the men for mercury poisoning. When the levels came back elevated, in excess of 20 mcg/L (normal value less than 5 mcg/L), the providers were able to initiate appropriate treatment. Madelyn also made a call to the county public health department to alert them to the cluster of cases.

Mercury poisoning has been around for centuries and noted as early as 1500 BC in Egyptian tombs. In the manufacture and processing of felt hats in the 18th and 19th centuries, chronic exposure of workers to the mercury used to process the felt led to the term "mad as a hatter." Mercury in any form is toxic. Exposure can be via ingestion, vapor inhalation, injection, and absorption through the skin.[46,47] The presentation of symptoms relates to the most commonly affected systems, which are the neurological, gastrointestinal, and renal systems. The concentration of mercury is very low in most foodstuffs (below 0.02 mg Hg/kg). However, certain types of marine fish (such as shark, swordfish, and tuna) and certain fish taken from polluted freshwaters (such as pike, walleye, and bass) may contain high concentrations of mercury (Fig. 16-4).[47] In this setting, mercury is almost completely in the form of methylmercury. It is not uncommon that concentrations of methylmercury in these fish are 1 mg/kg or even higher.[46] Organic mercury can be found in three forms—aryl, short-chain, and long-chain alkyl compounds. Once absorbed, the aryl and long-chain alkyl compounds convert to their inorganic forms and possess similar toxic properties to inorganic mercury. The short-chain alkyl mercurials are readily absorbed in the gastrointestinal tract (90%–95%) and remain stable in their initial forms. Alkyl organic mercury has high lipid solubility and distributes uniformly throughout the body, accumulating in the brain, kidney, liver, hair, and skin. Organic mercurials also cross the blood-brain barrier and placenta and penetrate erythrocytes, attributing to neurological symptoms, teratogenic effects, and high blood to plasma ratio, respectively.[46]

The presentation of acute mercury poisoning includes burning of the throat, edema of oral mucous membranes, abdominal pain, vomiting, bloody diarrhea, and shock.[46] Chronic mercury poisoning, which these men were experiencing, causes weakness, ataxia, intentional tremors, irritability, and depression. Exposure to alkyl (organic) mercury derivatives from contaminated fish or fungicides used on seeds has caused ataxia, convulsions, and catastrophic birth defects.[46] Without a complete history, mercury toxicity, especially in older adults, can be misdiagnosed as Parkinson's disease, senile dementia, metabolic encephalopathy, depression, or Alzheimer's disease.[48] It is imperative to do a thorough history that includes occupation, hobbies, and level of seafood intake if clinical suspicion includes mercury exposure.

Based on her own research and her discussion with the public health department, Madelyn found that the Environmental Protection Agency (EPA) (see Chapter 6) released regular reports on the safety of freshwater fish with recommended levels of consumption (Table 16-3).[49] For the river flowing through Rivertown, the recommendation for consumption of Rock Bass, Smallmouth Bass, and Yellow Bullhead was one meal per month. These men were consuming 12 to 16 times more than the recommended amounts.

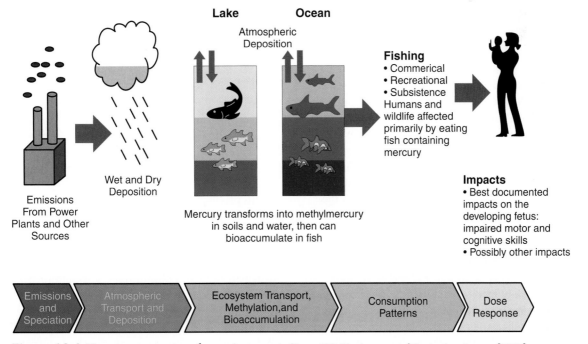

Figure 16-4 How mercury enters the environment. (*From U.S. Environmental Protection Agency [2012]. Mercury: Human exposure. Retrieved from http://www.epa.gov/hg/exposure.htm.*)

TABLE 16–3 EPA Advisory Table: Selected Bodies of Water in Ohio

Body of Water	Area Under Advisory	Species	One Meal per Month or Two Months	Contaminant
East Branch Black River	Richman Road (Lodi) to Foster Road (Lorain, Medina Counties)	Rock Bass, Smallmouth Bass, Yellow Bullhead	Month	Mercury
Great Miami River	Harrison Pike (Miamitown) to mouth (Ohio River) (Hamilton County)	Largemouth Bass 15" and over, White Bass	Month	Mercury
Cuyahoga River	State Route 87 (Russell Park) to Ohio Edison Dam Pool (Geauga, Portage, Summit Counties)	Common Carp Black Crappie, White Sucker 16" and over	Month	Polychlorinated biphenyls (PCBs) and mercury
Lake Erie	All Waters (Ashtabula, Cuyahoga, Erie, Lake, Lorain, Lucas, Ottawa, Sandusky Counties)	Channel Catfish, Common Carp 27" and over, Lake Trout	2 Months	PCBs
		Chinook Salmon 19" and over, Coho Salmon, Common Carp under 27", Freshwater Drum, Smallmouth Bass, Steelhead Trout, White Bass, Whitefish, White Perch	month	PCBs
		Brown Bullhead, Largemouth Bass	Month	Mercury

Source: See reference 49.

Madelyn was concerned that although this information was available on the Web site, the information was not getting out to the community.

Madelyn decided to contact the other two primary care groups in Rivertown and ask them whether they have seen anyone with similar complaints. The two other offices reported that they had, for a total of eight more patients, all male and all between aged 35 to 60. She joined forces with the nurses in these two clinics and proposed to the health department that a public campaign be launched locally to alert fishermen to the potential danger of eating a large quantity of fish caught in the local river. One of the men being treated told Madelyn that he belonged to a local fish and game club that had recently organized in the community. The nurses asked this club to help spread the word, thus reducing the risk of mercury poisoning in their community. Madelyn provided a valuable service to her community, not only because she solved the problem of the wobbly men, but also because she took it to the next step and worked at preventing more cases.

Emerging Primary Care Public Health Issues

Public health issues that challenge primacy care continue to emerge. For example, the swine flu pandemic presented problems related to limited quantities of the vaccine, which made it problematic when deciding who was at greatest risk. This required that primary care nurses remain on top of the public health information.

Some public health issues reflect the emergence of health problems that had appeared to be solved but come back with a vengeance, for example, the bedbug outbreak. In August 2010, the CDC and the EPA issued a joint statement on bed bug control.[50] The purpose of this statement was to highlight emerging public health issues associated with bed bugs in communities throughout the United States It provided information on the increase in bed bugs, implications of infestations, and the integrated approach to controlling them. This is a perfect example of agencies that interact with the community in which the patient lives coming together to handle a widespread problem. The bed bug has been around for centuries. Where do you think the childhood saying "Don't let the bed bugs bite!" comes from? This formerly funny saying is now a reality for many people across the country. The *Cimex lectularis* (bed bug) feeds on its host's blood, leaving behind an area of irritation that itches. The EPA, CDC, and the USDA consider the bed bug a public health pest, but it is not known as a vector for transmission or spread of disease.

The role for primary care is to educate the patient about what they look like, where to find them, and how to eradicate them. The adult bed bug is ¼ to ⅜ of an inch long, brown, with a flat, oval-shaped body (Fig. 16-5). Younger bed bugs, called nymphs, are smaller and lighter in color. Where are these critters? When not feeding, bed bugs hide in many places and, unlike scabies, which borrow under the skin, the bed bug may be found around the piping or seams of the mattress, box spring, or in the cracks in a headboard or footboard. With a heavy infestation, you will find them in every nook and cranny of the room because, being only the width of a credit card, they can squeeze in anywhere.

Prevention is a cornerstone of the defense against bed bug infestation. Educate the community to use caution when buying second-hand furniture (do a bed bug check), luggage, or bedding. Bed bugs need to feed every 5 to 10 days but they are very resilient and are capable of surviving more than a year without feeding. Educate patients to reduce clutter, places where bed bugs can hide and, when traveling, to check mattresses, bedding, and furniture so people don't bring home any extra guests from their trips. Treating bed bug infestation requires an integrated approach with washing and drying at high temperatures and discarding infested bedding

and furniture. Other approaches include the infusion of dry heat for at least 1 hour or cool treatments (below 0°F) for at least 4 days. The core treatment for a community with an invasive problem, no matter the cause, revolves around identification, education, and eradication.

Ongoing Use of Public Health Science in the Primary Care Setting

Nurses working in primary care consistently apply public health science to their practice. This includes trending disease and risk factors in the community they serve. They do not have to collect the data themselves. They can use local, state, and national public health surveillance data to help identify significant trends in the population they serve. In addition, primary care nurses who actively employ public health communication skills will build a partnership with the community and key stakeholders.

Tracking Health Trends in the Community Served

Many issues, such as the bed bug situation, require a population perspective in order to effectively treat the individual. For example, recent trends show a rise in emergency room admission for exacerbations of asthma. Members of the community, such as parents, school teachers, or PHNs, raise the question—Why is there an increase? Upon investigation by these members of the community, it's discovered that a new factory has opened up that manufactures aromatics that are released in the air. There is a direct correlation between this change in the environment and the rise in asthma exacerbations. A community seems to have a higher incidence of a certain cancer than another and the cause must be addressed.

A rise in the population complaining of back and foot pain because they started a new job at a warehouse is evidence that education on proper body mechanics is needed. The community-focused approach to problems has patient/public education at its heart, and nurses as educators are foundational to the success of these programs. Knowing the community means understanding their needs, values, education level, and what is important to them. When this part of the community can be identified, the best approach can be developed and success will occur. To develop a plan without the input and buy-in from a community will cause a weak foundation and result in failure.

Health-Care Policy and Primary Care

Let's now look to the future and where health care will be taking place as we enter the new era of health-care reform. There is much discussion on the utilization of community

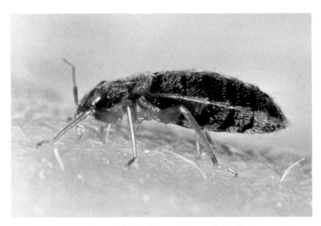

Figure 16-5 An adult bedbug, *Cimex lectularius,* ingesting a blood meal from the arm of a "voluntary" human host. *(From the CDC. Donated by the World Health Organization, Geneva, Switzerland, 1976.)*

health centers (CHCs) when reviewing the estimated 32 million Americans who will be seeking primary care. The ACA underwrites the CHCs and enables them to serve nearly 20 million new patients while adding an estimated 15,000 providers by 2015.[51] The CHCs were launched in 1965 by the office of Economic Opportunity as part of Lyndon Johnson's War on Poverty. They were designed to reduce or remove the health-care disparities among the poor, racial and ethnic minorities, and the uninsured. The plan was that the governance of these facilities was centered in the host community. There are more than 8,000 urban and rural sites in every state and territory. They are federally funded but must meet budget requirements and offer services according to an economic sliding scale. CHCs are dedicated to the delivery of primary medical, dental, behavioral, and social services to the underserved populations and have demonstrated their ability to provide care in a comprehensive fashion.[51] This

may explain the influx of patients. The CHC core values coincide with the **patient centered medical home (PCMH)** concept. The PCMH is built on the premise of a holistic approach that encompasses accessible, coordinated, and team-driven delivery of primary care that relies on outcome measurement and evidence-based practice.

Another issue is inclusion of the medical home in the ACA. The patient centered medical home (PCMH) includes (1) personal physicians; (2) whole person orientation; (3) coordinated and integrated care; (4) safe and high-quality care through evidence-based practice; appropriate use of health information technology and continuous quality improvements; (5) expanded access to care; and (6) payment that recognizes added value from additional components of patient-centered care. The five functions of a medical home are listed in Box 16-1.[52] The ACA includes the medical home as one of the required quality measures. Individuals with an NCD covered

---

BOX 16–1   Association for Health Care Research and Quality: The Medical Home Encompasses Five Functions and Attributes

The five functions and attributes of the medical home are as follows:

1. **Patient-centered:** The primary care medical home provides primary health care that is relationship-based with an orientation toward the whole person. Partnering with patients and their families requires understanding and respecting each patient's unique needs, culture, values, and preferences. The medical home practice actively supports patients in learning to manage and organize their own care at the level the patient chooses. Recognizing that patients and families are core members of the care team, medical home practices ensure that they are fully informed partners in establishing care plans.

2. **Comprehensive care:** The primary care medical home is accountable for meeting the large majority of each patient's physical and mental health-care needs, including prevention and wellness, acute care, and chronic care. Providing comprehensive care requires a team of care providers. This team might include physicians, advanced practice nurses, physician assistants, nurses, pharmacists, nutritionists, social workers, educators, and care coordinators. Although some medical home practices may bring together large and diverse teams of care providers to meet the needs of their patients, many others, including smaller practices, will build virtual teams linking themselves and their patients to providers and services in their communities.

3. **Coordinated care:** The primary care medical home coordinates care across all elements of the broader

health-care system, including specialty care, hospitals, home health care, and community services and supports. Such coordination is particularly critical during transitions between sites of care, such as when patients are being discharged from the hospital. Medical home practices also excel at building clear and open communication among patients and families, the medical home, and members of the broader care team.

4. **Superb access to care:** The primary care medical home delivers accessible services with shorter waiting times for urgent needs, enhanced in-person hours, around-the-clock telephone or electronic access to a member of the care team, and alternative methods of communication such as e-mail and telephone care. The medical home practice is responsive to patients' preferences regarding access.

5. **A systems-based approach to quality and safety:** The primary care medical home demonstrates a commitment to quality and quality improvement by ongoing engagement in activities such as using evidence-based medicine and clinical decision-support tools to guide shared decision making with patients and families, engaging in performance measurement and improvement, measuring and responding to patient experiences and patient satisfaction, and practicing population health management. Sharing robust quality and safety data and improvement activities publicly is also an important marker of a system-level commitment to quality.

Source: Association for Health Care Research and Quality. (n.d.). *What is the PCMH?* Retrieved from http://www.pcmh.ahrq.gov/page/
    what-pcmh.

under Medicaid may choose a PCMH, which can be an individual provider (such as a community health center or comprehensive primary care clinic) or a health team. This PCMH would provide the care needed to manage the NCD and could include care management, care coordination, health promotion, transitional care, family support, and referral to community and social support services when needed. The medical home should also use health information technology to link services.[52]

EVIDENCE-BASED PRACTICE
Patient Centered Medical Home (PCMH)

Practice Statement: A PCMH is based on the integration of patients as active participants in their own health and well-being.

Targeted Outcome: Improved health outcomes, increased ability to self-manage NCDs, prevention of both NCDs and communicable diseases, improved quality of health care, and decreased health-care costs.

Evidence to Support: The move to a PCMH is a core concept in the ACA. The evidence to support a specific organizational model for the delivery of patient-centered care is limited. Crabtree and colleagues[1] pointed out that based on their own 15-year program of research, successful transformation of primary care settings to a PCMH model is unlikely to be successful unless a stronger theoretical foundation is established. Primary care practices use only about a fifth of the recommended PCMH processes.[2] However, the evidence to support PCMH is growing.[3] There is now a major resource for funding research that will help determine whether a patient-centered approach improves outcomes. The purpose of the recently established Patient Centered Outcomes Research Institute (PCORI) is to provide the evidence that will direct best practices for patients and providers related to making better-informed health-care decisions.[4]

Sources

1. Crabtree, B.F., Nutting, P.A., Miller, W.L., McDaniel, R.R., Stange, K. C., Jaen, C.R., & Stewart, E. (2011). Primary care practice transformation is hard work: Insights from a 15-year developmental program of research. *Medical Care, 49*, S28-S35. doi:10.1097/MLR.obo13e318cad65c.
2. Rittenhouse, D.R., Casalino, L.P., Shortell, S.M., McClellan, S.R., Alexander, J.A., & Drum, M.L. (2011). Small and medium size physician practices use few

patient centered medical home processes. *Health Affairs, 30*(8), 1575-1584. doi:10.1377/hltaff.2010.1210.
3. Nutting, P.A., Miller, W.L., Crabtree, B.F., Jaen, C.C.R., Stewart, E.E., & Stange, K.C. (2009). Initial lessons from the national demonstration projects on practice transformation to a patient-centered medical home. *The Annals of Family Medicine, 7*(3), 254-260. doi:10.1370/afm.1002.
4. Patient Centered Outcomes Research Institute. (n.d.). *Mission and vision.* Retrieved from http://www.pcori.org/about-us/mission-and-vision/.

Communication and Collaboration

One of the standards in public health nursing is collaboration. One of the characteristics of collaboration is that the nurse partners with key individuals, group, coalition, and organizations to effect change in public health policies, programs, and services to generate positive outcomes.[53] This standard holds true for the primary care nurse. Nurses working in primary care settings enhance their practice when they build collaborative relationships with all of these entities. As evidenced by the cases provided in this chapter, each of the situations encountered by primary care nurses required communication and collaboration with members of the community, organizations, and other stakeholders. The building of these relationships takes time and requires a conscious effort to do so that goes beyond creating a list of referrals for patients. It means building strong partnerships and requires specific skills. Although this is not unique to primary care nurses, there are particular partnerships that should be a part of every primary care nurse's practice.

Community Organizations

A good starting point is the local public health department (see Chapter 14). Primary care health providers are required to report certain diseases to the public health department (Table 16-4). This system is a good starting point and can be a two-way street. For example, some communicable diseases are rare enough that they may be missed during the first assessment, but if the primary care nurse knows that there has been an increase in a particular disease, the level of suspicion increases. Then, if a patient comes into the primary care clinic, the nurse is more apt to be on the alert for symptoms that match that disease.

Many initiatives begin with the local public health department and require buy-in by primary care providers. Developing a relationship with the public health department brings a primary care clinic into the public health arena and increases the likelihood that the

| TABLE 16–4 | **Classification of Common Class A Notifiable Diseases Into Disease Type** | | | |

Bloodborne (Excludes HIV/AIDS)	Enteric/Food-Borne	Vaccine Preventable	Sexually Transmitted	Other
Hepatitis B	Campylobacteriosis	Hepatitis A	AIDS	Aseptic meningitis
Hepatitis C	Cryptosporidiosis	Measles	Chlamydia	Meningococcal disease
	Giardiasis	Mumps	Gonorrhea	*Haemophilus influenzae*
	Escherichia coli 0157:H7	Pertussis	Syphilis (primary, secondary, latent, congenital)	Tuberculosis
	Listeriosis			Legionellosis
	Salmonellosis			Streptococcal group A, invasive
	Shigellosis			
	Yersiniosis			

clinic's patients will benefit from these initiatives. Primary care nurses are in the "trenches" and often have a good grasp of the health issues faced by their patients. Collaborating with the public health department can result in the building of population-level initiatives that build on the experiences of the primary care nurses. This two-way communication can have a powerful effect on community-level public health that will actually work in the field.

There are a multitude of organizations with which primary care nurses can build a relationship to help better serve their patients. These include but are not limited to governmental organizations, other health-care providers, churches, community groups, and other primary care providers. Most student nurses learn how to conduct a community assessment (see Chapter 4), but once the course is completed, they fail to apply it when they move out into the real world of nursing care. In primary care, the community assessment component is essential. Consider the cases presented in this chapter. The nurses in these cases tapped into the resources available from various organizations such as the housing authority and the EPA.

Often, the collaboration can result in the building of coalitions. The role a primary care clinic can play in these coalitions is substantial. If a community wishes to address a particular health issue such as lead poisoning or secondary smoke exposure, the primary care setting is ideal for screening, distribution of health educations materials, and other health protection and promotion activities.

Community Members

The primary care setting is not an island, but exists within a community. Again, the lessons learned related to community assessment are essential to the primary care setting. The success of a primary care clinic depends on the trust built between the clinic and the population it serves. This requires reaching out to the community, not just persons in leadership positions such as a mayor or a school superintendent, but residents of the community. What is the nature of the community? Is it rich, poor, urban, suburban, or rural? How many people live in the community served by the clinic and what proportion uses the clinic? What are the age groups? What is the ethnic background of the community? These questions and more help to build a picture of the community and help primary care nurses tailor the services provided to the patients being served.

A case in point is a public primary care clinic located in a community of subsidized housing. This clinic operates on a first come, first served basis, using a sliding scale fee. The community is on the city bus line but is on the outskirts of the city and built next to the city landfill. It is also located close to a major interstate. The population is made up primarily of younger families and there are no major grocery stores within walking distance. The nearest grocery store requires a transfer from one bus to another. The clinic is the only one in the community and other clinics require at least one bus transfer to get to, but many residents opt to go to other clinics rather than to the clinic in their neighborhood.

The nurses working in the clinic struggle with a full waiting room, crying children, and clients who complain about the long waits. What can the nurses do? Where should they start? Contacting a few members in the community is a good place to start. This is the first step to looking outside the clinic, finding out what the residents think about the clinic, and beginning to work on ways to solve the problems. In this example, potential issues could include the long waiting times for mothers who do not have access to day care and must bring their children with them. The nurses providing the care might not fully understand the culture within the community. Another possibility is the perception of public assistance. If the nurses at the clinic begin to build a relationship with the community, they will include the community in solving these issues and truly form a partnership. These partnerships can result in multiple interventions that improve the health of all, not just those who come in for care on a given day. Without these partnerships, the primary care nurses may continue to create barriers to care without realizing it.

Public health science makes a strong contribution to the effectiveness of primary care nursing. It provides primary care nurses with the skills needed to be full members of the public health team, even if their focus is care of the individual and the family. Through active participation in disease surveillance and the building of partnerships with other organizations and the community itself, primary care nurses contribute to the health of the community in powerful ways.

Culture and Primary Care

As in any setting where nursing care is provided, culture is an important aspect in the provision of primary care. Cultural issues not only play a part in the assessment and development of a plan of care, but also affect the availability of resources for the family and the community. Because primary care clinics are located in a community, it is important for the primary care providers to learn about the culture of their community. Learning about the culture of a community can be challenging, especially if the community is made up of culturally diverse populations. However, this process is essential in order to meet cultural competence requirements (see Chapter 23).

Immigration presents another cultural issue for primary care settings. For example, in Cincinnati, Ohio, a group of refuges from the small country of Burundi settled in a poor, largely African American community within the city. These refugees came from a different climate and did not share in the culture of the predominant group in the community. They experienced acculturation issues as they tried to fit in to their new country. For the most part, they were young families and needed primary care services. However, they did not speak English and had low literacy in their own language. This group provides an example of the complexity of dealing with cultural issues in a primary care setting. The primary caregivers located in the community must not only locate an interpreter, but also become knowledgeable about the health practices and beliefs of the Burundians. This learning requires a population perspective and, if done carefully, will result in positive health outcomes over time.

Application of the community assessment approach described in Chapter 4 is essential if primary care–level interventions are going to be effective. The primary care provider, located in the community, is in an excellent position to gather this information and gain partners in developing culturally relevant interventions. Each day coming to work, the provider can observe the community by performing a brief windshield survey (see Chapter 4). Individuals and families can develop trusting relationships with the nurses who work in primary care settings, because this is often their only interaction with the health-care system. This is where they come for their physical checkups, where they bring their children for care, and where they go to first when they do not feel well. Having an understanding of the cultural context of the persons seeking primary care enhances nurses' ability not only to provide care to individuals and families, but also to develop programs such as an immunization program. Failure to take into account the culture of the persons served can result in poor follow-up care, miscommunication, and failure to build that essential trusting relationship (see Chapter 23).

■ Summary Points

- Primary care in the United States is a delivery system and primary health care from the WHO perspective is a movement to bring about health-care reform that will result in achieving equitable health care for all.
- Primary care encompasses all levels of prevention: primary, secondary, and tertiary.
- In the United States, primary care occurs in public settings such as health clinics run by public health departments as well as in private settings such as private practices and hospital-run clinics.
- Primary care is often the first line of action for emerging health issues such as the swine flu epidemic of 2009.
- Primary care involves policy, advocacy, and collaboration in the effort to address public health issues and enhance the health of populations.
- The importance of primary care is growing because of the ACA and the provision for a PCMH.

▲ CASE STUDY
Pertussis Vaccination Program for Parents
Learning Outcomes

At the end of this case study, the student will be able to:

- Apply principles of descriptive epidemiology to trend disease over time.
- Describe the steps taken to develop an intervention.
- Discuss national current recommendations for vaccination.

In 2010, there was an increase in pertussis cases across the United States, particularly in California, with predictions that the incidence rate would be the highest it had been in that state for 50 years. Across the United States, efforts were made not just to immunize children, but also to immunize adults. You have been assigned the task of developing a vaccination program for the parents and children who attend your public health well-baby clinic. Begin with the current incidence rates in the city or county nearest to you for pertussis in both children and adults. Then determine the recommendations for immunizations on the CDC Web site located at http://www.cdc.gov/vaccines/vpd-vac/pertussis/default.htm.

Based on your findings and building on what you learned about health assessment and planning in Chapters 4 and 5, develop a vaccination program for the clinic. Be sure you include the following:

- A summary of the incidence rates for your city or county compared with those for the state and the nation
  - Have the incidence rates increased or declined in the past 5 years?
  - Which population is at greatest risk?
- Current immunization recommendations from the CD
- A plan to inform clinic patients and their families about vaccination that includes:
  - Communication methods (e.g. TV, flyers, school newsletters)
  - Cultural considerations
  - Other communication strategies?
- A mechanism for handling potential increase in demand
- A plan to deal with a possible outbreak

REFERENCES

1. World Health Organization. (2008). *Primary health care: Now more than ever.* Geneva, Switzerland: Author.
2. US experiencing primary care shortage "likes of which we have not seen." *USA Today.* Retrieved from http://www.eurekalert.org/pub_releases/2009-03/acop-uep032409.php#.
3. American Medical Association. (2010). *Are primary care physicians an endangered species?* Retrieved from http://www.ama-assn.org/ama/pub/education-careers/graduate-medical-education/question-of-month/primary-care-endangered-species.page.
4. Bindman, A.B., & Majeed, A. (2003). Organization of primary care in the United States. *British Medical Journal, 326,* 631-634.
5. American Academy of Family Physicians. (2010). *Primary care.* Retrieved from http://www.aafp.org/online/en/home/policy/policies/p/primarycare.html.
6. U.S. Department of Health and Human Services. (2012). *Healthy People 2020 topics and objectives: Access to health services.* Retrieved from http://www.healthypeople.gov/2020/topicsobjectives2020/overview.aspx?topicid=1.
7. UNICEF. (2008). *Prioritizing maternal health in Sri Lanka.* Retrieved from http://www.unicef.org/devpro/46000_48498.html?q=printme.
8. Centers for Disease Control and Prevention. (2001). State-specific prevalence of current cigarette smoking among adults, and policies and attitudes towards secondhand smoke—United States, 2000. *Morbidity and Mortality Weekly Report, 50*(49), 1101-1105.
9. American Lung Association. (2010). *Trends in tobacco use.* Retrieved from http://www.lungusa.org/finding-cures/our-research/trend-reports/Tobacco-Trend-Report.pdf
10. O'Donnell, M.P. (2008). Evolving definition of health promotion: What do you think? *American Journal of Health Promotion, 23*(2). Retrieved from http://www.healthpromotionjournal.com/publications/journal/en2008-11.htm.
11. Centers for Disease Control and Prevention. (2012). *Children and diabetes—more information.* Retrieved from http://www.cdc.gov/diabetes/projects/cda2.htm.
12. Pathfinders for Health. (n.d.). *The Pima Indians.* Retrieved from http://diabetes.niddk.nih.gov/dm/pubs/pima/pathfind/pathfind.htm.
13. Krakoff, J., Funahashim, T., Stehouver, C.D.A., Tanaka, S., Matsuzawa, Y., ... Lindsay, R.S. (2003). Inflammatory markers, adiponectin, and risk of type 2 diabetes in the Pima Indian. *Diabetes Care, 26*(6), 1745-1751.
14. Centers for Disease Control and Prevention. (2012). *Vaccine recommendations: Health care workers.* Retrieved from http://www.cdc.gov/vaccines/spec-grps/hcw.htm.
15. Centers for Disease Control and Prevention. (2012). *Vaccines and immunizations schedules.* Retrieved from http://www.cdc.gov/vaccines/schedules/easy-to-read/adult.html.

16. U.S. Department of Health and Human Services. (2012). *Healthy People 2020 topics and objectives: Immunizations and infectious diseases.* Retrieved from http://www.healthypeople.gov/2020/topicsobjectives2020/overview.aspx?topicid=23.

17. Lane A., Martin, M., & Neuman, M.E. (2009). Breast cancer screening program targeting rural Hispanics in southeastern Indiana: Program evaluation. *Hispanic Health Care International, 7*(3), 153-159.

18. Centers for Disease Control and Prevention. (2010). *HIV screening: Standard care.* Retrieved from http://www.cdc.gov/actagainstaids/hssc/index.html.

19. Centers for Disease Control and Prevention. (2010). *Screening for breast cancer.* Retrieved from: http://www.cdc.gov/cancer/breast/basic_info/screening.htm.

20. Centers for Disease Control and Prevention. (2010). *Colorectal screening program.* Retrieved from http://www.cdc.gov/cancer/crccp/.

21. Kemper, P., Savage, C.L., Niederbaumer, P., & Anthony, J. (2005). A study of the level of knowledge about diabetes management of low income persons with diabetes. *Journal of Community Health Nursing, 22*(4), 231-239.

22. Case Management Society of America. (2012). *Glossary: Case management.* Retrieved from http://www.cmsa.org/Consumer/GlossaryFAQs/tabid/102/Default.aspx.

23. Zander, K. (2002). Nursing case management in the 21st century: Intervening where margin meets mission. *Nursing Administration Quarterly, 26,* 58-67.

24. Taylor, P. (1999). Comprehensive nursing case management: an advanced practice model. *Nursing Case Management, 4,* 2-13.

25. Kaiser, K.L., Miller, L.L., Hays, B.J., & Nelson, F. (1999). Patterns of health resource utilization, costs, and intensity of need for primary care clients receiving public health nursing case management. *Nursing Case Management, 4,* 53-62.

26. Pellitier, K.R. (2011). A review and analysis of the clinical and cost effectiveness studies of comprehensive health promotion and disease management programs at the worksite: Update VIII 2008–2010. *Journal of Occupational and Environmental Medicine.* doi:10.1097/JOM.obo13e3182337748.

27. Pimouguet, C., Le Goff, M., Thiebaut, R., Dartigues, J.F. & Helmer, C. (2011). Effectiveness of disease-management programs for improving diabetes care: A meta-analysis. *Canadian Medical Association Journal, 183*(2). doi:10.1503/cmaj.091786.

28. VanLandeghem, K., & Brach, C. (2009, March). *Impact of primary care case management (PCCM) implementation on Medicaid and SCHIP* (CHIRI Issue Brief No. 8). Rockville, MD: Agency for Healthcare Research and Quality. AHRQ Pub. No. 090020.

29. U.S. Department of Health and Human Services. (2012). *Federally qualified health centers.* Retrieved from https://www.cms.gov/center/fqhc.asp.

30. National Association of Free Clinics. (n.d.). *What is a free or charitable clinic.* Retrieved from http://www.nafcclinics.org/about-us/what-is-free-charitable-clinic

31. Cummins, S., & Macintyre, S. (2002). "Food deserts"—evidence and assumption in health policy making. *British Medical Journal, 325,* 436-438.

32. *The public health effects of food deserts: Workshop summary* (p 1). (n.d.). Retrieved from http://books.nap.edu/catalog/12623.html.

33. U.S. Department of Agriculture. (2009). *Access to affordable and nutritious food-measuring and understanding food deserts and their consequences.* Retrieved from http://www.ers.usda.gov/publications/ap-administrative-publication/ap-036.aspx.

34. *The public health effects of food deserts: Workshop summary* (p 3). (n.d.). Retrieved from http://books.nap.edu/catalog/12623.html.

35. Olendzki, B. (2012). *Dietary and nutritional assessment in adults.* Retrieved from http://www.uptodate.com/contents/dietary-and-nutritional-assessment-in-adults.

36. Fung, T.T., Rimm, E.B., Spiegelman, D., Rifai N., Tofler G.H., Willett W.C., & Hu F.B. (2001). Association between dietary patterns and plasma biomarkers of obesity and cardiovascular disease risk. *American Journal of Clinical Nutrition, 73,* 61.

37. Phillips, S., & Jensen, C. (2012). *Dietary history and recommended dietary intake in children.* Retrieved from http://www.uptodate.com/contents/dietary-history-and-recommended-dietary-intake-in-children.

38. National Restaurant Association. (n.d.). *Facts at a glance.* Retrieved from http://www.restaurant.org/research/facts/.

39. Harrison, K., & Marske, A. (2005). Nutritional contents of foods advertised during the television programs children watch most. *American Journal Public Health, 95,* 1568.

40. Powell, S., Szczypka, G., Chaloupka, F., & Braunschweig, C.L. (2007). Nutritional content of television food advertisements seen by children and adolescents in the United States. *Pediatrics, 120,* 576.

41. American Psychology Association. (2012). *The impact of marketing on childhood obesity.* Retrieved from http://www.apa.org/topics/kids-media/food.aspx?item=1.

42. U.S. Department of Health and Human Services. (2012). *Healthy People 2020 topics and objectives: Nutrition and weight status.* Retrieved from http://www.healthypeople.gov/2020/topicsobjectives2020/objectiveslist.aspx?topicId=29.

43. Parsons, R. (2006, May 24). The idea that shook the world. *The Los Angeles Times.* Retrieved from http://articles.latimes.com/2006/may/24/food/fo-farmer24.

44. U.S. Department of Agriculture. (2012). *Farmers markets and local food marketing.* Retrieved from http://www.ams.usda.gov/AMSv1.0/FARMERSMARKETS.

45. Greenmarket. (2012). *Greenmarket farmers.* Retrieved from http://www.grownyc.org/greenmarket.

46. Olsan, D.A. (2011). *Mercury toxicity.* Retrieved from http://emedicine.medscape.com/article/819872-overview.

47. U.S. Environmental Protection Agency. (2012). *Mercury: Human exposure.* Retrieved from http://www.epa.gov/hg/exposure.htm.

48. McPhee, S., & Papdakus, M. (2010). *Current medical diagnosis & treatment* (49th ed., pp 1439-1440). New York, NY: McGraw-Hill.

49. Ohio Environmental Protection Agency. (2014). 2014 *Ohio Sport Fish Health and Consumption Advisory.* Retrieved from http://www.epa.ohio.gov/dsw/ fishadvisory/index.aspx.

50. Centers for Disease Control and Prevention & U.S. Environmental Protection Agency. (n.d.). *Pesticides: Controlling pests. Joint statement.* Retrieved from http://www.cdc.gov/nceh/ehs/Publications/Bed_Bugs_ CDC-EPA_Statement.htm.

51. Adashi, E., Geiger, J., & Fine, M. (2010). Health care reform and primary care—the growing importance of the community health center. *New England Journal of Medicine, 362,* 2047-2050. doi:10.1056/NEJp1003729.

52. Shin, P., Ku, L., Jones, E., Finnegan, B., & Rosenbaum, S. (2009). *Financing community health centers as patient and community centered medical home: A primer.* Washington, DC: The George Washington University. Retrieved from http://publichealth.gwu.edu/ departments/healthpolicy/CHPR/downloads/ PCMH_CHC.pdf.

53. American Nurses Association. (2013). *Public health nursing: Scope and standards of practice.* Silver Springs, MD: Author.

Chapter 17

Health Planning With Rural and Urban Communities

LEARNING OUTCOMES

After reading this chapter, the student will be able to:

1. Define and implement the concepts of community partnership, community linkage, and community collaboration.
2. Describe the unique characteristics of rural and urban environments.
3. Identify specific health needs of rural communities and of urban communities.
4. Discuss potential solutions to decrease disparities in rural areas.
5. Describe the steps in community organizing and coalition building, and identify how these activities can be a useful tool for positive community change.
6. Discuss the potential role of the nurse and the impact on the health-care system in community-based participatory research, parish nursing, healthy communities/healthy cities, nurse-managed clinics, and community academic partnerships.

KEY TERMS

Broken window theory
Coalition building
Collaboration
Community-based participatory research (CBPR)
Community empowerment
Community organizing
Community partnerships
Federally qualified health centers (FQHC)
Metropolitan statistical area (MSA)
Patient centered medical homes
Rural
Telehealth
Urban
Urban agglomeration

Nursing in Partnership With Communities

Communities want to create a more positive environment for their residents. Chicago with its Walking School Bus program has discovered a way to protect children from the dangers of drugs, guns, strangers, and speeding traffic but lets them continue to be active by walking daily to and from school.[1] The communities have not done this alone. They have formed partnerships with identified collaborators to make it happen. A partnership was built between the community, the schools, the city of Chicago, and the police department through its Chicago Alternative Policing Strategy (CAPS). Children need a safe, secure environment not just within the school but also in the community on the way to and from school, and creating partnerships with stakeholders can make it happen. The program provides a consistent, supervised system in which children can walk to school under the watchful eyes of adults. Instead of carpooling to drive children to school, parents share the responsibility of walking children to school with a carefully managed volunteer program. By taking the same route each day, the parent volunteer can pick up children at identified areas as they walk, similar to school bus stops. The positive outcomes have included reduced traffic congestion and dangers around schools, physically active and healthier children and adults, reduced noise and air pollution, increased community interaction with more "eyes on the street" to reduce crime, introduction of positive adult role models, healthier relationship between adults and children, and decreased incidence of bullying.[1] These partnerships create mutual benefits that are greater than what an individual alone can create.

Definition of *Partnership*

Community partnerships, as defined by the U.S. State Department, are collaborative working relationships "in which the goals, structure and governance, as well as roles and responsibilities, are mutually determined and decision-making is shared. Successful partnerships are characterized by complementary equities, openness and transparency, mutual benefit, shared risks and rewards, and accountability."[2] Services in the community that promote health are often fragmented. Health delivery services frequently do not communicate with the education system, work opportunities, or housing. This calls for more collaboration among these agencies, working on reaching outcomes together that couldn't be reached alone.

Collaboration is an essential component of successful nursing interventions. **Collaboration** as defined in the Minnesota Wheel (Chapter 2) as an activity that "commits two or more persons or organizations to achieve a common goal through enhancing the capacity of one or more of the members to promote and protect health."[3] On a family basis, a collaborative relationship exists when clients and nurses see each other as partners, with both providing expertise and knowledge that will help the family reach its goals. Interpersonal and communication skills are critical for successful collaboration at all levels of intervention.

A successful partnership is based on respect and equity in the collaboration whether it is the nurse and family or multiple organizations. A successful partnership has been described as having synergy, making it larger than the sum of its parts. The collaboration not only benefits the work of one agency and the clients they serve, but also benefits the other agencies and the clients they serve. Success is built on clear roles, responsibilities, shared vision about outcome and process, open and frequent communication among all the stakeholders, and better use of resources which increases what can be accomplished.

The Center on Education and Training for Employment at Ohio State University created a six-step guide to facilitate the development of community collaboration through linkage programs.[4] By agencies linking together, they better serve clients with emphasis on the community needs and not the individual agency.

1. **Step 1:** Assess the need to work in partnership with other agencies. The first step involves assessing the need and climate for interagency partnerships in your local area. Some problems are best solved by a single agency. However, many problems or needs cannot be accomplished by an agency acting alone or cannot be accomplished as effectively. Questions to ask could include: How might closer relationships with other agencies help improve outcomes for our clients? What problems or issues could be addressed more effectively through interagency linkages?
2. **Step 2:** State the key problems and issues; articulate why they are better addressed by multiple agencies; and name who the key players might be. Recognize current linkages and establish internal administrative support.
3. **Step 3:** Identify the key players. An important consideration is who should actually represent the organization on the team. Experience has demonstrated that team members should either be or have access to decision makers within their agencies.
4. **Step 4:** Establish a collaborative relationship and not just a cooperative one. Funders want collaborative efforts not only because such coalitions stretch resources, but also because they produce better results.
5. **Step 5:** Establish mutual goals and objectives and a plan, create an effective planning environment, formulate the plan, and develop administrative support for the plan.
6. **Step 6:** Implement the plan.[4]

Importance of Partnerships

This partnership and linkage of agencies into collaborative relationships can improve client access to appropriate programs, promote referrals between agencies, coordinate limited resources, improve working relationships, increase knowledge of the functioning of the partner agencies, and provide a more realistic expectation of how to work together.[4] In recent research, linkages among local health departments and the community are usually directed at a specific purpose or a specific program. It appears from the limited research available that local boards have a wide range of collaborative involvement (from low to high) with their communities and that most would benefit from working more collaboratively with communities in setting community health status priorities and in meeting those health objectives.[5]

In forming a partnership the U.S. Department of Education in the Regional Education Network suggests three important components.[6] First, make certain that the members of the partnership are as diverse as the community in culture, race, experience, and perspective. You need to be inclusive. Second, as soon as you have a beginning partnership start to move forward, you will have new partners join as the collaboration coheres. Third, make sure the partners commit to the process. In general, it is most effective and efficient when the same people attend the meetings and are the same people who can make decisions/commitments from their organization.

● APPLYING PUBLIC HEALTH SCIENCE

The Case of Community Organizing

Public Health Science Topics Covered:

- Organized community effort
- Environmental science

Public Health Nursing Skills

- Assessment
- Program planning
- Intervention: Advocacy

A public health nurse (PHN) was working in an inner-city **federally qualified health center (FQHC)**. FQHCs are a critical component of the health-care safety net and receive this designation and funding under Section 330 of the Public Health Service Act. There are over 1,000 FQHC health centers in the United States serving more than 20 million clients. The clinics are community based and provide comprehensive primary care and behavioral and mental health services to patients regardless of their ability to pay. The FQHCs will be continued under the Affordable Care Act.[7]

The PHN was interested in identifying additional resources and increasing services to the lower-income urban community whose members attended the FQHC where she worked. She talked with the clinic staff, primarily family nurse practitioners (FNPs) and primary care physicians. They were very supportive, mentioned some of their concerns, and encouraged her to discover what linkages could be made. She identified multiple agencies serving the community from Head Start programs to social service agencies to schools and local community organizers. She repeatedly asked what she could do to link with these agencies to provide better service to the clients at the FQHC.

The agencies all agreed that it would be good to have partnerships and several had suggestions concerning what could take place. However, they all shared with her information about a newly formed group that met every 2 weeks and included not only the agencies she had identified, but also the representatives of people who lived in the community, business owners, and religious leaders. The agencies said the group was quite diverse; everyone was welcomed, but if you attended, you made a commitment to make the process work. A social worker had initiated the group; after meeting with her, the PHN attended the meetings.

She participated in this group for more than 4 years and learned a great deal about linkages and partnerships. With everyone around a table, it was obvious that communication was clearer and actual decisions could be made. However, it was also clear that forming partnerships took considerable time, trust was not easy to establish, and the larger organizations were generally less flexible in their participation. The commitment to making the process work was time consuming and frequently frustrating.

Early on in her participation, one of the community organizers with representatives from his smaller community discussed the concern about a city incinerator that was polluting their area. The participants from this smaller community felt no one in the larger community had challenged the location of this incinerator because the residents were poor and disenfranchised, with little leverage in city hall. The residents of the community had tried to show their city representative the dangers, but had been ignored. Likewise, the city health department did not respond to their data. Everyone around this larger community table agreed that it was a public health menace and that as a group they might have an impact. Because of the diversity of the partnership, it took many directions. The community organizers looked at how the community could show the city leadership how they felt through very public demonstrations. Others sought assistance from the local university to measure air quality and identify potential health problems. Others sought out public relation resources and got the message out in the newspapers, on the radio, and on television. An issue that had been successfully hidden became quite public, and the city leadership shut down the incinerator. It didn't happen quickly, but it did happen. The group was energized. They had taken on a specific issue and had made a difference for their community.

People who had thought the group was a waste of time recommitted to it. By working together on community issues people got to know each other and more trust and communication resulted. Now that the group was organized around one issue, they could see the possibilities of organizing around others. During the time this PHN worked with the group, they were able to convince the police department to resume foot patrol in designated high-crime areas, especially streets where robberies, aggravated assaults, and homicides were the most frequent. The police patrolled in pairs starting at 10 a.m. and stopping at 2 a.m. in two shifts.

They frequently involved themselves in community work while on patrol but also were likely to stop suspicious cars and individuals. The crime rate dropped by 24% and there was very little displacement of crime to nearby areas. All the partners declared it a success.

The partnership in another linkage set up monitoring in the high schools to decrease violence, but also facilitated tutoring volunteers at the school. The community group was always particularly sensitive to equity within the community members. When it was clear that before a funded teenage violence prevention program could be implemented, other community concerns needed to be first met, everyone agreed. The needs were met and then the new program was implemented.

This organization is still in existence, has become a respected model in the community, and is enmeshed in working toward a healthier community that includes all the immediate and distal causes of poor health. No one agency could have done this; it took partnerships, linkages, dedicated work, and true community participation to make it work.

As seen in The Case of Community Organizing, the process of building a collaborative partnership is multidimensional. One thing that was especially true in the urban partnership just described is the development of a vision for long-term change. It took considerable time to develop trust among the collaborators, to develop the appropriate group structure, and to recognize and mobilize people to create the change. It is also important to have a wide variety of participants to form a complete view of the community strengths and needs, since it is essential to have participants who are invested in the goals and activities of the partnership.[6]

Rural Communities

People living in rural communities have particular strengths and needs that are different from those in the urban environment. Multiple statistical data show increased health disparities among residents of rural communities. These are a reflection of the variation in the economic and educational systems, differences in the social and cultural factors, and physical and political isolation. Rural individuals tend to be poorer, sicker, older, and to have less health insurance than those in metropolitan areas.[8]

Characteristics of Rural Residents

Individuals who live in the rural and frontier areas of the United States:

- Are more likely to smoke and drink excessive alcohol
- Have more dental problems, with 40 dentists per 100,000 persons in rural areas versus 60 per 100,000 in urban areas; this disparity is increasing and total number of dentists is decreasing
- Age faster and die younger; the age-adjusted death rates in rural counties are about 17% higher than those in urban counties for males and about 23% higher for females.
- Have different age proportion in their population, with 18% over age 65, a larger proportion under 18, and much smaller proportion in the age range who work, which creates a high dependency ratio
- Live at further distances from state-of-the-art healthcare facilities, and in general have more limited access to health care, often resulting in part from no or very limited public transportation
- Have less education with more not completing high school (23.5% in rural areas vs. 18.8% in urban areas) and fewer completing college (15.1% in rural areas vs. 26.4% in urban areas)
- Have a higher rate of poverty with the per capita income almost $10,000 lower in rural areas in 2011 ($31,415 in rural areas vs. $41,244 in urban areas), with nearly 24% of rural children living in poverty[9,10]

In 2004, more than 500 state and local rural health workers responded to a survey to help identify what component should be included in *Rural Healthy People 2010 (RHP 2010)*. This was a companion document to *Healthy People 2010 (HP 2010)* and identified the unique needs of the rural population in the United States Each respondent was asked to check five of the 28 *HP 2010* concerns that they considered to have the highest priority in rural health. The top five concerns selected were (1) access to quality health care, (2) heart disease and stroke, (3) diabetes, (4) mental health and mental disorders, and (5) oral health.[11] According to the designers of *RHP 2010*, the document has provided policy makers, rural providers, and rural communities with a valuable resource for planning and policy making. It was so useful that the process was repeated with *HP 2020*. A repeat survey was conducted from 2009 to 2010 to help determine rural health priorities for the *RHP 2020*. This resulted in some changes from the 2010 top five concerns, with access to quality health care still the number one priority (Table 17-1).[12]

TABLE 17–1	Top 10 Priorities Based on *Rural Healthy People 2020 Survey* Rank
Rank	**Priority**
1	Access to Quality Health Care
2	Diabetes
3	Mental Health and Mental Illness
4	Nutrition and Weight Loss
5	Heart Disease and Stroke
6	Substance Abuse
7	Physical Activity and Health
8	Older Adults
9	Cancer
10	Maternal, Infant, and Child Health

Source: See reference 12.

■ RURAL HEALTHY PEOPLE (RHP 2020)
The Promotion of the Health of Americans Living in Rural Communities

Goal: To identify rural health priorities and strategies
Purpose: The purpose of *Rural Healthy People 2020* (RHP 2020) is to advance the promotion of the health of Americans living in rural communities by identifying rural health priorities, supporting rural health leaders and researchers, and promoting effective rural health programs. Through the coordinated RHP 2020 initiative, rural communities will benefit by increased ability to identify and implement right-sized, effective health programs for rural residents. Like *Rural Healthy People 2010* a decade ago, RHP 2020 will provide policymakers, rural providers, and rural communities with an invaluable resource for documenting successes as well as challenges and for planning, thereby contributing to the rural health infrastructure for improving the health of rural populations. Specifically, RHP 2020 will identify and promote rural-specific health priority areas, document what is known about health in rural areas, identify rural evidence-based best practice programs, community practices and interventions, and promote rural healthy communities.[12]

Health providers have additional challenges working in rural communities.[9] In the United States, as in most countries, there is unequal distribution of health-care providers. Most often health-care providers stay in the metropolitan areas after they complete their education or purposefully select to settle in urban areas, attracted by the well-resourced health-care centers, cultural and recreational opportunities, better housing, better work option for other family members, and in general a perceived higher quality of life for the family. In 2000, the Health Resource and Service Administration reported that 19.2% of the U.S. population lived in rural area while 11.2% of physician practiced in rural area with 66% of the primary care health professional shortage areas located in rural areas.[9,12,13]

Definition of *Rural Communities*

Rural is defined based on population size, population density, or by proximity to larger metropolitan areas. Federal agencies, in defining a rural community, frequently first define an urban area and then, by exclusion, the remaining area is considered rural. The three most commonly used definitions of *rural* come from the U.S. Bureau of the Census, the Office of Management and Budget (OMB), and the U.S. Department of Agriculture (USDA). They all have slightly different definitions of *rural*. The U.S. Bureau of the Census defines *urban* by population density (Fig. 17-1). An urbanized area (UA) has a central city or core and a surrounding area that contains at least 50,000 people. There is a population density of at least 1,000 people per square mile and adjoining areas with at least 500 persons per square mile. Areas are considered rural that are composed of open country and settlements with less than 2,500 residents. Areas designated as rural can have population densities as high as 999 per square mile or as low as 1 person per square mile.[14,15] The OMB uses metropolitan statistical areas (MSA). Each MSA must include a city with 50,000 or more inhabitants or an urbanized area with at least 50,000 inhabitants and a total MSA population of 100,000. An MSA region contains the county with the urban area and all contiguous counties related to the city. All areas not included in the MSA are rural.[16] The USDA uses a code of 0 to 9 to differentiate urban and rural. Metropolitan counties are distinguished by size with a ranking of 0 to 3, and nonmetropolitan counties with 4 to 9 with 9 equal to completely rural or a population of fewer than 2,500 and not adjacent to a metropolitan area. In 2011 only 16% of the population was considered rural (51 million living in rural areas and 258 million in urban areas), the lowest ever; in 2000, 20% was rural, compared with 72% back in 1910.[10,17] Rural areas include open spaces and longer distances between neighbors (Fig. 17-2).

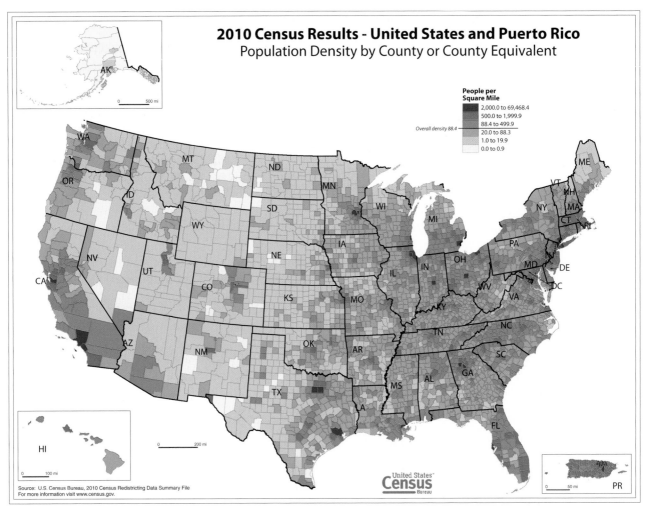

Figure 17-1 2010 Population density by county—United States and Puerto Rico. *(Retrieved from http://www.census.gov/geo/maps-data/maps/pdfs/thematic/us_popdensity_2010map.pdf.)*

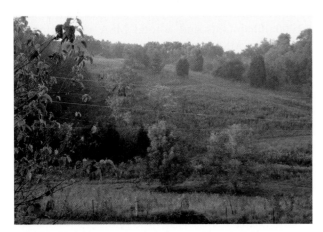

Figure 17-2 Rural Kentucky landscape. *(Photo by Christine Savage.)*

Specific Health Needs of Rural Communities

The biggest impediment to rural health care is the actual ability to access care. One factor is the long distances that individuals must travel to access care, especially state-of-the-art facilities (Fig. 17-2). Many rural health facilities are underfunded and understaffed, and many have had to close because of inadequate numbers of nurses and other health-care providers.[18] In addition, a larger percentage of rural dwellers have no or limited health insurance. Also, if there is an emergent situation, people in rural areas must wait on average 30 minutes or longer for ambulance service, whereas in urban areas the average wait is closer to 10 minutes.[19] Local governments often do not have the capabilities to provide safety net programs. Rural dwellers also have less access to ways to promote primary prevention such as exercising at gyms; and bike and walking trails are generally not available or some distance away.

Potential Solutions to Decrease Health Disparities

One solution to part of the problem of health disparities in rural areas is to provide more health care with an increase in physicians and health-care providers in the rural areas. Researchers have found that to retain health workers in rural areas it is important to have providers who come from small towns and who have a rural upbringing and an interest in becoming primary care physicians or nurse practitioners. One midwestern university has been proactive in identifying potential rural providers and giving them background in population health and a special rural-based curriculum. Collaboration and partnerships have formed the core of the program working with hospitals and family practitioners in the selected communities. It is important that universities recognize the need to purposely accept students from rural areas both in medicine and nursing who are likely to return to these areas to practice.[20] The Affordable Care Act (2010) does provide incentives for educating and training more health-care providers to work in rural areas, including nurses and primary care nurse practitioners in areas such as the Indian Health Service Centers.[21]

Another way to meet the challenge of providing care in rural areas, especially for those with noncommunicable diseases, is the use of the **patient centered medical home (PCMH)** model. The PCMH is an approach to primary care that aims to make care accessible, continuous, coordinated, family centered, comprehensive, compassionate, and culturally competent. The main components of the models as defined in the Bolin article[22] include:

- Patient- and family-centered full scope of care
- Access in time and location
- Coordinated, team-based (integrated) care
- Medication coordination and management
- Community linkages with transition
- Electronic records and other information systems support[22]

Bolin and colleagues suggest that this model used in rural communities would help address such issues as access, efficiency, quality, and sustainability while at the same time increase linkage with more integration and interdisciplinary practice. The Affordable Care Act of 2010 is designed to contribute resources to facilitating this medical home model in the rural setting.[21,22] This is an innovative example of partnerships and linkages that can decrease rural health disparities.

Telehealth, first developed in the 1970s, has also been shown in a variety of situations to be useful in increasing health access, decreasing some of the costs of health care, and increasing efficiency of providing the care. **Telehealth** is defined as providing health-related service where there is a distance between client and health-care provider, using electronic information and telecommunication technology. In addition to its other usefulness, Telehealth is important to nursing by improving the capacities of nurses in regions where there is a nursing shortage. It has been shown to decrease frequency of hospital visits and emergency hospital admissions and better management of noncommunicable diseases. Nurses use Telehealth in a variety of settings including home care, health clinics, schools, prisons, and hospitals to augment the existing clinical services.

Telehealth nursing has been defined and explained in an excellent fact sheet created by nurses who are members of the American Telemedicine Association[23] and supported by the International Council of Nurses.[24] The association lists multiple ways nurses employ telemedicine in a variety of settings. For example, nurses working in rural or isolated areas can telepresent a patient to a health-care provider for assessment and treatment for both emergent and nonemergent situations. Home health nurses use a monitoring system via phone or Internet wherein patients can send physiological data (e.g., blood pressure, pulse, respiratory peak flow) and images for review. Patients can call nurses to review how to give insulin or change a dressing. It provides an excellent resource for health education and counseling. Nurses also play an important role in creating, designing, developing, and implementing telehealth and e-health sites for the community. They are also active participants in researching the implementation of telehealth.[24]

Urban Communities

The shift from rural to urban is happening worldwide. In 2008, half of the world population was urban and half rural; by 2030, more than three-quarters of the world will be urbanized (Fig. 17-3). Much of the current shift is coming from the more rural low- and middle-income countries. As noted, the United States continues its trend toward urban living, as does the rest of the industrialized world, but currently at a slower rate than in Africa, Asia, and Latin America. Today, the largest metropolitan areas are identified as **urban agglomerations,** each an urban cluster that includes all of the built-up continuous

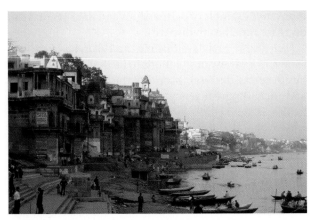

Figure 17-3 Urban cityscape: Varanasi, India. *(Photo by Chris Zahniser, BSN, R., MPH, 2000, Centers for Disease Control and Prevention.)*

urbanized area within a region. The region may include other distinct municipalities, which frequently results in the inconsistent identification of an agglomeration and the resulting population from one location to another. Some agglomeration may cross country borders as in San Diego–Tijuana (United States and Mexico) and Lille–Kortrijk (France and Belgium). Table 17-2 gives examples of the 10 largest agglomerations in 1975 and 2000, and projecting to 2025. It is interesting to note the changes in location of the largest agglomerations and the significant increase in population for each of them.[25]

Urbanization and the growth of the large central city in the United States accelerated in the 1800s with industrialization, immigration, and the Civil War. By the 1920s, there was a new landscape of high-rise buildings, and more than half of the U.S. population lived in cities. With changes in availability of mortgages for new homes, better roads, and more cars, after World War II the urban centers again shifted. Reflected in the 1970 U.S. census, it was clear the urban population had dispersed from the concentrated central city environment to the suburbs as a result of easier transport, economic ability to own single-family homes, and the desire of many to get away from the intense population concentration.[25] One of the factors contributing to the migration from urban settings was the phenomenon of "white flight." The majority of the population that left the urban setting for the surrounding suburbs were whites in higher

TABLE 17–2	Top 10 Largest Urban Agglomerations 1975, 2000, and Projected for 2025				
Cities 1975	Millions of Inhabitants	Cities 2000	Millions of Inhabitants	Cities 2025	Projected Millions of Inhabitants
1. Tokyo, Japan	26.6	1. Tokyo, Japan	34.5	1. Tokyo, Japan	36.4
2. New York, Newark, USA	15.9	2. Mexico City, Mexico	18	2. Mumbai (Bombay), India	26.4
3. Mexico City, Mexico	10.7	3. New York, Newark, USA	17.9	3. Delhi, India	22.5
4. Osaka-Kobe, Japan	9.8	4. São Paulo, Brazil	17.1	4. Dhaka, Bangladesh	22
5. São Paulo, Brazil	9.6	5. Bombay, India	16.1	5. São Paulo, Brazil	21.4
6. Los Angeles, Long Beach, Santa Ana, USA	8.9	6. Shanghai, China	13.2	6. Mexico City, Mexico	21
7. Buenos Aires, Argentina	8.8	7. Calcutta, India	13.1	7. New York, Newark, USA	20.6
8. Paris, France	8.6	8. Delhi, India	12.4	8. Calcutta, India	20.6
9. Calcutta, India	7.9	9. Buenos Aires, Argentina	11.9	9. Shanghai, China	19.4
10. Moscow, Russian Federation	7.6	10. Los Angeles, Long Beach, Santa Ana, USA	11.8	10. Karachi, Pakistan	19.1

Source: United Nations World Urbanization Prospects: the 2007 Revision.

income brackets, resulting in a negative impact on the city through a direct reduction in the tax base as well as a deterioration of both the social and physical environment of the city.[26] Today, these suburban towns have again shifted from being bedroom communities for the central city to having their own commercial areas, industry, and jobs within their own community.

Bradley and Katz point out that many Americans idealize the values of rural living where life is less frenetic, but in actuality the majority of Americans choose to live in the metropolitan areas where the economy is, the community is, and where they see their future—not in the small towns. Urban life was initially painted as unhealthy and very isolating. Today, people see that community and interconnectedness, important American values, occur in metropolitan areas as well as in more rural areas, and that American values are not tied to small towns but occur everywhere.[27]

Definition of *Urban*

From the perspective of the U. S. Census Bureau, what constitutes an **urban** area is defined for each census. For the 2010 U.S. census, the definition used is tied to population density (Box 17-1). As identified in defining *rural,* the area surrounding an urban core is a **metropolitan statistical area (MSA)**. The U.S. Census Bureau delineates an MSA as one or more adjacent counties or county equivalents that have at least one urban core area of at least 50,000 residents, plus adjacent territory that has a high degree of social and economic integration, with the

core as measured by commuting ties. A central urbanized area represents a contiguous area of relatively high population density. The counties containing the core urbanized area are known as the central counties of the MSA. Additional surrounding counties (known as outlying counties) can be included in the MSA if these counties have strong social and economic ties to the central counties as measured by commuting and employment. Some areas within these outlying counties are actually rural in nature.

These metropolitan areas are ranked by population. For example, using 2010 census data the New York–Northern New Jersey–Long Island, NY–NJ–PA, MSA was the largest, with a population of 18,897,109 and the Carson City, Nevada, MSA was the smallest, with a population of 55,274.[28]

Those living in these MSAs are tied to the social and economic climate of the urban core. Today, the country is quite urbanized with 67% of the population living in the largest 100 MSAs and 84% living in one of the 363 metropolitan statistical areas (see Fig. 17-1).[28] Urban living increases the density of population and currently in the United States a little more than 80% of the population live on 20% of the land.[25] Although there are more documented health issues with higher morbidity and mortality in the rural areas of the United States, there continue to be serious health problems that reflect on the conditions of our cities and are specific to urban living. The medical historian David Rosner wrote, "One lesson from history is that we create our own environment and hence we create the conditions within which we live and die."[29] Many of our health problems are of our own making, which can include communicable diseases (HIV/AIDS, tuberculosis, and Severe Acute Respiratory Syndrome [SARS]), poverty, homelessness, racism, and other social determinants of health. Creating a more positive environment for the public's health, whether it is rural or urban has the potential to benefit all.

Characteristics of the Urban Population

With our concern about how the public's health is related to urbanization, it is important to consider not only the number of people in an urban environment but also the size/density and economic status of the cities in which these individuals are living. As nurses, when we take a public health perspective to examine the issue, we can look at what influences urban living conditions from a perspective of both upstream and downstream factors. There are urban pockets of health needs that are as significant as those in the rural areas. We see this in areas with abandoned housing and community disorganization

---

BOX 17–1   2010 U.S. Census Bureau Definition of an Urban Area

For the 2010 U.S. Census, an urban area comprised a densely settled core of census tracts and/or census blocks that met minimum population density requirements, along with adjacent territory containing nonresidential urban land uses as well as territory with low population density included to link outlying densely settled territory with the densely settled core. To qualify as an urban area, the territory identified according to criteria had to encompass at least 2,500 people, at least 1,500 of which reside outside institutional group quarters. The Census Bureau identifies two types of urban areas:
• Urbanized areas (UAs) of 50,000 or more people;
• Urban clusters (UCs) of at least 2,500 and less than 50,000 people. *Rural* encompasses all population, housing, and territory not included within an urban area.

Source: See reference 14.

and their associated higher rates of sexually transmitted infections (STIs), drug addiction, homicide, and suicide.[30]

The needs themselves may be quite different and demand different solutions, but health disparity also persists in the urban environment. There is marked disparity in socioeconomic status (see Chapter 7), higher rates of crime and violence (see Chapter 12), prevalence of different but significant social and psychological stress, and the presence of marginalized populations groups.[31] Mental health needs and excessive exposure to violence and trauma are also part of the urban environment and can cause increased mental illness (see Chapter 10). In the densely populated areas, there may be a lack of affordable places to exercise and the air quality may be poor, especially for those with chronic respiratory disease (Chapter 6). The 10th annual American Lung Association *State of the Air* report found that 6 out of 10 Americans, 186.1 million people, live in almost exclusively major metropolitan areas where air pollution levels endanger lives.[32] Some of the urban population also lacks adequate health insurance, especially the poor, minorities, and undocumented immigrants. These individuals experience some of the same barriers to care that the rural population experiences, although access through emergency departments may be somewhat easier. In general, this marginalized population receives less and poorer quality care with few preventive health-care measures than do those urbanites with adequate health insurance. There are generally more available safety nets in urban areas such as FQHCs, health department clinics, community health centers, and specialty clinics, but this puts an enormous strain on the local metropolitan economic system, especially if it provides uncompensated care.[33]

Some of the things that may contribute to better health in cities is the exposure to more variance among the population including more economic and educational opportunities, more diverse social networks, more engaged civil society, and more and better health and social resources in closer proximity to the population. In addition, the new immigrants to the United States have brought with them their own culture, values, and sense of community, which changes the dynamic of community partnerships. The way communities mobilize is influenced by the culture and history of the residents. This can make the communities vibrant and open to change.[34]

Role of the Public Health Nurse

Community assessment, diagnosis, program planning, interventions, and evaluation are essential public health nursing skills for the urban environment (see Chapters 4 and 5). As no two rural areas are the same, identification of the problems and the interventions selected are community-specific. It is important for the PHN to look for and build the collective efficacy of the community. A community with residents who are willing to intervene on behalf of the common good provides a neighborhood cohesion that can promote health. Working as a cohesive group, a community can access resources not available to individuals, and as a group it can respond to threats from inside and outside the community, something that is not possible on an individual level. The community can form partnerships and links with local government, other organizations, and other communities, making it easier to produce positive change. This is an example of the development of social capital where resources become available through their social connections. Some studies have shown better health outcomes in communities with increased social capital when the social capital is measured as reciprocity, trust, and civic participation.[35]

A common environmental experience in the poor urban areas is community upheaval. Buildings are abandoned and subsequently torn down; then urban renewal takes over—all creating urban disruption. When people lose their homes and social network, they experience significant stress and grief at what they have lost. With building destruction, the community may be exposed to different ecological environmental threats, for example, increased lead and other potential dangerous particulates in the air, such as asbestos. With an increase in abandoned buildings, the rodent population may find a new niche in the ecosystem. With community disorganization, there may be more homelessness, and more drug use in the neighborhood. The whole social milieu changes and resources once easily available disappear. Managing daily life becomes difficult. The informal ties of a community are important to the functioning of the community, and when these are destroyed, most frequently in poor minority areas, the neighborhood system suffers and health disparities increase.[35]

Living in a disordered urban community where there is more crime, violence, and drug use may influence the activities of the community residents, especially those who are adolescents or just reaching adulthood. Furr-Holden and colleagues examined how increasing neighborhood disorder, measured by numbers of abandoned buildings, affected marijuana use among adolescents maturing into adulthood. They also found that those living in increasingly deteriorating neighborhoods were more likely to use marijuana than those who were living in a more ordered community. They used several theories in developing their research. One was specific to disordered society and family incivility. A component of this theory is the **broken window theory:** Broken windows that remain unrepaired signal that there is disrespect for the property and for the community in general. Further damage appears to be sanctioned and disorder ensues, with the feeling that no one will intervene, official or otherwise, to stop the disorder in the community. This allows people to violate social norms they would otherwise respect. The laws of the street rather than the laws of society now govern the neighborhoods.[36]

Community Organization and Public Health Nursing

Whether the public health need is in the rural or urban environment, the development of partnerships and linkages can be the difference between ongoing sustained success and short-term programs that produce few long-lasting outcomes

Community Organizing

Community organizing is an identified public health nursing activity in both the rural and urban communities. It has proved to be a useful tool for creating positive change domestically and internationally.

Definition of Community Organizing

Using the knowledge and definition of **community organizing** by experts in the field, the Minnesota Wheel defines this activity as "helping community groups to identify common problems or goals, mobilize resources, and develop and implement strategies for reaching the goals they collectively have set."[37,38]

Minkler and colleagues point out the importance of including the concept of community empowerment as a logical component of community organizing. Without empowering the community, the organizing has not been successful.[38] **Community empowerment** is defined as the social action process of increasing the capacity of individuals or groups to make choices and to transform those choices into desired actions and outcomes.[39] This empowerment occurs when the community has adequate access to information and the community members are included and participate in decision-making forums. The community must have the power to hold the decision makers accountable and have the capacity and resources to organize, to take on roles as partners with government and private agencies, and to make decisions about things that affect their interests.[40] The process of empowerment, especially with low-income and marginalized groups, can

be expected to take place only over an extended time period. By collaborating with organizations that have community settings that promote empowerment, the nurse can facilitate the development of empowerment by partnering with congregations, community centers, neighborhood organizations, educational settings, and civil rights and social justice organizations.[41]

Usefulness as a Tool for Change

Community organizing can be important in many facets of public health nursing. When providing health education or when you want to introduce a new intervention program into the community, you are more successful if you start with what the community wants and address their perceived needs, which are identified through community organizing. Likewise, simply the process of organizing a community with member participation and social involvement can in itself lead to a healthier community.[42]

Community organizing is not new in the United States and was used in the 1800s in a variety of communities. Women successfully got the right to vote and workers a 40-hour workweek through local organizing. However, the major focus of organizing until the middle of the 20th century was to help the community solve problems through cooperation, collaboration, and consensus. In the 1950s, the community organizer in Chicago, Saul Alinsky, and others introduced the community organizing strategy of conflict and confrontation to creat dissatisfaction to try to solve power imbalances. In the 1960s and 1970s, organizing took on the broader focus to create social change throughout the whole country, as reflected in the civil rights movement, the protest against the war in Vietnam, women's rights, gay rights, and the dwindling of our natural resources in the environment. Today, there are even newer changes with the introduction of the Internet as a tool for organizing.

The World Health Organization (WHO) has utilized a community organizing approach in interventions focused on improving the health of communities.[39] An example is the use of the community-directed intervention (CDI) strategy used in Africa to help combat the Onchocerciasis also known as river blindness caused by a parasitic worm.[43] In their tool box, *Resources for Organizing and Social Change*, a community organizing group in Maine suggests seven basic principles for creating social change through community organizing:

1. Use nonviolence in creating the change.
2. Find the root causes of the problems, look upstream, and create solutions that will improve things for everyone.

3. Provide communities the opportunity and support to work with each other to solve their problems.
4. Be concerned about economic equity throughout the community.
5. Help the community to gain power to control their own lives, and maximize their access to the decision-making processes that affect them.
6. Promote social equality with participation and leadership roles for those who frequently experience discrimination.
7. Be concerned about the sustainability of the environment.[44]

Other suggestions on how to organize a community include doing something interesting or unique to attract the attention of community members to engage them in the process. Always reach out for new members, keeping active lists of how individuals wish to participate. Recruit face-to-face, follow-up consistently, and encourage diverse leadership.[45] Make fundraising a regular part of the program, involve as many people in the group as possible, plan on more than one source of income, and keep good records. Throughout the literature, there is a repeated word of caution: A community has the capabilities, given the resources, to make its own decisions and it is important for those assisting with the organizing and providing the resources not to become part of the leadership of the organization, dictating policy and action, but rather to help to amplify the voices of the community.

Although community organizing is often a tool for community change, frequently over a contentious topic such as the removal of an incinerator or the use of a street patrol to decrease crime, it can also be used as part of a program intended to mobilize the community to initiate public health programs such as reducing smoking or limiting cardiovascular risk.[46, 47] In one study, community organizing was used as a tool to form coalitions between the university and different components of the surrounding community with the purpose of decreasing indicators of high-risk drinking by college students. Particular attention was paid to equity in the partnerships, because universities frequently appear to have more power than the communities in which they exist and tend to drive the relationships. As a result of this community organizing the interventions, schools compared with the control schools demonstrated at the end of 3 years decreased severe consequences resulting from the students' own drinking and alcohol-related injuries to others. The community organizing approach implemented new programs, changed institutional policies, and increased law enforcement efforts to prevent underage drinking on campus and in the community.[48]

Process of Community Organizing

As indicated, there are several steps in the process of community organizing. The PHN can immerse herself in the community, participating in activities, talking with residents, making home visits, and meeting the formal and informal leaders. This takes time because mutual respect and trust do not develop rapidly. The nurse will get to know the structure of the community, the issues discussed in the community, the strengths, and the problems. It is all part of community assessment, but it is more than community assessment because the nurse is really trying to assimilate into the community. It is only after doing so that the nurse can start to understand the strengths and problems the community has identified and begin to understand what role she might play in helping the community to organize, become empowered, and help create social change.

After the nurse has begun to understand the community, it is important to integrate the local leaders into a core group that can help identify and organize the community around public health needs. Next, the group can motivate others to respond to the same issues, encouraging collective action. After the problems have been identified and there is an interested group with leadership skills, the core group is ready to take action and mobilize the community. It is important that, before there is action, the group has clear goals, knows the resource availability, and has identified who will hinder and who will support the action. After every action is taken, the group reflects and evaluates to measure the successful outcomes and determine what still needs to be done. A more permanent organization may be formed with shared leadership under a simple structure. Also, after building the organization with multiple actions and reflection and building good leadership (good community capacity), it is time to step back and let the community independently own the organization.[49]

Coalition Building

Coalition building is another tool that the nurse can use to enhance community capacity.

Definition of Coalition Building

Coalition building is, according to the Minnesota Wheel, "promoting and developing alliances among organizations or constituencies for a common purpose. It builds linkages, solves problems, and/or enhances local leadership to address health concerns."[49] Key factors in coalition building are the readiness of the community to solve its problem, its willingness to work with multiple organizations to do that, and the motivation to solve the problem coming from within the community. Strong personal links to individuals and organizations within the community have been shown to create more successful coalitions.[50] Coalitions bring together community resources and have been most successful when mobilizing and focusing resources. Coalitions are less successful at actual implementation of programs, and communities have found it best to delegate the actual service delivery to community organizations that have the capacity to do it.[51, 52] McKay and Hewlett, two nurses who have participated in grassroots coalition building, suggest that nurses have the education and experience to formulate health delivery models and workforce solutions through successful coalition building. They offer 10 success strategies for building successful grassroots coalitions (Box 17-2).[53]

▶ SOLVING THE MYSTERY
The Case of the Mysterious Rise in Sexually Transmitted Infections

Public Health Science Topics Covered

- Epidemiology
  - Surveillance
  - Comparison of rates
- Health planning
  - Community organizing
  - coalition building

BOX 17–2 McKay and Hewlett's 10 Success Strategies for Coalition Building

1. Rally around a common issue/cause that has an impact on the public's health.
2. Establish and maintain key relationships.
3. Create a central entity and brand identity.
4. Fund the coalition's work.
5. Identify and support your champions.
6. Craft and disseminate the message.
7. Recognize roadblocks and develop plans to remove them.
8. Gain momentum and reach a tipping point.
9. Close the loop.
10. Share credit for successes.

Source: See reference 53.

- PHN Skills
  - Assessment
  - Health planning
  - Community diagnosis
  - Organization and management
  - Community partnerships

Health-care providers from two FQHCs, three private clinics, and one university-sponsored clinic in an underserved urban community formed a partnership to better serve the community. They met monthly to discuss innovative strategies and shared programs, especially in the area of primary prevention. The agenda for the current meeting was how to best serve the increasing number of clients without health insurance. Each of the clinics was approaching the problem from a slightly different direction and they thought a more unified plan seemed ideal. While talking about this, one of the nurses from the university clinic mentioned in passing that they were seeing a marked increase in the number of clients with no health insurance and who tested positive for STIs. One of the FNPs at the FQHC said she was also seeing more STIs in the family planning clinic. At the end of the meeting, the health-care providers had both a plan for how to better serve the uninsured and a surveillance plan for each clinic to gather data on current levels of STIs with a comparison of STI rates 1 year ago.

At the next meeting, all six clinics reported that they had seen between a 6% and 15% increase in STIs, especially gonorrhea and Chlamydia. It was almost exclusively in the young adult population between 18 and 28. The PHN at the clinic suggested that they contact other agencies in the community to see whether they would form a linkage to help solve the problem. The health-care providers agreed and said they would ask their patients, now that the problem was identified, about why they thought there was an increase. Others suggested a collaboration with the health department and other official agencies.

The next week, the PHN was talking with one of the community police officers. He said there had been a raid on a gambling operation in the community and several young community residents had been arrested. As part of the arrest processing, the young men received several health screenings. This police officer was shocked at the number of young men who had tested positive for STIs. It was higher than in any other community.

The PHN worked with a group of community organizers who were helping empower the community to achieve better health. When she met with them later in the week, she mentioned the increase in the number of young men and women with STIs in the neighborhood. They said they would put this on the agenda for their next community meeting. This group had been meeting over the past 2 years, had developed a shared vision and mission, and had successfully created positive change for the community. The PHN from the university clinic and two of the health-care providers from the FQHCs attended the next community meeting. The problem of the increased STIs was presented. The health-care providers reported that their patients were surprised that there was an increase in numbers, but said they were glad that they could be seen without insurance as the free health department STI clinic had closed 9 months ago. Some of the community leaders spoke up and said the health department downsized and closed the clinic even though community members had wanted it to stay open. They stated that the closest free STI clinic was now more than 10 miles away in a different ethnic and racial community and required two bus transfers to reach it. The group voted to work on solving this problem.

Using linkages and collaborative relationships, various community members collected and analyzed the soaring STI data, figured out the cost benefit of reopening a local health department clinic, and talked to key informants in the community and people who had used the clinic in the past. The community reported that it had been a well-subscribed walk-in clinic, and now community members were waiting much longer to seek care, trying to find money for treatment to avoid going to the another community for care, and waiting for an appointment. Without the local health department clinic, there rarely was active follow-up on sexual contacts and it seemed that the STIs were here to stay. Two community residents were chosen to represent the community at the next health department meeting. The health department listened respectfully to the community presentation and was both receptive and surprised by all the information. Within 8 weeks, the health department formally agreed that it was appropriate to reopen the clinic, and concurred that a member of the community organization could be on the board of the new STI clinic to enhance communication, service, and evaluation.

Community-Based Participatory Research

Community-based participatory research (CBPR) adds the community to research. Partnerships and coalition building are tools employed in CBPR, using shared power, respect, and equity between the researchers and the community. Public health nurses, already active in communities, are excellent resources to introduce community members to the researchers, participate in developing the research protocols, and help in interpreting the collected data. Actively engaging the community equitably in all aspect of the research process, frequently starting with a topic of importance to the community, promotes shared knowledge, expertise, and responsibility. It makes the outcome of the research more valid and useable in translating the research into practice. At the same time, it also can promote community development related to health disparities, as was demonstrated in a study that decreased environmental hazards and increased community health.[54,55]

When used in public health, CBPR has been defined as "a collaborative approach to research that equitably involves all partners in the research process and recognizes the unique strengths that each brings."[56] Partnerships can lead to sustainable changes.[57]

To address health disparities, an important part of *HP2020,* the Centers for Disease Control and Prevention has funded REACH 2010 projects (Racial and Ethnic Approaches to Community Health by 2010). These CBPR projects occur across the United States and address one of the following health priority areas: infant mortality, diabetes, cardiovascular disease, child/adult immunization, HIV/AIDS, and breast and cervical cancers. Wynn and colleagues acknowledge nine foundational principles of CBPR, similar to the principles of coalition building and linkages:

1. Community is the unit of identity.
2. Utilize the community strengths and resources.
3. Partner equity in all components of the research.
4. Provide opportunity for capacity building and co-learning.
5. Balance the research of knowledge generation and intervention
6. Identify the relevant public health problem.
7. Involve system development using a cyclical and iterative process.
8. Disseminate findings to all partners.
9. Start the project with plans for sustainability.[58]

Another emphasis in CBPR is building community capacity. Different definitions of community capacity building emphasize the community's capacity to identify and create change to address public health problems with the use of knowledge, skills, and resources. In one CBPR study, the collaboration of community and researcher increased community capacity to decrease environmental triggers for asthma.[54]

Public health nurses who practice in the community can help introduce researchers to the community. One of the challenges for the nurse who engages in CBPR is addressing the ethical issues that arise. Typically, ethical considerations in the conduct of human subject research focus on protecting the individual, but CBPR requires addressing ethical issues related to protecting the community.[59] These issues include ensuring that there is a benefit to the community related to the research, that there is a true sharing of the leadership roles, and that there is protocol established on sharing data collected on members of the community with community members who are on the research team. Bastida, Tseng, Mckeever, and Jack (2010) provide six principles that address these ethical issues and can help guide the nurse participating in this type of research (Box 17-3).[60]

Population Nursing Roles in the Community

In public health nursing, there are many types of employment in which the primary client is the community. We will examine three such areas for work as exemplars of what PHNs do in the community. All three of these can take place in both the urban and rural environments.

Parish Nursing/Faith Community Nursing

Faith community nursing is a specialty practice with its own scope and standards. Although parish nursing began in Christian congregations, it has grown to encompass

---

BOX 17–3   Six Principles for the Ethical Conduct of Community-Based Participatory Research

Principle 1. Respect the voice of the community and build on their contribution
Principle 2. Fiduciary transparency
Principle 3. Fairness among all stakeholders
Principle 4. Informed consent: always voluntary
Principle 5. Reciprocity with shared goals, dedication, and responsibility
Principle 6. Equal voice and full disclosure at each meeting for all members with study findings presented and shared with the community in respectful and understandable way

Source: See reference 60.

---

an inclusive approach to nursing within the context of a spiritual community. It is defined as follows:

> Faith community nurses are licensed, registered nurses who practice wholistic health for self, individuals, and the community using nursing knowledge combined with spiritual care. They function in paid and unpaid positions as members of the pastoral team in a variety of religious faiths, cultures, and countries. The focus of their work is on the intentional care of the spirit, assisting the members of the faith community to maintain and/or regain wholeness in body, mind, and spirit.[61]

As the practice of faith community nursing continues to evolve, the roles and organizational arrangements mature. The faith community nurse frequently provides population-centered individual care, with the congregation the population of service. The faith community nurse activities are, therefore, specific to the uniqueness of each congregation. The community needs assessment within the congregation is one action that assists the nurse in identifying these distinctive and appropriate activities. Assessment is the first core public health function and the first step in the planning process for program design, implementation, and evaluation for the unique congregation (see Chapter 4).[62]

Parish nursing was first envisioned by Reverend Dr. Granger Westburg, and first practiced in 1985 as a pilot project in Park Ridge, Illinois, a suburb of Chicago. The specialty has grown rapidly and now more than 12,000 nurses in the United States have received specialty education to practice faith-based nursing.[62] These nursing activities, some generally not found in more traditional practice sites, include:

- Health promotion, health education, and personal health counseling for the congregation
- Monitoring and screening for health problems
- Advocacy for individuals and groups
- Collaboration within the church and with organizations outside the church. Frequently, it involves establishing linkages with government and health-care agencies and local nongovernmental organizations. Establish new needed service for the congregation
- Congregational health assessment of the faith community, followed with analysis and program implementation
- Spiritual care through shared faith beliefs individually and in groups, such as grief counseling, substance abuse[62]

Qualifications for parish nursing for these activities include being both organized and flexible, a good communicator, and self-regulating. Specific requirements in most congregations also include:

- An active nursing license in the state where the person will practice as a parish nurse
- Baccalaureate degree in nursing preferred, with the concomitant public health nursing education. Experience in public health nursing is an advantage
- Graduate of a preparatory course about the specialty practice of parish nursing
- Mature and spiritual in nursing practice
- Have a clear understanding and support the spiritual teaching of the faith organization[63]

One of the unique components of this role is the spiritual care practice that integrates health and faith. For Christians, this involves a combination of health care and the Gospel, with a view of health from a biblical perspective. One study found that within the whole experience of receiving spiritual care from a Christian nurse, there were four phases. First, the patients found a safe place to tell their story and to be accepted. A relationship of trust was very important. In the second phase, patients were able to release their burden and reorient their thoughts. In the third phase, they revised their self-perception. In the fourth phase, they were able to find a new place with God and in the church community.[64]

Healthy Cities and Healthy Communities

The Healthy Cities movement is a WHO global project that resulted from the Alma-Ata Declaration in 1978 that emphasized social justice and equity with local community participation in health program design and implementation. Since 1987, there have been about 90 participant cities in Europe that have as their goal emphasizing equity and health in all the government sectors, especially at the local level with community participatory governance and emphasis on the determinants of health.[66] This local involvement can promote public health leadership and create environments that allow for healthier living. In Europe, this has been a structured, five-phased process with cities working to meet a range of health indicators that are defined in each phase. In other cities around the world and in the United States (Boston, Baltimore, and Denver), the same doctrines have been supported, but with less overriding structure.[67] The opportunity for community participation is there for nurses and especially for PHNs who are already a working part of the community. This is a real opportunity to work at decreasing disparities, especially health disparities.

Nurse-Managed Health Centers

Nurse-managed primary health-care centers are an important part of our health-care system. They are staffed by advanced practice nurses who can help provide the much-needed primary care for Americans (Fig. 17-4). Currently, they serve as a significant safety net for the medically underserved. With the implementation of the Affordable Care Act, there is a marked increase in need for primary care providers, as many of the 31 million currently uninsured are able to seek care. In 2011 it was estimated that there were over 200 nurse-managed health centers,[65] with 2 million patient encounters annually. They are known to provide high-quality, cost-effective care with the endorsement of the community. These clinics have the capacity to expand in order to provide care for many more.

● APPLYING PUBLIC HEALTH SCIENCE

The Case of the Family That Had Nowhere to Go

Public Health Science Topics Covered:

- Health service systems
- Intervention: advocacy

Mary and James Wilson and their two young children lived in a small rural community and had received primary care from a health maintenance organization through James's health insurance plan at work. When James lost his job because the manufacturing company closed, moving its operation overseas, the family lost their health insurance. Both Mary and James eventually

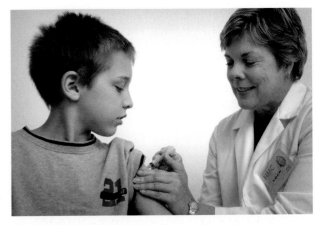

Figure 17-4 Nurse-managed care. *(From Centers for Disease Control and Prevention, courtesy of Judy Schmidt, #9423. Photographer, James Gathany, 2006.)*

found part-time work, but neither received any benefits with their jobs. They were able to meet most of their financial expenses if they were very careful, but would have to pay out of pocket for their health care. There was only one private clinic, and it was 20 miles from their home and very expensive. Even though it meant missing a day from work, Mary took the children to the local health department for well childcare, including immunizations. Because Mary and James were young and healthy, they thought they could get by without seeking any medical care. They had nowhere to go for health care that they could afford.

Things were fine for about 9 months, but then one of the children got sick and then the second. The health department did not provide sick care, and the private clinic was just too expensive. However, Mary was quite concerned when the children did not improve with over-the-counter medication, and finally got the courage to approach the PHN at the health department for assistance. The nurse was concerned about the health of the whole family, but she was pleased that there was a solution. Several weeks earlier, a rural nurse-managed primary care clinic had opened in a neighboring small town, and the providers there saw uninsured patients using a sliding scale for payment.

Mary and James were uncertain about the quality of care received in a nurse-managed clinic. The PHN introduced them to two families that were using the clinic. The families reassured the Wilsons, who felt they had little choice with no other accessible primary care. They were easily able to get an appointment and were relieved that the cost would be manageable. Mary was pleased when she met the pediatric nurse practitioner who cared for the children. The nurse practitioner seemed competent in her examination and treatment, was very friendly, and took time to talk with the children to relieve their anxiety. She spoke with Mary about what she could do to help manage the problem and to prevent it in the future. Mary felt that the nurse practitioner really listened to the issues and concerns of the family and understood their economic limitations. The nurse practitioner even suggested that they should apply for the State Children's Health Insurance Program, because they qualified and it would cover the medical care cost for the children (see Chapter 19). Mary was so reassured that she made an appointment for herself to receive a Papanicolaou smear and a breast examination. When she got home that night, she told James that she felt that they once again had a medical home and a practitioner upon whom they could rely.

Community-Academic Partnerships

An example of a partnership between a university and a community organization can take on the appearance of an educational program for minority students in the community, with the added benefit of providing an opportunity for the students to do community outreach and learn firsthand with the community organization about program planning, implementation, and addressing health disparities.[68]

In a different example, forming a partnership between a university and a variety of community groups leads to an increased awareness of how complex diabetes is in the community and unites the partners to work together to create social change and place emphasis on prevention. This includes partners not only in the health and social sectors, but also in the business and religious sectors. It emphasizes the importance of community research to create social action and positive change.[69]

■ EVIDENCE-BASED PRACTICE
Providing Supportive Housing for Individuals and Families With Special Needs

Practice Statement: Center for Urban Community Services (CUCS) is a supportive housing model aimed at increasing housing stability for urban-dwelling individuals and families.

Targeted Outcomes: The targeted outcomes include decreasing: (1) homelessness, (2) use of emergency room services, (3) acute care and, (4) mental health services.

Evidence to Support: Supportive housing interventions were introduced in the 1980s, with the goal of providing both housing and support services to homeless individuals. It has since expanded to include other vulnerable populations including at-risk families, seniors, people living with HIV/AIDs, and veterans. The intervention includes the provision of affordable apartments that blend with the community and provide access to support services needed, including health care. Permanent supportive housing is supported by the Substance Abuse and Mental Health Services Administration as an evidence-based approach, and it has published a tool kit for getting started. Evidence demonstrates not only that the individuals and families who receive supportive house have improved outcomes, but also that communities benefit.

References

1. Centers for Urban Community Services. (2013). *Supportive housing.* Retrieved from http://www.cucs.org/training-and-consulting/evidence-based-practice-offerings/supportive-housing.
2. Supportive Housing Network of New York. (2013). *Neighborhood impact.* Retrieved from http://shnny.org/research-reports/research/neighborhood-impact/.
3. Substance Abuse and Mental Health Services Administration. (2010). *Permanent supportive housing evidence-based practices kit.* Rockville, MD: U.S. Department of Health and Human Services.
4. Forman Center for Real Estate and Urban Policy, New York University, School of Law. (2008). *The impact of supportive housing on surrounding neighborhoods: evidence from New York City.* Retrieved from http://shnny.org/uploads/Furman_Center_Policy_Brief.pdf.

■ Summary Points

- Partnerships among community agencies, health-care providers, and community residents, even though it takes considerable time and work, create mutual benefits that are far greater than an individual agency or community residents can do alone.
- The health of rural and urban dwellers have much in common, including the fact that both experience health disparities.
- Rural Americans (16% to 19% of the population) have more problems accessing health and dental care, paying for health care, and having adequate income for education, transportation, food, and other necessities than do other Americans.
- Some solutions to health disparity in rural communities include retaining and increasing the number of health-care providers, a patient centered medical home, and telehealth.
- Poor urban communities frequently experience community upheaval, with community disruption leading to decreased community health.
- Community organizing with community empowerment and coalition building is a useful tool for positive change. Community-based participatory research can build community capacity, which can also lead to positive change.
- There are several roles that PHNs can play in providing population-based care at the community

level in both urban and rural environments: parish nursing, care in nurse-managed clinics, and as members of community academic partnerships.

▲ CASE STUDY
Health Partnerships to Increase Primary Health-Care Service in a Rural Community

1. In a small rural town in Wisconsin there was no primary health care. The closest physician was 35 miles away; the nearest hospital was 45 miles away. The health department provided immunization and well-child clinics once a month at the local library. All other health department clinics were located in the county seat 26 miles away. The community of 4,000 organized themselves and formed a partnership with the regional health-care services to explore the possibilities of primary care coming to their town. Explore the actual crisis in rural primary health care.
   http://depts.washington.edu/uwrhrc/uploads/Rural_Primary_Care_PB_2009.pdf
   http://www.healthreform.gov/reports/hardtimes/
2. Determine how other rural communities have solved this problem.
   Mission-focused health care: http://blog.rwjf.org/humancapital/2012/02/13/recruiting-primary-care-physicians-away-from-specialties-and-into-rural-areas/
   Solution in rural areas in other countries: http://www.health.gov.au/internet/nhhrc/publishing.nsf/content/16f7a93d8f578db4ca2574d7001830e9/$file/primary%20health%20care%20in%20rural%20and%20remote%20australia%20-%20achieving%20equity%20of%20access%20and%20outcomes%20through%20national%20reform%20(j%20humph.pdf
3. Who can provide the primary care?
   Rural Health Care: New Delivery Model Recommendations
   http://www.health.state.mn.us/divs/orhpc/pubs/delivery.pdf
4. Using this information about rural health primary care needs and health-care delivery alternatives, suggest two ways for this small town to attract primary care practitioners to the area.

REFERENCES

1. Chicago's walking school bus: Protecting our children. (n.d.). Working together for a safer healthier Chicago. Retrieved from www.thinkactbehealthy.org/saferoutes/pdfs/ChiWalkingSchoolBus.pdf.
2. U.S. Department of State Diplomacy in Action. (n.d.). *Guide to partnering.* Retrieved from http://www.state.gov/s/partnerships/guide/index.htm.
3. Heinemann, E.A., Lee, J.L., & Cohen, J.I. (1995). Collaboration: A concept analysis. *Journal of Advanced Nursing, 21,* 103-109.
4. *A guide for developing local interagency linkage teams.* (2009). Retrieved from http://literacy.kent.edu/CommonGood/Guide/foreward.html.
5. Studnicki, J., Platonova, E., Eiechelberger, C., & Fisher, J. (2011). Extent and patterns of community collaboration in local health departments: An exploratory survey. *BMC Research Notes, 4,* 387.
6. U.S. Dept of Education and Regional Education Laboratory Network. (2004). *Putting the pieces together, comprehensive school linked strategies for children and families.* Retrieved from http://www.ncrel.org/sdrs/areas/issues/envrnmnt/css/ppt/chap1.html.
7. Doty, M., Abrams, M., Hernandez, S., Stremikis, K., & Beal, A. (2010). *Enhancing the capacity of community health centers to achieve high performance: Findings from the 2009 Commonwealth Fund National Survey of Federally Qualified Health Centers. The Commonwealth Fund.* Retrieved from ttp://www.commonwealthfund.org/Publications/Fund-Reports/2010/May/Enhancing-the-Capacity-of-Community-Health-Centers-to-Achieve-High-Performance.aspx?page=all.
8. National Rural Health Association. (2007). *What's different about rural health care?* Retrieved from http://www.ruralhealthweb.org/go/left/about-rural-health/what-s-different-about-rural-health-care.
9. Health Resource and Service Administration, U.S. Department of Health and Human Services. (2011). *Designated health professional shortage areas (HPSA).* Retrieved from http://ersrs.hrsa.gov/ReportServer?/HGDW_Reports/BCD_HPSA/BCD_HPSA_SCR50_Smry&rs:Format=HTML3.2.
10. U.S.D.A. (2011). *Economic research service, data sheet 2011, state fact sheets: United States.* Retrieved from http://www.ers.usda.gov/statefacts/US.HTM.
11. Gamm, L. (2007). Keynote address: Rural *Healthy People 2010* and sustaining rural population In L. Morgan, & P. Fahs, P. (Eds.), *Conversations in the disciplines: Sustaining rural populations* (pp 1-12). Binghamton University: Global Academic Publishing.
12. Bolin, J., & Bellamy, G. (2012). *Rural Healthy People 2020.* Retrieved from http://sph.tamhsc.edu/srhrc/docs/rhp2020.pdf.
13. Health Resource and Service Administration, U.S. Department of Health and Human Services. (2011). *Office of Rural Health Policy, rural guide to federal health, professional funding.* Retrieved from http://www.hrsa.gov/ruralhealth/pdf/ruralhealthfundingguidance.pdf.
14. U.S. Census Bureau. (2013). *The urban and rural classification.* Retrieved from http://www.census.gov/geo/reference/urban-rural.html.
15. U.S. Department of Agriculture. (2014). *What is rural?* Retrieved from http://www.nal.usda.gov/ric/ricpubs/what_is_rural.shtml.
16. U.S. Census Bureau. (2013). *Metropolitan and Micropolitan Statistical Areas Main.* Retrieved from http://www.census.gov/population/metro/
17. Ingram, D., & Franco, S. (2009). *CDC: 2006 NCHS urban-rural classification scheme for counties.* Retrieved from http://wonder.cdc.gov/wonder/help/cmf/urbanization-methodology.html.
18. Rural US disappearing? Population share hits low. (2011). *Bloomberg Business Week.* Retrieved from http://www.businessweek.com/ap/financialnews/D9OODUPG1.htm.
19. Butterfield, P., Postma, J., & ERRNIE Team. (2009). The TERRA framework. Conceptualizing rural environmental health inequities through an environmental justice lens. *Advance in Nursing Science, 32*(2), 107-117.
20. Glasser, M., Hunsaker, M., Sweet, K., MacDowell, M., & Meuer, M. (2008). A comprehensive medical education program response to rural primary care needs. *Academic Medicine, 83*(10), 952-961.
21. Patient Protection and Affordable Care Act. (2010). *124 Stat. 119 thru 124 Stat. 1025 H.R. 3590.* Retrieved from http://www.gpo.gov/fdsys/pkg/PLAW-111publ148/content-detail.html.
22. Bolin, J., Gamm, L., Vest, J., Edwardson, N., & Miller, T. (2011). Medical homes. Will health care reform provide new options for rural communities and providers? *Family Community Health, 34*(2), 93-101.
23. American Telemedicine Association. (2011). *Telehealth nursing fact sheet.* Retrieved from http://www.americantelemed.org/docs/default-document-library/fact_sheet_final.pdf?sfvrsn=2.
24. International Council of Nurses. (2013). *Telenursing network.* Retrieved fromhttp://www.icn.ch/networks/telenursing-network/.
25. Auch, R., Taylor, J., & Acevedo, W. (2004). *Urban growth in American cities: Glimpses of U.S. urbanization.* Washington, DC: Geological Survey, U.S. Department of the Interior.
26. Frey, W.H. (1980). Status selective white flight and central city population change: A comparative analysis. *Journal of Regional Science, 20*(1), 71-89.
27. Bradley, J., & Katx, B. (2008, October 8). Village idiocy: Enough with small-town triumphalism. *New Republic.* Retrieved from http://www.tnr.com/article/urban-policy/village-idiocy?page=0,2.
28. U.S. Census Bureau. (2011). *Population: Estimates and projections—states, metropolitan areas, cities.* Retrieved from http://www.census.gov/compendia/statab/cats/population/estimates_and_projections—states_metropolitan_areas_cities.html.
29. Rosner, D. (2006). Public health in U.S. cities, a historical perspective. In N. Freudenberg, S. Galea, & D. Vlahov. (Eds.), *Cities and the health of the public* (p. 140). Nashville, TN: Vanderbilt University Press.

30. Coutts, A., & Kawachi, I. (2006). The urban social environment and its effects on health. In N. Freudenberg, S. Galea, & D. Vlahov. (Eds.), *Cities and the health of the public.* Nashville, TN: Vanderbilt University Press.

31. Unite for Sight. (2013). *Urban versus rural health.* Retrieved from http://www.uniteforsight.org/global-health-university/urban-rural-health.

32. American Lung Association. (2009). 60 percent of Americans live in areas where air is dirty enough to endanger lives. *Science Daily.* Retrieved from http://www.sciencedaily.com_ /releases/2009/04/090429131158.htm.

33. Freudenberg, N., Galea, S., & Vlahov, D. (Eds.). (2006). *Cities and the health of the public.* Nashville, TN: Vanderbilt University Press.

34. Lochner, K.A., Kawachi, I., Brennan R.T., & Buka, S.L. (2003). Social capital and neighborhood mortality rates in Chicago. *Social Science and Medicine, 56,* 1797-1805.

35. Fullilove, M. (2003). Fifty ways to destroy a city. Undermining the social foundation of health. In N. Freudenberg, S. Galea, & D. Vlahov. (Eds.). *Cities and the health of the public.* Nashville, TN: Vanderbilt University Press.

36. Furr-Holden, C.D.M., Lee, Y.H., Milam A., Johnson, R., Lee, K., & Ialongo, N. (2011). The growth of neighborhood disorder and marijuana use among urban adolescents: A case for policy and environmental intervention. *Journal of Studies on Alcohol and Drugs, 72,* 371-379.

37. Minnesota Department of Public Health, Office of Public Health Practice. (2006). *Wheel of Public Health Intervention.* Retrieved from http://www.health.state.mn.us/divs/cfh/ophp/resources/docs/wheelbook2006.pdf.

38. Minkler, M. (Ed.). (2012). *Community organizing and community building for health and welfare* (3rd ed.). New Brunswick, NJ: Rutgers University Press.

39. World Bank. (2011). *Empowerment.* Retrieved from http://web.worldbank.org/WBSITE/EXTERNAL/TOPICS/EXTPOVERTY/EXTEMPOWERMENT/0,,contentMDK:20245753~pagePK:210058~piPK:210062~theSitePK:486411,00.html.

40. Brinkerhoff, D., & Azfar, O. (2006). *Decentralization and community empowerment: Does community empowerment deepen democracy and improve service delivery? U.S. Agency for International Development Office of Democracy and Governance.* Retrieved from http://pdf.usaid.gov/pdf_docs/PNADH325.pdf.

41. Maton, K. (2008). Empowering community settings: Agents of individual development, community betterment and positive social change. *American Journal of Community Psychology, 41,* 4-21.

42. Wallerstein, N. (2006). *What is the evidence on effectiveness of empowerment to improve health?* (Health Evidence Network report). Copenhagen, Denmark: WHO Regional Office for Europe. Retrieved from http://www.euro.who.int/__data/assets/pdf_file/0010/74656/E88086.pdf.

43. World Health Organization, CDI Study Group. (2009). *Community-directed interventions for priority health problems in Africa: Results of a multicountry study.* Retrieved from http://www.who.int/bulletin/volumes/88/7/09-069203/en/.

44. Marysdaughter, K., & Dansinger, L. (2000). *Community organizer's guide.* Monroe, ME: Resources for Organizing and Social Change.

45. de Souza, R. (2009). Creating "communicative spaces": A case of NGO community organizing for HIV/AIDS prevention. *Health Communication, 24*(8), 692-702.

46. American Lung Association. (2014). *Community organizing.* Retrieved from http://center4tobaccopolicy.org/community-organizing/.

47. Villablanca, A.C., Arline, S., Lewis, J., Raju, S., Sanders, S., & Carrow, S. (2009). Outcomes of national community organization cardiovascular prevention programs for high-risk women. *Journal of Cardiovascular Translational Research, 2,* 306-320. doi:10.1007/s12265-009-9118-5.

48. Wagoner, K., Rhodes, S., Lentz, A., & Wolfson, M. (2010). Community organizing goes to college: A practice-based model to implement environmental strategies to reduce high-risk drinking on college campuses. *Health Promotion Practice, 11,* 817. doi:10.1177/1524839909353726.

49. Wisconsin Department of Public Health. (2001). *Public health interventions: Applications for public health nursing practice.* Retrieved from http://www.health.state.mn.us/divs/opi/cd/phn/docs/0301wheel_manual.pdf.

50. Mendoza, M. (2007). 10 Basic Steps in community organizing. In *TIPS: Tools insights and practices on strengthening RPOs in Asia.* Quezon City, Philippines: Asian NGO Coalition for Agrarian Reform and Rural Development. Retrieved from http://www.angoc.org/portal/wp-content/uploads/2010/07/19/ideas-in-action-for-land-rights-advocacy/13-10-Basic-Steps-in-Community-Organizing.pdf.

51. Wolff, T. (2001). A practitioner's guide to successful coalitions. *American Journal of Community Psychology, 29*(1), 173-191.

52. Chavis, D. (2001). The paradoxes and promise of community coalitions. *American Journal of Community Psychology, 29*(2), 309-319.

53. McKay, M., & Hewlett, P. (2009). Grassroots coalition building: Lessons from the field. *Journal of Professional Nursing, 25*(6), 352-357.

54. Parker, E., Chung, L., Israel, B., Reyes, A., & Wilkins, D. (2010). Community organizing network for environmental health: Using a community health development approach to increase community capacity around reduction of environmental triggers. *The Journal of Primary Prevention, 31,* 41-58. doi:10.1007/s10935-010-0207-7.

55. Savage, C., Xu, Y., Lee, B., Rose, B., Kappesser, M., & Anthony, J. (2006). A case study in the use of community-based participatory research in public health nursing. *Public Health Nursing, 23*(5), 472-478.

56. Community Health Scholars Program. (2002). *The Community Health Scholars program: Stories of impact.* Ann Arbor, MI: Author.
57. Minkler, M., Breckwich, V., Warner, J., Steussey, H., & Facente, S. (2006). Sowing the seeds for sustainable change: A community-based participatory research partnership for health promotion in Indiana, USA and its aftermath. *Health Promotion International, 21*(4), 293-300.
58. Wynn, T., Johnson, R., Fouad, M., Holt, C., Scarinci, I., Nagy, C., . . . Parham, G. (2006). Addressing disparities through coalition building: Alabama REACH 2010 lessons learned. *Journal of Health Care for the Poor and Underserved, 17,* 55-77.
59. Flicker, S., Travers, R., Guta, A., McDonald, S., & Meagher, A. (2007). Ethical dilemmas in community-based participatory research: Recommendation for institutional review board. *Journal of Urban Health, 84*(4), 478-493.
60. Bastida, E., Tseng, T., McKeever, C., & Jack, L., Jr. (2010). Ethics and community-based participatory research: Perspective from the field. *Health Promotion Practice, 11*(1), 16-20. doi:10.1177/1524839909352841.
61. Church Health Center. (n.d.). *What is faith community nursing?* Retrieved from http://www.parishnurses.org/.
62. Swinney, J., Anson-Wonkka, C., Maki, E., & Corneau, J. (2001). Community assessment: A church community and the parish nurse. *Public Health Nursing, 18*(1), 40-44.
63. King, M., & Pappas-Rogich, M. (2011). Faith community nurse: Implementing healthy people standards to promote the health of elderly clients. *Geriatric Nursing, 32*(6), 459-464.
64. Acting globally, inspiring locally. (2012). *International Parish Nurse Resource Center.* Retrieved from http://www.parishnurses.org/WhatisaParishNurseFaithCommunityNurse_299.aspx.
65. Kovner, C. & Walani, S. (2011). *Nurse Managed Health Centers (NMHCs).* Initiative on the Future of Nursing. Retrieved from http://www.thefutureofnursing.org/resource/detail/nurse-managed-health-centers-nmhcs.
66. World Health Organization. (2012). *Healthy cities.* Retrieved from http://www.euro.who.int/en/what-we-do/health-topics/environment-and-health/urban-health/activities/healthy-cities.
67. Dooris, M., & Heritage, Z. (2011). Healthy cities: Facilitating the active participation and empowerment of local people. *Journal of Urban Health: Bulletin of the New York Academy of Medicine.* doi:10.1007/s11524-011-9623-0.
68. Glazer, G., Ponte, P., Stuart-Shor, E., & Cooley, M. (2009). The power of partnership: Addressing cancer health disparities through an academic-service partnership. *Nursing Outlook, 57,* 123-131.
69. Giachello, A., Arrom. J., Davos, M., Sayad, J., Ramirez, D., Nandi, C., & Ramos, C. (2003). *Reducing diabetes health disparities through community-based participatory action research: The Chicago southeast diabetes community action coalition.* Retrieved from http://www.uic.edu/jaddams/csdcac/.

Chapter 18

Health Planning for Maternal-Infant and Child Health Settings

LEARNING OUTCOMES

After reading this chapter, the student will be able to:

1. Describe maternal, infant, and child health from a global and national perspective.
2. Identify key concerns for public health planning for maternal, infant, and child health.
3. Apply health promotion planning to maternal, infant, and child health.
4. Integrate cultural perspectives into planning for maternal, infant, and child health interventions.
5. Discuss strategies for community engagement and consensus building for maternal, infant, and child health planning.

KEY TERMS

Infant mortality rate
Fishboning
Low birth weight
Mainstream smoke
Maternal health

Maternal mortality rate
Preterm birth
Preterm labor
Secondhand smoke
Sidestream smoke

Sudden infant death
  syndrome (SIDS)
Sudden unexplained
  infant death
Teen pregnancy

Teen pregnancy birth rate
Under-five mortality rate
Upstream approach
Very low birth weight

◼ Introduction

Maternal, infant, and child health is a global health priority. According to the World Health Organization (WHO), the number of children under the age of 5 who die each year is about 7 million, or approximately 800 per hour.[1] Malnutrition and insufficient suboptimal breastfeeding are the leading risk factors leading to death in children under 5 years. These risk factors contribute to the leading specific causes of death such diarrheal diseases, pneumonia, measles, and severe neonatal infections. Most of these deaths are preventable simply by providing affordable interventions.[1] Nurses working in settings that provide care to mothers and their children play a key role in the interventions aimed at improving the health of mothers and their children.

Approximately 800 pregnant women and women giving birth die of preventable causes per day, or more than half a million a year. In addition, more than 10 million women a year suffer injury, infection, or disease related to pregnancy and childbirth.[2] Most common causes are bleeding, pregnancy-related hypertension (eclampsia), infections and sepsis, and labor-related problems such as cephalic pelvic disproportion, a condition in which the head of the fetus is larger than the maternal pelvic opening, usually requiring a cesarean section.

Maternal health specifically refers to the woman's health during pregnancy, childbirth, and the postpartum period. Infant health includes the health of newborns, that is, infants up to 28 days of age and children younger than 1 year. In this chapter, child health focuses on the health of children under the age of 5. This age group is the recipient of much of the focus on child health because of the high risk of morbidity and mortality during this age span.[1] The issue of maternal, infant, and child health spans the globe, with major public health initiatives aimed at improving the health of this vulnerable population.

Historical Perspectives

Lillian Wald was one of the earliest pioneers in population approaches to health and is considered the founder of public health nursing (see Chapter 1). Her work at the Henry Street Settlement addressed health disparities among expectant mothers and children. The interventions she planned and implemented focused on the health priorities of the population living in the Lower East Side of New York City during the last decades of the 19th century and the first decades of the 20th century. Through this work, she developed maternity services at Henry Street, including health classes for mothers and home visits for maternal-infant health assessment and teaching. She addressed health reform for sanitation and public health and developed prevention programs for mothers, infants, and children. Considered the founder of school health services and visiting nursing, she also developed what became known as the Children's Bureau.[3]

Unfortunately, more than a century later, health disparities and high rates of morbidity persist for pregnant women and their infants worldwide. Although the leading causes of mortality and morbidity have changed somewhat during the past 100 years, there is a continued need for nurses to use public health science to address maternal child health issues. Nurses use the science of epidemiology to examine morbidity and mortality data and identify priorities for maternal and infant health.

Trends in Maternal, Infant, and Child Health

In the United States, maternal, infant, and child health remains central to the improvement of the health of the country's population as a whole. It is a key topic area in *Healthy People 2020 (HP 2020)* with 33 objectives.

■ HEALTHY PEOPLE 2020
Health Planning for Maternal Infant and Child Health Settings

Targeted Topic: Maternal, infant, and child health
Goal: Improve the health and well-being of women, infants, children, and families.
Overview: Improving the well-being of mothers, infants, and children is an important public health goal for the United States. Their well-being determines the health of the next generation and can help predict future public health challenges for families, communities, and the health-care system. The objectives of the Maternal, Infant, and Child Health topic area address a wide range of conditions, health behaviors, and health systems indicators that affect the health, wellness, and quality of life of women, children, and families.
Source: See reference 4.

To help understand the trends in maternal, infant, and child health, it helps to begin with three indicators often used to evaluate the maternal, infant and child health of a population, infant mortality rate, maternal mortality rate, and under-five mortality rate. **Infant mortality rate** (IMR) is calculated by dividing the number of infant deaths following a live birth in a given year by the total number of live births for that year. It does not include fetal demise or miscarriage. The **maternal mortality rate** (MMR) is calculated by dividing the number of maternal deaths by the number of during a live births (or by the number of live births plus fetal deaths) in that year. To be classified as a maternal death, the woman must be pregnant or within 42 days of the termination of a pregnancy and the death must be directly related to pregnancy, not including accidental or incidental causes. The **under-five mortality rate** of children is technically is not an actual rate, but rather represents the probability of a child born in a specific year dying before the age of 5. It is calculated per 1,000 births.

Across the world, IMR is used as an indicator of population health. It reflects the quality of pre- and postnatal care in that population and is an indicator of access to medical care, socioeconomic conditions, and public health practices.[5-6] Although some have challenged the legitimacy of IMR as an indicator of the health of an entire population, it has withstood the test of time. In addition, in countries with few resources to monitor other health indictors, IMR is an easily calculated indicator.[7] As of 2014 based on estimated infant mortality data, the United States ranked 55th worldwide for infant mortality with a rate of 6.2 per 1,000 live births (Fig. 18-1).[8,9] Within the United States, there are differences among ethnic/racial groups in relation to IMR. For example, in 2012 the IMR for babies whose mothers were non-Hispanic black women was double the IMR for babies whose mothers were white non-Hispanic women (11.42 per 1,000 live births versus 5.33 per 1,000 live births).[10,11] The leading causes of infant death in the United States are congenital malformations, preterm birth and low birth weight (LBW), and sudden infant death syndrome (SIDS).[4] Globally, the leading causes of death are preterm birth, birth trauma, and infections.[1] Preterm birth is defined as a birth occurring less than 37 weeks gestation. Low birth weight is defined as a birth weight less than 2,500 grams (5 lbs. 8 oz.). Preterm birth is a serious problem. The

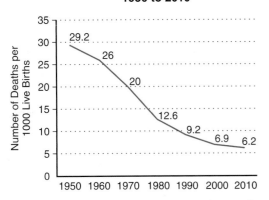

U.S. Infant Mortality Rate 1950 to 2010

Figure 18-1 Infant mortality in the United States from 1950 to 2010. *Source: National Center for Health Statistics. National Vital Statistics Reports (NVSR).*

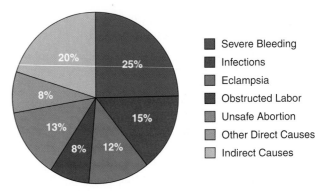

Figure 18-2 Leading causes of maternal death worldwide. *Source: See reference 2.*

TABLE 18–1	**Leading Causes of Death in Children Aged 1 to 4**
United States	**Worldwide**
Injury, intentional, and nonintentional	Diarrhea
Developmental/genetic disorders present at birth	Pneumonia
Cancer	Malaria

Sources: See reference 6 and Centers for Disease Control and Prevention. (2011). *Health United States.* Retrieved from http://www.cdc.gov/nchs/data/hus/hus11.pdf.

number of preterm babies worldwide is 15 million, with 1 million infants dying annually as a result of preterm births. Countries in Asia and Africa are most significantly affected, with almost 85% of all preterm births occurring in those areas.[12,13]

Globally, the MMR is declining.[14] However, this is not the case in the United States. The United States ranks lower than other high-income countries in relation to maternal deaths, with an MMR in 2008 of 17 per 100,000 live births. In comparison, other high-income countries such as Sweden and Italy have an MMR of 4 to 6.[15] According to the Health Resources and Services Administration, the downward trend in U.S. MMR reversed from a low of 6.6 in 1987 to 17 in 2008.[16] Some of the change is due to changes in coding and some of the upward trend is due to the HIV epidemic.[14,16] Other risk factors associated with MMR include the higher preeclampsia rate in U.S. women, possibly due to the increase in obesity and diabetes in U.S. women of childbearing age.[17] The most common causes of maternal mortality worldwide are severe bleeding, infections, eclampsia, unsafe abortions, and obstructed labor (Fig. 18-2).[2]

The mortality rate for children under the age of 5 has improved since 1990, with a drop from 12 million to 7.6 million in 2012.[18] In 2011, in the United States the under-five mortality rate was 8 per 1,000 live births.[18] Globally, the primary causes of death for children under the age of 5 that are not birth related are pneumonia, diarrheal diseases, and malaria.[18] In contrast, in the United States the leading causes of death in children between the ages of 1 and 4 are accidents, developmental/genetic conditions present at birth, and cancer (Table 18.1).[19]

International and National Maternal, Infant, and Child Health Goals and Objectives

National and international organizations have set goals that address the health of mothers, infants, and children under the age of 5. Because poverty is strongly associated with poorer maternal, infant, and child health, in 2000 the United Nations set the Millennium Development Goals (MDGs) to reduce poverty and improve health worldwide. For this reason, two of the MDGs address both maternal and child health. Three of the eight goals directly address health, whereas others indirectly address prevention of disease by targeting social and economic factors that contribute to the global burden of disease. Millennium Development Goal 4 is "Reduce by two thirds, between 1990 and 2015, the under-five mortality rate." This goal includes infant mortality as part of its focus. Millennium Development Goal 5 is "Improve Maternal Health," which specifically targets maternal mortality, including not only safer pregnancy and birth but also adolescent pregnancy and access to safe contraception.[20] As noted above, the *HP 2020* objectives offer target objectives related to the improvement of maternal, infant, and child health across 33 key areas. Among the objectives that address maternal child health, several help to illustrate ways that nurses using a population focus can plan and implement programs to improve health for maternal-child populations. The objective for reduction of LBW (less than 2,500 grams) and very low birth weight (VLBW) (less than 1,500 grams) for 2010 was not met, and the number of preterm births continues to exceed the goals set for *HP 2020*. The current target is to reduce the number of preterm births by 10%.[4]

■ HEALTHY PEOPLE 2020
Maternal Infant Child Health Objectives.

Objective: MICH 9.1 Reduce total preterm births.
Baseline: 12.7 percent of live births were preterm in 2007.
Target: 11.4 percent
Target-Setting Method: 10 percent improvement
Source: See reference 4.

Population Focus in Maternal, Infant, and Child Health

A population focus to improving the health of mothers, infants, and children under the age of 5 is essential. The following examples are reminders of the importance of this perspective for maternal, infant, and child health. Using principles of epidemiology, changes in clinical practice and policies greatly reduced the leading causes of death for pregnant women and infants. In the first example, during the 1840s, Dr. Ignaz Semmelweis, a Hungarian working in Austria, discovered that hand washing reduced the incidence of puerperal fever (also called childbed fever) or septicemia that follows delivery. This serious condition caused deaths among 30% of those women who delivered their newborns in the hospital. He had observed that women who delivered their babies at home where a midwife assisted at the birth had much better outcomes than did those who delivered in the hospital. Noting that the medical students came to the delivery ward directly from the autopsy room at the hospital without washing their hands, Semmelweis ordered a change in hand washing policy. Once the policy change took place, the maternal death rate decreased from 12% to 1% within 2 years.[21] His work is an early

record of the importance of epidemiology for improving health outcomes.

The second example is more recent. Sudden infant death syndrome (SIDS) is the third leading cause of death for all infants in the United States and the leading cause of death for infants from 1 to 12 months of age. **Sudden infant death syndrome (SIDS)** or the more recent term **sudden unexplained infant death** is defined as the sudden death of an infant less than 1 year of age, which cannot be explained after an extensive examination that includes a review of the clinical history, a complete autopsy, and complete assessment of the site where the death occurred. In the 1980s, the prevalence rate for SIDS in the United States was approximately 1.4 per 1,000 live births. The results of population-based studies conducted in the late 1980s and 1990s established that babies placed on their backs were at a much lower risk of SIDS than those placed on their stomachs.[22, 23,24]

In response to these findings, in the United States a national Back to Sleep campaign was instituted in 1992 that encouraged parents to place infants in the supine position (Fig. 18-3). Currently, this campaign is sponsored by the Eunice Kennedy Shriver National Institute of Child Health and Human Development, the Maternal and Child Health Bureau, the American Academy of Pediatrics, the SIDS Alliance, and the Association of SIDS and Infant Mortality Programs.[25] Following the initiation of the Back to Sleep campaign, the SIDS national mortality rates fell dramatically so that by 2006, in the United States the total number of SIDS-related infant deaths fell from more than 5,000 in prior years to a total of 2,323 infant deaths, an IMR of 0.54 per 1,000 live births.[26,27] From 1980, the rate fell by 66% with the majority of the decrease occurring the ten years following the institution of the Back to Sleep campaign.[27,28]

Upstream to Prevention Across the Maternal-Child Health Continuum

The population approach calls for what is often called the **upstream approach**.[29] The upstream approach is a metaphor for looking at the upstream factors that contribute to illness and disease. It is based on the idea that if you only focus on pulling drowning people out of the river, you may miss the fact that they are falling off the bridge upstream. If you keep them from falling off the bridge in the first place, you will not have to save them from drowning further down the stream. Nurses and other health providers are urged to focus upstream on the social, political, economic, and behavioral causes of

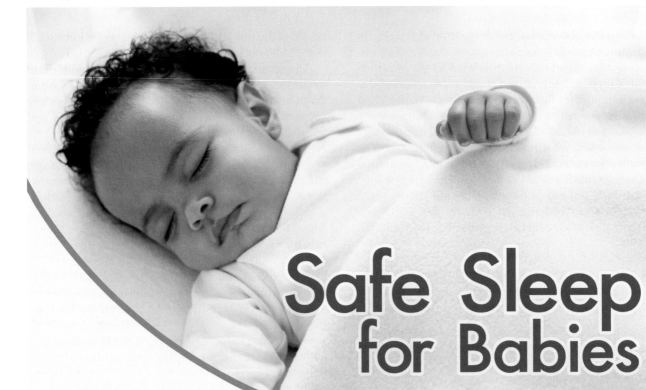

Safe Sleep for Babies

Safe Sleeping Tips For Baby

☑ **Place infant(s) to sleep on their backs**

☑ **Use firm, tight-fitting mattress**

☑ **Never use extra padding, blankets, or pillows under baby**

☑ **Remove pillows or thick comforters**

☑ **Positioning devices are not necessary and can be deadly**

☑ **Regularly check crib for loose, missing or broken parts or slats**

☑ **Do not try to fix a broken crib**

☑ **Place cribs or playpens away from windows to avoid window covering or fall hazards**

Safe Sleep

Check www.cpsc.gov to find out if your crib, bassinet, or
play yard has been recalled.

U.S. Consumer Product Safety Commision
CPSC Hotline: (800) 638-2772
(301) 595-7054 (TTY)

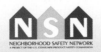
NEIGHBORHOOD SAFETY NETWORK
A PROJECT OF THE U.S. CONSUMER PRODUCT SAFETY COMMISSION

Sign up to receive free NSN
Safety Alerts and Posters at:
www.cpsc.gov

Figure 18-3 Safe Sleep Tips for Babies. *(From the U.S. Consumer Product Safety Commission, Back to Sleep campaign promotional advertisement, 2012.)*

disease and unhealthy health events to prevent poor health outcomes for mother and child.

The health and safety of the mother, the health of the developing fetus, safe birth for the newborn, and continued healthy development of the child are the top priorities for nurses who work in maternal-child health. If the mother is healthy throughout the pregnancy and delivers a healthy child, the nurse working in the hospital only interacts with the mother/child dyad (group of two) for a brief time along this continuum. Therefore, it is essential for nurses to think upstream to the root causes of health problems and to prepare new mothers and families for their future health back in the community. The maternal-child health continuum spans the time from preconception and continues as the child develops. The health and well-being of the woman throughout her pregnancy and perinatal period and the healthy growth and development of the fetus and child continue for decades. The potential impact of upstream approaches to health and safety for the maternal-child health continuum is significant in health, social, and economic terms, particularly for children. For this reason, nurses use public health approaches to ensure adequate nutrition, appropriate prenatal care, safe delivery for the newborn, and care of mother and child during the postpartum period.

Review of Assessment and Planning in Maternal, Infant, and Child Health Settings

Nursing approaches to improve health for maternal-child populations often involve interdisciplinary teams that bring the breadth of expertise necessary for strong programs. As a key member of that team, the nurse is vital for success in creating successful and effective programs. Assessment at the population level involves analysis of data from national, state, and local data sources (see Chapters 4 and 5). Such data allow the nurse planner to identify risks and protective factors related to maternal-child health. International, national, state, and local data that track risks and adverse outcomes are available through numerous governmental and nongovernmental agencies such as the Centers for Disease Control and Prevention (CDC), the National Center for Health Statistics, and the Office of Minority Health. Another excellent source of data at the state level is the Pregnancy Risk Assessment Monitoring System, which is available at http://www.cdc.gov/prams/. These data help nurses identify risks related to the population for which they are caring. Another useful example is the PeriStats data, available from the March of Dimes at http://www.marchofdimes.com/PeriStats/about.aspx. Once risks are identified, then other assessment strategies such as

interviews, community forums, and identification of local resources can follow to aid in the planning process.

Models for community assessment, discussed in Chapter 4, illustrate the need to include social, political, economic, and cultural contextual perspectives in epidemiological investigations. In addition, the strengths or assets are always identified in any population-level assessment. Data collected for the assessment can include archival data, health indicator data, interviews, observational surveys, formal surveys, focus groups, and community forums. Other sources of local data include hospital records, local health surveys, and agency records.

Health problems as well as community or organizational assets can be identified from the analysis of the data collected in the needs assessment. A variety of methods for prioritization exist. Most are based on the perceived severity of the health problem and importance placed on the problem by the community or organization. In the case of maternal-child health, serious immediate risks for maternal or infant mortality often rank higher than do long-term morbidity risks. Although obesity is an important risk factor related to maternal, neonatal, and child health,[30,31] other immediate risks can take priority. For example, in the fall and winter of 2009–2010, the H1N1 pandemic became the immediate priority because of the high risk to the health of pregnant women and their fetuses, resulting in a nationwide effort to immunize pregnant women.[32] Another example is the pertussis outbreak that began in 2012 and was responsible for 18 deaths as of January 2013.[33] This has resulted in pertussis immunization becoming a priority for infant and child health. In addition, the feasibility and likelihood of positive change as a result of the planned interventions is important for prioritization. Short-term programs with a greater likelihood of success often receive a higher prioritization ranking for funding.

Once the priority needs for the maternal-child population of interest are identified, planning can begin (Chapter 5). As reviewed in Chapter 5, goals and objectives are created. The goals must be both long and short term and must address positive health outcomes; the objectives must be measurable. The identified goals guide the evaluation process. Planning must include the exploration of resources as well as constraints to the planned interventions, which include political, economic, and time constraints. Before any interventions can begin, a budget must be developed; staffing needs must be met; supplies, equipment, and space need to be obtained; required protocols must be followed; permissions must be granted. Interventions that are well planned can be completed successfully. Clear evaluation plans that include both process and outcome measures document the success of the program.

In maternal-child health, the challenge is to identify significant health risks in maternal-infant populations across different health settings, set priorities for planning, suggest strategies for interventions to address the risks, and discuss evaluation plans for the selected interventions. For the nurse working in maternal-child health acute care and primary care settings, this requires building alliances with other disciplines, agencies, and members of the community. There are a variety of risks for the mother and child across the continuum from preconception to childhood.

Health promotion with this population begins with prevention of high-risk pregnancy and reduction of shared exposures to risk for both the pregnant mother and the developing fetus. These efforts to promote the health and safety of mother and developing fetus can reduce the incidence of preterm birth, low birth weight, birth defects, and infant mortality rate. Nurses who seek to address health risks for maternal-infant settings must apply assessment and planning strategies of public health science.

● APPLYING PUBLIC HEALTH SCIENCE

The Case of the Teenage Pregnancy Epidemic

Public Health Science Topics Covered:
• Assessment
• Program development
• Program evaluation

Nurses in the local hospital in City A, a moderate-sized city in an economically depressed area, responded to a state health department call for funding for teen pregnancy prevention and the initiation of a community program to address the a growing teen pregnancy rate. **Teen pregnancy** is defined as a pregnancy in which the mother is between 15 and 19 years of age and the **teen pregnancy birth rate** is calculated as the number of births per 1,000 women in this age group.[34] The nurses felt they could contribute to the development of a teen pregnancy program because of their expertise in working with pregnant teens who came to their hospital for care across the perinatal period and through their infants' first year of life. These nurses included those working in the labor and delivery room, the hospital-run prenatal clinic for teens, the neonatal unit, and the pediatric unit. They felt that addressing teen pregnancy would also address the larger issue of the high IMR in the community as recommended by authorities in the field.[34,35]

The nurses began by reviewing the literature related to teen pregnancy. They found that commonly reported teen pregnancy adverse outcomes increased risk for both the mother and infant. These adverse outcomes included maternal death, risk for sexually transmitted infections, and greater risk for cephalopelvic disproportion, wherein the infant's head is too large to fit through the mother's pelvis. In addition, they found that teen mothers are less likely to seek prenatal care early and more likely to deliver low-birth-weight infants.[34,36] Based on these national statistics, the team became curious about the teens who were served by their hospital and decided further assessment was needed.

The team also recognized the importance of the various legal and ethical concerns when working with adolescents who are minors in the eyes of the law. Nurses who work with programs to prevent teen pregnancy face a number of ethical concerns. Because teens are often under the age of 18 and must have parental consent for most of their interactions with health-care providers, the nurse must consider whether a planned intervention will require parental consent. In addition, many school settings where teens spend most of their days also control the content of information made available to students.[37] Various issues should be addressed up front from an ethical perspective to best protect this vulnerable population (Box 18-1).

To begin the work, these nurses created an interdisciplinary team of key stakeholders to help identify critical issues related to teen mothers in the community they served and to develop a program based on those findings. These stakeholders included key personnel from the hospital's maternal-child health services and community-based health service providers such as the federally qualified community health center, the director of the teen clinic at the health center, the director of the Planned Parenthood center, and the nursing director from the local department of public health. They also felt it was important to invite representatives from the public and private schools in the community, the director of immigrant services, leaders of the four ethical/cultural groups in the community, and the director of the U.S. Department of Agriculture's

BOX 18–1	Legal and Ethical Issues Related to Preventing Teen Pregnancy

Females under the age of 21 come under the definition of a vulnerable population. In addition, women who are pregnant are also considered vulnerable. Caution must be taken to protect their privacy and the confidentiality of their information. There are differing laws in relation to emancipation of minors and the dispensing of information related to pregnancy. Community buy-in is an important issue and various community groups, including parents, political bodies, and religious groups, have differing opinions on:

• Sexual behaviors
• Abstinence
• Safer sexual practices
• Use of illegal substances
• Use of tobacco and alcohol products
• Contraception options
• Abortion counseling
• Birth options

Source: See reference 37.

Women, Infants, and Children nutrition program. In addition, the nurses reached out to the community and invited women living in the community to join the nurse team to help complete the assessment and create a program based on their findings.

The team believed that they needed to begin with a focused assessment to identify the risk factors associated with the problem of teen pregnancy specific to their community (see Chapter 4). Their approach included a mapping of community assets related to maternal, infant, and child health and identification of adolescent programs that included females.

They began their assessment using a technique referred to as **fishboning,**[38] which is an easy and fast method of identifying root causes of a complex issue or problem. This technique begins with the forming of a root cause diagram (Fig. 18-4). The planning team assembled their diagram with a facilitator leading the process. In this case, the team identified social causes such as poverty, minority status, and access to adequate prenatal care. They also identified maternal behavioral risk factors including substance use and maternal stress. Finally, they identified issues related to teen maternal health and pregnancy outcomes, including nutrition and prior birth history.[39–41] The effect they wished to address was preterm birth and low birth weight, with teen pregnancy as one of the root causes.

Using the results of the fishbone diagram process based on national data, the team then searched the epidemiological data from their community to identify whether the issues they found were significant in their community. First, they reviewed the overall demographics of the city. They found that in City A, 50.1% of the residents had less than a high school education compared with 20% of the state residents. The city reported that 25.7% of the households were below the poverty line, whereas in the state in general, only 13.2% of households were below the poverty line. Thirty percent of high school female teens reported using tobacco in City A, compared with 22.5% at the national level, and 28% met the definition for obesity, compared with 17% nationally. Next, they looked at the publically available birth data and discovered that the teen birth rate was 49.5 per 1,000 births, compared with 31.9 at the national level and 35.2 at the state level. Also, teen mothers in City A had a preterm birth rate of 17.8%, which was significantly higher than the 11.6% rate for all pregnancies at the national level. Another key issue was access to prenatal care, with teen mothers 20% less likely to receive adequate prenatal care or breastfeed their babies than women in the state overall.

They then requested information from the city health department on the rates of low birth weight, IMR, prenatal care, maternal obesity, prematurity, and tobacco use among teen moms based on the birth certificate data. The city agreed to provide this information and reported back that the IMR for teen mothers overall was 8.7 per 1,000 births, and for African American teen mothers it was 16.8 per 1,000 births. The health department reported similar disparities in relation to preterm birth and low birth weight. Tobacco use in white teen mothers (25%) was higher than in African American teen mothers (10%), compared with 23.8% and 8.4%, respectively, of female teens at the national level. There was a slight difference in the initiation of prenatal care between the two groups, with 71% of white teen mothers and 68% of African American teen mothers initiating prenatal care in the first trimester. The percentage of obese teen moms was similar in both groups, with a 27.5% prevalence of obesity in white teen mothers and 29.3% in African American teen mothers.

Based on the data they gathered, the team concluded that for their community, City A, the teen pregnancy rate was the highest in the state and represented a significant health problem. In addition, tobacco use and

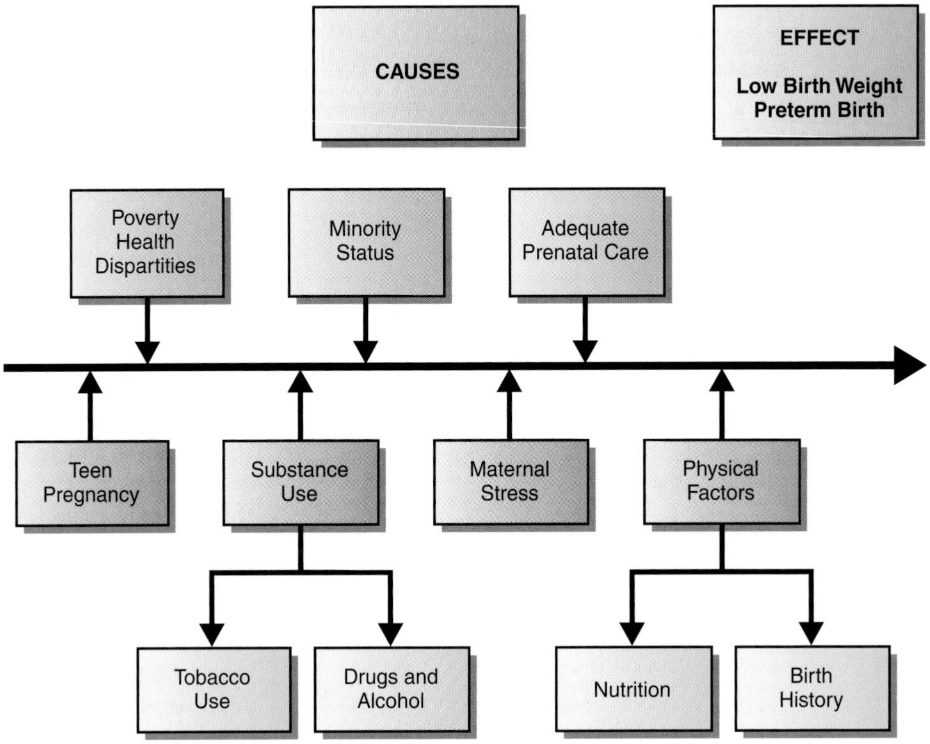

Figure 18-4 Ishakawa fishbone template for low birth weight and prematurity outcomes.

obesity among adolescent females during pregnancy was a problem. The team decided that obesity and tobacco use would be the target of their program.

Obesity and Pregnancy

Based on these facts, the team next took a closer look at the link between maternal obesity and neonatal outcomes. Based on the studies they read, they found that obesity has been linked to multiple adverse outcomes for both the mother and the baby. Researchers have demonstrated that babies born to obese mothers are at greater risk for mortality during their first month and also their first year of life. In one study, the risk of fetal death was found to be about three times greater among women who gained the most weight (up to 1 pound per week) than that of mothers who gained the recommended weight.[42] Infants born to obese mothers were more likely to have macrosomia, that is, they have an excessive birth weight. This often resulted in higher rates of cesarean section delivery and birth injury, VLBW, and neural tube defects.[43] Mothers who were obese during pregnancy were also found to be at greater risk of developing gestational diabetes, hypertension, and preeclampsia.[43] Children born to mothers with gestational diabetes were found to have

an elevated body mass index (BMI) during their lifetime. In addition, women who were obese during pregnancy were also more likely to use medical services, have longer hospital stays, and were twice as likely to have a cesarean section delivery with an increase in health-care costs.[43]

Tobacco Use and Pregnancy

They next examined the issue of tobacco use among pregnant teens. Smoking poses risks for both the mother and the infant. Women who smoke during pregnancy are about two times more likely to have premature rupture of membranes, placenta previa, or placental abruption than women who do not smoke. Further, among pregnant nonsmokers, those who are exposed to secondhand tobacco smoke are 20% more likely to give birth to a low-birth-weight baby than are those pregnant mothers who are not exposed to secondhand tobacco smoke during pregnancy.[44] **Secondhand smoke** includes **sidestream smoke,** which is defined as smoke from the lighted end of a tobacco product, and **mainstream-smoke,** which is defined as smoke exhaled by the smoker.

Tobacco use also poses a significant health risk for the baby. Babies born to women who use tobacco are

30% more likely to be born prematurely and are more likely to be born with low birth weight (less than 2,500 grams or 5.5 pounds). Overall, babies born to mothers who use tobacco weigh 200 grams less on average than babies born to nonsmoking mothers.[45,46] In addition, babies born to mothers who smoke are anywhere from one and a half to three times more likely to die of SIDS.

Infants and children exposed to secondhand smoke related to tobacco use are more likely to experience adverse health issues.[47,48] Exposure to secondhand smoke causes premature death and disease in children exposed in their home or daycare environment. These children experience higher rates of ear infections and respiratory problems that include bronchitis, asthma, and pneumonia. Although campaigns have reduced the prevalence of smoking and consequently the exposures in the home setting, in 2007–2008 approximately half of all children aged 3 to 11 years were exposed to secondhand smoke.[49]

Based on their findings, the team decided on a multifaceted approach. Programs that address issues such as teen pregnancy, healthy weight preconception, appropriate weight gain during pregnancy, and tobacco use generally focus on outcomes such as reduction in number of pregnant teens, reduction in rate of obesity among childbearing women, recommended weight gain during pregnancy, and reduction in tobacco use by pregnant mothers. Achieving the target measures for these outcomes should improve the health of teenage mothers and infants in City A. A more significant outcome would be the actual decline in the maternal mortality or infant mortality rates.

In the case of City A, the team considered a variety of approaches that had been successful in other locations, such as community programs that strengthened parent-child communication and school-based programs.[50,51] From their assessment, they elected to work with the hospital outreach program and the local neighborhood health center. In particular, the nurses at the hospital would serve as the hospital's representatives on the team. The nurses' role included two aspects. First, they provided nutrition education to pregnant teens attending the teen pregnancy clinic based in their hospital, with a focus on healthy eating and achieving a healthy weight gain over the course of the pregnancy. They also put together a smoking cessation program that included the development of a smoking cessation peer-led support group. The hospital provided space for the teens to meet and the nurses

filled the role of facilitator. Once again, the support program was put in place in conjunction with the teen pregnancy clinic. The hospital agreed to give the nurses time within their workweek to provide this service. In addition, the nurses worked with community members and stakeholders on the team to look for opportunities to extend the nutritional education program out into community settings and link it back to the care given in the prenatal clinics. Finally, the nurses agreed to take the responsibility for collecting the needed evaluation data to establish whether the program was successful. They collected baseline and outcome data using specific outcome measures. For the teens who participated in the program, the nurses collected data on overall weight gain during the pregnancy, the percentage of participants who smoked and were able to quit, as well as recording maternal birth outcomes such as pregnancy complications, birth weight, gestational age, and other physical outcome measures related to maternal and neonatal outcomes chosen by the team.

Based on the statistics for City A, the team decided that they should also seek funding to expand the program to address other key areas they had identified during their assessment. They hoped by demonstrating success with their teen pregnancy clinic program, they would be able to secure funding to expand the program and thus have a bigger impact on the problem of teen pregnancy in City A.

Before submitting a grant, the nurses reconvened the larger team and discussed the need for community buy-in and consensus in order to expand the program. After demonstrating the success of their original program, they received funding from the hospital and some of the stakeholders to support a communitywide forum to be held at the city high school. The team held five work meetings prior to the community meeting, in which logistics and format were planned, donated refreshments were solicited, and meeting details and advertising were arranged. Representatives of all community service agencies would be invited to the planning meeting.

During the community forum planning, the team scheduled the mayor to speak to the assembly of 110 attendees, followed by local politicians at the state and national levels. This confirmed the importance of the work. Then, the audience broke into five small workgroups. Members of the planning team who were skilled in consensus building used the *nominal group process*.[52] Nominal group process or technique refers to the process wherein a larger group can come to consensus for prioritizing needs in a fairly brief meeting time. To be successful, all participants must be in agreement that they will accept the results of the group process to represent their position for program planning. The first step is often called brainstorming, in which each participant is given a pad of paper and instructed to write down every important issue he or she can think of related to the broad topic of the forum. After about 5 to 8 minutes for this brainstorming, the participants post their written papers in clusters on a white board. With input from the group, the facilitator arranges the clusters into smaller categories. In this particular community forum, the smaller groups contained about 22 participants. Next, the 90 ideas that were generated were consolidated into 12 categories. Through a process of voting to rank order the topics/categories, the group was able to identify their top three concerns or problems:

1. Teen pregnancy prevention
2. High rates of smoking by pregnant adolescents
3. Obesity among adolescent females

They also concluded that low birth weight was an issue, but low birth weight was being addressed in another program. Based on the initial success of the nurses' tobacco cessation and healthy nutrition program with pregnant teens, the community felt the team had the experience to take on a more comprehensive primary prevention program that focused on preventing pregnancy, tobacco use, and obesity in females under the age of 20.

The nurses were now working with a larger community team. They were able to secure support from the chief nursing officer at their hospital by demonstrating the value of the potential program to the hospital and its community outreach initiative. Together with the community team, the nurses developed the following goals for females aged 12 to 19 in City A:

1. Reduce the number of pregnancies.
2. Reduce the rate of obesity.
3. Reduce the initiation of tobacco use.

For both goals 1 and 2, the team developed a healthy living program that used the school-based health clinic system. They based the program on evidence from other programs.[50,51] The nurses on the team brought the school nurses into the planning process. The program extended over the academic year and included support groups for female students aimed at building self-esteem and healthy lifestyles with a focus on healthy sexual practices and healthy eating. There was some resistance from certain members of the community related to the information that might be provided in the support groups, so materials used in the program were developed in conjunction with parent groups. The program was expanded to include faith-based settings for alternative support groups that would provide the same intervention but with an emphasis on abstinence from sexual relations for parents and teens who were only willing to consider abstinence-based approach.

The nurses established three measurable outcome objectives:

- 75% of the teens who participate in the healthy lifestyles program will demonstrate an increase in self-esteem.
- 75% of participants who report they are not sexually active at the beginning of the program will report they are still abstinent at the end of the program, and 75% of those who report that they are sexually active will report that they are practicing safe sex.
- 75% of the participants will demonstrate healthy eating habits and daily exercising; 50% of participants with a BMI above normal will have a BMI within the normal range within 5 months of starting the program.

When developing the nutrition intervention, they took into account the fact that there may be cultural issues that should be addressed in the program. Food is fundamental to a person's social and racial identify. In many parts of the world, health is determined by traditional dietary rules and practices. Recommendations given by a nurse or health-care provider are often in direct conflict with cultural rules. As a result, women make food choices before conception, during pregnancy, when planning feeding for their newborn, and during their postpartum period based on their cultural and social history. To address this, they included a cultural assessment related to the nutritional aspect of their program prior to implementing the program (see Chapter 23).

For goal 2, the community team chose to take a universal approach and target enforcement of existing laws in City A. The nurses helped the team develop a campaign to stop sales of tobacco products to underage customers, targeting stores selling tobacco located close to schools and playgrounds. The team's objectives were that 100% of all these stores in City A would comply with laws that prohibit sales of tobacco products to minors. The community team also decided to initiate a media campaign aimed at female middle school children, using social networking sites at the beginning of the school year. Their objective was that there would be no change in the percentage of students who reported they did not use tobacco from the beginning of the school year to the end.

During the entire process, the nurses who had initiated the project had the opportunity to work with an interdisciplinary team that included key stakeholders and members of the community. They personally implemented the team's first intervention as a result of their expertise and their ability to evaluate the success of the program. They were then able to work with a larger community team to develop a more ambitious primary prevention program that they titled the Healthy Teens and Healthy Families program. They were able to partner with nurses in a school setting to deliver part of the program. They had actively advocated for their patients and helped to fill a gap in their community while building on available community resources, such as the hospital-affiliated prenatal clinic for teens and the school-based health clinics.

■ EVIDENCED-BASED PRACTICE
Culture and Nutrition During Pregnancy

Practice Statement: Food is fundamental to a person's social and racial identity. In many parts of the world, health is determined by traditional dietary rules and practices. Recommendations given by a nurse or health-care provider are often in direct conflict with cultural rules. As a result, women make food choices during the preconception period, during pregnancy, for feeding for their newborn, and during their postpartum period based on their cultural and social history.

Targeted Outcome: Healthy nutrition throughout pregnancy that is congruent with cultural practices

Evidence to Support: Development of a nutritious diet plan for pregnant women requires that nurses learn about and respect the food practices of the diverse clients with whom they work. Strong evidence exists that early nutrition has a positive effect on the growth and development of the fetus and the child. However, limited nursing research has been conducted on the cultural aspect of nutrition during pregnancy. Nurses who plan health promotion programs

for maternal-infant settings must consider race, ethnicity, and culture in order to plan culturally appropriate interventions. Differences exist from a cultural perspective in relation to weight gain and nutrition. Two qualitative studies were found that supported the importance of cultural considerations during prenatal care, one with Mexican American women and one with African American women. Cultural issues were seen as both support for and barriers to healthy nutrition. Other issues that emerged were economic and food security. Kannan and associates used a focus group approach to assess the cultural issues related to nutrition during pregnancy. Their study provides guidance on how to do a similar assessment within a community. Further evidence is needed that evaluates the effectiveness of cultural tailoring of pregnancy nutrition curriculum for diverse populations.

Recommended Approaches: Conducting a cultural assessment prior to implementing a nutritional program for pregnant women is a critical first step. Understanding the cultural norms for nutrition can help in the development of a pregnancy nutrition curriculum that incorporates cultural supports and addresses possible cultural barriers.

Sources
1. Koletzko, B., Brands, B., & Demmelmair, H. (2011). The Early Nutrition Programming Project (EARNST): 5 y of successful multidisciplinary collaborative research. *American Journal of Clinical Nutrition, 94*(Suppl.), 1749S-1753S.
2. Ramakrishnan, U., Grant, F., Goldenberg, T., Zongrone, A., & Martorell, R. (2012). Effect of women's nutrition before and during early pregnancy on maternal and infant outcomes: A systematic review. *Paediatric and Perinatal Epidemiology, 26*(Suppl. 1), 285–301. doi:10.1111/j.1365-3016.2012.01281.x.
3. Monti, D. (2000). Nutrition news. Food customs and their role in pregnancy and infant feeding. *International Journal of Childbirth Education, 15*(4), 18 (7 ref).
4. Brooten, D., Youngblut, J.M., Golembeski, S., Magnus, M.H., & Hannan, J. (2012). Perceived weight gain, risk and nutrition in pregnancy in five racial groups. *Journal of the American Academy of Nurse Practitioners, 24*(1), 32-42.
5. Berry, A.B. (1999). Mexican American women's expression the meaning of culturally congruent prenatal care. *Journal of Transcultural Nursing, 10*(3), 203-212.

6. Kannan, S., Webster, D., Sparks, A., Acker, C.M., Greene-Morton, E., Tropiano, E. & Turner, T. (2009). Using a cultural framework to assess the nutrition influences in relation to birth outcomes among African American women of childbearing age: Application of the PEN-3 theoretical model. *Health Promotion Practice, 10*(3), 349-358.

Prematurity and Low Birth Weight

As discovered by the nurses in City A, preterm birth and low birth weight are associated with increased morbidity and mortality during the first year of life as well as developmental delays that can extend across childhood. **Low birth weight (LBW)** is defined as a weight that is less than 5.5 pounds, or 2,500 grams, whereas **very low birth weight (VLBW)** is defined as a weight that is less than 3.3 pounds, or 1,500 grams. Babies born with a low birth weight have a variety of morbidities that correspond to the severity of their low birth weight.[53]

There are racial disparities in the United States in relation to LBW, with the African American low birth weight rate almost two times higher than that of white infants (14% vs. 7.4%). In some areas of the country, the rate can be three times as high.[54]

Strongly associated with LBW is preterm birth. **Preterm birth** is defined as a birth of a live infant before 37 weeks of gestation, whereas a very preterm infant is born at less than 32 weeks gestation (Fig. 18-5). Frequently, babies born prematurely face health problems

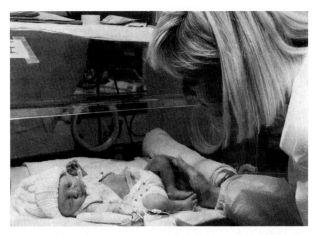

Figure 18-5 Nurse caring for premature infant. *(From the CDC public health awareness campaign to promote prenatal care; Centers for Disease Control and Prevention Public Health Images Library #8291.)*

such as respiratory distress owing to immature lungs and respiratory system; problems with feeding; difficulty with thermoregulation; jaundice; neurological problems with brain development; cerebral palsy; and risk for learning disabilities, blindness, and hearing loss. They are also at greater risk of death.[55,56] In addition, there are significant costs. In the United States, those costs amount to approximately $26 billion per year.[56]

Most infants born prematurely meet the definition of LBW, but not all infants with an LBW are premature. A way to help separate out the two terms is to evaluate the infant's weight, head circumference, and length against standardized growth charts based on gestational age. An infant born at 30 weeks who weighs 1,490 grams may meet the definition of VLBW, but is actually close to the 50th percentile for his gestational age. But an infant born at 38 weeks who weighs 2,400 grams not only meets the definition of LBW, but also is in the 5th percentile for his gestational age. Therefore, there are differences between preterm birth and LBW. From an epidemiological perspective, both prematurity and LBW are used as measures of the overall neonatal health of a population despite the overlap between the two terms.

The difficulty is determining the risk factors associated with each of these health indicators. In almost one-half of all preterm births, the cause is unknown. Risks associated with preterm labor include bacterial infection in the mother. It is thought that the infectious process sets off an immune response in the body of the pregnant mother that contributes to preterm labor and delivery. Another risk is psychological stress in the mother and fetal stress that trigger early uterine contractions. Corticotrophin-releasing hormone (CRH), a stress-related hormone, can be triggered by chronic psychosocial stress in the mother or physical stress to the fetus. The release of CRH is thought to precipitate uterine contractions that lead to premature labor and delivery. Maternal complications such as placental abruption are also linked to prematurity. In response to the bleeding, blood clotting stimulates uterine contractions. When there are multiple fetuses or abnormalities of the uterus or placenta, the uterus can be overstretched and premature contractions may occur. Infants born as multiple births are about nine times more likely be premature and have an LBW than singleton (one baby) births. Other medical risks include diabetes, hypertension, the mother being underweight before pregnancy, obesity, and short time between pregnancies. Finally, interventions such as inductions and cesarean sections can also lead to preterm births.[53-57] *HP 2020* includes target goals for the reduction in preterm births.

■ HEALTHY PEOPLE 2020
Maternal Infant Child Health (MICH) Objectives Related to Low Birth Weight

MICH objective 8.1 Reduce low birth weight (LBW)

Baseline: 8.2 percent of live births were low birth weight in 2007
Target: 7.8 percent
Target-Setting Method: Projection/trend analysis
Source: National Vital Statistics System–Natality (NVSS–N), CDC, NCHS

MICH objective 8.2 Reduce very low birth weight (VLBW)

Baseline: 1.5 percent of live births were VLBW in 2007
Target: 1.4 percent
Target-Setting Method: Projection/trend analysis

March of Dimes Prematurity Campaign

In 2003, the March of Dimes initiated the Prematurity Campaign with a goal of reducing the U.S. preterm birth rate by 15%.[54] This campaign includes funding for basic research to improve practice both in the United States and globally; provides information and services for families of newborns in neonatal intensive care units; and creates community intervention programs to increase awareness of the problem. In addition, the campaign helps health-care providers to identify risks for premature birth and increase their ability to detect these risks in pregnant women. Since the initiation of the campaign, the March of Dimes has awarded millions of dollars for research and advocated for the PREEMIE Act (Prematurity Research Expansion and Education for Mothers Who Deliver Infants Early) that became law in 2006. The work of the campaign also led to the 2005 publication of the Institute of Medicine report entitled *Preterm Birth: Causes, Consequences and Prevention.* Following the PREEMIE Act, the Surgeon General's office sponsored the first conference on Prevention of Preterm Birth in 2008. The March of Dimes sponsored a Symposium on Quality Improvement to Prevent Prematurity to address quality improvement strategies for prematurity prevention and published a white paper, *The Global and Regional Toll of Preterm Birth,* in 2009.[57] This white paper was in response to the fact that the rate of premature birth increased by 36% between the early 1980s and 2006. This trend and the dynamics underlying it underscored

the critical importance and timeliness of the March of Dimes Prematurity Campaign. Since then, the premature birth rate fell to 12.7 per 100 live births in 2006 and continued to decline, though at a slower rate, to 12.2 in 2011.[54] The campaign focuses on modifiable factors that also increase the risk of having an LBW infant, including prepregnancy weight, maternal age, and tobacco and other substance use.[57]

Knowledge of strategies to effect change in the modifiable risk factors for infant mortality, specifically preterm birth and LBW, include education of women about preconception health, and the risks of smoking, alcohol use, and illegal drug use. In addition, all health-care providers involved with pregnant women as well as pregnant women themselves must be aware of the signs of **preterm labor,** defined as the presence of uterine contractions between 20 and 37 weeks that result in progressive dilation and effacement of the cervix. Nurses must reach out to diverse population groups and integrate culturally sensitive messages into the educational materials and programs that they promote, advocate for legislation, and support federal and state legislation to increase research on prematurity and expand maternity care services.

● APPLYING PUBLIC HEALTH SCIENCE
The Case of the Small Babies
Public Health Science Topics Covered:

- Epidemiology
- Focused assessment
- Health planning
- Coalition building

In order to determine additional priority areas for nursing interventions, epidemiological and demographic data should be used for assessment. In response to the work begun with the Healthy Teens and Healthy Families program, the nurse team from City A also worked to obtain funding to address the preterm birth rate in the city. They were aware that their city had not met the *HP 2020* objective to reduce LBW and VLBW. To further evaluate the data, the nurse team compared the local rates with the state's, using the national morbidity data set. Their findings confirmed that the rate of preterm births exceeded the state and national rates as well as the *HP 2020* goals and had increased over the past decade from 15.5% to 22.2%. This was a little under double the national rate. The team decided to conduct a more in-depth epidemiological investigation to identify determinants of this health issue as well as strategies for addressing the problem in City A. To plan an intervention that would address preterm birth and LBW, the team partnered with the state department of maternal-child health and the local chapter of the March of Dimes. Both of these entities had a long-standing commitment to the improvement of maternal and infant outcomes and were able to provide some funding. Partnerships are essential to the success of programs that address population health issues for a variety of reasons. They adopted a model of partnership proposed by two public health nurses (PHNs), Leffers and Mitchell, that included the following components:[58]

- *Participation* by a number of constituencies strengthens the community support for the interventions.
- *Collaboration* that is necessary to address health problems is fundamental to partnerships.
- *Issues of diversity* can only be addressed respectfully and appropriately with representation of the various diverse groups in the community.
- *Expertise and resources* are stronger with broad partners working together.
- *Partnership relationships* are essential for the sustainability of interventions.

Another issue that the team addressed was disparities in preterm births and LBW related to ethnicity. At the national level, both the LBW rate and the preterm birth rate were higher for African American mothers than they were for any other ethnic group, with the LBW rate almost double in these mothers compared with non-Hispanic white mothers (13.3% vs. 7.1% in 2011) (Fig. 18-6). In the city where Leffers and Mitchell implemented this program, the LBW rate for African American mothers was 20.2%, compared with 6.8% for non-Hispanic white mothers, almost three times higher.

When they examined the literature to help understand the underlying causes of the disparity, two of the obvious possible causes were access to care and lower income among the minority populations, who are more often living in poverty and have less access to appropriate care. In a classic study, researchers dispelled the notion of the likelihood of genetic differences based on findings from their study that the rates of LBW and VLBW for first generation African American women were similar to the rates for U.S.-born, non-Hispanic white women and significantly less than the rate for U.S.-born, African American women.[59] Since then, much of the evidence supports a strong link between LBW and VLBW infants and social determinants,

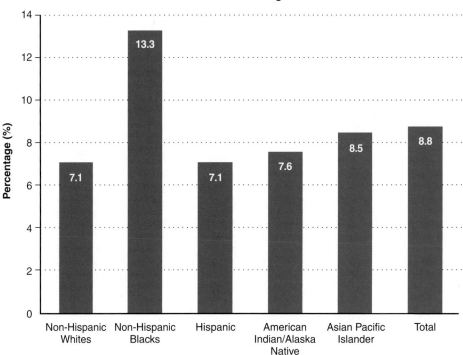

Percent of Low Birth Weight Births 2011

Figure 18-6 Low-birth-weight rates for 2011. *Source: National Center for Health Statistics. National Vital Statistics Reports (NVSR).*

poverty, racial discrimination, and chronic stress.[60] In addition, other minority-status mothers were also more likely to have LBW infants.[61]

Based on their analysis of the data that confirmed significant disparities among racial and ethnic groups in City A, the team developed a citywide Healthy Babies, Healthy Families program with two major goals that used the *HP 2020* objectives as their targets:

• **Goal 1** Reduce Preterm Births
• **Goal 2** Reduce the number of LBW and VLBW infants

The program included multiple interventions, including a media campaign and an outreach to underserved neighborhoods within the community using trained lay health workers, aimed at increasing prenatal care and promoting healthy living. The risk factors targeted by their program included the issues addressed in their first program with pregnant teens, tobacco use, and obesity, because these are associated with preterm births and LBW, while adding an intervention aimed at improving access to and utilization of prenatal care. They planned to expand their intervention to all women of childbearing age. In addition, to reach their goals to reduce preterm births and LBW, they needed to assess outcomes over a longer period of time to identify changes that could be attributed to the program in City A. The goals and objectives for the prematurity and LBW initiatives would be measured by both immediate outcomes and long-term impact evaluation (see Chapter 5).

In addition to the impact evaluation, the nurses were involved with a process evaluation (see Chapter 5). For the citywide Healthy Babies, Healthy Families program, the team created an advisory committee to strengthen the collaboration with the community and provide feedback. In the process evaluation, issues of implementation such as efficiency and effectiveness for the components of the program were addressed. In this case, the team evaluated the performance by team personnel, the lay health workers, educational resources and process, program participation and compliance with program elements, degree of fidelity to program interventions, timeliness, and budget expenditures. They located a number of resources for protocols and tools for evaluation.[62,63] The main long-term outcome of the Healthy Babies, Healthy Families program was a reduction in the number of preterm births and LBW and VLBW infants in City A, with a subsequent reduction in IMR as well.

Applying Public Health Science to Acute Maternal, Infant, and Child Health Settings

The use of a population-level approach is helpful in acute maternal-infant health settings as well. Often, the nurses are the first to pick up a trend in the health of infants and small children and reach out to the community to implement a prevention program. For example, as mentioned in Chapter 13, the trauma nurses at the Cincinnati Children's Hospital Medical Center developed and implemented a child passenger safety program based on their exposure to severe trauma in children who were not properly restrained in a car. The program was offered to low-income families at 46 fitting stations located in the community, including fire stations and health departments, so that parents could receive help on car seat installation. In other cases, nurses implement changes in procedures within the hospital setting to help provide better care, as illustrated in the use of an intensive care approach to care for children with polio in the 1950s (see Chapter 15). This requires applying public health science to the problem and determining whether the intervention was effective.

● APPLYING PUBLIC HEALTH SCIENCE
The Case of Toxins in the Nursery
Public Health Science Topics Covered:

• Epidemiology
  • Surveillance
  • Rates
• Health planning

In the neonatal intensive care units (NICU) at a tertiary care hospital, Nurse Franco became involved with a group of nurses from the Alliance of Nurses for Healthy Environments. They were specifically interested in addressing health risks to vulnerable newborns in the hospital setting. She began to engage her nurse colleagues in learning more about the environmental hazards specific to these infants. They met with the nurse manager for maternal-child health services and formed a small task force to identify and address the hazards. The nurses working in the nursery units had already been setting an agenda for the hospital system to decrease the rate of hospital-acquired infections in the nurseries, to promote a healthy maternity unit experience for both mother and baby, and to improve outcomes for low-birth-weight and preterm infants. When Nurse Franco added her concern about environmental hazards, the team wanted to learn more.

The team began with a needs assessment to identify the specific risks to newborn health in the nursery setting. They first learned more about the risks by consulting governmental and nongovernmental sources such as the National Library of Medicine (NLM), Health Care Without Harm, and Toxipedia. In particular, their TOXLINE and TOXNET data sources were very helpful to the team as they learned more about hazards. The Health Care Without Harm advocacy group, which was cofounded by nurses, not only provided information about the importance of safe hospital environments, but also provided links to advocacy and educational efforts for health promotion. At the NLM and Toxipedia Web sites, the nurses learned more about toxicology and the specific hazardous chemicals used in the nursery through a series of basic, useful introductory learning modules (Box 18-2). They learned that infants in the hospital nurseries were being exposed to harmful chemicals in the plastics used in tubing, bags, and plastics bottles used for feeding and medical interventions.[64] The most common chemical

---

BOX 18–2 Chemical Hazards in the Nursery

- Medical products made of polyvinyl chloride (PVC) include IV bags, tubing, catheters, and other plastic devices. Plasticizers are often used to soften the plastic and make it more flexible and durable during bending.
- Di(2-ethylhexyl)phthalate (DEHP) is a phthalate used to soften PVC. It is used in the nursery for tubing and plastic materials such as umbilical vessel catheters, peripherally inserted central catheter (PICC) lines, and enteral feeding products but can also be found in teethers, rattles, and other plastic baby toys.
  - It is absorbed into the body through leaching from the plastic into the body fluids.
  - In the neonate, it can damage the lungs, liver, kidneys, and reproductive nervous and immune systems
- Bisphenol A is a phenol that is used to make plastic more rigid and is found in baby bottles and water bottles.
  - BPA is generally absorbed into the body through diet.
  - According to the National Toxicology Program, there is a danger for the newborn and infant to experience adverse effects the brain, behavior, and prostate gland.

Source: See references 65–70.

---

hazards in the nursery were phthalates, particularly DEHP and bisphenol A (BPA).[65,66] Most alarming was the fact that newborn exposure to phthalates can be 20 times greater than the Food and Drug Administration's tolerable intake of 0.6 mg/kg per day.[67] As an endocrine disrupting toxicant, DEHP increases the risk to infants that can result in long-term adverse health effects.[66,68,69] Further, they found that in a study population, all infants had BPA in their urine at eight times the CDC median level for children aged 6 to 11 years.[65,70]

The direct effects of the harmful chemical exposures in the nursery for child development are difficult to measure for a variety of reasons. First, the determination of cause is difficult to prove owing to the long time span between exposure and effects as well as the multiple exposures that a child experiences before any health effects are noted. The nurse team learned that, as a part of the Children's Health Act of 2000 and funded by the federal government, the National Institute of Child Health and Development launched the National Children's Study to research the effects of environmental exposures on a study population of 100,000 children from preconception until age 21. By examining the influence of genetic, biological, chemical, and psychosocial factors, researchers will be able to better understand the effects of the specific exposures.[71]

Consequently, the nurse team discovered that the usual epidemiological data they would use to support a needs assessment were not available. Nurse Franco asked her nurse colleagues to read the precautionary principle developed by a team of experts at the Wingspread Center in January 1998 that states, "When an activity raises threats of harm to human health or the environment, precautionary measures should be taken even if some cause and effect relationships are not fully established scientifically. In this context the proponent of an activity, rather than the public, should bear the burden of proof."[72] The Alliance of Nurses for Healthy Environments reaffirmed this for nursing in their 2009 Wingspread Statement, developed by a team of environmental health nursing experts at Wingspread. In addition, they state, "Nurses have a role in protecting human health, especially of the most the vulnerable populations—the fetus, young children, the frail and elderly—from harm associated with environmental exposures."[73]

For further assessment, the nurses contacted the purchasing department of the hospital to identify all materials used in the nursery that might be likely to contain phthalates or other hazardous substances. Seeking to gain partners for the task force in the hospital system, they identified key informants for their work. Partners included nurse managers of the various maternal-child health units, directors of neonatal care and pediatrics, and personnel from the purchasing departments and occupational health. They supplied a resource list that included information about Practice Greenhealth[74] so that the hospital leaders would be able to learn what hospitals in other communities were doing to promote health in their workplace and community. The nurse team contacted all obstetricians and pediatricians on staff at the hospital to invite them to join the nurses in their efforts. The interdisciplinary composition of the partners is essential to successful collaboration for change in large systems such as that of a hospital.

The task force developed priorities for their work. First, for Goal 1 they planned an advocacy campaign to change the hospital purchasing policy to replace harmful materials containing phthalate and BPA alternatives. Second, for Goal 2 they planned an educational campaign about Green Nursing and how nurses can be change agents in their work settings. *Green Nursing* is a term used to identify ways that nurses can be involved in promoting environmentally friendly policies in their work settings while also promoting health to the populations they care for. Holly Shaner, a nurse who began the Nightingale Institute for Nursing and the Environment in 1996, urged hospital staff to identify ways to reduce the negative impact of hospital practices on the environment and to actually save money by doing so. One initiative was referred to as "Green Birthdays," in which harmful exposures for newborns were addressed.[75]

To expand their knowledge of how best to advocate for policy change, they consulted the Health Care Without Harm group,[76] the Maryland Hospitals for a Healthy Environment (MDH2E), and the Women's Environmental Health Network. The nurses and other experts who work with these organizations offered a number of strategies to achieve their goals.

With the resources available from these organizations and information provided by the purchasing department, the nurse team and Newborn Nursery Task Force developed a cost-benefit analysis to be used in the intervention phase of their work. They gathered information to demonstrate that hospital expenses could actually be reduced by the adoption of environmentally safe alternatives referred to as Environmentally

Friendly Purchasing. Citing the initiatives begun in 1996 by Health Care Without Harm and the Nightingale Institute for Nursing and the Environment,[76] they showed that waste segregation, safe disposal of hazardous materials, and toxic substance use reduction could actually save thousands of dollars annually.[77] Once they could demonstrate to the hospital administration that the use of DEHP and BPA alternatives would not cause excessive expenses, they were better able to prepare their policy recommendations.

They created several measurable objectives to meet each goal. For Goal 1, they set the following objectives:

- Objective 1: By the end of month 1, the team will create a letter signed by nurses, obstetricians, and pediatricians working with pregnant mothers and newborns to support their goals.
- Objective 2: By the end of month 3, the team will develop a business plan with the purchasing department that will replace the hazardous materials from the nursery and use safer alternatives. The recommendations include PVC-free products such as silicone, ethylene vinyl acetate (EVA), polypropylene, or polyurethane. In addition, safer alternatives are reported on the Sustainable Hospitals Project Web site and the Health Care Without Harm Web site.
- Objective 3: By the end of month 3, the team will develop supportive materials from their consultation with the Health Care Without Harm and Maryland Hospitals for a Healthy Environment to provide supportive evidence available for members of the Newborn Nursery Task Force to use when meeting with the hospital administration.
- Objective 4: By the end of month 4, the team will meet with the hospital administration to advocate for purchasing policy change.

Using their assessment information and prioritization of the plans, they formulated a timeline to implement the plans. Once they were able to address Objectives 1 through 4 and meet with the hospital administration, they would begin work on Goal 2. They met with the hospital administration only when they were prepared to strongly advocate for the proposed change. The hospital administrators elected to change the hospital purchasing policy to non-DEHP and non-BPA products because the nurse team had developed a sound proposal using public health science planning principles for advocacy.

Building on the success of the advocacy campaign, the nurse team developed objectives to meet Goal 2, which addressed how nurses can be change agents in their work settings through an educational campaign about Green Nursing.

- Objective 1: "By the end of month 1 the nurse team will establish a 'Green Team' in the hospital."
- Objective 2: "By the end of month 2, the nurse team will identify four key areas of the hospital for implementation of policy change for safer alternatives." From the Green Team examination of published research, they chose to implement change for hospital use of mercury, dioxin, and latex as well as policy for operating room and oncology unit exposures.
- Objective 3: "By the end of month 3, the Green Team will make application to Health Care Without Harm for one of the minigrants to create an educational seminar for staff nurses at the hospital. By the end of month 12, the Green Team will offer their first Green Nursing Seminar." Once these intermediate objectives were met, the Green Team would develop strategies for expanding their advocacy efforts.

The team consulted with the Women's Health & Environmental Network to learn more about their Environmentally Responsible Health Care program.[78] In addition to the creation of the Green Team, the nurses began to address their practice role in environmental health. Each nurse obtained an environmental assessment tool, I-PREPARE, that was developed by the Agency for Toxic Substances and Disease Registry.[79]

The nurses at this hospital were empowered by their success in addressing population health concerns for newborns in their work setting and building a Green Team to expand their work in environmental health in their city. In order to build programs, they established goals, objectives, and evaluation plans for all their activities, and sought program funding from Health Care Without Harm and other sources to continue the work of health promotion and prevention for their hospital and for their community.[80]

Maternal-Infant and Early Childhood Home Visiting

Home visiting has been a key component of public nursing since the turn of the last century as exemplified in the work done by Lillian Wald in New York City in the early 1900s (see Chapter 1). Nursing home health visits have traditionally included the delivery of health care in the home. It is not a specific, single intervention but rather represents a systematic approach to the delivery of services within the home setting that combines resources and supports available in the community. Common elements across home visiting programs for mothers and children include provision of social support to parents, connecting families to community services, and providing education to parents on childhood development.[81]

The Affordable Care Act and Maternal, Infant, and Early Child Home Visiting

Prior to the implementation of the Affordable Care Act (ACA), approximately 450,000, or about 2% of U.S. children and their families, received home visiting services. To help increase the number of children and families receiving these services, the 2010 ACA authorized federal funding for Maternal Infant and Early Child Home Visiting (MIECHV) programs. These were defined as programs that included home visiting as a primary service delivery strategy.[82] These programs were set up to be offered on a voluntary basis to pregnant women of children age 5 or under. The goal was to improve maternal-child health outcomes.[83] In 2012, $71,900,246 was awarded to 10 state-level organizations. The purpose was to implement home visiting programs that provide links to services as well as early childhood education for at-risk pregnant mothers and children aged 5 or under.[84] As part of the grant application process, organizations had to conduct a needs assessment (Chapter 4) using a public health approach to identify the needs of the population and tailor the program to the population and the specific needs of that population.

Home Visiting Program Models: What Works?

Astero and Allen[82] pointed out the evidence is divided over what works, but across studies there is evidence that home visiting programs have resulted in positive outcomes. Central to the effectiveness of programs is the inclusion of a systematic approach to the delivery of services. Kahn and Moore[81] completed a systematic review of 66 studies that included a home visiting component. They found that high-intensity, early childhood programs were effective for one or more childhood outcomes. The Health Resources and Services Administration has compiled a list of home visiting programs and encourages the collection of further evidence to support the use of a home visiting approach.[85]

Many of these interventions are delivered by PHNs. For example, in Washington County, Oregon, the Web site related to maternal-child home visits states that "the Field Team consists of experienced public health nurses who make home visits to pregnant or postpartum women and families with newborn infants or young children with special health care needs."[86] These nurses meet with families in their homes, provide education, and help to link the families with needed resources. The focus is to help decrease the disparity in childhood outcomes related to socioeconomic status.[82]

The Health Resources Services Administration (HRSA) published a list of evidence- based programs that meet their criteria (Box 18-3). The benchmarks chosen for the MIECHV programs are consistent with the goal of the program to reduce disparity in health outcomes in children. They include six areas (Box 18-4). The evidence-based programs listed by the HRSA are, for the most part, based on a developmental theoretical framework. For example, the Child First program is based on research related to early brain development. The program focuses on building a nurturing environment for at-risk children based on the hypothesis that nurturing is protective in relation to brain development.

Public health nurses providing maternal, infant, and child home visits are actively engaged in prevention using a selective approach (Chapter 2), providing interventions to mothers and children at greater risk for

BOX 18–3	**Evidence-Based Home Visiting Service Delivery Models**

Home Visiting Evidence of Effectiveness (HomVEE), a program within the U.S. Department of Health and Human Services, has reviewed 12 home visiting models that meet the HHS criteria for evidence-based models, including at least one high- or moderate-quality impact study with favorable, statistically significant impacts in two or more of the eight outcome domains; at least one of the impacts is from a randomized controlled trial and has been published in a peer-reviewed journal; and at least one of the impacts was sustained for at least 1 year after program enrollment.
- Child FIRST
- Early Head Start—Home Visiting
- Early Intervention Program for Adolescent Mothers
- Early Start (New Zealand)
- Family Check-Up
- Healthy Families America (HFA)
- Healthy Steps
- Home Instruction for Parents of Preschool Youngsters (HIPPY)
- Nurse Family Partnership (NFP)
- Oklahoma Community-Based Family Resource and Support Program
- Parents as Teachers (PAT)
- Play and Learning Strategies (PALS) Infant
- SafeCare Augmented

Source: See reference 85.

BOX 18–4	**Benchmark Areas to Demonstrate Improvement to Reduce Health Disparities in Children**

The six benchmark areas in which to demonstrate improvement among eligible families participating in the Maternal, Infant, and Early Childhood Home Visiting Program (MIECHV) are:
1. Improved maternal and newborn health
2. Prevention of child injuries, child abuse, neglect, or maltreatment, and reduction of emergency department visits
3. Improvement in school readiness and achievement
4. Reduction in crime or domestic violence
5. Improvements in family economic self-sufficiency
6. Improvements in the coordination and referrals for other community resources and supports.

Source: Health Resources and Services Administration. (n.d). *Maternal, Infant, and Early Childhood Home Visiting Program.* Retrieved from http://mchb.hrsa.gov/programs/homevisiting/.

poorer childhood outcomes. The effectiveness of the MEICHV programs will be tracked over the next decade, with the goal of a reduction of the disparity between children living in poverty and those more economically advantaged.

■ Summary Points

- Maternal, infant, and child health is a major indicator of the health of populations.
- Globally, the infant mortality and maternal mortality rates continue to be a major health issue.
- Preterm birth is a leading cause of infant mortality worldwide.
- Nurses working in maternal-child health settings can actively engage in efforts to improve the health of mothers and children through the implementation of programs at the community level and within an acute care nursing unit.

▲ CASE STUDY
Planning a Breastfeeding Promotion Program
Learning Outcomes
At the end of this case study, the student will be able to:

- Apply assessment strategies for accessing secondary data.
- Describe assessment strategies for obtaining primary data.

- Identify evidenced-based practice relevant to perinatal health promotion.
- Describe strategies for the development of a health program.

The nurses in an urban hospital in Rhode Island attended a professional development program that emphasized the role of nurses working in perinatal settings to promote breastfeeding. On return to work, they decided to review their current breastfeeding promotion program to identify opportunities for improvement and ways to connect with resources in the community. They invited the maternal-child health nurse at the city public health department to help them review the existing data about breastfeeding. She directed them to available Web sites including the Annie E. Casey Kid's Count Web site located at: http://datacenter.kidscount.org/data/bystate/Rankings.aspx?state=RI&ind=2881. They also consulted the Rhode Island data available at the Kaiser Family Foundation at http://www.statehealthfacts.org/profileind.jsp?cat=10&sub=117&rgn=41. Next, they identified evidence in the literature to guide their investigation and planning.

Using their approach, answer the following questions that apply to assessment and planning.

1. How does the state of Rhode Island's data compare with other national data?
2. Do the data indicate a need for breastfeeding support programming?
3. Where else can you search for data that are important for assessment?
4. What other information will help the needs assessment?
5. Consult nursing research to determine evidence-based strategies for nurses working in maternal-infant settings to improve breastfeeding support.
6. How will the problems be prioritized?
7. Describe the process of partnership. Who will be likely partners for the nurse team?
8. Develop a plan for one intervention in a maternal-infant setting.
9. Develop one goal and related objectives for the plan.

REFERENCES

1. World Health Organization. (2012). *What are the key health dangers for children?* Retrieved from http://www.who.int/features/qa/13/en/index.html.
2. World Health Organization. (2012). *Maternal mortality.* Retrieved from http://www.who.int/mediacentre/factsheets/fs348/en/index.html.
3. Buhler-Wilkerson, K. (1993). Bringing care to the people" Lillian Wald's legacy to public health. *American Journal of Public Health, 83,* 1778-1786.
4. *Healthy People 2020.* (2014). *Maternal, infant, and child health.* Retrieved from http://www.healthypeople.gov/2020/topicsobjectives2020/objectiveslist.aspx?topicId=26.
5. Hossain, M.M., & Islam, M.R. (2009). Socio-economic variables affecting infants and children mortality in Bangladesh. *The Internet Journal of Health, 9*(2). Retrieved from http://www.ispub.com/journal/the-internet-journal-of-health/volume-9-number-2/socio-economic-variables-affecting-infants-and-children-mortality-in-bangladesh.html#sthash.esk3O3Fy.dpbs. doi:10.5580/8f5.
6. World Health Organization. (2012). *Probability of dying under the age of five.* Retrieved from http://www.who.int/healthinfo/statistics/indunder5mortality/en/.
7. Reikpath, D.D., & Allotey, P. (2003). Infant mortality as an indicator of population health. *Journal of Epidemiology and Community Health, 57*(5), 344-346.
8. Central Intelligence Agency. (2014). *The World Fact Book: infant mortality rate.* Retrieved from https://www.cia.gov/library/publications/the-world-factbook/rankorder/2091rank.html.
9. United Nations. (2009). *World mortality.* Retrieved from http://www.un.org/esa/population/publications/worldmortality/WMR2009.htm.
10. MacDorman, M.F., & Mathews, T.J. (2009). *Behind international rankings of infant mortality: How the U.S. compares with Europe.* Retrieved from http://www.cdc.gov/nchs/data/databriefs/db23.htm.
11. Hamilton B.E., & Sutton, P.D. (2012). Health—E-stat recent trends in birth and fertility rates through June 2012. *National Vital Statistics Report, 61*(6).
12. March of Dimes. (2009). *March of Dimes white paper on preterm birth: The global and regional toll. March of Dimes Foundation.* Retrieved from http://www.marchofdimes.com/files/Global_white_paper.pdf.
13. World Health Organization. (2012). *Preterm birth.* Retrieved from http://www.who.int/mediacentre/factsheets/fs363/en/.
14. World Health Organization. (2012). *Trends in maternal mortality 1990–2010: WHO, UNICEF, UNFPA & World Bank estimates.* Geneva, Switzerland: Author. Retrieved from http://www.who.int/reproductive-health/publications/monitoring/9789241503631/en/index.html.
15. Hogan, M.C., Foreman, K.J., Naghavi, M., Ahn, S.Y., Wang M., Makela, S.M., & Murray, C.J.L. (2010). Maternal mortality for 181 countries, 1980–2008: A systematic analysis of progress towards Millennium Development Goal 5. *The Lancet, 375,* 1609-1623.
16. U.S. Department of Health and Human Services, Health Resources and Services Administration, Maternal and Child Health Bureau. (2010). *Child*

health USA 2010. Rockville, Maryland: Author. Retrieved from http://www.mchb.hrsa.gov/chusa10/hstat/hsi/pages/205mm.html.

17. Preeclampsia Foundation. (2014). *Accelerating preeclampsia research.* Retrieved from http://www.preeclampsia.org/research.

18. UNICEF, World Health Organization, the World Bank & United Nations. (2012). *Level and trends in child mortality report 2012.* New York, NY: The United Nations Children's Fund.

19. Centers for Disease Control and Prevention. (2012). *Child health.* Retrieved from http://www.cdc.gov/nchs/fastats/children.htm.

20. World Health Organization. (2012). *Millennium development goals.* Retrieved from http://www.who.int/mediacentre/factsheets/fs290/en/.

21. Potter, P. (2001). About the cover: Ignaz Philipp Semmelweis (1818–65). *Emerging Infectious Diseases, 7*(2). doi:10.3201/eid0702.AC0702.

22. Dwyer, T., & Ponsonby, A.L. (1995). SIDS epidemiology and incidence. *Pediatric Annals, 24*(7), 350-352; 354-356.

23. Fleming, P.J., Blair, P.S., Bacon, C., Bensley, D., Smith, I. Taylor, E. et al. (1996). Environment of infants during sleep and risk of sudden infant death syndrome: Results of 1993–5 case-control study for confidential inquiry into stillbirths and deaths in infancy. Confidential Enquiry into Stillbirths and Deaths Regional Coordinators and Researchers. *British Journal of Medicine, 313*(7051), 191-195.

24. Mitchell, E.A., Tuohy, P.G., Brunt, J.M., Thompson, J.M., Clements, M.S., Stewert, A.W. et al. (1997). Risk factors for sudden infant death syndrome following the prevention campaign in New Zealand: A prospective study. *Pediatrics, 100*(5), 835-840.

25. Anderson, M.E., Johnson, D.C., & Batal, H.A. (2005). Infant sleep position practices 2 years into the "Back to Sleep" campaign. *Clinical Pediatrics, 39*(5), 285-289.

26. Martin J.A., Hamilton, B.E., Sutton, P.D., Ventura, S.J., Menacker, F., Kimeyer, S., & Mathews, T.J. (2009) Births: Final data for 2006. *National Vital Statistics Reports, 57*(7). Hyattsville, MD: National Center for Health Statistics.

27. American SIDS Institute. (2014). *Incidence.* Retrieved from http://sids.org/what-is-sidssuid/incidence/.

28. Heron, M.P., Hoyert, D., Murphy, S.L., Xu, J.Q., Kochanek, K.D., & Tejada-Vera, B. Deaths: Final data for 2006. (2009) *National vital statistics reports, 57*(14). Hyattsville, MD: National Center for Health Statistics.

29. McKinley, J.B. (1994). A case for refocusing upstream: The political economy of illness. In P. Conrad & R. Kern. (Eds.). *The sociology of health and illness: Critical perspectives* (4th ed., pp. 509-523). New York, NY: St. Martin's Press.

30. Watkins, M.L., Rasmussen, S.A., Honein, M.A., Botto, L.D., & Moore, C.A. (2003). Maternal obesity and risk for birth defects. *Pediatrics, 111*(5), 1152-1158.

31. Chen, A., Feresu, S.A., Fernandez, C., & Rogan, W.J. (2009). Maternal obesity and the risk of infant death in the United States. *Epidemiology, 20*(1), 74-81.

32. Lieberman, R.W., Bagdasarian, N., Thomas, D., & Van De Ven, C. (2011). Seasonal Influenza A (H1N1) infection in early pregnancy and second trimester fetal demise. *Emerging Infectious Disease, 17*(1). Retrieved from http://wwwnc.cdc.gov/eid/article/17/1/09-1895_article.htm.

33. Centers for Disease Control and Prevention. (2013). *Pertussis outbreak trends.* Retrieved from http://www.cdc.gov/pertussis/outbreaks/trends.html.

34. Centers for Disease Control and Prevention. (2012). *Teen pregnancy.* Retrieved from http://www.cdc.gov/reproductivehealth/AdolescentReproHealth/index.htm.

35. Fluhr, J.D., Oman, R.F., Allen, J.R., Lanphier, M.G., & McLeroy, K.R. (2004). A collaborative approach to program evaluation of community-based teen pregnancy prevention programs. *Health Promotion Practice, 5*(2), 127-137.

36. Chen, X., Wen, S.W., Fleming, N., Demissie, K., Rhoads, G.G., & Walker, M. (2007). Teenage pregnancy and adverse birth outcomes: A large population based retrospective cohort study. *International Journal of Epidemiology, 36*(2), 1-6.

37. Koshar, J.H., & Catlin, A.J. (2001). Pediatric ethics, issues, & commentary: Teen pregnancy 2001: Still no easy answers. *Pediatric Nursing, 27*(5), 505-509.

38. Hewitt-Taylor, J. (2012). Identifying, analyzing and solving problems in practice. *Nursing Standard, 26*(40), 35-41.

39. Smith, S., Hulsey, T., & Goodnight, W. (2008). Effects of obesity on pregnancy. *Journal of Obstetric and Gynecological Nursing, 37,* 176-184.

40. Sangalang, B.B., Barth, R.P., & Painter, J.S. (2006). First-birth outcomes and timing of second births: A statewide case management program for adolescent mothers. *Health and Social Work, 31*(1), 54-64.

41. Porter, L.S., & Holness, N.A. (2012). Breaking the repeat teen pregnancy cycle: how nurses can nurture resilience in at-risk teens. *Nursing for Women's Health,* 369-381. doi:10.1111/j.1751-486X.2011.01661.x.

42. Simmons, R. (2008). Perinatal programming of obesity. *Seminars in Perinatology, 32*(5), 371-374.

43. Centers for Disease Control and Prevention. (2008). *Press release: Pregnant women who are obese linked with greater health care services use; also have longer hospital stays* Retrieved from http://www.cdc.gov/media/pressrel/2008/r080402.htm.

44. Centers for Disease Control and Prevention. (2009). Trends in smoking before, during and after pregnancy—Pregnancy Risk Assessment Monitoring System (PRAMS), United States, 31 sites, 2000–2005. *Morbidity and Mortality Weekly Report Surveillance Summaries, 58*(SS04), 1-29.

45. March of Dimes. (2012). *Prematurity research.* Retrieved from http://www.marchofdimes.com/research/prematurityresearch.html.

46. Centers for Disease Control and Prevention. (2012). *Tobacco use and pregnancy.* Retrieved from http://www.cdc.gov/reproductivehealth/TobaccoUsePregnancy/.

L

47. Centers for Disease Control and Prevention. (2012). *Smoking and tobacco use: Secondhand effects.* Retrieved from http://www.cdc.gov/tobacco/data_statistics/fact_sheets/secondhand_smoke/general_facts/#children.

48. American Cancer Society. (2012). *Secondhand smoke.* Retrieved from http://www.cancer.org/cancer/cancercauses/tobaccocancer/secondhand-smoke.

49. Centers for Disease Control and Prevention. (2013). *Secondhand smoke facts.* Retrieved from http://www.cdc.gov/tobacco/data_statistics/fact_sheets/secondhand_smoke/general_facts/#children.

50. Green, H.H., & Documet, P.L. (2005). Parent peer education: lessons learned from a community-based initiative for teen pregnancy prevention. *Journal of Adolescent Health, 37*(Suppl. 3), S100-S107.

51. Hoyt, H.H., & Broom, B.L. (2002). School-based teen pregnancy prevention programs: A review of the literature. *School Nurse, 18*(1), 11-17.

52. Van de Ven, A.H., & Delbecq, A.L. (1972). The nominal group as a research instrument for exploratory health studies. *American Journal of Public Health, 62*(3), 336-342.

53. Health Resources Services Administration. (2012). *Child health 2011: Low birth weight.* Retrieved from http://mchb.hrsa.gov/chusa11/hstat/hsi/pages/201lbw.html.

54. Health Resources Services Administration. (2012). *Child health: Premature birth.* Retrieved from http://mchb.hrsa.gov/chusa11/hstat/hsi/pages/203pb.html.

55. March of Dimes. (2012). *March of Dimes prematurity campaign.* Retrieved from http://www.marchofdimes.com/mission/prematurity_campaign.html.

56. Centers for Disease Control and Prevention. (2012). *Reproductive health: Preterm birth.* Retrieved from http://www.cdc.gov/reproductivehealth/MaternalInfantHealth/PretermBirth.htm.

57. March of Dimes. (2009). *White paper on the preterm birth: The global and regional toll.* Retrieved from http://www.marchofdimes.com/mission/globalprograms_pretermbirthreport.html.

58. Leffers, J., & Mitchell, E.M. (2011). Conceptual model for partnership and sustainability in global health. *Public Health Nursing, 28*(1), 91-102.

59. David, R.J., & Collins, J.W. (1997). Differing birth weight among infants of US born blacks, African born blacks and US born whites. *New England Journal of Medicine, 337*, 1209-1214.

60. Rowley, D.L. (2001). Closing the gap, opening the process: Why study social contributors to preterm delivery among black women. *Maternal & Child Health Journal, 5*(2), 71-74.

61. Acevedo-Garcia, D., Soobader, M., & Berkman, L.F. (2005). The differential effect of foreign born status on low birth weight by race/ethnicity and education. *Pediatrics, 1215*(Suppl. 1), e20-e30.

62. McKenzie, J.F., Neiger, B.L., & Thackeray, R. (2009). *Planning, implementing & evaluating: Health promotion programs* (5th ed.). San Francisco, CA: Pearson/Benjamin Cummings.

63. Griffin, F., Reininger, R.M., Parra-Medina,D., Evans, A.E., Sanderson, M., & Vincent, M. (2005). Development of multidimensional scales to measure key leader's perceptions of community capacity and organizational capacity for teen pregnancy prevention. *Family and Community Health, 28*(4), 307-319.

64. Shea, K.M. (2003). Pediatric exposure and potential toxicity of phthalate plasticizers. *Pediatrics, 111*(6), 1467-1474.

65. Calafat, A.M., Weuve, J., Ye, X., Jia, L.T., Hu, H., Ringer S., Huttner, K., & Hauser R. (2009). Exposure to bisphenol A and other phenols in neonatal intensive care unit premature infants. *Environmental Health Perspectives, 117*(4), 639-644.

66. Pak, V.M., Nailon, R.E., & McCauley, L.A. (2007). Controversy: Neonatal exposure to plasticizers in the NICU. *American Journal of Maternal Child Nursing, 32*(4), 244-249.

67. Jaeger, R.J., Weiss, A.L., & Brown, K. (2005). Infusion of di-2-ethylhexylphthalate for neonates: A review of potential health risk. *Journal of Infusion Nursing, 28*(1), 54-60.

68. Calafat, A.M., Needham, L.L., Silva, M.J., & Lambert, G. (2004). Exposure to di-(2-ethylhexyl)phthalate among premature neonates in a neonatal intensive care unit. *Pediatrics, 113*(5), e429-434.

69. Sattler, B., & Malkan, S. (2005). Toxic chemicals in IV tubing. *New Jersey Nurse, 35*(4), 7.

70. Green, R., Hauser, R., Calafat, A., Weuve, J., Schettler, T., Ringer, S., et al. (2005). Use of di(2-ethylhexyl) phthalate-containing medical products and urinary levels of mono(2-ethylhexyl) phthalate in neonatal intensive care unit infants. *Environmental Health Perspectives, 113*(8), 1222-1225.

71. U.S. Department of Health and Human Services. (2009). *The national children's study: Health, growth, environment.* Retrieved from http://www.nationalchildrensstudy.gov/Pages/default.aspx.

72. Raffensperger, C., & Tickner, J. (1999). *Protecting public health and the environment: Implementing the precautionary principle.* Washington, DC: Island Press.

73. Afzal, B., Gilden, R., Sattler, B., Smith, C., Choiniere, D., Anderko, L., et al. (2009). *ANHE Wingspread Statement. Alliance of Nurses for Healthy Environments.* Retrieved from http://e-commons.org/anhe/files/2009/07/anhe-wingspread-statement-2009.pdf.

74. *Practice Greenhealth.* (n.d.). Retrieved from http://www.practicegreenhealth.org/.

75. Shaner, H. (2002). Green birthdays. *Journal of Pediatric Nursing, 17*(3), 222-225.

76. Hall, A.G. (2006). Nurses: Taking precautionary action on a pediatric environmental exposure: DEHP. *Pediatric Nursing, 32*(1), 91-93.

77. Shaner-McRae, H., McRae, G., & Jas, V. (2007). Environmentally safe health care agencies: Nursing's responsibility, nightingale's legacy. *Journal of Issues in Nursing, 12*(2) online. Retrieved from http://www.medscape.com/viewarticle/561370.

78. Women's Environmental Health Network. (2009). *Environmentally responsible health care.* Retrieved from http://www.when.org/index.php?option=com_content&

view=article&id=116:environmentally-responsible-healthcare&catid=64:health-care&Itemid=106.

79. Agency for Toxic Substances and Disease Registry. (n.d.). *Environmental exposure history: I-PREPARE card.* Retrieved from http://www.atsdr.cdc.gov/asbestos/site-kit/docs/IPrepareCard.pdf.

80. Schlettler, T. (2002). DEHP exposures during the medical care of infants: A cause for concern. In *Going Green: A resource kit for pollution prevention in health care.* Reston, VA: Health Care Without Harm. Retrieved from https://noharm-uscanada.org/sites/default/files/documents-files/100/DEHP_Exposure_of_Infants.pdf.

81. Kahn, J., & Moore, K.A. (2010). What works for home visiting programs: Lessons from experimental evaluations of programs and interventions. *Child trend fact sheets* (Publication No. 2010). Retrieved from http://www.childtrends.org/wp-content/uploads/2005/07/2010-17WWHomeVisit.pdf.

82. Astero, J., & Allen, L. (2009). Home visiting and young children: An approach worth investing in? *Social Policy Report, 23*(5), 3-21.

83. Health Resources and Services Administration. (n.d.). *Maternal infant and early childhood home visiting program.* Retrieved from http://mchb.hrsa.gov/programs/homevisiting/.

84. U.S. Department of Health and Human Services news release. (2012). *Health care law expands support for children and families.* Retrieved from http://www.hhs.gov/news/press/2012pres/04/20120403b.html.

85. Health Resources and Services Administration. (n.d) *Home visiting models.* Retrieved from http://mchb.hrsa.gov/programs/homevisiting/models.html.

86. Washington County, OR. (n.d.). *Field team—maternal child health home visiting.* Retrieved from http://www.co.washington.or.us/HHS/PublicHealth/field-team-maternal-child-health-home-visiting.cfm.

Chapter 19

Health Planning for School Settings

LEARNING OUTCOMES

After reading this chapter, the student will be able to:

1. Define *school nursing*.
2. Discuss the contribution of school health to the achievement of *Healthy People 2020* objectives.
3. Describe the components of a coordinated school health program.
4. Describe the roles, responsibilities, and interventions of school nurses in providing wellness care, episodic care, and care to children with noncommunicable illnesses or behavioral health problems.

5. Discuss other school nursing interventions focused on health teaching, advocacy, and policy development.
6. Discuss the role of school nurses in addressing health disparities among school-age children in the United States.
7. Discuss the role of policy in understanding school nursing practice.
8. Discuss challenges to school health nursing for the future.

KEY TERMS

Asthma action plan
Body mass index (BMI)
Coordinated school
   health program
Cyberbullying
Delegation

Disabilities
Individualized education
   program
Individualized family
   service plan

Individualized Healthcare
   Plan
Least restrictive
   environment
National Health Education
   Standards

School-based health
   center
School nursing
Title I

■ Introduction

The National Association of School Nurses (NASN) defines **school nursing** as:

> a specialized practice of professional nursing that advances the well-being, academic success and life-long achievement and health of students. To that end, school nurses facilitate positive student responses to normal development; promote health and safety including a healthy environment; intervene with actual and potential health problems; provide case management services; and actively collaborate with others to build student and family capacity for adaptation, self-management, self-advocacy, and learning.[1]

School nurses use the nursing process to provide individual and population-based care in schools to facilitate the school nurse's goal of supporting the health and academic achievement of students:

- Assessment
- Diagnosis
- Outcome identification
- Planning
- Implementation
- Evaluation

School nurses may be employed by local school districts, health departments, hospitals, or other entities.

Health priorities and educational goals converge in school nursing, requiring the school nurse to understand and function in two cultures: the worlds of health and education. Translation of these two cultures is a vital role for school nurses as they advocate for students. The school nurse is knows both education and health priorities, goals, policies, and legal requirements in the implementation of school health services. This knowledge places school nurses in a central role as coordinators and connectors in the school setting. The NASN published the Code of Ethics to set forth "a commonality of moral and ethical conduct" for school nurses. The code of ethics for school nurses focuses on three aspects: client care, professional competency, and professional responsibilities (Box 19-1).[2]

▶ SOLVING THE MYSTERY
An Outbreak of Mild Febrile Illness

Public Health Science Topics Covered:
- Outbreak investigation
- Collaboration

On Thursday, April 23, 2009, the school bell rang, and within minutes there were six students who reported to the school nurse's office. This was slightly above the norm. The students reported sore throats and high fevers. Once the school nurse, Mary, finished with these six students, she became aware of a growing number of students who were lined up outside her office waiting to be seen. The symptoms were very similar. Most of the students had fevers of 101°F. Some had headaches. She was used to seeing a large number of students per day, often with similar types of complaints. This was different. There were at least a dozen students in line. Although it was a large school of 2,700 students, the number of sick children was alarming. Mary decided that she should notify the doctor on

---

BOX 19–1   National Association of School Nurses: Code of Ethics for School Nurses

Client Care:
The school nurse is an advocate for students, families, and members of the school community.
- School nurses deliver care in a manner that promotes and preserves student, family, and community client autonomy, dignity, and rights.
- School nurses support and promote individuals' and families' ability to achieve the highest quality of life as understood by each individual and family.
- School nurses deliver care in an inclusive, collaborative manner that embraces diversity in the school community.
- School nurses maintain client confidentiality within the legal, regulatory, and ethical parameters of health and education.
- School nurses advocate on behalf of clients' needs.

Professional Competency:
The profession of nursing is obligated to provide competent nursing care.
- The school nurse must be aware of the need for continued professional learning and must assume personal responsibility for currency of knowledge and skills.
- School nurses must evaluate their own nursing practice in relation to professional practice standards and relevant statutes, regulations, and policies.
- School nurses must have knowledge relevant to meet the needs of clients within the school setting. Because individual expertise varies, nurses consult with peers and other health professionals with expertise and recognized competencies in various fields of practice. When in the client's best interest, the school nurse

refers clients to other health professionals and community health agencies.
- Nurses are accountable for judgments made and actions taken in the course of nursing practice. The scope and standards of school nursing practice reflect a practice rounded in ethical commitment. The school nurse is responsible for establishing and maintaining a practice based on these standards.

Professional Responsibilities:
The school nurse:
- Is obligated to demonstrate adherence to the profession's standards by monitoring these standards in daily practice, participating in the profession's efforts to improve school health services, and promoting student health and academic success.
- Utilizes available research in developing the health programs and individual plans of care and interventions.
- Participates in and promotes research activities as a means of advancing school health services and the health of students. This is done as appropriate to the nurse's education, position, and practice environment and in adherence to the ethics that govern research, specifically:
  - Right to privacy and confidentiality
  - Voluntary and informed consent
  - Awareness of and participation in the mechanisms available to ensure the rights of human subjects, particularly vulnerable populations (minors, disabled, etc.)
- Recognizes that practice environments impact the quality of client care and is cognizant of the need to work with others to improve these environments.

Source: See reference 2.

call for the Bureau of School Health. Within a short time, the city health department was there to investigate. By the next day, the number of sick children was even greater. Mary acted swiftly, engaging the public health department to help explain this crisis in this school. Her quick thinking helped launch a global investigation into an emerging life-threatening disease.

In this real-life case, the school nurse, Mary Pappas, became known for her role in identifying a large outbreak of influenza A, or the HINI influenza, at her school (see Chapters 8 and 13).[3,4] The majority of the 124 students and employees with the confirmed HINI had a mild, febrile disease, with a median incubation period of 2.2 days. Several students had returned from Mexico where they had gone for spring break, which was evidence of the link to a new respiratory illness that had emerged in Mexico and quickly spread throughout the United States and 21 countries by May 6, 2009. By June 11, 2009, the World Health Organization (WHO) declared a worldwide pandemic.[5] The actions of school nurses in cases similar to the HINI outbreak illustrate the role of nurses in case finding, surveillance, and providing the leadership needed within schools and communities to address continuing and emergent health issues.[6]

Historical Foundations of School Nursing

School nursing emerged as a specialty within the broader field of public health nursing. In the beginning of the 20th century, the convergence of compulsory education laws in the United States and medical exclusion of students with contagious diseases paved the way for Lillian Wald (see Chapter 1) to collaborate with the New York City Board of Education and Board of Health to hire a school nurse to work with students and families in four schools where there were high numbers of student absenteeism and medical exclusions.[7] On October 1, 1902, Lina Rogers Struthers's work began as a month-long experiment when she took the role of a school nurse in those four New York City schools. By December, Lina Rogers Struthers's use of school nurse assessments, planning, interventions, evaluations, and documentation yielded increased school time for children and an expansion of the school nurse staff from one nurse to 12.

Lina Rogers Struthers, who became the superintendent of school nurses for New York City schools, and the school nurses who worked with her were the first school nurses hired by a municipality. The advent of school nursing resulted in students being able to remain in schools if possible and only excluded children with communicable diseases.[7] The presence of school nurses proved effective. From October 1902 to October 1903, student health-related exclusions from New York City public schools decreased by more than 90%, from 10,567 students to 1,101 students.[8] Based on this groundbreaking work by the New York City school nurse demonstration project, school nursing spread throughout the United States and Canada. From the inception of school nursing, school nurses focused on whole school populations and individual student case coordination. They assisted in the delivery of school health programs from that point on such as the 1920s movement to increase the consumption of milk by school-age children (Fig. 19-1) and are an integral part of school-based health programs in the 21st century.

Healthy People 2020 and School Nursing

Two new topics were identified in *Healthy People 2020 (HP 2020)* that have particular relevance to school nursing—those of early and middle childhood and adolescent health. Both of these topics emphasize the link between behavioral patterns established in either early childhood or adolescence to adult health and the

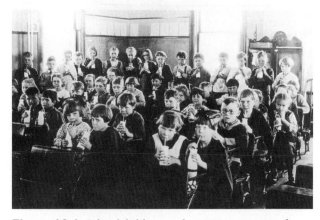

Figure 19-1 Schoolchildren and a 1920s campaign for drinking milk. *(From the Centers for Disease Control and Prevention/Minnesota Department of Health, R.N. Barr Library; Librarians Melissa Rethlefsen and Marie Jones, 1922.)*

role of the school setting in promoting health. Thus, school nurses have a very important role to play in influencing health outcomes in children and adolescents as well as the long-term health of these children in the future.

■ HEALTHY PEOPLE 2020
School Health

HP 2020 Topic relevant to School Health: Early and Middle Childhood

Goal: Document and track population-based measures of health and well-being for early and middle childhood populations over time in the United States.

Overview: There is increasing recognition in policy, research, and clinical practice communities that early and middle childhood provide the physical, cognitive, and social-emotional foundation for lifelong health, learning, and well-being. Early childhood, middle childhood, and adolescence represent the three stages of child development. Each stage is organized around the primary tasks of development for that period.

Selected *HP 2020* Objectives: Early and Middle Childhood

EMC–1: (Developmental) Increase the proportion of children who are ready for school in all five domains of healthy development: physical development, social-emotional development, approaches to learning, language, and cognitive development.
EMC–4: Increase the proportion of elementary, middle, and senior high schools that require school health education.
Source: See reference 9.

HP 2020 Topic relevant to School Health: Adolescent Health

Goal: Improve the healthy development, health, safety, and well-being of adolescents and young adults.
Overview: Adolescents (aged 10 to 19) and young adults (aged 20 to 24) make up 21% of the population of the United States. The behavioral patterns established during these developmental periods help determine young people's current health status and their risk for developing noncommunicable diseases in adulthood.

Selected *HP 2020* Adolescent Health Objectives

AH–2: Increase the proportion of adolescents who participate in extracurricular and out-of-school activities.

AH–5: Increase educational achievement of adolescents and young adults.
AH–6: Increase the proportion of schools with a school breakfast program.
AH–7: Reduce the proportion of adolescents who have been offered, sold, or given an illegal drug on school property.
AH–8: Increase the proportion of adolescents whose parents consider them to be safe at school.
Source: See reference 10.

HP 2020 also includes a topic on educational and community-based programs. This topic includes schools as one of the targeted settings for delivery of these programs aimed at improving health.[11] An important objective under this topic is objective number 5: "Increase the proportion of elementary, middle, and senior high schools that have a full-time registered school nurse-to-student ratio of at least 1:750 per student."[11] Currently, the ratio varies by states and regions with some school districts providing one school nurse for every 1,500 students. Though at the national level this target was met, by 2011, 38 states had improved their school nurse-to-student ratio in a 10-year period.[12] This *HP 2020* topic also includes objectives related to the provision of health-related educational programs including such topics as unintentional injury; violence; suicide; tobacco use and addiction; alcohol or other drug use; unintended pregnancy, HIV/AIDS, and sexually transmitted infections (STIs); unhealthy dietary patterns; and inadequate physical activity.[11]

Coordinated School Health Programs

With 50 million students spending a significant portion of their lives in school, schools are one of the most powerful social institutions shaping the next generation. The primary mission of schools is education, but health is also important as educational outcomes are intricately linked to health. Consequently, a coordinated school health program is important and the school nurse is a vital link in this effort (Fig. 19-2). **A coordinated school health program** is an integral set of planned, sequential, school-affiliated strategies, activities, and services designed to promote the optimal physical, emotional, social, and educational development of students.[13–15] The concept of a comprehensive school health program is not new. The model is built on the inclusion of four main supportive structures:

- School health advisory council
- School health coordinator

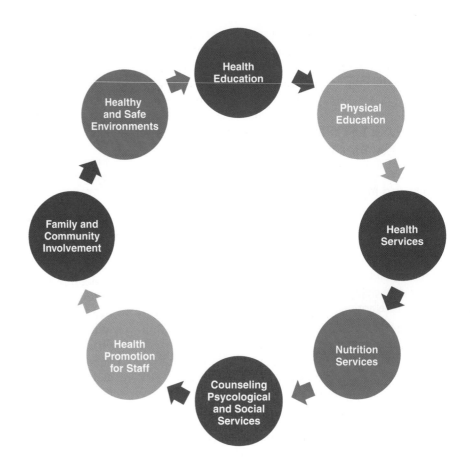

Figure 19-2 Coordinated school health program.

- School-based health teams
- School board policy[16]

Members of the team include teachers, principals, administrators, school board members, nurses, psychologists, counselors, and other health and education experts and researchers. A coordinated school health program is made up of eight components:

- Health education
- Physical education
- Health services
- Nutrition services
- Counseling—for both psychological and social services
- Healthy school environment
- Health promotion for staff, family, and community involvement[15,16]

Health Education Component

The heath education component consists of a planned, sequential, K–12 curriculum that addresses the physical, mental, emotional, and social aspects of health.[16] The goal is to motivate and assist students in maintaining and improving their health, preventing disease, and reducing health-related risk behaviors. It allows students to develop and demonstrate health-related knowledge, attitudes, skills, and practices. The comprehensive health education curriculum includes a variety of topics such as personal health, family health, community health, consumer health, environmental health, sexuality education, mental and emotional health, injury prevention and safety, nutrition, prevention and control of disease, and substance use and abuse. Qualified, trained teachers provide health education.

The School Health Policies and Practices Study (SHPPS) is a national survey that is conducted regularly at the state and district levels. It was conducted in 1994, 2000, 2006, 2012 and again in 2014 at all levels (state, district, school, and classroom).[17] In 2012, three-quarters (74%) of states had adopted the 2007 **National Health Education Standards** (NHES) that includes eight areas.[18] According to the Centers for Disease Control and Prevention (CDC), the NHES "were developed to establish, promote and support health-enhancing behaviors for students in all grade levels—from pre-Kindergarten through grade 12."[18] These standards provide the framework for the curricula and the methods used to deliver the curricula. They also provide guidelines for assessing student progress as well as expectations for school-based health education programs.[18] In a 2007 review of the 2006 SHPPS data, school nurses were responsible for teaching content in approximately 40% of the elementary schools and 20% of middle and high schools.[19] Based on the 2012 data, at the state level, only 5.4% of state health education coordinators had a bachelor of science in nursing (BSN) compared with 43% with a bachelor's degree in health education and 14% with a bachelor's degree in physical education.[17]

Physical Education Component

The physical education component consists of a planned, sequential K–12 curriculum that provides cognitive content and learning experiences in a variety of activity areas such as basic movement skills; physical fitness; rhythms and dance; games; team, dual, and individual sports; tumbling and gymnastics; and aquatics. Quality physical education should promote, through a variety of planned physical activities, each student's optimal physical, mental, emotional, and social development, and should promote activities and sports that all students enjoy and can pursue throughout their lives. It is recommended that qualified, trained teachers teach physical activity.[20]

Almost two-thirds of the nation's high school students do not meet recommended levels of participation in physical activity (being physically active 60 minutes per day, 5 days a week).[21] There is also a disparity in physical activity by race and ethnicity. About 20% more white high school students meet this criterion than do black or Hispanic high school students.[21] In addition, few schools provide daily physical education for students in all grades in the school for the entire school year. Specifically, only 3.8% of all elementary schools, 7.9% of all middle schools, and 2.1% of all high schools provide daily physical education per school year.[21]

A growing body of evidence shows that increased time for physical activity programs is associated with a neutral or positive impact on academic outcomes.[22] The school nurse can play an important role in promoting increased physical activity either inside school or outside school. Children can be encouraged to bike or walk to school or walking programs can be initiated. Within the classroom, creative approaches are being used and a recent review of a classroom-based physical activity program called Take 10—integrating academics and physical activity—shows promise.[22] Take 10 was found to

increase levels of physical activity among elementary-level students, improve academic scores, and decrease **body mass index (BMI)** Z scores (the number that results from the BMI calculation). BMI is a score that is calculated by dividing a person's body mass (expressed in kilograms) divided by the square of their height (expressed in meters) (see below).

Health Services Component

The health services component is a service provided to students that assesses, protects, and promotes health. These services are designed to ensure access or referral to primary care services, foster appropriate use of primary care services, prevent and control communicable disease, provide emergency care for illness or injury, promote and provide optimal sanitary conditions for a safe school facility and school environment, and provide educational and counseling opportunities for promoting and maintaining individual, family, and community health.[16] Qualified professionals such as physicians, nurses, dentists, health educators, and other allied health personnel provide these services.

School nurses play a significant role in delivering health services within the health suite or in school-based clinics. These health services included emergency services, acute care evaluation, noncommunicable disease management, health education, and preventive services. These services can occur within a health suite or a **school-based health center.** There are currently 1,900 school-based health centers in 48 states and territories providing services to approximately 2 million children and youth.[23] Forty-one percent of these centers are located in **Title I** schools.[24] Title 1 schools are federally funded through the No Child Left Behind Act of 2001 that serve economically disadvantaged students. The services provided in the school-based health center include primary care, mental health, immunizations, and STI testing. The impact of these centers on both academic and health outcomes has been studied. One study found that students who used school-based health centers were more satisfied with their health and were more involved with health-promoting behaviors than students not using them.[25] Another study found that school-based health center use was associated with academic improvements over time.[26]

Nutrition Services Component

Nutrition services promote access to a variety of nutritious and appealing meals that accommodate the health and nutrition needs of all students. School nutrition programs reflect the U.S. Dietary Guidelines for Americans and other criteria to achieve nutrition integrity. The school nutrition services offer students a learning laboratory for classroom nutrition and health education, and serve as a resource for linkages with nutrition-related community services. It is recommended that qualified child nutrition professionals provide these services.[16]

Fewer than one in three children and adolescents meet dietary recommendations for limiting intake of saturated fat, fewer than one in five eats enough fruits and vegetables, and fewer than one in five adolescent girls has an adequate intake of calcium.[27] Several studies and reports indicate that a substantial proportion of American youth do not eat breakfast on any given day.

School-based programs can influence the extent to which youth eat breakfast. In 2007–2008, the nationwide School Breakfast Program provided breakfast for approximately 8.5 million low-income children.[28] However, on an average day, less than half (46%) of the children who participated in free or reduced-price lunch also participated in the School Breakfast Program for which they were eligible.[29] There are no definitive conclusions regarding the effects of breakfast on learning, although there are numerous studies that report findings suggesting that breakfast consumption favorably affects learning outcomes.[30-33] What is less equivocal is that eating a high-quality breakfast is associated with improved school attendance.[34-36]

One of the factors thought to influence the growing problem of obesity in children and youth is the availability of junk food in vending machines and the lack of nutritious foods in school lunches. In 2008, the CDC reported that nationwide, 11.9% of all elementary schools, 25.4% of all middle schools, and 48% of all high schools allowed students to purchase food and beverages high in fat, sodium, or added sugars from a vending machine school store, canteen, or snack bar during school lunch periods.[36] A recent study also found that offering French fries and dessert more than once per week in subsidized school meals was associated with a greater likelihood of obesity. In addition, the availability of low-nutrient, energy-dense food in vending machines was associated with higher BMI Z scores.[37]

In 2010, the Healthy Hunger-Free Kids Act was signed into law. The bill allows the U.S. Department of Agriculture (USDA) to update nutritional standards for all food sold in schools including vending machines. It also provides an increase in funding for school lunch programs The three broad initiatives of the bill are to (1) improve nutrition with a focus on reducing childhood obesity; (2) increase access to school health meals; and (3) increase program monitoring and integrity.[38] School nurses played a significant role in advocating for this law.

Counseling and Psychological Services

Counseling and psychological services are provided to improve students' mental, emotional, and social health. It is estimated that the overall prevalence of any mental health disorder for children aged 8 to 15 in the past 12 months is 13.1%.[39] These disorders include attention deficit-hyperactivity disorder (ADHD), which is the most prevalent (8.4%) as well as mood disorders, anxiety disorders, behavioral disorders, major depression, and eating disorders. Over a lifetime, approximately 46% of 13- to 18-year-olds will experience a prevalence of any disorder, with 21.4% experiencing a severe disorder.[39,40] Services to address these disorders include individual and group assessments, interventions, and referrals. Organizational assessment and consultation skills of counselors and psychologists contribute not only to the health of students but also to the health of the school environment. Professionals such as certified school counselors, psychologists, and social workers provide these services.[14]

The need to expand mental health services in schools goes back to several reports. These reports include the 1999 Surgeon General's Report,[41] the 2003 President's New Freedom Commission on Mental Health,[42] and No Child Left Behind Act in 2001 (U.S. Department of Education Office of Elementary and Secondary Education, 2002).[43] These federal initiatives were designed to address the need to align mental health and education and the need to develop models integrating social-emotional learning into school settings.[44]

Counseling programs provide education, prevention, and intervention services, which are integrated into all aspects of the students' lives. Early identification and intervention with academic and personal/social needs is essential in removing barriers to learning and in promoting academic achievement. The knowledge, attitudes, and skills that students acquire in the areas of academic, career, and personal counseling serve as a foundation for the successful transition to an independent and self-sufficient adulthood.

Healthy School Environment

The healthy school environment is focused on providing the physical and aesthetic surroundings as well as the psychosocial climate and culture of the school to promote an environment conducive to learning. Factors that influence the physical environment include the school building and the area surrounding it, any biological or chemical agents that are detrimental to health, and physical conditions such as temperature, noise, and lighting. The psychological environment includes the physical, emotional, and social conditions that affect the well-being of students and staff.[16]

Indoor air quality is one example of a physical condition that has gained significant attention. It has particular relevance to asthma.[45] The Environmental Protection Agency (EPA) developed a tool kit, the Indoor Air Quality Tools for Schools Action Kit, which guides schools on developing a practical plan to improve air problems.[46] Some of the sources of problems are classroom pets and plants, water/moisture accumulation, eating facilities attracting vermin, secondhand smoke, combustion problems from furnace rooms and kitchens, and ventilation systems.[45,46] Select interventions have been outlined by the EPA.[46] In addition, the Healthy Schools Campaign, a national nonprofit organization advocating for green cleaning in schools, publishes a guide focused on the practical steps in implementing a green program.[47]

Another intervention aimed at providing a safe environment for students is the safe walk to school national program. A federal safe route to school program started in 2005. Then, in 2012, the new transportation bill MAP-21 combined this program with safe transportation programs related to walking and bicycle use, giving more discretion to the states for funding these programs.[48] Thus, safety for schoolchildren exists both inside the school and in the community surrounding the school (Fig. 19-3).

The psychosocial environment is equally important in schools. Violence within schools is one factor that can undermine academic learning within a school (see Chapter 12). Violence can take the form of bullying behavior in schools, but also includes other forms of peer victimization. These include physical assault, physical intimidation, emotional victimization, sexual victimization, property crime, and Internet harassment.[49] This victimization can also occur within the context of a dating relationship. Overt signs of violence within schools also include carrying weapons, an act that can intimidate students from attending school. In some cases, children are exposed to extreme acts of violence, as in Newtown, Connecticut, at the Sandy Hook Elementary School (see Chapter 12). Based on the data collected from the Youth Risk Behavior Surveillance System survey in 2013, 17.9% of the students reported carrying a weapon to school and 5.5% had carried a gun in the past 30 days. In the past 12 months, 8.1% reported being in a fight on school property, and 8.1% reported not going to school in the past 30 days because of concern for safety.[50]

Health Promotion for Staff

The school consists of teachers as well as students. In a coordinated school health initiative, the school nurse provides opportunities for school staff to improve their health status through health assessments, health education, and health-related fitness activities. Consider the following example. Every year, the high school nurse holds a teacher wellness day on a day before the students return to class in the fall. The nurse, with the help of the teachers, picks a different topic each year based on health issues that would be prevalent in this age group of high school students.[14-17] A variety of teaching tools to engage the teachers are used in these health promotion activities.

These opportunities encourage school staff to pursue a healthy lifestyle that can contribute to their improved health status, improved morale, and a greater personal commitment to the school's overall coordinated health program. Health promotion activities among staff have improved productivity, decreased absenteeism, and reduced health insurance costs.[51] A guide that provides information, practical tools and resources for school employee wellness programs is the School Wellness Guide.[52]

Family/Community Involvement

The eighth component is concerned with involving and integrating the parents and community with school efforts for purposes of enhancing the well-being of the students. This can be accomplished through school health advisory councils, coalitions, and other constituencies to promote school health. It includes the active involvement of the school in soliciting parent involvement and engaging

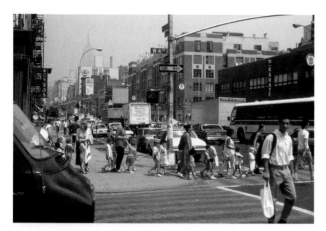

Figure 19-3 Safe Routes to School, New York City. *(From the Centers for Disease Control and Prevention/ Dr. Edwin P. Ewing Jr., 1988.)*

community resources and services to respond to student needs.[16]

The importance of this component cannot be underestimated. It represents an ecological extension of the coordinated school health program and includes connections with the family as well as the community resources available for school-based wellness. These community resources include faith communities, businesses, service clubs, foundations, medical organizations, government and public health departments, to name a few. Change can occur when the school-based interventions are connected to families and the community. It also includes the importance of local school district infrastructure (school policies, administrative procedures, budgetary resources, and operating systems).[53]

Public Health Interventions and School Nursing Roles

The role of the school nurse in coordinated school health can be one of leadership or one of supporting the effort of other team members.[54] The role can vary, but school health nurses have a core set of roles and responsibilities outlined by the National Association of School Nurses (Box 19-2).[55] These roles can be clearly seen in coordinated school health efforts and are also depicted in the interventions outlined in the Minnesota model for public health nursing practice known as the *Intervention Wheel* or the *Minnesota Wheel* (see Chapter 2).[56] The Intervention Wheel describes 17 public health interventions that are population based. A population-based approach considers intervening at three possible levels of practice. Interventions may be directed at the entire population within the school's community, the systems

that affect the health of those populations, and/or the individuals and families within those populations known to be at risk.

Surveillance and Vaccinations

Providing wellness child services has been an important role of school nurses since the development of the specialty. Monitoring vaccinations among children and adolescents to assure compliance with state mandates is an important school nurse role related to surveillance. School nurses support the use of state registries to identify fully immunized children as well as those who are not fully immunized and consequently at risk. This also helps to prevent duplication of vaccinations. The school nurse also increases an awareness of other recommended vaccinations.

There are many resources related to vaccinations for both health professionals and parents and the CDC keeps an updated list on its Web site.[57,58] Other sources of current vaccine recommendations include the National Network for Immunization Information and the American Academy of Pediatrics immunization schedules, also available online. These recommendations are updated on a yearly basis because of changes in risk, changes in pathogens such as the flu virus, and changes in the evidence related to best practices for different vaccines. School nurses play a key role in counseling families and staff about immunizations across the lifespan. The CDC urges school nurses to specifically promote preteen vaccines.[59] The recommended vaccinations for preteens include but are not limited to:

- Meningococcal conjugate vaccine (MCV4), which protects against meningococcal disease
- Tdap, a booster against tetanus, diphtheria, and pertussis
- HPV for girls and boys, which protects against the four types of HPV that cause 70% of cervical cancer and 90% of genital warts

To address the recommendation from the CDC, the school nurse can apply health-planning principles to help develop school-located immunization programs.[59]

The seasonal influenza vaccine is of particular interest in school nursing practice. The main resource for nurses is the Advisory Committee on Immunization Practices, a division of the CDC. The committee periodically updates the influenza vaccine recommendations including recommendations for school-age children.[60] In 2013, the committee recommended annual influenza vaccination for everyone aged 6 months or older.[60] Seasonal influenza is a source of significant

| BOX 19–2 | **National Association of School Nurses: Roles of the School Nurse** |

- Facilitate normal development and positive student response to interventions
- Provide leadership in promoting health and safety, including a healthy environment
- Provide quality health care and intervene with actual and potential health problems
- Use clinical judgment in providing case management services
- Actively collaborate with others to build student and family capacity for adaptation, self-management, self-advocacy, and learning

Source: See reference 55.

morbidity and mortality, with a range in mortality from 3,000 to 49,000 each season and a mean of 226,000 influenza-associated hospitalizations per annual flu season.[60] In addition, the annual influenza attack rates among children are estimated to be 20% to 30%.[61] School-located vaccination programs have become a viable option for reaching the target populations and are likely to continue. The models for providing this care vary; sometimes school nurses administer the vaccines, and in other cases the public health department administers the vaccine in the schools.[62] The roles of school nurses vary in this endeavor from that of providing direct care to working at a community and systems levels to assure coverage from a population perspective.

Health Screening of Children and Adolescents

Screening is another important role of school nurses in addressing the actual and potential health problems of children. School nurses conduct vision and hearing screenings as well as BMI screenings, depending on the regulations within the jurisdictions. Other screenings can include postural or scoliosis screening; blood pressure reading; drug abuse screening; and screening for mental health problems, type 2 diabetes, cholesterol level, asthma, tuberculosis, and head lice. In all of these cases, it is important to assess the value of the screening program, to assess the costs versus the benefits, and to assure that there is not any inadvertent harm that evolves from the program. The sensitivity and specificity of the screening tools are also important to evaluate (see Chapter 2).

Some screening procedures, such as screening for scoliosis, have fallen out of favor over the past decade in some areas. A recent meta-analysis in 2010 found that the use of the forward bending test in school scoliosis screening is insufficient and there is a need for more research to assess the clinical effectiveness of school scoliosis screening.[63] In 2004, the U.S. Preventive Services Task Force changed its prior determination of the forward bending test as "insufficient evidence for or against" to "recommends against the routine screening of asymptomatic adolescents."[64] Screening guidelines can vary by state and it is important for school nurses to access information on requirements at both the national and state levels. One resource is the National Association of State Boards of Education Web site, State School Healthy Policy Database, which lists mandated screening tests by state.[65]

Vision Screening

Vision screening in schools has a history dating back to 1899, when the Snellen eye chart was first used. Although the Snellen chart continues to be prominent in the toolbox of school nurses, there is a need to evaluate the vision screening tools used by school nurses, based on national and international eye chart design guidelines, and to use best practices based on research.[66] It is equally important to use an eye chart that matches the cognitive level of the child. Young children, at-risk children, and children who were never screened should be screened for near, distance, binocular, and color visual function. This should be followed up by periodic appraisal of older, previously screened children.

Audiometric Screening

Screening for hearing problems is another important school nursing activity. The American Academy of Audiology has specific childhood hearing screening guidelines. Minimum grades for screening include preschool, kindergarten, and grades 1, 3, 5, and either 7 or 9. It is also important to screen any student who enters a new school system without evidence of having had a previous hearing screening (Box 19-3).[67] Although these criteria are specific to hearing screening, the principles of proper communication, referral, follow-up and effective treatment are equally important for any type of screening program.

BOX 19–3   Position Statement: American Academy of Audiology

The position statement on early childhood and school-age population screening is as follows:

"The American Academy of Audiology endorses detection of hearing loss in early childhood and school-aged populations using evidence-based hearing screening methods. Hearing loss is the most common developmental disorder identifiable at birth and its prevalence increases throughout school-age due to the additions of late-onset, late identified and acquired hearing loss. Under identification and lack of appropriate management of hearing loss in children has broad economic effects as well as a potential impact on individual child educational, cognitive and social development. The goal of early detection of new hearing loss is to maximize perception of speech and the resulting attainment of linguistic-based skills. Identification of new or emerging hearing loss in one or both ears followed by appropriate referral for diagnosis and treatment are first steps to minimizing these effects. Informing educational staff, monitoring chronic or fluctuating hearing loss, and providing education toward the prevention of hearing loss are important steps that are needed to follow mass screening if the impact of hearing loss is to be minimized."

Source: See reference 67.

Screening for Obesity

It is evident from the National Health and Nutrition Examination Survey (NHANES) that obesity is a significant problem among U.S. adolescents and children. There was a slight decline in the prevalence rate of obesity among low-income children from 15.2% in 2003 to 14.94% in 2010. However, the rate remains up from the prevalence rate of 13.05% in 1998.[68] In 2013, the CDC reported that for all U.S. children aged 2 to 19 years, the prevalence rate for obesity was approximately 17%. The increasing prevalence of childhood obesity cuts across every demographic group in the United States; however, Mexican American, non-Hispanic black, and Native American children and adolescents are particularly at high risk, along with lower socioeconomic status and living in the southern region of the country.[68,69] This disparity in obesity rates is the result of a complex set of risk factors including genetics, cultural nutritional practices, environments, and socioeconomic differences, The increase in obesity adversely affects children and adolescents through increasing the risk for type 2 diabetes, hypertension, and depression, as well as throughout their lives with the possibility of arthritis, cancer, and cardiovascular disease. Prevention and intervention efforts rely on multiple factors and partnerships.

The primary screening method for obesity in children is the calculation of BMI. As noted above, BMI is a number calculated from a child's weight and height and is a reliable indicator of body fatness. To screen for obesity in children, the BMI by itself is not sufficient. The BMI number is plotted on a growth chart specific to girls or boys and a percentile ranking is obtained. This percentile indicates where the child is in relationship to other children of the same age and sex.[70] The categories are further broken down into underweight, healthy weight, overweight, and obese (Box 19-4).[70] A tool that can be used by school nurses to calculate the BMI as well as the percentile ranking in children is the CDC Body Mass Index: Child and Teen Calculator. In addition to height and weight, the calculator uses information on sex, date of birth, and date of measurement to calculate the percentile.[71] Communication of the results of the BMI to the family as well as a health-care provider is important as well as a challenge in designing effective tailored prevention and intervention plans, because cultural norms and perceptions must be taken into consideration.[72] In addition, examining obesity trends within one's school allows the school nurse to be an advocate at a community and systems level through his or her involvement in school wellness policies related to nutrition and physical activity.

BOX 19–4 BMI-for-Age Weight Status Categories and the Corresponding Percentiles

After BMI is calculated for children and teens, the BMI number is plotted on the CDC BMI-for-age growth charts (for either girls or boys) to obtain a percentile ranking. Percentiles are the most commonly used indicator to assess the size and growth patterns of individual children in the United States. The percentile indicates the relative position of the child's BMI number among children of the same sex and age. The growth charts show the weight status categories used with children and teens (underweight, healthy weight, overweight, and obese). BMI-for-age weight status categories and the corresponding percentiles are shown in the following table:

Weight Status Category	Percentile Range
Underweight	Less than the 5th percentile
Healthy weight	5th percentile to less than the 85th percentile
Overweight	85th to less than the 95th percentile
Obese	Equal to or greater than the 95th percentile

Source: See reference 70.

Outreach to Immigrant Populations

Student populations are becoming increasingly diverse in the United States, given the growing number of immigrant parents. The percentage of all children living in the United States with at least one foreign-born parent rose from 15% in 1994 to 24% in 2012.[73] Children of immigrants often face many challenges, including cultural differences, poverty, lack of health insurance, lack of access to public assistance, limited English proficiency, and high levels of psychological distress in those who have experienced war and other adverse events. Outreach to these populations is one intervention in which a school nurses can play an integral role. The multiple roles connected with outreach might include those of developing a welcoming orientation for the student, developing student support teams, facilitating the integration of the student into after-school activities, and serving as an overall advocate for the families. In the Minneapolis public school system, for example, a school nurse coordinates the Welcome Center Healthy Learners project with goals of identifying health barriers to learning, providing on-site immunizations needed for entry into school, connecting families to health-care providers, and assisting families in applying for health-care insurance.[74]

Episodic Care in the School Setting

An important role of the school nurse is to provide episodic care and to conduct a diseases and health investigation. In a survey of 384 school nurses in the United States, the most common types of school nursing procedures reported were episodic care including first aid (97.1%), inhaler administration (94.8%), and nebulizer administration (85.7%).[75] A study of 12,947 school-based health clinics encounters in eight school districts or subdistricts that implemented new school-based health clinics in 2000–2001 found that the largest *International Statistical Classification of Diseases and Related Health Problems (ICD-9)* codes (see chapter 15) were respiratory problems, physicals, follow-ups, and wellness checks.[76] Only 14.8% of the students seen in these clinics were actually dismissed from school, an important outcome with educational implications. School nurses spend a significant portion of their day caring for acute injuries and illnesses as well as providing episodic care for minor illnesses, such as headaches, stomachaches, pain, and hay fever, and medication administration.

● APPLYING PUBLIC HEALTH SCIENCE

The Case of the Unknown Asthmatic

Public Health Science Topics Covered:

- Surveillance
- Health planning

Janet had just taken a job as a school nurse in an inner-city school. During her second week on the job, Janet met John. The physical education (PE) teacher had sent John to the nurse's office because he had heard John wheezing during a physical assessment test, which required running for a specific amount of time. When Janet looked in John's file, she found that he had no treatment orders and no inhaler in the health room to treat his asthma.

Janet observed John sitting quietly in her office. His breathing was shallow, regular, and tachypneic. John answered Janet's questions politely, but looked toward the ground during most of the interview. He said that he did have an inhaler but used it infrequently and had never brought it to school. John reported that he wheezed when he exercised but that wasn't a real problem because he had avoided exercise such as running or walking for a long time. He had no symptoms of an upper respiratory infection, no cough, and no fever or chills.

On exam Janet recorded the following:

Vital Signs: BP 130/80, P 80, R 24, Temp 98.8°F, BMI greater than 40.
Neck: the trachea midline, nontender. No stridor, no bruits, no adenopathy.
Chest: No use of accessory muscles, lungs sounds distant, vesicular breath sounds present over most of lungs, no wheezes no rales, PF 400 L/min.
Heart: Normal S_1, S_2, no extra sounds, no murmur, RRR.

Janet called John's mother, Juanita, and discussed the findings. Juanita confirmed that John had a history of infrequent wheezing associated with exercise and had experienced a number of colds this past year. Janet and Juanita agreed that John should finish the day at school since he was no longer wheezing. In addition, Juanita agreed to ask John's primary care provider (PCP) to order an inhaler with a spacer and make sure he had one at school. Janet also told Juanita about the **asthma action plan** and asked her to have John's PCP complete one. This could then be used at school when symptomatic and before exercise. The asthma action plan is an education and communication tool used by health-care providers, patients, families, and caregivers to properly manage asthma and respond to asthma episodes. The use of an asthma action plan helps increase the use of the peak flow meter, the recognition of warning signs, and the appropriate administration of asthma medicines.[77]

Janet also raised the question of John's weight and elevated blood pressure with Juanita. She told Juanita that she would recheck John's blood pressure two more times and let her know the results and asked her whether she would be interested in learning more about how to help John lose weight. Juanita stated that she would. Janet assured her that she would get back to her with some suggestions. When she was done talking with Juanita, Janet informed John that he could go back to class. She gave him an order form for an inhaler to be signed by the PCP and told him she would meet with him again when he brought in his inhaler with the order. She scheduled two blood pressure checks right after lunch in the coming week.

Over the next few days, Janet thought further about this quiet, very polite boy who looked so out of place. She had many questions. She questioned why she had not known about this child's asthma. At the start of each year, an information card is sent home with each student for the guardian to complete details on emergency contacts, allergies, disabilities, acute and noncommunicable illnesses, and medications. Using these data, Janet created a master sheet for each grade level with a list of illnesses, allergies, treatments, and plans of care. John was not on the list. There was no information on John, including no written indication of medications, allergies, or medical issues. She wondered who else might be missing from the list.

Based on John's visit to her office and her review of the school-level data, Janet knew she needed to do two things: (1) Complete a plan of care for John and (2) complete a plan of care for the school on how to address the multiple issues presented by John (obesity, asthma, and hypertension). To help build a plan of care for John, Janet met with him when he brought in his medication order, asthma action plan, inhaler, and spacer. She asked what his normal peak flow was. He was not sure that had been established. Janet and John talked about asthma, his triggers, the frequency of wheezing, and how often he used the inhaler. As John talked, he reported that he often wheezed at nighttime when he lay in bed and sometimes experienced short-ness of breath. He reported using his inhaler, but it often did not relieve his symptoms. When Janet asked how he slept, he stated that he did not sleep well and woke up frequently. He also reported wheezing when he walked quickly, so he usually avoided any activity that resulted in wheezing and shortness of breath. Janet observed John use his inhaler correctly with the spacer and recorded another peak flow reading. Janet discussed with John the importance of completing a mutually agreed-on contract in relation to his inhaler use at school. The signed contract included John's commitment not to share his inhaler, to let the school nurse know if he forgot his inhaler and needed it, and to let the school nurse know if his symptoms became more frequent or were nor relieved by two puffs.

Once she had completed an individual-level plan of care with John, she also shared it with John's mother as promised, and put in place reminders for following up on John's progress over the next few months. Provid-ing episodic care and investigating illness are important roles for the school nurse; another role is developing programs at the population level, in this case, the school or groups of students within the school. In addi-tion, the underlying cause of the acute care episode may be a noncommunicable disease such as asthma. In John's case, Janet became aware of an underlying health problem that required her to shift from providing episodic care to case management.

School nurses also provide support to the students and parents in the management of noncommunicable diseases that are chronic (see below). Janet used her experience at the individual level with John to develop a schoolwide program to address obesity and asthma. Janet accessed the EPA's Web site and found a na-tional-level, evidence-based program called *Managing Asthma in the School Environment: Indoor Air Quality Tools for Schools*.[78] She also found a wealth of information on evidence-based, school-based obesity prevention pro-grams. She was able to get administrative support to adapt these programs to the school using the knowl-edge she had acquired related to program planning and program evaluation (Chapter 5). To assist with evalua-tion, she revised the process of tracking student health issues over time. The long-term outcome for her school was improved surveillance of health issues, an obesity prevention program, an asthma management protocol for the school, and a special program for students who were obese.

Life-Threatening Emergencies in the School Setting

School nurses can also be confronted with life-threatening emergencies, including cardiac arrest, head injuries, over-dose, seizures, and heat stroke.[79] In addition, following the Sandy Hook shooting in 2012, there has been increased awareness of the potential for school-based violence (see Chapter 12). The CDC reported that only 1% to 2% of child homicides occur on school grounds or on the way to school.[80] Despite the low incidence rate, the school nurse must be prepared for the potential of a life-threatening violent act occurring at a school. These life-threatening emergencies require well-equipped schools, training and skills in first aid and cardiopulmonary resuscitation, and lay rescuer automated external defibrillator (AED) pro-grams.[79,80] There has been recent attention paid to the value of having a nurse present when a life-threatening event occurs within a school.[81] One approach has been to have a designated medical emergency response plan on record in every school. A recommendation is that schools practice the plan at least a few times each year. The other recommendation is to identify who within the system is authorized to make emergency medical decisions and to make sure AEDs are available in the school.[82]

Food Allergies

Food allergy is one example of a potential life-threatening illness. Between 1997 and 2007, reported food allergies increased 18% among children under age 18 years.[83] In a recent national survey of U.S. households with children, food allergy prevalence was 8.0%. The food allergens most often noted among allergic children in this survey were peanuts (25.2%), milk (21.1%), and shellfish (17.2%).[84] Among these same children with a food allergy, 38.7% had a history of severe reactions and 30.4% had multiple food allergies. The symptoms of an allergic reaction can range from skin symptoms to gastrointestinal symptoms, to respiratory symptoms, and to life-threatening anaphylaxis.

Fatal allergic reactions most often occur outside the home, which has implications for school nurses.[85] In fact, 16% to 18% of children with a food allergy have experienced a reaction in school.[86] The National Association of School Nurses created a tool kit for school nurses that provides guidance for creating a comprehensive program that includes prevention as well as steps to take in the event a child has a mild or severe food allergy reaction.[87] It is obvious that prevention is crucial in thinking about this role and demands adequate management plans, successful food allergy avoidance, recognition of food allergy reactions, preparation for appropriate treatment of acute allergic reactions, knowledge of treatments, and access to self-injectable epinephrine (EpiPens).[85,86,88] The Food Allergy and Anaphylaxis Management Act (FAAMA) was signed into law by President Obama on January 4, 2011. This bill calls for voluntary national guidelines to help schools manage students affected by food allergies. In 2013, the School Access to Emergency Epinephrine Act (also known as the EpiPen Act) was enacted. These bills are aimed at improved management of anaphylaxis and access to epinephrine auto-injectors in a school setting.

Resources to guide the development of school plans can be found at the Food Allergy and Anaphylaxis Network Web site.[88]

Case Management of Noncommunicable Diseases and Mental Health Disorders

Noncommunicable disease affects 10% to 25% of children and adolescents in schools and has the potential to have a great impact on school outcomes.[89] Noncommunicable diseases (see Chapter 9) include asthma, diabetes, allergies, cancer, and other medical disorders (see Chapter 11). Often, the health-care needs of children with a noncommunicable disease are complex and require careful planning, appropriate referrals, safe management, and delegation of nursing tasks to licensed and unlicensed assistive personnel (UAP).[90] Mental disorders are also common among children. According to the National Institute of Mental Health, almost half of 13- to 18-year-old children have a lifetime prevalence of a mental health disorder (46.3%), with ADHD being the most prevalent (Fig. 19-4).[91–93]

Both noncommunicable diseases and mental health disorders in children and adolescents require coordination between family members, school personnel, and health-care providers. Case management of noncommunicable diseases and mental health disorders in the school setting can contribute to positive academic and health outcomes. Case management is defined as:

a process by which the school nurse identifies children who are not achieving their optimal level of health or academic success because they have a chronic illness that is limiting their potential. Case management is based on

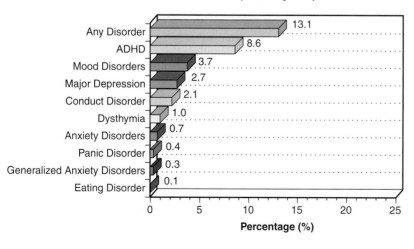

12-month Prevalence for Children (8 to 15 years)

- Any Disorder: 13.1
- ADHD: 8.6
- Mood Disorders: 3.7
- Major Depression: 2.7
- Conduct Disorder: 2.1
- Dysthymia: 1.0
- Anxiety Disorders: 0.7
- Panic Disorder: 0.4
- Generalized Anxiety Disorders: 0.3
- Eating Disorder: 0.1

Percentage (%)

Figure 19-4 Twelve-month prevalence of mental health disorders for children aged 8 to 15 years. *(From the National Institute of Mental Health. [n.d.]. Any disorder among children. Retrieved from http://www. nimh.nih.gov/statistics/1anydis_child.shtml, data from the CDC.)*

a thorough assessment by the school nurse and involves activities that not only help the child deal with problems but also prevent and reduce their occurrence. Case management includes nursing care directed toward the child and coordination and communication with parents, teachers, and other care providers. The interventions are goal oriented, based on the specific needs of the child, and evaluated based on their impact.[94]

Several researchers have evaluated the effectiveness of case management in the school setting and have found improvement in quality of life, skills, and knowledge to manage their illness as well as classroom participation, grades, and participation in extracurricular activities.[94,95]

Case management begins when the PCP confirms a diagnosis, for example, of ADHD. Symptoms of ADHD in school-age children can be marked by academic difficulties, inattention, impulsiveness, oppositional behavior, poor self-esteem, excessive motor activity, low frustration tolerance, increased risky behavior, aggressive and antisocial behavior, and less adaptive behaviors.[94] The overall prevalence in school-age children is about 8.5%.[92] The school nurse is often the designated professional to help bridge the gap between teachers, who often first see the behaviors suggestive of a diagnosis of ADHD, and the PCP, who can make an appropriate diagnosis. The school nurse also oversees the delivery of medications.[96]

In addition to providing individual care, the application of a population perspective allows the school nurse to develop programs at the school level to help identify and provide evidence-based approaches to the care of students with ADHD. One evidence-based approach is the Dang school–based framework.[97] The Dang framework provides the steps and standardized practice for the early identification and management of ADHD children. The role of the school nurse is significant in bridging the gap between the teacher and the health professional making a diagnosis.[98] A part of the process in this framework is to encourage an assessment by parents and teachers using the Connors Rating Scale, a child behavior rating scale that has good reliability, validity, accessibility, and ease of administration.[99] In addition, the school nurse performs behavioral classroom observations and documents how often the child is off task. All of these combined efforts are focused on early diagnosis and treatment of ADHD for purposes of decreasing academic failure, social isolation, high-risk behaviors, family conflict, and adversity later in life for these children.[100]

Asthma

In 2011, 14% of children under 18 had been diagnosed with asthma.[89] Asthma is a significant noncommunicable health problem among adolescents. Over the past 20 years, asthma in children has increased when measured by prevalence, ambulatory visits, morbidity, and mortality.[101] The presence of a full-time registered school nurse is important to provide care and care coordination for students with asthma. In addition, the school nurse provides instruction to school staff concerning the recognition of and action steps for severe respiratory symptoms. School nurses also take a lead in providing school based education to improve asthma management. A recent review found that school based asthma educational programs improved knowledge, self-efficacy, and self-management behaviors, although actual asthma outcomes (symptom days, symptom nights, absences) were not affected.[102] Another review of asthma education programs published between 1998 and 2009 found that the programs were associated with a decrease in school days missed but not with a decrease in emergency department visits or hospital admissions.[103]

Diabetes

Diabetes is another noncommunicable disease that requires self-management and coordination of care within the school setting. There are two types of diabetes. Type 1 is an autoimmune disease in which the body forms antibodies to insulin, thus affecting the body's ability to produce insulin, known as insulin-dependent disease. It is one of the most common noncommunicable diseases in children younger than 20 years, with a rate in the United States between 18.6 to 19 per 100,000, depending on age. Type 2 occurs when cells do not respond correctly to insulin, resulting in insulin resistance. Type 2 diabetes has a rate of eight per 100,000.[104] The prevalence of type 1 diabetes has remained relatively unchanged over the past two decades, but type 2 diabetes is on the rise in children.[105] About one in every 400 children under the age of 20 is diagnosed with type 1 or type 2 diabetes.[104] Type 2 diabetes is a complex metabolic disorder with social, behavioral, and environmental risk factors including being overweight, a family history of type 2 diabetes, or other conditions such as high blood pressure, polycystic ovary syndrome, abnormal cholesterol, or acanthosis nigricans.[106]

One of the roles of the school nurse is to identify children with diabetes or who are at risk of developing type 2 diabetes and refer them to care. Once a diagnosis has occurred, the school nurse has an important role in encouraging self-care, which includes increasing knowledge and skills such as blood glucose testing, insulin injection, preparation of the insulin, diet management, and hypoglycemic treatment.[107,108] In addition, assessing for signs of stress and providing needed support are important. The school nurse works closely with student, family, and community-based health-care providers to develop a plan for managing children with diabetes.[108]

Disabilities

Students with disabilities represent another population that requires case management from the school nurse.[109] The Individuals With Disability Education Act of 2004 provides a comprehensive definition of a child with **disabilities** (Box 19-5).[110]

BOX 19–5	**Individuals With Disabilities Education Act—Definitions of a Child With a Disability**

Child with a disability.—

"(A) In general.—The term 'child with a disability' means a child—

"(i) with mental retardation, hearing impairments (including deafness), speech or language impairments, visual impairments (including blindness), serious emotional disturbance (referred to in this title as 'emotional disturbance'), orthopedic impairments, autism, traumatic brain injury, other health impairments, or specific learning disabilities; and

"(ii) who, by reason thereof, needs special education and related services.

"(B) Child aged 3 through 9.—The term 'child with a disability' for a child aged 3 through 9 (or any subset of that age range, including ages 3 through 5), may, at the discretion of the State and the local educational agency, include a child—

"(i) experiencing developmental delays, as defined by the State and as measured by appropriate diagnostic

Child With a Disability: (A) In general.—The term "child with a disability" means a child—(i) with mental retardation, hearing impairments (including deafness), speech or language impairments, visual impairments (including blindness), serious emotional disturbance (referred to in this title as 'emotional disturbance'), orthopedic impairments, autism, traumatic brain injury, other health impairments, or specific learning disabilities; and (ii) who, by reason thereof, needs special education and related services."

Child Ages 3 Through 9 (or any subset of that age range): May, at the discretion of the State and the local educational agency, include a child (i) experiencing developmental delays, as defined by the State and as measured by appropriate diagnostic instruments and procedures, in 1 or more of the following areas: physical development; cognitive development; communication development; social or emotional development; or adaptive development; and (ii) who, by reason thereof, needs special education and related services."

Source: See reference 110.

School health services enable students with disabilities to attend school. The needs may include medication administration, treatments, emergency care plans, individualized health-care plans, health teaching, and health counseling. School nurses maintain referral sources so that students and families may be appropriately referred for care and services. In addition, the school nurse is responsible for providing a safe and healthy environment. In the case of children with disabilities, this may mean wheelchair access; special furniture; elevators; and restroom accommodations or dedicated space in the health room for diaper changes, tube feedings, medication administration, or rest.

National policy has resulted in the integration of children with disabilities into the school setting. These laws help to define the rights of children with disabilities as well as to define the role of the school nurse. One law that had a significant impact on school nursing is the Education for All Handicapped Children Act (EAHCA) of 1975.[111] The ages covered under this law include birth to 2-year-olds in infant and toddler programs, as well as 3- to 21-year-old students. EAHCA appropriated federal funding to states for the provision of free appropriate public education in the **least restrictive environment.** The purpose of a least restrictive environment is to provide disabled students with the opportunity to be educated with their nondisabled peers.[111] This was followed by the Individuals With Disabilities Education Act (IDEA), passed in 2004.[112] This law builds on the original 1974 legislation and provides a mechanism for continual updating of available resources. It addresses the same issues for children as the EAHCA does, but encompasses the issues for all individuals with disabilities. Thus, the needs of people with disabilities are now covered across the life span. IDEA has undergone several amendments, with the most current in 2004. The current iteration of IDEA specifies school nursing as one of the related services that will meet the needs of the student.[112]

A central component of these laws is the **individualized education program.** An individualized education program is the individualized plan for a child with disability with the goal of helping the child meet educational goals. School nurses are integral members of the team. If the student's disability requires the services of a nurse, the school nurse contributes to the individualized education program, which is both a process and a plan. School nurses, as part of the team, provide resources and information when transition planning begins for students with special educational services. An **individualized family service plan** is indicated for qualified birth to 3-year-old children. It is similar to an individualized education program and is provided to children with developmental delays to help address the delays. Once a child turns 3, an individualized education program is implemented instead.

Other laws, including Section 504 and the Americans With Disabilities Act, that affect children with disabilities are seen in Table 19-1.[113,114] Although school administrators are required to accommodate children with disabilities, school administrators, faculty, and staff are not required to accommodate limitations due to other characteristics such as poor literacy skills (that are not due to learning disabilities), low educational levels, inability to meet the minimum entrance requirements of the learning environment, or lack of credentials. Parents and students can ask for reasonable accommodations based on functional limitations secondary to a medical condition. These accommodations are made by teachers and other staff via adjustments to their standard practices in order to meet specific needs of the student.

Mental Health Disorders

The prevalence of mental health disorders in children and adolescents on average is about 13%, with ADHD being the most common at around 8.5%.[92] A comprehensive school-based health program must incorporate mental health care. One approach is to provide a minimum elementary school counselor-student ratio to help improve the overall school climate to reduce disruptions within classrooms that result from fighting, cutting class, stealing, or using drugs.[115]

Integrating learning and behavioral health with an overall focus on improving functioning and not just symptom reduction is a topic that is receiving increased emphasis.[43,116] Integrating social-emotional learning into school health education is needed. This can be accomplished on an individual basis or by developing and implementing schoolwide programs to address positive behavioral support.[116]

School nurses also have a very important role in the early identification of mental health needs. Some children frequently visit the school nurse's office with unexplained physical symptoms. These frequent visitors ("frequent flyers," or what some have called "somatizers") actually account for a disproportionate use of resources in the school.[117] Pediatric somatization is described as cases in which children present with medically unexplained symptoms that

TABLE 19–1	Description of Federal Laws for Children With Special Needs	
Law	Description	Special Considerations
Pub. L. No. 94-14 Education for All Handicapped Children Act (EAHCA) of 1975. Renamed the Individuals With Disabilities Education Act (IDEA) in 1990. Source: http://www.scn.org/~bk269/94-142.html.	This law appropriated federal funding to states for the provision of free appropriate public education in the least restrictive environment to certain students with disabilities who qualified for the service.	Individualized education program (IEP) was mandated for each student in special education. An individualized family service plan (ISFP) is indicated for qualified birth to 2-year-old children.
Section 504 of the Rehabilitation Act of 1973 and current amendments (2008). 29 U.S.C. § 794. Source: http://www2.ed.gov/about/offices/list/ocr/504faq.html.	This is a civil rights law that prohibits discrimination based on disabilities by entities receiving federal funds, including local education agencies; several amendments to the law expanded provisions in Section 504.	Public elementary and secondary schools must provide Free Appropriate Public Education for qualified students with a disability.[30] A 504 plan is written by the team. Section 504 expands disabilities beyond learning to a mental or physical impairment that substantially limits one or more life activities.
Americans With Disabilities Act (ADA) 1990 Americans With Disabilities Act (ADA) Amendment 2008. P.L. 110-325. Source: http://www.ada.gov/pubs/adastatute08.pdf.	The ADA is another civil rights law that prohibits discrimination based on disability.	The provisions of this law apply to agencies with or without the receipt of federal funds.

are believed by the family and child to be making the child unwell.[118] Once a physical etiology has been ruled out, somatization should be recognized as an early identifier of potential mental health needs and stress in school-age children. The school nurse can monitor school-based mental health care; act as a case manager; advocate for the student; and act as a liaison between the family, school, clinic, and primary provider for these children.[116,118,119] In addition, the nurse develops the health portion of the individualized education program and the **Individualized Healthcare Plan** for children with identified mental health needs. The nurse may be the first person to recognize the need for counseling. Consider the following examples of student visits to the school nurse:

Example 1: The first example illustrates how the school nurse can identify a problem that can be addressed with a simple solution. Jason came to the health room on a regular basis with complaints of coughing and shortness of breath due to asthma. His physical examination often did not correlate with his complaints. After recognition of a pattern of these complaints, it was found that these visits to the health room occurred only during math class. During consultations with the counselor, family, and his math teacher, it was learned that Jason was not getting good grades and was anxious about not doing well in class. Referral to tutoring services recommended by the counselor was an acceptable solution to this problem to all concerned, including Jason. After a few weeks, Jason was better prepared for class and did not complain of asthma symptoms during class.

Example 2: The second example is more complex. Annie, a 14-year-old middle school student, was referred to the school nurse by the PE teacher. Annie was at the point of failing PE because she could not participate in the activities because she forgot to bring her PE clothes to school. The PE teacher asked whether the nurse could talk to Annie. Annie and the nurse talked in private to discuss PE. Annie felt uncomfortable undressing and changing her clothes in front of other girls. There were no private dressing areas. She was self-conscious about her weight. When the nurse talked to Annie's mother, she discovered that Annie had not asked her mother for money for the PE clothes. Her mother did not have a lot of money and Annie did not want to be an additional financial burden. The final plan was to allow Annie to change her clothes in the privacy of the health room and then go to PE. There were extra used but clean PE clothes available that were given to Annie. When Annie got dressed, the nurse noted

healed and new linear wounds on both her upper forearms. They sat and talked. The nurse shared her assessment of the old scars and new wounds as being self-inflicted. Annie agreed. She had not wanted her classmates or teachers to know. The school counselor, the nurse, the mother, and Annie met to discuss the implications of the self-inflicted wounds. Annie and her mother agreed that Annie would see a psychologist and she would attend PE with a long-sleeved PE shirt. The nurse met with Annie weekly to discuss healthy eating habits and daily physical activity. Along with counseling by a trained psychologist, increased daily exercise, and a change in dietary habits, Annie began to lose weight, passed PE, and had a group of friends by the end of the year.

These two examples differ in the severity of the issues. Jason did not have a mental health disorder, but Annie's symptoms were indicative of a possible mental health disorder. The right decision was to refer her for further assessment and possible treatment. Both examples exemplify a very important point: Although the mental health field has traditionally focused on psychopathology, the absence of mental illness does not necessarily equate with positive mental health.[120,121] Children who have low psychopathology and low subjective well-being are also at risk for academic and behavior problems and can benefit from counseling.

The links between mental health and academic achievement have been well established.[121] In addition, the CDC has stated that if mental health disorders are left untreated, adolescents are more likely to experience higher rates of suicide, violence, school dropout, family dysfunction, juvenile incarceration, alcohol, drug use, and unintentional injuries.[121] These examples support the role of the school nurse in providing counseling and in conducting programs focused on prevention.

Delegation

Delegation is an intervention that has particular relevance to the school nurse in addressing noncommunicable diseases and mental health disorders in the schools. According to the National Council of State Boards of Nursing (1995), **delegation** is defined as transferring to a competent individual the authority to perform a selected nursing task in a selected situation.[122] Because of budgetary constraints resulting in the lack of school nurses, delegation is given to UAPs to meet the health needs of student populations. One of the challenges of delegation is the fact that laws, regulations, scopes of practice, and standards vary by state and there is the potential conflict between state laws and nurse practice acts. Another challenge is that of assuring safe and effective delegation in school settings. The school nurse must consider "the needs of the student, the stability of the student, the complexity of the task, the competence of the UAP, the expected outcomes, and the needs of other students in determining the appropriateness of delegating a specific task to a UAP."[123]

School Nurses and Health Education

School nurses have an important role to play in selecting, implementing, and evaluating comprehensive educational efforts at the school level. At least four of the *HP 2020* Healthy Educational and Community Based Programs objectives address the provision of comprehensive health education in schools to prevent health problems.[11] Areas of importance to school health include sexuality, mental health promotion, including substance abuse/violence prevention, and an evidence-based example of health education called *life skills*.

Sexuality and Sex Education

Half of all sexually transmitted infections (STIs) occur in those aged 15 to 24.[124] Primary prevention of high-risk behaviors related to sexuality is a priority for school populations. It is estimated that 47.4% of high school students have had sexual intercourse and most adolescents who have ever had sexual intercourse remain sexually active.[125] About 15% have had multiple partners. The prevalence of being currently sexually active (past 30 days) varies across ethnic and gender groups, with a third of white females (35.0%) reporting current sexual activity compared with 30% of white males. Black males were more apt to be sexually active than black females (46.0% vs. 36.9%), and Hispanic males (35.3%) were more active than Hispanic females (31.6%).

One approach to prevention within a school setting is sex education. The topic of sex education is value laden. At the local, state, and national levels, educational experts have discussed who should decide what will be taught in schools. Factors that play into those decisions are parental concerns, public health prevention concerns, and issues concerning the role the educational system plays in public health prevention versus parental rights. School nurses can help inform the discussion through the presentation of empirical data related to magnitude and consequences of teen births and sexual activity among adolescents in their own school district and suggest evidence-based practices related to prevention. In addition, the school nurse must take into consideration

cultural and environmental issues specific to their school and the children who attend their school. Standard 5 of the National Health Education Standards from the CDC provides a sound basis for curriculum development in this area. Standard 5 states: "Students will demonstrate the ability to use decision-making skills to enhance health."[126] Once general content is outlined, there are many resources available to assist local educators in selecting appropriate curricula to promote healthy sexuality.[127-130]

Violence Prevention

Cyberbullying

Student-to-student violence takes various forms within the school setting. Recently, there has been increased coverage in the media of cyberbullying and dating violence. In 2013, a 12-year-old girl jumped to her death from a water tower after being cyberbullied. Two other girls, one 12 and one 14, were arrested in the case. In 2012, a high school girl was repeatedly sexually assaulted by members of the high school football team in Steubenville, Ohio. Pictures of the assault were posted on social media. These cases demonstrate the extensive harm that can occur through bullying and violence to school-age children. The school nurse has the potential to play a role in the prevention, early identification, and provision of treatment to victims of violence.

● APPLYING PUBIC HEALTH SCIENCE
The Case of the Frequent Flyer

Public Health Science Topics Covered:

- Assessment
- Program planning
- Program evaluation

Carly, an eighth grader, recently entered a new middle school when her family moved midyear from a rural area to a large urban center after her father obtained a job transfer. Carly had spent her entire life in the rural area and was apprehensive about the move. For the first few weeks, things seemed to go well. She was welcomed by a group of girls who were the "popular" girls in the class. They offered to include her in activities outside of class, including football games and parties. To Carly's surprise, within a month she had received an upsetting e-mail from someone she did not know accusing her of sexual behavior. She learned that a number of derogatory remarks about her had been posted on a social media site that left her feeling alone and depressed. As these postings continued, her enthusiasm about school decreased and she became more withdrawn. She was afraid to log on to her computer for fear that she would be bullied or picked on online.

Bob, the school nurse, began to suspect something was going on when Carly kept showing up in the health suite with nondescript, vague symptoms. Because he had heard through the student grapevine that a new girl was being bullied online he wondered whether it might be Carly. After some initial probing about her adjustment to her new school, he learned about Carly's situation. Bob began to provide direct care to Carly to help her address the bullying and with Carly's permission included her parents. He also included the school administration. Bob took this case very seriously given the recent cases in the news in which cyberbullying had resulted in the victim committing suicide. Counseling was sought for Carly and she began to show improvement,

Helping Carly was only half of the problem; preventing further bullying was the other half. The school administration asked Bob to spearhead the school team with the charge to provide an educational program for the school. Bob found evidence-based programs and decided to include students, teachers, and parents on his team to help choose the program most appropriate for his school. The team agreed that in addition to putting in place an educational program, they should also make an assessment to help establish the extent of the problem. Bob located a resource with tools to measure bullying, published by the CDC.[131] The team conducted a survey of the students and discovered that it was more widespread than they had initially thought.

To help the team, Bob found a definition of *bullying* that helped them understand the broad scope of the problem. According to Olweus, "A student is being bullied or victimized when she is exposed, repeatedly and over time to negative actions on the part of one or more other students."[132] Bob explored the issue further and found that the phenomenon of bullying includes three groups: the bully, the victim, and persons who are both bully and victim. He found that the prevalence varies but has been found to be 15% in elementary and lower secondary schools in Norway; and among 11- to 15-year-olds in 40 countries, 26% have been involved in bullying.[133–135]

Because the school was specifically concerned with cyberbullying, Bob looked for a clear definition. Based on what he read, he reported to the team that

cyberbullying is the purposeful and repeated harm inflicted through the use of computers, cell phones, and other electronic devices.[136–138] To help the team understand the seriousness of the problem, Bob explained to them that bullying can result in severe consequences for the victim, including elevated levels of depression, anxiety, poor self-esteem, psychosomatic problems, suicide ideation, and actual suicide attempts, some of which can be successful.[125,135] Using an ecological understanding of the bullying behavior and Bob's help, the team concluded that the program they implemented should be based on the components of the Olweus Bullying Prevention Program. This program consists of school-level, classroom-level, individual-level, and community-level components.[134] The principles guiding this evidence-based program are that adults should:[134]

- Show warmth and positive interest in their students
- Set firm limits to unacceptable behavior
- Use consistent nonphysical, nonhostile negative consequences when rules are broken
- Function as positive roles models

The team completed their assessment and, based on their findings, put together an antibullying campaign at the school. The campaign included educational sessions for students, teachers, and parents; public service announcements posted throughout the school; an anonymous hotline for reporting suspected bullying; and the institution of a bullying intervention program to help with early identification and intervention with victims. Because the team had collected initial assessment data, they were able to demonstrate significant improvement over time after the implementation of the campaign.

Dating Violence

Dating violence is another form of violence that is not unfamiliar to adolescents and, unfortunately, is a common occurrence, with 10% of a national sample reporting it.[138] There is a need to screen adolescents for teen dating violence, especially those with certain high-risk behaviors, including alcohol and drug use and high-risk sexual behaviors.[139] Social-emotional skills are particularly important in addressing healthy relationships, and school-based interventions are increasingly being designed and tested.[140] Different methods of engaging adolescents in these educational efforts are being explored. Creative approaches using peers and the arts are ways of addressing these difficult topics. Fredland reports on the use of community-based research in developing a theater script that was used in 7th grade health classes to address the promotion of healthy relationships.[140]

■ EVIDENCE-BASED PRACTICE
Risky Adolescent Behaviors

Practice Statement: Risky behaviors in adolescents can lead to adverse consequences including injury and violence.

Targeted Outcome: Prevention of alcohol use, tobacco, marijuana use, and violence

Evidence to Support: There are many curricula for mental emotional health, tobacco, substance use, and violence. One that addresses both substance use and violence is Life Skills Training. Life Skills Training is a universal program that targets social and psychological factors that promote risky behaviors. It is based on enhancement models of prevention that focus on both social influence and enhancing competence. It teaches personal and social skills that build resilience. The program has been implemented in all 50 states and in 32 countries. It is estimated that 10,000 schools/sites, and 3 million students have participated in the program. Life Skills Training has been extensively evaluated in more than 30 scientific studies. Lower rates of alcohol, tobacco, marijuana, and polydrug use were found in comparison with control schools. Reductions in violence and delinquency have also been found.

Recommended Approaches: There are three separate programs: elementary school (grades 3 to 6), middle school (grades 6 to 9), and high school (grades 9 to 12). The curriculum encourages facilitated discussion, structured small group activities, and role-playing scenarios, which are used to stimulate participation and promote the acquisition of skills.

Sources

Substance Abuse Mental Health Services Administration. (2008). *Evidence-based programs and practices: Life skills training.* Retrieved from http://www.nrepp.samhsa.gov/ViewIntervention.aspx?id=109.

Botvin, G.J., Baker, E., Dusenbury, L., Botvin, E.M., & Diaz, T. (1995). Long-term follow-up results of a randomized drug abuse prevention trial in a white middle-class population. *JAMA, 273*(14), 1106-1112.

Botvin, G.J., Griffin, K.W., & Nichols, T.D. (2006). Preventing youth violence and delinquency through a universal school-based prevention approach. *Preventive Science, 7*(4), 403-408.

Spoth, R.L., Randall, G.K., Trudeau, L., Shin, C., & Redmond, C. (2008). Substance use outcomes 5½ years past baseline for partnership-based, family-school preventive interventions. *Drug Alcohol Dependence, 96*(1-2), 57-68.

There is a need to identify and use evidence-based programs in school health. The two registries of evidence-based programs that address violence are located in the National Registry of Effective Programs and Practices and Blueprints for Violence Prevention.[141,142] In addition, the Community Prevention Services Task Force has a Web site that also provides a review of evidence-based violence prevention programs.[143] The guide recommends universal programs or programs that teach all students in a given school or grade about the problem of violence. The recommendation is that the program should address one or more of the following topics or skills intended to reduce aggressive or violent behavior: emotional self-awareness, emotional control, self-esteem, positive social skills, social problem-solving, conflict resolution, or teamwork. In this review, violence refers to both victimization and perpetration.[143]

Consultation

Because of health expertise, the school nurse is likely to provide consultation within schools to address health issues. This can be seen in the role of the school nurse on individualized education program evaluations, in which nurses have a critical role in determining student eligibility for 504 plans, especially since new Americans With Disabilities Act amendments went into effect in January 2009, making more health-related functions fit the criterion of major life activities. The list now includes reading, concentrating, thinking, sleeping, eating, performing manual tasks, and other major bodily functions.[144]

In addition to local school nurses, there is a state school nurse consultant in 40 states. This person provides consultation to nurses practicing in schools and is in a position to advocate for state-level policies and local school nursing practices.[145] The National Association of State School Nurse Consultants (NASSNC) has a position paper that provides the rationale for having a state school nurse consultant in every state. The NASSNC rationale for having a state school nurse consultant (SSNC) is as follows: The SSNC "is responsible for promoting statewide quality standards for school health policies, nursing scope of practice and clinical procedures, documentation, and for initiating and coordinating a quality assurance program for accountability. S/he works in collaboration with the state board of nursing, provides guidance in health program development and planning, establishes a continuum of staff development, and serves as a liaison and resource expert in school nursing practice and school health program(s)."[145] The position paper goes on to outline the responsibilities of the SSNC (Box 19-6).

Advocacy

Advocacy for the school nurse occurs on multiple levels. The school nurse can advocate for the student population and their families through efforts to influence policy at the local, state, and/or national levels.[146] The school nurse also serves as direct advocate for the health-care consumers, in this case students, families, and school communities. This can include advocating for culturally competent and developmentally appropriate care, optimal utilization of resources, and promotion of a healthy environment.[147]

BOX 19–6	Responsibilities of State School Nurse Consultants

The responsibilities of the state school nurse consultant include:

- Serving as liaison and resource expert in school nursing and school health program areas for local, regional, state, and national school health care providers, and policy setting groups;
- Providing consultation and technical assistance to local school districts, parents, and community members;
- Coordinating school health program activities with public health, social services, environmental, and educational agencies as well as other public and private entities;
- Monitoring, interpreting, synthesizing, and disseminating relevant information associated with changes in health and medical care, school nursing practice, legislation, and legal issues that have an impact on schools;
- Facilitating the development of policies, standards, and/ or guidelines. Interprets updates and disseminates policies, standards, guidelines, and/or procedures to enhance coordinated school health programs;
- Fostering and promoting staff development for school nurses. This may include planning and providing orientation, coordinating, and/or providing educational offerings and networking with universities and other providers of continuing education to meet identified needs;
- Promoting quality assurance in school health services by initiating and coordinating a quality assurance program that includes needs assessment, data collection and analysis, and evidence-based practice;
- Participating in state-level public interagency/private partnerships with statewide stakeholders to foster a coordinated school health program, representing school nurses in multidisciplinary collaborations;
- Initiating, participating in, and utilizing research studies related to a coordinated school health program, the health needs of children and youth, school nursing practice, and related issues; and
- Serving as legislative liaison regarding school health issues with the state department of health.

Source: See reference 145.

▶ SOLVING THE MYSTERY

The Case of the Missing Student Assessment

Public Health Science Topics Covered:

- Interdisciplinary collaboration
- Program planning

Tameka, the school nurse in a large inner-city charter high school, served on the attendance review committee. Because attendance in school is critical to learning, the school administration had convened the committee with those who could provide the most insight into underlying factors that might contribute to attendance problems. The current emphasis on academic achievement of all students mandated by the No Child Left Behind (NCLB) Act provided the initial rationale for convening the committee. The school administration understood that academic achievement is linked to students being present in class,[148,149] and reduction of absenteeism was a major strategic goal for the school. The committee was composed of the vice principal, two teachers, the school social worker, and Tameka. During one meeting, the committee discussed one student, Aisha, who was in danger of losing credits for courses she was passing because of excessive absenteeism. Aisha had recently moved into the school district and had no record of a health problem. The committee decided that Tameka would contact the student and parent or guardian for additional information

As a first step, Tameka asked Aisha to come to the health suite. Aisha told Tameka that she was an only child and her mother, Monique, was a single parent who had a night-shift job that paid the minimum wage. To make up for the low wages, Monique worked as much overtime as she could get. They had moved to the city to be closer to extended family. Aisha had made a few friends in school and in her neighborhood. She worked hard at staying current with her schoolwork, despite school absences.

After some probing, Aisha explained that she had juvenile rheumatoid arthritis (JRA), specifically, polyarticular disease, but had not reported it because she was sure she could cope with it on her own. She was diagnosed with JRA 4 years ago. She described a typical morning on school days: it took her about 2 to 3 hours to get dressed and ready for school because of extreme discomfort in her joints. Her mother usually did not return from her shift until after the time Aisha needed to leave for school. Aisha sometimes gave up trying to get ready in time to make the walk to school. Although it was only four blocks, some mornings the pain made it very difficult to walk.

When Tameka spoke with Aisha's mother, Tameka discovered that they did not have a car and traveling on the city bus to see her primary care provider was difficult for Aisha as it required two bus changes. The mother then admitted that Aisha had not actually seen a PCP since they had moved to the city. The prescribed medication regimen was abandoned by the family because of a lack of finances. Aisha primarily relied on over-the-counter NSAIDs for pain relief she described as "okay, sometimes."

Tameka concluded that her priority regarding Aisha was to help connect her health care, including support for medication costs. Tameka referred Monique to the local health department for assistance with completing the state children's health insurance plan application. With approval of the application, Aisha began visits to health-care providers.

The absentee committee helped to set up a class schedule to allow Aisha a first period study hall so that she could get to school in time for classes. The social worker also worked with Aisha and Monique to get documentation approved for the possibility of Aisha receiving home instruction in the event of exacerbation of JRA. Tameka also arranged for Aisha to receive transportation to school if needed. It was hoped that with proper management as well as accommodations within the school setting, Aisha would not miss school.

Again, intervening on Aisha's behalf was only the beginning of the Tameka's job as advocate. Through a collaborative approach, the school team had helped address an issue for Aisha and also identified a gap in how they collected health information on new students. Tameka proposed that they develop a new student process that would help to identify students at risk for adverse educational outcomes due to health issues such as Aisha's. The team identified other team members who needed to be on their committee, including the

staff who did the initial intake. In Aisha's case, she had not reported the problem, but when the team reviewed her transcript form from the other school, they found a notation on Aisha's condition that had been missed. Changing the intake process was a crucial step for the school in the process of advocating for their students who needed additional support services.

Tameka modeled the nurse's role by illustrating the importance of health services that support learning, health, and student achievement. She began by focusing on individual student advocacy and then helped to lead the team in advocating for the student body as a whole.

Policy Development and Enforcement

Policy plays a significant role in influencing school health and the health services provided to students. This can be seen in the focus on school health in *HP 2020*, federal and state laws, and local regulations governing services. The advocacy role of school nurses includes advancing school health policy, whether it is local school policy, state policy, or national policy affecting children and adolescents.[146]

Local Laws and Regulations

From a local school perspective, implementing wellness policies and practices reflecting the goals of *HP 2020* is one example of how nurses intervene at this level. In Wisconsin, a guide has been published, *What Works in Schools: Healthy Eating, Physical Activity, and Healthy Weight*, which provides approaches that nurses can perform for prevention of obesity.[150] School nurses play an important role on school health advisory councils (wellness committees, school wellness advisory councils) where they can advocate for comprehensive health programs and recommend, review, and facilitate the implementation of district policies.[151] These policies relate to key components that support school health including the built environment, school wellness policies, delegation of nursing care in schools, or changing longstanding policies that are no longer supported by evidence.[152–154] Changing head lice management policies is an example of the challenge of translating evidence-based practice into a school setting. Past policies of "no nits" in schools contributed to school absences. This belief in exclusion from schools is no longer warranted based on evidence, but changing practice and policy is difficult. Changing practice involves changing beliefs, which requires collaborative community relationships, identification of hierarchy structures in school policy development, and system education.[155]

State Laws and Regulations

Variations in legislative mandates for school nurses occur within and among states in the United States. School nurses are mandated in 51% of states and of those states, 69% of the laws protect the title "school nurse."[156] School nurses practice under state nurse practice acts and codes, which requires that nurses not only understand the scope and standards of school nursing practice but also the specific state level regulations related to their scope of practice, required level of education, and other relevant laws. For example, school nurses need to know if state nurse practice acts provide for delegation of certain nursing tasks to UAP or the minimum level of education required to practice as a school nurse.

State immunization regulations govern the criteria for required vaccines for enrollment in schools. School nurses must be alert to changes in immunization regulations and requirements so that parents and guardians can be informed and review of compliance may be accomplished.

States vary on what is mandated in student screening of certain health conditions. Over 70% of states require hearing and vision screening in order to detect potential hearing or vision problems; over 50% of states require scoliosis screening.[157] School nurses conduct these screenings in schools. In some school districts, technicians, not school nurses, are responsible for conducting hearing and vision screenings.

Federal Laws

School nurses also play a significant role in adhering to federal laws and promoting the development of federal policies. The laws with particular relevance to children with disabilities are reviewed in preceding sections. Other laws are also important to the role of the school nurse are discussed here

Elementary and Secondary Education Act: School health services are influenced by a number of federal laws, beginning with the Elementary and Secondary Education Act (ESEA), also referred to as the NCLB Act. This legislation provides federal funding for improved academic achievement for students, including students with disabilities. NCLB sets the stage for education policy and reform from the federal, state, and local levels and sets the atmosphere in which schools work, including school health services. The act has come under some criticism owing to the requirement of standardized testing. Under President Obama, the act was modified to allow states to apply for waivers from the requirements of the act. States need to apply and demonstrate how they will improve academic achievement.[158] Title I of the NCLB is aimed at improving the academic outcomes of the

disadvantaged. It provides a mechanism for local education agencies to apply for grants to fund programs aimed at improving the academic achievement of students. If funded, the grantee school districts are required to evaluate outcomes.[159]

Child Abuse Prevention and Treatment Act: The Child Abuse Prevention and Treatment Act (CAPTA) was first passed into law in 1974 as Public Law 93-247 and has undergone numerous amendments over the years. CAPTA includes provisions for funding state child welfare agencies, among other provisions.[160] School nurses, along with other school staff, are required to report suspected child abuse and neglect according to state laws and regulations.

Family Educational Rights and Privacy Act: The **Family Educational Rights and Privacy Act (FERPA)** provides for the protection of privacy for parents and eligible students as related to education records in educational agencies and institutions that receive funds from the U.S. Department of Education. Because private and religious schools do not generally receive funds from the U.S. Department of Education, they would not be subject to FERPA. With FERPA, parents and students have certain rights to review, inspect, and request amendments to a student's education record. FERPA sets forth the parameters for educational agencies and institutions for disclosure of personally identifiable information from education records.[161] For example, student health records are often considered part of the education record and the school nurse must maintain the privacy of the records under FERPA. According to FERPA, "At the elementary or secondary level, a student's health records, including immunization records, maintained by an educational agency or institution subject to FERPA, as well as records maintained by a school nurse, are 'education records' subject to FERPA."[161] From this perspective, school health records are considered education records. In some cases, they are considered medical records and therefore come under the **Health Information Privacy Protection Act (HIPPA).**[162] HIPAA sets out requirements for electronic healthcare transactions and to protect the privacy and security of individually identifiable health information.[161] Thus, it is important for school nurses to know which act applies in their school district.

Children's Health Insurance Program: In 1997, the U.S. Congress passed legislation titled the **Children's Health Insurance Program (CHIP),** which was reauthorized as the Children's Health Insurance Reauthorization Act of 2009 (Pub. L. 111-3).[163] CHIP provides health insurance to approximately 8 million children whose family incomes are too high to qualify for Medicaid and too low to afford health insurance. The federal government provides matching funds to states. The states can implement the program as an extension of Medicaid, a separate program from Medicaid, or a combined CHIP-Medicaid program[164] The CHIP programs are maintained under the Affordable Care Act (ACA) through 2019 and requires states to maintain eligibility standards through 2019. CHIP funding is extended until October 1, 2015, at which time the federal matching rate will increase by 23 percentage points. There is an extra $40 million in federal funding in the ACA aimed at promoting enrollment in Medicaid and CHIP.[164]

School nurses serve a vital role in facilitating student enrollment in CHIP. School nurses are often the only health-care providers who see students on a regular basis. They collaborate with local health departments to provide information and outreach to parents and families of children about enrolling in CHIP. School nurses work one-on-one with families with ill children who need to seek primary health care but are hesitant to do so because of a lack of or inadequate health-care insurance.

Another recent example of a federal law is the Healthy Hunger Free Kids Act of 2010 (Pub. L. 111-296), which was signed into law on December 13, 2010. This law allows the USDA to update the school nutrition standards and provides funding to increase the national school lunch program.[165] School nurses have taken leadership in testifying for and supporting this new law.

Challenges for the Future

Time spent in childhood poverty has been linked with poor child health status, with African American children disproportionately affected.[166] Poor health status plays a role in limiting educational achievement of adolescence.[167] Addressing health disparities that have an impact on education, such as vision, asthma, teen pregnancy, aggression and violence, physical activity, breakfast, and inattention and hyperactivity has a role in promoting educational attainment among low-income and minority adolescents.[168] School nurses are in a position to lead health-promoting efforts and reform to help address health disparities in school-age children and to transform educational and health systems to achieve health and educational equity.

Health-Care Reform

With the passage of the federal ACA as Public Law 111-148, school nursing will have a role in certain provisions.

Highlights of those provisions of Public Law 111-148 include:[169]

• Access to health insurance for people with preexisting conditions
• Streamlined enrollment procedures for Medicaid and CHIP
• Development of standards and protocols for health information technology
• Teen pregnancy prevention strategies and services
• Increased access to clinical preventive services through school-based health centers
• Oral health-care prevention activities
• Funding for a childhood obesity demonstration project

School nurses must remain aware of activities related to health-care reform. Partnerships with local health departments enable school nurses to know what resources exist for children and families.

School Health Services Funding

With few funded mandates for school nursing, financing school health services generally occurs with local government dollars: education or public health. What would it take for both health and education to support funding for school health services? The health needs of schoolchildren must be met. The answer may require the building of creative and collaborative linkages between schools and community health services.[170]

Data on the cost-effectiveness of school nursing will allow critical and strategic decision making related to funding school health services. A study of the economic value of hospital nurses concludes that while "only a portion of the services that professional nurses provide can be quantified, . . . partial estimates of economic value . . . illustrate the economic value to society of improved quality of care achieved through higher staffing levels."[171] Demonstrating the economic value of professional nursing in the school setting may facilitate the provision of appropriate school nurse staffing to meet the health needs of students.

▪ Summary Points

• School nursing provides care to individuals, families, and communities within the educational system.
• *HP 2020* sets specific goals related to promotion of optimal health in school-age children and adolescents.
• The coordinated school health program provides a model for school nurses to follow in providing care to children and adolescents within a school setting.

- Public health science informs school nursing practice, especially in relation to surveillance, case management, screening, health education, and program planning.
- Specific federal, state, and local laws apply to school nursing practice. School nurses serve as advocates for students, their families, and their communities in the obtaining resources, protecting rights, and promoting reform.

▲ CASE STUDY
The Case of the New Nurse
Learning Outcomes

At the end of this case study, the student will be able to:

- Discuss how to prioritize steps for building a health program.
- Identify opportunities for collaboration.
- Apply evidence-based school health programs to a specific population.
- Identify applicable education related regulations.
- Apply components of health planning, assessment, and program development to the school setting.

Nesrin started her new job as a school nurse in a K–5 charter school in New York City that had just been established and was due to open its doors in 3 months. The school was located in a district where the population was 40% non-black Hispanic, 30% African American, and 10% non-Hispanic white, and had a growing Arabic population. She took the job because the charter schools in New York have more freedom to create their own programs. She was included as part of the leadership team charged with creating a healthy learning environment. Based on her recommendation, the team decided to construct their program using the elements of coordinated school health programs as recommended by the CDC as well as a newer model, Whole School, Whole Community, Whole Child (WSCC) model created in collaboration with CDC.[172]

1. What would her first steps be from a public health perspective?
2. Compare your answers with your classmates' answers, make a master list, and prioritize the steps.
3. Once you have completed these first steps, put together a comprehensive health program for the school.
   a. Who would you put on your planning team?
   b. What essential elements are needed for the program?
   c. What resources are needed?

4. Put together a draft program based on available evidence of best practices.
5. Be sure to address the different developmental needs of the students.
6. How will you address special health needs, including accommodations for students with disabilities?
7. How will health education play a part in your plan?
8. What federal, state, and local regulations must you include in the plan?

REFERENCES

1. National Association of School Nurses. (2015). *Definition of School Nursing.* Retrieved from http://www.nasn.org/RoleCareer/PlanningaCareerinSchoolNursing.
2. National Association of School Nurses. (2010). *Code of Ethics.* Retrieved from http://www.nasn.org/RoleCareer/CodeofEthics.
3. Woo, T.M. (2010). 2009. H1N1 influenza pandemic. *Journal of Pediatric Health Care, 24*(4), 258-266.
4. Lessler, J., Reich, N.G., & Cummings, D.A.T. (2009). Outbreak of 2009 pandemic influenza A (H1N1) at a New York City School. *The New England Journal of Medicine, 361,* 2628-2636.
5. World Health Organization. (2015). *Pandemic (H1N1) 2009.* Retrieved from http://www.who.int/csr/disease/swineflu/en/.
6. Sheetz, A.H. (2010). The H1N1 pandemic: Did school nurses assume a leadership role? Some thoughts on leadership. *NASN School Nurse, 25,* 108-109.
7. Zaiger, D. (2006). Historical perspectives of school nursing. In J. Slelekman (Ed.), *School nursing: A comprehensive text.* Philadelphia, PA: F.A. Davis.
8. Struthers, L.R. (1917). *The school nurse.* New York, NY: Putnam.
9. U.S. Department of Health and Human Services. (2013). *Healthy People 2020: Early and middle childhood.* Retrieved from http://www.healthypeople.gov/2020/topicsobjectives2020/overview.aspx?topicid=10.
10. U.S. Department of Health and Human Services. (2015). *Healthy People 2020: Adolescent health.* Retrieved from http://www.healthypeople.gov/2020/topicsobjectives2020/overview.aspx?topicid=2.
11. U.S. Department of Health and Human Services. (2015). *Healthy People 2020: Educational and community-based programs.* Retrieved from http://www.healthypeople.gov/2020/topicsobjectives2020/overview.aspx?topicId=11.
12. National Research Council and Institute of Medicine, Committee on Adolescent Health Care Services and Models of Care for Treatment, Prevention, and Healthy Development. (2009). *Adolescent health services: Missing opportunities.* Washington, DC: National Academies Press. Retrieved from http://books.nap.edu/openbook.php?record_id=12063&page=.

13. Centers for Disease Control and Prevention. (2015). *The case for coordinated school health.* Retrieved from http://www.cdc.gov/healthyyouth/cshp/case.htm.

14. Maine Department of Education and Department of Health and Human Services. (2013). *Coordinating school health programs: Introduction—guidelines for coordination.* Retrieved from http://www.mainecshp.com/guidelines.html.

15. Centers for Disease Control and Prevention. (2015). *Components of a coordinated school health program.* Retrieved from http://www.cdc.gov/healthyyouth/cshp/components.htm.

16. Allensworth, D.D., & Kolbe, L.J. (1987). The comprehensive school health program: Exploring an expanded concept. *Journal of School Health, 57,* 409-412.

17. Centers for Disease Control and Prevention. (2013). *School health policies and practices study 2012.* Retrieved from http://www.cdc.gov/healthyyouth/shpps/2012/factsheets/pdf/FS_Overview_SHPPS2012.pdf.

18. Centers for Disease Control and Prevention. (2015). *National Health Education Standards.* Retrieved from http://www.cdc.gov/HealthyYouth/SHER/standards/.

19. Kann, T., Telliohan, S.K., & Wooley, S.F. (2007). Health education: Results from the School Health Policies and Programs Study 2006. *Journal of School Health, 77*(8), 408-434.

20. Kahn, J.A., Huang, B., Gillman, M.W., Field, A.E., Austin, S.B., Colditz, G.A., et al. (2008). Patterns and determinants of physical activity in U.S. adolescents. *Journal of Adolescent Health, 42*(4), 369-377.

21. Centers for Disease Control and Prevention. (2010). *The association between school based physical activity, including physical education, and academic performance.* Atlanta, GA: U.S. Department of Health and Human Services.

22. Kibbe, D.L., Hackett, J., Hurley, M., McFarland, A., Schubert, K.G., Schultz, A., & Harris, S. (2011). Ten years of TAKE 10!: Integrating physical activity with academic concepts in elementary school classrooms. *Preventive Medicine, 52*(Suppl. 1), S43-S50. Advance online publication.

23. Tucker, C. (2011, April). School-based health centers improving access for youth. *The Nation's Health,* 1.

24. Richardson, J.W. (2010). Advancing school-based health care policy and practice. *American Journal of Public Health, 100*(9), 1561.

25. McNail, M.A., Lichty, L.F., & Mavis, B. (2010). The impact of school-based health centers on the health outcomes of middle school and high school students. *American Journal of Public Health, 100*(9), 1604-1610.

26. Walker, S.C., Kerns, S.E.U., Lyon, A.R., Bruns, E.J., & Cosgrove, T.J. (2010). Impact of school-based health center use on academic outcomes, *Journal of Adolescent Health, 46,* 251-257.

27. Stewart, J.A., Dennison, D.A., Kohl, H.W., & Doyle, J.A. (2004). Exercise level and energy expenditure in the TAKE 10! in-class physical activity program. *Journal of School Health, 74,* 397-400.

28. Food Research and Action Center. (2009). *School breakfast scorecard school year 2007–2008.* Washington, DC: Author. Retrieved from http://frac.org/pdf/breakfast08.pdf.

29. Benton, D., & Jarvis, M. (2007). The role of breakfast and a mid-morning snack on the ability of children to concentrate at school. *Physiology & Behavior, 90*(2-3), 382-385.

30. Gajre, N.S., Fernandez, S., Balakrishna, N., & Vazir, S. (2008). Breakfast eating habit and its influence on attention-concentration, immediate memory and school achievement. *Indian Pediatrics, 45*(10), 824-828.

31. Mahoney, C.R., Taylor, H.A., Kanarek, R.B., & Samuel, P. (2005). Effect of breakfast composition on cognitive processes in elementary school children. *Physiology & Behavior, 85*(5), 635-645.

32. Widenhorn-Muller, K., Hille, K., Klenk, J., & Weiland, U. (2008). Influence of having breakfast on cognitive performance and mood in 13- to 20-year-old high school students: Results of a crossover trial. *Pediatrics, 122*(2), 278-284.

33. Pollitt, E., & Mathews, R. (1998). Breakfast and cognition: An integrative summary. *American Journal of Clinical Nutrition, 67*(4), 804S-813S.

34. Rampersaud, G.C., Pereira, M.A., Girard, B.L., Adams, J., & Metzl, J.D. (2005). Breakfast habits, nutritional status, body weight, and academic performance in children and adolescents. *Journal of the American Dietetic Association, 105*(5), 743-762.

35. Taras, H. (2005). Nutrition and student performance at the school. *The Journal of School Nursing, 21*(2), 199-213.

36. Centers for Disease Control and Prevention. (2008). Competitive foods and beverages available for purchase in secondary schools—selected sites, United States, 2006. *Morbidity and Mortality Weekly Report, 57*(34), 935-938. Retrieved from http://www.cdc.gov/mmwr/preview/mmwrhtml/mm5734a2.htm.

37. Fox, M.K., Dodd, A.H., Wilson, A., & Gleason, P.M. (2009). Association between school food environment and practices and body mass index of US public school children. *Journal of American Dietetics Association, 109*(Suppl. 2), S108-S117.

38. U.S. Department of Agriculture, Food and Nutrition Service. (2014). *Healthy Hunger-Free Kids Act.* Retrieved from http://www.fns.usda.gov/school-meals/healthy-hunger-free-kids-act.

39. National Institute of Mental Health. (n.d). *Any disorder in children.* Retrieved from http://www.nimh.nih.gov/statistics/1ANYDIS_CHILD.shtml.

40. Merikangas, K.R., Jian-ping, H., , Burstein, M., Swanson, S.A., Avenevoli, S., Cui, L. et al. (2010). Lifetime prevalence of mental disorders in U.S. adolescents: Results from the National Comorbidity Study-Adolescent supplement (NCS-A). *Journal of American Academy Child Adolescent Psychiatry, 49*(10), 980-989.

41. U.S. Department of Health and Human Services. (1999). *Mental health: A report of the Surgeon General.* Rockville, MD: Substance Abuse and Mental Health Services, National Institutes of Health, National Institute of Mental Health.

42. President's New Freedom Commission on Mental Health. (2003). *Achieving the promise: Transforming*

mental health care in America. Final report (DHHS Publication No. SMA-03-3832). Rockville, MD: U.S. Department of Health and Human Services.

43. U.S. Department of Education, Office of Elementary and Secondary Education. (2002). *No Child Left Behind: A desktop reference.* Washington, DC: Author.

44. Atkins, M.S., Hoagwood, K.E., Kutash, K., & Seidman, E. (2010). Toward the integration of education and mental health in schools. *Administrative Policy Mental Health, 37,* 40-47.

45. Dishop, M.L. (2002). Maintaining environmental cleanliness in school. *Journal of School Nursing, 18*(Suppl. 4), 23–26. doi:10.1177/105984050201800406.

46. Environmental Protection Agency. (2015). *Creating healthy indoor environments in schools.* Retrieved from http://www.epa.gov/iaq/schools/.

47. Healthy Schools Campaign. (2013). *The quick and easy guide to green cleaning in schools.* Retrieved from http://www.greencleanschools.org/.

48. Safe Routes to School. (n.d.). *National policy and advocacy.* Retrieved from http://www.saferoutes partnership.org/national.

49. Turner, A., Finkelhor, D., Hamby, S.L., Shattuck, A., Richard, K., & Ormrod, N. (2011). Specifying type and location of peer victimization in a national sample of children and youth. *Journal of Youth Adolescence, 40,* 1052-1067. doi:10.1007/s10964-011-9639-5.

50. Centers for Disease Control and Prevention (2014). *1991-2013 High School Youth Risk Behavior Survey Data.* Retrieved from http://nccd.cdc.gov/ youthonline/.

51. Ryan, K.M. (2008). Health promotion of faculty and staff: the school nurse's role. *The Journal of School Nursing, 24*(4), 183-189.

52. *Directors of Health Promotion and Education. (n.d). School wellness—a guide for protecting the assets of our nation's schools.* Retrieved from https://c.ymcdn. com/sites/dhpe.site-ym.com/resource/group/ 75a95e00-448d-41c5-8226-0d20f29787de/Download able_Materials/EntireGuide.pdf.

53. Lohrmann, D.K. (2010). A complementary ecological model of the coordinated school health program. *Journal of School Health, 80*(1), 1-9.

54. National Association of School Nurses. (2013). *Position statement—coordinated school health programs Revised 2013.* Retrieved from PolicyAdvocacy/ PositionPapersandReports/NASNPositionStatements FullView/tabid/462/ArticleId/19/Coordinated-School-Health-Programs-Revised-2008.

55. National Association of School Nurses. (2011). *Issue brief—the role of the school nurse.* Retrieved from http://www.nasn.org/PolicyAdvocacy/PositionPaper-sandReports/NASNPositionStatementsFullView/ tabid/462/ArticleId/87/Role-of-the-School-Nurse-Revised-2011.

56. Public Health Nursing Section. (2001). *Public health interventions—applications for public health nursing practice.* St. Paul: Minnesota Department of Health.

57. Centers for Disease Control and Prevention. (2013). Vaccination coverage among children in kindergarten—United Stated, 2012–2013. *Morbidity and Mortality Weekly Report, 62*(30), 607-612.

58. Centers for Disease Control and Prevention. (2015). *Immunization requirements for child care and school.* Retrieved from http://www.cdc.gov/vaccines/parents/ record-reqs/childcare-school.html.

59. Wharton, M., & Bobo, N. (2010). CDC urges school nurses to promote pre-teen vaccines. *NASN School Nurse, 25*(5), 214-215.

60. Centers for Disease Control and Prevention, Advisory Committee for Immunization Practices. (2013). Prevention and control of seasonal influenza vaccines: Recommendations of the ACIP—United Stated, 2013–2014. *Morbidity and Mortality Weekly Report, 62*(RR07), 1-43.

61. World Health Organization. (2015). *Influenza.* Retrieved from http://www.who.int/biologicals/ vaccines/influenza/en/.

62. Jenlink, C.H., Kuehnert, P., & Mazyck, D. (2010). Influenza vaccinations, Fall, 2009: Model school-located vaccination clinics. *The Journal of School Nursing, 26*(Suppl. 1), 7S-13S.

63. Fong, D.Y., Lee, C.F., Cheung, K.M., Cheng, J.C., Ng, B.K., Lam, T.P., et al. (2010). A meta-analysis of the clinical effectiveness of school scoliosis screening. *Spine, 35*(10), 1061-1071.

64. U.S. Preventive Task Force Services. (2015). *Screening for idiopathic scoliosis in adolescents.* Retrieved from http://www.uspreventiveservicestaskforce.org/Page/ Topic/recommendation-summary/idiopathic-scoliosis-in-adolescents-screening.

65. National Association of State Boards of Education. (n.d.). *State school healthy policy database.* Retrieved from http://nasbe.org/healthy_schools/hs/bytopics. php?topicid=4100&catExpand=acdnbtm_catD.

66. Chaplin, P.K.N., & Bradford, G.E. (2011). A historical review of distance vision screening eye charts. *NASN School Nurse, 26*(4), 221-228.

67. American Academy of Audiology. (2011). *Childhood hearing screening guidelines.* Retrieved from http:// www.cdc.gov/ncbddd/hearingloss/recommendations. html

68. Centers for Disease Control and Prevention. (2012). Trends in the prevalence of extreme obesity among U.S. preschool-aged children living in low-income families, 1998–2010. *JAMA, 308*(24), 2563-2565.

69. Centers for Disease Control and Prevention. (2013). *Childhood overweight and obesity.* Retrieved from http://www.cdc.gov/obesity/childhood/.

70. Centers for Disease Control and Prevention. (2015). *About BMI for children and teens.* Retrieved from http://www.cdc.gov/healthyweight/assessing/bmi/ childrens_bmi/about_childrens_bmi.html.

71. Centers for Disease Control and Prevention. (n.d.). *BMI percentile calculator for child and teen, English version.* Retrieved from http://nccd.cdc.gov/dnpabmi/ Calculator.aspx.

72. Daniels, S.R., Arnett, D.K., Eckel, R.H., Gidding, S.S., Hayman, L.L., Kumanyika, S., et al. (2005). Over-weight in children and adolescents: Pathophysiology, consequences, prevention, and treatment. *Circulation,*

111, 1999-2012. doi:10.1161/01.CIR.0000161369. 71722.10 Retrieved from http://circ.ahajournals.org/ cgi/reprint/111/15/1999.

73. Childstats.gov. (2013). *America's children: Key indicators of well being, 2013; Children of at least one foreign-born parent.* Retrieved from http://www. childstats.gov/americaschildren/famsoc4.asp.

74. Mendonca, L., Selser, K., Teskey, C., & Butler, S. (2009). Immigrant and refugee youth: Challenges and opportunities for the school nurse. *NASN School Nurse, 24*(6), 250-252.

75. Krause-Parello, C.A., & Samms, K. (2011). School nursing in a contemporary society: What are the roles and responsibilities? *Issues in Comprehensive Pediatric Nursing, 34*, 26-39.

76. Wade, T.J., Mansour, M.E., Guo, J.J., Huentelman, T., Line, K., & Keller, K.N. (2008). Access and utilization patterns of school-based health centers at urban and elementary and middle schools. *Public Health Reports, 123*, 739-750.

77. U.S. Department of Health and Human Services. (2007). *Asthma action plan* (Publication No. 07-5251). Retrieved from http://www.nhlbi.nih.gov/files/docs/ public/lung/asthma_actplan.pdf.

78. U.S. Environmental Protection Agency. (2010). *Managing asthma in the school environment: Indoor quality for schools* (EPA 402-K-10-004). Retrieved from http://files.eric.ed.gov/fulltext/ED524615.pdf.

79. Olympia, R.P., Wan, E., & Avner, J.R. (2005). The preparedness of schools to respond to emergencies in children: A national survey of school nurses. *Pediatrics, 116*(6), e738-e745.

80. Centers for Disease Control and Prevention. (2013). *School violence: Data and statistics.* Retrieved from http://www.cdc.gov/violenceprevention/youthviolence/ schoolviolence/data_stats.html.

81. Monsalve, L. (2010). NASN membership survey: Developing and providing leadership to advance the school nursing practice. *NASN School Nurse, 25*(4), 176-181.

82. American Heart Association. (2009). *Medical emergency response plan for schools.* Retrieved from http://bethebeat.heart.org/media/pdfs/KJ-0781_ECC_ BTB_Flyer.pdf.

83. Centers for Disease Control and Prevention. (2008). *NCHS brief. Food allergy among U.S. children: Trends in prevalence and hospitalizations.* Retrieved from http://www.cdc.gov/nchs/data/databriefs/ db10.htm.

84. Gupta, R.S., Springston, E.E., Warrier, M.R., Smith, B., Kumar, R., Pongracic, J., & Holl, J.L. (2011). The prevalence, severity, and distribution of childhood food allergy in the United States. *Pediatrics, 128*(1), e9-e17. doi:10.1542/peds.2011-0204.

85. Pumphrey, R.S. (2000). Lessons for management of anaphylaxis from a study of fatal reactions. *Clinical and Experimental Allergy, 30*, 1144-1150.

86. Young, M.C., Munoz-Furlong, A., & Sicherer, S.H. (2009). Management of food allergies in schools: A perspective for allergists. *Clinical Review in Allergy and Immunology, 124*, 175-182.

87. National Association of School Nurses. (2013). *Saving lives at school: Anaphylaxis and epinephrine.* Retrieved from http://portal.nasn.org/media/Saving LivesatSchool_Handbook.pdf.

88. Food Allergy and Anaphylaxis Network. (2015). *Resources for schools.* Retrieved from http://www. foodallergy.org/resources/schools.

89. Bloom, B., Cohen, R.A., & Freeman, G. (2012). Summary health statistics for U.S. children: National Health Interview Survey. National Center for Health Statistics. *Vital Health Statistics, 10*(254).

90. Children's Health Fund. (2010). *Chronic illness and school performance.* Retrieved from http://www. childrenshealthfund.org/sites/default/files/ chronic-illness-and-school-performance.pdf.

91. Merkangas, K.R., He, J., Burstein, M., Swanson, S.A., Avenevoli, S., & Swendses, J. (2010). Lifetime prevalence of mental disorders in US adolescents: Results from the National Comorbidity Study—Adolescent supplement. *Journal of the American Academy of Child & Adolescent Psychiatry, 49*(1), 980-989.

92. National Institute of Mental Health. (n.d.). *Any disorder among children.* Retrieved from http://www. nimh.nih.gov/statistics/1anydis_child.shtml.

93. National Heart, Lung, and Blood Institute. (n.d). *Students with chronic illnesses: Guidance for families, schools, and students.* Retrieved from http://www. nhlbi.nih.gov/health/public/lung/asthma/guidfam.pdf.

94. Engelke, M.K., Guttu, M., Warren, M.B., & Swanson, M. (2008). School nurse case management for children with chronic illness: Health, academic, and quality of life outcomes. *The Journal of School Nursing, 24*(4), 205-214.

95. Bonaiuto, M.M. (2007). School nurse case management: Achieving health and educational outcomes. *The Journal of School Nursing, 23*(4), 202-209.

96. Johnson, K.H. (2010). School-based referrals for attention deficit hyperactivity disorder: School nurses bridge the gap. *NASN School Nurse, 25*(4), 167-169.

97. Dang, M.T., Warrington, D., Tung, T., Baker, D., & Pan, R.J. (2007). A school-based approach to early identification and management of children with ADHD. *The Journal of School Nursing, 23*, 2-12.

98. Vierhile, A., Robb, A., & Ryan-Krause, P. (2009). Attention-deficit/hyperactivity disorder in children and adolescents: Closing diagnostic, communication, and treatment gaps. *Journal of Pediatric Health Care, 23*(Suppl. 1), S5-S21.

99. Connors, C.K. (2000). *Connors' rating scales-revised: Instruments for use with children and adolescents.* Niagara Falls, NY: Multi-Health System.

100. Salmeron, P.A. (2009). Childhood and adolescent attention-deficit hyperactivity disorder: Diagnosis, clinical guidelines, and social implications. *Journal of the American Academy of Nurse Practitioners, 21*, 488-497.

101. Lear, J.G. (2007). Health at school: A hidden health care system emerges from the shadows. *Health Affairs, 26*(2), 409-419.

102. Coffman, J.M., Cabana, M.D., & Yelin, E.H. (2009). Do school-based asthma education programs

improve self-management and health outcomes? *Pediatrics, 124*(2), 729-742. doi:10.1542/peds. 2008-2085.

103. Ahmad, E., & Grimes, D.E. (2011). The effects of self-management education for school-age children on asthma morbidity: A systematic review. *The Journal of School Nursing, 27(4),* 282-292.

104. Centers for Disease Control and Prevention. (2011). *Fast facts on diabetes.* Retrieved from http://www.cdc.gov/diabetes/pubs/pdf/ndfs_2011.pdf.

105. U.S. Department of Health and Human Services, National Institutes of Health. (2015). *Diabetes, type 2.* Retrieved from http://report.nih.gov/NIHfactsheets/ViewFactSheet.aspx?csid=121&key=D#D.

106. *National Diabetes Information Clearinghouse (NDIC).* Retrieved from http://diabetes.niddk.nih.gov/

107. Brown, R. (2010). To catch a thief. Recognizing diabetes. *NASN School Nurse, 25*(4), 164-167.

108. Kelo, M., Martikainen, M., & Eriksson, E. (2011). Self-care of school age children with diabetes: An integrative review. *Journal of Advanced Nursing, 67*(10), 2096-2108.

109. Maughan, E. (2003). The impact of school nursing on school performance: A research synthesis. *The Journal of School Nursing, 19*(3), 163-171.

110. *Individuals With Disabilities Education Act of 2004, Pub. L. No. 108–446* (2006). Retrieved from http://idea.ed.gov/download/statute.html.

111. *Education for All Handicapped Children Act of 1974, Pub. L. No. 94–142* (1975). Retrieved from http://www.scn.org/~bk269/94-142.html.

112. U.S. Department of Education. (2013). *Building the legacy: IDEA 2004.* Retrieved from http://idea.ed.gov/explore/home.

113. Wrightslaw. (n.d,). *Section 504, the Americans With Disabilities Act, and Education Reform.* Retrieved from http://www.wrightslaw.com/info/section504.ada.peer.htm .

114. Sampson, C.H., & Galemore, C.A. (2012). What every school nurse needs to know about section 504 eligibility. *NASN School Nurse, 2*(2), 89-93.

115. Reback, R. (2010). Schools' mental health services and young children's emotions, behavior, and learning. *Journal of Policy Analysis and Management, 29*(4), 698-725.

116. Atkins, M.S., Hoagwood, K.E., Kutash, K., & Seidman, E. (2010). Toward the integration of education and mental health in schools: Administrative policy. *Mental Health, 37*(1-2), 4047.

117. Shannon, R.A., Bergren, M.D., & Matthews, A. (2010). Frequent visitors: Somatization in school-age children and implications for school nurses. *The Journal of School Nursing, 26*(3), 169-182.

118. Campo, J.V., & Fritz, G. (2001). A management model for pediatric somatization. *Psychosomatics, 42,* 467-476.

119. National Association of School Nurses. (2008). *Position statement: Mental health of students.* Retrieved from http://www.nasn.org/PolicyAdvocacy/PositionPapersandReports/NASNPositionStatementsArticle View/tabid/462/ArticleId/36/Mental-Health-of-Students-Revised-2008.

120. Puskar, K.R., & Bernardo, L.M. (2007). Mental health and academic achievement: Role of school nurses. *Journal of Specialists in Pediatric Nursing, 12*(4), 215-223.

121. Centers for Disease Control and Prevention. (2015). Mental health basics. *Healthy youth mental health.* Retrieved from http://www.cdc.gov/mentalhealth/basics.htm

122. National Council of State Boards of Nursing. (2005). *Working with others: A position paper.* Retrieved from https://www.ncsbn.org/Working_with_Others.pdf.

123. Resha, C. (2010). Delegation in the school setting: Is it a safe practice? *The Online Journal of Issues in Nursing, 15*(2), 5. doi:10.39 12/OJIN.Vol15No.02Man05.

124. Centers for Disease Control and Prevention. (2013). *CDC fact sheet: Incidence, prevalence and cost of sexually transmitted infections in the United States.* http://www.cdc.gov/std/stats/STI-Estimates-Fact-Sheet-Feb-2013.pdf.

125. Centers for Disease Control and Prevention. (2012). Youth Risk Behavior Surveillance—United States 2011. *Morbidity and Mortality Weekly Report, 61*(4).

126. Centers for Disease Control and Prevention. (2012). *Adolescent and school health: Standard 5.* Retrieved from http://www.cdc.gov/healthyyouth/sher/standards/5.htm.

127. The National Campaign to Prevent Teen and Unplanned Pregnancy. (2010). *What works: 2010 curriculum-based programs that help prevent teen pregnancy.* Retrieved from http://www.thenational-campaign.org/resources/pdf/pubs/WhatWorks.pdf.

128. Advocates for Youth. (2008). *Science and success. Sex education and other programs that work to prevent teen pregnancy, HIV, and sexually transmitted infections.* Retrieved from http://www.advocatesforyouth.org/storage/advfy/documents/sciencesuccess.pdf.

129. Colen, C.G., Geronimus, A.T., & Phipps, M.G. (2006). Getting a piece of the pie? The economic boom of the 1990s and declining teen birth rates in the United States. *Social Science & Medicine, 63,* 1531-1545.

130. Office of Adolescent Health. (2011). *Healthy People 2020.* Retrieved from http://www.hhs.gov/ash/oah/resources-and-publications/healthy-people-2020.html.

131. Centers for Disease Control and Prevention. (2012). *Measuring bullying victimization, perpetration, and bystander experiences: A compendium of assessment tools.* Retrieved from http://www.cdc.gov/violenceprevention/pub/measuring_bullying.html.

132. Olweus, D. (1993). *Bullying at school: What we know and what we can do.* Oxford, England: Blackwell.

133. Craig, W., Harel-Fisch, Y., Fogel-Grinvald, H., Dastaler, S., Hetland, J., Simons-Morten, B., et al. (2009). A cross-national profile of bullying and victimization among adolescents in 40 countries. *International Journal of Public Health, 54,* S216-S224.

134. Olweus, D., & Limber, S.P. (2010). Bullying in school: Evaluation and dissemination of the Olweus Bullying Prevention Program. *American Journal of Orthopsychiatry, 80*(1), 124-134.

135. Hinduja, S., & Patchin, J.W. (2009). *Bullying beyond the schoolyard: Preventing and responding to cyberbullying.* Thousand Oaks, CA: Sage.

136. Patchin, J.W., & Hinduja, S. (2006). Bullies move beyond the schoolyard: A preliminary look at cyberbullying. *Youth Violence and Juvenile Justice, 4*(2), 148-169.

137. Hinduja, S., & Patchin, J.W. (2010) Bullying, cyberbullying, and suicide. *Archives of Suicide Research, 14,* 206-221.

138. Cutter-Wilson, E., & Richmond, T. (2011). Understanding teen dating violence: Practical screening and intervention strategies for pediatric and adolescent healthcare providers. *Current Opinion in Pediatrics, 23*(4), 379-383.

139. Foshee, V.A., Reyes, H.L., Ennett, S.T., Suchindran, C., Mathias, J.P., Karriker-Jaffe, K.J., et al. (2011). Risk and protective factors distinguishing profiles of adolescent peer and dating violence perpetration. *Journal of Adolescent Health, 48*(4), 344-350. Advance online publication.

140. Fredland, N.M. (2010). Nurturing healthy relationships through a community-based interactive theater program. *Journal of Community Health Nursing, 27,* 107-118.

141. Substance Abuse Mental Health Services Administration. (2013). *Evidence-based programs and practices.* Retrieved from http://www.nrepp.samhsa.gov/.

142. University of Colorado Boulder, Center for the Study and Prevention of Violence. (2013). *We know what works.* Retrieved from http://www.colorado.edu/cspv/blueprints/.

143. Community Prevention Services Task Force. (2013). *Violence prevention.* Retrieved from http://www.thecommunityguide.org/violence/index.html.

144. U.S. Department of Education, Office for Civil Rights. (2011). *Protecting students with disabilities.* Retrieved from http://www2.ed.gov/about/offices/list/ocr/504faq.html.

145. National Association of State School Nurse Consultants. (2008). *State school nurse consultant position.* Retrieved from http://www.schoolnurseconsultants.org/wp-content/uploads/2013/05/NASSNC-Position-Statement-Need-for-State-School-Nurse-Consultants.pdf.

146. Chau, E.A. (2013). Advocacy and the role of the school nurse. *NASN School Nurse, 28*(3), 124-125.

147. National Association of School Nurses & American Nurses Association. (2011). *School nursing: Scope and standards of practice* (2nd ed.). Silver Spring, MD: American Nurses Association.

148. Fiscella, K., & Kitzman, H. (2009). Disparities in academic achievement and health: The intersection of child education and health policy. *Pediatrics, 123*(3), 1073.

149. Pennington, N., & Delaney, E. (2008). The number of students sent home by school nurse compared to unlicensed personnel. *The Journal of School Nursing, 24,* 290-297.

150. Dworak, L.M. (2009). From paper to practice: A look at Healthiest Wisconsin 2010 and the development of local school wellness policies that aid in the prevention of child overweight. *NASN School Nurse, 24*(2), 85-89.

151. Sheetz, A.H. (2011). Why is a school health (wellness) advisory council important for school nursing practice? *NASN School Nurse, 26*(5), 280-282.

152. Pontius, D.J. (2011). Hats off to success. Changing health lice policy. *NASN School Nurse, 26*(6), 357-362.

153. Spriggle, M. (2009). Developing a policy for delegation of nursing care in the school setting. *The Journal of School Nursing, 25*(2), 98-107.

154. Hoxie-Setterstrom, G, & Hoglund, B. (2011). School wellness policies: Opportunities for change. *The Journal of School Nursing, 27*(5), 330-339.

155. Andresen, K., & McCarthy, A.M. (2009). A policy change strategy for head lice management. *The Journal of School Nursing, 25*(6), 407-416.

156. National Association of School Nurses. (2007). *School nursing in the United States: A qualitative study.* Silver Spring, MD: Author.

157. Aud, S., Hussar, W., Planty, M., Snyder, T., Bianco, K., Fox, M., et al. (2010). *The condition of education 2010* (NCES 2010-028). Washington, DC: National Center for Education Statistics, Institute of Education Sciences, U.S. Department of Education.

158. U.S. Department of Education. (2011). *No Child Left Behind.* Retrieved from http://www2.ed.gov/nclb/landing.jhtml.

159. U.S. Department of Education, Office of Planning, Evaluation and Policy Development. (2013). *Evaluation reports.* Retrieved from http://www2.ed.gov/about/offices/list/opepd/ppss/reports.html.

160. U.S. Department of Health and Human Services, Children's Bureau. (2011). *The Child Abuse Prevention and Treatment Act (CAPTA) 2010.* Retrieved from http://www.acf.hhs.gov/programs/cb/resource/capta2010.

161. U.S. Department of Health and Human Services, U.S. Department of Education. (2008). *Joint guidance on the application of Family Educational Rights and Privacy Act (FERPA) and the Health Information Portability and Accountability Act (HIPAA) of 1996 to student health records.* Retrieved from http://www.hhs.gov/ocr/privacy/hipaa/understanding/coveredentities/hipaaferpajointguide.pdf.

162. National Association of School Nurses. (2013). *Issue brief: Privacy standard for student health records.* Retrieved from http://www.nasn.org/portals/0/briefs/2004briefprivacy.pdf.

163. *Children's Health Insurance Program Reauthorization Act of 2009, Pub. L. No. 111-3 (2010).* Retrieved from http://frwebgate.access.gpo.gov/cgi-bin/getdoc.cgi?dbname=111_cong_public_laws&docid=f:publ003.111.pdf.

164. Medicaid.gov. (n.d.). *Children's health Insurance Program (CHIP).* Retrieved from http://www.medicaid.

gov/Medicaid-CHIP-Program-Information/By-Topics/Childrens-Health-Insurance-Program-CHIP/Childrens-Health-Insurance-Program-CHIP.html.

165. U.S. Department of Agriculture Food and Nutrition Services. (n.d.). *Local wellness policy.* Retrieved from http://www.fns.usda.gov/tn/healthy/wellnesspolicy.html.

166. Malat, J., Oh, H., & Hamilton, M. (2005). Poverty experience, race, and child health. *Public Health Reports, 120*, 442-447.

167. Hass, S.A., & Fosse, N.E. (2008). Health and the educational attainment of adolescents: evidence from the NLSY97. *Journal of Health and Social Behavior, 4*(2), 178-192.

168. Basch, C.E. (2010, March). Healthier students are better learners: A missing link in school reforms to close the achievement gap. *Equity Matters: Research Review No. 6.* New York, NY: Teachers College, Columbia University.

169. *Patient Protection and Affordable Care Act of 2010, Pub. L. No. 111-148* (2010). Retrieved from http://frwebgate.access.gpo.gov/cgi-bin/getdoc.cgi?dbname=111_cong_bills&docid=f:h3590enr.txt.pdf.

170. Lear, J.G. (2007). Health at school: A hidden health care system emerges from the shadows. *Health Affairs, 26*(2), 409-419.

171. Dall, T.M., Chen, Y.J., Seifert, R.F., Maddox, P.J., & Hogan, P.F. (2009). The economic value of professional nursing. *Medical Care, 47*(1), 97.

172. Whole School, Whole Community, Whole Child (WSCC). Retrieved from http://www.cdc.gov/healthyyouth/wscc/index.htm.

Chapter 20

Health Planning for Older Adults

LEARNING OUTCOMES

After reading this chapter, the student will be able to:

1. Describe demographic and social trends in an aging America.
2. Define successful aging and determinants of health in the older population.
3. Describe the main health issues facing older adults.
4. Apply current frameworks related to prevention of illness and injury in older adults.

5. Characterize priorities for chronic disease management in the aging population.
6. Identify community resources for helping older adults age in place.
7. Describe age-specific models of health-care delivery across the continuum from wellness to end-of-life care.
8. Articulate key ethical issues related to aging in our society.

KEY TERMS

Aged dependency ratio
Ageism
Aging
Baby boomers
Caregiver
Centenarians
Continuing care
    communities

Core end-stage indicator
Dependency ratio
Early onset at-risk
    substance use
Elder maltreatment
Elderly
Elderly persons
Geriatrics

Gerontology
Hospice care
Late onset at-risk
    substance use
Life expectancy
Life span
Naturally occuring
    retirement community

Old old
Older adult
Palliative care
Population aging
Rectangularization
    of aging
Super centenarians

■ Introduction

The current aging of the world's population is unprecedented.[1] In the first half of the last century, the increase in older populations was largely due to improvements in life expectancy. **Life expectancy** is defined as the probable number of years a person will live based on the birth and mortality statistics of the population. In the United States, life expectancy increased from 49 years at the beginning of the 20th century to 78.2 years in 2010.[2] In 2012, 32 high-income countries had a life expectancy that exceeded 80 years of age.[3] Factors that have influenced this increase in life expectancy during the last half of the 20th century include decreased fertility rates and increased urbanization.[1] The fact that we are living longer has had a direct impact on public health, allocation of health resources, and demand for nursing services. Understanding this phenomenon from a public

health perspective provides nurses with the context in which aging occurs and the factors that can contribute not only to living longer, but also to maintaining an optimal health related quality of life as we age. This understanding in turn helps nurses develop, implement, and evaluate nursing interventions across settings from a public health prevention framework that will improve the health-related quality of life experienced by older adults and reduce the need for more costly tertiary care.

Health of Aging Populations

Who Is Old?

In the United States, the commonly accepted definition of **older adult** is a person aged 65 or older and is used in this chapter to be consistent with language used in *Healthy People 2020 (HP 2020)*.[4] The age of 65 was chosen because in high-income countries, most persons are eligible at this age for retirement benefits. The World Health Organization (WHO) pointed out that this definition is somewhat arbitrary and may not be applicable in lower-income countries.[5] The problem is that chronological age may not accurately reflect a similar biological age of persons living in a low-income country compared with someone the same age living in a high-income country. For example, the WHO argued that a person aged 50 or 55 living in a low-income country may be comparable biologically with a person aged 65 living in a high-income country. People who live in low-income countries age faster owing to inadequate nutrition, exposure to communicable diseases, and poorer living conditions.[5] Thus, the aging process is a product not only of chronological age but also of biological age.

Aging occurs differently in individuals and populations. Rather than viewing aging as an inevitable decline, it can instead be viewed as the later stages of continuous growth and development that occur across the life span. The quality and length of life depends on factors that improve the biological response to growth and development experienced across the life span. This includes not only individual healthy habits embraced in youth and followed across the life span, but also the environment in which an individual lives. The term **life span** is used to describe the measure of a life from birth to death. It also refers to the genetically based limit to the length of life. In humans, the documented maximum life span achieved was 122 years.

Though chronological age as a marker for aging has some limitations, it provides a way to compare populations. Other terms commonly used are **elderly** or **elderly persons** but the preferred term is *older adult*. These terms are also defined using chronological criteria and are typically used to describe persons aged 65 years or older.[5] There are also terms for subpopulations, as evidenced by terms such as **old old,** defined as those 85 years of age or older. As life expectancy lengthens, another chronological group is also emerging, those over the age of 100. This population is referred to as **centenarians. Super centenarians** are those who live to be 110 years of age or older.

Nurses provide needed care for older adults and are educated to view aging as a lifelong process, not simply a particular chronological age or an end stage of life. Understanding the specific needs of the older adult from a population perspective provides nursing with an opportunity to actively participate in the public health initiative reflected in the *HP 2020* objective to improve the quality of life for older adults.[4] For nurses providing care to older adults, there is an opportunity to reduce risk and enhance function at the individual level, even in the face of age-related changes. When this is expanded to include groups of individuals, communities, and populations, the impact of nursing interventions is greater.

Regardless of clinical practice settings, most nurses are likely to provide care to older family members, friends, or members of their communities. Providing care to older adults requires examining the phenomenon of aging from a population perspective that includes:

- The demographic, social, and health trends associated with aging
- Public health issues
- Impact on individual care delivery systems
- Resources for health prevention and promotion
- Implications for policy and research

Thus, aging is not adequately measured by chronological age. Instead, the quality of life experienced as individuals age is a product of our chronological and biological age and is affected by the environments in which we live.[5]

An Aging America

In 2012, the U.S. Census Bureau estimated that 13.8% of the U.S. population was 65 years old or older.[6] By 2050, the estimated number of persons aged 65 or older will be 83.3 million, and 60% of these older Americans will be over the age of 74 (Figs. 20-1 and 20-2).[7] On average, those who are 65 years of age will now live another 18 years, and those aged 85 years will live on average into their early 90s.[8] This phenomenon is referred to as **population aging,** which is defined as a shift in the distribution of a country's population toward older ages. In other words, the proportion of

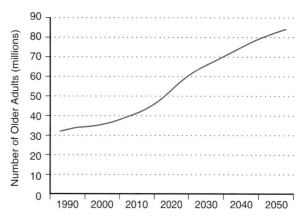

Figure 20-1 Increase in the number of U.S. older adults expressed in millions, 1990–2050. *(From the U.S. National Institutes of Health, National Institute on Aging [2009]).[7]*

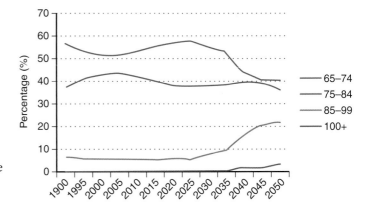

Figure 20-2 Distribution of U.S. older adults over age groups, 1990–2050. *(From the U.S. National Institutes of Health, National Institute on Aging [2009]).[7]*

the population that is older has increased. This is usually reflected in an increase in the population's mean and median ages, a decline in the proportion of the population composed of children, and a rise in the proportion of the older adult population. Population aging is widespread across the world, and is most advanced in the high-income countries.[9,10] This aging of the population globally, according to the WHO, is a cause for celebration because it reflects the positive effect of interventions aimed at improving health. It also offers opportunities, because older adults are a wonderful resource. However, this trend puts strains on pension funds and the demand for health-care services;[10] thus, it is imperative to tailor health-care resources and systems to the unique needs of an aging population.

What accounts for the population aging in the United States? One of the reasons is improvement in the environment. In the first half of the 20th century, diseases that previously led to death in early life became less threatening owing to the development of antibiotics and other medications. In addition, improvements in sanitation, diagnostic advances, the application of technology, and improved prenatal and obstetrical care contributed to longer living.[11] Prior to these innovations in the United States, nearly half of the people born in the year 1900 died before they reached age 50. Contrast this with our current situation, wherein people born today can expect to live beyond their 75th year, and an increasing number are living to be 100. In 1900, about one in 25 Americans was over 65; today one in eight is over 65. The older adult population in the United States is expected to double from 40.2 million in 2010 to 88.5 million in 2050. Increases in longevity can also be seen in the fastest growing age group in our society, the old old. By the middle of this century, there will be 15 to 18 million persons over the age of 85. We also can expect to see nearly a million centenarians, or people 100 years or older.[12,13]

Along with changes in life expectancy, a main reason for the dramatic increase in the number of older adults in the United States is the effect of the baby boomer generation. **Baby boomers** are those members of the U.S. population born between 1945 and 1964. In 2010, the first of this generation turned 65. Growth in the number of older adults will continue as this cohort moves through the upper age groups and will begin to stabilize after 2050.[13] According to the U.S. Census Bureau, in 2010 a little more than 14% of the older population was over the age of 85 but by 2050, when all of the baby boomer generation is over the age of 85, that proportion is expected to increase to over 21%.[13] A good way to visualize this cohort is through a comparison of population pyramids over time. Figure 20-3 includes four population pyramids for the United States 20 years apart, starting with 1990. The 1990 pyramid shows the baby boomer bump clearly when the baby boomers were between 25 and 45 years old. By 2050, this cohort is 85 years of age or older and accounts for the change in the top of the pyramid (Fig. 20-3).[13]

Another term that describes the shift in our population toward the older ages is the **rectangularization of aging.** This describes the population trend toward increased numbers of healthy years before decline or, more exactly, a reduction in variability of age of death.[14] With a steady or slightly declining birthrate and reductions in early deaths, a population's tendency to move toward older ages emerges, which is what we are seeing in the United States today.

The face of aging in the United States is changing dramatically. People are living longer, achieving higher levels of education, living in poverty less often, and experiencing lower rates of disability.[12] Even with this positive outlook, there are still significant public health challenges. For example, the old old age group is not only increasing in numbers, but is also prone to the development of serious chronic conditions such as dementia, placing a

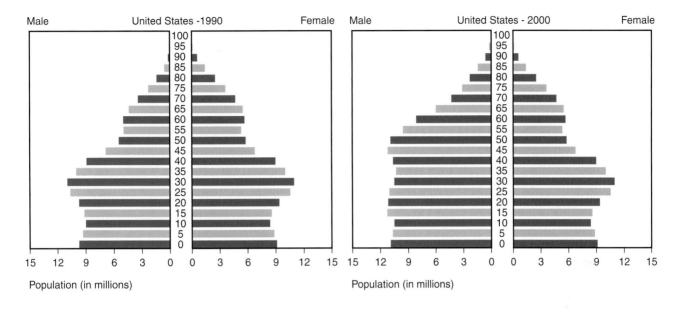

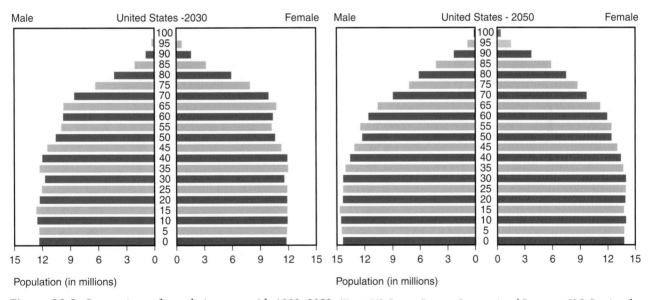

Figure 20-3 Comparison of population pyramids 1990–2050. *(From US Census Bureau, International Programs U.S. Retrieved from http://www.census.gov/population/international/data/idb/informationGateway.php/.)*

disproportionate demand on health-care resources.[15] This group is also more likely to be living in poverty, and to experience functional declines. Also, the epidemic of obesity will have an impact on the development of cardiovascular disease and diabetes in the aging population, with implications not only for longevity, but also for health-care utilization and quality of life.[16]

Aging and the Workforce

In our daily lives, our joint activities and interactions with older adults demonstrate the valuable contributions to family life, workplaces, and communities. Consider the greeter at Walmart, the volunteer at the library, our elected officials serving as senators and representatives well into their 70s and sometimes 80s. As more people over the age of 65 participate in the workforce,[8,17,18] we encounter more and more persons actively contributing to the health and well-being of our communities who are over 65.

From 1977 to 2007, the number of persons over the age of 65 increased by 101%. This graying of the workforce is not just the result of the increase in the numbers of older adults staying in the workforce; also, younger Americans are entering the workforce at an older age.[18] Older adults are staying in the workforce for a variety of reasons. One factor was the economic recession of 2008 to 2010 that reduced the savings of older adults, with more than half of those 62 and over in 2009 citing the recession as their reason for staying in the workforce. Other reasons for staying in the workforce included feeling productive, needing social interaction, and having something to do.[18]

One of the things the increased life expectancy of a population affects is the dependency ratio. The **dependency ratio** is the proportion of dependents (those aged 0 to 14 years plus those 65 years of age and older) per every 100 members of the population aged 15 to 64. In relation to the older population, the ratio is referred to as the **aged dependency ratio** and reflects the ratio of the number of persons age 65 and older per every 100 members of the population aged 15 to 64 (Box 20-1). Because of the aging population, there is an expected rise in the dependency ratio as well.[18] Factors that may improve the aged dependency ratio include the increased age of full retirement for Social Security benefits for baby boomers increasing from 65 to 67 and the graying of the U.S. workforce. However, as the number of those who live past the age of 65 increases, any possible benefits from the increased number of those over 65 who work may be wiped out by the increasing number of the person aged 75 and older.[18]

BOX 20-1	**Aged Dependency Ratio**

Total Dependency Ratio =

$$\frac{\text{Number of people aged 0 to 14} + \text{number of people aged 65 and older}}{\text{Number of people aged 15 to 64}} \times 100$$

Aged Dependency Ratio =

$$\frac{\text{Number of people aged 65} +}{\text{Number of people aged 15 to 64}} \times 100$$

HP 2020 and Older Adults

As life expectancy increases along with the proportion of the society living over the age of 85, society is confronted with both challenges and opportunities for people of all ages. The challenge for the 21st century is to make these added life span years as healthy and productive as possible and to continue the current trend of decline in disability across all segments of the population. Many older adults experience hospitalizations, nursing home admissions, and low-quality care, and may lose the ability to live independently at home. Chronic conditions are the leading cause of death and disability among older adults. Because of these concerns, HP 2020 added a new topic area, Older Adults.[4]

■ HEALTHY PEOPLE 2020
Older Adults

Healthy People Topics Relevant to Health Planning for Older Adults

Targeted Topic(s): Older adults
Goal: Improve the health, function, and quality of life of older adults.
Overview: Older adults are among the fastest growing age groups, and the first baby boomers (adults born between 1946 and 1964) will turn 65 in 2011. More than 37 million people in this group (60%) will manage more than one chronic condition by 2030.
Source: See HP 2020 for background, objectives, interventions, and resources.[4]

Why Is the Health of Older Adults Important? According to HP 2020, more than 60% of older adults manage more than one chronic condition. To address this growing burden on our health-care system, population-level approaches are needed to reduce the morbidity and mortality associated with chronic diseases (see Chapter 9) and improve the health-related quality of life experienced by older adults. HP 2020 supports population approaches that will increase prevention initiatives while improving access to services. Emerging issues for improving the health of older adults include efforts to:[4]

- Coordinate care
- Help older adults manage their own care
- Establish quality measures
- Identify minimum levels of training for people who care for older adults
- Research and analyze appropriate training to equip providers with the tools they need to meet the needs of older adults[4]

Culture: The Changing Diversity in the Older Adult Population

Another changing demographic for older adults in the United States is the changing ethnicity of this population. Although those over 64 are less ethnically and racially diverse compared with younger groups, this is projected to dramatically change over the next four decades. The number of white older adults is projected to decrease by 10% and all other ethnic/racial groups will increase, with 42% of older adults being members of a minority population by 2050. The number of persons 65 years of age or older that are of Hispanic origin will nearly double from 37.4 million in 2010 to 71 million in 2050.[19,20] The increasing ethnic diversity of the older adult population has implications for the development of culturally relevant interventions that take into account the diverse cultural heritage of the population. Thus, conducting a cultural assessment and maintaining cultural competency is an essential skill for nurses working with older adult populations (see Chapter 23).

Determinants of Aging and Health

To begin to think about the public health implications of an aging population, it is important to understand what it means to age. **Aging** is the process of becoming chronologically and biologically older. This process is determined by genetics and modulated by the environment. It can also be viewed from a perspective that moves beyond the physiology of aging. As noted by the WHO, aging is a concept that encompasses more than counting years or the physiological and psychosocial features that change over time.[5] It is often defined as a feeling or a state of mind or as a product of what an individual is able to do, in other words, a functional definition of aging. Simply viewing aging in terms of the number of years lived or specific age-associated signs limits a true definition of an older adult, for individuals of a given age may exhibit widely varied characteristics. Older adults are a diverse group of people moving across the life course with many heterogeneous and unique features. Indeed, there are more and more differences among individuals as they grow older. Important indicators of age are physical health, psychological well-being, socioeconomic factors, functional abilities, and social relations. Goals of nursing care are to modify physiological and cognitive changes and help people stay healthy, functional, and independent longer.

Theories of Aging

The processes of aging have long intrigued scientists and philosophers. However, finding an explanation for the many complex changes associated with aging, both predictable and random, has presented a formidable challenge. Many ideas have been proposed and tested, but the only certainty is that no single theory can explain everything about the process of aging. Theories encompass biological, immunological, psychological, and developmental realms. Even these widely ranging ideas about aging have some key features in common.

One theoretical approach to aging is that signs of aging emerge when demands exceed resources, that is, the person no longer independently has the resources needed to meet the demands of everyday life. Some of the biological theories provide examples of this imbalance. Another theory is that aging occurs when there is a loss of effectiveness in maintaining equilibrium at the biological level, such as what occurs in heart failure. Other theories are based on the loss of the ability to adapt to change, which becomes more pronounced with the advance of time.[21]

Biological Theories of Aging

The biological theories of aging regard the body as a collection of cells and materials that are subject to mechanical or architectural failure as they grow older. Biological failure with aging may result from genes, such as when harmful genes "turn on" and become active in later life, or when some older adults exhibit youthful vigor and well-being in older adulthood, which seems to run in their families. It is also thought that some genes actually promote functional decline and structural deterioration, thereby producing the outward and organic signs of aging. In genetic studies of worms, scientists have been able to isolate the specific gene that controls longevity, and by manipulating that gene, can cause the worms to live a greatly extended life span.[21] The excitement that accompanied the mapping of the human genome was coupled with the hope that by decoding genetic material, we would be able to understand, and ultimately influence health and longevity. However, many more questions have developed from our knowledge thus far, including the mysterious forces that cause a gene to turn on or turn off.

Another theoretical viewpoint of aging suggests that aging occurs as a result of the accumulation of errors in protein synthesis over time, leading to impaired cell function. In aging, it is thought that successive generations of faulty cells eventually lead to impaired biological function. However, despite evidence of declines in cell replication, amino acid sequencing does not change with age, and there is no evidence that RNA becomes defective with age. Once again, this biological theory cannot fully explain the dynamics and differences of aging organisms.[21]

Another theory is that aging is related to mutations that occur when cells are exposed to environmental factors, such as radiation or chemicals, causing the DNA to be damaged and altered. Thus, genetics are modulated by the environment. This is based on the observation that accumulations of mutations are time-dependent, and it is possible that faulty cells from youth are replicated and harbored, increasing in numbers with age. This is one explanation for the deleterious effects that can show up later in life.[21]

The *free-radical* theory is another major idea in the biological realm, stemming from the observation that older adults are more prone to the damaging effects of free radicals and have lower levels of protectant free-radical scavengers, such as vitamin A, vitamin C, and niacin. Free-radical damage to cells and organs occurs as a result of oxidative stress, and is thought to have cumulative effects. There are both internal and external sources for oxidative stress, as free radicals are a by-product of oxygen metabolism. Some research into the effects of free-radical damage has uncovered the accumulation of harmful pigmented proteins called *lipofuscins* that are associated with aging. The key idea is that cells are repeatedly aggravated by harmful stressors that may be metabolic by-products, and in aging the DNA cannot keep up with needed repairs, resulting in a decline in function and numbers of cells. Serious problems occur when nonreplaceable cells are damaged, such as muscle, heart, nerve, and brain.[22]

Another major biological theory of aging is the *cross linkage* or *connective tissue* theory, which describes the chemical reactions that create strong bonds between molecular structures that are normally separate, particularly in collagen, elastin, and ground substance. Increased numbers of cross-links in collagen yield stiffness and loss of resilience. In elastin, cross-links affect movement and elasticity. Evidence of these processes might be seen in stiffening of blood vessels or skin changes associated with aging. One of the reasons that caloric restriction and steroids have been associated with the slowing of the aging process may have to do with the formation of fewer cross-linkages on a molecular level.[23]

Some of the physiologically based theories of aging describe relatively random events, but there are also some key ideas about programmed aging, or a biological or genetic clock that determines how an individual's original pool of genetic material is played out in an orderly manner. Examples of this can be seen in human development, maturation, and the expected cessation of certain body functions, for example, menopause, graying of hair, or thymus atrophy. The programmed aging theory is based on the concept that cells double a limited number of times before they die, or that there is an expected life span for every cell.

Psychosocial Theories of Aging

Psychosocial theories of aging revolve around three major and somewhat conflicting ideas: disengagement, activity, and continuity. Early theorists offered the observation that older adults tend to disengage from pursuits and roles that they enjoyed in earlier life, and suggested that this process was a mutual withdrawal of the individual from society. In a classic article, Cumming[24] proposed that this process of disengagement was accepted and actually desired by older adults, and that it was a natural and universal feature of a long life. From their perspective, disengagement was the "correct" way to age.

However, a clearly opposing theory was at work. Older adults who resisted withdrawal and remained active and engaged in life were observed to age more optimally. In fact, the more active they were, the greater satisfaction they expressed with the quality of their lives. They were more likely to be able to substitute new roles for those lost through changing function or social circumstances. Many community-based programs for older adults are based on the activity theory, and offer many activities that help older adults to keep busy and socially engaged. For many older adults, activity is a vital coping strategy, as they face inevitable losses and changes in their lives.

Perhaps strongest of all is the theory that people are basically consistent throughout their lives, and their personalities remain constant through the passing years. This is described as continuity,[25] and can be an important consideration for nurses as we assist individuals in managing health issues or dealing with new challenges associated with aging. We can help older adults use their past experiences to frame new situations, and work from the strengths within their perspectives and personalities.

Key Aging Research

Despite the fact that we live in a rapidly aging society, the truth is that many people have a limited understanding of what it means to grow older. Some people may have misconceptions about the natural processes of aging, and may view the world of aging according to their own experiences and even prejudices. Some may lack understanding of the trials and triumphs that older adults experience in their everyday lives. It is imperative that nurses are open in their views of aging. Older adults are not "the other;" they are a preview for those who are younger, moving along life's continuum ahead of them.

Formal study of the aging process has developed over the past several decades. With a growing population of aging adults, the National Institutes of Health established the National Institute of Aging specifically to conduct research about the processes of aging. Research projects range from examinations of minute molecular, genetic, and biochemical mechanisms, all the way to entire populations, and every aspect in between. Exciting discoveries and insights that are revealed today will inform nursing practice as nurses care for older adults in our society. In the following sections, three major longitudinal studies are discussed that have shaped our understanding of the processes and challenges of aging, have helped to define the determinants of health in aging, and help to identify health priorities for an aging population.

Baltimore Longitudinal Study of Aging

The Baltimore Longitudinal Study of Aging (BLSA) began in 1958, and is the longest running scientific study of human aging.[26] It is an excellent example of a longitudinal cohort study (see Chapter 3). The focus of this study is to discover what happens as people age, and to distinguish changes that are due to natural aging from those that are due to diseases or other causes. More than 1,400 individuals have been followed from age 20 to 90 and older. Over the course of the study, important aspects of the aging process and determinants of health have been uncovered, including:

- Normal age-related circulatory system changes and the development of cardiovascular disease
- Impact of lifestyle choices on the development of disease
- Brain and memory changes that predict declines
- Stability of personality in older years, coping strategies, and perceived happiness
- Organic changes, such as prostate enlargement and diagnostic parameters for disease
- Sensory changes, such as alterations in hearing and taste
- Metabolism and nutrition in aging, including body composition, predictors for the development of diabetes, and age-related changes in renal function

A fundamental aim of the BLSA is to differentiate which changes are a normal part of aging and which are the result of disease processes. The study has been able to demonstrate that slower reaction speed and some changes in short-term memory are associated with aging in the absence of disease. However, sudden losses, such as those that accompany heart attacks or strokes, are clearly the result of disease, but can be worsened by the changes that occur naturally with aging. The good news is that lifestyle decisions can affect the occurrence or progression of age-associated disease.

New England Centenarian Study

One fascinating way to look at aging is through the extremes of longevity, for example, by examining the features of very long-lived individuals, or the super centenarians. The oldest documented living person was Jeanne Calment of Arles, France, who attained the age of 122 years. Her extremely long life span was carefully studied, as it pushed the boundaries of what we thought could be possible in human survival and suggested some traits and behaviors that might contribute to longevity.[27] For example, Madame Calment remained physically active through most of her life. She kept a lean weight. But contrary to the accepted wisdom about healthy behaviors, she smoked cigarettes from the age of 21 until the age of 117. She ascribed her longevity and relatively youthful appearance to olive oil, wine, and chocolate.

Serious research about the features and commonalities of people who live to 100+ years is reflected in the ongoing New England Centenarian Study. Scientists have observed that individuals who age well into the extremes of the life span have a marked delay in the development of age-associated disability. Among the study subjects, about 15% have no significant disease at age 100, and these people are characterized as "escapers." About 43% of the group has age-related disease that did not show up until around age 80, and these are called the "delayers." The remaining people can be described as "survivors," as they have clinically demonstrable disease prior to age 80, but they manage to survive and continue to live even with these diseases.[28] Basically, longevity trends support a hypothesis of compression of morbidity, wherein older adults experience more years of health prior to the development of disease. Researchers suggest that in aging, as stated by Hilt, Young-Xu Silver, and Perls, ". . . the older you get, the healthier you've been."[28–30]

Normative Aging Study

The Normative Aging Study began in 1963 and has followed male veterans longitudinally to evaluate changes in their physical health, health-related behaviors such as smoking and dietary intake, and other factors that may influence health.[31] For example, during certain years of the study, measurements were collected of lead and cadmium content in participants' bodies. Neurocognitive tests have been tracked, along with tests of motor function, memory, and learning. Other psychosocial variables that can have a strong effect on aging and health include depression, negative life events, optimism, and perceived stress. This study also has a large bank of DNA samples to look at genes associated with the development of Alzheimer's disease.[31] With such a wide range of variables collected over a long period of time, investigators may be able to identify specific relationships among genetic, environmental, physiological, and psychosocial variables.

These ongoing studies and many others continue to reveal important information about the normal processes of aging and to identify important roles for nurses in the community to promote health, reduce risk factors for disease, and support and enhance optimal management of chronic conditions associated with aging.

Program Planning and Successful Aging

As demonstrated in the major aging research studies, longevity and health are influenced by complex interactions among biological, psychological, and sociological factors. Past research about aging has often emphasized the extent to which health problems, such as diabetes or osteoporosis, could be attributed exclusively to age. Such research tended to exaggerate the homogeneity of older adults. However, researchers are now reporting some important elements that contribute to healthy aging overall, and have helped to identify preventive health-care goals for older adults and 10 keys to healthy aging (Box 20-2).[32]

Changing demographic trends related to an aging population have driven many changes in health care, requiring specialized knowledge and application of **gerontology** (the study of the effects of time on human development or the study of the aging process) and **geriatrics** (specialized medical care of older adults). Nursing has been a leader in the field of gerontology, as it was the

first profession to offer advanced certification, in recognition of the specialized skills and knowledge required in the care of older adults.[33]

The Rowe and Kahn Model of Successful Aging

While absence of disease is important, it is not the entire story of successful aging. Successful prevention programs include more than the avoidance or management of disease. Rowe and Kahn[34,35] examined the phenomenon of successful aging and compared it with usual aging in the general population. They determined that successful aging contained three key components:

- Low probability of disease or disability
- High cognitive and physical function capacity
- Active engagement with life

The Rowe and Kahn model of successful aging is a highly valuable framework for promoting health and self-management into older years. Besides the avoidance of disease, older adults can learn to optimize the management of chronic disease and continue to age successfully even when they do have health problems. The goal is to promote and protect their well-being and autonomy and to prevent excess disability, while controlling symptoms and disease progression. This entails health education, screening and prevention activities, and specific management strategies to optimize function, independence, and quality of life.

For example, an older woman with osteoporosis and hypertension can follow a plan that includes medications, regular exercise, and nutrition, which allows her to maintain the activities that she enjoys. Another example of optimizing management of a problem is an older adult who needs to give up driving because of a vision problem. He can work with family and community to find alternative transportation resources to allow him to continue to get out as safely and independently as possible, supporting his social engagement.

The first consideration in promoting successful aging is the importance of enhancing and encouraging healthy life choices at all ages. Nurses may be involved in health promotion initiatives at any age that may protect health, reduce risk factors, and lay the groundwork for optimal health in aging. For example, the health programs that are focused on eliminating childhood obesity, promoting physical activity, and stopping smoking may have far-reaching effects on the aging process. This is because healthy weight is associated with less hypertension and healthier glucose metabolism, activity is associated with strength and mobility, and smoking cessation reduces the risk of developing respiratory and cardiovascular

| BOX 20-2 | **Ten Keys to Healthy Aging** |

1. Controlling hypertension
2. Stopping smoking
3. Screening for cancer
4. Keeping current on immunizations
5. Regulating blood glucose
6. Lowering cholesterol
7. Being physically active
8. Preventing bone loss and muscle weakness
9. Maintaining social contact
10. Combating depression

Source: See reference 32.

disease. Thus, healthy and/or unhealthy behaviors practiced during the younger years contribute to the health, function, and well-being of the older adult.

Many of the risk factors for the development of disease and disability in aging can be modified through changes in behavior or changes in environment.[4] Such modifications are a key focus for public health nurses working with older populations, whether in the form of public health education, screening programs, surveillance, exercise, diet, immunization programs, and sanitation, as well as for nurses who provide individualized care. Another priority in nursing care of the older adult is providing care with consideration of factors that are uniquely important to older adults' quality of life. For example, health conditions that affect mobility can have significant consequences in terms of independence and autonomy and can threaten older adults' ways of living. Or, older adults may have specific motivations for managing a health condition, such as being able to participate in a special family event, or to complete a personal goal.

Finally, when we look at risk factors for the development of disease and disability in aging, we recognize that most can be modified through changes in behavior or changes in environment. Such modifications are a key focus of community health nursing, whether in the form of public health education, screening programs, surveillance, exercise, diet, immunization programs, sanitation, or individualized care.

▶ SOLVING THE MYSTERY
The Case of the Lonely Women
Public Health Science Topics Covered:

- Community assessment
  - Face-to-face interviewing
  - Field observations
- Health planning
  - Engaging stakeholders
  - Applying program models
  - Adapting interventions to the population being served

At St. John's parish in a small New England town, the newly hired parish nurse, Barbara, reviewed her recent community assessment of the parish. She had used a comprehensive approach (see Chapter 4) and had lots of information including data on the demographics obtained from the U.S. Census Bureau and other town and state data sources. She had even sent out a health survey to the parishioners and received a decent response. The majority of the parish reported that their

health was good to excellent and that they were most interested in programs that would help them lose weight. However, the mean age of the respondents was 36 and only 5% of the surveys returned were from people over 65 and none from those over 75, yet the parish census showed that 19% of the parish was over the age of 65. This percentage was similar to the census data on the town (18.5%) and higher than the U.S. percentage (12.4%). When she looked at the community data and the parish membership, she discovered that there was a subpopulation of older females in the community and the parish who were living alone. These facts, coupled with the projected increase in this population over the next three decades, concerned Barbara.

Barbara decided to supplement the demographic data with some basic field observations. For the next 2 weeks, she attended every Mass and watched who attended services. During Sundays, the church was full and the demographic mix related to age was encouraging, with many young families as well as older adults. The Sunday announcements were about the parish schoolchildren, the parish picnics, and the fund-raising for the new church. But during weekday Masses, the church was quiet and the attendees were almost always older women who came in alone, sat quietly during Mass, and left alone. She then looked for these same women on Sundays and began to see them as isolated islands in the sea of busy families and chatty parishioners.

Barbara wondered why these women had not returned their surveys and what their needs were. At the next health ministry meeting, she raised this topic. The members of the ministry who had lived in the parish longer than Barbara agreed that there was a population of women in the parish who were living alone and for the most part they were not actively engaged in the parish.

Barbara remembered what she had learned about successful aging in a recent class she had taken and looked up the Rowe and Kahn model of successful aging. At the next meeting of the health ministry, she came armed with the information she had found. She explained the model to the members of the ministry and suggested that they use the model as a guide in the development of a program specifically for these women.

Barbara explained that other additions to the Rowe and Kahn model include the importance of positive spirituality,[33] social support, inner strength or the spirit to age successfully, exercise, and activity.[35–37] She felt that the common themes were minimal disease and disability, and active engagement with life. In the presence of disease, the key to success hinges on the ability of the older adult to manage and cope with disease so that disability is minimized. Barbara thought the parish could sponsor a program that would reach out to the older women in the parish and engage them in parish activities. She thought she could then add to this intervention a chronic disease self-management program (see Chapter 9).

One of the members of the health ministry asked how they could actually go about engaging the women in the parish in a way that would be respectful and draw on what they could contribute to the parish. Barbara thought the best approach would be an intervention that would tie these women to the vibrant family life so apparent in the parish. She proposed a program that would match the women to the children in the parish. She thought the parish could model their program after other adopt-a-grandparent programs.

The health ministry committee liked Barbara's idea and the chair of the committee brought the suggestion to the parish council. The council approved the idea, so the health ministry approached the parish school. The school asked whether the program could be a two-way process. They explained that they had students in need of tutoring, but many of the students' parents worked and it was hard for the parents to help with homework. Could the program expand to include an after-school tutoring program given by older parishioners? They presented Barbara with a number of other ideas, including music lessons and art classes.

Barbara took all the ideas back to her office feeling very pleased with herself and then the thought struck her. She had not asked the women themselves what they thought of the idea. She was amazed that she had missed a key principle in public health, working *with* the community and not *for* the community, which includes all stakeholders in the process (see Chapter 4). Chagrined, she set about talking with the women she had seen at the weekday Masses. The first woman she approached, Eleanor, was surprisingly helpful. Eleanor happily sat down and chatted with Barbara and told her all about herself. She said it was so nice to have someone to talk to. She was 76 and had been widowed last year. Her daughter and son lived in other states and visited only occasionally. She was doing okay except for arthritis, but she was lonely. She

found the church a comfort; however, as soon as Mass was over, she went right home. She loved watching all the young families on Sundays. Her joy was music, but she could no longer play the piano. Would she be interested in helping out at the school? Well, she wasn't sure. She had never worked and didn't know what she could do.

After talking with Eleanor, Barbara spent the next 2 weeks talking with women after Mass, or calling them and visiting them in their homes. She kept a record of what they told her. She found that most of them were happy to talk to her and many talked of being lonely, especially those who had been recently widowed. After interviewing over 30 women, she reported back to the health ministry and the school that the women were interested and would love to be more engaged in the parish activities, but so many of those activities seemed to be for families with children. Some of the women needed transportation but would love to get out. Others hoped that the children would visit them. A few agreed to serve on the health ministry, thus bringing key stakeholders to the planning process.

The health ministry concluded that they could develop a multilayered program that included services the women could provide the schoolchildren, and services the parishioners could provide the women. In addition, Barbara found that some of the women were struggling to manage a chronic disease, such as type 2 diabetes, arthritis, and hypertension. Barbara said her next step was to develop a chronic disease self-management program (see Chapter 9) that incorporated the Rowe and Kahn model of successful aging.

Barbara had successfully applied a number of community assessment approaches to the issue. As presented in Chapters 4 and 5, she built on initial community assessment data and collected primary data through face-to-face interviews and field observations. She engaged key stakeholders in the planning process and adapted existing evidence-based programs such as the "adopt a grandparent" program used by other agencies and a chronic disease self-management program to the specific needs of their parish (Fig. 20-4). Barbara's program addressed a number of key issues for successful aging with the central component being engagement with others. Over time, both the older women and the children of the parish felt an increase in their self-worth as they actively engaged in helping one another. It wasn't long before the older men in the parish also wanted to get involved.

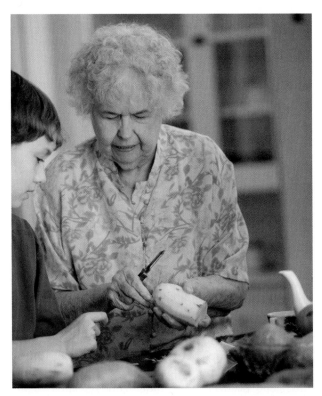

Figure 20-4 The Adopt-a-Grandparent program. *(From the Centers for Disease Control and Prevention, Dawn Arlotta; Cade Martin, photographer, 2009.)*

Aging, Health, Disability, and Disease

As we age, our risk for development of disease and disability increases. Aging decreases the ability to ward off communicable diseases and increases the likelihood of developing a noncommunicable disease. For example, as we age, our risk increases for diabetes mellitus, arthritis, heart failure, and dementia.[4] Prior to World War II, this was accepted as part of the aging process, and there was little focus on prevention. Today, there is clear evidence that healthy behaviors across the life span, beginning in utero, increase the chances of a longer life with reduced disease and disability. Because of this, the older adult was added to the *Healthy People* topics in 2020.[4] From 2000 to 2011, heart disease was the leading cause of death for those 65 years of age or older, accounting for a little under a third of all deaths in this age group.[38]

Communicable Disease

Older adults are more vulnerable to acquiring a communicable disease and at greater risk for morbidity and mortality related to communicable diseases. (See Chapter 8 for more information on communicable diseases.) There

are three main reasons for increased vulnerability to communicable diseases in the older adult:

- Decreased immunity
- Existence of comorbid illness
- Undernutrition

All of these reasons are host specific. Decreased immunity occurs as a result of the aging process and poor antibody production. Another issue for decreased immunity is alteration in the skin integrity because of drying and thinning of the epidural layer. The existence of comorbid conditions actually has a greater impact on the immune function than does aging, leading to more complex infections and reduced ability of the body to recover from infection. Finally, undernutrition has an impact on the body's defense system. Undernutrition in the older adult occurs for various reasons, including psychosocial issues and medication side effects.

The main communicable diseases of concern in the older adult are influenza, pneumonia, shingles with influenza symptoms, and tuberculosis. For 2000 to 2010 influenza with pneumonia was the sixth leading cause of death in adults 65 years or older and the fifth leading cause of death for those 85 years of age or older. Pneumonia and influenza infection occurs due to exposure to the pathogen.[39] On the other hand, shingles occurs from the reactivation of the varicella zoster virus years after initial exposure to the virus that resulted in chickenpox. Any adults who have had chickenpox are at risk for shingles, because the virus remains in a dormant state in the body following a case of chickenpox. Seventy percent of all cases occur in persons over the age of 50 and over 50% of those age 80 or older will get shingles.[40] Mycobacterium tuberculosis (TB) can occur in older people from both routes, either through exposure to a person with an active TB infection or due to reactivation of the mycobacterium related to an earlier exposure. In addition to increased susceptibility, older adults living in group living facilities such as long-term care facilities are at increased risk for exposure.

Emerging Communicable Disease Issues in Older Adults

There are three emerging issues for the baby boomer generation and older adults related to communicable diseases. These are the increase in human immunodeficiency virus (HIV), sexually transmitted infections (STIs), and the increased prevalence of chronic hepatitis C in those over the age of 50.[41–43] These two issues will take on increased importance as more of the baby boomer generation passes the 65-year milestone.

The increase in the number of older adults diagnosed with an STI is attributed to two issues: changes in sexual activity in this population and the increased vulnerability to exposure to the pathogens. In today's society, there is a higher rate of divorce and an increase in partner changes among older adults. In addition, older adults are less apt to use condoms based on decreased perception of risk.[42] There is concern that health-care providers are not adequately screening for STIs in this population.[41] Although the reported increased prevalence in HIV among older adults includes those 50 or older, as this population ages, there is a predicted increased prevalence of HIV. In addition to the increase in at-risk sexual activity among the older adult population, the other issue is that patients with HIV infection are living longer.

In 2012, the Centers for Disease Control and Prevention (CDC) released recommendations for screening for chronic hepatitis C in those born between 1945 and 1965. Over the next two decades, this population will meet the current definition of older adult. Currently, three-quarters of all persons diagnosed with chronic hepatitis C are over the age of 50.[43] The CDC used epidemiological data to develop their recommendations for this targeted cohort. They considered the weighted, unadjusted anti-HCV prevalence, the size of the population, and the differences in prevalence among racial/ethnic groups.[43] Based on their extended analysis of the data, the CDC made the following recommendations:

In addition to testing adults of all ages at risk for HCV infection, CDC recommends that:

- Adults born during 1945–1965 should receive one-time testing for HCV without prior ascertainment of HCV risk (Strong Recommendation, Moderate Quality of Evidence), and

- All persons identified with HCV infection should receive a brief alcohol screening and intervention as clinically indicated, followed by referral to appropriate care and treatment services for HCV infection and related conditions (Strong Recommendation, Moderate Quality of Evidence).[43]

Prevention of Communicable Diseases in Older Adults

Based on the epidemiology triangle (see Chapter 3), public health interventions for preventing communicable diseases in older adults for the most part focus on primary prevention through vaccination aimed at improving the ability of the host to resist infection. This includes vaccination for prevention of pneumonia, influenza, and shingles. For that reason, there are specific recommendations for vaccination in the older adult population to prevent these infections (Table 20-1).[44]

An example of this primary prevention focus is the public health campaign to have all adults over the age of 64 vaccinated for influenza. This campaign is aimed at reducing the burden of disease related to influenza. Annually, there are approximately 90,000 hospitalizations and 5,000 deaths among older adults related to influenza.[45] One concern is that, although over the past few decades the influenza vaccine rate increased from 15% to 65%, there was no significant decrease in the death rate. To address this, new flu vaccines for older adults are now available with increased immunogenicity (the ability of a substance to provoke an immune response needed for the vaccine to be effective).[45]

Population-level initiatives aimed at reducing communicable disease in the older adult population require a broad perspective. If vaccines alone are not effective in reducing morbidity and mortality, then other strategies to improve an older adult's resistance to disease are

TABLE 20–1	Vaccine Recommendations for Older Adults	
Vaccine	Age	Dose and Schedule
Trivalent inactivated influenza vaccine (TIV) IM	65 yr and older	Give standard-dose TIV every year in fall or winter.
Pneumococcal polysaccharide vaccine (PPSV) Give IM or SC	65 yr and older	Give one dose if unvaccinated or if previous vaccination history is unknown Give a one-time revaccination to people Age 65 yr and older if 1st dose was given prior to age 65 yr and 5 yr have elapsed since dose #1.
Herpes zoster (shingles) (Zos) Give SC	60 yr and older	Give one-time dose if unvaccinated, regardless of previous history of herpes zoster (shingles) or chickenpox.

Source: See reference 44.

also needed. As noted above, the older adult is at increased risk for communicable diseases because of his or her increased vulnerability. Efforts aimed at decreasing vulnerability include better self-management of noncommunicable disease (NCD) improved nutrition, and physical exercise.

For communicable diseases such as influenza, pneumonia, and shingles, the rapid progression from infection to disease requires a primary prevention focus. For other communicable diseases, a secondary prevention approach should also be implemented. For example, the new recommendation to screen all those born between 1945 and 1965 for hepatitis C underlines the importance of identifying subclinical cases of a chronic infection so that treatment can begin, thus reducing the morbidity and mortality associated with hepatitis C, especially liver disease. Increasing screening for STIs could also result in earlier identification of these communicable diseases, earlier initiation of treatment, and subsequent reduction in morbidity and mortality.

Noncommunicable Diseases (NCD)

The risk for developing a NCD increases over the life span owing to genetics, the physiology of aging, health behaviors, and the environment. The majority of older adults with NCDs have more than one.[46] Thus, a single disease approach to care of the older adult may not work. Instead, the challenge is to develop programs for older adults that address a combination of NCDs. Risk factors associated with cardiovascular disease, the leading cause of death in older adults, include obesity and hypertension. These risk factors also increase the risk for diabetes and other NCDs. The prevalence of these risk factors increases with age. Over a quarter of the older adult population is obese and the prevalence of hypertension ranges from 64% to over 81% (Table 20-2).[38]

In addition to vaccination, primary prevention models focus on reduction of behavioral risk factors associated with obesity and hypertension. These include improving nutrition, increasing physical activity, and social support.

TABLE 20-2	Health Risk Factors for Older Adults—2010	
	Obese	Hypertension
Men 65–74	41.5%	64.1%
Men 75+	26.6%	71.1%
Women 65–74	40.3%	69.3%
Women 75+	28.7%	81.3%

Source: See reference 38.

HP 2020 has a link to community approaches for addressing these issues with older adults.[4] Secondary prevention approaches for older adults focus on screening and early intervention. Ten of the areas listed by the CDC under prevention indicators and recommended interventions include screening (Box 20-3).[47] (For more information on screening for NCDs, see Chapter 9.)

Evidence-based tertiary prevention programs include those aimed at self-management of NCDs. *Healthy People 2020* has a link to community preventions aimed at the self-management of diabetes.[4] According to the chronic disease self-management model discussed in Chapter 9, the basic elements of self-management include the ability to communicate with a health-care provider, proper use of medications, nutrition, regular exercise, and disease-specific activities such as foot care for those with diabetes. Management of NCDs can become a challenge for the older adult. Older adults may be home-bound and/or no longer able to drive, resulting in difficulty getting to their health-care provider or obtaining resources. If they have more than one NCD, such as heart failure and diabetes, they may need to access two separate providers that are not located in the same practice. Grocery stores are increasingly located in areas that require access by car. Regular exercise may be difficult for the city dwelling older adult because of an unsafe

BOX 20-3	Centers for Disease Control and Prevention: Clinical Prevention Services for Older Adults

Eight indicators that provide a baseline of data through which to monitor progress in ensuring that recommended services reach this key population:

1. Vaccinations that protect against influenza
2. Vaccinations that protect against pneumococcal disease
3. Screening for early detection of breast cancer
4. Screening for colorectal cancer
5. Screening for diabetes
6. Screening for lipid disorders
7. Screening for osteoporosis
8. Counseling service for smoking cessation
   Recommended services for older adults:
1. Alcohol misuse screening and counseling
2. Aspirin use
3. Blood pressure screening
4. Cervical cancer screening
5. Depression screening
6. Obesity screening and counseling
7. Zoster vaccination

Source: See reference 47.

environment. The lack of safety can include lack of sidewalks and/or street crime and some neighborhoods that are unsafe for regular exercise.

▶ SOLVING THE MYSTERY
The Case of the Failing Hearts
Public Health Science Topics Covered:

- Focused assessment
  - Chart review
  - Geographic information systems
- Health planning
  - Adapting interventions to the population being served

Cathy worked as a nurse at the heart failure clinic for a few months and was becoming increasingly frustrated with the patients at the clinic who also had type 2 diabetes. She had spent time doing health education with them and had even developed a pamphlet on managing your diabetes, to no avail. They were missing their appointments at the diabetes clinic and continued to have elevated blood sugars. She explained to them that tight glucose control was essential to the management of their heart failure, but week after week these patients were not following through with what she had mapped out for them.

In desperation she contacted her friend Adele, a family nurse practitioner who specialized in diabetes and also had completed a public health nursing master's program. Adele came to the clinic and asked her to explain the problem. After listening to Cathy, Adele suggested that they do a focused assessment of the patients who were not following through with their diabetes care. Adele explained the importance of doing assessments prior to implementing an intervention. Together they conducted a chart review of the patients that Cathy identified as having difficulty. Most of them were over the age of 60 and all of them had limited transportation options. They plotted the addresses of these patients on a city map. They then located the heart failure clinic on the map as well as the diabetes clinic. These two clinics were located a number of miles apart. The heart failure clinic was close to a bus route, but the diabetes clinic was a few blocks from the nearest bus stop. By tracing the travel routes they found that the effort needed to make two appointments in the same week for the majority of the patients was a main barrier for Cathy's patients.

Together Cathy and Adele developed a one-stop approach for the patients at the heart failure clinic who also had diabetes. Adele arranged to be present at the heart failure clinic one day a week and Cathy scheduled the patients with type 2 diabetes for that day. Adele developed a special diabetes self-management program for these patients who, for the most part, were over 65 years of age and had decreased access to transportation. This program included aspects of case management (see Chapter 9). With her knowledge of the resources in the community, Adele was able to assist these patients in various aspects of diabetes management. For example, for some of the patients she contacted Meals on Wheels to deliver meals that fit within the patients' dietary restrictions.

These two nurses used basic public health skills to identify an older population at risk for increase morbidity and mortality including assessment and health planning. Their intervention reduced the number of clinic visits these patients needed to make and, over time, Cathy and Adele saw an improvement in the majority of these patients. They also were able to demonstrate a decrease in hospitalizations. Their decision to not take a one-disease approach but rather incorporate two specialties had positive results.

Injury and Violence in the Older Adult

Injury and violence are issues for the older adult and include both unintentional and international injury (Box 20-4). Consistently unintentional injury ranks as the ninth leading cause of death in older adults.[48] Unintentional injuries that pose the greatest threat include falls, motor vehicle crashes, and residential fire. Intentional injuries include elder maltreatment and suicide. Reducing injury in older adults is a national public health priority as evidenced by the CDC National Resource Center for Safe Aging, the National Center for Injury Prevention and Control, and others. These

BOX 20-4	Injury and Violence That Pose the Greatest Threat to Older Adults in the United States

- Falls
- Older adult drivers
- Elder abuse and maltreatment
- Residential fire
- Sexual abuse
- Suicide

Source: See reference 48.

resources focus not only on reducing the morbidity and mortality related to injury in the older adult, but also on helping older adults maintain an independent lifestyle.

Unintentional Injury

Falls are the most common form of unintentional injury in the older adults. One in every three adults over the age of 65 falls every year.[49] Falls are one of the leading causes of injury and death in the population. The risk factors associated with falls in the older adult are well understood and help in the design of prevention activities. Based on the key risk factors the CDC has dedicated a whole Web site to the prevention of falls. Risk factors include muscle weakness, unsteady gait, osteoporosis, failing eyesight, and hypotension. Many of these risk factors are associated with NCDs. Other risk factors are associated with the home environment and the community environment. Within the home are issues such as scatter rugs, lack of grab bars in the bathroom, and other hazards that contribute to falls. In the community, sidewalk safety, well lit streets, and other factors are key to prevention of falls. Prevention strategies are aimed at these risk factors and can be applied at the individual, group, or community level.[49]

■ EVIDENCE-BASED PRACTICE
Fall Prevention With Older Adults

Practice Statement: Improve the gait and balance of older adults through a regular exercise program.
Targeted Outcome: Decrease the number of falls.
Evidence to Support: According to the CDC, there are interventions that can reduce falls and help older adults live better and longer.[49] Based on evidence, exercise is one of the possible approaches because it appears to have statistically significant beneficial effects on balance ability in the short term. However, there is less evidence to support long-term balance because many of the studies they reviewed were small studies and often had methodological weaknesses. They recommend further research to help standardize the timing of outcome assessments and more long-term follow-up of outcomes.
Recommended Approaches: The CDC has two downloadable guides that provide in-depth review of population-level strategies:

• Preventing Falls: What Works; A CDC Compendium of Effective Community-based Interventions From Around the World
• Preventing Falls: How to Develop Community-based Fall Prevention Programs for Older Adults

Sources: See references 50 and 51.

Intentional Injury: Elder Maltreatment

Intentional injury is also a concern with the older adult population. Older adults are often victims of abuse and neglect that can result in serious injury and/or debilitation. An estimated 2.1 million older Americans are victims of physical, psychological, or other forms of maltreatment. The actual incidence of elder maltreatment is likely to be underestimated. It is thought that for every case of maltreatment that is reported to the authorities, as many as 5 cases have not been reported. While there is rightful concern about the direct effects of abuse or neglect, there are also health-related consequences that place victims at high risk. Elder maltreatment and self-neglect are associated with shorter survival after adjusting for other factors associated with increased mortality in older adults.[52,53] Various terms are used in the literature including elder abuse, elder mistreatment, and elder maltreatment. For this chapter the term *elder maltreatment* is used and refers to both abuse and neglect.

The CDC has compiled a comprehensive definition of elder maltreatment:

> *Elder maltreatment is any abuse and neglect of persons aged 60 and older by a caregiver or another person in a relationship involving an expectation of trust. Forms of elder maltreatment include:*
>
> • *Physical abuse occurs when an elder is injured (e.g., scratched, bitten, slapped, pushed, hit, burned, etc.), assaulted or threatened with a weapon (e.g., knife, gun, or other object), or inappropriately restrained.*
> • *Sexual abuse or abusive sexual contact is any sexual contact against an elder's will. This includes acts in which the elder is unable to understand the act or is unable to communicate. Abusive sexual contact is defined as intentional touching (either directly or through the clothing), of the genitalia, anus, groin, breast, mouth, inner thigh, or buttocks.*
> • *Psychological or emotional abuse occurs when an elder experiences trauma after exposure to threatening acts or coercive tactics. Examples include humiliation or embarrassment; controlling behavior (e.g., prohibiting or limiting access to transportation, telephone, money or other resources); social isolation; disregarding or trivializing needs; or damaging or destroying property.*
> • *Neglect is the failure or refusal of a caregiver or other responsible person to provide for an elder's basic physical, emotional, or social needs, or failure to protect them from harm. Examples include not providing adequate nutrition, hygiene, clothing, shelter, or access to necessary health care; or failure to prevent exposure to unsafe activities and environments.*

- **Abandonment** *is the willful desertion of an elderly person by caregiver or other responsible person.*
- **Financial abuse or exploitation** *is the unauthorized or improper use of the resources of an elder for monetary or personal benefit, profit, or gain. Examples include forgery, misuse or theft of money or possessions; use of coercion or deception to surrender finances or property; or improper use of guardianship or power of attorney.*[54]

Risk Factors for Elder Maltreatment

Elder maltreatment is a complex problem that affects over 500,000 older adults each year in the United States.[55] There is no single pattern of elder maltreatment. Elder maltreatment is an equal opportunity issue that crosses all walks of life and social strata. Victims are not just infirm or mentally impaired people who are vulnerable to abuse. Elder maltreatment can occur in situations such as the case of Mickey Rooney, a movie actor who testified before Congress in 2011 that he was the victim of maltreatment from his son.

A combination of individual-, relationship-, community-, and social-level factors are associated with increased risk for elder maltreatment (Box 20-5).[56,57] Individual-level risk factors include both the perpetrator and the victim. The interaction of these individual risk factors occurs at the relationship level. However, both community and societal factors also influence risk. On the flip side, there are protective factors as well (see Box 20-5).[56] These protective factors provide areas that nurses can work to strengthen not only with individuals and their families but in combination with the community.

BOX 20-5	Centers for Disease Control and Prevention: Elder Maltreatment—Risk and Protective Factors

A combination of individual, relational, community, and societal factors contribute to the risk of becoming a perpetrator of elder maltreatment. They are contributing factors and may or may not be direct causes. Understanding these factors can help identify various opportunities for prevention.

Risk Factors for Perpetration

- Individual Level
  - Current diagnosis of mental illness
  - Current abuse of alcohol
  - High levels of hostility
  - Poor or inadequate preparation or training for caregiving responsibilities
  - Assumption of caregiving responsibilities at an early age
  - Inadequate coping skills
  - Exposure to maltreatment as a child
- Relationship Level
  - High financial and emotional dependence upon a vulnerable elder
  - Past experience of disruptive behavior
  - Lack of social support
  - Lack of formal support
- Community Level
  - Formal services, such as respite care for those providing care to elders, are limited, inaccessible, or unavailable
- Societal Level
  - A culture where:
  - There is high tolerance and acceptance of aggressive behavior

- Health-care personnel, guardians, and other agents are given greater freedom in routine care provision and decision making
- Family members are expected to care for elders without seeking help from others
- Persons are encouraged to endure suffering or remain silent regarding their pains
- There are negative beliefs about aging and elders.

Protective Factors for Elder Maltreatment

Protective factors reduce risk for perpetrating abuse and neglect. Protective factors have not been studied as extensively or rigorously as risk factors. However, identifying and understanding protective factors are equally as important as researching risk factors. Several potential protective factors are identified below. Research is needed to determine whether these factors do indeed buffer elders from maltreatment.

Relationship Level
- Having numerous, strong relationships with people of varying social status

Community Level
- Coordination of resources and services among community agencies and organizations that serve the older population and their caregivers.
- Higher levels of community cohesion and a strong sense of community or community identity
- Higher levels of community functionality and greater collective efficacy

Source: See reference 56, 57.

Primary, Secondary, and Tertiary Prevention For Elder Maltreatment

It is essential that nurses identify those who may be victims of elder maltreatment and provide evidence-based interventions at the individual and community levels. Perel-Levin argues that prevention efforts should include two levels of intervention: screening as a routine part of primary care and working with the community to provide services. Interventions should seek to decrease the incidence of elder maltreatment, improve early identification, and provide proper management of those who were victims of maltreatment. According to Perel-Levin, interventions should be interdisciplinary and take into account the context of the person. Key components for overcoming barriers to prevention are building trust and effective communication among all persons involved.[58]

A number of screening tools are available, such as the geriatric assessment instrument (GAI).[59] The challenge for the nurse is to build a screening program that includes not only training in the use of the screening tool, but also establishing links with resources for those who screen positive for elder abuse.[60] Another approach at the community level is providing information to both professional health-care providers and members of the community. For example, the Florida Department of Elder Affairs has a Web site dedicated to prevention of elder abuse. Another example is the information and links available through the U.S. Administration on Aging National Center on Elder Abuse (NCEA).[61] Community initiatives to address elder abuse and neglect include programs to:

- Increase public awareness and shift public attitudes toward recognizing and reporting abuse
- Improve identification and triage of cases.[62]
- Increase integrated service models
- Improve justice system response
- Leverage and utilize emerging and untapped resources

Other community-based activities focus on disseminating promising practices in the courts, creating elder law clinics, educating older adults about such things as predatory mortgage lending, building new response systems for complaints of abuse and neglect, and convening clergy and lay leader groups to work within faith communities to make a difference in elder abuse and neglect.[63]

Policy

Policy-level interventions have been undertaken to prevent and address elder maltreatment. The Elder Justice Act of 2010 (Pub. L. 111-148) is part of the Affordable Care Act and provides specific benefits to elders.[64] In addition, at the state level is the Adult Protective Services (APS) that facilitate the protection of vulnerable adults including the older adult. The role of APS is to prevent, correct, or discontinue maltreatment (Box 20-6).[65]

Reporting suspected elder abuse or neglect cases to APS agencies provides access to services that address the social, medical, and legal needs of older persons.[63,64] Once a report is made to APS, a process of investigation and support begins. Based on the information APS receives, caseworkers determine whether there is imminent danger. They make contact with the victim and further evaluate the situation, looking at the risk factors

BOX 20-6 Principles of Adult Protective Services

- **Freedom Over Safety:** The client has a right to choose to live at risk of harm, providing she or he is capable of making that choice, harms no one else, and does not commit a crime.
- **Self-Determination:** The client has a right to personal choices and decisions until a time that she or he delegates, or the court grants, the responsibility to someone else.
- **Participation in Decision Making:** The client has a right to receive information to make informed decisions and to participate in all decision making affecting his or her circumstances to the extent able.
- **Least Restrictive Alternative:** The client has a right to service alternatives that maximize choice and minimize lifestyle disruption.
- **Primacy of the Adult:** The worker has a responsibility to serve the client, not the community's, family members', or landlord's concerns.
- **Confidentiality:** The client has a right to privacy and secrecy.
- **Benefit of Doubt:** If there is evidence that the client is making a reasoned choice, the worker has a responsibility to see that the benefit of doubt is in his or her favor.
- **Do No Harm:** The worker has a responsibility to take no action that places the client at greater risk of harm.
- **Avoidance of Blame:** The worker has a responsibility to understand the origins of any maltreatment and to commit no action that would antagonize the perpetrator and so reduce the chances of terminating the maltreatment.
- **Maintenance of the Family:** The worker has a responsibility to deal with the maltreatment as a family problem, if the perpetrator is a family member, and to try to find the necessary family services to resolve the problem.

Source: See reference 65.

and the victim's capacity to understand. They develop a care plan that may include services provided directly by caseworkers, through arrangements with community-based resources, or contracted by APS on a short-term emergency basis. Victims of abuse may receive short-term services, such as emergency shelter, home repair, meals, transportation, help with financial management, home health services, and medical and mental health services. The APS caseworker may continue to monitor the service provision to make sure that victim risk is reduced or eliminated.[63]

A geriatric interdisciplinary team can be involved to provide a comprehensive medical, functional, and social assessment. Based on the findings from the assessment and in collaboration with the APS team, an individualized intervention plan can be formulated. Some cases of elder abuse or neglect may require intervention from the criminal or civil justice system for serious legal issues such as sexual assault, financial exploitation, or guardianship. Other resources, such as Area Agencies on Aging, local women's shelters, and the National Center for Elder Abuse, are available to help manage elder abuse and neglect cases in the community.[64,66]

Substance Use in Older Adults

Obtaining an accurate picture of substance use in the older population is difficult. Of concern is the baby boomer cohort that has a higher rate of substance use compared with other cohorts. The concern is that as this cohort ages, there will be a substantial increase in the number of older adults with health problems associated with substance use, with the main issue related to alcohol use and an estimated doubling of the prevalence of substance use disorders in those over age 50 by 2020.[67] This increase includes alcohol and licit and illicit drugs. However, we know little about age-specific interventions to promote recovery and reduce morbidity and mortality. Population-level approaches are required to address this issue rather than relying on individual behavior modification. This requires population-level interventions based on a clear picture of the problem (Box 20-7).[68]

For older adults, there are two separate issues related to substance use disorders: early onset and late onset substance misuse, clearly defined in the 1990s.[69] **Early onset at-risk substance use** reflects older adults who have a history of regular alcohol consumption above the recommended limits or problem illicit/licit drug use that began early in their adult lives. This group of older adults is often referred to as hardy survivors. **Late onset at-risk**

BOX 20-7	**Public Policy Recommendations to Prevent Licit and Illicit Substance Use in Older Adults**

Informed and active policy will require new approaches and investment in the following:

- Data and analysis, with increased emphasis on documenting substance abuse in the elderly, in addition to the historical emphasis on alcohol abuse and mental health problems
- Expanded literature review that encompasses studies not considered in this report,* some of which may not be specific to substance abuse but can offer new conceptual and methodological insights
- Prevention, treatment, and management strategies specifically tailored for older adults from different ethnic, gender, and racial groups, including immigrant populations
- Monitoring of demographic shifts in heterogeneous older populations
- Long-term projections of the demand for expanded clinical and public health services for substance abusers
- Traumatic brain injury

*Report by the Substance Abuse and Mental Health Services Administration that addressed the projected demand for substance abuse services over the next 20 to 30 years for those born during the baby boomer years.

Source: See reference 68.

---

substance use is defined as at-risk substance use that began later in life, often triggered by a sentinel event such as widowhood.[69]

Alcohol and Older Adults

Although heavy alcohol use was reported by only 2.1% of those over 65 in 2013,[70] these figures may not be the true picture because of underreporting of alcohol use in this population.[71] As the baby boomer generation continues to turn 65, there may be a cohort effect in relation to prevalence of risky drinking, because more than 60% of baby boomers (aged 45 to 64) are current drinkers. Therefore, the prevalence of alcohol use disorders in the older population may increase over the next few decades.

Alcohol use disorders are not the only issue. As we age, our ability to metabolize alcohol also changes. Alcohol has a more potent effect owing to the physiological changes of aging. There is less body water to dilute the alcohol as a result of a decrease in the ratio of body water to fat as well as a decrease in the hepatic blood flow and a reduction in the efficiency of liver enzymes, resulting in a decreased ability to metabolize alcohol. This, in turn, affects the duration of elevated blood alcohol and increases the risk of liver damage.[72] Another issue for the older adult is medication interaction with alcohol. In one large study, 19% of older adults using medications with potential alcohol interactions reported concomitant alcohol use.[73]

As explained in Chapter 11, the recommended drinking limits are less than five standard drinks per day or 14 per week for men or less than four standard drinks per day or eight per week for women. However, healthy people aged 65 and older should consume no more than three standard drinks per day and no more than seven drinks per week.[74] The older adults who exceed the recommended daily limits are at increased risk for alcohol related problems due to differences in metabolism and physiology. Changes include a decrease in the ratio of body water, to fat leaving less body water to dilute the alcohol. As we age there is also a decrease in the hepatic blood flow resulting in a reduction in the efficiency of liver enzymes. This then reduces the ability of the body to metabolize alcohol. These two changes in turn affect the duration of elevated blood alcohol and an increased risk of liver damage.[69]

Medication Interactions

The issue of adverse interactions between alcohol and prescribed medication is a special concern in older adults, because up to 75% are using medications with potential alcohol interactions[73] and approximately a fifth of these persons reported concomitant alcohol use. Two types of interactions occur: pharmacokinetic interaction, wherein alcohol interferes with the body's ability to metabolize the medications, and pharmacodynamic interaction, wherein alcohol enhances the effects of the medication.[69] The growing recognition of the potential harm related to alcohol and medication interactions in older adults underscores the need for a population perspective. Though both the National Institute on Alcohol Abuse and Alcoholism and the Substance Abuse and Mental Health Services Administration have highlighted the issue, few public health approaches are available for increasing awareness of the problem leaving the burden on the individual practitioner to inform individual adults.

Substance Use and Physical Health

Both licit and illicit drug use increase the risk for adverse health outcomes. Alcohol consumption in older adults increases their risk for injury and increased risk for NCDs and communicable diseases. Alcohol may be the underlying cause for up to half of older trauma patients. Early onset substance users, even those who are currently abstinent but have a history of consuming alcohol or other drugs above the recommended limits for a long period of time, often have serious health problems that may be mistaken for symptoms of aging, such as dementia or depression.[69]

An example of how important it is to evaluate early onset users for physical complications is the negative impact of long-term alcohol use on the ability to absorb thiamine (vitamin B_1), an essential, water soluble vitamin. Untreated thiamine deficiency in older adults with a history of early onset alcohol use may result in Wernicke-Korsakoff syndrome, a brain disorder. However, the prevalence of Wernicke-Korsakoff syndrome at autopsy exceeds recognition during life.[75] Thus, clinicians may fail to screen for long-term alcohol use in this population. Owing to the long-term impact on the human body, alcohol use above the recommended limits increases the risk for other adverse outcomes that occur as the person ages, including alcohol-related cardiomyopathy; liver cirrhosis; pancreatitis; various cancers including cancers of the liver, mouth, throat, larynx (the voice box), and esophagus; high blood pressure; and psychological disorders.[69]

One possible public health intervention might be to initiate a universal screening approach aimed at helping clinicians identify both early and late onset alcohol use that places the older adult at increased risk for alcohol-related NCDs as well as injury. A five-step process was recommended by Savage that includes information not only on current use but also on prior use and duration of use over the lifetime.[76]

Aging in Place

During the past three decades, there has been an increase in the emphasis of an aging-in-place approach that includes implementation of community-based programs that include health promotion, prevention of disease, improvement of functioning, and enhancement of quality of life in older adults while maintaining them in their homes.[77,78] This emphasis mirrors a decline in the percentage of the population 65 years of age or older living in skilled nursing facilities from 5.1% in 1990 to 3.1% in 2010. The decline was also seen in the population 85 years of age or older. In 1990, almost 25% were living in skilled nursing facilities. That dropped to 10.4% in 2010.[79]

Barriers to aging in place include funding for home modifications, delivery of needed services, and consumer awareness.[78] Because of changing health status, some older adults need special services beyond the basics to maintain themselves safely in their own home settings.

Likewise, issues of environmental safety and security can impinge on aging successfully in place. One community-based approach is the Community Aging in Place Advancing Better Living for Elders (CAPABLE) program developed by a team of nurse researchers from Johns Hopkins University School of Nursing. This innovative program combines health-care services with home modifications and links to services within the community to meet the needs of disabled older adults so that they can remain in their homes.[80]

Aging in place requires an understanding of the community in which older adults live.[80] The built environment surrounding the older adult has a direct impact on quality of life. Changing lifestyles in older adults means that they may have more time to enjoy amenities in the community such as recreation facilities. However, biological changes, such as decrease in vision and mobility, alter their ability to enjoy these facilities. To achieve aging in place the CDC states:

> Affordable, accessible and suitable housing options can allow older adults to age in place and remain in their community all their entire lives. Housing that is convenient to community destinations can provide opportunities for physical activity and social interaction. Communities with a safe and secure pedestrian environment, and near destinations such as libraries, stores, and places of worship, allow older adults to remain independent, active, and engaged. Combined transportation and land-use planning that offers convenient, accessible alternatives to driving can help the older adults reach this goal of an active, healthy lifestyle.[81]

The concept of aging in place is growing in popularity. There is now a National Aging in Place Council and the American Association of Retired Persons has a guide to livable communities and a Web page dedicated to the subject. The process includes a match between affordable housing, access to services, and a healthy built environment. Housing options for older adults span a continuum from complete independence to dependence, with many gradations in between. Many people can remain at home completely independently throughout a long life, or with just a little help getting around or keeping house. Care ranges from help with household tasks and running errands to round-the-clock care for someone who is seriously ill.

Naturally Occurring Retirement Community

With the aging of the American population, a new phenomenon is emerging: the **naturally occurring retirement community** (NORC). Federal funding was established in 2010 for NORC with more than $25 million in federal and matching funds that have resulted in the establishment of more than 50 supportive service programs.[82] A NORC is defined by the Administration on Aging as a community that provides:

- Residential housing with supports
- Transportation for appointments and shopping
- Individual assessment of those at risk, followed by referral and follow-up of service
- Coordination of nonprofessional services[82]

NORCs take many different forms. They can exist in subsidized housing complexes, condominiums, apartments, or single-family neighborhoods. Closed or vertical NORCs are geographically confined, such as apartment buildings or complexes. The open or horizontal form of NORC refers to one- and two-family homes in age-integrated neighborhoods. By capitalizing on the valuable contributions of experience and skill from older residents, and making use of the density and proximity of older adults in NORCs, resources and economies of scale (factors that cause the average cost of producing something to decrease as its output increases) make it possible to organize and deliver services that promote healthy aging in place. Instead of service delivery that is reactive to a crisis, is time limited, and is disconnected from the communities in which older residents have built their lives, NORC programs seek to deepen the connections that older adults have to their communities before problems arise.

Continuing Care Retirement Communities

In anticipation of changing needs, some older adults arrange to become part of **continuing care retirement communities** (CCRCs), a relatively new phenomenon in the United States that have appeared during the past three decades. A CCRC is defined as a community that provides housing and health care across the continuum from independent living, to assisted living, to skilled nursing care. Residents are required to sign a contract on entrance into the community. They are charged an entry fee as well as a monthly maintenance fee.[83] The advantage of such communities is the ability for older adults to remain within the CCRC over the long term. The disadvantage is the costliness of such facilities. Entrance into these communities requires the financial ability to pay the entrance fee and the monthly payment. In the 1990s and early 2000s, approximately 10 to 20 units were established per year. After the 2008 recession, there was a sharp decline in the industry, because many older adults could not sell their homes and therefore did not have the money necessary to pay the entrance fee.

All of these models are aimed at keeping the older adult in a community setting and as independent as possible as long as possible. With the aging of the population, the need for viable community-based living for older adults will increase. Nurses such as the researchers at Johns Hopkins School of Nursing are key to helping this population achieve optimal health within their own communities.

Ageism in Our Society

Defined in 1991 by Robert Butler,[85] **ageism** describes bias toward older adults that is based on stereotypes. Butler defined ageism as a combination of three connected elements: prejudicial attitudes toward older people, old age, and the aging process; discriminatory practices against older people; and institutional practices and policies that perpetuate stereotypes about older people. Ageism, like racism and sexism, is a way of judging or categorizing people and not allowing them to be individuals with unique ways of living their lives. It is a set of beliefs, attitudes, norms, and values used to justify age-based prejudice and discrimination.[84] It can actually have an impact on patient outcomes. For example, older adults with cancer who experience ageism have poorer outcomes.[85]

Ageism may occur when health-care providers incorrectly attribute pathology to normal aging. These assumptions can influence screening procedures, information exchanges, and treatment decisions. Ageism may manifest itself through the use of patronizing language, or by dismissing symptoms as "all part of growing older." Even unintentionally, health-care providers may hold attitudes, beliefs, and behaviors that are associated with ageism against older patients. This is why it is so important to have a good working knowledge of age-related physiological and psychological changes, so that signs of disease or disability can be differentiated and treated appropriately.

Dementia and Alzheimer's Disease: Impact on the Older Adult Population

During the past two decades, Alzheimer's disease (AD) has received much attention from the media and is a growing public health issue because of the increase in the older adult population. It accounts for 50% to 70% of all dementia cases. Other dementia diagnoses include vascular dementia, mixed dementia, dementia with Lewy bodies, and frontotemporal dementia. It is estimated that more than 5 million Americans have Alzheimer's

disease.[86] The central issues for those with Alzheimer's are the problems with memory and the impact on cognition. Both Alzheimer's and dementia severely affect people's ability to work, care for themselves, or engage in social activities. AD is the sixth leading cause of death in adults in the United States.[87,88]

Prevention

From a primary prevention perspective, prevention of AD and other types of dementia is challenging, because there is no clear evidence that specific interventions actually prevent AD or cognitive decline.[89] However, secondary prevention through memory screening programs has helped identify those in the early stages. Early identification has the potential to slow the progression of the disease with emerging pharmaceutical treatments for those with AD and dementia. There are currently five drugs approved by the Food and Drug Administration for the treatment of AD (donepezil, galantamine, memantine, rivastigmine, and tacine) that have shown a temporary slowing of the progression of the disease over 6 to 12 months.[90] These treatments also provide the person with AD to plan for the future while still able to do so. Tertiary prevention focuses on active management of AD with the goal of achieving an optimal quality of life within the realities of the disease.[89,90]

Centers for Disease Control and Prevention's Healthy Brain Initiative

Another element in health promotion/prevention is the Healthy Brain Initiative: The Public Health Road Map for State and National Partnerships, 2013–2018, which was jointly developed by the Alzheimer's Association and the CDC Healthy Aging Program to advance cognitive health as a public health goal.[91] See Box 20-8 for details of this program.

Caregiving

One of the primary challenges facing the older population, especially those with AD, dementia, or a chronic NCD, is the need for caregiving when physical and or mental disorders affect the ability to perform the activities of daily living. A **caregiver** is defined as anyone who provides assistance to someone else who is incapacitated in some way and needs help.[92] Informal caregivers or family caregivers are unpaid family members, friends, and neighbors who provide such care. Formal caregivers are volunteers or paid caregivers associated with a service system. It is estimated that there are 34 million unpaid caregivers in the United States who provide 90% of all long-term care. A little over 20% of households are

| BOX 20-8 | **Healthy Brain Initiative: The Public Health Road Map for State and National Partnerships, 2013–2018** |

The role of public health in enhancing the physical health of older adults is well-known. Public health's role in maintaining cognitive health, a vital part of healthy aging and quality of life, is emerging. The need for a clearly delineated public health role comes at a critical time given the dramatic aging of the U.S. population, scientific advancements in knowledge about risk behaviors (e.g., lack of physical activity, uncontrolled high blood pressure) related to cognitive decline, and the growing awareness of the significant health, social, and economic burdens associated with cognitive decline. The Healthy Brain Initiative is a multifaceted approach to cognitive health that includes the following:

- The Healthy Brain Initiative: A National Public Health Road Map to Maintaining Cognitive Health
- Surveillance
- Research
- Policy and Partnerships
- Reports and Resources

The lack of cognitive health—from mild cognitive decline to dementia—can have profound implications for an individual's health and well-being. Older adults and others experiencing cognitive decline may be unable to care for themselves or conduct necessary activities of daily living, such as meal preparation and money management. Limitations with the ability to effectively manage medications and existing medical conditions are particular concerns when an individual is experiencing cognitive decline or dementia. If cognitive decline can be prevented or better treated, lives of many older adults can be improved.

Opportunities for maintaining cognitive health are growing as public health professionals gain a better understanding of cognitive decline risk factors. The public health community should embrace cognitive health as a priority, invest in its promotion, and enhance our ability to move scientific discoveries rapidly into public health practice.

Source: See reference 91.

caring for an older adult[91] and in 2007 $375 billion was spent on caregiving.[93]

There can be significant consequences to caregivers' health. The long hours, physical tasks, stress, and relentless responsibility can take a toll on caregivers, and can show up in health problems such as increased blood pressure, hyperinsulinemia, impaired immune system function, and cardiovascular disease. Health consequences relate to the number of hours spent providing care. Two-thirds do not take advantage of preventive health services for themselves. Twenty-five percent of caregivers have health problems, such as back injuries, resulting directly from caregiving activities. They may also experience mental and emotional effects as a result of their caregiving, which can include depression and isolation.[92,93]

Because of the toll that caregiving exacts from the caregivers, the CDC has declared caregiving a public health priority. To address this priority, the CDC developed the Reach Effectiveness Adoption Implementation Maintenance (RE-AIM) framework.[94] The framework is aimed at helping communities and organizations develop programs for caregivers. The RE-AIM publication provides case examples for interventions aimed at assisting the caregiver. This is an example of how evidence can be translated into practice at the population level to address an important public health issue.

The caregiving relationship can be a very complicated one and often requires engaging the community to help plan interventions. Nurses should recognize the warning signs of caregiver stress early. Nurses can help caregivers look at the sources of stress, identify what they can and cannot change, and identify resources within the community that can relieve the stress, such as respite care for the caregiver. The RE-AIM publication from the CDC provides case studies that can help nurses build programs for caregivers and underlines the importance of working at the population level to help individuals deal with the large task of caring for a loved one.[94]

Hospice and End-of-Life Care

Traditionally, **hospice care** has come under the domain of community health care, because the goal is to provide care to persons at the end of life within the community setting. Many older adults have an ideal picture of the way that they would choose to die, although frank discussions about these wishes and preferences are far too rare, and specific actions that will assure that wishes are respected are sometimes difficult to articulate and communicate. Common descriptions of the preferred circumstances of death include being free of pain and suffering, being in the company of loved ones, and being in one's own home. **Hospice** care was formally developed to address this need. It is usually defined as the provision of care to persons who have less than 6 months to live that reflects the provision of care and comfort rather than cure or treatment.

Originally the term *hospice* was used to describe a place of shelter for weary and sick travelers returning from religious pilgrimages. During the 1960s, Dr. Cicely Saunders began to develop hospice care in the United Kingdom and was invited by the dean of the Yale School of Nursing to become a faculty member and help build hospice care in the United States. There, an organized professional team approach to end-of-life care was established, the first program to formalize the use of modern pain management techniques to care for the dying. The first hospice in the United States was established in New Haven, Connecticut, in 1974, and now there are many thousands of such programs across the country.[95]

Hospice is not a physical place but rather a philosophy of care. Eighty percent of hospice care is provided in the patient's home, a family member's home, and in nursing homes. Specialized inpatient hospice facilities are also available to assist with end-of-life care. If a person has a terminal illness or disease that is no longer responding to treatment, the person is eligible for hospice care. Two physicians must certify that the person has a terminal illness and that if the disease were to run its normal course survival would be 6 months or less.[96] In 2012, between 1.5 and 1.6 million people received hospice care. The majority were 65 years of age or older (83%). Most had a primary diagnosis of cancer (36.9%) and the mean length of stay in hospice care was 71.8 days.[97]

Unique to the hospice philosophy is the recognition that there is potential for growth for the patient and family, even at the end of life, and that there is such a thing as a good death. Hospice programs seek to support living through the dying process, and include family as part of this process. Hospice programs provide state-of-the-art palliative care and supportive services according to unique individual and family needs.

Palliative Care

A key component of hospice is the use of palliative care. At some point in life, it becomes unreasonable to expect cure or reversal of disease processes or to restore a previous level of functioning and independence, and it is clear that life is nearing its end. Death is a natural process, and older adults go through developmental tasks as they approach death, with the goal of life closure. As death approaches, adaptation to a new state allows beings to remain whole: to interact with their environments, to experience human relationships, and to achieve personally meaningful goals.

The WHO defines **palliative care** as "an approach that improves the quality of life of patients and their families facing the problem associated with life-threatening illness, through the prevention and relief of suffering by means of early identification and impeccable assessment and treatment of pain and other problems, physical, psychosocial and spiritual."[98] According to the WHO, palliative care has specific aspects (Box 20-9).

End-of-life nursing care may focus on symptom control and solving functional, physical, or psychological problems to optimize the older adult's quality of life, regardless of the amount of time that remains. Patient/family-centered care is clearly appropriate for the unique experience of dying. Many nursing actions center on supporting physiological function and preventing complications, goals that are still appropriate at the end of life. Appreciating each person as a unique individual is extremely important in assuring optimal care at end of life. While it may be evident to health-care providers that certain goals and interventions would suit the patient's needs, even more important is finding congruence with the patient's own perceived and stated goals and values, and upholding his or her rights to self-determination. For example, the presence and involvement of family and friends may have great importance at the end of life. Family members may seek involvement in the caring activities as an expression of feelings of closeness and love. They may try to find understanding of, resolution to, or closure of past issues. For the person nearing the end of life, the presence of family, friends, and even pets may be a powerful affirmation of the continuity of life.[99]

Palliative care for older adults focuses on issues surrounding the geriatric syndromes and on the provision

---

BOX 20-9 WHO Components of Palliative Care

By the WHO definition, palliative care
- Provides relief from pain and other distressing symptoms
- Affirms life and regards dying as a normal process
- Intends neither to hasten or postpone death
- Integrates the psychological and spiritual aspects of patient care
- Offers a support system to help patients live as actively as possible until death
- Offers a support system to help the family cope during the patient's illness and in their own bereavement
- Uses a team approach to address the needs of patients and their families, including bereavement counseling, if indicated
- Will enhance quality of life, and may also positively influence the course of illness
- Is applicable early in the course of illness in conjunction with other therapies that are intended to prolong life, such as chemotherapy or radiation therapy, and includes those investigations needed to better understand and manage distressing clinical complications

Source: See reference 98.

of care in a variety of long-term care settings. Common geriatric syndromes occurring at the end of life include dementia, delirium, urinary incontinence, and falls.[100] The decision to initiate palliative care in geriatrics is based on the presence of several markers that indicate that curative approaches are no longer appropriate. **Core end-stage indicators** that characterize the terminal phase of a chronic NCD include physical decline, weight loss, multiple comorbidities, and a serum albumin of less than 2.5 g/dL, along with dependence on assistance with most activities of daily living.[101] Nondisease-specific indicators for palliative care include frailty or extreme vulnerability to morbidity and mortality owing to progressive decline in function and physiological reserve. Frequent falls, disability, susceptibility to acute illness, and reduced ability to recover are examples of frailty. Issues such as functional dependence, cognitive impairment, and family/caregiver support needs can enter into the decision to take a palliative approach to care.

Culture: End-of-Life Decisions

A key issue in end-of-life decisions is the cultural perspective of the patient and family making the decision. For example, African Americans are less likely to accept do-not-resuscitate (DNR) status than whites. In other cultures, such as Asian cultures, care of the older members of a family is a cultural responsibility. When planning and implementing end-of-life policies and procedures in any setting caring for the older adult, it is important to know the culture of the population receiving care. The health-care provider who expresses an interest in the cultural heritage of the older adult receiving care will be able to establish rapport and assist the family and the patient in making end-of-life decisions that match their cultural perspective and beliefs.[102]

Life Closure

At the end of a long life, the personal experience of death can be viewed as an opportunity, or even an achievement. Older adults in the dying process may examine their lives outwardly and deal with their worldly affairs as a way to interface with the world and find some meaning from their lives. The outward aspects of their lives include their relationships with their community, organizations, and other social groups. Older adults may take actions to assure they leave a legacy. They also may reflect on the impact their lives have had on others. They may make choices and plans about how they are leaving this world.

As they move further into the process of life closure, they step into an inner world, where they seek to derive meaning, affirm love of self, love of others, and complete family and friend relationships. This may involve some form of saying goodbye, knowing this is the last time, and accepting the finality of life. Surrendering to the unknown and letting go may be very difficult, but it is part of achieving a peaceful death.

As nurses involved in end-of-life care, we are faced with the fact that there are some things we cannot fix. We cannot stop death. We cannot find the perfect words, erase the anguish, or take away the depth of loss. But it may be enough to be present for the person and the family, respond with compassion and kindness, and keep a realistic perspective that to everything there is a season.

■ Summary Points

- The aging population is growing with an increased need for health-care services.
- Both biological and psychosocial factors play a role in healthy aging.
- More than 50% of older adults experience more than one NCD, resulting in a new focus in *Healthy People 2020* that includes the improvement of the ability of the older adult to self-manage NCDs.
- Older adults experience issues related to communicable diseases and substance use.
- Health planning for older adults is key to meeting *Healthy People 2020* objectives.
- Substance use is a growing issue among the older population.
- Alzheimer's disease and dementia have an impact on the quality of life for the older population and their families.
- The hospice model allows for the delivery of compassionate end-of-life care for the older adult population.

▲ CASE STUDY

Health Planning to Improve Self-Management of Noncommunicable Diseases

The members of the nursing department in a large urban public health department were challenged with developing a program for older adults with more than one NCD, which resulted in increased confidence to manage their diseases. To complete this case study, do the following:

1. Access the *HP 2020* Web site related to objectives for older adults at http://healthypeople.gov/2020/topicsobjectives2020/objectiveslist.aspx?topicid=31.

2. Examine the literature and determine what baseline data are available related to the objective from a national perspective.
3. Critique possible population-level approaches in relation to their utility in meeting the objectives including but not limited to:
   a. Policy initiatives
   b. Development of a health program
   c. Public service announcements
4. Determine what data are available in the city nearest you that would help determine the prevalence of NCDs in that city among older adults.
5. Come to a conclusion on the how the nurses can complete the assignment. Be sure to include in your conclusion the following:
   a. Assessment needs
   b. Types of population-level interventions best suited to meet the objective
   c. Health-planning steps needed specific to the chosen intervention(s)

REFERENCES

1. Kinsella, K., & Wan, H. (2009). *In an aging world 2008* (U.S. Census Bureau, International Population Reports P95/09-1). Washington, DC: U.S. Government Printing Office. Retrieved from http://www.census.gov/prod/2009pubs/p95-09-1.pdf.
2. Centers for Disease Control and Prevention. (2013.) *FastStats: Life expectancy.* Retrieved from http://www.cdc.gov/nchs/fastats/lifexpec.htm. http://www.cdc.gov/nchs/data/hus/hus2009tables/Table024.pdf.
3. Central Intelligence Agency. (n.d.). *The world fact book.* Retrieved from https://www.cia.gov/library/publications/the-world-factbook/rankorder/2102rank.html.
4. U.S. Department of Health and Human Services. (2013). *2020 topics and objectives: Older adults.* Retrieved from http://www.healthypeople.gov/2020/topicsobjectives2020/overview.aspx?topicid=31.
5. World Health Organization. (2010). *Definition of an older or elderly person.* Retrieved from http://www.who.int/healthinfo/survey/ageingdefnolder/en/index.html.
6. U.S. Census Bureau. (2013). *USA quick facts.* Retrieved from http://quickfacts.census.gov/qfd/states/00000.html.
7. U.S. Department of Health and Human Services, Administration on Aging. (2013). *Projected future growth of older adults.* Retrieved from http://www.aoa.gov/Aging_Statistics/future_growth/future_growth.aspx.
8. Federal Interagency Forum on Aging Related Statistics. (2011). *Older Americans 2010: Key indicators of wellbeing.* Retrieved from http://www.agingstats.gov/agingstatsdotnet/Main_Site/Data/2010_Documents/Docs/OA_2010.pdf.
9. Gavrilov L.A., & Heuveline, P. (2003). Aging of the population. In P. Demeny P., & G. McNicoll (Eds.). *The encyclopedia of population.* New York, NY: Macmillan Reference USA.
10. World Health Organization. (2013). *Aging and the life course.* Retrieved from http://www.who.int/ageing/about/ageing_life_course/en/index.html.
11. Department of Health and Human Services, Administration on Aging. (2010). *Projected future growth of the older populations.* Retrieved from http://aging.senate.gov/crs/aging1.pdf.
12. Grayson, V.K., & Velkoff, V.A. (2010). The next four decades: The older population in the United States: 2010 to 2050. In *Current population reports* (P25-1138). Washington, DC: U.S. Census Bureau. Retrieved from http://www.aoa.gov/aoaroot/aging_statistics/future_growth/DOCS/p25-1138.pdf.
13. U.S. Census Bureau. (2011). *International data base.* Retrieved from http://www.census.gov/ipc/www/idb/country.php.
14. Wilmoth, J.R., & Horiuchi, S. (1999). Rectangularization revisited: Variability of age at death within human populations. *Demography, 36*(4), 475-495.
15. Kawas, C.H., & Corrada, M.M. (2006). Alzheimers and dementia in the oldest-old: A century of challenges. *Current Alzheimer Research, 3*(5), 411-419.
16. Sommers, A.C. (2009). Obesity among older Americans. *Congressional research service report for Congress.* Retrieved from aging.senate.gov/crs/aging3.pdf.
17. Pew Research Center. (2009). *Recession turns a graying office grayer: America's changing workforce.* Retrieved from http://pewresearch.org/pubs/1330/american-work-force-is-graying.
18. U.S. Department of Labor, Bureau of Labor Statistics. (2008). *Older workers.* Retrieved from http://www.bls.gov/spotlight/2008/older_workers/.
19. U.S. Census Bureau. (2010). *Aging boomers will increase dependency ratio, Census Bureau projects.* Retrieved from http://www.census.gov/newsroom/releases/archives/aging_population/cb10-72.html.
20. U.S. Census Bureau. (2010). *The next four decades: The older population in the United States: 2010-2050.* Retrieved from http://www.census.gov/prod/2010pubs/p25-1138.pdf.
21. Miller, C. (2000). *Nursing for wellness in older adults: Theory and practice* (4th ed.). Baltimore, MD: Wolters Kluwer Health.
22. Hekimi, S., Lapointe, J., & Wen, Y. (2011). Taking a "good" look at free radicals in the aging process. *Trends in Cell Biology, 21*(10), 569-576.
23. Martin, G.M. (2007). Biology of aging. In L. Goldman & D. Ausiello (Eds.), *Cecil medicine* (23rd ed.). Philadelphia, PA: Saunders Elsevier.
24. Cumming, E. (1975). Engagement with an old theory. *International Journal of Aging and Human Development, 6*(3), 187-191.
25. Atchley, R.C. (1989). A continuity theory of normal aging. *Gerontologist, 29*(2), 183-190.
26. Ferrucci, L. (2008). The Baltimore Longitudinal Study of Aging (BLSA): A 50-year-long journey and plans for the future. *Journal of Gerontology, 63,* 1416-1419.
27. Allard, M., Lebre, V., Robine, J-M. & Calment, J. (1998). *Jeanne Calment: From Van Gogh's time to*

ours; 122 extraordinary years. New York, NY: W.H. Freeman.

28. Boston University School of Medicine. (2012). *New England Centenarian Study.* Retrieved from http://www.bumc.bu.edu/centenarian/.

29. Evert, J., Lawler E., Bogan, H., & Perls, T. (2003). Morbidity profiles of centenarians: Survivors, delayers, and escapers. *Journal of Gerontology, 58,* 232-237.

30. Hilt, R., Young-Xu, Y., Silver, M., & Perls, T. (1999). Centenarians: The older you get the healthier you've been. *Lancet, 354*(9179), 652.

31. Mroczek, D.K., & Spiro, A. (2003). Modeling intra individual change in personality traits: Findings from the Normative Aging Study. *Journal of Gerontology, 58,* 153-165.

32. Newman, A.B., Bayles, C.M., Milas, C.N., McTigue, K., Williams, K., Robare, J.F., & Kuller, L.H. (2010). The 10 keys to healthy aging: Findings from an innovative prevention program in the community. *Journal of Aging and Health, 22*(5), 547-566.

33. American Nurses Credentialing Center. (n.d.). *Gerontological nursing certification.* Retrieved from http://www.nursecredentialing.org.

34. Rowe, J.W., & Kahn, R.L. (1997). Successful aging. *Gerontologist, 37,* 433-440.

35. Crowther, M.R., Parker, M.W., Achenbaum, W.A., Larimore, W.L., & Koenig, H.G. (2002). Rowe and Kahn's model of successful aging revisited: positive spirituality—the forgotten factor. *Gerontologist, 42*(5), 613-620.

36. Hazzard, W.R. (1997). Ways to make "usual" and "successful" aging synonymous: Preventive gerontology. *West Journal of Medicine, 167*(4), 206-215.

37. Morely, J.E. (2009). Successful aging or aging successfully. *Journal of the American Medical Directors Association, 10*(2), 85-86.

38. Centers for Disease Control and Prevention. (2013). *FastStats: Older person's health.* Retrieved from http://www.cdc.gov/nchs/fastats/older_americans.htm.

39. Centers for Disease Control and Prevention. (2013). *FastStats: Pneumonia.* Retrieved from http://www.cdc.gov/nchs/fastats/pneumonia.htm.

40. Centers for Disease Control and Prevention. (2011). *Protect yourself against shingles.* Retrieved from http://www.cdc.gov/features/shingles/.

41. Wilson, N.M. (2006). Sexually transmitted diseases in older adults. *Current Infectious Disease Reports, 8*(2), 139-147.

42. Minichiello, V., Hawkes, G., & Pitts, M. (2011). HIV sexually transmitted diseases and sexuality in later life. *Current Infectious Disease Reports, 13*(2), 182-187.

43. Smith, B.D., Morgan, R.L, Becket, G.A., Falck-Ytee, Y., & Ward, J.W. (2012). Recommendations for the identification of chronic hepatitis C virus infection among persons born during 1945–1965. *Morbidity and Mortality Weekly Reports, 61*(RR04), 1-18.

44. Centers for Disease Control and Prevention. (2012). *Immunization schedules for adults.* Retrieved from http://www.cdc.gov/vaccines/schedules/easy-to-read/adult.html.

45. Talbot, H.K., Libster, R., & Edwards, K.M. (2012). Influenza vaccination for older adults. *Human Vaccine Immunotherapy, 8*(1), 96-101.

46. Weiss, C.O., Boyd, C.M., Yu, Q., Wolff, J.L., & Leff, B. (2007). Patterns of prevalent major chronic disease among older adults in the United States. *JAMA, 298*(10), 1160-1162.

47. Centers for Disease Control and Prevention. (2011). *Clinical preventive services for older adults.* Retrieved from http://www.cdc.gov/Features/PreventiveServices/.

48. Centers for Disease Control and Prevention. (2007). *Injuries among older adults.* Retrieved from http://www.cdc.gov/ncipc/olderadults.htm.

49. Centers for Disease Control and Prevention. (2011). *Falls among older adults: An overview.* Retrieved from http://www.cdc.gov/HomeandRecreationalSafety/Falls/adultfalls.html.

50. Centers for Disease Control and Prevention. (2011). *Injury prevention and control: Home and recreational safety.* Retrieved from http://www.cdc.gov/HomeandRecreationalSafety/Falls/FallsPreventionActivity.html.

51. The National Council on Aging. (n.d.) *Fall prevention.* Retrieved from http://www.ncoa.org/improve-health/center-for-healthy-aging/falls-prevention/.

52. *U.S. Administration on Aging, National Center on Elder Abuse.* (2012). Retrieved from http://www.ncea.aoa.gov/Main_Site/index.aspx.

53. Lachs, M.S., Williams, C.S., O'Brien, S., Pillemer, K.A., & Charlson, M.E. (1998). The mortality of elder mistreatment. *JAMA, 280*(5), 428-432.

54. Centers for Disease Control and Prevention. (2012). *Elder maltreatment definition.* Retrieved from http://www.cdc.gov/features/elderabuse/.

55. Centers for Disease Control and Prevention. (2012). *Elder maltreatment prevention.* Retrieved from http://www.cdc.gov/ViolencePrevention/eldermaltreatment/definitions.html.

56. Centers for Disease Control and Prevention. (2010). *Elder maltreatment: Risk and protective factors.* Retrieved from http://www.cdc.gov/ViolencePrevention/eldermaltreatment/riskprotectivefactors.html.

57. U.S. Administration on Aging, National Center on Elder Abuse. (2011). *Risk factors for elder abuse.* Retrieved from http://www.ncea.aoa.gov/Main_Site/FAQ/Basics/Risk_Factors.aspx.

58. Perel-Levin, S. (2008). *Discussing screening for elder abuse at the primary care level. Aging and life course family and community health.* Geneva, Switzerland: World Health Organization.

59. Fulmer, T. (n.d.). *Elder mistreatment: Training manual and protocol.* Retrieved from http://hartfordign.org/uploads/File/Fulmer_EM_full.pdf.

60. Stark, S. (2012). Elder abuse: Screening, intervention and prevention. *Nursing 2012, 29*(10), 24-29. doi:10.1097/01.NURSE.0000419426.05524.45. Retrieved from http://www.nursingcenter.com/prodev/ce_article.asp?tid=1434093&Journal_ID=54016&Issue_ID=1433745,%20Issue%201.

61. National Center on Elder Abuse. (n.d.). *Resources.* Retrieved from http://www.ncea.aoa.gov/resources/index.aspx.

62. Giles, L., Brewer, E.T., Mosqueda, L., Huba, G.L., & Melchoir, L.A. (2010). Vision for 2020. *Journal of. Elder Abuse and Neglect, 22*(3-4), 375-386.

63. Dyer, C.B., Heisler, C.J., Hill, C.A., & Kim, L.C. (2005). Community approaches to elder abuse. *Clinical Geriatric Medicine, 21*(2), 429-447.

64. Falk, N.L., Baigis, J., & Kopac, C. (2012). Elder mistreatment and the Elder Justice Act. *OJIN: The Online Journal of Issues in Nursing, 17*(3). Retrieved from http://www.nursingworld.org/MainMenuCategories/ANAMarketplace/ANAPeriodicals/OJIN/Tableof-Contents/Vol-17-2012/No3-Sept-2012/Articles-Previous-Topics/Elder-Mistreatment-and-Elder-Justice-Act.html.

65. *Principles of Adult Protective Services.* (n.d.). Retrieved from http://www.morrowjfs.com/Principles.pdf.

66. Malks, B.F., Strobel, D.M., Leung, Y., Court, M.W., Morris, J.R., May, G., et al. (2010). Changing systems to address elder abuse: Examples from aging services, the courts, the long-term care ombudsman, and the faith community. *Journal of Elder Abuse and Neglect, 22*(3-4), 306-327.

67. Gfroerer, J.C., Penne, M.A., Pemberton, M.R., & Folsom, R.E. (2008). *The aging baby boom cohort and future prevalence of substance abuse.* Retrieved from http://www.oas.samhsa.gov/aging/chap5.htm.

68. Substance Abuse and Mental Health Services Administration. (2008). *Substance abuse by older adults: Impact on the treatment system.* Retrieved from http://www.oas.samhsa.gov/aging/chap3.htm.

69. Blow, F.C. (1998). *Substance abuse among older adults. Treatment Improvement Protocol 26.* Rockville, MD: Substance Abuse and Mental Health Services Administration. Retrieved from http://www.ncbi.nlm.nih.gov/books/NBK14467/.

70. Substance Abuse and Mental Health Administration. (2014). *Results from the 2013 national survey on drug use and health: Summary of national findings.* Retrieved from http://www.samhsa.gov/data/sites/default/files/NSDUHresultsPDFWHTML2013/Web/NSDUHresults2013.pdf.

71. O'Connell, H., Chin, A., Hamilton, F., Cunningham, C., Walsh, J.B., Coakley, D., & Lawlor, B.A. (2004). A systematic review of the utility of self-report alcohol screening instruments in the elderly. *International Journal of Geriatric Psychiatry, 19,* 1074-1086.

72. National Institute on Aging. (2013). *Health and aging.* Retrieved from http://www.nia.nih.gov/health.

73. Pringle, K.E., Heller, D.A., & Brown, T.V. (2005). Potential for alcohol and prescription drug interactions in older people. *Journal of the American Geriatric Society, 53*(11), 1532-1554.

74. National Institute on Alcohol Abuse and Alcoholism. (2005). *Helping patients who drink too much: A clinician's guide.* Retrieved from http://pubs.niaaa.nih.gov/publications/Practitioner/CliniciansGuide2005/guide.pdf.

75. Sechi, G., & Serra, A. (2007). Wernicke's encephalopathy: New clinical settings and recent advances in diagnosis and management. *The Lancet, 6,* 441-455.

76. Savage, C.L. (2008). Screening for alcohol use in older adults. *Directions in Addiction Treatment and Prevention, 12*(2), 17-26.

77. Morely, J.E. (2009). Successful aging or aging successfully. *Journal of American Medical Directors Association, 10*(2), 85-86.

78. Vasunilashorn, S., Steinman, B.A., Leibig, P.S., & Pynoos, J. (2012). Aging in place: Evolution of a research topic whose time has come. *Journal of Aging Research, 17.*

79. U.S. Census Bureau. (2010). *Census brief: The older population.* Retrieved from http://www.census.gov/prod/cen2010/briefs/c2010br-09.pdf.

80. Szanton, S., Thorpe, R.J., Boyd, C., Tanner, E.K., Liff, B., & Gitlin, L. (2011). Community aging in place, advancing better living for elders: A bio-behavioral environmental intervention to improve functioning and health related quality of life in disabled older adults. *Journal of the American Geriatrics Society, 59*(12), 2314-2320.

81. Centers for Disease Control and Prevention. (2012). *Healthy aging and the built environment.* Retrieved from http://www.cdc.gov/healthyplaces/healthtopics/healthyaging.htm.

82. Department of Health and Human Services, Administration on Aging. (2011). *Naturally occurring retirement communities.* Retrieved from http://www.aoa.gov/AoARoot/AoA_Programs/HCLTC/NORC/index.aspx.

83. Zarem, J. (Ed.). (2010). *Whitepaper: Today's continuing care communities.* Retrieved from https://www.seniorshousing.org/filephotos/research/CCRC_whitepaper.pdf.

84. Butler, R.N. (2009). Combating ageism. *International Psychogeriatric, 21*(211).

85. Simkins, Chelsea L. (2007). Ageism's influence on health care delivery and nursing practice. *Journal of Nursing Student Research, 1*(1), Article 5.

86. National Institute on Aging. (n.d.). *Prevalence of Alzheimer's disease.* Retrieved from http://www.nia.nih.gov/alzheimers/publication/2011-2012-alzheimers-disease-progress-report/prevalence-alzheimers-disease.

87. Centers for Disease Control and Prevention. (2009). *Healthy aging: Alzheimer's disease.* Retrieved from http://www.cdc.gov/aging/aginginfo/alzheimers.htm.

88. Centers for Disease Control and Prevention. (2011). *FastStats: Leading causes of death.* Retrieved from http://www.cdc.gov/nchs/fastats/lcod.htm.

89. Williams, J.W., Plassman, B.L., Burke, J., Holsinger, T., Benjamin, S. (2010, April). *Preventing Alzheimer's disease and cognitive decline.* Washington, DC: Agency for Healthcare Research and Quality, Department of Health and Human Services.

90. Alzheimer's Association. (2014). *Medications for memory loss.* Retrieved from http://www.alz.org/alzheimers_disease_standard_prescriptions.asp.

91. Centers for Disease Control and Prevention. (2012). *Healthy brain initiative.* Retrieved from http://www.cdc.gov/aging/healthybrain/index.htm.

92. Centers for Disease Control and Prevention. (2012). *Healthy aging: Family caregiving—the facts.* Retrieved from http://www.cdc.gov/aging/caregiving/facts.htm.

93. American Psychological Association. (2013). *The financial costs of family caregiving.* Retrieved from http://www.apa.org/pi/about/publications/caregivers/faq/financial-costs.aspx.

94. Centers for Disease Control and Prevention & the Kimberly-Clark Corporation. (2008). *Assuring healthy caregivers: A public health approach to translating research into practice; The RE-AIM framework.* Neenah, WI: Kimberly-Clark Corporation.

95. National Hospice and Palliative Care Organization. (2014). *History of hospice care.* Retrieved from http://www.nhpco.org/i4a/pages/index.cfm?pageid=3285.

96. National Hospice and Palliative Care Organization. (2014). *Hospice eligibility requirements.* Retrieved from http://www.nhpco.org/hospice-eligibility-requirements.

97. National Hospice and Palliative Care Organization. (2013). *NHPCO's facts and figures: Hospice care in America.* Retrieved from http://www.nhpco.org/sites/default/files/public/Statistics_Research/2013_Facts_Figures.pdf.

98. World Health Organization. (2012). *WHO definition of palliative care.* Retrieved from http://www.who.int/cancer/palliative/definition/en/.

99. Michael, K. (2006). Rehabilitation and palliative care. In B. Ferrell & N. Coyne (Eds.), *Oxford textbook of palliative nursing* (2nd ed.). New York, NY: Oxford University Press.

100. Kapo, J., Morrison, L.J., & Liao, S. (2007). Palliative care for the older adult. *Journal of Palliative Medicine, 10*(1), 185-209.

101. Matzo, M.L. (2004). Palliative care: Prognostication and the chronically ill; Methods you need to know as chronic disease progresses in older adults. *American Journal of Nursing. 104*(9), 40-49.

102. Searight, J.R., & Gafford, H. (2005). Cultural issues at the end of life: Issues and guidelines for family physicians. *American Family Physician, 5*(13), 515-522. http://www.marianjoylibrary.org/Diversity/documents/CulturalDiversityattheEndofLifeIssuesandGuidelines.pdf.

Chapter 21

Health Planning for Occupational Health

LEARNING OUTCOMES

After reading this chapter, the student will be able to:

1. Define *occupational health* and *occupational and environmental health nursing*.
2. Describe the relationship between the work environment, workplace exposures, and worker health and safety.
3. Discuss the concept of toxicology and the relevance to understanding and preventing occupational diseases.
4. Discuss controlling hazards and reducing injuries in the workplace.
5. Identify vulnerable worker populations.
6. Explain the role of the occupational and environmental health nurse in the development, management, and evaluation of occupational health programs.
7. State methods of worker protection and safety as well as health promotion strategies in the occupational health setting.

KEY TERMS

Case management
Disability
Employee assistance program (EAP)
Engineering controls
Environmental monitoring
Epidemiological triangle
Ergonomics
Hazard Communication Standard
Health risk appraisal (HRA)

Hierarchy of controls
Material safety data sheet (MSDS)
National Institute for Occupational Safety and Health (NIOSH)
National Occupational Research Agenda (NORA)
Occupational and environmental health history

Occupational and environmental health nurse (OEHN)
Occupational and environmental health nursing
Occupational Safety and Health (OSH) Act
Occupational Safety and Health Administration (OSHA)

Personal protective equipment (PPE)
Toxicology
Vulnerable worker populations
Workers' compensation
Work-family interface
Workplace assessment/ workplace walkthrough

Introduction

Every week, 245 million Americans go to work.[1] Construction workers can be seen during the day at a new building site or doing repairs on a busy highway in the middle of the night. Health-care providers are present around the clock in hospitals and emergency departments. Behind the scenes are nutrition services, plant facilities staff, laundry workers, and hazardous waste workers. In an office building, top executives are in the boardroom, while administrative assistants spend hours in front of a computer, telephones ringing in the background. When the workday is over, the housekeeping staff cleans bathrooms, polishes floors, and removes trash for another new day. The goal of occupational health is to ensure that each worker returns home safely at the end of the workday. Unfortunately, not all workers do. Fatalities and injuries occur: mine explosions, deaths of truckers, collapses at construction sites, loss of limbs among soldiers, and violent incidents in the health-care workplace. Every work setting presents its own unique exposures and hazards and its own mix of worker demographics that may affect the health and well-being of employees. The **occupational and environmental health nurse (OEHN)** is a key member of the interprofessional team responsible for the assessment and detection of occupational hazards and the implementation of interventions to protect the health of worker populations (Box 21-1).

Focus of Occupational Health

The Joint International Labour Organization/World Health Organization describes the focus of occupational health as the following:

- Follow a systems approach to promoting safe and healthy work environments
- Afford prevention the highest priority
- Develop work cultures in a direction supporting health and safety at work while preventing and controlling hazards and risks, and in doing so promoting a positive social climate and smooth operation that may enhance productivity and quality[2]

The **Occupational Safety and Health Administration (OSHA)** is a federal agency that was formed in 1970. OSHA is charged with protecting coworkers, family members, employers, customers, suppliers, nearby communities, and other members of the public who are affected by the workplace environment.[3]

The Workplace and the Epidemiological Triangle

The workplace is only one component of the overall environment, but the workplace is where adults spend approximately one-third of their time.[4] The incorporation of the **epidemiological triangle** (Chapter 3) provides a framework to describe the complex relationships between an agent (the exposure(s) in the workplace), the host (worker/employee), and the environment (workplace)—the setting in which the agent and host come together.[5] This chapter clarifies how these three components relate to one another.

Occupational and Environmental Health Nursing

The profession of occupational health nursing evolved during the 19th century, when industry hired nurses to decrease the spread of communicable disease among workers and to reduce injury and promote safety. The landmark events in the evolution of the profession are described in Box 21-2. Today's OEHN has expanded this specialty practice into management areas, consultation with government and industry, policy setting at the local, state, and national levels, and education and research. Nevertheless, a major role for the OEHN is the provision of direct care to employees in the workplace.

BOX 21-1	Members of the Interprofessional Occupational and Environmental Health Team	
Occupational Health Professionals	**Primary Focus**
Occupational and environmental health nurse	Prevention of occupational disease and injury, restoration of employee health and return to work, protection from occupational hazards
Occupational health physician	Diagnose, treat, and manage occupational disease and injury
Occupational and environmental hygienist	The recognition, evaluation, and control of chemical, biological, or physical factors or stressors arising in the workplace; and the utilization of analytical techniques to detect exposures and implement engineering controls to correct, reduce, or eliminate exposure
Ergonomist	Evaluate, design, and promote the interface between the worker, the tools used, and their work
Occupational psychiatrist/psychologist	Diagnose, treat, and manage mental and behavioral disorders secondary to exposures in the workplace
Toxicologist	Evaluate and describe the toxic properties of chemical and physical agents used during work
Injury prevention/safety specialist	Develop procedures, standards, or systems to achieve the control or reduction of hazards, injuries, and exposures
Health promotion educator	Develop educational strategies and methods to promote the health of worker(s) in the occupational setting

BOX 21–2	Landmark Events in the Evolution of Occupational and Environmental Health Nursing

1888	Betty Moulder of Pennsylvania was the first reported occupational health nurse who cared for coal miners and families.
1942	American Association of Industrial Nurses established.
1970	The Occupation Safety and Health Act is passed creating the Occupational Safety and Health Administration (OSHA) and the National Institute for Occupational Safety and Health (NIOSH). NIOSH Occupational Safety and Health Education and Resource Centers are created to educate occupational health professionals (nurses, physicians, industrial hygienists, and safety specialists), now called NIOSH Occupational Safety and Health Education and Research Centers.
1972	The Accreditation Board for Occupational Health Nursing is established, creating certification of nurses in the specialty practice of occupational and environmental health nursing.
1977	The American Association of Industrial Nurses name changed to the American Association of Occupational Health Nurses.
1993	The Office of Occupational Health Nursing (OOHN) was established at OSHA

Source: Adapted from Institute of Medicine. Committee to Assess Training Needs for Occupational Safety and Health Personnel in the United States, 2000.

In 1993, the Institute of Medicine conducted a workshop to discuss the growing need to enhance occupational and environmental health content in the practice of nursing. The workshop resulted in the establishment of the Committee on Enhancing Environmental Health Content in Nursing Practice and competencies for this nursing specialty.[6] Today, the importance of occupational health is also evident in the *Healthy People 2020 (HP 2020)* objectives.[7]

■ HEALTHY PEOPLE 2020
Health Planning for Occupational Health

Healthy People Topic Relevant to Health Planning for Occupational Health

Targeted Topic: Occupational Health and Safety
Goal: Promote the health and safety of people at work through prevention and early intervention.

Overview: The intent behind the occupational safety and health topic area is to prevent diseases, injuries, and deaths that result because of working conditions. Work-related illnesses and injuries include any illness or injury incurred by an employee engaged in work-related activities while at or away from the worksite.

Workplace settings vary widely in size, sector, design, location, work processes, workplace culture, and resources. In addition, workers themselves are different in terms of age, gender, training, education, cultural background, health practices, and access to preventive health care. This translates to great diversity in the safety and health risks for each industry sector and the need for tailored interventions.

Occupational safety and related *HP 2020* objectives are primarily addressed through the **National Occupational Research Agenda (NORA)**. NORA was established by the Centers for Disease Control and Prevention (CDC), **National Institute for Occupational Safety and Health (NIOSH),** and its partners to stimulate research and improve workplace practices. Now in its second decade (2006–2016), NORA focuses on occupational safety and health in 10 sectors:

1. Agriculture, Forestry, and Fishing
2. Construction
3. Health Care and Social Assistance
4. Manufacturing
5. Mining
6. Oil and Gas Extraction
7. Public Safety
8. Services
9. Transportation, Warehousing, and Utilities
10. Wholesale and Retail Trade[7]

Occupational and environmental health nursing is defined by the American Association of Occupational Health Nursing (AAOHN) as "the specialty practice that provides for and delivers health and safety programs and services to workers, worker populations and community groups."[8] The AAOHN is the professional organization that develops and approves standards of practice, supports education and research, and provides political consultation to state and national legislatures related to OEHN. The Accreditation Board for Occupational Health Nursing certifies nurses in the specialty practice of occupational and environmental health nursing.

The practicing OEHN focuses on promotion and restoration of health, prevention of illness and injury, and protection from work-related and environmental hazards. The profession is guided by a code of ethics (Box 21-3) that provides an ethical framework for decision making and nursing actions.[9] Another important document developed by the AAOHN is the Standards of Occupational and Environmental Health Nursing.[10] The standards include a definition of and scope of practice for OEHNs. Because OEHNs frequently have a combined knowledge of health and business, they are equipped with the skills to incorporate their experience in health care with their knowledge of establishing safe and healthful working environments.

Key Agencies in Occupational Health

The passage of the **Occupational Safety and Health (OSH) Act** in 1970 created two government organizations, OSHA and NIOSH.[3] The work of both agencies has a profound effect on the work environment and the health and safety of workers in this country.

Occupational Safety and Health Administration

OSHA, which is part of the Department of Labor, is the main federal agency charged with the regulation and enforcement of the OSH Act. The mission at OSHA involves the development and enforcement of safety and health standards to assure safe and healthful working conditions for working men and women. The OSH Act includes the General Duty Clause, which requires an employer to "furnish to each of his [*sic*] employees employment and a place of employment which are free from recognized hazards that are causing or are likely to cause death or serious physical harm." Most employees who work for private employers in the United States are protected by federal OSHA or through an OSHA-approved state program. Federal agencies must have a safety and health program that meets the same standards as required under federal OSHA. The self-employed, family members of family farms, employers

BOX 21–3	Code of Ethics and Interpretive Statements for the American Association of Occupational Health Nurses

Preamble

The American Association of Occupational Health Nurses, Inc. (AAOHN) Code of Ethics has been developed in response to the nursing profession's acceptance of its goals and vales and the trust conferred upon it by society to guide the conduct and practices of the profession. As professionals, occupational and environmental health nurses (OHNs) accept the responsibility and inherent obligation to uphold these values.

The Code of Ethics is based on the belief that the goal of occupational and environmental health nurses is to promote the worker, worker population and community health and safety. This specialized practice focuses on promotion and restoration of health, prevention of illness and injury and protection from occupational and environmental hazards. The occupational and environmental nurse has a unique role in protecting the integrity of the workplace and the work environment.

The client can be workers, workers' families/significant others, worker populations, community groups and employers. The purpose of the AAOHN Code of Ethics is to serve as a guide for registered professional nurses to maintain and pursue professionally recognized ethical behavior in providing occupational and environmental health and safety services.

Ethics is synonymous with moral reasoning. Ethics is now law, but a guide for moral action. Professional nurses, when making judgments related to the health and welfare of the client, utilize these significant universal moral principles.

There principles are:
• Right of self-determination
• Confidentiality
• Truth telling
• Doing or producing good
• Avoiding harm
• Fair and nondiscriminatory treatment

Occupational and environmental health nurses recognize that dilemmas may develop that do not have guidelines, data or statutes to assist with problem resolution; thus, occupational and environmental health nurses use problem-solving, collaboration and appropriate resources to resolve dilemmas.

The Code is not intended to establish nor replace standards of care or minimal levels of practice. In summary, the Code of Ethics and Interpretative Statements provide a guiding ethical framework for decision-making and evaluation of nursing actions as occupational and environmental health nurses fulfill their professional responsibilities to society and the profession.

Source: From the AAOHN, used with permission.

who do not employ outside employees, and workers who are protected by regulations of another federal agency (for example, the Mine Safety and Health Administration, the Federal Aviation Administration, and the Coast Guard) are not covered by the OSH Act.[11] Additionally, the act requires businesses with more than 10 employees to keep records of fatalities, injuries, and illnesses on the OSHA 300 form. This record-keeping is critical to an employer's safety and health program for several reasons. Identification and description of the causes of work-related illness and injury assist in identifying problem areas that need corrective action to reduce hazardous workplace conditions. The data collected on these logs are used by the Department of Labor and OSHA to develop workplace statistics, including fatality, morbidity, and incidence rates for workplace illnesses and injuries for U.S. industries. These statistics are available to the public and provide a yearly accounting of the injuries and illnesses occurring among U.S. worker populations. The data in OSHA 300 logs provide information for OSHA to monitor the progress that is being made to reduce workplace health and safety problems.[12] OSHA also uses these logs to target the need for enforcement activities in industries in which the majority of workplace illnesses and injuries occur.

National Institute for Occupational Safety and Health

The second agency created by the OSH Act was NIOSH, an agency of the Department of Health and Human Services, whose mission is to conduct research and to provide information, education, and training in the field of occupational safety and health. In 1996, NIOSH created NORA.[7,13] NORA is a partnership program between governmental agencies, large and small businesses, universities, worker organizations, and professional groups that work in collaboration to develop innovative research with the ultimate goal of improving workplace practices.[7,14] Ultimately, the research partnerships formed seek to provide recommendations for safer, healthier workplaces.

Occupational Safety and Health (OSH) Program

The formal OSH program is an essential tool for the OEHN. According to a rule originally proposed by OSHA to ensure compliance with OSHA standards but later withdrawn, each employer is responsible for developing an OSH program that will manage health and safety at the worksite to reduce injuries, illnesses, and fatalities by complying with OSHA standards and the General Duty Clause.[15] An additional requirement in this draft law is that the OSH program will address the unique hazards and conditions found at each worksite.

The OSH program provides a systematic process that evaluates the workplace, recognizes the exposures and hazards found in each area of the worksite, provides a plan to control these exposures and hazards, and evaluates the effectiveness of these controls through routine **environmental monitoring** of the worksite and routine medical screening to assess for any adverse health conditions of the workforce. Environmental monitoring is the assessment of the workplace to identify risks and other hazards, whereas screening refers to identifying individual risks within individual workers such as heart disease and high blood pressure. The OEHN is part of an interprofessional team that provides information on the health data collected during the medical screening process in order to assist in the evaluation of the effectiveness of the OSH program. If a problem is found, corrective action is taken and the workers are reevaluated.

Primary, Secondary, and Tertiary Prevention

In most workplaces, an occupational safety and health program focuses on primary, secondary, and tertiary prevention of occupational illnesses and injuries, and promotes worker health. Through primary prevention, workers are protected from exposure to hazards, or exposures are limited to levels that are considered safe. Examples of primary prevention interventions in the workplace include **engineering controls,** such as use of less hazardous chemicals, or **personal protective equipment (PPE),** such as masks, gloves, or earplugs, or tethering a roofing worker to prevent a fall.

Secondary prevention requires the early recognition of a disease before the disease becomes irreversible or is no longer easily treatable. Screening and monitoring of workers are examples of secondary prevention activities designed to detect early signs of disease (e.g., audiometric screening to detect hearing loss for workers in a noisy environment, or spirometry screening to detect a reduction of lung function due to work in a closed, dusty environment). Tertiary prevention involves the treatment of the disease. The diagnosis of an occupational illness, such as work-related asthma, may require that the worker be removed from the exposure and transferred to another job. For nonoccupational illnesses that occur, the OEHN must coordinate with the worker's family physician or nurse practitioner regarding the timing of work return, particularly if accommodations in the workplace are needed. For example, an employee recovering from a myocardial infarction may require a gradual return to physically demanding work, or an employee being treated for cancer may require flexibility of the work schedule to accommodate chemotherapy or radiation.

Worker Populations

The demographic characteristics of workers vary by age, race, gender, culture, ethnicity, and functional ability. These factors may influence a worker's vulnerability and susceptibility to exposures in the workplace and must be incorporated into the OSH program. In the United States, employment is often begun during adolescence and young adulthood. Approximately 57% of young individuals are employed in their first job at 14 or 15 years old. As the American workplace becomes more diverse, OEHNs must focus on the vulnerable worker. The U.S. workforce is changing in a variety of ways. As many traditional service and manufacturing jobs migrate to other countries, the workforce is becoming much more dependent on "knowledge" workers.[16] Occupational health providers also need to direct attention toward this rapid movement toward a knowledge-based economy that relies heavily on the creativity, mental stamina, and intellectual capacity of workers. This trend will likely change the pattern of disease and injuries that occur. For example, fewer physical injuries such as falls and crush injuries are likely to occur as factory-worker jobs are relocated to other countries. A higher rate of sedentary lifestyle diseases such as high blood pressure, diabetes, and obesity may occur as employees spend more time sitting at a computer versus physically moving during the course of their workday.

Emerging issues in the workplace are tied to the trend of longer working hours, greater participation of women in the workforce, couples having children later in life, and increasing responsibility for care of aging family members and families with dual career families. Workers are increasingly finding themselves sandwiched between work and domestic responsibilities.[17-19] Today, researchers at NIOSH are focused on the associations between work-life balance, well-being, and functioning.[20] Examples of research needed in this field include the effects of telecommuting and other organizational practices that meld work and family life, and the benefits of increased job flexibility and control over family obligations.

Unions

Unions have played an important role in the evolution of occupational safety and health in the United States. In 1890, the United Mine Workers of America (UMWA) was formed with the primary purpose of preventing miner deaths.[21] The UMWA was instrumental in the passage of the Coal Mine Health and Safety Act of 1969 as a result of their constant effort taken to describe the dangerous conditions in coal mines that lead to black lung disease and fatalities.[21] Over the years, labor unions have used collective bargaining agreements to help improve worker health and safety at union worksites. An example of this type of initiative was demonstrated in the 1974 contract agreement between the U.S. Steel Corporation and the United Steel Workers of America that addressed the adverse health effects caused by exposure to coke oven emissions during steel production.[21] Unions assist their members with day-to-day issues at work; participate in legislative and regulatory policies; and conduct collective bargaining for workers over wages, working conditions, and benefits. Unions also conduct education and training programs for their members. They provide workers with a voice in workplace decisions and provide a mechanism for resolving workplace issues that are unavailable to a worker in a nonunionized workplace.

Over the years, the number of union members in the United States has fallen dramatically, from 20.1% of American workers in the private sector in 1983 to 11.3% of wage and salary workers in 2012.[22] Yates discusses several reasons for the decline of American unions. External forces include the shift of the economy from the production of goods to a service economy and the lack of demand by workers for the services offered by unions.[21] An internal force that has affected unions is the way in which union leaders are chosen. They are no longer selected from rank-and-file members, but from delegates far removed from the average rank and file union member.[21]

The OEHN must establish a working relationship with a union that has a presence in the workplace. Health and safety meetings should involve the union so that trust and mutual respect are developed among members of the health and safety program. Despite the fact that their numbers have decreased in the United States, unions such as the Service Employees International Union, the American Federation of Labor-Congress of Industrial Organizations, and others remain important organizations representing workers in many high-risk industries.

● APPLYING PUBLIC HEALTH SCIENCE

The Case of the Contaminated Home

Public Health Science Topics Covered:

- Epidemiology and biostatistics

Juan, a Mexican immigrant to the United States, works in California and Oregon during the harvest season as a migrant/seasonal farmworker. His 8-month work experience includes the harvesting of strawberries, asparagus, and naval oranges in California. In Oregon, he works in the berry and celery fields, usually for 6-week periods and often for many different owners. In one of these jobs, he experienced a puncture wound to his foot, resulting in the need for a tetanus shot, after which he traveled back to California to work in the raisin grape harvest.

Depending on the season, Juan spends up to 12 hours per day working in the fields, planting or harvesting crops, and unloading trucks. At the end of the day, his clothes are often covered with dust. He sometimes brings his wife and children into the field to assist him with the picking of fruit or vegetables.

Juan and his family are often provided substandard housing with a communal bathroom and shower and a shared kitchen in the local shantytowns. The location of the housing is often directly across from the fields and inhabitants may be exposed to the pesticides with which the fields are sprayed.

The public health nurse (PHN) from the local health department provides care to the migrants. As a part of this role, the PHN sees Juan in the nearby free clinic as a follow-up to his foot injury. The puncture wound to his foot has healed and has no signs of infection. The PHN realizes that exposures in the worksite are critical to Juan's health and interviewed him about his work and current health status. Juan reports leaving the fields late every day and eating dinner before removing his work clothes or taking a shower. He also complains of slight abdominal discomfort and diarrhea that has lasted for the past 7 days. After further inquiry, the PHN learns that although 1,3-dichloropropene is the most common pesticide used locally to control pests from eating the roots of grape plants, local farmers may be spraying several other pesticides and fungicides.

The pesticide 1,3-dichloropropene is a sweet-smelling, colorless liquid that dissolves in water and evaporates quickly.[23] The pesticide that is released into the atmosphere takes several days to break down. After learning of the proximity of Juan's home to the fields, the PHN develops an exposure risk-reduction plan in collaboration with Juan. The plan includes Juan wearing a facemask and dusting off his clothing prior to entering his home. He will then remove his clothing at the door and put them in a bag to keep them from contaminating the rest of the home. Juan will then shower before eating. When the fields are being sprayed, Juan's children will wait 5 days before playing outside near the fields or their home. The PHN then asks Juan to return in 2 to 3 weeks for a reevaluation of his symptoms.

Exposures in the Workplace

Exposures for any worker can include physical, chemical, biological, or psychological hazards. These hazards may have a profound effect on the short- and long-term health of workers. It is important for OEHNs to identify hazards in their work environments so that mitigation plans can be implemented to reduce the potentially harmful effect to workers.

Physical Exposures

Physical hazards in the workplace, such as noise, excessive hot or cold temperatures, vibration, and nonionizing and ionizing radiation, cause harm or injury to body tissues through energy transfer.

Noise is an exposure frequently found in workplaces where construction, welding, or work with heavy machinery or power tools is performed. After years of exposure to loud noises, hearing loss can occur due to damage of the hair cells in the inner ear and failure of sound wave transmission to the auditory nerve. Loudness and duration of noise exposure are two important factors that affect hearing loss. Nonwork exposure to loud noise by workers can occur at music concerts, in sports such as hunting or target practice, and without use of hearing protection such as ear buds, all of which may lead to hearing loss. OSHA has developed a standard that regulates noise exposure and requires a hearing protection program in the workplace.[24] This standard requires monitoring of noise levels within the work environment, use of hearing protection, training and education of employees in the proper use of hearing protection, creation of baseline audiograms for each employee, and annual hearing tests.

Excessive heat exposure can be found in foundries, pottery-making plants with kilns, and in the road construction and fishing/agriculture industries during the summer months. In the case of Juan, health outcomes of working in hot environments can be debilitating and potentially life threatening when heat stress, heat exhaustion, and heat stroke occur. Industries that require outdoor work during the summer months also expose workers to nonionizing radiation from the sun and increased risk for skin cancer.[25] Jobs with winter-month cold exposures include construction and police and fire service work, although food industry workers may spend time in freezers or stock frozen foods year-round. Cold exposure results in the stimulation of the sympathetic nervous system, potentially resulting in frostbite and hypothermia.[26]

Workers are exposed to vibration in manual tasks that involve two main mechanisms: hand-arm vibration, in which the main exposure is associated with power tools, such as a jackhammer; or whole-body vibration transferred to the body by large machinery, such as a bulldozer. These types of vibration exposures place workers at risk for acute and chronic musculoskeletal disorders.[27]

The Agency for Toxic Substances and Disease Registry defines ionizing radiation as any one of several types of particles and rays given off by radioactive material, high-voltage equipment, nuclear reactions, and stars. The types of ionizing radiation normally important to health are alpha particles, beta particles, x-rays, and gamma rays.[28,29] Ionizing radiation can have significant health effects, including skin burns, hair loss, nausea, birth defects, illness, and death. Certain types of cancer have been associated with ionizing radiation, although a person's risk may be influenced by dose and the age of the person when exposed.[28,29] For example, hospital x-ray technicians can be exposed to ionizing radiation during radiological procedures. However, most hospitals employ comprehensive safety protocols to prevent ionizing radiation exposure.

Chemical Exposures

According to OSHA, there are approximately 650,000 existing chemical products and hundreds of new products being introduced into the workplace annually. These chemical exposures may cause health effects to our body systems and may act as carcinogens. As a result of these findings, OSHA issued the **Hazard Communication Standard**.[30] This policy requires both employers and employees to be knowledgeable about hazards and to take action to protect themselves from illness or injury. This standard also requires the producers of chemicals to be responsible for reviewing the scientific evidence related to chemical hazards and for generating and communicating information to chemical users in the form of a **material safety data sheet (MSDS)**. An MSDS accompanies the hazardous chemical and describes the physical and chemical properties (e.g., acid, solvent) and health hazards, the routes of exposure, safe handling and use, emergency and first aid procedures, and control measures.

Heavy Metals

Lead, mercury, cadmium, beryllium, nickel, and aluminum are examples of heavy metals that may be found in an occupational environment.[31] Information on chemical exposures may be obtained at the Agency for Toxic Substances and Disease Registry's Web site. An example of a chemical hazard in the workplace is beryllium, a metal naturally found in mineral rocks, coal, soil, and volcanic dust. Beryllium compounds are mined and purified for use in nuclear weapons and reactors, aircrafts, satellites, and x-ray machines. Workers who are exposed to beryllium may develop an inflammatory respiratory condition known as chronic beryllium disease years after exposure. Lung cancer screening for these workers is also recommended because beryllium is a human carcinogen.[32]

Pesticides

Migrant/seasonal farmworkers such as Juan and pest control workers are exposed to pesticides when they enter fields where pesticides have been applied or they mix or apply them. Organophosphates, one type of pesticide, are powerful cholinesterase inhibiters. Cholinesterase is an enzyme important for the proper functioning of the nervous system in humans, other vertebrates, and insects.[33] Inhibition of this enzyme can cause a buildup of acetylcholine within nervous and skeletal smooth muscle systems, leading to signs and symptoms affecting the respiratory system, cardiovascular system, central nervous system, eyes, and skin.

Organic Solvents

Organic solvents (e.g., benzene, toluene, carbon disulfide, carbon tetrachloride, trichloroethylene or TCE) are volatile hydrocarbons found in a variety of industries. These chemicals are used in degreasing and dry cleaning operations and in the manufacturing of paints, paint strippers, lacquers, rubber products, plastics, and textiles. Health effects of these agents are caused by central and peripheral nervous system damage, kidney and liver damage, reproductive effects, as well as skin lesions and cancer. An example is benzene, a product derived from coal and petroleum and found in gasoline, is a known carcinogen. Chronic exposure to benzene affects bone marrow and blood production and can lead to leukemia. Short-term exposures may cause drowsiness, unconsciousness, dizziness, and death.[34]

Biological Exposures

Biological agents include bacteria, viruses, and other microorganisms that can be transmitted by air, food, water, soil, or direct contact.[35] Health-care providers in hospitals, clinics, and community health settings can be exposed to bloodborne pathogens such as HIV and hepatitis B and C. OSHA's Bloodborne Pathogen Standard, first introduced in the early 1990s, provides strict regulations for health-care settings to prevent and manage exposures by use of needleless devices, sharps containers, nonrecapping of needles, and proper disposal of body fluids.

OSHA also provides guidelines for the protection of employees exposed to tuberculosis. Employees must have a respiratory protection program outlining when an employee needs to use a respirator as protection against tuberculosis, the proper selection and fit of respirators, fit testing and medical evaluation of workers who use respirators, and training for respirator use.[36] A respirator is a personal protective device (PPD) worn on the face and covers at least the nose and mouth. It is used to reduce the wearer's risk of inhaling hazardous airborne particles (including dust particles and infectious agents such as tuberculosis), gases, and vapors.[37] Prior to using a respirator, a worker must have a medical evaluation to ensure that he or she is able to use the respirator, a fit test must be done to determine the proper dimensions of the respirator on the worker, and the worker must be trained in the proper use and handling of a respirator.

Biological exposures are also common among workers who provide animal care in zoos, farms, or research facilities where studies are completed on animals such as rats, mice, and monkeys. Work in wet environments (such as chicken- or meat-processing facilities) may increase exposure to fungal diseases.

Psychological Exposures

Work has changed dramatically in the United States as a result of greater competition for goods and services. Globalization is increasing the speed and demand for products, and the information technology field has altered communication practices. Outsourcing of jobs to developing countries, layoffs, and downsizing have changed job security. These changing trends affect the physical and psychological well-being of workers, and outcomes may include hypertension, cardiovascular disease, gastrointestinal disease, alcoholism, difficulty sleeping, workplace violence, hostility, depression, low productivity, and absenteeism.[38]

Job Stress

Job stress is the harmful physical and emotional response that occurs when the requirements of the job do not match the capabilities, resources, or needs of the worker.[20] Two job-stress models demonstrate strong associations between work stress and disease. The Demand Control Model developed by Karasek and colleagues describes the relationship between job demands and job control.[39] The job demands variable examines the pace and intensity of work, and job control relates to the ability of the worker to direct and manage work. When work involves a high level of demand with low level of control, job strain can result in physiological and psychological changes in the worker, particularly cardiovascular disease risk.[39-41]

A third variable, social support at work, added to the Demand Control Model by Johnson and Hall, affirms that the level of job strain may be reduced by the protective effect of social support from coworkers and supervisors.[42] Examples of situations that are stressful include the employee in a supermarket who must check and bag groceries quickly and efficiently (high demand) under the watchful eye of a supervisor, who records the number of customers assisted without the development of long lines (control). Another example is the catalogue "800" operator, who is recorded and timed for speed and courtesy when taking orders (high demand/low control).

A second work stress model, the Effort-Reward-Imbalance Model, builds on the concept of job demands and includes the amount of effort invested by a worker in the job.[43] It is hypothesized that mental distress and negative health outcomes develop when a high degree of effort is not returned by any reward such as a promotion, a pay raise, or increased status in the company.

To assist workers in coping with stressful conditions at work or within the family, workplaces may employ psychologists, social workers, counselors, or psychiatric-mental health clinical nurse specialists, or they may contract with an **employee assistance program (EAP)**.[44] The benefit of an EAP is that it allows employees to discuss work, financial, or social issues in a confidential setting. Health promotion programs may also assist the worker to cope with stressful situations by encouraging regular physical exercise, relaxation, or meditation to reduce workers' psychosocial stress.[45]

Routes of Exposure

There are three body systems that can serve as routes of exposure to hazardous substances found in the workplace:

- Lungs
- Skin
- Gastrointestinal tract

Inhalation of substances (i.e., gases, particles, carbon monoxide, solvents) into the lungs may cause local or systemic effects. The upper respiratory tract protects the lungs by filtering large particles in the nose and via the cilia, but respirable particles that range from 1 to 10 microns in diameter still can be inhaled into the lower respiratory tract. Factors that may increase absorption of respirable particles include faster respiratory rate and greater depth of respiration.

Pesticides, solvents, and cleaning agents are examples of agents absorbed through inhalation as well as through the skin (dermatological absorption). Damage to the epidermis or exposure to a lipid soluble substance (solvent) increases absorption. Ingestion of particles into the gastrointestinal tract may occur by eating or smoking in the workplace. Providing a separate location for workers to consume meals and take breaks reduces this exposure. Although ingestion is the least common source of exposure, transfer of toxins by hand-to-mouth activity can be reduced by proper hand hygiene.

Controlling Hazards and Injuries in the Workplace

An effective OSH program can be accomplished by controlling hazards and preventing injuries in the workplace. Two strategies to achieve this goal are incorporating principles of ergonomics and adopting a **hierarchy of controls.**

Ergonomics

One approach to reducing injuries is to apply the field of **ergonomics,** which incorporates the science of biomechanics, to design work that is less demanding of a worker's joints, back, and muscles to prevent injury. An ergonomist designs the job to fit the worker, rather than physically forcing the worker's body to fit the job. There is increased ergonomic risk associated with jobs that require repetitive, forceful, or prolonged exertions of the hands; frequent heavy lifting, pushing, pulling, or carrying of heavy objects; or prolonged awkward postures. Workers with these types of jobs have greater risk of developing musculoskeletal problems such as back pain, carpal tunnel syndrome, and tendonitis. Examples of workers who may have ergonomic risks are meat and poultry processors; grocery store checkout personnel; and nursing home staff whose jobs involve bathing, turning, and walking patients. Workstations, tools, and equipment can be adapted to fit the worker and reduce the physical stress on a worker's body. Additional examples of tasks that have ergonomic risks include the following:

- Lifting heavy or awkward items
- Pushing or pulling heavy loads without assistance
- Being exposed to excessive vibration
- Using excessive force to perform tasks
- Repeating the same motion throughout the workday
- Working in awkward or stationary positions
- Maintaining the same posture for long periods of time
- Using the body or a body part to press against hard or sharp edges
- Cold temperatures
- Combined exposures to several risk factors[46]

In addition to chemical, psychological, and physical exposures for our case study individual, Juan, ergonomic issues also are of concern. Repeatedly lifting heavy baskets of fruits and vegetables can result in musculoskeletal problems, possibly leading to long-term problems.

Hierarchy of Controls

Occupational health providers can use a systematic process known as the hierarchy of controls to control workplace hazards. There are five levels of control: (1) elimination or substitution, (2) engineering controls, (3) warning, (4) administrative controls, and (5) PPE.[47]

The most effective level of control is the elimination or substitution of a hazardous material, task, or process. For example, benzene is an aromatic solvent used in many industrial products such as glues, paints, gasoline, and rubber, and can cause changes in the production of white cells in the bone marrow, leading to leukemia. Benzene can be eliminated by substituting toluene, a less toxic solvent.

If elimination or substitution is not possible, the next most effective strategy is the implementation of engineering controls. Isolation of a hazard is an example of an engineering control. For example, in the past, antineoplastic agents were mixed by nurses at workstations without ventilation hoods. Based on research findings that cited reproductive effects, these agents are now mixed under properly ventilated hoods in the pharmacy.[48]

A third-line strategy is warnings. OEHNs can place warning signs in higher risk areas. For example, a yellow-taped walkway on the floor of a bottling plant can remind forklift operators of the potential for employees to be walking along a given path. Another example is a mandated sign that warns of radioactive exposures found in hospitals where radioactive isotopes or radiation producing machines are located.

Use of administrative controls is a fourth strategy of hazard control. Job rotation is an example of how one may reduce overexposure of workers in the nuclear power industry to radiation. Hygienic work practices and good housekeeping, such as frequent floor washing in dust-producing industries, reduce the hazard of respirable particles from entering the air. The most important administrative control may be the training and education of workers so that they are knowledgeable about hazards present in the workplace. Educational materials must be culturally sensitive and produced at an appropriate cognitive and literacy level for workers. In addition, materials may need to be provided in multiple languages.

The least effective level of control, yet still important, involves the use of PPE. Hard hats, masks, respirators, gloves, hearing protection (ear muffs or ear plugs), gowns, metal-toed shoes, and head gear are examples of PPE. In the hierarchy of controls, PPE is least effective, primarily because worker compliance is difficult to ensure. Equipment may interfere with movement, hearing, and comfort, and may be cumbersome and hot if worn properly for 8 hours, leading workers to use PPE incorrectly or not at all. Therefore, close supervision of worker compliance with PPE is important.

Workplace Assessment (Workplace Walkthrough)

As an OEHN, regularly scheduled assessments with members of the occupational health team are important. The purpose of the **workplace assessment** or **workplace walkthrough** is to observe the operations taking place in a facility, to observe workers performing their jobs, to identify the use of engineering controls, to view the use of equipment (moving and stationary) in work areas, and to observe the physical layout and cleanliness of the facility including locker rooms, hand washing stations, changing facilities, and break and lunch rooms. During the walkthrough, the OEHN should also engage managers, supervisors, and individual workers in discussions about their work and safety and health issues.

● APPLYING PUBLIC HEALTH SCIENCE

The Case of the Pottery Factory Walkthrough

Public Health Science Topics Covered:

- Epidemiology and biostatistics

John is an OEHN at a large pottery-making facility with 452 workers. The building is located in a rural area and is the size of three football fields. It includes the kiln, storage of sand and silica, machines for pottery production, paints and glazes, heavy equipment, workstations and an inventory of finished pottery. The occupational health clinic is located in a separate administration building adjacent to the main facility.

As he walks to the plant on a beautiful summer day, John observes a truck being loaded with boxes of pottery. At the plant, the kiln is in use and the plant temperature is 91°F. Machines are mixing the clay and workers are providing the materials for this process. (Many of the materials are stored in 50-pound bags.) The clay is then transferred to machines that form plates, cups, and other items, which are then stored on drying racks. Once the pottery is dry, small teams of four to six workers stand at a workstation and manually place handles on the cups or smooth the edges of the pottery to prepare the items for glazing. The last process he observes is the decoration of the pottery in a clean room where workers sit at large tables applying decals or painting the pottery with small brushes. As John walks through the plant, he observes continuous activity and notices that a pathway is painted to denote safe travel routes by machinery and walkers. Small electric carts transfer materials to workstations throughout the plant and honk their horns at workers on foot. The plant is noisy and it is not air conditioned; John can hear the loud ventilation system.

Production in this plant occurs around the clock. However, the night shift employs only 25 workers to repair equipment in the plant. Workers on the day shift and evening shift are allowed 30 minutes for lunch or dinner and an additional 20-minute break.

Following the walkthrough, management requests that John write a summary report of his findings (Box 21-4). The report would consist of a summary and recommendations regarding the strengths and weakness of the OSH program, medical surveillance, emergency response, and record keeping. It would be followed by an action plan for management.

A summary of John's report and action plan follows:

No obvious hazardous substances were identified. There is a risk that small molecules known as particulates are being released into the air during the manufacturing process of the pottery. Measurements need to be taken by the industrial hygienist to determine whether employees are inhaling the particulates. If particulates are found, masks will need to be fitted to and worn by workers to prevent the inhalation of particulates. Employees are at risk for low back injuries while lifting bags of pottery

The OEHN report needs to address the following questions:

1. What are the hazardous exposures (physical, biological, chemical, and psychosocial) present in the plant?
2. What are the specific mechanisms of exposure (inhalation, ingestion, dermal) in the plant?
3. What physical and chemical exposures should be evaluated by the occupational/environmental hygienist who accompanied the OEHN on the walkthrough?
4. What types of accidents and injuries would the OEHN anticipate in this plant? What are the potential causes?
5. Are hierarchies of control followed in this plant? What PPEs are appropriate?
6. What is the level of housekeeping within the plant? (For example, are floors wet or cluttered? Are there other fall hazards?)
7. Are workers provided training and information regarding the hazards of their work? Do employees demonstrate the safety practices that they received training on?

materials. Optimally, 25-pound bags will be purchased in the future. Workers with lifting responsibilities need to start an exercise program to strengthen their low back muscles and undergo education on proper body mechanics when lifting to prevent a low back injury. Industrial hygienist also needs to take noise measurements to determine whether the noise is excessive and places workers at risk for noise-induced hearing loss. Based on facts reported by the OEHN 72% of all hearing-related illnesses occurs in the manufacturing sector, so a hearing protection program may need to be implemented.[49]

Occupatonal and Environmental History

Another tool used by the OEHN is a comprehensive **occupational and environmental health history**. A physical assessment is conducted on an employee after a formal offer of employment is made. The objective of a history is to identify factors that would increase the health or safety risk of the new employee in performing the new job. Findings from the history may require work accommodations, an in-depth physical exam, and/or further screenings. For example, a new employee who worked in a plant assembling small toys by hand for the past 15 years is at risk for carpal tunnel syndrome. Further assessment of carpal tunnel syndrome and possibly job rotation may be necessary to prevent the onset or worsening of the disorder. The health history must

remain confidential and accessible only to the occupational health team.

To perform an adequate history, the OEHN needs a formal job description that identifies the job tasks required of the employee and the job exposures that the worker will have. A careful analysis of the job description and the worker's capabilities and current health status facilitates the proper placement of the new employee. For example, an individual who had a prior back injury should not be placed in a position requiring heavy lifting. An individual with well-controlled diabetes may not do well with frequent alternating shift work. An individual with cardiovascular disease should avoid work in confined spaces as well as exposure to carbon monoxide and solvents. When a worker returns to work after an injury or the diagnosis and treatment of an acute or chronic disease, a new history and assessment are necessary to determine the need for accommodation.

Key components of the history are:

- The review of systems
- A personal and family health history
- A psychosocial history
- Past medical history

Following the occupational history, a physical assessment is performed by a licensed occupational health practitioner. Specialized exams may be required for different job descriptions. For example, if a worker drives trucks across the country, the Department of Transportation requires an annual exam that includes an audiometric exam, vision testing, depth perception, a complete blood count, blood chemistry, urinalysis for drugs, and an electrocardiogram.

Finally, when the history and physical exam are completed, a discussion of the results with the employee should occur and recommendations regarding safety and health practices should be provided. The new employee should be encouraged to use the resources provided by the occupational health program to maintain, protect, and promote his/her health during employment.

Vulnerable Workers

With the increasing diversity in the U.S. workforce, not everyone goes to work healthy, not everyone goes to work free of stress, and not everyone goes to work in a friendly, accepting environment. This next section describes **vulnerable worker populations** who may be affected by demographic, social, physical, psychological, and economic factors that lead to potential susceptibility and health disparities in the workplace.

● APPLYING PUBLIC HEALTH SCIENCE

The Case of Adolescent Workers

Public Health Science Topics Covered:

• Social sciences

Stephen is a 17-year-old employed by a heavy equipment rental agency on weekends. He is a reliable and hard-working adolescent and his employer regularly requests him to return equipment to the storage lot and to service and prepare it for rerental. At times, Stephen also drives large tractors and feels privileged to be given the responsibility to do so. Two questions to think about in this case are whether Stephen's employer is compliant with the Fair Labor Standards Act (FLSA) and what developmental issues the employer should consider when assigning Stephen to these more complex tasks.

Adolescence is commonly the first time an individual becomes employed, unless he or she works for parents on a family farm or business. The U.S. Congress passed the FLSA in 1938, which governs the number of hours an adolescent can work and what types of jobs adolescent workers can safely perform.[50] Despite these regulations, approximately 70 adolescents die every year in work-related situations, which are the result of adolescents performing tasks that are not in compliance with the FLSA, including operating hazardous equipment, such as motor vehicles or meat slicers; working late at night or alone; handling hot liquids and grease; and lifting heavy objects.[51,52] In Stephen's case, is his employer compliant with the FLSA? In actuality, this type of work is considered hazardous work and is restricted by the FLSA until a worker is 18 years old.

A cross-sectional study conducted by Runyan and colleagues documented risks to adolescents that included exposures to chemical, physical, and biological agents.[53] Of note in this study are significant findings related to the absence of use of PPE, even after work orientation and training of the adolescents.[54] In general, adolescents are employed in part-time, temporary, low-paying jobs in the service sector. As new workers, they are often inexperienced, are unfamiliar with job tasks, lack knowledge of workplace hazards, and are frequently unaware of their rights as workers. Assessment of the physical characteristics of an adolescent is an important consideration, because growth spurts occur between the ages of 14 and 17, especially among males. Taller and more muscular males may be given adult tasks with minimal regard to

experience or maturity. The common psychological characteristics of the adolescent include enthusiasm; however, a sense of invulnerability may increase risk for injury. Communication skills and self-esteem may also be underdeveloped and interactions with customers and supervisors may be challenging.[55,56] Stephen's physical size, coordination, sense of invulnerability, and responsible demeanor may give his employer a false sense of security. Stephen may not have the skills and decision-making ability to work with heavy equipment, even though it may seem like an exciting opportunity to him.

The benefits of employment for adolescents include the development of self-reliance, self-esteem, and discipline as well as organizational and communication skills. However, research by educators has demonstrated that negative effects occur when an adolescent works more than 20 hours per week and has less time for participation in extracurricular school activities and limited time for interaction with peers and family activities.[57] Educators have also found that work among adolescents leads to fatigue and inadequate time for completion of homework.[55]

It has been documented that working adolescents may not enroll in rigorous courses such as math and science because busy work schedules or long work hours may result in absenteeism. Increased disposable income also may promote the use of alcohol, illicit drugs, and smoking. Exposures to hazardous agents (e.g., carcinogens, noise, or heavy physical labor) early in life may have acute or long-term (latent) effects on disease development later in life. For the OEHN, education and training of working adolescents can be facilitated by communicating with employers, parents, school personnel, and the teen. OSHA developed a Web site for teen workers that promotes health and safety and provides information regarding hazards, PPE, and the details of the FLSA.[55]

Aging Workers

The baby boomer generation, those individuals born between 1946 and 1964, are contributing to the aging pool of workers. The healthy lifestyles of many of these workers has improved life expectancy and extended working life. The trend of working beyond age 65 years is also influenced by the 1983 Social Security Amendment, which raised full retirement age (eligibility for 100% Social Security benefits) beginning with individuals born in 1938 or later. For example, an individual born in 1960 would not be eligible for full Social Security retirement until age 67.[58,59]

Older workers may be motivated to remain employed owing to various factors such as financial need, family responsibilities, a sense of job satisfaction and purpose, productivity, social engagement, and the ability to use skills and knowledge developed over the years. Alternatively, an individual with fewer years of education may select retirement at an earlier age because they began working in their early teens and twenties and have saved for retirement. Or, a physically demanding job (such as construction, mining, or farming) may have resulted in musculoskeletal injury or the development of a chronic disease that stimulates early retirement.[60]

The physical and psychological changes that occur with the aging process may have an impact on the duration of work life, such as decreased physical strength and endurance, loss of bone density and flexibility, fatigue, slower reaction time, increased vision and hearing deficits, and changes in balance and coordination.[61] In addition to the normal anatomical and physiological changes of aging, older workers may have a chronic disease as a result of their past work exposures or lifestyle behaviors, which may limit their employment opportunities. Older workers may be more vulnerable to falls and trauma. Frequently among injured older workers, recovery time for an injury is lengthened and return to work is delayed. The OEHN needs to assess risk of injury and recommend ergonomic changes that adjust the work environment to the aging worker's capability, such as improved lighting, audible or flashing safety signals, reduction of repetitive tasks and use of force.[62]

Enrollment of older workers in fitness programs also preserves and builds muscle strength, prevents loss of bone density, and improves aerobic capacity and cardiopulmonary function. Workplace health promotion programs provide nutrition education, weight control instructions, risk factor reduction guidelines for cardiovascular disease and cancer, and assistance for individuals to adapt to and manage noncommunicable disease.[63]

Women Workers

Approximately 51% of workers in the United States are women, of whom 75% work full-time. Median earnings of women are gradually increasing; however, on average their salaries are 80% of a man's earnings. The number of working women with college degrees has more than tripled since 1970, allowing women to enter professional and management positions.[64] The majority of women are employed in the service and health-care sectors, where multiple hazards exist, including ergonomic hazards (lifting), chemicals (antineoplastics, anesthetic gases, latex), biological agents (bloodborne pathogens), and psychosocial hazards (stress, violence).

As women have entered nontraditional employment, such as construction, engineering, and forestry, their vulnerability to injury has increased. PPE is often designed for the average-sized man, so fit of the equipment often becomes an issue for women workers. In addition, a woman's total body strength is generally two-thirds of a man's (being lower than a man's in the upper extremities and similar to a man's in the lower extremities), placing many women workers at risk for musculoskeletal injuries. Women workers are often employed in sedentary jobs with computer and keyboarding responsibilities, and proper ergonomic assessment of a workstation identifies modifications to prevent musculoskeletal and repetitive motion disorders.[65] Social stressors such as sexual harassment and gender-based discrimination are sometimes problematic.

Finally, as with all workers, the **work-family interface** must be considered. Women workers, in particular, remain the predominant individuals balancing work and family life. As such, shift work, weekend work, and the total number of hours worked frequently present challenges.[66]

Disabled Workers

The Americans With Disabilities Act (ADA) of 1990 (amended in 2008) is landmark legislation that prohibits workplace discrimination of a qualified individual with a **disability.** [67] It has promoted the hiring of individuals with disabilities and has mandated accommodations for disabled workers. The ADA defines disability as meeting three criteria.[67] First, there must be a physical or mental impairment that substantially limits one or more major life activities of such individual. For example, military personal returning from war may have one or more amputated extremities that prevent their ability to independently perform activities of daily living. Second, there needs to be a record of such impairment. Records can be obtained from the worker's personal physician or nurse practitioner or from a state agency that certified the disability. Third, the person needs to be regarded as having impairment, meaning that the disability would affect the person's ability to perform a job without accommodation.

According to the U.S. Bureau of Labor Statistics, approximately 5 million people with disabilities were employed in 2009.[68] These workers represent about 4% of the employed population, and are employed predominately in the service sector and in professional occupations.

Work eligibility for an individual with a disability is defined as the ability to perform the essential functions of the job. These functions must be defined by each workplace and be on record. After a job offer is made, a disabled individual may request accommodations from the employer. Examples include job restructuring, so that long periods of standing do not occur, or the provision of a large computer monitor for an individual with visual impairments. The ADA also provides for workers who become disabled during the course of employment, after which the worker may request an accommodation (e.g., change in hours worked).

A primary role of the OEHN is to support an individual with a disability to maintain work and to assist the worker who has developed an acute or chronic injury or illness to return to work. Assessing the social, demographic, occupational, clinical, and psychological factors unique to the worker will facilitate maintenance of employment. For example, an individual with diabetes and hypertension who is recovering from a myocardial infarction may need an accommodation to participate in a cardiac rehabilitation program. An older worker may require assistance with lifting and walking duties following a hip replacement, or a worker with a leg thrombosis might be allowed to telecommute 2 to 3 days per week to reduce commuting time.

Immigrant or Foreign-Born Workers

In 2012, the U.S. labor force included 25 million immigrant workers who made up 16.1% of the labor force.[69] These workers are predominantly men and foreign born (48.3% Hispanic and 23.7% Asian) and account for one-half of the labor force increase in 2007. In addition, about 25% of these workers are not high school graduates.

Individuals and families migrate for many reasons: to provide a better life for their family, to escape war, to seek political asylum, or to obtain a job as a scientist or health-care provider. Approximately 25% of working immigrant men work in agricultural or production jobs, and 33% of working immigrant women are employed in service sector occupations (hotel workers, cooks, servers, dry-cleaning workers). These workers are a vital part of the labor force in the United States, although the Bureau of Labor Statistics predicts a job decline of these workers in the coming decade because of changes in immigration laws.[70]

As members of the U.S. labor force, immigrant workers often have physically demanding jobs that expose them to hazards such as pesticides, cleaning agents, farm animals, infectious diseases, or excessive heat or cold, which place them in jeopardy of sustaining poisonings, disease, and physical injuries.[71] In general, immigrants are poorly paid and many live below the poverty level. For further investigation of the factors that influence immigration, see the U.S. Department of State, U.S. Citizenship

and Immigration Services, and the U.S. Department of Labor Web sites. Having the knowledge to assist immigrants with the basic needs of shelter, food, health care, and employment helps with major issues related to this worker population.[71] Another important consideration is the cultural needs of foreign-born workers. There are special considerations for OEHNs when working at organizations employing immigrants. First, health and safety outreach training programs need to be in compliance with OSHA standards for immigrant workers. Outreach training programs educate workers on their rights and responsibilities for helping create a safe workplace.[72] Programs also show workers how to file complaints. Education and signage in the workplace needs to be provided in the native languages of workers for whom English is a second language. In addition, the education and signage should be culturally appropriate. Assessment of understanding may need to be conducted through the use of interpreters, language phone lines, written or oral surveys written in the workers' native languages, and observation of adherence to safe work practices. Ideally, education and on-the-job training will be conducted by bilingual coworkers.

Minority Workers

In general, workers of minority, ethnic, and racial populations are disproportionally exposed to poor working conditions, limited health-care access, and reduced career opportunities. Factors associated with such disadvantages include lack of educational and economic opportunities as well as the unfortunate persistence of discriminatory practices by some employers. There are greater proportions of minority workers in some of the most dangerous industries, such as construction and agriculture, where there is a heavy reliance on the labor of recent immigrants. Additionally, there are several historical and current examples of manufacturing settings that pose greater risks to minority worker populations. Examples from the past include textile factories, in which cotton dust caused increased rates of byssinosis in workers who were primarily African American, and uranium mining, which placed Native American miners at risk for pulmonary cancer.

Even within a single industry, it is often the minority workers who hold the dirtiest, highest risk jobs. An example comes from the hospitality industry, a work setting that may not immediately come to mind as one that is risky to a worker's health. But if one looks at the demographic distribution of hotel workers by job title, minority workers are overrepresented in the lowest paid jobs with the highest exposures to hazards. The tasks of a hotel housekeeper include handling trash and working with cleaning products as well as the ergonomic stressors of lifting, bending, and working in awkward postures to change linen.[73] Furthermore, these job activities must be carried out under working conditions that impose even more stress—time pressures related to meeting quotas, questionable social support, and threatened job security—with little power to advocate for an improved working environment.

Workers of minority groups are also disproportionately represented among those who are unable to find employment. The unemployment rates in the United States vary from 13.7% for African Americans, 9.1% for Latinos, to 6.6% for whites and 5% for Asians.[74] There is a clear need to promote fair employment practices and safe and equitable working conditions for all who are eligible to be part of the workforce.

Roles of the OEHN

Occupational Disease Surveillance

The OEHN has important responsibilities for assessing, monitoring, and providing surveillance for occupational diseases. A working knowledge of **toxicology,** "the study of the adverse effects of chemical, physical or biological agents on living organisms and the ecosystem, including the prevention and amelioration of such adverse effects," and the common diseases unique to the specific occupational health settings is essential.[75] Tables 21-1 and 21-2

TABLE 21–1	Examples of Occupational Exposures and Effects	
Symptoms and Diseases *Immediate or Short-Term Effects*	**Agent**	**Potential Exposures**
Dermatoses (allergic or irritant)	Metals (chromium, nickel), fibrous glass, solvents, caustic alkali, soaps	Electroplating, metal cleaning, plastics, machining, leather tanning, housekeeping
Headache	Carbon monoxide, solvents	Firefighting, automobile exhaust, wood finishing, dry cleaning
Acute psychoses	Lead, mercury, carbon disulfide	Removing paint from old houses, fungicide, wood preserving, viscose rayon industry
Asthma or dry cough	Formaldehyde, toluene diisocyanate, animal dander	Textiles, plastics, polyurethane kits, lacquer, animal handling
Pulmonary edema, pneumonitis	Nitrogen oxides, phosgene, halogen gases, cadmium	Welding, farming, chemical operations, smelting
Cardiac arrhythmias	Solvents, fluorocarbons	Metal cleaning, solvents use, refrigerator maintenance
Angina	Carbon monoxide, methylene chloride	Car repair, traffic exhaust, foundry, wood finishing
Abdominal pain	Lead	Battery making, enameling, smelting, painting, welding, ceramics, plumbing
Hepatitis (may become a long-term effect)	Halogenated hydrocarbons (e.g., carbon tetrachloride)	Solvents use, lacquer use, hospital workers
Latent or Long-Term Effects		
Chronic dyspnea, pulmonary fibrosis	Asbestos, silica, beryllium, coal, aluminum	Mining, insulation, pipefitting, sandblasting, quarrying, metal alloy work, aircraft or electrical parts
Chronic bronchitis, emphysema	Cotton dust, cadmium, coal dust, organic solvents, cigarettes	Textile industry, battery production, soldering, mining, solvent use
Lung cancer	Asbestos, arsenic, nickel, uranium, coke oven emissions	Insulation, pipefitting, smelting, coke ovens, shipyard workers, nickel refining, uranium mining
Bladder cancer	β-naphthylamine, benzidine dyes	Dye industry, leather, rubber-workers, chemists
Peripheral neuropathy	Lead, arsenic, hexane, methyl butyl ketone, acrylamide	Battery production, plumbing, smelting, painting, shoemaking, solvent use, insecticides

TABLE 21–1 Examples of Occupational Exposures and Effects—cont'd

Symptoms and Diseases	Agent	Potential Exposures
Behavioral changes	Lead, carbon disulfide, solvents, mercury, manganese	Battery makers, smelting, viscose rayon industry, degreasing, manufacture/repair of scientific instruments, dental amalgam workers
Extrapyramidal syndrome	Carbon disulfide, manganese	Viscose rayon industry, steel production, battery production, foundry
Aplastic anemia, leukemia	Benzene, ionizing radiation	Chemists, furniture refinishing, cleaning, degreasing, radiation workers

Source: Adapted from the Agency for Toxic Substances and Disease Registry. (2008). *Case studies in environmental medicine: Taking an exposure history.* Retrieved from http://www.atsdr.cdc.gov/csem/exphistory/docs/exposure_history.pdf.

TABLE 21–2 Organ Systems Often Affected by Toxic Exposure

Organ/System	Exposure Risks
Respiratory	Asbestos, radon, cigarette smoke, glues
Skin	Dioxin, nickel, arsenic, mercury, cement (chromium), polychlorinated biphenyls (PCBs), glues, rubber cement
Liver	Carbon tetrachloride, methylene chloride, vinyl chloride
Kidney	Cadmium, lead, mercury, chlorinated hydrocarbon solvents
Cardiovascular	Carbon monoxide, noise, tobacco smoke, physical stress, carbon disulfide, nitrates, methylene chloride
Reproductive	Lead, carbon disulfide, methylmercury, ethylene dibromide
Hematological	Arsenic, benzene, nitrates, radiation
Neuropsychological	Tetrachloroethylene, mercury, arsenic, toluene, lead, methanol, noise, vinyl chloride

Source: Adapted from the Agency for Toxic Substances and Disease Registry. (2008). *Case studies in environmental medicine: Taking an exposure history.* Retrieved from http://www.atsdr.cdc.gov/csem/exphistory/docs/exposure_history.pdf.

provide descriptions of common occupational and environmental exposures, the organ systems that are affected, the signs and symptoms, and diseases that are caused by these agents. Latent and long-term effects of these exposures and the organ systems involved are described.

Preventing Injuries and Fatalities

Approximately 3.9 million workers are injured on the job annually and about 12 workers die each day as a result of traumatic injuries they have sustained.[76] In the United States alone, 3.9 million nonfatal work-related injuries/illnesses occur annually, with more than 2 million injuries/illnesses requiring a job transfer, work restrictions, or time away from the job. Among all workers, 2.6 million are treated in emergency departments annually, and approximately 110,000 of these workers are hospitalized. Fatalities among workers result from transportation incidents, contact with objects and equipment, assaults and violent acts, falls, and exposure to harmful substances or environments.

During work, nonfatal and fatal injuries occur. Figure 21-1, which displays the causes of nonfatal injuries in the private industry in 2011, shows that the leading sectors where injuries occur are manufacturing, health care, the retail trade, and construction. In Figure 21-2, fatal work injuries are described by cause, with transportation incidents being the highest source of fatality.

Case Management

Case management is an approach to deliver health care in a cost-effective manner.[77] After an employee is injured and/or is recovering from an acute or chronic disease, OEHNs assume a case management role in assessing the worker's disability and rehabilitation needs to promote return to work. The case manager assists with the transition from hospital to home and works with the employee, family members, and rehabilitation specialists (if applicable) in the coordination of the employee's successful return to work.

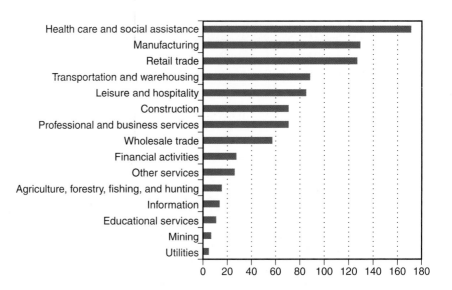

Figure 21-1 Number of nonfatal occupational injuries and illnesses involving days away from work in the private industry (in thousands). *(Data from the Bureau of Labor Statistics, U.S. Department of Labor. [2012, November 8]. News release: Nonfatal occupational injuries and illnesses requiring days away from work, 2011. Retrieved from http://www.bls.gov/news.release/archives/osh2_11082012.pdf.)*

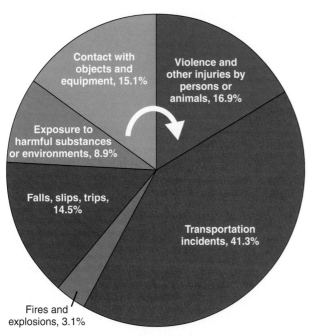

Figure 21-2 Fatal occupational injuries by industry and event or exposure, all U.S., 2011 (total 4,693). *(Data from Bureau of Labor Statistics, U.S. Department of Labor. [2013, April 25]. Fatal occupational injuries by industry and event or exposure, all U.S., 2011. Retrieved from http://www.bls.gov/iif/oshwc/cfoi/cftb0259.pdf.)*

Workers' Compensation

Workers' compensation provides income benefits, medical payments, and rehabilitation payments to workers injured on the job, as well as benefits to surviving families of fatally injured workers. Workers' compensation laws are considered to be no-fault laws. Because these laws ensure that employees who suffer injuries or fatalities as a result of work are provided fixed monetary awards, they eliminate the ability for employees to sue employers for pain and suffering, even if the employer was negligible.[78] However, not all injuries may be identified in the law and may require filing suit to determine reasonable compensation. Each state workers' compensation law regulates the amount and duration of compensation for workers who are injured or who die. In general, most state workers' compensation laws cover medical expenses related to a disability and the cost of job retraining following an injury. A disabled worker receives two-thirds of the normal monthly salary during the disability, and may receive more for permanent physical injuries or if the worker has dependents.[79] The act provides compensation for survivors of employees who die. Although workers' compensation laws are complex, OEHN case managers frequently assist injured workers and families in negotiating the laws.

Workplace Health Promotion

Health promotion programs in the workplace are designed to identify and prevent both occupational and nonoccupational disease and injury, and to educate workers about behaviors that influence health and wellness. The goals of health promotion are designed to:

- Reduce absenteeism
- Increase productivity
- Sustain or increase the level of well-being, self-actualization, and personal fulfillment of a given worker or worker group

The OEHN plays an important part in initiating, conducting, and evaluating health promotion programs. Both employees and employers derive benefits from the participation in and the initiation of a health promotion program, including:

- Reduction in health-care costs and improved injury care
- Increased productivity
- Reduced absenteeism
- Improved sense of well-being among workers
- Management viewed as proactive and invested in workers[80]

The number of health promotion programs being developed by corporations and industries has grown considerably. This increase is believed to be associated with the rising cost of health benefits and services that employer-based health-care programs have experienced over the past decade. Many of these programs are designed to manage noncommunicable health conditions that workers may bring to the workplace. It is also important to educate employers that the top five disease groups (cardiovascular, cancers, cerebrovascular, chronic respiratory disease, and unintentional injuries) are preventable and responsive to behavior change.[81,82]

The workplace provides a stable and captive audience (workers) for health promotion programs. In addition, the workplace can serve as a source of coworker and supervisor social support for positive behavior change.[83] The CDC's report *The Healthier Worksite Initiative* strongly recommends that reducing morbidity associated with behavioral and biological risk factors is a public health priority for the country.[84] The majority of studies completed to date show positive health and financial impacts of worksite health promotion programs over the past three decades.[85–87]

■ EVIDENCE-BASED PRACTICE
Improving the Health-Promoting Activities of Workers[87]

Practice Statement: Employees need to be aware of their health risks in order to make health-promoting lifestyle changes.

Targeted Outcome: Adoption of health-promoting activities such as increased physical activity and reduced tobacco use.

Evidence to Support: Soler and colleagues conducted a systematic review evaluating worksite health promotion programs that used the Assessment of Health Risks with Feedback (AHRF) methodology to determine health program effectiveness.[87] AHRF includes three components: (1) the collection of information about two or more personal health behaviors; (2) a translation of these behaviors into a risk score; and (3) feedback to the employee regarding their risk status, either overall or related to a specific risk behavior.

The effectiveness of the studies was assessed on the basis of change in health behaviors, such as physical activity, dietary behaviors, tobacco use, and physiological indicators (reduction in blood pressure), change in risk estimates, health-care service use, and worker productivity. Fifty-one out of 127 workplace health promotion programs met the criteria for review. Strong or sufficient evidence for meaningful effects was identified on the following outcomes: tobacco use, alcohol use, dietary fat intake, blood pressure, cholesterol, summary health risk estimates, worker absenteeism, and health-care service use.

Recommended Approaches: It is important for an OEHN to consider interventions at the individual and population levels to maximize the adoption of health-promoting behaviors. AHRF may be useful as a component of a comprehensive workplace health promotion program.

Source: Soler, R.E., Leeks, K.D., Razi, S., Hopkins, D.P., Griffith, M., Aten, A., et al. Task Force on Community Preventive Services. (2010). A systematic review of selected interventions for worksite health promotion. The assessment of health risks with feedback. *American Journal of Preventive Medicine,* 38(Suppl. 2), S237-S262.

A **health risk appraisal (HRA)** is frequently the initial component of many successful health promotion programs in the workplace. HRAs are questionnaires completed by employees to assess personal health habits and behavioral risk factors, such as smoking and alcohol or seat belt use. An individual's actual age is compared with an estimate of their risk age, an overall measure of risk for morbidity and mortality as identified by epidemiological research. An example of an individual with a decreased risk age is one who maintains a healthy body mass index, exercises regularly, does not smoke tobacco products, drinks moderately, and complies with an age-appropriate screening schedule as defined by a health-care provider. A worker with an increased risk age may not exercise, is overweight, drives without a seat belt, and does not have a health provider. If a worker is identified with a high-risk age and he or she incorporates healthy lifestyle behavior changes, such as physical exercise or weight reduction, a reduced risk age could be achieved. It is essential that the HRA results are communicated to employees by the OEHN. The worker with the reduced risk age should be commended and encouraged to maintain a healthy lifestyle. The worker at increased risk will need a health assessment, education, and counseling to assist with behavior change, if desired.[88] Effective workplace health promotion programs require a strong leadership and management team that is committed to initiating an effective, evidence-based educational program focused on an individual or worker group. Resources to run an effective program, educators, incentives, and equipment are also essential. Finally, outcome evaluations of the efficacy of the program must be conducted.[88]

Because the occupational health provider is working with adult learners, several important concepts should be considered:[89,90]

- Workers need to volunteer and be receptive to the learning process, rather than a passive recipient.
- Selection of the education content should address the worker's self-identified needs.
- Selection of the education schedule needs to accommodate the worker and eliminate distractions.
- Use active listening.
- Engage in change talk.
- Repetition is a useful teaching technique.
- The learning environment should be pleasant, with progress recognized and encouragement provided.
- Information provided should progress from the simple to the complex, and should be paced appropriately and examples given.

● APPLYING PUBLIC HEALTH SCIENCE

The Case of the Ethical Dilemma

Public Health Science Topics Covered:

- Health service systems

Jorge is a 45-year-old man with a history of diabetes, cardiovascular disease, and obesity. He was recently hospitalized for a myocardial infarction. During his return-to-work assessment, the occupation physician instructed Jorge to begin light exercise daily and start a low-fat, low salt, 2,000 calorie per day diet. Jorge comes to the OEHN clinic for guidance on exercise and diet. The OEHN negotiates with the plant manager to allow Jorge to return from his lunch period 20 minutes late each day so that he can walk on the trail next to the plant. Jorge is also permitted to be "on the clock"

during his walks. Several times during the past week, the OEHN sees Jorge sitting on a bench playing games on his telephone and not walking.

- What is the ethical dilemma posed in this case study?
- What options does the OEHN have to resolve this dilemma?
- What is the best option? Provide a rationale for this option.

OEHNs have a responsibility to their employers to manage employees' illnesses and injuries while reducing overall health-care expenditures. Once the OEHN becomes aware that Jorge is not using the time away from the plant as agreed to by Jorge and the plant manager, the OEHN has a responsibility to notify the plant manager. Prior to notifying the plant manager, the OEHN reviews the American Association of Occupational Health Nurses' Code of Ethics and Interpretive Statements. The code has six principles: (1) right of self-determination, (2) confidentiality, (3) truth telling, (4) doing or producing good, (5) avoiding harm, and (6) fair and nondiscrimatory treatment.[9] The OEHN realizes that there is an ethical dilemma resulting from being aware that Jorge is not taking the walks. The dilemma results from the employer's right to cancel the walk periods if they are not being used appropriately and Jorge's rights to self-determination and confidentiality.

The OEHN considers several options in this case. First, the OEHN could notify the employer that Jorge is not taking the walks. This option violates Jorge's confidentiality. Second, the OEHN could follow Jorge to the walking trail daily and instruct him that he needs to take the walk. This option violates Jorge's right of self-determination. Third, the OEHN could meet with Jorge in the clinic and discuss the current treatment and options. The third option is chosen by the OEHN. During the discussion, the OEHN asks Jorge about his adherence and barriers to walking each day while at work. The OEHN openly shares the rationale for the conversation: They are talking precisely because the OEHN saw him sitting on a bench and not walking. Speaking privately with Jorge also provides for his confidentiality. A new treatment plan is devised that allows for Jorge's right of self-determination. Jorge reports that it is too hot for him in the afternoon to walk. He has agreed to arrive to work early and take his walk before his shift starts. The OEHN will follow up with him in 2 weeks to evaluate his progress.

Emerging Issues in Occupational Health

Emerging issues in occupational health highlight the need for the OEHN to remain current and knowledgeable about the ever-changing trends in the field. OEHNs can remain up to date on emergency issues by joining professional societies, belonging to occupational-focused online mailing lists, and attending professional conferences dedicated to emerging issues in occupational health. Following the next case study, two significant issues for the future are discussed.

● APPLYING PUBLIC HEALTH SCIENCE

The Case of Popcorn Lung

Public Health Science Topics Covered:

- Epidemiology and biostatistics

Many people like eating microwave popcorn when watching movies at home. Most people would never consider that the flavoring in their microwave popcorn has made some workers very sick. In 2000, the Missouri Department of Health and Senior Services received a report about eight cases of lung disease in workers who had formerly all worked in the same microwave popcorn factory between 1992 and 2000. Four of these workers were on waiting lists for lung transplants.[91] After a Health Hazard Investigation by NIOSH, it was determined that the fixed obstructive lung disease, or bronchiolitis obliterans (BO), was caused by exposure to the food flavoring diacetyl.

Diacetyl is a water-soluble di-ketone found naturally in butter, coffee, wine, and beer. The chemical diacetyl has butter-flavored characteristics and is used in candies, pastries, and frozen foods. The problem occurs in the manufacturing of the microwave popcorn, because diacetyl easily vaporizes when heated. The workers with the highest rates of BO were the mixers and the microwave-packaging workers. The mixers worked around large mixing tanks, where visible dust, aerosols, and vapors were produced. The microwave packers worked within 5 to 30 meters from the mixing tanks. On inspection, NIOSH required these groups of workers to use respirators.[91,92] In December 2003, a NIOSH alert was sent to more than 4,000 businesses that use food flavorings in their manufacturing processes, advising employers to reduce vapors in the mixing room and to warn workers of the hazard.[93]

Emergency Preparedness and Disaster Management

Frequently, a business will ask its OEHN to prepare an emergency response plan to respond to human-created and natural disasters. In large corporations, this planning is usually done by a committee that includes the OEHN as well as management, human resources, security, and other support services staff. Whether the OEHN works at a large company or a small business, emergency preparedness or "all hazards" preparedness is a continuous and coordinated process that must be constantly evaluated and redefined as needed to ensure the safety of the workforce in response to a disaster.[94]

Knowledge of the five components of disaster preparedness is an important element for planning a disaster response. Four of the five components include (1) the preparedness phase, in which the capacity to respond to a disaster is evaluated and assured; (2) the response phase, in which support is provided to persons and communities; (3) the recovery phase, which describes the time when systems are returned to a predisaster functional state; and (4) the mitigation phase, in which a disaster may be prevented or the effects of an event may be minimized.[95] The following questions serve to provide basic assessment information:

- How will the OEHN communicate with employees who are onsite and off-site?
- Are there employees with disabilities and what are their needs in an emergency situation?
- What types of emergency supplies are needed and for what period of time?
- If everyone must leave the site, how will the OEHN evacuate the area?
- If it is necessary for everyone to shelter in place, what supplies are needed to accommodate everyone?
- Are fire plans up to date?
- Is the OEHN prepared for all types of medical emergencies?
- Has the OEHN coordinated plans with other businesses in the area?

The fifth component is evaluation. At the conclusion of a disaster event, it is important to conduct a formal evaluation to identify areas for further improvement and preparedness prior to another disaster.

An OEHN should review and evaluate an emergency preparedness plan at least once every year and ensure that employees' families have a plan for their home. It is often necessary for employees to remain at the worksite as a result of an emergency, and fear for the location of and safety of family members is often of concern.

Another important component of the disaster is the psychological effect that each employee may experience, and an awareness that symptoms of acute anxiety and post-traumatic stress may be outcomes for workers and for workers providing disaster care to victims. The U.S. Federal Emergency Management Association offers a comprehensive guide for businesses that want to develop a preparedness plan.[96] An additional resource for the OEHN is Wisniewski et al.'s *Areas of Competency for Emergency Preparedness*.[97]

"Green" Jobs

The term "green jobs" represents the effort to create employment in the field of renewable and efficient energy production. The topic of green jobs has evolved from two important issues facing the United States in the 21st century: (1) the need to rebuild the economy after the worst economic crisis since the Great Depression; and (2) the need to develop strategies that will respond to the threat of global climate change. Green jobs are designed to preserve or enhance environmental quality and build a clean energy environment, but green jobs are not always new jobs. The goal of this movement is to build a clean energy environment by several methods: (1) to invest in sources of renewal energy, such as wind turbines and solar power generation; and (2) to increase energy efficiency by investments in mass transit and modern infrastructure.[98] Because many of the concepts described above must be done locally by local workers, another important goal of the clean energy economy is to prevent jobs from moving out of the United States. The most important goals of the clean energy economy are job creation, economic growth, the growth of new industries, and innovation that will end the dependence of the United States on polluting and costly fossil fuels, as well as creating strategies for solving global climate change.[98] Many of the occupational risks associated with green jobs may not be known for years, indicating the need for the OEHN to be vigilant in risk assessments of the worker population and remaining current with notices on new risk patterns.

■ Summary Points

- Occupational health is focused on the maintenance and promotion of workers' health, improving working environments, and developing work organizations and cultures to support health and safety.
- Occupational and environmental health nursing (OEHN) is a specialty nursing practice focused on health and safety programs and services to workers.

- Two federal agencies that have had an impact on worker health are the National Institute for Occupational Safety and Health (NIOSH) and the Occupational Safety and Health Administration (OSHA).
- Occupational nurses have responsibilities for promoting the health within the workplace by conducting workplace assessments and occupational and environmental health histories.
- Preventing injuries and hazards is dependent on knowledge of exposures, vulnerable worker populations, and using hierarchy of controls.
- Toxicology is the study of adverse effects of chemical, physical, or biological agents on living organisms and the ecosystem.
- The roles of the OEHN include disease surveillance, preventing fatalities and injuries, case management, and health promotion within the workplace.
- Emerging issues in occupational health include emergency preparedness and disaster management and the creation of green jobs.

▲ CASE STUDY
The Case of Tidy Cleaners
Learning Outcomes:

At the end of this case study, the student will be able to:

- Discuss ways to conduct an employee health assessment of the workplace environment.
- Identify potential physical and chemical hazards in the workplace.
- Identify potential peer assistance issues.
- Apply components of health planning, assessment, and program development to the occupational health setting.

As a member of an interprofessional occupational health team, an OEHN, Nancy, was asked to assess the employees working for Tidy Cleaners, a well-respected dry-cleaning business in a large metropolitan area. Initially, Nancy consulted with the manager to obtain the list of chemicals used in the dry-cleaning process and to ascertain the demographics of the employees. During a workday, Nancy then conducted a walkthrough of the site. There were 22 workers who have worked for Tidy Cleaners for an average of 15 years and who ranged in age from 18 to 54 years; the workers were predominantly female. The women frequently sort garments, remove stains, and repair and press clothing after the dry-cleaning process. The males were responsible for the operation (loading and emptying machines) and the repair of the dry-cleaning equipment. One to two employees were available to assist customers when they dropped off or picked up their cleaning and to manage the cash registers. The workforce was composed of Hispanics, many of whom spoke Spanish only, and whites. The hours of operation were from 9 a.m. to 8 p.m., 6 days a week, and employees worked rotating shifts. Ladders were used to transfer cleaned clothing from overhead electric racks when being claimed by customers. The buildings were windowless, except for the entrance, and a series of powerful stationary fans supplemented an old ventilation system.

The manager of Tidy Cleaners reported that the most effective dry cleaning solvent used in his business was perchloroethylene ("perc"), along with carbon tetrachloride.[99] One of the employees, Mr. T, has been absent from work and the manager suspects that Mr. T. is an alcoholic because he frequently arrives at work late and seems to be forgetful. The manager also remarked that he thinks Mr. T.'s suspected heavy alcohol consumption is related to family stress. As a conscientious business owner, the manager stated that he would like Nancy to do an occupational assessment of the plant and to assess the workers for occupational exposures and risks. He stressed that prior to conducting an assessment, consent from each employee must be obtained in writing and the data remain confidential. Nancy was also requested to make recommendations to improve the health and safety in the plant.

1. What hazardous exposures (physical, biological, chemical, and psychosocial) are present in the plant?
2. What are the potential mechanisms of exposure (inhalation, ingestion, dermal) in the plant?
3. What physical and chemical exposures should be further evaluated by an occupational/environmental hygienist?
4. What types of accidents and injuries could Nancy anticipate occuring in this workplace setting? What are the potential causes?
5. Are hierarchies of control followed in this plant? What PPEs are appropriate?
6. What training and information should be provided to workers regarding the hazards of their work? Do employees demonstrate the safety practices that they received training on?

After completing her assessment, Nancy reported the results of screening tests conducted with the workers. After consultation with the occupational physician, Nancy noted that two of the employees have elevated liver enzyme tests: One employee was identified with chronic musculosketal problems, and several workers have chronic skin rashes.

7. What actions could Nancy take to intervene for the workers?
8. Whom would Nancy consult with concerning the elevated liver enzymes, and why?
9. What alterations in the work environment and work processes would Nancy recommend, and why?

REFERENCES

1. Bureau of Labor Statistics, U.S. Department of Labor. (2013). *Economic news release: Employment situation summary table A. Household data, seasonally adjusted.* Retrieved from http://www.bls.gov/news.release/empsit.a.htm.
2. International Labour Office. (2004). *Global strategy on occupational safety and health.* Retrieved from http://www.ilo.org/wcmsp5/groups/public/---ed_protect/---protrav/---safework/documents/policy/wcms_107535.pdf.
3. Occupational Safety and Health Administration, U.S. Department of Labor. (1970). *Occupational Safety and Health Act of 1970, Pub. L. No. 91-596, 84 Stat. 1590, 91st Congress, S.2193.* Retrieved from https://www.osha.gov/pls/oshaweb/owadisp.show_document?p_table=OSHACT&p_id=2743.
4. Taneja, S. (2013). Sustaining work schedules: Balancing leisure and work. *Academy of Strategic Management Journal, 12*(2), 113-122.
5. Gordis, L. (2009). *Epidemiology* (4th ed.). Philadelphia, PA: Elsevier/Saunders.
6. Pope, A.M., Snyder, M.A., Mood, L.H., & Institute of Medicine Committee on Enhancing Environmental Health Content in Nursing Practice. (1995). *Nursing, health & the environment: Strengthening the relationship to improve the public's health.* Washington, DC: National Academies Press.
7. *Healthy People 2020.* (2015). *Topics & objectives: Occupational safety and health.* Retrieved from http://www.healthypeople.gov/2020/topicsobjectives2020/overview.aspx?topicid=30.
8. Salazar, M.K., & American Association of Occupational Health Nurses. (2006). *Core curriculum for occupational & environmental health nursing* (3rd ed.). Philadelphia, PA: Saunders.
9. American Association of Occupational Health Nurses. (2004). AAOHN code of ethics and interpretive statements. *AAOHN Journal, 52*(4), 140-142.
10. American Association of Occupational Health Nurses. (2012). *Standards of occupational & environmental health nursing.* Retrieved from http://www.aaohn.org/aaohn-practice-files.html?download=11:standards-of-practice.
11. Occupational Safety and Health Administration. (2013). *All about OSHA. The 2010 OSHA guide.* Retrieved from http://www.allaboutosha.com/2010-osha-guide.

12. Occupational Safety and Health Administration, U.S. Department of Labor. (2005). *OSHA recordkeeping handbook: The regulation and related interpretations for recording and reporting occupational injuries and illnesses* (OSHA Publication No. 3245-01R). Washington, DC: Author.

13. Centers for Disease Control and Prevention. (2012). *About NORA . . . partnerships, research and practice.* Retrieved from http://www.cdc.gov/niosh/nora/about.html.

14. Centers for Disease Control and Prevention. (2013). *NORA sector agendas.* Retrieved from http://www.cdc.gov/niosh/nora/comment/agendas/.

15. Occupational Safety & Health Administration, U.S. Department of Labor. (n.d.). *Draft proposed safety and health program rule: 29 CFR 1900.1, Docket No. S&H-0027.* Retrieved from http://www.osha.gov/dsg/topics/safetyhealth/nshp.html.

16. Wolff, E.N. (2005). The growth of information workers in the U.S. economy. *Communications of the ACM, 48*(10), 37-42.

17. Winslow, S. (2005). Work-family conflict, gender, and parenthood, 1977–1997. *Journal of Family Issues, 26*(6), 727-755.

18. Bond, J.T., Galinsky, E., & Swanberg, J. (1997). *The 1997 national study of the changing workforce.* New York, NY: Families and Work Institute.

19. Harrington, B.H., Van Deusen, F., & Ladge, J. (2010). *The new dad: Exploring fatherhood within a career context.* Chestnut Hill, MA: Boston College Center for Work & Family.

20. National Institute for Occupational Safety and Health. (2011). *Work organization and stress-related disorders.* Retrieved from http://www.cdc.gov/niosh/programs/workorg/.

21. Yates, M.D. (2009). *Why unions matter* (2nd ed.). New York, NY: Monthly Review Press.

22. Bureau of Labor Statistics, U.S. Department of Labor. (2013). *Economic news release: Union members summary.* Retrieved from http://www.bls.gov/news.release/union2.nr0.htm.

23. Agency for Toxic Substances and Disease Registry, U.S. Department of Health and Human Services. (2015). *Toxicological profile for dichloropropenes.* Retrieved from http://www.atsdr.cdc.gov/toxprofiles/tp40.pdf.

24. Occupational Safety & Health Administration. (n.d.). *Occupational noise exposure.* Retrieved from http://www.osha.gov/SLTC/noisehearingconservation/.

25. Cardarelli, J.J. (2011). Ionizing and non-ionizing radiation. In B.S. Levy, D.H. Wegman, S.L. Baron, & R.K. Sokas (Eds.), *Occupational and environmental health: Recognizing and preventing disease and injury* (6th ed., pp. 345-365). New York, NY: Oxford University Press.

26. Krake, A.M. (2011). Extremes of temperature. In B.S. Levy, D.H. Wegman, S.L. Baron, & R.K. Sokas (Eds.), *Occupational and environmental health: Recognizing and preventing disease and injury* (6th ed., pp. 332-344). New York, NY: Oxford University Press.

27. Cherniack, M.G. (2011). Vibration. In B.S. Levy, D.H. Wegman, S.L. Baron, & R.K. Sokas (Eds.), *Occupational and environmental health: Recognizing and preventing disease and injury* (6th ed., pp. 228-239). New York, NY: Oxford University Press.

28. Cardarelli, J. (2011). Ionizing and nonionizing radiation. In B.S. Levy, D.H. Wegman, S.L. Baron, & R.K. Sokas (Eds.), *Occupational and environmental health: Recognizing and preventing disease and injury* (6th ed., pp. 258-280). New York, NY: Oxford University Press.

29. Agency for Toxic Substances & Disease Registry. (2015). *Toxic substances portal—ionizing radiation.* Retrieved from http://www.atsdr.cdc.gov/toxfaqs/tf.asp?id=483&tid=86.

30. Occupational Safety & Health Administration. (n.d.). *Hazard communication in the 21st century workplace.* Retrieved from http://www.osha.gov/dsg/hazcom/finalmsdsreport.html.

31. Gochfeld, M., & Laumbach, R. (2011). Chemical hazards. In B.S. Levy, D.H. Wegman, S.L. Baron, & R.K. Sokas (Eds.), *Occupational and environmental health: Recognizing and preventing disease and injury* (6th ed., pp. 192-226). New York, NY: Oxford University Press.

32. Agency for Toxic Substances & Disease Registry. (2015). *Toxic substances portal – beryllium.* Retrieved from http://www.atsdr.cdc.gov/toxfaqs/TF.asp?id=184&tid=33.

33. EXTOXNET: Extension Toxicology Network (n.d.). *Toxicology information briefs: Cholinesterase inhibition.* Retrieved from http://pmep.cce.cornell.edu/profiles/extoxnet/TIB/index.html

34. Occupational Safety & Health Administration. (n.d.). *Safety and health topics: Benzene.* Retrieved from http://www.osha.gov/SLTC/benzene/.

35. Russi, M. (2011). Biological hazards. In B.S. Levy, D.H. Wegman, S.L. Baron, & R.K. Sokas (Eds.), *Occupational and environmental health: Recognizing and preventing disease and injury* (6th ed., pp. 281-295). New York, NY: Oxford University Press.

36. Occupational Safety & Health Administration (n.d). *Respiratory protection: Personal protective equipment (1910.134).* Retrieved from https://www.osha.gov/pls/oshaweb/owadisp.show_document?p_id=12716&p_table=STANDARDS

37. National Institute for Occupational Safety and Health. (2014). *Respirator trusted-source information.* Retrieved from http://www.cdc.gov/niosh/npptl/topics/respirators/disp_part/RespSource.html

38. National Institute for Occupational Safety and Health. (1999). *Stress . . . . at work* (NIOSH Publication No. 99-101). Retrieved from http://www.cdc.gov/niosh/docs/99-101.

39. Karasek, R., & Theorell, T. (1990). *Healthy work: Stress, productivity, and the reconstruction of working life.* New York, NY: Basic Books.

40. Schnall, P., Belkic, K., Landsbergis, P., & Baker, D. (2000). Why the workplace and cardiovascular disease? *Occupational Medicine, 15*(1), iii, 1-6.

41. Sauter, S.L., Murphy, L.R., Hurrell, J.J., & Levi, L. (1998). Psychosocial and organizational factors. In J.M. Stellman (Ed.), *ILO encyclopedia of occupational health and safety* (pp. 34.2-34.3). Geneva, Switzerland: International Labour Office.

42. Johnson, J.V., & Hall, E.M. (1988). Job strain, work place social support, and cardiovascular disease: A cross-sectional study of a random sample of the Swedish working population. *American Journal of Public Health, 78*(10), 1336-1342.

43. Siegrist, J. (2000). Place, social exchange and health: Proposed sociological framework. *Social Science & Medicine, 51*(9), 1283-1293.

44. The Employee Assistance Trade Association. (2013). *Employee Assistance best practices.* Retrieved from http://www.easna.org/research-and-best-practices/.

45. Wright, J. (2007). Stress in the workplace: A coaching approach. *Work: A Journal of Prevention, Assessment & Rehabilitation, 28*(3), 279-284.

46. Occupational Safety & Health Administration. (n.d.). *Identify problems.* Retrieved from http://www.osha.gov/SLTC/ergonomics/.

47. International Labour Oganization. (n.d.). *Controlling hazards.* Retrieved from http://actrav.itcilo.org/actrav-english/telearn/osh/hazard/hamain.htm.

48. Connor, T.H., & McDiarmid, M.A. (2006). Preventing occupational exposures to antineoplastic drugs in health care settings. *CA: A Cancer Journal for Clinicians, 56*(6), 354-365.

49. National Institute for Occupational Safety and Health. (2010). *Occupationally-induced hearing loss* (DHHS-NIOSH Publication No. 2010-136). Retrieved from http://www.cdc.gov/niosh/docs/2010-136/pdfs/2010-136.pdf.

50. Wage and Hour Division, U.S. Department of Labor. (n.d.). *Compliance assistance—Wages and Fair Labor Standards Act (FLSA).* Retrieved from http://www.dol.gov/whd/Flsa/index.htm.

51. Windau, J., & Meyer, S. (2005). Occupational injuries among young workers. *Monthly Labor Review Online, 128*(10), 11-23.

52. Morisi, T. (2008). Youth enrollment and employment during the school year. *Monthly Labor Review Online, 131*(2), 51-63.

53. Runyan, C.W., Schulman, M., Dal Santo, J., Bowling, J.M., Agans, R., & Ta, M. (2007). Work-related hazards and workplace safety of U.S. adolescents employed in the retail and service sectors. *Pediatrics, 119*(3), 526-534.

54. Runyan, C.W., Vladutiu, C.J., Rauscher, K.J., & Schulman, M. (2008). Teen workers' exposures to occupational hazards and use of personal protective equipment. *American Journal of Industrial Medicine, 51*(10), 735-740.

55. Steinberg, L.D. (2010). *Adolescence* (9th ed.). New York, NY: McGraw-Hill.

56. Fitzgerald, S.T., & Laidlaw, A.D. (1995). Adolescents and work: Risks and benefits of teenage employment. *AAOHN Journal, 43*(4), 185-189.

57. Barling, J., & Kelloway, E.K. (Eds.). (1999). *Young workers: Varieties of experience.* Washington, DC: American Psychological Association.

58. Occupational Safety & Health Administration. (n.d.) *Young workers: You have rights!* Retrieved from http://www.osha.gov/SLTC/teenworkers/.

59. U.S. Social Security Administration. (n.d). *Retirement age calculator.* Retrieved from http://www.ssa.gov/planners/retire/ageincrease.html

60. Toossi, M. (2009). Labor force projections to 2018: Older workers staying more active. *Monthly Labor Review Online, 132*(11), 30-51.

61. Choi, S.D. (2009). Safety and ergonomic considerations for an aging workforce in the US construction industry. *Work: A Journal of Prevention, Assessment & Rehabilitation, 33*(3), 307-315.

62. Sanders, M.J., & McCready, J. (2009). A qualitative study of two older workers' adaptation to physically demanding work. *Work: A Journal of Prevention, Assessment & Rehabilitation, 32*(2), 111-122.

63. Silverstein, M. (2007). Will you still need me when I'm 64? Designing the age-friendly workplace. *EHS Today.* Retrieved from http://ehstoday.com/safety/ehs_imp_77115/.

64. U.S. Bureau of Labor Statistics. (2013, February). *BLS reports: Women in the labor force: A databook* (BLS Publication No. 1040). Washington, DC: Author.

65. Pierret, C.R. (2006). The "sandwich generation": Women caring for parents and children. *Monthly Labor Review Online, 129*(9), 3-9.

66. U.S. Bureau of Labor Statistics. (2009). *Women in the labor force: A databook* (2009 ed.). Retrieved from http://www.bls.gov/cps/wlf-intro-2009.htm.

67. *United States Department of Justice, Civil Rights Division. Americans With Disabilities Act of 1990, as amended.* Retrieved from http://www.ada.gov/pubs/adastatute08.htm.

68. Bureau of Labor Statistics, U.S. Department of Labor. (2010). *Data on the employment status of people with a disability.* Retrieved from http://www.bls.gov/cps/cpsdisability.htm/.

69. Bureau of Labor Statistics, U.S. Department of Labor. (2013). *News release: Foreign-born workers: Labor force characteristics—2012.* Retrieved from http://www.bls.gov/news.release/pdf/forbrn.pdf.

70. Bureau of Labor Statistics, U.S. Department of Labor. (2012). *Agricultural workers.* Retrieved from http://www.bls.gov/oco/ocos349.htm.

71. McCauley, L.A. (2005). Immigrant workers in the United States: Recent trends, vulnerable populations, and challenges for occupational health. *AAOHN Journal, 53*(7), 313-319.

72. Occupational Safety and Health Administration. (2013). *Outreach training program requirements.* Retrieved from https://www.osha.gov/dte/outreach/program_requirements.pdf.

73. Frumin, E., Moriarty, J., Vossenas, P., Halpin, J., Orris, P., Krause, N., & Punnett, L. (2006). *Workload-related musculoskeletal disorders among hotel housekeepers: Employer records reveal a growing national problem.* Retrieved from http://www.hotelworkersrising.org/pdf/hskpr_analysis0406.pdf.

74. Bureau of Labor Statistics, U.S. Department of Labor. (2013). *News release: The employment situation—June 2013. USDL Publication No. 13-1284.*

75. Society of Toxicology. (2013). *Communiqué*. Retrieved from http://www.toxicology.org/AI/PUB/si05/Si05_Define.asp.

76. National Institute for Occupational Safety and Health. (2013). *Workplace safety & health topics: Traumatic occupational injuries.* Retrieved from http://www.cdc.gov/niosh/injury/.

77. Wassel, M.L., Randolph, J., & Rieth, L.K. (2006). Disability case management. In M.K. Salazar & American Association of Occupational Health Nurses (Eds.), *Core curriculum for occupational & environmental health nursing* (3rd ed., pp. 331-364). Philadelphia, PA: Saunders.

78. Zichello, C., & Sheridan, J. (2008). Occupational health nurses and workers' compensation insurance programs. *AAOHN Journal, 56*(11), 455-458.

79. Strasser, P.B. (2010). Workers' compensation management—changes in Medicare regulations *AAOHN Journal, 58*(5), 217-219.

80. Goetzel, R.Z. (2005). *Policy and practice working group: Examining the value of integrating occupational health and safety and health promotion programs in the workplace.* Retrieved from http://www.google.com/url?sa=t&rct=j&q=&esrc=s&source=web&cd=1&ved=0CCwQFjAA&url=http%3A%2F%2Fwww.saif.com%2F_files%2FCompNews%2FCNexamining.pdf&ei=Q0zzUcCxDJTb4AO-oYHACQ&usg=AFQjCNGXxQoSA-gD3PYmpd32AarFv6v5gg&bvm=bv.49784469,d.dmg&cad=rja.

81. Goetzel, R.Z., Shechter, D., Ozminkowski, R.J., Marmet, P.F., Tabrizi, M.J., & Roemer, E.C. (2007). Promising practices in employer health and productivity management efforts: Findings from a benchmarking study. *Journal of Occupational and Environmental Medicine, 49*(2), 111-130.

82. Sparling, P.B. (2010). Worksite health promotion: Principles, resources, and challenges *Preventing Chronic Disease, 7*(1), A25.

83. Fabius, R., & Frazee, S.G. (2008). The "trusted clinician": An alternative approach to worksite health promotion? *American Journal of Health Promotion, 22*(Suppl. 3), iii, 1-7.

84. Centers for Disease Control and Prevention. (2015). *Healthier worksite initiative: Introduction.* Retrieved from http://www.cdc.gov/nccdphp/dnpao/hwi/index.htm.

85. Pelletier, K.R. (2005). A review and analysis of the clinical and cost-effectiveness studies of comprehensive health promotion and disease management programs at the worksite: Update VI 2000-2004. *Journal of Occupational and Environmental Medicine, 47*(10), 1051-1058.

86. Chapman, L.S., & *American Journal of Health Promotion.* (2005). Meta-evaluation of worksite health promotion economic return studies: 2005 update. *American Journal of Health Promotion, 19*(6), 1-11.

87. Soler, R.E., Leeks, K.D., Razi, S., Hopkins, D.P., Griffith, M., Aten, A., & Task Force on Community Preventive Services. (2010). A systematic review of selected interventions for worksite health promotion: The assessment of health risks with feedback. *American Journal of Preventive Medicine, 38*(Suppl. 2), S237-S262.

88. Anderson, D.R., & Staufacker, M.J. (1996). The impact of worksite-based health risk appraisal on health-related outcomes: A review of the literature. *American Journal of Health Promotion, 10*(6), 499-508.

89. O'Donnell, M., Bishop, C., & Kaplan, K. (1997). Benchmarking best practices in workplace health promotion. *The Art of Health Promotion, 1*(1), 1-8.

90. Huffman, M.H. (2010). Health coaching: A fresh approach for improving health outcomes and reducing costs. *AAOHN Journal, 58*(6), 245-250.

91. Centers for Disease Control and Prevention. (2002). Fixed obstructive lung disease in workers at a microwave popcorn factory—Missouri, 2000–2002. *Morbidity and Mortality Weekly Report, 51*(16), 345-347.

92. Kanwal, R. (2008). Bronchiolitis obliterans in workers exposed to flavoring chemicals. *Current Opinion in Pulmonary Medicine, 14*(2), 141-146.

93. National Institute for Occupational Safety and Health. (2003). *NIOSH alert: Preventing lung disease in workers who use or make flavorings* (DHHS-NIOSH Publication No. 2004-110). Retrieved from http://www.cdc.gov/niosh/docs/2004-110/pdfs/2004-110.pdf.

94. Katz, R., & Mauery, D.R. (2010). Women and public health emergency preparedness. *Women's Health Issues, 20*(1), 3-6.

95. Jakeway, C.C., LaRosa, G., Cary, A., Schoenfisch, S., & Association of State and Territorial Directors of Nursing. (2008). The role of public health nurses in emergency preparedness and response: A position paper of the association of state and territorial directors of nursing. *Public Health Nursing, 25*(4), 353-361.

96. Federal Emergency Management Association. (2013). *Preparedness planning for your business.* Retrieved from http://www.ready.gov/business.

97. Wisniewski, R., Dennik-Champion, G., & Peltier, J.W. (2004). Emergency preparedness competencies: Assessing nurses' educational needs. *Journal of Nursing Administration, 34*(10), 475-480.

98. Hendricks, B., Light, A., & Goldstein, B. (2009). *A green jobs primer: Job creation in a clean energy economy.* Retrieved from http://www.americanprogress.org/issues/2009/04/green_jobs_primer.html.

99. National Institute for Occupational Safety and Health. (2013). *NIOSH pocket guide to chemical hazards.* Retrieved from http://www.cdc.gov/niosh/npg/default.html.

Chapter 22

Public Health Policy and Finance

LEARNING OUTCOMES

After reading this chapter, the student will be able to:

1. Discuss the role of policy in optimizing health for populations.
2. Describe the role of policy in the delivery of health care in the United States.
3. Apply public health principles to public health policy planning.
4. Identify ethical issues related to public health policy.
5. Examine the role of nurses in public health policy.
6. Describe U.S. governmental policies related to the financing of health care.

KEY TERMS

Advocacy
Affordable Care Act
Children's Health Insurance Program (CHIP)
Culturally acceptable health policies
Economics
Effectiveness

Efficiency
Equity
Grants
Health economics
Market economy
Medicaid
Medicare
Policy

Public health economics
Public health finance
Public health policy
Social Security Disability Insurance
Supplemental Nutrition Assistance Program (SNAP)

Supplemental Security Income (SSI)
Temporary Assistance for Needy Families (TANF)
Woman, Infants, and Children (WIC)

■ Introduction

Universal health care for all U.S. citizens may soon be a reality despite much political debate and lobbying. The Patient Protection and **Affordable Care Act** (ACA) was signed into law by President Obama in March 2010 and represents the largest change in the federal health policy since the passing of Medicare and Medicaid legislation in 1965. This major health policy reform was designed to reduce the cost of health care to both individuals and the government by mandating health insurance coverage for all citizens.[1] Some might wonder how anyone could argue with improving access to health care, but as with any policy of this magnitude, the freedom to choose and

individual rights versus government mandates are causes for great debate.

Longest defines **policy** as authoritative governmental decisions that are intended to direct or influence the actions, behaviors, or decisions of others.[2] When authoritative decisions made by agencies and organizations are included, policy is defined as authoritative decisions made in government, agencies, or organizations that are intended to direct or influence the actions, behaviors, or decisions of others. **Public health policy** refers to policies that are specifically intended to direct or influence actions, behaviors, or decisions that influence the health of populations.

For the nursing profession, public health policy is a two-way street. It not only affects nurses in their own personal and professional lives; it is also an explicit part of the nurse's professional role of advocacy. **Advocacy** often takes the form of actively engaging in strategies to effect policies that improve the health of populations, especially those who are experiencing disparity. As noted in Chapter 1, nurses are responsible for identifying, interpreting, and implementing public health laws, regulations, and policies.[3] Public health policy activities engaged in by nurses across settings and specialties include investigations of situations reported to public health officials, or monitoring and inspecting regulated entities such as nursing homes. It also includes educating the public on relevant laws, regulations, and policies. For example, a nurse working in a pediatric clinic is required to report to the local public health department a case of shigellosis and can help monitor for additional cases to help determine whether there has been an outbreak (see Chapter 9). Knowledge of public health policy is necessary for the nurse not only to educate the parents of the children infected with shigellosis, but also to partner with the public health department's outbreak investigation aimed at reducing the spread of the infection.

Nurses are affected by state nurse practice acts that determine the scope of practice for registered nurses (RNs). These policies come under the umbrella of public health policy since they are designed to protect the public who are the recipients of nursing care. Nurses who provide direct care to patients are also affected in their day-to-day life by public health policies designed to protect both them and the patients they care for. These policies include the use of personal protective equipment and procedures for handling and disposing of sharps such as hypodermic needles or blades and mandated vaccinations.

Public health policy includes local and county policies mandating recycling of certain materials or special recycling procedures for hazardous materials and medications that hold special pollution risks in an effort to reduce environmental health risks. Other examples of public health policies include the fluoridation of the water to prevent dental carries, mandatory vaccinations for schoolchildren, regulations related to pharmaceuticals, and the Surgeon General's warnings on cigarette packages. Public health policies may involve mandating single interventions or comprehensive programs. For example, a school district might set a policy that all seventh graders attend a specific educational session about drug abuse. A comprehensive policy may include mandating educational sessions for various grades, mandatory drug testing for student athletes, community-based programs for parents, and the presence of a police liaison officer in the school.

We are all affected by governmental policies such as taxes that fund government including the federal income tax, payroll taxes, and state and local taxes. Although taxes are not regularly thought of as public health policy, the policy of exempting employer-sponsored health benefits from income and payroll taxes has influenced employers to offer health benefits in lieu of increased salaries. With the 2010 health-care reform law, new mandates are now in place to require that employers provide health-care coverage. The purpose of the reform was to improve access to health care. Therefore, from a public health perspective, a broad range of policies are instituted to directly or indirectly protect or promote the health of populations through the passing of laws and the setting of regulations based on the greatest good for the greatest number.

Public Health Policy and the U.S. Health-Care System

Public health policies directly affect our health-care system and its underlying philosophies. The U.S. health-care system is a complex combination of privately funded and provided, publicly funded and provided, and publicly funded and privately provided services. Why is our health-care system so complex? In part, it is complex because of the economic culture within the United States that supports an open market for the exchange of goods/services and payments, including health-care services. When the government attempts to intervene in the market system to promote quality, fairness, and equity, a tension is created between allowing and even facilitating the market and the principles of an open market system. This tension was evident in the debate over health-care reform that took place between 2009 and 2010. Of the 33 developed countries, the United States was the last to implement a universal health-care system that was completely enacted by 2014, despite continued attempts by Congress to rescind it.

In a **market economy,** the prices of goods and services are set by supply and demand. A well-functioning market economy is one in which there are many buyers, many sellers, and complete information about the goods and services that are being exchanged. In many ways, the U.S. health-care market does not meet the criteria of a free market. Buyers often do not have complete information about goods and services. For instance, after an auto crash, injured persons or their families do not have time to evaluate the quality and cost of ambulance and emergency room services in the area. In addition, because health-care decisions, such as whether to undergo a screening exam or what kind of cancer treatment to initiate, are often based on interpretation of technical information, individuals rely on advice given by health-care providers, the media, and significant others. In some areas, there are few "sellers" of specific services. For example, in 2008, 87% of counties in the United States did not have an abortion provider.[4]

Whereas government intervenes in the market economy to ensure quality, supply, and equity, the U.S. governmental role in the health-care market has been restrained owing to cultural factors that emphasize individual rights and a relatively unfettered market system. Early government intervention included conducting research into the adulteration and misbranding of food and drugs, providing health care to the merchant marines, and developing and enforcing quarantine laws.

The idea of health insurance took root in the 1930s in the private market whereby individuals could take out an insurance policy to defray the cost of health care if they became ill or suffered an accident.[5] Today, employer-based health insurance is the norm owing to Internal Revenue Service (IRS) rulings (i.e., policies) since the 1940s that allowed for health insurance expenses to be tax favored.[6] An employer-based model was retained in the ACA.

In the 1960s, federal health insurance policies became the norm with the development of Medicare to aid older adults and Medicaid to aid the poor and disabled. These two groups were generally not covered by employer-based health care. Despite the existence of these large programs, and with movement toward health reform, it was not until 2010 that the United States passed into law universal health insurance by mandating health insurance that took effect in 2014.

Health expenditures in the United States are far above those of other industrialized countries, and health outcome performance lags behind those countries in many areas.[7] For example, the United States ranked 18th in the world for the prevalence of adult obesity rates with 33% of adults having a Body Mass Index (BMI) greater to or equal to 30.0.[8] Despite the high expenditure on health care, in 2013 the United States ranked 51st in life expectancy.[8]

Within the United States, there are great disparities in the leading health indicators such as access to care and immunizations.[9] Prior to the ACA, fewer than half of U.S. adults received preventive tests and screenings recommended for their age and sex and nearly one-third of adults under age 65 were either under- or uninsured.[7]

These indicators are particularly poor for members of minority groups and those living in poverty. In 2010, less than half of African Americans used employer-sponsored health insurance compared with 62% of non-Hispanic whites.[10] Only 20.8% of African Americans were uninsured compared with 11.7% of non-Hispanic whites. African Americans were more likely to die from heart disease, stroke, cancer, asthma, influenza and pneumonia, HIV/AIDS, and homicide than non-Hispanic whites. Even in the category of adult immunization rates, often provided free or at a reduced rate through local public health departments, African Americans aged 65 and older were almost one-third less likely to have received a flu shot than their white counterparts.[10] When one looks more closely at infant mortality rates for African Americans and other minority groups, the differences are dramatic. Infant mortality rates for African Americans were 2.3 times higher than those of non-Hispanic whites.[11] The difference was less dramatic for Hispanic Americans whose overall infant mortality rate was 5.6 deaths/1,000 live births.[12]

Patient Protection and Affordable Care Act (ACA) of 2010

The passage and enactment of the Affordable Care Act (ACA) in 2010 by the federal government was a first step in the nation's effort to reform the health-care delivery system in the United States. The purpose of the ACA is to improve access to affordable health coverage for everyone, including the most vulnerable, to provide ways to bring down health-care costs, and to improve quality of care by improving health outcomes. The ACA already provides no denial of coverage for preexisting conditions, and young adults can stay on their parents' plan until age 26 if they don't have insurance through their job. There is currently confusion and lack of understanding by the general public about the new law, and support generally follows party lines.

The main provisions in 2014 are the following:

• Access to care has been expanded, with the requirement that most U.S. citizens and legal residents have health insurance. Individuals without coverage will pay a tax penalty.
• Employers with 50 or more employees will need to offer insurance coverage or pay a fine.
• Medicaid will expand to all non-older adults under 133% of the federal poverty level.
• There will be the creation of a state-based American Health Benefit Exchange and Small Business Health Option Program Exchanges to allow individuals and

small businesses to purchase health insurance more economically.

- More preventive health care will be provided at no additional cost (e.g., annual exams, flu shots, cancer screenings).[13]

There are components of public health programs in the ACA, with significant potential implications for public health nursing.[14] Some of these are authorized, mandatory funds for evidence-based early childhood home visitation, an authorized CDC national diabetes prevention program, loan repayment to increase public health workforce, programs to help educate more public health professionals, public health and preventive medicine training programs through HRSA funding, more school-based health centers, public/private partnerships to do education and outreach campaigns, increase in community health centers and nurse managed clinics, workplace wellness programs, and national quality improvement strategies to improve population health.[15]

The Affordable Care Act also established the Prevention and Public Health Fund. It provides increased and sustained national resources for prevention and public health, improves health outcomes, and enhances health-care quality. The USDHHS summarizes the investments as a "broad range of evidence-based activities including community and clinical prevention initiatives; research, surveillance and tracking; public health infrastructure; immunizations and screenings; tobacco prevention; and public health workforce and training.[15]

The ACA provides for greater access to preventive services and low cost medications as well as eliminates the denial of coverage for preexisting conditions.[16] With the full implementation of the ACA in 2014, insurance companies coverage of preventive services is mandated for both adults and children with no out of pocket costs. Covered preventive services for adults include risk-based screenings for abdominal aortic aneurysm, alcohol misuse, hypertension, cholesterol, colorectal, depression, HIV, obesity, tobacco use, and syphilis. Additional preventive services include access to aspirin therapy, diet counseling, and immunizations.[16]

While some might suggest that race and ethnicity is the primary reason for the dramatic disparities in health indicators, current research suggests that socioeconomic status plays a larger role.[17–20] The relationship between health and socioeconomic status is very complex. Despite the fact that individuals living at or below the federal poverty level may qualify for public insurance programs, they also frequently lack other resources, such as transportation, making access to health-care services challenging. Lack of resources, whether financial, educational

(literacy), or health-care related, or even social marginalization result in chronic stress. Certainly exposure to chronic stress is linked to greater incidence of stress related illnesses such as cancer, heart disease, and other chronic diseases. This combined with absence of insurance and reduced access to quality health care results in increasing mortality among minority groups and all individuals living in poverty.[21]

In the United States, most health-care goods and services are exchanged in the private market with individuals choosing their care provider and directly or indirectly paying for services. Often, the type of indirect payment (e.g., particular health insurance policies that pay for medical or health-related expenses) affect individual choices regarding care. For instance, the contractual agreement between an individual or a group and a health insurer may not cover particular screenings such as mammography. The extent of coverage of a particular insurance policy is in itself a policy that affects health-care choices. Individual health insurance is mainly regulated at the state level, and most states have a special office that is sometimes led by a state insurance commissioner.

Although some states use model acts and model regulations as guides, policies that govern private health insurance vary greatly from state to state. For instance, inclusion of mental health services in private insurance policies varies greatly. Some states prohibit insurers from discriminating in coverage for mental health and other health problems, some states require a minimum level of coverage of mental health expenses, and some do not require insurance companies to cover mental health services at all.[22]

In addition to the publicly funded programs that cover older adults and the poor through Medicare and Medicaid, respectively, the U.S. government both provides and pays for care for certain specific populations. The federal government is deemed to have responsibility for providing and paying for services for soldiers, veterans, prisoners in federal facilities, and American Indians/Native Americans.

There are many laws and regulations that guide health policy at the national level. The constitutional basis of federal involvement in health care resides in Article 1, Section 8, of the U.S. Constitution. This article gives the federal government certain authority including providing for the general welfare and regulating commerce among the states and has been interpreted as the basis for a variety of federal powers and activities.

National Health Policy

At the national level, *Healthy People* is a prevention agenda for the nation to guide interventions for the improvement of health outcomes in areas such as infant mortality, years of healthy life, and racial and ethnic health disparities.[23] Federal, state, and local health officials together with health-care providers and consumers developed national health goals and objectives for the United States. Since 1979, goals and objectives have been reevaluated about every 10 years.[23] *Healthy People* includes targets that are examples of federal health policy. *Healthy People* also includes specific goals and objectives for policy changes (see Chapter 1). It is an example of setting policy agendas at the national level using a consensus-building approach. That is, the agenda was built based on the input from numerous stakeholders.

■ HEALTHY PEOPLE 2020
History of Healthy People

Healthy People 2020 (HP 2020) is based on the accomplishments of four previous *Healthy People* initiatives:

- 1979 Surgeon General's Report, *Healthy People: The Surgeon General's Report on Health Promotion and Disease Prevention*
- *Healthy People 1990: Promoting Health/Preventing Disease; Objectives for the Nation*
- *Healthy People 2000: National Health Promotion and Disease Prevention Objectives*
- *Healthy People 2010: Objectives for Improving Health*

Development of *HP 2020*

HP 2020 is the result of a multiyear process that reflects input from a diverse group of individuals and organizations.[24]

Federal Government and Medicare

Where *HP 2020* is an example of agenda setting, other policies at the national level represent laws passed to help improve the health of populations. An important national health policy is the **Medicare** program. Since 1965, Medicare has provided payment for hospital care; long-term care; and pharmaceutical, physician, and other services to individuals 65 and older, and specified groups of people with disabilities under 65 including individuals with end-stage renal disease. Medicare is not a care delivery system, but rather a social insurance system administered by the Centers for Medicare & Medicaid Services (CMS), a federal governmental agency within the U.S. Department of Health and Human Services. Concerns about financial viability of Medicare have led to discussions about funding, eligibility, and fraud reduction.[25]

Federal Government and Medicaid

Medicaid, another national health policy administered by the CMS, provides financial assistance to states and counties for low-income families with dependent children, low-income older adults, and disabled individuals. Unlike Medicare, a federal program, Medicaid is jointly financed by matching funds from federal and state governments. Medicaid is described in more detail in the State Health Policy section.

Occupational Safety and Health Administration

The federal Occupational Safety and Health Administration (OSHA), part of the U.S. Department of Labor, regulates safety and health for workers. "OSHA's mission is to prevent work-related injuries, illnesses, and deaths."[26] Since the agency was created in 1971, occupational deaths have been cut by 62% and injuries have declined by 42%. For example, OSHA's bloodborne pathogens standard requires an exposure control plan that includes components such as observance of universal precautions to prevent contact with blood or other potentially infectious body fluids; engineering and work practice controls to minimize exposure; and vaccination, postexposure evaluation, and follow-up.

Special Populations

As mentioned earlier, the U.S. government directly provides health care for soldiers, veterans, members of federally recognized American Indian/Native American tribes, and inmates of federal prisons. Special agencies are charged with providing health care to these populations. For instance, the Department of Veterans Affairs provides health care for veterans through Veteran's Administration (VA) hospitals and programs. Indian Health Services (IHS) is a federally funded program to provide health services to Native populations based on treaties established during the early development of the United States. Nurses who work in the armed forces, VA, IHS, and federal prisons are usually employees of the federal government.

Affordable Care Act

The most recent national health-care legislation is the ACA, discussed throughout this book. This federal statute resulted in the most significant overhaul of the U.S. health-care regulatory system since the passage of Medicare and Medicaid legislation in 1965. An important goal of the ACA was the reduction in the number of uninsured individuals in the U.S. through two means: (1) the expansion of Medicaid eligibility to individuals at 138% of the federal poverty level (see Chapter 24) and

(2) the creation of state-based insurance exchanges. Opponents of the ACA challenged the constitutionality of the individual insurance mandate, suggesting it amounted to a tax; however, the U.S. Supreme Court upheld the legislation.[27]

The major provisions of the ACA contain changes to insurance standards including the development of an online marketplace, or health insurance exchange, in every state where individuals and businesses can purchase health insurance, minimum standards for health insurance policies (e.g., coverage for preventive care, mandatory contraceptive coverage, childhood and adult immunizations, and medical screenings), and guaranteed coverage regardless of preexisting medical conditions. In addition to changes in insurance regulations, the ACA also includes an individual mandate that every person must purchase health insurance or pay a penalty. Persons who purchase insurance via the exchanges and whose incomes fall between 100% and 400% of the federal poverty level are eligible for federal subsidies to help pay the cost of premiums. Finally, the ACA provided financial incentives and/or penalties to health-care systems to provide high-quality, cost-effective care. For example, all health-care systems were required to implement an electronic medical record or pay a penalty.

State Health Policy

States and Medicaid

Medicaid is jointly financed and administered by federal and state governments. States set their own guidelines for eligibility and services but must include certain federally mandated basic services: inpatient and outpatient hospital care; laboratory and radiology services; skilled care at home or at a long-term care facility; early periodic screening, diagnosis, and treatment for those younger than 21 years of age; and family planning services.[28] The federal government mandates that participating states include federally determined categories (low-income families with dependent children, low-income older adults, and disabled individuals) in their Medicaid eligibility criteria. Participating states may choose to provide Medicaid coverage to other groups such as the medically needy, individuals with income levels above Medicaid cutoffs but who have extraordinary medical costs. Many states have received waivers from the federal government to use Medicaid funds in a different way.[29] For instance, Wisconsin used Medicaid funds in a demonstration project, BadgerCare Plus, to pay for health-care services for low-income adults without dependent children.

A related federal/state program is the state Children's Health Insurance Program (CHIP) (see Chapter 19). The federal government provides matching funds to states for coverage of children in families having incomes too high to qualify for Medicaid, yet unable to afford private insurance. States have some latitude in determining covered services and eligibility levels.

Some states have decided on policies that incrementally moved toward universal health-care coverage for their residents. For instance, Oregon initiated a plan to provide health insurance to low-income residents while holding down costs through explicitly rationing certain services.[30] Ballooning costs resulted in limitation of services and severe limitations in eligibility, even institution of a lottery for remaining spots in the plan. In 2006, Massachusetts passed a statute requiring all state residents to obtain health insurance coverage.[31] Free and subsidized health insurance was made available to low-income residents. States are experimenting with a variety of policies to address health insurance coverage especially for low-income people.

Another important health policy at the state level is the regulation of health-care services through ensuring predetermined criteria for both health-care providers and facilities. For example, in Wisconsin, the Department of Regulation and Licensing is responsible for ensuring the safe and competent practice of licensed professionals in health care and other professions.[32] The department sets licensing requirements, establishes professional practice standards, and enforces occupational licensing laws. The department also regulates educational programs for licensed professionals. The Wisconsin Division of Quality Assurance is charged with, among other responsibilities, assuring the safety and quality of health-care facilities. This division is also responsible for ensuring that hospitals meet CMA standards for receiving reimbursement from Medicare and Medicaid. Each state takes responsibility for ensuring the safe regulation of health-care services.

Each state has an official state public health agency that deals with public health and is headed by a chief executive officer, often called the state health commissioner. These agencies, funded by state legislatures, monitor health status, enforce public health laws and regulations, and distribute federal and state funds for public health activities to local public health agencies. The form and structure of state public health agencies vary greatly from state to state, with some states merging the state public health agency with social services.

For example, the official state public health agency in Wisconsin has created a secure Web site and emergency messaging system called the Health Alert Network for communication about bioterrorism and other public health threats. This initiative was funded by a grant from the U.S. Centers for Disease Control and Prevention (CDC). This system connects local health departments with hospitals, clinics, law enforcement, firefighters, and emergency medical providers, and is used for multiple kinds of notifications.

Local Health Policy

Local public health agencies derive their authority from state and local laws and regulations. They deal with issues such as water safety and fluoridation, sanitation, infectious diseases, sanitary food and beverages, and they sometimes regulate and/or own health-care facilities such as hospitals, clinics, or nursing homes.[33] The form and structure of local public health agencies vary with centralized models operated directly by the state or decentralized models under county, city, or other local jurisdictions. Local public health agencies have a chief executive officer who generally works with local boards of health that are appointed or elected.

Local Health Department Personnel

Health department personnel are influential in developing, monitoring, and enforcing local health laws and regulations (see Chapter 14). For instance, local health agency advocacy has resulted in many local jurisdictions passing ordinances restricting use of tobacco in public settings. Local health agencies have policies whereby sanitarians inspect restaurants, convenience stores, food vendors at county fairs, and other public facilities that serve food to enforce guidelines such as food holding temperatures. These establishments can be closed if they do not meet certain standards. Another example of health-related policy at the local level involves zoning ordinances. A community in need of a shelter for homeless families was having difficulty securing a permit to open a shelter in a residential area because of zoning laws and property owners' fear of decreasing property values. Advocates for the homeless along with public health representatives met with residents to determine a plan for the shelter that would minimally affect the neighborhood. Advocates also petitioned the elected city board for a change in the zoning laws to allow a homeless shelter in that area of the city.

In order to promote equity and efficiency, a local health agency may have a policy about services offered to residents. For instance, one local health agency may decide to offer free home visits to families of newborns who meet certain risk criteria, whereas another local health agency decided to offer one free home visit to all families of newborns. As public health agency budgets are reduced, it is important to base local policy decisions on scientific evidence.

Likewise, local health agencies need to determine policies for payment for services such as immunizations or clinics that treat sexually transmitted infections. Should clients pay the full or partial (sliding fee) cost of each unit of service, should the agency request a donation, or should these services be free of charge? Sometimes, state or federal policy influences these decisions, but often these kinds of policy decisions are left to the local health agency. These decisions would potentially affect access to care, utilization rates of the service, and resources available for other services.

Local jurisdictions or even regions need to coordinate emergency services such as 911 call centers, ambulance, fire and rescue dispatch, and routing to local hospitals. Development of policies regarding emergency response services requires extensive coordination of multiple stakeholders within multiple jurisdictions.

Emergencies involving disasters, such as a flood, collapse of a bridge, chemical spill, or act of bioterrorism, require extensive planning. Public health agencies are often involved in primary prevention, but some disasters cannot be prevented, such as a tornado. Public health agencies work cooperatively with other agencies and community stakeholders to develop an emergency management plan that includes preparedness, response, and recovery (Chapter 25). An emergency management plan is an example of a policy. Many counties and other jurisdictions hold disaster drills to test aspects of their emergency disaster plans.

Business/Organizational Health Policy

Federal, state, and local laws affect health, but so do policies of businesses and organizations. Organizations and businesses may choose to develop policies for their employees or customers such as a hospitals and universities that establish smoke-free campuses. Likewise, the decision to offer health insurance and/or paid sick leave to employees beyond which might be specified by state or local law is an important health-related policy decision of businesses. Nutrition information provided by restaurants is another example of a health-related business decision policy. A local amateur hockey league may require that all players wear protective headgear while on the ice. Some schools have implemented health policies that restrict vending choices during school hours. Such initiatives at the organizational or business level can build into governmental policies such as recent policies by school districts to change to healthier foods in the school lunch programs.[34] Various stores, including a number of national chains, have established policies about not selling inhalants to minors and/or have moved inhalants to a secure area to prevent shoplifting.

Principles of Public Health Policy

Important principles guide public health policy. First, public health policy must be grounded in the health planning process. It focuses on promoting and protecting the health of populations. It should be based on evidence and be ethically sound and culturally appropriate.

Health Policy Assessment and Planning Process

Effective public health policy is grounded in the health assessment and planning process, a problem-focused process (Chapters 4 and 5). The health planning process, the policy process, and the nursing process use similar terms.

Assessment of health status, social data, needs, and resources is an important first step in the policy process. Goals and objectives for the policy are established with input from stakeholders, those directly or indirectly affected by the policy. Think of a school nurse who needs to make an authoritative decision about which children will be screened for vision problems. The school has limited resources and the state does not have a definitive policy about which children or grade levels to screen. Discussion with other school nurses shows that the majority of schools screen children in first and second grades. The nurse will use the policy process to decide on an authoritative decision about vision screening. What evidence-based standards exist regarding vision screening of school-age children? What evidence is there about the yield (new cases discovered) of vision screening at various grades? What else would be needed besides screening for an effective vision health program? Where can the nurse refer children who lack the means to pay for the services of an optometrist or for glasses?

In the health policy assessment and planning process, much attention is given to the development of the policy. Specific policy alternatives are posited and analyzed regarding factors such as cost, likely effectiveness, social and political feasibility, and equity. A school nurse making policy about vision screening would specify policy alternatives regarding vision screening. One policy might be to require vision checkups as a prerequisite to entering or transferring to the school.

Using Explicit Evaluation Criteria for Policy Planning

Policy alternatives can be judged according to explicit evaluation criteria. Three criteria most often used are effectiveness, efficiency, and equity (Table 22-1). **Effectiveness** involves the likelihood of achieving the goals and objectives of the policy. Increasing physical activity in a population might include requiring daily physical education classes for all schoolchildren, which may be more effective than open access to a community fitness center for residents of a school district. **Efficiency** involves achievement of policy goals relative to cost. The cost of providing daily physical education classes to school-age children (hiring teachers, increased facility requirements, lengthening the school day to accommodate the requirement, and lost opportunity costs of a required class in physical education vs. math or music, etc.) would be compared with the cost of providing access to physical fitness facilities for all residents (facility capital costs, additional staff, liability insurance, etc.). **Equity** involves fairness or justice in the distribution of a policy's costs, benefits, and risks. Using the prior example, the requirement of daily physical fitness courses provides a benefit exclusively for the school-age population, whereas open access to fitness facilities potentially benefits all age groups. The costs for both policy choices would be incurred by taxpayers. Weighing these three key criteria helps policy makers in deciding which policy approach to implement. Of course, the status quo is always another policy approach to take, in this case, the third unstated policy is to continue "business as usual" with students having physical education classes twice a week and those with the financial means and desire joining a fitness facility. Other important criteria for evaluating policy include liberty/freedom, political feasibility, social acceptability, administrative feasibility, and technical feasibility (Table 22-1).[5]

A theory links the proposed policy with the actions, behaviors, and/or decisions of others. Many public health policies are based on psychological or economic theories. A law imposing a penalty for being detected by police for not wearing a seat belt raises the potential cost of that action. This policy is based on at least two theories: rational action choice theory and the theory of reasoned action. Rational action choice theory assumes that individuals will make choices that benefit them the most with the least cost.[35–37] In this scenario, the theory suggests that individuals will buckle up in order to avoid the financial penalty. Barjonet, Ajzen, and Fishbein's (1975, 1980) theory of reasoned action also explains and supports this policy.[38] The theory suggests that behavioral intentions

TABLE 22–1	Selected Criteria for Evaluating Public Policy Proposals	
Criterion	Definition	Limits to Use
Effectiveness	Likelihood of achieving policy goals and objectives or demonstrated achievement of them.	Estimates involve uncertain projection of future events.
Efficiency	The achievement of program goals or benefits in relationship to the costs. Least cost for a given benefit or the largest benefit for a given cost.	Measuring all costs and benefits is not always possible. Policy decision making reflects political choices as much as efficiency.
Equity	Fairness or justice in the distribution of the policy's costs, benefits, and risks across population subgroups.	Difficulty in finding techniques to measure equity; disagreement over whether equity means a fair process or equal outcomes.
Liberty/ Freedom	Extent to which public policy extends or restricts privacy and individual rights and choices.	Assessment of impacts on freedom is often clouded by ideological beliefs about the role of government.
Political feasibility	The extent to which elected officials accept and support a policy proposal.	Difficult to determine. Depends on perceptions of the issues and changing economic and political conditions.
Social acceptability	The extent to which the public will accept and support a policy proposal.	Difficult to determine even when public support can be measured. Depends on saliency of the issues and level of public awareness.
Administrative feasibility	The likelihood that a department or agency can implement the policy well.	Involves projection of available resources and agency behavior that can be difficult to estimate.
Technical feasibility	The availability and reliability of technology needed for policy implementation.	Often difficult to anticipate technological change that would alter feasibility.

Source: Adapted with permission from Kraft, M., & Furlong, S.R. (2010). *Public policy: Politics, analysis, and alternatives* (3rd ed.). Washington, DC: CQ Press.

depend on a person's attitude about the behavior and subjective norms. Because subjective norms, perceived expectations from others, and intention to comply with those expectations guide personal behavior, policies have the potential to influence behavior by influencing how others behave and, more specifically, by changing the social norm of using seat belts.

Policies are formulated, interpreted, and implemented. It is difficult to differentiate between the planning and implementation phases of policy development.[39] Implementing policy is a complex activity that involves determining and enacting the various activities that will put the policy into effect. For instance, laws are interpreted by the executive branch of government and implemented by numerous agencies and organizations including employers, health-care providers, service agencies, and public health departments. States may interpret and implement the federal laws differently. Specifically, implementation involves developing the details of the process that will allow for the intended outcome to take place.

This could include such things as hiring personnel, establishing fines or penalties for those who do not follow the policy, and disseminating information about the policy.

Stakeholder Involvement

Like the nursing process, in which it is important to involve the client as much as possible, stakeholder involvement is important in the policy process. In assessment, or identification of the policy issue, sometimes stakeholders identify the need for a policy and sometimes they identify a problem but are not sure what type of policy will best address the problem. In Chapter 5, you read about the Elmwood Senior residence and concerns for isolation because of violence in their neighborhood. Community members, parents of young children, and the elders living in a senior residence facility felt that community violence kept them from physical activity such as walking outside and spending time in the park. The community health nurse obtained information from religious organizations, school representatives, seniors, and other community stakeholders to plan a program to address the perceived barrier to physical activity. At the organizational level, Elmwood residential facility organized an escort service for the residents. At the community level, local law enforcement could increase their presence through periodic patrolling of this neighborhood. The school recognized the need for increased after-school activities for the youths. The nurse worked with community organizers to obtain funds for after-school activities for teens.

Focus on Health Determinants

Health status is a complex interaction of environmental, socioeconomic, genetic, health service, and behavioral determinants. Public health policy attempts to change health status by influencing these determinants as precursors to morbidity and mortality. Public health policy emphasizes intervention in environmental protection, health promotion, and specific disease prevention. The concept of influencing determinants of health prior to the development of poor health or even physiological changes that would lead to poor health is known as *upstream thinking*. Examples of public health problems or issues that benefit from upstream policies designed to prevent those problems or issues from occurring in the first place include lead poisoning and dental caries (Table 22-2). Note that some upstream policies directly change the physical environment, whereas some policies require behavioral change.

Federal laws such as Medicaid that provides health services to poor families and the Family Medical Leave Act (FMLA) that guarantees continuation of work for those experiencing a health event in their families are examples of policies affecting socioeconomic determinants. The decision of an employer to provide paid sick leave for workers is a type of socioeconomic policy that, in most states and communities, is left to the employer.

Health-care provider decisions to expand primary care services to weekend and evening hours improve access to care, increasing primary care utilization and thus better health. Public health departments providing free vaccinations in schools increases immunization rates and herd immunity. State laws mandating certain vaccinations for school entry are also examples of policies having an impact on health through health services.

A school district's decision to implement a tooth brushing program for preschool and elementary students is intended to influence oral hygiene behavior of children and families and improve overall oral health. A construction company's decision to implement random drug testing for employees who operate heavy equipment may reduce drug use and injuries among employees. Mandating certain vaccinations for health-care workers is another example affecting worker behavior.

Evidence-Based Practice

Do the health policies described above really affect health? While anecdotal evidence exists for many health policies, some health policies are not supported by a body

TABLE 22–2	Examples of Upstream Policies Addressing Specific Public Health Problems or Issues
Public Health Problem/Issue	**Upstream Policy**
Lead poisoning in children	Federal and state restrictions on use of leaded paint in residential use
Exposure to secondhand smoke	Restaurant association's endorsement of smoke-free facilities among its members
High rates of cardiovascular disease	Health insurance policy to co-fund gym or weight-reduction club memberships Local zoning laws requiring sidewalks and bike paths in area of new development
Infant and maternal health	Employer providing onsite lactation room in workplace
Poor nutrition among poor	Supplemental Nutrition Assistance Program, previously known as Food Stamps, that provides assistance to low- and no-income individuals and families living in the United States
Dental caries	Municipality adding fluoride to drinking water
Herd immunity or individual immunity	School entry vaccination laws
Unintentional injuries of children	Child seat use laws

of scientific evidence. For example, although there is fairly good evidence that a sedentary lifestyle combined with extreme obesity is related to increased morbidity and mortality, the evidence that mandating sidewalks or including nutrition information on restaurant menus results in positive changes in individual actions, behaviors, and decisions is less clear. It is difficult if not impossible to randomly assign individuals or even communities to these interventions. Therefore, it is difficult to evaluate the impact of these interventions on health.

Another example is the evidence that drinking fluoridated water reduces the number of dental caries. While theoretically it would be possible to randomly assign communities supplied by separate water systems to fluoridated or nonfluoridated water status, in the United States a decision such as fluoridation of water is under local control and is often a political decision. There is often no authority to give permission for random assignment. In this case, the evidence of the success of the program is based on population data over time. Based on the evidence, there has been a decline in dental carries overall in countries that fluoridate water and those that do not.[40] This is because other changes have been introduced, including topical fluoride applications, fluoridated toothpastes, and salt and milk fluoridation. With 100 years of accumulated population-level evidence that fluoride in many forms reduces dental carries, the World Health Organization (WHO) recommends that public health policy support the use of fluoridated toothpastes and, where economically, technically, and culturally feasible, water fluoridation.[41] In the United States, in addition to fluoridation of water supplies, fluoride varnish programs have been implemented. This intervention involves the application of a thin layer of fluoride to the teeth of children.[42] School districts concerned with dental health may adopt other related policies such as limiting sugar-laden vending choices. Evaluating the effectiveness of one policy, such as a varnish policy, is difficult owing to the other interventions in current use.

There are a number of good sources of reviews for evidence-based practice on which to base policy decisions. The Agency for Healthcare Research and Quality's (AHRQ) U.S. Preventive Services Task Force publishes a *Guide to Clinical Preventive Services (Clinical Guide)* that recommends clinical preventive services based on systemic review of clinical practices.[43] This guide includes dozens of reviews in areas such as alcohol and drug abuse, cancer screening, nutrition, and exercise and is updated regularly. A second source is the CDC's *Guide to Community Preventive Services: The Community Guide: What Works to Promote Health* referred to as the *Community Guide*.[44] An excellent source that complements the AHRQ guide, the *Community Guide* was developed by the Task Force on Community Preventive Services. The *Community Guide* includes more than 200 systematic reviews and recommendations for interventions that promote population health (Table 22-3). For instance, regarding skin cancer prevention, the *Community Guide* recommends a wide variety of interventions focused on promotion of sun protection behaviors and environmental protections."[45]

TABLE 22–3	Task Force on Community Preventive Services		
	Systematic Reviews on Policy Interventions Conducted by the *Guide to Community Preventive Services*		
Topic	**Policy Setting**	**Intervention Title**	**Recommendation**
Preventing Excessive Alcohol Use	Community	Enhanced enforcement of laws prohibiting sales to minors	Recommended (Sufficient Evidence)
		Regulation of outlet density	Recommended (Sufficient Evidence)
		Privatization of retail sales	Insufficient Evidence
Preventing Skin Cancer	Education	Educational and policy: childcare centers	Insufficient Evidence
		Educational and policy: primary school settings	Recommended (Strong Evidence)
		Educational and policy: secondary schools and colleges	Insufficient Evidence
	Community	Educational and policy: outdoor recreation settings	Insufficient Evidence
	Worksite	Educational and policy: outdoor occupation settings	Insufficient Evidence

Continued

TABLE 22–3	Task Force on Community Preventive Services—cont'd		
Topic	Policy Setting	Intervention Title	Recommendation
Motor Vehicle–Related Injury Prevention	Community	Reducing alcohol-impaired driving: sobriety checkpoints	Recommended (Strong Evidence)
		Reducing alcohol-impaired driving: lower legal blood alcohol concentrations for young and inexperienced drivers	Recommended (Strong Evidence)
		Reducing alcohol-impaired driving: 0.08% blood alcohol concentration (BAC) laws	Recommended (Strong Evidence)
		Reducing alcohol-impaired driving: minimum legal drinking age	Recommended (Strong Evidence)
		Use of child safety seats: laws mandating use	Recommended (Strong Evidence)
		Use of safety belts: laws mandating use	Recommended (Strong Evidence)
		Use of safety belts: primary (vs. secondary) enforcement laws	Recommended (Strong Evidence)
Oral Health	Community	Dental caries (cavities): community water fluoridation	Recommended (Strong Evidence)
	Education	Dental caries (cavities): school-based or -linked sealant delivery	Recommended (Strong Evidence)
Promoting Physical Activity	Community	Community-scale urban design and land use policies	Recommended (Sufficient Evidence)
		Street scale urban design/land use policies	Recommended (Sufficient Evidence)
		Transportation and policies and practices	Insufficient Evidence
Tobacco Use	Community	Increasing tobacco use cessation: increasing the unit price of tobacco products	Recommended (Strong Evidence)
		Reducing tobacco use initiation: increasing the unit price of tobacco products	Recommended (Strong Evidence)
		Reducing exposure to environmental tobacco smoke: smoking bans and restrictions	Recommended (Strong Evidence)
		Restricting minors' access to tobacco products: community mobilization with additional interventions	Recommended (Sufficient Evidence)
		Restricting minors' access to tobacco products: active enforcement of sales laws directed at retailers	Insufficient Evidence
		Restricting minors' access to tobacco products: laws directed at minors' purchase, possession, or use of tobacco products	Insufficient Evidence
	Education	School tobacco-free policies	Insufficient Evidence
	Worksite	Smoke-free policies to reduce tobacco use among workers	Recommended (Sufficient Evidence)
Vaccine Preventable Diseases	Education	Vaccination requirements for childcare, school, and college attendance	Recommended (Sufficient Evidence)

TABLE 22–3	Task Force on Community Preventive Services—cont'd		
Topic	Policy Setting	Intervention Title	Recommendation
Violence Prevention	Community	Firearms laws • Bans on specified firearms or ammunition • Restrictions on firearm acquisition • Waiting periods for firearm acquisition • Firearm registration and licensing of firearm owners • "Shall issue" concealed weapons carry laws • Child access prevention laws • Zero tolerance of firearms in schools • Combinations of firearms laws	Insufficient Evidence
		Transfer of juveniles into adult court system to reduce violence	Recommended Against (Strong Evidence)
Worksite Health Promotion	Worksite	Smoke-free policies to reduce tobacco use among workers	Recommended (Sufficient Evidence)

Source: Adapted from the Centers for Disease Control and Prevention, on Community Preventive Services Task Force. (2014). Topics. Retrieved from http://www.thecommunityguide.org/.

A third good source is the Cochrane Reviews, a database of systematic reviews of the effects of health-care interventions (Table 22-4).[46] The reviews are conducted by a global collaboration of volunteers and a small staff in London, United Kingdom. While many of the Cochrane Reviews are clinically focused, there are a number that have a public health emphasis. For instance, in the area of injury control, there are reviews on interventions for promoting smoke alarm ownership and use and interventions for preventing injures in the construction industry.

Ethical and Cultural Implications of Policy

Public health policy ethics involve principles and values that guide authoritative decisions made in government, agencies, or organizations that are intended to influence population health. A basic assumption of public health policy is that society has the right and even obligation to collectively assure conditions for healthy people. An additional assumption is that the collective can sometimes impose on individual rights for the sake of the common good. There is debate about the balance between the autonomy, privacy, and liberty interests of individuals and collective interests and a debate about the appropriate role of government involvement in promoting population health.

An example is the Community Preventive Services Task Force recommendation for universal helmet laws. The recommendation was based on strong evidence of the effectiveness of motorcycle helmet laws.[47] Some argue that requiring the use of helmets violates a person's individual rights. Despite the strength of the evidence, a few states did not have helmet laws as of 2014 and a number of states only required the use of helmets for those who were 17 and younger.

TABLE 22–4	Good Sources for Reviews of Evidence-Based Practice for Basing Public Health Policy	
Community Guide	Centers for Disease Control and Prevention, Task Force on Community Preventive Services	http://www.thecommunityguide.org/index.html#topics
Clinical Guide	Agency for Healthcare Research and Quality, U.S. Preventive Services Task Force	http://www.ahrq.gov/clinic/uspstfix.htm
Cochrane Reviews	Cochrane Collaboration	http://www.cochrane.org/reviews/index.htm

Culture in its broadest sense refers to learned knowledge, attitudes, and behaviors of groups of people, which often are accepted without question. We often think of the culture of various ethnic and racial groups; however, all groups, including communities and workplaces, have culture. Most people are members of multiple cultural groups, and policy makers are influenced by their own cultural groups as well as the culture of their constituents and other stakeholders.

Public health policies can affect culture by changing knowledge, attitudes, and behaviors of individuals and groups (Fig. 22-1). For example, changes in the social acceptability of tobacco use allowed for smoking restriction policies that would have been unacceptable in the 1960s. Smoking restriction policies in turn affect knowledge, attitudes, and behaviors regarding smoking.

Culturally acceptable health policies are those that make sense to the people they affect. For example, many of the *HP 2020* objectives are aimed at reducing health disparities.[48] It is critical to consider the unique cultural makeup of the community in determining appropriate programmatic and policy decisions. A policy prohibiting individuals from serving foods prepared in their home for general consumption at large social gatherings (e.g., funerals and weddings) may help reduce the incidence of foodborne illness but would be met with resistance by groups that traditionally prepare foods in the home for such occasions. Conversely, a policy allowing individuals and families to rent a small area of land within a community garden in an urban area would be well received by individuals from cultures with a tradition for consuming homegrown produce. These examples demonstrate the importance of obtaining stakeholder input during the policy planning process.

Many public health policies target vulnerable groups. Poverty and unemployment disproportionately affect people of color and many rely on public health insurance for coverage.[10] Policies specifically benefiting impoverished individuals have the potential to benefit minority groups to a greater degree. For instance, CHIP has the potential to improve the health of minority populations by improving access to health services, leading, it is hoped, to fewer illnesses and resulting in decreased school absenteeism and increased high school graduation rates.

The Legislative Process and Public Health Policy

Advocating for the best interest of patients is second nature to nurses, but advocating for health-care policies is often unfamiliar territory. In order to affect policy change for the profession and for patient care, it is important that nurses be familiar with the legislative process and how to make their opinions count regarding specific legislation. Nurses should have a grasp of how a bill becomes law in the U.S. Congress (Fig. 22-2). Similar processes take place in state legislatures.

Through the U.S. Constitution, a series of checks and balances are created to ensure adequate opportunity for consideration and debate of an issue. Congress, made up of the House of Representatives and the Senate, is the official body through which all legislation is presented. The Senate is composed of 100 members, two from each of the 50 states, regardless of population or area, who serve for 6 years. The House of Representatives is composed of 435 members elected every 2 years from among the 50 states, apportioned by their population. The Constitution limits the number of representatives to not more than one for every 30,000 population. Each member of the Senate or House of Representatives has one vote.

The chief function of Congress is making laws. Both the Senate and House of Representatives have equal legislative functions and powers with just a few exceptions. Ideas for legislation come from members of Congress, from their constituent groups, and from executive communication from the President, a member of the President's Cabinet, or a head of an independent agency such as the Agency for Toxic Substances and Disease Registry.[49]

Once an idea or concern is presented, the elected official can introduce a bill to Congress. The representative or senator becomes its sponsor and other legislators can cosponsor the piece of legislation. The bill is given a number (preceded by H.R. if proposed in the House of Representatives and S. if a bill is introduced by the Senate) and referred to the appropriate committee or committees (i.e., House Ways and Means or Senate Appropriations Committee).

Perhaps the most important phase of the legislative process is the action taken by committees. Once in committee, the bill undergoes extensive consideration and debate. It is during this phase that government officials, industry experts, and anyone with interest in the bill can give testimony. The period when a bill is being considered in committee is an important time to contact legislative staff and legislators who are on the committee considering

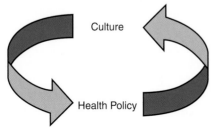

Figure 22-1 Relationship of culture and health policy.

From Bills to Laws: The Course of Legislation in Congress

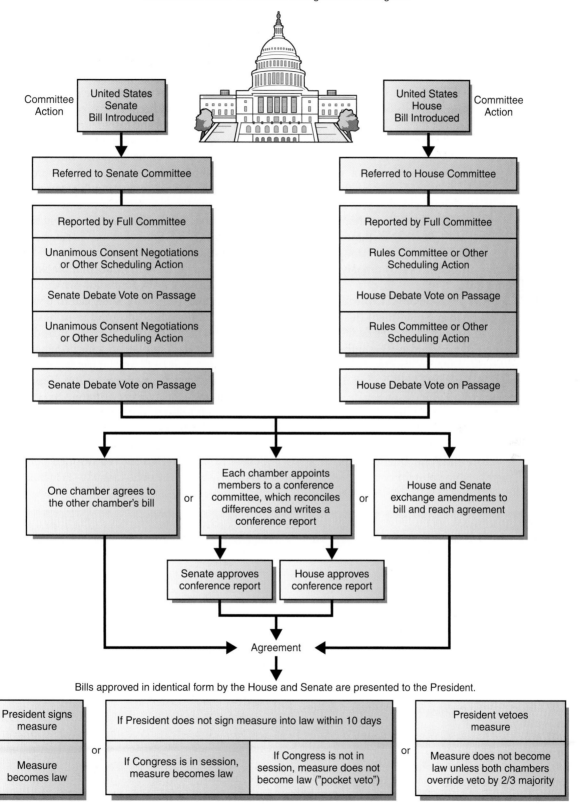

Figure 22-2 How a bill becomes law. *(Adapted from Congressional Research Service, A division of the Library of Congress.)*

the bill. For example, in 2009 the American Nurses Association Board of Directors provided testimony before the Democratic Steering and Policy committee of the House of Representatives Forum on the urgent need for health care reform. Individuals and organizations who testify before a committee must file a written statement of their proposed testimony before they appear. Once before the committee, testimony is limited to a brief summary of their arguments. A transcript of their testimony is printed and distributed to committee members as well as made available to the public.

After hearings are completed, the bill enters a "markup" phase in which a vote is taken to determine the action of the committee. The committee can approve the bill, amend the bill, "table" (postpone indefinitely), or reject the bill. If the committee approves the bill, it moves on in the legislative process. Bills can be rejected through a vote or simply by not acting on them; this is commonly referred to as "dying in committee."

Once a bill is approved, it is reported to the full House or Senate, where it is written and published. This includes the impact on existing law, budgetary considerations, any tax implications (increases or decreases) required by the bill, and the opinions of the committee either for or against the legislation. A reported bill is then placed on the legislative calendar of the House or Senate, where it is scheduled for floor action and debated before the full membership. Once general debate has ended, a second reading of the bill begins, during which amendments may be offered. Once debate ends and amendments are approved, the full membership votes for or against the bill.

Depending on the congressional body in which the bill originates, after a bill is approved it is sent to the other chamber where the same process is repeated. Once both chambers of Congress have approved the bill in identical form, it is sent to the President of the United States for action. The President may sign the bill into law, take no action on the bill for 10 days while Congress is in session, at which time it automatically becomes law, or veto the bill. If no action is taken on a bill and Congress adjourns, the bill dies. This is referred to as a "pocket veto."[49] Congress may override a veto by the President by a two-thirds vote in favor of the bill in both houses of Congress. Once a presidential veto is overridden, it is written as a binding statute and becomes law. All laws of the United States are published in the *U.S. Code*, a listing of the general and permanent laws organized according to subject matter under 50 title headings.[50]

To illustrate the process by which a bill becomes law, the history of the Genetics Information Nondiscrimination Act (GINA), signed into law on May 21, 2008, is a good example. Legislation designed to prohibit the improper use of genetic information in health insurance and employment decisions was first introduced in both the House of Representatives and the Senate during the 104th Congress in 1995. Similar legislation was then reintroduced in both houses again in 1996. The bill was reintroduced under its current name in 2003 and again in 2005 in both houses and eventually was signed into law during the 110th session of Congress. The bill eventually passed in the House of Representatives in 2007 and Senate in 2008. GINA moved through both houses to eventually become Public Law 110-233 (Box 22-1).[51]

BOX 22–1	How a Bill Goes Through the Legislative Process: The Genetic Information Nondiscrimination Act (GINA) of 2007

House
1/16/07 Introduced by a bipartisan team (Representatives Biggert, Eshoo, & Walden)
1/30/07 Heard in House Education and Labor Subcommittee on Health, Employment, Labor, and Pensions
2/14/07 Approved by House committee by unanimous vote
3/5/07 Reported by subcommittee (H. Rept. 110-28, Part 1)
3/8/07 Heard in House Energy & Commerce Subcommittee on Health
3/14/07 Heard by House Ways & Means Subcommittee on Health
3/21/07 Approved by House Ways & Means Subcommittee on Health
4/25/07 Passes the House 420–3
5/1/08 Passes House by vote of 414–1

Senate
1/22/07 Introduced by a bipartisan team (Senators Snowe, Kennedy, Enzi, & Dodd)
1/31/07 Approved by Senate Committee on Health, Education, Labor, & Pensions

3/29/07 Placed on the Senate legislative calendar
4/24/08 Passes Senate by vote of 95–0

5/21/08 Signed by President

Source: National Human Genome Research Institute. (2009). *Genetic information Nondiscrimination Act (GINA) of 2008*. Retrieved from http://www.genome.gov/24519851.

Participation of Nurses in Health Policy

There is power in numbers. Based on the 2008 National Sample Survey of Registered Nurses, there was an estimated 3,063,162 licensed registered nurses who are dispersed in every voting district in the nation.[52] Individual nurses, like all citizens, have the right and some would argue the duty to be politically active, yet results of studies demonstrate that nurses do not participate politically as much as they could. Reasons for a lack of political involvement range from professional demands (e.g., increasing workloads, understaffing), personal responsibilities (e.g., family roles, childcare), and the very nature of political activity which can be viewed as aggressive.[53,54]

The implications of lack of political involvement by nurses are extensive. Those who engage the system through voting and expressing their views are the individuals and groups that receive the attention of policy makers. Policy makers hear from individual physicians, pharmacists, and health insurance leaders. Policy makers also hear from lobbyists and organizations representing these professional groups such as the American Medical Association, Pharmaceutical Research and Manufacturers of America, and America's Health Insurance Plans. Whether as individuals or through their representative groups, information, views, and opinions help to shape policy. Because the 3 million nurses in the United States (more than three times the number of physicians) constitute the largest segment of the health workforce, imagine the impact if every nurse participated in advocating for health policy. Health policy, one of the most debated issues among political candidates, is influenced by the efforts of individuals but even more so by the efforts of organized groups and professional lobbyists. Nurses can affect policy through their individual efforts and utilizing their collective power.

Individual Participation

When nurses engage the political system, politicians will see them as a powerful voting group to whom they must pay attention in order to be successful in seeking reelection to office. Advocacy activities can include active involvement in policy such as providing testimony, writing letters and meeting with your state and federal legislators.[55] Nurses engage in advocacy on behalf of their patients every day; however, advocating for health policy has the potential to affect entire populations. Nurses interested in influencing the policy process, even those with limited time and resources, can become advocates for health policy legislation.[56] They can advocate for particular policies (Box 22-2). It helps to follow certain guidelines for communicating with policy makers (Box 22-3).

BOX 22–2 Advocacy for Particular Health Policies

- Communicating with legislators through letters, e-mail, face-to-face communications (personal visit), phone calls—providing your name and address during these communications in case the legislator wishes to seek additional information about his/her viewpoint
- Participating in annual state legislative days (i.e., Day at the Capital)
- Joining organizations that use collective power to influence policy such as the American Nurses Association (ANA), state/local nursing association, or specialty nursing associations
- Seeking out policy workshops, internship, or fellowships.
- Attending a town hall meeting

BOX 22–3 Tips for Communicating With Policy Makers

- **Keep it short.**
  Effective letters are brief and direct.
- **Focus on one topic.**
  Limit your letter to one topic/subject. Clearly state your topic/subject in the opening paragraph.
- **Share experiences.**
  Although form letters provide a template to work from, they don't carry the same weight as does a letter in your own words. Providing personal experiences and views gives the issue a human face.
- **Provide your name and contact information, including address.**
  Legislators and policy makers pay most attention to letters that come from individuals who have the potential to vote for them. Including your contact information also enables them to contact you with questions or for clarification.
- **Persistence pays off.**
  Contact legislators and their staff frequently, particularly if they have not taken a position on an issue.

Members of Congress are most responsive to people from their own jurisdictions. They and their staffers need and want to have input from well-informed nurses in order to be aware of priority problems and the ramifications of changes in policy. Many nursing organization Web sites provide a link at which you can enter a ZIP code to find contact information for legislators in a particular area. Many nursing organization Web sites also contain specific policy agendas and sample letters. Nurses can increase their expertise in policy analysis and development through workshops, internships, and fellowships (Box 22-4).

Collective Participation

Most changes in policy are the result of intentional activity of many individuals and groups. Because the policy process is influenced by the knowledge, attitudes, and actions of elected officials, influencing policy necessitates influencing the knowledge, attitudes, and actions of those elected officials. Strategies range from joining an organization that uses its collective powers to influence policy such as the Association of Operating Room Nurses (AORN), American Association of Critical Care Nurses (AACN), Oncology Nurses Society (ONS), or a state or national nursing organizations like the American Nurses Association (ANA), writing a letter or making a call about an issue, to getting elected to public office.

Nurses can affect policy through the efforts of professional organizations like the ANA, National League for Nurses, and specialty organizations such as AORN and AACN. However, RNs in the United States do not always become members of organizations. This is a disheartening finding, considering that nurses who are in professional organizations are more likely to be politically active.[57] Professional organizations not only employ professional lobbyists who influence legislators through sustained activity over months and years but they also form political action committees whose very function is to engage in political advocacy and fundraising. Although individual advocacy efforts are important, invitations to testify to Congress are typically offered to larger, organized groups that may have taken a position on an issue. The advocacy of the professional organization combined with individual advocacy efforts cannot be underestimated.[58]

Nursing has a legacy of political advocacy. Florence Nightingale, Lillian Wald, and Mary Breckinridge were all instrumental in shaping public health policy during their time. Today, political involvement by nurses continues to shape public health policy and contribute to the solutions to improve population health. Nursing has the potential to affect health policy in any country owing to its large numbers in the health workforce. Institution of sound public health policy improves the health of the patients whom nurses care for and the communities in which their patients live.

Public Health Finance

To further understand the public health system, it is important to understand how public health services are funded. **Public health finance** is a complex system involving funding streams, economic factors, and policy and political changes. This complexity along with the lack of transparency and the wide variation in local public health discretionary spending make it difficult to establish a consistent blueprint of public health agency funding. In the 1955 issue of the *American Journal of Public Health*, Burney and Yoho suggested that "the economic status of local government has been the most important single deterrent to the expansion of community health services" (p. 976).[59] They posited that as local health departments strive to meet the needs identified in communities, they must also convince people that the benefits of the services required to meet those needs are worth the cost. This necessitates a realistic evaluation of all public health programs and a degree of fiscal scrutiny, which promotes selection of those programs that are predicted to have the greatest impact on the population for the costs involved (see Chapter 14).[59] Unfortunately, there appears to be little progress made in connecting the relationship between public health funding/expenditures to the health of populations.

Finance Terms

There are basic terms associated with health-care funding. Broadly speaking, **health economics** is a field that encompasses the process for understanding the supply and demand of health-care services.[60] As stated by the CDC, "*Economics [is] the study of decisions—the incentives that lead to them, and the consequences from them—as they relate to production, distribution, and consumption of goods and services when resources are limited and have alternative uses.*" The CDC then

BOX 22–4	**Examples of Public Policy Internships of Interest to Registered Nurses**

Congressional Fellows Program
Congressional Fellowships on Women and Public Policy
Coro Fellows Program in Public Affairs
Kellogg Fellows in Health Policy Research
Nursing Organization Alliance: Nurses in Washington Internship (NIWI)
Presidential Management Fellows Program
Robert Wood Johnson Health Policy Fellows Program
Watson Fellowships
The Wellstone Fellowship for Social Justice
White House Fellows Program

applies economics to the process for conducting cost benefit analysis as it applies to preventive strategies. That is they compare the costs and the outcomes between alternative strategies aimed at preventing adverse injury and disease.[61] Public health finance is specific to population-level health care and includes the acquisition, utilization, and management of the resources needed to deliver public health services provided by public health agencies and departments. It also includes an examination of how those resources affect both population health and the public health system.[62] **Public health economics** examines the financing of public health from a governmental perspective with a focus on the delivery of public health goods and services and the financing of public health programs.[63] Public health economists are concerned with the cost analysis, economic evaluation, modeling, and analysis of health-care regulation on the cost, burden, health, effectiveness, and efficiency of health programs.[61]

Public Health Funding

People in every community in the United States have come to expect a basic level of public health services, including food and water safety and control of communicable disease outbreaks. These services come with a price tag and require a well-trained, well-equipped, and well-prepared public health system. Funding levels and sources of public health and disease prevention programs vary dramatically from neighborhood to neighborhood, community to community, city to city, and state to state. To adequately provide these services requires stable and adequate funding.[64]

Federal Funding

Historically, the federal government funded programs to ensure the health of specific groups of people. In 1798, the federal government created the Marine Hospital Service, under the direction of the Surgeon General, to provide health care for sick and disabled sailors and to protect the nation's borders against the importation of disease through seaports.[65] Funds for these services came from a per-month charge of 20 cents taken from the wages of American sailors.[65] In 1879, the federal government established the National Board of Health, charged with overseeing the health of the public. Due to contention around the authority of the U.S. government and other concerns it ceased to exist in 1893.[66] Currently the United States Public Health Service (USPHS) is charged with protecting the health of the nation. Within the USPHS, many laws were created to protect the public from disease. The federal government, in cooperation

with the health department, established quarantine rules along with a means to record vital information (e.g., births, deaths, and specified diseases).[66] Funding for state and local municipalities to support these efforts continues to come primarily from federal and state sources to this day.

The CDC, established in 1946, continues to provide a significant source of public health funding through grants and contracts to state and local public health departments. In 2013, they reported that with a budget of about $7 billion they awarded approximately 85% of it through their grant programs and contracts. They awarded over 14,000 separate grant and contract actions to promote health and quality of life by preventing and controlling disease, injury, and disability.[67] The CDC funds health-related and research organizations that contribute to the CDC's mission through health information dissemination, preparedness, prevention, research, and surveillance.[67]

All federal funds are categorical in nature and address specific programming. Many local health departments receive federal dollars to fund programs. Examples of federal funds that help fund programs include the Title V Maternal Child Health program; Women, Infants, and Children (WIC), and the Well Women HealthCheck Program. Changes in federal funding levels affect the local health department to provide categorical programming. Examples of the changing federal revenue streams includes the discontinuation of Prevention Grant dollars included in Consolidated Contracts to local health departments effective October 1, 2011, and the addition of Pandemic funds, which were made available in 2009 and 2010.

State Funding

State health departments are central to the public health system. The U.S. Constitution identifies the states as primarily responsible for the health of their citizens and authorized to carry out these functions through a variety of state agencies.[68] The official state public health agency is often a freestanding department reporting to the governor of the state. In many cases, the state health departments rely on regional or district offices to carry out their responsibilities as well as support the local health departments.[68] State statutes and policies dictate the programs and services offered and include regulatory, program, and service mandates. Funding for state health departments and programs varies widely in the United States, primarily coming from a combination of federal grants and contracts, program fees, and tax revenues. Examples of state public health programs include administering the Women, Infant, and Children (WIC) program, collection of vital statistics, tobacco use prevention, public health laboratories, food safety, and health facility regulation.[68]

Local Funding

The local health department is where most direct public health service delivery occurs providing the majority of the community prevention and clinical preventive services. Counties provided care for more than 40 million people accessing local health departments and contracted facilities and spent more than $30 billion in local tax revenues on health services. Local sources (26%) provided the greatest source of funding, followed by state funds (21%), federal dollars passed through the state department (14%), and federal dollars provided directly to the state. Medicaid, Medicare, private grants, and fees make up the majority of local health department funding.[68,69]

Significant variation exists in local health department per capita revenues and expenditures throughout the United States. In 2010, the local health department median per capita expenditure was $41, whereas the median per capita revenue was $44. In six states, the median per capita expenditure was less than $20, whereas in 10 states it was more than $55.[69] Reasons for this variation are multifaceted, ranging from geographical size, population size and characteristics, variation in tax base among counties and municipalities, types of services offered, and type of governance (i.e., city, county, regional, state, or shared governance).

Health department structure and governance can affect the amount and source of funding for programming (Box 22-5). In 2010, 68% of local health departments in the United States were county based, with 21% based in city or townships and governed by a local board of health or county commission or executive.[68,69] The remainder of the health departments served a regional or multicounty jurisdiction or a mixed jurisdiction serving both a county and a city located outside the county boundaries.[69] These differences may affect the revenue sources and per capita funding levels that fund a local health department. For example, health departments using a state/regional model may not receive local levy as a revenue source.

Another important factor in local health department funding is the size of the population served and the type and array of programs and services provided. The median annual expenditures for health department funding was $1.5 million, with a range of $512,000 for local health departments serving fewer than 25,000 people to $58.5 million for those serving 1 million or more residents.[69] This

---

BOX 22–5 Investing in America's Health: A State-by-State Look at Public Health Funding and Key Facts

The National Association of County & City Health Officials provided four overarching recommendations related to public health funding:

1. Core funding for public health—at the federal, state, and local levels—be increased
2. Funding be considered strategically, so funds are used efficiently to maximize effectiveness in lowering disease rates and improving health
3. The Prevention Fund, identified as part of the Affordable Care Act enacted on March 23, 2010, be implemented quickly and strategically to effectively and efficiently reduce rates of disease. For more information about the fund, please go to http://www.healthcare.gov/news/factsheets/2011/02/prevention02092011a.html.
4. Accountability must be a cornerstone of public health funding—the use of funds and the outcomes achieved from the use of the funds be transparent and clearly communicated with the public

Source: See reference 69.

---

variation in funding may lead to differences in service availability and delivery across geographical locations. Also, greater funding from both public and private sources is generally available to departments that demonstrate increased community health needs (i.e., high morbidity and mortality rates, poverty levels) and are able to prove positive program outcomes. The types of services most often provided include immunizations for children and adults, communicable disease surveillance, tuberculosis screening, inspection/licensing of retail food establishments, environmental health programming, and tobacco use prevention.[68]

This may all seem abstract, but the financing of public health is a complex issue. In 2009 during the H1N1, outbreak the CDC put forward a campaign to deliver vaccine to those most at risk through a mobilization of the public health system. How the vaccine program was implemented and how it was paid for varied from state to state. To provide a mechanism to implement an emergency vaccine program, federal 2009 H1N1 vaccine implementation funds were made available by the federal government to public health departments. Specific guidelines for the use of those funds were provided to help ensure that those at highest risk (pregnant women, children, and care givers of children) had priority for receiving the vaccine This outbreak demonstrates that financing of public health in the United States includes a combination of federal, state, local, and private insurance funds.

Grants

Grants are monetary awards given by an organization or government agency to plan and implement a program or project. Often grant dollars are distributed via a competitive process with many agencies vying for the same dollars. Other grants may be noncompetitive but prescriptive in nature. With reduced budgets many public health agencies have turned to grants to offset reduced funding from local tax levies. National and local organizations such as the United Way help support local programs designed to serve some of the most vulnerable populations (e.g., health care for the homeless). Grant funds are often time limited, requiring the grantee to demonstrate sustainability and a plan to evaluate the outcomes of the project after the grant period ends.[70]

The Local Health Department Budget Process

Through the community health assessment process, local health department representatives along with community stakeholders (e.g., representatives from a variety of community organizations, police and fire departments, local health system) identify public health issues and action plans to address these. The resulting community health improvement plan identifies possible solutions to public health issues that influence programming and budget allocations. As public health budgets shrink, this process provides the critical justification for program revenues and expenditures.

The process of health department funding involves the complex interaction of government agencies, public/private partners, county officials, local taxpayers, and public health agency staff (see Chapter 14). Inherent in the process is the knowledge that public health funding, given these interdependent relationships, can vary greatly from one fiscal year to the next. Because the bulk of public health funding is supported by local taxpayers, economic instability can have a significant impact on the ability of health departments to deliver services. Many local health departments rely on local tax dollars or levies that are affected by both political and economic forces. For example, many municipalities collect taxes based on property values. This approach to taxation is vulnerable to the ups and downs of the economy. When the housing market is down and property values fall, tax dollars raised are also reduced. This results in budget shortfalls that are often compensated for through reducing or charging for services that were once free.

Health programs mandated by state statute must be provided regardless of budget concerns. Examples of mandatory programs may include inspections of establishments serving food to the public and communicable disease follow-up to limit the spread of illness. Others, however, such as prevention programs addressing issues such as child abuse or suicide prevention, may be vulnerable to reductions or elimination if there are no grant funds or partnerships to sustain them.

The public health nurse and other local health department staff play a critical role in the budget process. Local health departments typically operate on an annual fiscal year (January to December) budget cycle, with programs often funded through a combination of federal, state, and local tax dollars. Other sources of program funding such as grants may operate on a different fiscal cycle with reporting timelines from July to June or October to September. Public health nurses in charge of specific programs must provide the required reports to the funding source to ensure continued program funding.

Funding Access to Care

Low-income families face a web of problems that compromise their ability to financially seek out health care. These problems can include a lack of health insurance, unemployment, old age, incarceration, chronically ill or disabled family members, lack of child support, debt, and low educational level. Low minimum wages and unrealistic low federal poverty guidelines often leave these families with an inability to support themselves and without the knowledge of their eligibility for services. This section discusses some of the federal/state programs that offer a safety net for both health insurance and income.

Government Health Insurance Programs

Today, Medicare and Medicaid account for the greatest expenditure of federal governmental health-care spending. Through these programs, the federal government purchases health-care services for population groups via health-care organizations, including both private and public sector providers such as physicians, hospitals, health maintenance organizations (HMOs), community health centers, and health departments.

Medicaid

Medicaid is a federal and state partnership that covers health costs for certain groups of people, including those with lower incomes, disabilities, older people, and some families and children. Although the eligibility rules vary in each state, as a result of the ACA, in 2014 it is expected that adults under the age of 65 with incomes of about $15,000 per year will qualify for Medicaid in participating states.[71] Medicaid benefits and the contrasts with Medicare benefits are found in Table 22-5.

The Medicaid services that must be covered for children and sometimes for adults include: physical, occupational, or speech therapy; eye doctor visits, eyeglasses; audiology, hearing aids; prosthetic devices; mental health services; respite and other in-home, long-term care; case management; personal care services; and hospice services.[71]

Medicaid is an evolving program that was initially created in 1965 with the Social Security Amendments. It took 18 years for it to become available in every state.[72] Initially, it focused on children under the age of 21 and then was extended in the 1970s to those who were disabled. In the 1980s, there were inclusions for pregnant women, illegal immigrants for some emergency situations, and dental needs. In 1991, the Medicaid Drug Rebate Program was put into place to cover the cost of prescription drugs; in 2000, the Breast and Cervical Cancer Treatment and Prevention Act allowed any uninsured woman who had breast or cervical cancer to be treated.[72] The latest evolution is the possible expansion of Medicaid eligibility under the ACA beginning in January 2014. The minimum eligibility level for Medicaid is 133% of the federal poverty level ($31,322 for a household of four for 2013/2014) for almost all Americans under the age of 65.

Children's Health Insurance Program

Children's Health Insurance Program (CHIP) is also a federal and state partnership that provides coverage for children who live in families that have incomes too high to qualify for Medicaid, but cannot afford private health insurance. Basic eligibility is focused on three groups: children up to age 19, pregnant women, and other citizens and legal immigrants. Families of four with incomes up to $45,000 are considered eligible for CHIP; in some cases, families with higher incomes may also qualify. Pregnant women may be eligible and CHIP will generally cover lab testing, labor and delivery costs, and 60 days of care after delivery. Finally, U.S. citizens and some legal immigrants are covered but states have the option of providing this coverage. Undocumented immigrants are not eligible for CHIP.[73] The services provided are similar or identical to Medicaid and include routine checkups, immunizations, dental and vision

TABLE 22–5	Comparison of Medicaid and Medicare	
	Medicaid	Medicare
What is it?	A combined state and federal health insurance program for people with limited resources and income. Certain components of the program such as CHIP help certain populations.	A federal health insurance program for: • Individuals aged 65 and older • Certain disabled individuals, under age 65 • Individuals with end-stage renal disease
Who runs the program?	State government	Federal government
What does it cover?	• Laboratory tests and x-rays • Inpatient hospital care • Health screening • Dental and vision care • Long-term care and support in a skilled facility • Family planning and midwifery services • Doctor visits, outpatient health care • Prescription drugs • Home health-care services for certain people • Nursing home care even when custodial	Part A: Inpatient hospital care and some care in a skilled nursing facility Part B: Doctor's visit and care received as an outpatient, some preventive services Part D: Some pharmacy prescription coverage Does not cover long-term custodial care
What does it cost?	Depends on the rules in the state and the income and resources of the individual. Many are exempt from any out-of-pocket costs. Others have copayments, deductibles, and premiums.	Depends on which parts of Medicare the individual selects. It can include copayments, deductibles, and premiums.

Source: United Health Care. (n.d.). Medicare versus Medicaid. Retrieved from http://www.medicaremadeclear.com/about/medicare-vs-medicaid/.

care, inpatient and outpatient hospital care, and lab and x-ray services.[73]

Medicare

Medicare is health insurance that covers three groups of people: people aged 65 or older, people under 65 with certain disabilities, and people of all ages with end-stage renal disease (permanent kidney failure requiring dialysis or a kidney transplant). Medicare is also part of the Social Security Amendment signed into law on July 30, 1965, by President Johnson, providing the first federally funded health insurance for those 65 and older. The other significant change occurred in 2003 when President George W. Bush signed into law and added the outpatient prescription drug benefit to Medicare recipients.[74]

There are three parts to Medicare. Part A is Hospital Insurance that covers inpatient care in hospitals, hospice, some home health, as well as skilled nursing facilities that are not considered custodial or long-term care settings. Most people do not pay a premium because they have already paid for the insurance as part of their taxes. Part B is Medical Insurance that covers doctors' services, outpatient care, and some additional services of physical and occupational therapists, home health, and some medical supplies. For this portion, most people pay a monthly premium (about $100/month). If someone has Part A and Part B, that person can choose to enroll in Medicare Part C (Medicare Advantage). Then, she would receive all of her care through a selected private provider organization (such as an HMO or preferred provider organization) administered by Medicare. Part D is the Medicare prescription drug coverage, and is actually a separate policy that one must purchase from a private insurer. Beneficiaries choose a drug plan and pay a monthly premium for purposes of lowering prescription drug costs.[75]

Government Income Support Programs

Temporary Assistance for Needy Families

Temporary Assistance for Needy Families (TANF) is a cash assistance program that is generally limited to 60 months in an adult's lifetime. The money for this program is a block grant from the federal government that allows each state flexibility in developing its own program. The purpose of TANF is to make the assistance temporary, not permanent, by supporting economically needy families, helping parents complete their education, teaching job skills, and encouraging two-parent families. There are work requirements for the adult program participants, and teen parents must live with their parents or a supervising adult and remain in school. Most recipients of TANF also qualify for Medicaid.[76]

People With Disabilities

The federal government administers two income supplement programs that serve individuals with disabilities.[77] The first is **Social Security Disability Insurance (SSDI),** a federal program that provides income benefits to individuals (or in some cases, family members) if the disabled person has worked long enough in the past (40 quarters, 10 years) to pay Social Security tax, and is expected to be unable to work for at least 1 year. It can be provided on a temporary or permanent basis as defined by the disability. There is not an income or resource restriction.[78]

The **Supplemental Security Income (SSI)** is also a federal income supplement program, but it is funded by general tax revenues and not Social Security taxes. It covers adults and children who have a significant physical or mental disability that has lasted or is expected to last at least 12 months, have limited income level and resources, have not met the work requirement for SSDI, as well as people 65 and over without disabilities who meet the financial limits. The disabled individual must remain below the income threshold to continue to receive SSI. It provides cash to meet basic human needs such as food, shelter, and clothing. Most people who receive SSI also qualify for Medicaid.[78]

Supplemental Nutrition Assistance Program (SNAP) is the new name for the Food Stamp program and is administered by the Food and Nutrition Service of the U.S. Department of Agriculture. This program provides financial assistance for the purchase of food to help recipients maintain a healthy diet, and is the largest program in the domestic hunger safety net. People who are eligible for TANF and SSI are automatically eligible for SNAP, and others are eligible if they meet the financial requirements.[79] **Woman, Infants, and Children (WIC),** a federal grant program (not an entitlement program), also provides nutritional supplements to nutritionally at-risk, low-income pregnant women until 6 weeks postpartum, breastfeeding mothers until an infant's first birthday, and children up to the age of 5. WIC pays for essential items such as milk, eggs, and baby formula, and currently serves up to 53% of all infants born in the United States. The program also provides education and counseling at the WIC clinics, and screening and referrals to other health and social service agencies.[80]

■ Summary Points

- Public health policies are authoritative governmental decisions made in government, agencies, or organizations directed toward influencing actions, behaviors, or decisions that influence population health.

- Public health policy is intrinsically connected to our health-care system, values, and underlying philosophies about the place of government versus the market system.
- Public health policies are enacted at national, state, and local levels of government as well as by businesses and organizations.
- Public health policies are grounded in the health planning process. A policy's likely effectiveness, efficiency, and effect on equity should be considered.
- Public health policies focus on health determinants and are based on evidence.
- Nurses can be involved in the public health policy-making process through individual and collective actions.
- Public health departments receive funds from a variety of sources including federal, state, and local tax dollars as well as grants.
- The majority of funding for local health departments comes from local sources and per capita funding varies widely across the United States based on type of government structure (city, county, region), geography, population size and characteristics, tax base, and types of services offered.
- The greatest expenditure of federal health-care dollars is spent on Medicare and Medicaid.
- Government income support programs, including Social Security Disability, Supplemental Security Income, and Woman, Infants, and Children, provide support to persons whose income or health status makes them vulnerable to poor health.
- The Affordable Care Act of 2010, signed into law by President Obama, overhauls the U.S. health-care system and focuses on improving quality and reducing cost of health insurance for individuals. Notable changes in coverage include greater access to preventive care and services and the creation of health insurance exchanges to increase coverage and affordability.

▲ CASE STUDY
Reducing Exposure to Tobacco Smoke Through Health Policy
Learning Outcomes

At the end of this case study, the student will be able to:

- Gain understanding of the public health policy.
- Describe the role of policy in the promotion of the public's health.

In 2009, President Obama signed into law the Family Smoking Prevention and Tobacco Control Act (FSPTCA). It grants the Food and Drug Administration the authority to set national standards related to the tobacco industry and covers seven areas of regulation: (1) advertising and marketing, (2) product labeling, (3) preemption of state regulation, (4) development of "safer" cigarettes, (5) performance standards, (6) user fees and taxes, and (7) the creation of a scientific advisory committee. Globally, the WHO established an international tobacco treaty in 2005 that the U.S. Congress has not ratified.

Access information related to the law on the Internet and review the WHO treaty at http://www.who.int/mediacentre/news/releases/2005/pr09/en/print.html. Then answer the following questions:

1. How is this law related to public health?
2. How does the law align with *HP 2020* objectives?
3. What are the barriers to enactment of the law in the United States?
4. Are these the same barriers that have impeded the ratification of the WHO treaty?

REFERENCES

1. U.S. Dept of Health and Human Services, Office of Population Affairs. (n.d.). *Affordable care act.* Retrieved from http://www.hhs.gov/opa/affordable-care-act/index.html.
2. Longest, B.B. (2006). *Policymaking in the United States* (4th ed.). Chicago, IL: Health Administration Press; Washington, DC: Association of University Programs in Health Administration.
3. American Nurses Association. (2007). *Public health nursing: Scope and standards of practice.* Silver Spring, MD: Nursesbooks.org.
4. Guttmacher Institute. (2013). *Facts on induced abortion in the United States.* Retrieved from http://www.guttmacher.org/pubs/fb_induced_abortion.html.
5. Kraft, M.E., & Furlong, S.R. (2010). *Public policy: Politics, analysis, and alternatives* (3rd ed.). Washington, DC: CQ Press.
6. Richmond, J.B., & Fein, R. (2005). *The health care mess: How we got into it and what it will take to get out.* Cambridge, MA: Harvard University Press.
7. Commonwealth Fund Commission on a High Performance Health System. (2011). *Why not the best? Results from a national scorecard on U.S. health system performance 2011.* Retrieved from http://www.commonwealthfund.org/Publications/Fund-Reports/2011/Oct/Why-Not-the-Best-2011.aspx?page=all.
8. Central Intelligence Agency. (n.d.). *The world factbook: Country comparison; Obesity, adult prevalence rate.*

Retrieved from https://www.cia.gov/library/publications/the-world-factbook/rankorder/2228rank.html.

9. U.S. Department of Health and Human Services. (2013). *The leading health indicators.* Retrieved from http://healthypeople.gov/2020/LHI/infographicGallery.aspx.

10. U.S. Department of Health and Human Services, Office of Minority Health. (2012). *African American profile.* Retrieved from http://minorityhealth.hhs.gov/templates/browse.aspx?lvl=2&lvlID=51.

11. U.S. Department of Health and Human Services, Office of Minority Health. (2009). *Infant mortality disparities fact sheet—African Americans.* Retrieved from http://minorityhealth.hhs.gov/templates/content.aspx?ID=6903.

12. U.S. Department of Health and Human Services, Office of Minority Health. (2009b). *Infant mortality/SIDS and Hispanic Americans.* Retrieved from http://minorityhealth.hhs.gov/templates/content.aspx?ID=3329.

13. Food and Nutrition Service, FDA. (n.d.). *About WIC: WIC at a glance.* Retrieved from http://www.fns.usda.gov/wic/aboutwic/wicataglance.htm.

14. Kaiser Family Foundation. (n.d.). *Focus on health reform. Summary of Affordable Care Act.* Retrieved from http://kaiserfamilyfoundation.files.wordpress.com/2011/04/8061-021.pdf.

15. National Association of County and City Health Officials. (n.d.). *Public health and prevention provisions of the Affordable Care Act.* Retrieved from http://www.naccho.org/advocacy/upload/PH-and-Prevention-Provisions-in-the-ACA-Revised.pdf.

16. U.S. Department of Health and Human Services. (2012). *Preventive services covered under the Affordable Care Act.* Retrieved from http://www.hhs.gov/healthcare/facts/factsheets/2010/07/preventive-services-list.html#CoveredPreventiveServicesforAdults.

17. Wolfe, B. (2011-2012). Poverty and poor health: Can health care reform narrow the rich-poor gap? *Focus, 28*(2), 25-30. Retrieved from http://www.irp.wisc.edu/publications/focus/pdfs/foc282f.pdf.

18. Woolf, S.H., Johnson, R.E., & Geiger, H.J. (2006). The rising prevalence of severe poverty in America: A growing threat to public health. *American Journal of Preventive Medicine, 31*(4) 332-341. doi:10.1016/j.amepre.2006.06.022. Retrieved from http://www.ajpmonline.org/article/S0749-3797(06)00233-9/fulltext.

19. Kingston, R.S., & Smith, J.P. (1997). Socioeconomic status and racial and ethnic differences in functional status associated with chronic diseases. *American Journal of Public Health, 87*(5), 805-810.

20. Phelan, J.C., & Link, B.G. (2003). When income affects outcome: Socioeconomic status and health. *Research in Profile, 6.* Retrieved from http://www.investigatorawards.org/downloads/research_in_profiles_iss06_feb2003.pdf.

21. Fiscella, K., & Williams, D.R. (2004). Health disparities based on socioeconomic inequities: Implications for urban health care. *Academic Medicine 79*(12), 1139-1147.

22. National Conference of State Legislators. (2010). *State laws mandating or regulating mental health benefits.*

Retrieved from http://www.ncsl.org/IssuesResearch/Health/StateLawsMandatingorRegulatingMentalHealthB/tabid/14352/Default.aspx.

23. U.S. Department of Health and Human Services, Office of Disease Prevention and Health Promotion. (n.d.). *Healthy People.* Retrieved from http://www.healthypeople.gov/.

24. Department of Health and Human Services, Office of Disease Prevention and Health Promotion. (n.d.). *History & Development of Healthy People.* Retrieved from http://www.healthypeople.gov/2020/about/history.aspx.

25. U.S. Department of Health and Human Services, Centers for Medicare & Medicaid Services. (n.d.). *CMS programs & information.* Retrieved from http://www.cms.hhs.gov/.

26. U.S. Department of Labor, Occupational Safety & Health Administration. (n.d.). *Occupational Safety & Health Administration.* Retrieved from http://www.osha.gov/.

27. The Henry J. Kaiser Family Foundation. (2012). *A guide to the Supreme Court's decision on the ACA's Medicaid expansion.* Retrieved from http://kff.org/health-reform/issue-brief/a-guide-to-the-supreme-courts-decision/.

28. U.S. Department of Health and Human Services, Centers for Medicare & Medicaid Services. (n.d.). *Medicaid.* Retrieved from http://www.cms.hhs.gov/home/medicaid.asp.

29. U.S. Department of Health and Human Services, Centers for Medicare & Medicaid Services. (n.d.). *Medicaid waivers and demonstration lists.* Retrieved from http://www.cms.hhs.gov/MedicaidStWaivProgDemoPGI/MWDL/list.asp?listpage=53.

30. Pear, R. (1993, March 20). U.S. backs Oregon's health plan for covering all poor people. *The New York Times.* Retrieved from http://www.nytimes.com/1993/03/20/us/us-backs-oregon-s-health-plan-for-covering-all-poor-people.html.

31. Massachusetts Trial Court Law Library. (2009). *Massachusetts law about health insurance.* Retrieved from http://www.lawlib.state.ma.us/subject/about/healthinsurance.html.

32. State of Wisconsin DRL. (n.d.). *Registered nurse.* Retrieved from http://drl.wi.gov/profession.asp?profid=46&locid=0.

33. Novick, L.F., Morrow, C.B., & Mays, G.P. (2008). *Public health administration: Principles for population-based management* (2nd ed.). Sudbury, MA: Jones & Bartlett.

34. U.S. Food and Drug Administration, Food and Nutrition Service. (2013). *Nutrition standards for school meals.* Retrieved from http://www.fns.usda.gov/cnd/governance/legislation/nutritionstandards.htm.

35. Becker, G.S. (1990). *The economic approach to human behavior.* Chicago, IL: University of Chicago Press.

36. Abraham, C., & Michie, S. (2008). A taxonomy of behaviour change techniques used in interventions. *Health Psychology, 27*(3), 379-387.

37. National Institute for Health and Care Excellence. (2007). *Behavior change at population, community and individual levels* (NICE Public Health Guidance No. 6). London, England: Author.

38. Barjonet, P. (Ed.) (2001). *Traffic psychology today.* Dordrecht, the Netherlands: Kluwer.

39. Green, L.W., & Kreuter, M.W. (2005). *Health program planning: An educational and ecological approach* (4th ed.). Boston, MA: McGraw-Hill.

40. Fluoride Action Network. (n.d.). *Health effects: Tooth decay in fluoridated vs. unfluoridated countries.* Retrieved from http://www.fluoridealert.org/health/teeth/carries/who-dmft.html.

41. Peterson, P.E., & Lennon, M.A. (2004). Effective use of fluorides for the prevention of dental carries in the 21st Century: The WHO approach. *Community Dental Oral Epidemiology, 32,* 319-321.

42. American Dental Association Council on Scientific Affairs. (2006). Professionally applied topical fluoride: Evidence-based clinical recommendations. *Journal of the American Dental Association, 137,* 1151-1159.

43. Agency for Healthcare Research and Quality. (2014.). *The guide to clinical preventive services: 2014.* Retrieved from http://www.ahrq.gov/professionals/clinicians-providers/guidelines-recommendations/guide/cpsguide.pdf.

44. Centers for Disease Control and Prevention, Community Preventive Services Task Force. (2013). *The guide to community preventive services.* Retrieved from http://www.thecommunityguide.org/index.html.

45. Centers for Disease Control and Prevention, Community Preventive Services Task Force. (2014). *Preventing skin cancer: Primary and middle school-based interventions.* Retrieved from http://www.thecommunityguide.org/cancer/skin/education-policy/primaryandmiddleschools.html.

46. Cochrane Collaboration. (2014). *Cochrane Reviews.* Retrieved from http://www.cochrane.org/cochrane-reviews.

47. Centers for Disease Control and Prevention, Community Preventive Services Task Force. (2014). *Use of Motorcycle Helmets: Universal Helmet Laws.* Retrieved from http://www.thecommunityguide.org/mvoi/motorcyclehelmets/helmetlaws.html.

48. U.S. Department of Health and Human Services. (2014). *Healthy People 2020.* Retrieved from http://www.healthypeople.gov/hp2020/default.asp.

49. Johnson, C.W. (2003). *How our laws are made.* Washington, DC: U.S. Government Printing Office.

50. U.S. Government Printing Office (n.d) *United States code: Main page.* Retrieved from http://www.gpoaccess.gov/uscode/.

51. National Institutes of Health National Human Genome Research Institute. (2010). *Genetic nondiscrimination federal legislation archive.* Retrieved from http://www.genome.gov/11510239.

52. U.S. Department of Health and Human Services, Health Resources and Services Administration (2010). *The registered nurse population: Findings from the 2008 National Sample Survey of Registered Nurses.* Retrieved from http://bhpr.hrsa.gov/healthworkforce/rnsurveys/rnsurveyfinal.pdf.

53. Cramer, M.E. (2002). Factors influencing organized political participation in nursing. *Policy, Politics, & Nursing Practice 3*(2), 97-107.

54. Boswell, C., Cannon, S., & Miller, J. (2005). Nurses' political involvement: Responsibility versus privilege. *Journal of Professional Nursing, 21*(1), 5-8.

55. American Public Health Association. (2014). *Advocacy and policy: Advocacy activities.* Retrieved from http://www.apha.org/advocacy/activities/.

56. The Nursing Organization Alliance: Nurses in Washington Internship. (2013). *Health policy tool kit.* Retrieved from http://www.nursing-alliance.org/documents/NIWI_2013__Health_Policy_Toolkit_3086974_1.pdf.

57. Warner, J.R. (2003). A phenomenological approach to political competence: Stories from nurse activists. *Policy, Politics, & Nursing Practice, 4*(2), 135-143.

58. Abood, S. (2007). Influencing health care in the legislative arena. *OJIN: The Online Journal of Issues in Nursing, 12*(1). Retrieved from www.nursingworld.org/MainMenuCategories/ANAMarketplace/ANAPeriodicals/OJIN/TableofContents/Volume122007/No1Jan07/tpc32_216091.aspx.

59. Burney, L.E., & Yoho, R. (1955). Financing local health services. *American Journal of Public Health, 45,* 974-978. Retrieved from www.ncbi.nlm.nih.gov/pmc/articles/PMC1623122/pdf/amjphnational00348-0013pdf.

60. Santerre, R.E., & Neun, S.P. (2004). *Health economics: Theories, insights, and industry studies* (3rd ed.). Mason, OH: Thomson South Western.

61. Centers for Disease Control and Prevention. (2013). *Public health economics and tools.* Retrieved from http://www.cdc.gov/stltpublichealth/pheconomics/.

62. Honore, P.A., & Amy, B.W. (2007). Public health finance: Fundamental theories, concepts and definitions. *Journal of Public Health Management and Practice, 13*(2), 89-92.

63. Carande-Kulis, V.G., Getzen, T.E., & Thacker, S.B. (2007). Public goods and externalities: A research agenda for public health economics. *Journal of Public Health Management and Practice, 13*(2), 227-232.

64. Vandenhouten, C., Mrocek, T., Beinemann, J., Fryda, S., Behm, L., & Hansen, J. (2012). *Making sense of local health department funding: A public health finance toolkit.* Retrieved from http://www.dhs.wisconsin.gov/R_counties/HealthOfficerMaterials/NewHealthOfficers/O1_Making%20Sense%20of%20LHD%20Funding_PH%20Finance_Revised_06192012.pdf.

65. Michael, J.M, (2011). The national Board of Health: 1879-1883. *Public Health Reports, 126*(1), 123-129.

66. U.S. Department of Health and Human Services (2014). *Commissioned Corps of the U.S. Public Health Service.* Retrieved from http://www.usphs.gov/aboutus/history.aspx.

67. Centers for Disease Control and Prevention. (2013). *CDC's procurement and grants office.* Retrieved from http://www.cdc.gov/about/business/funding.htm.

68. Turnock, B.J. (2011). *Public health: What it is and how it works.* Boston, MA: Jones & Bartlett.

69. National Association of County & City Health Officials. (2011). *2010 national profile of local health departments.* Retrieved from http://www.naccho.org/

topics/infrastructure/profile/resources/2010report/
upload/2010_Profile_main_report-web.pdf.

70. Robert Wood Johnson Foundation, Trust for
America's Health. (2011). *Investing in America's
health: A state-by-state look at public health
funding and key health facts.* Retrieved from http://
healthyamericans.org/assets/files/Investing%20in%
20America's%20Health.pdf.

71. Tretmore, J., & Burke Smith, N. (2009). *The only writing series you'll ever need: Grant writing.* Avon, ME:
Adams Media.

72. U.S. Department of Health & Human Services. (n.d.).
Medicaid. Retrieved from http://www.healthcare.gov/
using-insurance/low-cost-care/medicaid/#howmed.

73. Go Medicare. (2013). *Medicaid history.* Retrieved
from http://www.gomedicare.com/medicare-
information/medicaid-history.html.

74. U.S. Department of Health & Human Services. (n.d.).
Children's Health Insurance Plan. Retrieved from
http://www.healthcare.gov/using-insurance/low-
cost-care/childrens-insurance-program/index.html.

75. Centers for Medicare & Medicaid Services. (2013). *History.* Retrieved from http://www.cms.gov/About-CMS/
Agency-Information/History/index.html?redirect=/
history/.

76. Centers for Medicare & Medicaid Services. (n.d.).
Eligibility. Retrieved from http://www.medicaid.
gov/AffordableCareAct/Provisions/Eligibility.
html.

77. U.S. Department of Health & Human Services. (2013).
*Temporary Assistance for Needy Families (TANF)
overview.* Retrieved from http://www.hhs.gov/recovery/
programs/tanf/tanf-overview.html.

78. Social Security Administration. (n.d.). *Benefits for people with disabilities.* Retrieved from http://www.ssa.
gov/disability/.

79. Social Security Administration. (2012). *Disability
benefits (SSA Publication No. 05-10029).* Retrieved
from http://www.ssa.gov/pubs/EN-05-10029.pdf.

80. Food and Nutrition Service, FDA. (n.d.). *Supplemental Nutrition Assistance Program (SNAP).* Retrieved
from http://www.fns.usda.gov/snap.

Chapter 23

Culture and Public Health Nursing

LEARNING OUTCOMES

After reading this chapter, the student will be able to:

1. Recognize the impact of culture on health promotion in populations, groups, and individuals.
2. Differentiate culture from related concepts of race, ethnicity, and minority groups.
3. Compare the difference between cultural competency and cultural humility.
4. Use cultural assessment skills to design effective primary, secondary, and tertiary interventions for populations, families, and individuals.
5. Identify cultural characteristics that are health promoting in populations, communities, groups, families, and individuals.
6. Discuss health system and provider barriers that may hinder the provision of culturally appropriate care.

KEY TERMS

Acculturation	Cultural humility	Ethnocentrism	Race
Core cultural values	Cultural imposition	Folk medicine	Stakeholders
Cultural assessment	Cultural safety	Key informants	Stereotyping
Cultural competency	Culture	Locus of control	Worldview
Cultural conflict	Ethnicity	Minority group	

■ Introduction

The influence of culture on the health of populations has been a topic of increasing interest in the health professions. Public health nursing, which has its focus on providing care for populations, aggregates, and communities, must be especially concerned about delivering care that reflects appropriate appreciation that the cultural context in which people live affects their health and is essential to the building of a trusting relationship between health-care providers and the communities they serve. The development of successful primary, secondary, and tertiary interventions in public health nursing are dependent on understanding and incorporating the cultural context. In this chapter, we explore the impact of cultural beliefs and practices on health and health-care decisions in selected groups.

Cultural Context In Public Health Nursing

In order to develop and provide nursing interventions that are effective, knowledge and understanding of this cultural context are essential. Various terms and concepts used in nursing for understanding culture and for providing care take culture into account:

- Cultural awareness
- Sensitivity
- Congruence
- Competency
- Safety
- Humility

The meanings of these terms overlap and indicate that health-care providers need to understand the impact of cultural differences and provide skillful care that recognizes, accepts, values, and incorporates these differences into an effective plan of care.

Traditionally, **culture** is defined as patterns of human behavior, beliefs, and values that have shared meanings among groups of people. According to Hall, culture has at least three components:[1]

1. What people think
2. What people do
3. The material products people produce

Culture can be depicted as a circular concept that includes family and kinship, language and tradition, health beliefs, and practices that help to form the worldview of groups of people (Fig. 23-1). Cultural patterns have been learned, not inherited, and passed from one generation to the next. They are manifest in the intangible, such as religious beliefs and family role expectations, as well as the tangible, such as the production of art, music, and dress. For example, in Pennsylvania Dutch country, the tradition of making *faustnaughts,* or German donuts, the Tuesday before Ash Wednesday has been passed down from family to family among the Amish and Mennonites who live in Lancaster County, Pennsylvania, and is part of their cultural tradition. It is considered bad luck not to have a faustnaught on Faustnaught Day. The culture of one group often extends to the community or region of a country they live in. Many of the Amish cultural traditions such as Faustnaught Day have become part of the regional culture in Lancaster County.

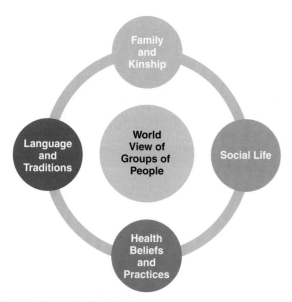

Figure 23-1 Model of culture.

Race

In contrast with culture, the concept of **race** is socially constructed and refers to the categorization of people with shared physical characteristics such as skin color and hair texture. This categorization is not scientifically based because there is no biological basis for placing one person or group of persons into one category or another as clearly demonstrated through the findings from the Human Genome Project. For thousands of years, the migratory habits of the human species resulted in humans traveling from one environment to another. Consequently, the gene pool was shared from one group to another and resulted in close genetic similarities among apparently different groups that do not share traditional physical characteristics such as skin color. Like sickle cell (caused by an abnormality in the hemoglobin gene), most traits are influenced by separate genes and inherited independently one from another. They are said to be nonconcordant. Someone with brown hair might have A, B, or O blood. Sub-Saharan Africans tend to have dark skin, but so do Dravidians from India, Aborigines from Australia, and Melanesians from the South Pacific. Large numbers of West Africans are lactose intolerant, as are Japanese, but East Africans are not. German and Papua New Guinean populations have almost exactly the same frequencies of A, B, and O blood. At one point on the genome, an individual might share a gene form that is common in Africa, at another site, East Asia, and still another, Europe. Jared Diamond points out that for each trait we can classify people into races by that trait, each giving us different and overlapping races depending on the trait selected.[2] According to Marks, racial categories represent "folk heredity." In other words, persons and their offspring are required to choose from one of a small number of designated groups. Biologically, these designations are useless and race does not reflect biological divisions in the human species.[3]

Membership in one racial category or another in the past has often been based on the current social climate. When immigrants from Mediterranean countries first migrated to the United States, they were placed in a different racial category and were not considered white. Over time, their assimilation into the mainstream culture and their lack of easily identifiable facial and skin color characteristics moved them from a separate racial category to the white category.

In the United States, the subject of race has proved to be divisive and used as a means to discriminate and deny certain groups the privileges of the larger group. The distribution of racial groups has changed over the past two decades, as illustrated by the census data from 2000 and 2010 and predictions for 2020 to 2050. For example, in 2010, 15.5% of the U.S. population identified themselves as Hispanic. The U.S. Census Bureau predicts that this will increase to over 24% by 2050 (Table 23-1). Within this larger group are numerous culturally diverse groups. For example, within the larger group of Hispanic Americans are diverse groups such as Mexican, Puerto Rican, Cuban, and Dominican Americans. Another group placed in a single category in the U.S. Census is Asian. Yet within this group, there are culturally very diverse groups such as Chinese, Japanese, and Korean. In addition, almost 18% of the residents of the United States report that English is not their primary language, highlighting the linguistic diversity in the United States. These numbers have huge implications for the ways in which we provide health care.

Ethnicity

Ethnicity refers to a shared heritage, which usually includes language and country of origin, such as Irish, Hispanic, or German. The term comes from the Greek word *ethnos,* normally translated as "nation." This shared heritage is usually based on a common history and ancestry related to a specific geographical area. It can be expressed through a shared language, food preferences, dress, religion, values, and health practices. It can represent a subset of the population from a specific country or the country as a whole or a group with shared heritage that crosses national borders. For example, Ashkenazi Jews are descended from medieval Jews who had settled along the Rhine in Germany. Over the next centuries, they migrated from Germany to eastern European countries, taking with them their culture and the Yiddish language that is a composite of the Germanic language and Hebrew. Members of this eastern European group were

conscious of their membership in the group and were recognized by others as a distinct ethnic group. There is an active East European Jewish Heritage Project aimed at preserving the rich ethnic heritage of this group (http://eejhp.netfirms.com/). A similar sense of identity was experienced by Irish immigrants in the United States, who maintained their cultural identity through song and celebrations such as St. Patrick's Day and Halloween. However, the sense of ethnic identity can change over time as groups become assimilated into other groups and new generations assimilate into the larger cultural group of their peers. Despite changes over time, ethnicity is an important factor in personal identity and reflects a person's or group's membership in a larger group with shared customs and values.

As it is used currently, the term *ethnicity* also implies minority status and is often blurred with the term *race*. However, racial categories such as white or black are inclusive of many different ethnic groups. Words presented as ethnic categories such as *Latino* or *Hispanic* again include diverse ethnic groups with different histories, ancestries, and cultural practices. There is a danger inherent in the use of broader categories such as Latino or even African American. These terms imply an underlying assumption that all of the groups including in the category are the same when they are actually quite different. For example, the category Hispanic includes populations from Spanish-speaking countries, including countries located in such diverse areas as the Caribbean islands and Central America and do not actually reflect a homogeneous ethnic group. What terms to use has been an issue in the wording of race/ethnicity categories in the U.S. Census Bureau, with changes occurring over time. To help with presenting population data, this book has adopted the U.S. Census Bureau terms. However, care must be taken when interpreting these data to develop public health interventions, so that the complexity of the groups contained within one of these categories is recognized.

TABLE 23–1	National Population Projections			
Population or Percentage and Race or Hispanic Origin	2020	2030	2040	2050
Population Total	333,896	358,475	380,016	399,803
White alone	255,346	267,604	276,438	282,959
Black alone	44,810	49,246	53,412	57,553
Asian alone	18,884	22,833	26,838	30,726
White alone, not Hispanic	199,313	198,817	193,887	186,334

Source: US Census Bureau. (2013). *2012 National population projections: summary tables, Table 4: projections of the population by sex, race and Hispanic origin for the United States 2015-2060.* Retrieved from http://www.census.gov/population/projections/data/national/2012/summarytables.html.

Minority Group

Minority group is another term that is commonly used to describe people in the United States who are not a part of the majority population of people of European descent. The continued use of this term is in question, as European Americans who have always represented the majority in the United States are projected to decline in numbers. The distribution of racial groups is projected to change over the next 40 years (see Table 23-1) In 2010, 56% of the population reported that they were white alone, not Hispanic, whereas 13% reported they were African American/black, 16% reported they were Hispanic Non Black, and 5% reported they were Asian. Six percent reported they were some other race and 3% reported they were more than one race. The smallest proportion of the population was American Indian/Alaska Native (0.9%) and Native Hawaiian/Other Pacific Islander (0.2%). By 2050, it is projected that 50.1% will report they are white alone and 24.4% will report they are Hispanic. This reflects a shift from a dominant majority population to a growing diverse population having no clear majority group. The term *minority group* describes groups who have less power, status, and advantage experienced by the majority population. Minority and majority do not simply represent numbers, but rather represent the locus of power. The changes in majority/minority that occur over this century status will also depend on closing the gap in education, household income, and personal achievement that have existed in the past between white Americans and other ethnic groups.

According to Healey, minority groups share the following characteristics:

- The experience of a pattern of disadvantage and inequality
- A visible trait or characteristic that differentiates them from other groups
- Self-consciousness as a social unit (awareness/view of world/society)
- Membership in the group is usually determined at birth
- Members tend to marry within the group[4]

Being able to clearly differentiate these terms is an important first step in understanding what culture *is* and what culture *is not*. It is also critical to understand the universality of culture in the human experience. Each person is shaped by his or her culture, and each sees the world through lenses that are colored by his or her own cultural programming. Those who share common ethnicity, racial categorization, or minority group status often share a common culture. However, this cannot be assumed. Making this assumption leads to **stereotyping** (assigning common negative or positive characteristics to everyone within a group without recognizing individual differences). Examples of negative stereotyping include making the assumption that all whites are racist or that all Muslims are terrorists. Examples of positive stereotyping include assuming that all African Americans are great basketball players, all Asians are smart, or all Italians are great cooks.

In the 21st century, the population of the United States continues to diversify at an astounding rate. We are moving away from a culture of assimilation in which diverse cultural groups are coerced into accepting and adopting the lifestyles of the dominant European American culture. Instead, we are moving toward a culture of inclusion wherein cultural diversity is accepted and even celebrated. Providing culturally based health care is essential. It is impossible and inappropriate to memorize facts about multiple cultures and apply them methodically to all within a cultural group. However, it *is* possible for nurses to commit themselves to transforming their thinking and their environments to improve health for all people while taking into account the cultural context. How nurses develop the skills to conduct cultural assessments and provide appropriate care is a conscious process that requires reflection, commitment, and experience. Nurses who have developed them and use these skills effectively can transform health-care environments into safe, effective places for people of all cultural backgrounds.

United States: Cultural Norms and Values

Although there is great cultural diversity within the United States, it is clear that there are overarching norms and values that can be distinctly identified as a part of the culture of the United States. Some of these cultural norms and values are political in origin, such as democracy and individual rights. Others stem from the puritanical culture of the first settlers, such as the work ethic, whereas others have evolved over time, such as materialism, competition, and the free market place. At times, these values lie in direct conflict with cultural groups whose norms are more collective and cooperative, or who do not place a high value on achieving material wealth.

Values and norms in the culture of the United States are changing rapidly as a result of advances in technology. Various computer technologies have altered the ways in which Americans live, influencing almost every aspect of their lives. Education, social networking, and obtaining health information are only a few aspects of living that occur frequently by way of computer, instead of by face-to-face encounters. These technologies in turn are changing the global culture as the Internet allows instant access to people in other countries. Knowledge can be shared and collaborations fostered internationally with the click of the mouse. It remains to be seen how technology will continue to influence and shape both American and global cultures (see Chapter 13).

Regional Cultural Norms and Values

People living in various regions of the United States are cognizant of the differences in culture from region to region. We are all familiar with the Cajun and Creole cultures of New Orleans and related cuisine and the New England region with its distinctive accent and fierce independence. Different regions of the country celebrate these kinds of rich cultural traditions and use them to promote tourism. Regional cultural differences are expressed in food, language, music (e.g., bluegrass music and New Orleans jazz), art, and even social norms.

Climate and topography are just two environmental influences on regional cultural differences. Those who live in temperate climates such as the Southeast and the Southwest spend more time outdoors, participate in more outdoor activities, and socialize more with those outside of the home. Lifestyles may also be more relaxed in regions with warmer year round temperatures. For example, casual clothing may be more acceptable even in professional environments in these areas. In contrast, those who live in colder climates may spend more time indoors and have less opportunity to meet community members in casual outdoor settings year-round. Very cold regions of the United States develop community gatherings indoors during the winter, such as the gathering around the wood stove in Vermont country stores. Over time, these practices can shape unique regional cultures related to social practices and how communities interact. For example, when persons from one climate immigrate to another climate, the ability to change clothing styles to adapt to the new climate is harder because of the cultural norms surrounding clothing styles. In the 1800s, missionaries to Hawaii continued to change into winter clothing in November based on the dictates of their New England culture and the seasonal changes of that region, despite the fact that the weather is warm year-round in Hawaii.

Cultural foods vary from region to region and are often developed based on environmental availability, economics, and ethnic origins. Examples include different types of seafood such as Maine lobster and Gulf Coast crawfish or Louisiana "cracklins" made from frying pork skins. Regional foods are rich in variety and have contributed to the tourist trade. What would Philadelphia be without the Philly cheesesteak, Baltimore without the Maryland crab cake, or New Orleans without jambalaya?

Various ethnic groups have settled in large numbers in different regions of the United States and have influenced the overall culture of that region through music, architecture, foods, dialects, and other customs As migration continues to occur, regional cultures will invariably change. For example, large numbers who fled New Orleans after Hurricane Katrina in 2005 have settled permanently in various regions of the United States, bringing their unique culture with them.

Because the shared learning, values, and traditions that make up culture guide and influence all aspects of human behavior, they shape individual and community health beliefs and responses to threats to health.

Cultural Competency and Cultural Humility

Over the past two decades, **cultural competency** has become a core aspect of care for health-care providers. It is traditionally defined as the attitudes, knowledge, and skills the health-care provider has to provide quality care to culturally diverse populations. It revolves around acquiring an understanding and capacity to provide care in a diverse environment. This implies an endpoint of acquired knowledge related to the culture of others. **Cultural humility,** conversely, acknowledges that the understanding of the multitude of diverse cultures in the world today may be too big a task. Cultural humility is a continual process of self-awareness about one's own culture and the acknowledgment of the requirement that we approach others as equals with respect for their prevailing beliefs and cultural norms.[5-7] One is not exclusive of the other. Rather, cultural competence is the standard to help guide the delivery of health care to individuals and to populations, whereas cultural humility is the underlying quality needed to truly implement interventions aimed at improving health in partnership with communities and populations.

Developing cultural humility takes self-reflection. This provides an essential beginning point for nurses to develop the insight and knowledge needed to provide care to those who differ culturally from themselves. How do nurses create health-care environments that are safe and welcoming for clients and patients from all backgrounds? The first step in this process for individual nurses should be a cultural self-assessment. Cultural self-assessment involves a critical reflection of one's own viewpoints, experiences, attitudes, values, and beliefs. When one can honestly identify learned stereotypes and ethnocentric attitudes, enlightenment can occur. Nurses cannot begin to effectively provide care taking into consideration the cultural context without first exploring their own cultures. The following questions can be used to guide cultural self-reflection:

- Where did I grow up? How did this environment influence my worldview (country, region, rural, urban)?
- What values were emphasized in my family of origin?
- Who were the people most influential to me in shaping my worldview?
- Who were the people within my circle of friends and acquaintances during my years of growing up? How did they differ from me?
- What privileges did I enjoy while growing up?
- What are some of the key experiences that have shaped my view of the world and the people in it?
- What are my religious beliefs, if any?
- What are the values and morals that I adhere to?
- What does "good health" mean to me? How do I obtain and maintain good health?
- How do I view those individuals whose values differ from my own?

Creating a culturally welcoming health-care environment requires purposeful action by health-care providers. This necessitates commitment to principles and practices on all levels that support inclusion. These principles and practices should be a part of the systemic workings of health-care organizations. There should be visible and tangible signs of culturally welcoming health-care environments. However, more important is the provision of care by those nurses who are skilled at cultural assessment and inclusionary care.

Nurses must be familiar with current research findings to guide their practice. Combining the knowledge gained from cultural communities with scientific evidence can help nurses develop interventions that are culturally appropriate and evidence based. Interventions that have been tested and found effective with various cultural groups can be considered for possible implementation in like communities. Nurses must become astute in scrutinizing research evidence for inclusion and applicability to various cultural, ethnic, and racial groups. A good example is the research that has been done related to health practices of African American men. Because this group is at high risk for preventable noncommuicable diseases such as diabetes and hypertension, researchers have explored the cultural contexts of health practices as well as the utility of certain settings that would provide an appropriate cultural context for interventions such as the use of African American barber shops as a setting for interventions. These studies form the basis of evidence-based practice in relation to the inclusion of culture into health interventions.

■ EVIDENCE-BASED PRACTICE
The Use of Barber Shops as a Cultural Space to Provide Interventions to African American Men

Practice Statement: The prevalence and severity of hypertension is higher in African Americans than in any other ethnic group in the United States, and men are more apt to have unrecognized hypertension than are women.[1]

Targeted Outcome: Reducing uncontrolled hypertension in African Americans

Evidence to Support: Numerous studies have been conducted to help identify possible interventions that would be culturally relevant to African American males. One culturally central place is the neighborhood barbershop.[1] Based on the findings from a number of studies, there is strong evidence to suggest that the barbershop is culturally appropriate setting for the delivery of interventions aimed at early identification and treatment of hypertension in African American males. These interventions deliver the screening and referral for treatments within the context of the daily life to the men. The barbers themselves become advocates for the intervention. This model has been subsequently adopted for implementing screening programs for prostate cancer and for HIV/AIDS.

References:
Agency for Healthcare Research and Quality (2014). *Barber-based monitoring, education, and referral support improve treatment rates and blood pressure control in African-American men.* Retrieved from http://www.innovations.ahrq.gov/content.aspx?id=3046.

Alexander, B.K. (2003). Fading, twisting and weaving: An interpretive ethnography of the black barbershop as cultural space. *Qualitative Inquiry, 9*(1), 105-128.

Hess, P., Reingold, J, Jones, J.,Fellman, M.A,, Kowles, P., Ravenell, J.E. . . . Victor, R.G.(2007). Barbershops as hypertension detection, referral, and follow-up centers for black men, *Hypertension. 49*(5):1040-1046. Apr 2.

National Standards for Culturally Appropriate Health Care

National standards for culturally and linguistically appropriate health care provide a framework for preferred practices for culturally competent care as well as guidelines for health-care organizations. The goal of these guidelines is to establish measures by which health-care organizations can evaluate their practices in providing competent and equal care. The Office of Minority Health of the U.S. Department of Health and Human Services has developed 14 standards organized by themes: Culturally competent care, language access services, and organizational supports for cultural competence (Box 23-1).[8]

To help guide the use of standards in practice, health-care providers can apply the National Quality Forum's four guiding principles for measuring and reporting cultural competency:

1. Cultural competency in health care embraces the concept of equity, with patients having equal access to quality care and nondiscriminatory, patient-centered practices delivered by health-care providers.
2. Cultural competency is necessary, but not sufficient, to achieving an equitable health-care system.
3. Cultural competency should be viewed as an ongoing process and a multilevel approach, with assessments and interventions needed at the system, organization, group, community, and individual levels. Cultural competency should not be viewed as an endpoint; rather, communities, organizations, and individuals should strive for continuous improvement.
4. The successful implementation of cultural competency initiatives to achieve high-quality, culturally competent, patient-centered care requires an organizational

---

BOX 23–1 National Standards on Culturally and Linguistically Appropriate Services (CLAS)

The National Standards for Culturally and Linguistically Appropriate Services in Health and Health Care (The National CLAS Standards) aim to improve health care quality and advance health equity by establishing a framework for organizations to serve the nation's increasingly diverse communities.

Principal Standard

1. Provide effective, equitable, understandable and respectful quality care and services that are responsive to diverse cultural health beliefs and practices, preferred languages, health literacy and other communication needs.

Governance, Leadership and Workforce

2. Advance and sustain organizational governance and leadership that promotes CLAS and health equity through policy, practices and allocated resources.
3. Recruit, promote and support a culturally and linguistically diverse governance, leadership and workforce that are responsive to the population in the service area.
4. Educate and train governance, leadership and workforce in culturally and linguistically appropriate policies and practices on an ongoing basis.

Communication and Language Assistance

5. Offer language assistance to individuals who have limited English proficiency and/or other communication needs, at no cost to them, to facilitate timely access to all health care and services.
6. Inform all individuals of the availability of language assistance services clearly and in their preferred language, verbally and in writing.
7. Ensure the competence of individuals providing language assistance, recognizing that the use of untrained individuals and/or minors as interpreters should be avoided.
8. Provide easy-to-understand print and multimedia materials and signage in the languages commonly used by the populations in the service area.

Engagement, Continuous Improvement and Accountability

9. Establish culturally and linguistically appropriate goals, policies and management accountability, and infuse them throughout the organizations' planning and operations.
10. Conduct ongoing assessments of the organization's CLAS-related activities and integrate CLAS-related measures into assessment measurement and continuous quality improvement activities.
11. Collect and maintain accurate and reliable demographic data to monitor and evaluate the impact of CLAS on health equity and outcomes and to inform service delivery.
12. Conduct regular assessments of community health assets and needs and use the results to plan and implement services that respond to the cultural and linguistic diversity of populations in the service area.
13. Partner with the community to design, implement and evaluate policies, practices and services to ensure cultural and linguistic appropriateness.
14. Create conflict- and grievance-resolution processes that are culturally and linguistically appropriate to identify, prevent and resolve conflicts or complaints.
15. Communicate the organization's progress in implementing and sustaining CLAS to all stakeholders, constituents and the general public.

Source: U.S. Department of Health and Human Services, Office of Minority Health (2014). Retrieved from http://minorityhealth.hhs.gov/omh/browse.aspx?lvl=2&lvlid=53.

commitment with a systems approach toward cultural competency. Addressing both organizational and clinical aspects when managing diversity and the needs of a diverse workforce, the surrounding community, and the patient population are important factors in providing culturally competent care.[9]

Public Health Nursing Standards for Cultural Competence

Cultural competency is one of the core competencies for all public health-care providers as well as public health nurses (PHNs). The core competencies in public health nursing were developed by the Quad Council and cover both generalist and advanced public health nursing practice. The Quad Council is made up of representatives from four organizations: (1) the American Nurses Association Council on Nursing Practice and Economics, (2) the Association of Community Health Nurse Educators, (3) the Public Health Nurses section of the American Public Health Association, and (4) Association of Public Health Nurses. These competencies demonstrate the importance of working with diverse groups and adapting public health interventions to cultural needs and differences. [10]

Applying these cultural competencies as well as cultural humility to real-life situations is essential to the success of interventions aimed at improving the health of populations. As pointed out by Levi,[6] cultural humility is essential to the delivery of ethical health care to diverse populations. It is a lifelong process of self-discovery conducted with a belief in equality and partnership between people of different cultures.

● APPLYING PUBLIC HEALTH SCIENCE
Cancer in a West Virginia Coal Mining Community
Public Health Science Topics Covered:
• Assessment

In the United States, the region known as Appalachia includes 410 counties in 13 states, extends from southern New York through northern Alabama and Mississippi, and includes significant portions of the states of Kentucky and Ohio, and all of West Virginia.[11] This region has long been recognized for its lower socioeconomic status, but more recently, distinct health disparities have been identified in Appalachia when compared with other regions of the United States The

elimination of health disparities in the United States is one of the overarching goals of the *Healthy People 2020 (HP 2020)* document that sets goals for the nation's health (see Chapter 7) (Box 23-2).

In addition to mortality from other causes, cancer has specifically been identified as a major cause of death in both white and black Appalachian people. Colorectal, breast, cervical, and lung cancers have been cited as especially high in Appalachia[11,12] and have been linked to the coal mining industry that has been a major employer in West Virginia for nearly a century (Fig. 23-2). Those who live in coal mining communities, where both surface and deep mining occur, have higher rates of various health problems such as cardiopulmonary disease, chronic obstructive pulmonary disease, hypertension, lung disease, kidney disease, and cancer. Although most miners are men, women are also subject to poorer health when compared with those who do not live in mining communities, which may be related to exposure to coal dust in the environment.[12]

The Cultural Assessment

To help illustrate the importance of culture, let's examine how PHNs can include **cultural assessment** as part of a focused assessment of a hypothetical community. As mentioned in Chapter 4, a focused community assessment starts with the problem and attempts to determine the underlying factors that either contribute to the problem or protect against it, which are specific to the community or population being assessed. A cultural assessment is defined as the assessment of the culture of the community and/or population of interest. It is part of the larger community assessment process described in Chapters 4 and 5. The results provide insight into the role this community's culture plays in health and disease and provides valuable information needed to develop a culturally appropriate intervention.

BOX 23–2	*Healthy People 2020* Overarching Goals

• Attain high quality, longer lives free of preventable disease, disability, injury, and premature death.
• Achieve health equity, eliminate disparities, and improve the health of all groups.
• Create social and physical environments that promote good health for all.
• Promote quality of life, healthy development and healthy behaviors across all life stages.

Source: US Department of Health and Human Services, *Healthy People 2020.* Retrieved from http://www.healthypeople.gov/2020/about/default.aspx.

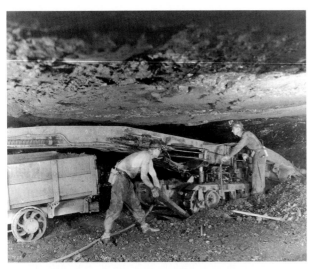

Figure 23-2 Coal miners in Appalachia. This image depicts two miners inside a coal mine as they are operating a mechanized coal bin loader. The loader is excavating raw ore from the walls of the mine shaft, and then dumps the ore into a wooden railcar. Of importance is the fact that neither miner is wearing protective breathing gear, which would have filtered the dust-laden air prior to inhalation by the miners. Owing to the inescapable presence of airborne coal dust in the small confines of a mine, miners are predisposed to the long-term, negative health effects of this profession, such as black lung disease, or coal-workers' pneumoconiosis. Today, the federal government's stringent regulations on the level of coal dust permissible in the air of a coal mine, and the requisite use of filtered breathing devices, have dramatically lowered the number of cases of black lung disease. *(From the Centers for Disease Control and Prevention, National Institute for Occupational Safety and Health.)*

This case involves three new PHNs recruited to practice in a medically underserved coal mining community in West Virginia. This community of about 5,000 lies in a county that is a major coal producer in the state. The closest major city is Charleston, the capital, which is about 50 miles away. The population is 90% white, with an average age of 41. About 52% of the population is married. The average income is about $28,000. Mortality rates from lung, breast, and cervical cancers in this community have continued to rise in spite of efforts to increase education about the value of cancer screenings. The nurses are asked to conduct a community assessment to help establish underlying risk factors and develop relevant programs. One of the nurses suggests that they include a cultural assessment in their overall community assessment.

They all agree that culture is important to developing an intervention, but they disagree on the value of a cultural assessment.

Three Approaches to the Community Cultural Assessment

The first nurse completed a master's degree in public health nursing and took a course on vulnerable populations. She and the other students in her class completed a special project on Appalachian culture. She believes that she is prepared to develop an effective program of interventions for the community based on the cultural knowledge she gained from her education. She is not sure that there is a need to conduct a cultural assessment.

The second nurse grew up in the Appalachian region of the United States, although not in this particular community. He left Appalachia to attend college and now has returned to use his knowledge and skills to improve health in this medically underserved region. He has personal knowledge of the Appalachian culture and believes that he is best prepared to develop interventions that will be effective in reaching the community for addressing cancer prevention. Like the first nurse, he believes he has sufficient cultural knowledge and is not sure a cultural assessment is needed.

In contrast, the third nurse has had little exposure to the culture of Appalachia. However, she has experience in working with various populations in medically underserved regions in the United States and abroad. She values the information from the other nurses but believes that they should conduct a cultural assessment that would provide insight into this specific Appalachian community. She believes that they should include community members as partners in the design of any program that they develop related to cancer prevention.

All three of the nurses bring needed skills to the table. The knowledge that the first nurse has acquired in her graduate program course is valuable and will provide useful information to help this team of nurses in addressing the problem of increasing cancer rates in this community. However, knowledge gained from textbooks and course work cannot alone be relied on as the basis for the design of appropriate intervention strategies. The second nurse has personal cultural knowledge about Appalachia that will benefit this team in developing intervention strategies. One individual's personal knowledge, however, cannot be relied on as the basis for the design of a program of intervention, because his knowledge is based on the culture of his own community and may differ from this community.

However, his Appalachian background may give him credibility and help him interface with the community. Knowledge emanating from the individuals who dwell in the community in combination with a systematic community assessment provide the best basis for developing an effective intervention for cancer prevention in this community.

The third nurse's strategy for conducting the cultural assessment will take into account the cultural history of the community as well as current norms, values, and health beliefs. This information will be part of their full focused assessment that includes other aspects of the community such as the physical environment, the political environment, education, health-care accessibility, and epidemiological data.

Conducting the Community Cultural Assessment

Next, an in-depth assessment of the culture of this community is warranted. Andrews and Boyle delineate the components of a cultural assessment:[13]

- Family and kinship systems
- Social life
- Political systems
- Language and traditions
- Worldview, value orientations, and cultural norms
- Religion
- Health beliefs and practices
- Environmental influences on culture

In addition to the seven components outlined by Andrews and Boyle, adding the environmental influences on culture to this list provides additional information needed to accurately describe the cultural domain. Often, cultural practices occur because of environmental aspects such as geographic isolation or climate. Using these eight components to guide the assessment will result in the knowledge of the culture of this coal mining community in West Virginia that is needed to develop effective interventions for prevention of cancer mortality.

To best develop an understanding of the cultural context of a community, spending time with community members is essential. Ideally, living in the community, attending community social functions, and becoming involved in the political system would give the nurse the best view of the cultural workings of the community. However, in most cases, this in-depth engagement with community members is not possible. Nurses often live in communities outside of the ones in which they work. They are challenged to find a way to develop insight into the culture of an entire community

without depending on stereotypical knowledge, or knowledge derived purely from textbook information. Public health nurses should also incorporate readings from evidence-based literature, culturally produced reading materials such as local newspapers or magazines, and historical readings about the culture.

Conducting a cultural assessment should begin with a review of the demographics of the community. How many people live in the community and what are their ages? Where do they live? The nurses used the guide in Box 23-3 to help guide their cultural assessment.

Key Informants and Stakeholders

They began by identifying **key informants** in the community. Key informants are people who are known to

---

BOX 23–3 Guide for Conducting a Community Cultural Assessment

- Identify the cultural community of interest:
  - Demographics
  - Environment
  - History in the community
  - Sociopolitical conditions
  - Language
- Explore the culture through reading:
  - Evidence-based literature
  - Local cultural publications (newspapers, magazines)
  - Historical literature about the culture
- Interact with members of the cultural community.
  - Participate in community cultural events.
  - Visit local churches, gathering places, and social activities.
- Connect and engage with community groups.
  - Identify community stakeholders.
  - Talk with key informants about cultural community issues.
  - Participate with local community councils, or attend meetings.
- Ask, listen, observe:
  - Customs
  - Traditions
  - Beliefs
  - Practices
  - Values and norms
  - Family structure and roles
- Identify cultural strengths.
- Identify risks, barriers, and untapped resources.
- Confirm assessment data with key members of the cultural community.
- Analyze data with members of the cultural group to begin community planning.

hold specific and accurate knowledge about the community or culture. Key informants usually share the **worldview** of the community, that is, the community culture and its view of reality about the world. They have been members of the community for a long period of time and can articulate the values, beliefs, and traditions of the culture.

Next, the PHNs identified the stakeholders in the community. **Stakeholders** in a community are those people who live, work, and interface with the community, and have a vested interest in the life, health, and maintenance of the community. They have a concern for its people, families, institutions, and traditions, and for the preservation of the community. Stakeholders always include community dwellers, and may include people of influence such as community leaders, clergy, health-care workers, teachers, community council members, and law enforcement officers. Community stakeholders have a unique insider's perspective into the "life ways" of the community. Their abilities to identify strengths, challenges, problems, and solutions are based on their participation in the culture and the daily life experiences in the community.

The stakeholders included not only members of the health-care community and residents of the community but also the employers, all of whom were experiencing lost work time owing to illness and a rise in their health insurance costs. As a group, the stakeholders and the key informants provided access to information for their broader focused assessment that included the collection of data across various aspects of the community. For the cultural assessment piece, the key informants and community stakeholders are essential because they often have the cultural knowledge that is hidden to outsiders, which can be the key to making an intervention effective.

After the community stakeholders were identified, a meeting was called to talk about the initial findings of their full focused assessment, which provided detail on the prevalence of cancer in their community and the cancer mortality rate. At the meeting, all of the community stakeholders revealed that they had family members and friends who had died of cancer, and were pleased that they were invited to participate in finding solutions. The stakeholders decided that they wanted to hold more meetings so that they could gain greater clarity about the scope of the problem and what the next steps should be.

Focus Groups

As part of the cultural assessment, the stakeholders, including the nurses, decided that they would invite community members to a series of focus groups to talk

about their culture and how what aspects of their culture may help to improve the success of an intervention aimed at reducing cancer in their community. They developed focus group questions that addressed the key aspects of the cultural assessment (family and kinship, social life, sociopolitical systems, language and traditions, worldview, value orientations, cultural norms, religion, health beliefs and practices, and cultural influences on the environment).

Focus group members were also asked how the health-care system might more adequately meet their health-care needs, taking into account their unique culture. From the broader assessment, they had already identified important key issues for the community such as lack of access to care, which included access to health information about cancer prevention, prevention and treatment services, and long distances to major medical centers. They had also learned that illness had a negative impact on the families' economic stability, as these families lived from paycheck to paycheck.

Findings From the Cultural Assessment

From the cultural assessment, the PHNs identified a strong cultural asset in the value placed on close family and community ties. Community members spoke about the closeness of family and friends who were the major support systems in both health and illness. Community pride was important and members of the community trusted those who lived and grew up in their community. The people in the community relied on each other and when a family member was ill, other members of the community stepped in and helped with the essentials such as food preparation and childcare. They were proud of their crafts and especially their music. Almost every family had a vegetable garden and every summer and fall canned vegetables from the garden, especially green beans, pickles, and tomatoes, providing a rich source of fresh vegetables during the summer and fall and a source of vitamins (especially vitamin C) during the winter months.

The nurses also found that the people in this community valued their churches and counted on their congregations to help them when they were sick, not only through actual assistance but also through prayer. Churches were the main gathering place and source of information for the members of the community. The focus group members believed that the greatest strength in their community was their religious faith. The nurses also discovered that their predominant belief about cancer was that it was God's will and had to be endured.

People in the community reported that they were reluctant to see the doctor not only because of cost and long distances, but also because it was a sign of weakness to admit that they were sick or felt any pain. Community members believed that they were isolated geographically from larger communities and cities. Traveling to receive health care was difficult and required a full day to do so. The community members also felt that their isolation kept them from receiving needed education and screenings.

The process took time, but as the PHNs progressed through the cultural assessment they not only gained knowledge about the culture of the community but also began to build trust between themselves and the people

of the community. They summarized their findings using the eight domains of a cultural assessment (Table 23-2). The community respected the nurses' dedication to learning about the people's culture and their willingness to listen and see the world through the eyes of the community. The nurses discovered that the community was also concerned about the growing cancer cases, but that they had been reluctant to seek help because they distrusted outsiders and felt it was their lot in life to suffer these illnesses.

Culturally Appropriate Interventions

After the completion of their cultural assessment, the three nurses met to discuss how to build on their new

TABLE 23–2 Findings From the Cultural Assessment of a Hypothetical Coal Mining Community in West Virginia

Cultural Domain	Findings
Family and Kinships	Strong family relationships and community networks Traditional nuclear and extended families Traditionally patriarchal Respect and honor for elders
Social life	Family-oriented and church-sponsored activities
Political systems	Mayor and police force viewed with respect because they all were raised in the community
Language and traditions	English with some regional variation
Worldview, value orientations, cultural norms	Personal and family privacy Regional loyalty Family and regional pride Suspicion of outsiders Trust earned over time through repeated encounters
Religion	Strong belief and faith in God Prayer is an important part of life and means of healing
Health beliefs and practices	Fatalism, especially with diagnosis of cancer Low expectations of good health because of the hazardous mountain life Parish nurses seen as credible care providers and one of the family doctors treated as one of their own New clinic sponsored by the regional hospital viewed with skepticism as the nurses and doctors are outsiders Most health-care information obtained from friends, neighbors, and family High rates of tobacco use Strong belief in folk medicine
Environment	Though environment is related to the broader comprehensive assessment, key issues for the culture of the community stem from environmental issues. There is a low population density in the community—that is, there is a large area with families scattered in valleys and "hollers," increasing the isolation within the community and therefore the reliance on family. The geographical isolation related to the valleys and the main river that separates the community from its neighbors contributes to the community's identification as a separate entity and increases the distrust of neighbors.

knowledge to develop a culturally relevant intervention aimed at reducing cancer rates in the community.

The first nurse believed that after the community assessment, including the cultural assessment, was completed, all of the health-care providers in the community should meet together to decide on the best way to address the rise of cancer in the community. She believed that knowledgeable professionals who were the caregivers in the community would have the skill, professional insight, and experience with members of the community to develop culturally appropriate interventions.

The second nurse suggested that they hold a large community forum to tell the community about the results of their community assessment, including the cultural assessment and the cancer problem and urge them to participate in health screenings and educational programs about cancer.

Although she thought these suggestions had merit, the third nurse felt strongly that the community assessment, cultural assessment, and community engagement should go hand in hand. She wanted to actively engage the community in solving its own health problems using members' own ideas that arose from their cultural knowledge. She suggested that they partner with the community throughout the development of the intervention, believing that this approach would help to apply the cultural knowledge they had gathered to the health problem they were addressing while building on the acceptance they had gained while doing their cultural assessment, thus increasing buy-in by the community for the intervention.

Through discussion, they agreed that the first nurse was correct in recognizing that the health-care providers in the community had a special insight into the health problems in the community and some of the barriers to health that existed. She was also correct in understanding the knowledge and skill related to prevention, care, and treatment that these health-care providers possessed. Despite this, they concluded that if their intervention was driven *only* by professional health-care providers without community input, then their program might not be successful. Their main concern was the possible misperception by the community that this program was being done *for* them rather than *with* them. Although the nurses concluded that all of the health-care providers in the community met the standard for culturally competent care, they agreed that the cultural assessment had identified some missing links related to cultural understanding that were vital to the

intervention, in particular that the community valued partnering with health-care providers as equals. This had implications for their view of the health-care providers at the new hospital clinic as outsiders.

The second nurse recognized the need for community members to be active participants in their own care. He believed that after collecting the cultural and community assessment data, the nurses became the cultural and community experts and would deliver its prescriptive solutions to the community. Through further discussion, the last nurse was able to explain that cultural knowledge dwelled within the community and the community members were the true experts. The three concluded that the community itself (professionals as well as lay members) should develop interventions aimed at reducing the high prevalence of cancer in their community as equal partners. Only in this way would the intervention be culturally relevant to the community.

The third nurse suggested that they continue to work with the group of stakeholders that had helped them conduct the cultural assessment. She also suggested that they identify additional community stakeholders who could help with the development and implementation of the program. In particular, she felt it was important to have a cultural mediator who was completely familiar with the Appalachian culture of this particular community and understood the health-care providers' perspective. A cultural mediator helps to translate the culture of the community and the culture of the health-care providers to each group, thus enhancing understanding between the two groups.[14] In this way, the mediator assists in the sharing of information and helps to create a relationship between the health-care providers and the community.

The PHNs chose as their cultural mediator a physician who had grown up in the community and had been practicing medicine in the community for 35 years. He was chosen because he was a valued member of the community with personal knowledge of the culture, was skilled in interpersonal relations, and also had a knowledge of the health-care community.

Development of a Culturally Relevant Intervention

The findings from the cultural assessment and the broader focused community assessment were reviewed by the community partnership and incorporated into the planned cancer prevention program. This program was multifaceted and included plans to make environmental changes to reduce exposure to coal dust, a smoking cessation program, and a cancer-screening program. The community partnership agreed that the interventions required a culturally appropriate approach. Specifically, the nurses made the following recommendations to the local health district related to the incorporation of the community's culture into the program:

- Train and hire community members as lay community health-care providers to conduct smoking and tobacco chewing cessation support groups.
- Use clergy, church leaders, and church activities to promote cancer screening and provide additional support to those wishing to quit tobacco chewing and/or smoking.
- Host a crafts and music festival as a kickoff event to the beginning of the cancer screening and tobacco chewing and smoking cessation program, with the proceeds going to a fund to help pay for cancer screening.
- Continue quarterly meetings of the community stakeholders' group to evaluate the inclusion of culture into the two health programs and make new recommendations as necessary.
- Hold open meetings for the community in the planning of the proposed environmental changes aimed at reducing exposure to coal dust to help reduce the possibility of distrust between community members and those implementing the changes.

The process of conducting a cultural assessment and developing a culturally relevant intervention must be conducted in concert with community members. In this scenario, the cultural assessment added needed information in the development of a health program aimed at addressing the high rates of cancer in a West Virginia coal mining community by providing essential cultural information that is required for a culturally relevant intervention. Cultural knowledge derived from those who share cultural values, norms, beliefs, and experiences has the potential to enhance the delivery of health information and prevention interventions. For health-care providers and nurses in particular, lack of knowledge of cultural health beliefs and practices can lead to cultural misunderstandings and conflict between health-care providers and the families they serve.

Cultures in Conflict

Cultural beliefs and practices surrounding health and illness are deeply entrenched in families and are often unknown to health-care providers who do not share a similar cultural background. The Western medical model of health care at times may be in direct opposition to the beliefs and practices of those from an Eastern perspective. This **cultural conflict** has the potential to lead to misunderstandings and inaccurate assessment data by the PHN. Cultural conflict can occur when values, beliefs, and practices of one cultural group are in variance with those of another. In the prior section, we discussed the role of the community and cultural assessment when working with a population or an aggregate. However, there are other situations in which the nurse must plan and provide care for a family who may live in isolation from their cultural community. When the nurse develops a plan of care based on his own cultural knowledge, an incorrect assessment may be the result.

Asian Pacific Islanders represent the fastest growing group of immigrants to the United States. Within this group of immigrants, the largest number are from China. The greatest numbers of Chinese immigrants are clustered in larger urban areas such as Chicago, New York, Boston, Philadelphia, and Washington, DC, and many live in the state of California. People known as Chinese American are quite diverse and range from recent immigrants to those who have been long-time U.S. residents and have become highly acculturated to Western society.[15]

▶ **SOLVING THE MYSTERY**

East Meets West: The Postpartum Predicament

Public Health Science Topics Covered:

- Assessment
- Advocacy
- Communication

Diane, a new PHN, has become a part of the maternal-child division of the health department in a small community in the midwestern United States. She makes home visits to new mothers at high risk for postpartum difficulties. She is scheduled to visit Ms. Wang, a recent immigrant from China and a first-time mother. Ms. Wang and her husband recently moved to Nebraska when her husband took a position with a large manufacturing company in the area after completing his degree at a major university.

Prior to her first visit with Ms. Wang, Diane reviewed the postpartum notes from Ms. Wang's hospital stay. She delivered a healthy baby boy. However, post-delivery, the nurses noted that Ms. Wang refused her meals, did not want to bathe or shower, and asked that her baby be given his bath in the newborn nursery. Ms. Wang was discharged with standard discharge instructions and was given an appointment for the baby's first well-baby visit in 2 weeks. Ms. Wang indicated that she understood the instructions. Because she did not show up for the scheduled appointment for the baby's checkup, she was referred to the maternal-child division of the health department. At 3 weeks postpartum, Diane called to make an appointment for a home visit. Ms. Wang answered the phone and very reluctantly agreed to have Diane visit.

When Diane arrived at the home, Ms. Wang's mother greeted her at the door and escorted her into the bedroom. Diane found Ms. Wang sitting in a chair next to the bed. Although it was a warm summer day, the house was unusually warm with no air-conditioning or fans. Diane noted that Ms. Wang was dressed in long pants with socks and a long-sleeved blouse.

Diane greeted Ms. Wang and explained that the purpose of her visit was to check both the baby and Ms. Wang to make sure that the baby was thriving and that Ms. Wang was recovering from the delivery. Diane used standard assessment tools and found that the baby was meeting appropriate physical and developmental milestones for 3 weeks of age. However, she ascertained that Ms. Wang's mother was providing most of the care for the baby except for feeding.

After receiving Ms. Wang's permission, Diane assessed her uterus for involution. She noticed a distinct body odor and inquired about Ms. Wang's activity including her bathing routines since the baby had been born. Ms. Wang indicated that she had neither bathed nor showered. Diane was concerned that the house temperature was too warm for a newborn baby. She documented the lack of Ms. Wang's self-care, especially the lack of bathing, and the limited infant care provided by Ms. Wang. Though Diane did not speak or understand Chinese and Ms. Wang spoke limited English, Diane gave Ms. Wang and her mother written instructions in English about postpartum and infant care as this was the only written instructional material she had available. She advised Ms. Wang to bathe regularly and wash her hair. She provided information for the family to obtain fans to cool their home. She reminded Ms. Wang of her 6-week postpartum visit. Diane also made a recommendation that Ms. Wang be evaluated for postpartum depression at the 6-week checkup. Ms. Wang nodded her assent to Diane's instructions, but felt worried and confused after Diane left. How could

Diane have included key cultural assessment pieces to her encounter with Ms. Wang? (Box 23-4).

At 6 weeks postpartum Ms. Wang was scheduled to come in for her appointment. Prior to the visit, Edith, the nurse working at the clinic, read the notes from Diane's home visit with the Wang family. After calling Ms. Wang to confirm her appointment, Edith arranged for a Chinese language interpreter to assist with Ms. Wang's visit. When Ms. Wang arrived at the clinic for her appointment, she was dressed in long pants, a long-sleeved shirt, and a jacket. She was pleasant and pleased to see a Chinese interpreter. Edith conducted a modified individual cultural assessment tailored specifically to childbearing beliefs and practices. This assessment, developed by the nurse, was based on specific cultural information that she needed to know to provide appropriate care related to childbearing. A brief individual cultural assessment can elicit needed cultural information at the point of care. This individual approach differs from an in-depth community cultural assessment, which is much broader in scope and can be used to develop a wealth of knowledge about a cultural group or community.

Speaking directly to Ms. Wang, she asked the following questions, which the interpreter reiterated in Chinese to Ms. Wang:

- What does it mean to you and your family to have a new baby boy?
- What are the special ways that you take care of yourself after having a baby?
- What are the things that you should avoid after having a baby?
- What kinds of foods should you eat after having a baby?
- Who makes the decisions about your and the baby's care?

BOX 23–4	East Meets West: The Postpartum Predicament

Questions for Consideration

- How could Diane have better prepared to conduct the home visit with Ms. Wang?
- What critical errors did Diane make in her postpartum assessment of Ms. Wang?
- How might Diane have been more effective in delivering care to the Wang family?
- How did cultural differences between Diane and the Wang family lead to an inaccurate and inappropriate assessment?

- What people are important to give you support after having the baby?
- What can we (your health-care providers) do to help you stay healthy?

These open-ended questions addressed issues of culture related to childbearing. Although it was not a complete cultural assessment, a targeted abbreviated assessment can be helpful when time is limited, as is often the case in health-care visits. From the abbreviated cultural assessment of Ms. Wang, Edith was able to ascertain the cultural meanings of childbearing and infant care as perceived by Ms. Wang. Her assessment included cultural contexts related to various issues including:

- Appropriate physical care after delivery
- Appropriate celebratory customs following childbirth
- Dietary needs and restrictions
- Family roles, including the role of health-care decision making
- Cultural support systems

Finally, her assessment included information on ways in which the health-care providers could provide culturally appropriate health care to Ms. Wang.

Cultural Meanings of Childbirth in the Chinese Culture

To help illustrate the importance of Edith's approach, it helps to understand the meanings of childbearing in the Chinese culture. For the Chinese, the birth of a child is a very important event and is a time of great celebration. The mother is considered to be very vulnerable during the postpartum period. It is customary for mothers to have a 1- to 3-month "sitting period." During this period, the mother stays in the house and even in bed during the first few days. Most traditional Chinese families adhere to the "hot/cold" theory. This theory suggests that certain physical conditions and foods are categorized as either hot or cold. A balance of hot and cold is needed to maintain health. Because pregnancy and childbirth is considered "cold," the mother must have no exposure to cold air, water, or foods. She must be kept warm with no exposure to air-conditioning or fans, and is sometimes forbidden to touch water. There is a strong belief that these exposures may lead to arthritis and other joint symptoms later in life. Therefore, the mother is kept in a warm environment and is dressed in a manner that covers her arms, legs, and feet. Immediately postpartum, she may request several blankets to keep warm in the traditional

air-conditioned American hospital. She also may refuse ice chips, ice water, sherbet, and other cold foods that are often offered in American hospitals. Mothers may refuse a shower or bath or pretend to take a shower to please the nurse.[16,17]

There are also dietary needs and restrictions. The postpartum diet should include warm foods such as soups, broths, and other traditional foods that are considered to be hot foods. These foods not only help protect the mother from illness but aid in ample milk production.

A central component of childbearing in the Chinese culture is the role the family plays and the cultural support systems that exist. The father may or may not take an active role, depending on the level of **acculturation** of the family. Acculturation refers to the degree to which one has assimilated into the dominant culture, adopting values, practices, and beliefs. Fathers with greater levels of acculturation may take a greater role in childcare. Reliance on family members, particularly the maternal grandmother, is of importance during the postpartum period. The mother gets advice and support from her mother about care for herself during this time. The family also is supported by Chinese American friends and organizations such as churches, which may provide food for the mother during her sitting month.

There are special cultural celebrations surrounding childbearing. After the traditional sitting month, the family may have a celebration at home to which family members and friends are invited to celebrate the birth of the baby.

From the abbreviated cultural assessment and the physical examination, Edith was able to conclude that Ms. Wang was experiencing a healthy postpartum recovery. Ms. Wang was beginning gradually to use water for bathing. Ms. Wang had concluded her sitting month and had begun to go out of the house for limited periods of time. Edith made the following additions to Ms. Wang's plan of care:

1. Provide information regarding contacts with Chinese American community organizations and groups.
2. Include family as requested by Ms. Wang in the provision of health care.
3. Provide written materials in Chinese to Ms. Wang.
4. Give information regarding contraception and allow Ms. Wang to choose a method of her preference.
5. Schedule follow-up clinic visits as indicated.

Ms. Wang and her family left the clinic visit pleased to have been able to communicate in their own language and to have had their customs understood and appreci-ated. They eagerly accepted the written materials and planned to contact a local Chinese American organiza-tion for social support.

The two nurses took different approaches to Ms. Wang's care. Diane took an ethnocentric approach to providing care. **Ethnocentrism** is the belief that one's own cultural beliefs and practices are correct and are the standard by which other beliefs and practices should be measured. Diane based her assessment on Western hygienic practices and comfortable environ-mental temperature. She therefore made the assump-tion that Ms. Wang's behavior might be evidence of postpartum depression. Diane's plan of care can also be seen as **cultural imposition.** When one places her cultural values upon others and expects them to be-have accordingly, cultural imposition has occurred. Diane gave directions for Ms. Wang to bathe and use cool air fans, imposing Western values and traditions inappropriately. Both Diane and Ms. Wang felt uncom-fortable owing to communication barriers that Diane failed to prepare for in advance. The cultural conflict between Diane and Ms. Wang led to an ineffective health-care encounter.

In contrast, Edith determined the cultural norms for childbearing and postpartum care through a modified targeted cultural assessment. She devel-oped her plan of care based on the cultural norms, beliefs, and practices of Chinese culture based on what Ms. Wang had explained to her through the aid of the interpreter. Edith prepared for Ms. Wang's visit in advance by calling her on the phone and de-termining that language interpretation would be ad-vantageous to facilitating clear communication. She secured written materials in Chinese. Edith also rec-ognized the importance of desired support by other Chinese Americans. She assisted Ms. Wang in finding a local support system of Chinese Americans. Edith fully incorporated culture into the plan of care, cre-ating a culturally safe health-care environment. **Cul-tural safety** refers to an environment in which individuals believe that their culture is valued and respected. They are able to trust their health-care providers and participate in an open exchange about their health without fear of being challenged or rep-rimanded. The term *cultural safety* was developed in New Zealand in the 1980s to address the need for health-care providers to deal with issues related to caring for patients and clients who were culturally different. It focused on creating a safe environment for all (Box 23-5).

| BOX 23–5 | **What Is Cultural Safety?** |

Cultural safety within a health-care context requires an understanding of the cultural differences in communica-tion as well as perception of health on both sides, the provider and the client:
- Examining power relations between care providers and patients/clients
- Avoiding cultural imposition in health-care provision
- Permitting clients/patients to decide if they feel safe in the health-care environment
- Recognizing broad explanations of culture for example, age, social class, ethnicity, sex, sexual identity, religious beliefs, and disability
- Focusing on competency in practice.

Sources: Papps, E., & Ramsden, I. (1996). Cultural safety in nursing: The New Zealand experience. *International Journal for Quality in Health Care, 8*(5) 491-497. See reference 13.

Addressing Cultural Issues in Childbearing at the Population Level

After speaking with the interpreter, Edith discovered that there was a growing Chinese American commu-nity with many young families in the geographical area. From her interaction with Ms. Wang, Edith suspected that the childbearing needs of this growing population might need to be addressed more effectively. She wanted to develop a plan to educate and inform health-care providers about Chinese American cultural beliefs, traditions, and practices surrounding childbearing. Edith began by collecting census data about the numbers of Chinese American families of childbearing age in the community. Using her cultural reference books, she conducted research related to Chinese American cul-ture and specifically health issues related to childbear-ing. She then contacted the Chinese American interpreter that she had met when working with Ms.Wang. She believed that the interpreter, Ms. Xu, could help her gain entry into the community. Ms. Xu in-troduced her to key informants in the Chinese American community, a group of young women from a local Chinese American church. Ms. Xu agreed to help set up a meeting with Edith and the women to discuss how best to educate local nurses about the childbearing needs of Chinese American women.

During the meetings, Edith confirmed the knowl-edge that she had obtained from her research. She also gained clarity about cultural traditions and practices that were previously not clear to her. After several meetings, the group developed and delivered a half-day seminar for maternal-child nurses in the region on

Chinese culture and its influence on childbearing. Nurses were guided in ways to appropriately incorporate traditional beliefs and practices into care. They were cautioned not to assume that all Chinese American mothers would adhere to these beliefs and practices. The group also designed an evaluative survey in Chinese for distribution at hospitals, health departments, and clinics, so that they could determine if the intervention was effective.

The group agreed to meet quarterly to discuss health-care challenges related to Chinese American culture, to invite other members of the Chinese American community to meetings, and to expand their attention beyond childbearing concerns. The story of East Meets West: The Postpartum Predicament demonstrates how a community-level problem related to cultural misunderstandings might first be identified through the interaction at the family level. Edith recognized that the goal of public health nursing is to address health for populations. She effectively moved a family-level intervention to the level of the population of Chinese American community members through community engagement.

Delivering nursing care based solely on one's ethnocentric values raises certain ethical concerns. The ethical principles of beneficence, autonomy, respect for persons, and justice can easily be violated when nurses fail to plan and provide care that takes into account cultural beliefs and values (Box 23-6). The case of the Wang family is an example of how the ethical principles of beneficence and respect for persons can easily be violated unknowingly. Providing care that is culturally appropriate is imbedded within ethical health-care delivery.

Keeping the Lid on High Blood Pressure: African American Culture

People of African descent in America have a rich cultural heritage. Having first arrived on the shores of America in the 1500s as slaves by way of the Middle Passage, they were a diverse group of people of differing tribes, customs, traditions, and languages. The common experience of life as slaves over a period of 400 years forged a new culture, rich from a variety of African ways of life and traditions combined with learned European culture. Life in America since slavery has continued to be challenging for those people now called African Americans because of the assaults of discrimination, legal segregation, and racism. African Americans have had a long and hard-fought battle

---

BOX 23-6 Ethical Considerations

Providing culturally appropriate care for individuals, groups, and communities is directly linked to the basic principles of ethics that are recognized in public health nursing.
- Beneficence—the requirement to do good and not harm
  Can the public health nurse actually harm individuals/families/communities when attempting to provide care without appropriate cultural knowledge?
- Autonomy—acknowledgment of people as free moral agents who can make independent decisions about their own lives
  When the nurse imposes her/his own cultural beliefs on individuals/families/communities, do they lose the ability to make independent decisions?
- Respect for Persons—valuing of each individual because of the person's humanity regardless of age, race, gender, socioeconomic status, or belief system
  When cultural beliefs are dismissed as irrelevant or purposeless, are nurses being disrespectful to individuals/families/communities?
- Justice—equal treatment for all persons
  When the nurse provides care to people who share his/her own culture, are people of differing cultures treated equally?

---

for equal rights and treatment in America. These experiences continue to shape their lives and culture. Many African American people may be reluctant to trust health-care providers and traditional medical treatment modalities because of issues of real and perceived racism and discrimination.

In the 21st century, African Americans remain diverse because of migration to various regions of the country, intermarriage with other groups, varied opportunities, and differing life experiences. Representing about 13% of the population of the United States, approximately 30% of African American people live in poverty compared with about 8.2% of non-Hispanic whites. The majority of African American people are clustered in the rural south or large urban areas.[18] Those African Americans who live in poverty are at increased risk for health threats. However, African Americans who live in midrange and upper socioeconomic groups still experience disparate health in many areas. People of African descent continue to immigrate to the United States and are often identified or grouped together as black/African American in health research and other types of data collection. This population is growing; 1.4 million people immigrated in 2007 compared with only 35,355 in 1960, and most of the growth has occurred since 1990.[18] On arrival in the United States, they find themselves grouped in with the African American population despite the fact that they do not share the same culture or history. This once again highlights the difficulty of placing persons into racial categories with other groups who are not only biologically dissimilar but who also do not share a cultural or ethnic background.

In spite of the internal diversity within the group called African Americans, there remain **core cultural values** that many people of African descent share. Core values are the deeply rooted beliefs that are part of the fabric of a culture. They are guiding principles that shape behaviors and practices. Some of these values are collective responsibility, spirituality, extended family, and kinship relationships including fictive kin (those people considered kin but who are not related by blood). These values have a tremendous impact on health, health care, and beliefs and practices of African American people. Core cultural values should be recognized as strengths and incorporated into an effective plan of health care for African American people.

● APPLYING PUBLIC HEALTH SCIENCE
Consequences of Missing Cultural Cues
Public Health Science Topics Covered:
- Assessment
- Screening
- Ethics

Ms. Boykin, a 40-year-old African American woman, attends an annual health fair in her community at which she receives screenings for diabetes, cholesterol, vision, hearing, and blood pressure. In previous years, her screenings had all been within normal range. However, this year, her blood pressure reading was 150/95. Ms. Boykin was advised to make an appointment with her health-care provider for the appropriate follow-up. Because she did not have a regular provider, she made an appointment with the provider to whom she was referred at the health fair.

Faith, a nurse at the ambulatory clinic, conducted a routine history and initial assessment with Ms. Boykin. Ms. Boykin tells Faith that her mother and grandmother both had high blood pressure. Her grandmother was on dialysis for many years before dying of kidney failure. Her mother continues to have problems

with her pressure. Ms. Boykin's blood pressure reading at this visit was 160/94. She was given a prescription for medication, instructed about a healthy dietary regimen and exercise, and was given an appointment to return for follow-up in 6 weeks.

Ms. Boykin did not keep her appointment, but a year later returned to the community health fair for blood pressure screening. Alarmingly, her blood pressure reading was 190/100. Gail, the nurse who conducted the screening, found out that Ms. Boykin lives with her mother and works as an administrative assistant at a real estate office during the day. She also works processing packages on the late shift at a shipping company. She does not have health insurance. She also discovered that Ms. Boykin purchased and took the prescribed medication for a month, but after receiving a bill from the ambulatory care clinic decided not to return for follow-up. Still concerned, she solicited advice from some of her family members and friends from church. They suggested daily apple cider vinegar mixed in water and raw garlic as a way that they have always been able to lower their pressure. After sending Ms. Boykin for emergency treatment to lower her blood pressure, the nurse referred her to the federally qualified health center for follow up and to develop a long-term treatment plan. However, Faith missed important cultural cues that might have prevented this health-care mishap.

The Modified Cultural Assessment

As in the case with Ms. Wang, time for a full cultural assessment may not be available at an office visit. However, key questions to elicit cultural beliefs and practices can always be incorporated in order to deliver culturally informed care. Too often, important cultural data are collected, but are not used in the plan of care. Key questions can be used to elicit pertinent cultural data in the case of Ms. Boykin (Box 23-7).

From this brief cultural assessment, Faith gleaned enlightening cultural information about Ms. Boykin. Health for Ms. Boykin meant that she was able to work and care for herself and her mother. Other family members also relied on her for financial help from time to time. Because neither of her jobs provided health insurance and she had not had any serious illnesses, home remedies passed down from her family were used for minor ailments.

Ms. Boykin obtained most of her information about health from television, friends, family members, women's magazines, and church members. She has been relatively healthy; however, she stated that she prays

Key Questions on Health Beliefs

Health Beliefs and Practices

- Where do you get your health information?
- What is your usual source of health care?
- What does it mean to be healthy?
- How do you care for yourself?
- How do you feel about taking medication?
- Who helps you make important decisions about your health care?

More Specifically

- What is the meaning of high blood pressure for you?
- What do you believe causes high blood pressure?
- How do you think high blood pressure can be treated?
- What would help you continue to follow a plan of care for treatment of your high blood pressure?

about all major decisions and also asks for advice from her mother, sisters, and her prayer group. Ms. Boykin believed that high blood pressure runs in her family and she was sure that her turn would come soon. She realized that "high blood pressure pills" would probably be needed, but believed because initially it "wasn't very high" she thought that she would try the cider vinegar and garlic because these remedies had worked for her family, and friends at church had recommended them.

Ms. Boykin indicated that she would like to eat healthier foods and exercise; however, her mother prepares traditional meals each day that are high in fat and salt. Ms. Boykin's mother takes great pride in her cooking and is glad that she can help her daughter out. She admitted that she has given up trying to exercise because of her exhausting work schedule. Ms. Boykin believed that she could best follow a plan of care with a provider who understands her busy lifestyle and who would not be judgmental about her familial obligations. She also wanted her health-care provider to treat her with respect by not applying negative stereotypes commonly attributed to African Americans. She also was in need of affordable health care and medications. Based on the cultural assessment, Faith identified cultural values, practices, and beliefs specific to Ms. Boykin.

Faith recognized that for Ms. Boykin, health was equated with being able to provide for not only herself, but also for her family. The importance of her extended family was evident by her commitment to help provide financially for them. Ms. Boykin and her mother shared living space and responsibility for taking care of their household. Faith recognized that

strong kinship relationships and strong work ethic were consistent with what she has read about African American culture.

Faith also understood that prayer, religious activities, and church were important and meaningful in Ms. Boykin's life experience. She received health information and advice from those she identified as church family. She also spoke of prayer as a help in making decisions about her life.

Faith appreciated the fact that **folk medicine** and home remedies are used as healing in many cultures.[19] Folk medicine involves using traditional remedies and treatments for health promotion or illness, which are usually passed down through cultural transmission. Faith's challenge lies in figuring out how to incorporate Ms. Boykin's use of folk medicine with evidence-based health care. Some of these African American traditional folk remedies include the insertion of a lock of hair into the ear to treat an earache or use of honey to treat a cold sore.[20]

To some extent, Faith believed that Ms. Boykin has an external **locus of control.** Those who have an external locus of control perceive that they have little power over their destiny or future. Ms. Boykin believed that becoming hypertensive is inevitable for her because of her family history. Primary prevention efforts may be less successful when people believe that healthy behavior changes may not necessarily lead to healthy outcomes.

Traditional ways of selecting and preparing food is a tangible expression of culture. In Ms. Boykin's life, the food prepared by her mother represented a shared relationship, familial affection, and cultural expression. Faith will try to help Ms. Boykin preserve cultural meanings of food while making healthy modifications.

Ms. Boykin admitted to Faith that she had concerns about being treated with respect, having her culture valued, and not being labeled with negative stereotypes. Faith recognized the history of discrimination and racism in all aspects of society, including the health-care system. She was sensitive to the experiences that Ms. Boykin may have had and wants to provide care in which Ms. Boykin feels culturally safe. Faith developed a prevention intervention plan, based on the cultural assessment and sound nursing practice (Table 23-3).

Addressing Hypertension Screening in the African American Community

Faith was confident that she had provided culturally appropriate care for Ms. Boykin, recognizing cultural

TABLE 23–3	Keeping the Lid on High Blood Pressure: African American Culture; An Individual Plan of Cultural Care		
Primary Intervention	**Secondary Intervention**	**Tertiary Intervention**	
Encourage continued participation in spiritual and church activities.	Continue annual screenings at community health fair.	Connect with resources to help purchase medications at a reduced rate.	
Provide a culturally safe environment at the ambulatory care center that can be a medical home for Ms. Boykin.	Assist Ms. Boykin in obtaining a home blood pressure monitor and encourage self-monitoring and record-keeping.	Discuss use of folk remedies and their use for hypertension if they are not known to be harmful.	
Encourage continued social networking for stress reduction and health promotion.	Provide screenings as recommended at future visits to the ambulatory care center, e.g., body mass index, cervical cancer, breast, lipids, and blood glucose.	Refer Ms. Boykin and her mother to the nutritionist at the ambulatory care center for healthy modifications to the cultural diet.	
Provide culturally acceptable written materials about management of hypertension and other preventable conditions.		Explore exercise opportunities that fit within Ms. Boykin's schedule.	
Collaboratively set goals for health promotion (diet, exercise, stress reduction) and give positive feedback for goal achievement.	Evaluate goal attainment and adjust plan of care accordingly.	Collaboratively set goals related to blood pressure maintenance and give continuous positive feedback for goal achievement.	

values as strengths and using them to develop interventions. However, Faith, as a PHN, knew the importance of using the knowledge that she had obtained to also address hypertension on the population level within the African American community. Faith learned that Ms. Boykin received health-care information and screenings through a community health fair each year and recognized that health fairs are an effective means of connecting community members with health-care resources and education and such fairs have gained popularity in African American communities. Faith understood that she could use the established intervention program of the community health fair to more effectively address hypertension in the African American community.

Faith already recognized that hypertension is pervasive in the African American population and leads to early death from stroke, end-stage renal failure, and heart disease.[21] Faith interacts frequently with African American patients and believes that she is reasonably knowledgeable of African American culture. However, she also recognizes that she remains a secondhand observer and not a cultural participant. Faith conducted her own research on evidence-based practice with African Americans as it relates to hypertension interventions. She also read relevant literature on African American culture and history. Next, Faith met with Gail, an African American public health nurse who is a colleague and who also shared an interest in reducing hypertension morbidity in the African American community. Gail introduced Faith at the next African American community stakeholders' meeting to discuss their concerns about providing effective follow-up for persons who obtain screenings at community health fairs (Fig. 23-3).

Faith became involved in the health and wellness subcommittee of the stakeholders' group. This subcommittee was composed of key members of the African American community who were interested in its health issues. Over several months, they collected information on the various health fairs conducted in their local community. They held a meeting with the organizers of the various groups that conducted health fairs to determine how to establish continuity, congruence, and collaboration among the community entities.

As a result of this collaborative effort, the group determined that through combining resources, they could provide a larger and more comprehensive health fair that would reach greater numbers of community members. An essential component of the health fair would be a to deliver a sociocultural screening program for

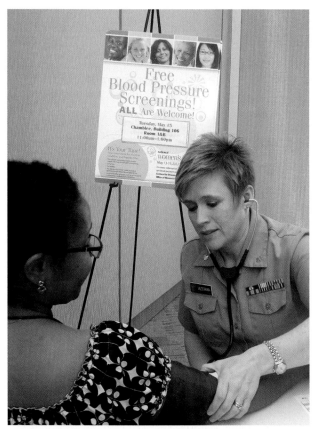

Figure 23-3 Screening for hypertension. *(From the Centers for Disease Control and Prevention, Courtesy of Nasheka Powell, 2012. Photography by Yvonne Green, RN, CNM, MSN.)*

hypertension with appropriate resources on site to meet the needs of the those who screened positive, that is, had a blood pressure reading at or greater than 140 over 90. These individuals would be advised to have an on-site sociocultural assessment for possible hypertension by a trained health-care provider and referral for treatment if needed. Individuals who followed the assessment for hypertension and were found to have high blood pressure would be followed up with a phone call in 1 month from a member of the health and wellness subcommittee to determine whether they had been able to receive treatment for hypertension. The subcommittee would use these data to determine whether this intervention was effective in providing early intervention for hypertension in the African American community. Faith continued her active involvement with the African American community through participation with the stakeholders' group and the health and wellness subcommittee.

The case we just discussed illustrates the role of the PHN in recognizing how sociocultural issues have an impact on the health of individuals in a cultural community. The PHN recognizes that this knowledge is a step toward developing population-level interventions that have large-scale impact. This story also emphasizes how direct involvement with the cultural community, when possible, can lead to an exchange of knowledge that is beneficial for the nursing community and the cultural community.

Summary Points

- A community assessment should include a cultural assessment.
- Engaging community members who know their own cultural realities best is the approach most likely to be successful.
- Designing an intervention through community engagement will result in a more culturally relevant program.
- Families of various types are units by which culture is transmitted, learned, shared, and enacted.
- Cultural beliefs surrounding childbearing are deeply imbedded within families and are often transmitted by the women elders.
- Ignoring cultural differences and imposing Western values can result in ineffective nursing encounters.
- Information from individual- and family-level encounters can result in the development of population-level interventions.
- Following individual care, engaging the community can result in population changes and long-term community partnerships.

▲ CASE STUDY
Getting to Know You
Objectives: At the end of this case study, the student will be able to:

1. Identify methods for obtaining secondary data related to the ethnicity of a population
2. Examine the relevance of cultural information to a specific public health activity.
3. Discuss differing cultural approaches to death.
4. Describe strategies that can be used improve cultural understanding.

Shirley Jones, RN, relocated from Maine to San Antonio, Texas, as a result of a change in her husband's job. She began to work for the San Antonio Metropolitan

Health District as a maternal and infant nurse. Her job included conducting all the interviews with mothers who had experienced the loss of an infant for the health department's fetal infant mortality review program. These interviews are conducted as part of the surveillance data collected to help the county understand contributing factors to fetal and infant death. Her husband wondered whether she was ready for the job, because a large portion of the population in San Antonio is Mexican American. Shirley responded that she felt confident in taking on the job because she had taken Spanish in college and had been brushing up on the language. However, her husband pointed out to her that when she was working in Maine she had not had any Hispanic/Latino patients. To help prepare for the job, where should she start?

1. Review the demographics of Texas and of San Antonio. What are the major ethnic groups in the state and in San Antonio?
2. Identify key cultural issues of which she will need to be aware.
3. How would she conduct a cultural assessment of the community? How will this inform her visits with mothers?
4. How will her increased understanding inform her responsibilities in the job?

REFERENCES

1. Hall, L.E. (2005). *Dictionary of multicultural psychology: Issues, terms, and concepts.* Thousand Oaks, CA: Sage.
2. Diamond, J. (1994). Race without color. *Discover, 15*(11). Retrieved from http://www.learntoquestion.com/resources/database/archives/001377.html.
3. Marks, J. (1996). Science and race. *American Behavioral Scientist, 40*(2), 123-133.
4. Healey, J.F. (2008). *Race, ethnicity, and class* (5th ed.). Thousand Oaks, CA: Sage.
5. Miller, S. (2009). Cultural humility is the first step to becoming global providers. *Journal of Obstetrical Gynecological and Neonatal Nursing, 38*(1), 92-93.
6. Levi, A. (2009). The ethics of nursing students' international clinical experiences. *Journal of Obstetrical Gynecological and Neonatal Nursing, 38*(1), 94-99.
7. Jewell, G. (2007). Bridging the gap: A curriculum to teach residents cultural humility. *Family Medicine, 38*(2), 97-102.
8. U.S. Department of Health and Human Services, Office of Minority Health. (2014). *National Standards on Culturally and Linguistically Appropriate Services (CLAS).* Retrieved from http://minorityhealth.hhs.gov/omh/browse.aspx?lvl=2&lvlid=53.
9. National Quality Forum. (2009). *Cultural competency: A comprehensive framework and preferred practices for measuring and reporting cultural competency.* Washington, DC: Author.
10. Quad Council of Public Health Nursing Organizations. (2011). *Quad Council competencies for public health nurses.* Retrieved from http://www.achne.org/files/Quad%20Council/QuadCouncilCompetenciesforPublicHealthNurses.pdf.
11. Behringer, B., Friedell, G.H., Dorgan, K.A., Hutson, S.P., Naney, C., Phillips, A., et al. (2007). Understanding the challenges of reducing cancer in Appalachia: Addressing a place-based health disparity population. *California Journal of Health Promotion, Health Disparities & Social Justice, 5,* 40-49.
12. Williams, W. (2008). Health risks greater in coal mining communities. *The State Journal.* Retrieved from http://www.statejournal.com/story.cfm?func=viewstory&storyid=36542.
13. Andrews M.M., & Boyle, J.S. (2003). *Transcultural concepts in nursing care.* Philadelphia, PA: Lippincott.
14. Colorado Department of Education. (2002). *Fast facts: Cultural mediators, translators and interpreters.* Denver, CO: Author.
15. Purnell, L.D., & Paulanka, B.J. (2008). *Transcultural health care: A culturally competent approach* (3rd ed.). Philadelphia, PA: F.A. Davis.
16. Liu, N., Mao, L., Sun, X., Liu, L., Chen, B., & Ding, Q. (2006). Postpartum practices of puerperal women and their influencing factors in three regions of Hubei, China. *BMC Public Health, 6*(274). doi:10.1186/1471-2458-6-274.
17. Xu, Y. (2009). Personal communication.
18. Terrazas, A. (2010). *Migration information source.* Retrieved from http://www.migrationinformation.org/USfocus/display.cfm?id=719.
19. Fletcher, A.B. (2000). African American folk medicine: A form of alternative therapy. *The Online Archive of American Folk Medicine.* (2001). Retrieved from http://www.folkmed.ucla.edu/index.html.
20. Ostchega, Y., Yoon, S.S., Hughes, J., & Louis, T. (2008). *Hypertension awareness, treatment and control: Continued disparities in adults; United States, 2005–2006* (NCHS Data Brief). Hyattsville, MD: National Center for Health Statistics.

Chapter 24

Vulnerable Populations

LEARNING OUTCOMES

After reading this chapter, the student will be able to:

1. Describe the concept of vulnerability from a population perspective.
2. Distinguish groups in our society who are traditionally considered vulnerable.
3. Demonstrate an understanding of the individual and social determinants of health and their contribution to population vulnerability.
4. Apply the multiple determinants of a vulnerability approach in determining levels of vulnerability of a particular population.
5. Develop strategies for reducing vulnerability among various groups.
6. Differentiate the various roles and responsibilities of the nurse when caring for vulnerable populations.

KEY TERMS

Asylee
Discrimination
Food security
Health disparity
Homelessness
Immigrant
Legal permanent resident (LPR)

Marginalization
Migrant agricultural worker
Migrant worker
Point in time estimate
Poverty
Poverty guidelines
Poverty threshold

Primary homelesness
Refugee
Secondary homelessness
Social capital
Socioeconomic status (SES)
Stereotype
Stigma

Sustainability
Tertiary homelessness
Unauthorized immigrant
Vulnerability
Vulnerable populations

■ Introduction

Vulnerable populations are populations at substantially greater risk for poor physical, mental, and social health, and have higher rates of morbidity and mortality than the remainder of the population. Their vulnerability may be associated with their socioeconomic status, where they live, gender, age, disability status, or sexual orientation.[1] The Urban Institute Health Policy Center defines vulnerable populations as those "that are not well integrated into the health-care system because of ethnic, cultural, economic, geographic, or health characteristics."[2] These groups have certain characteristics or experiences such as poverty, disabilities, inadequate housing, marginal education, less secure jobs, increased stress, multiple noncommunicable diseases, and less social capital that increase their risk of vulnerability, and in turn contribute to poorer health than found in the general population.[1,2]

In the words of Lou Ann Aday,[3] "Both the origins and remedies of vulnerability are rooted in the bonds of human communities." This means that the very system that creates vulnerability also possesses both the knowledge and skills necessary for reducing vulnerability.

The words *vulnerable* and *vulnerability* stem from the Latin word *vulnus*, which means "wound."[4] Webster's dictionary defines *vulnerability* as the capability of being physically wounded; open to attack or damage.[5] From a public health perspective, **vulnerability** can be thought of as the increased susceptibility to poor health of an individual or group stemming from exposure to multiple risk factors.[6] To understand vulnerable populations is a step in understanding and then decreasing health disparities (see Chapter 7).

In 2011, the United States spent two and a half times more per capita on health care than did other high-income countries (HICs). Despite this high level of spending, the U.S. life expectancy that used to be one and a half times higher than the average in other HICs is now one and a half times lower.[7] Some of this drop is due to the persistent and growing inequalities in mortality, morbidity, and disability between the higher socioeconomic status and other groups that are more vulnerable.[8] One saying that conveys health disparity and vulnerability is that "when America catches a cold, vulnerable groups catch pneumonia."[9] This statement is a simple way of expressing a complex phenomenon known as health disparities. As defined in Chapter 7, **health disparity** is a difference or inequality in some aspect of health. Disparities reflect particular types of differences in health status or outcomes, or in the most important influences on health that can be shaped by health and social policies.[10] Not only are these differences unnecessary and avoidable, they are also unfair and unjust, and as such violate the ethical principles that serve as the foundation of our society. In other words, health disparities typically are present in vulnerable social groups such as people living in poverty, minority populations, women, populations with substance abuse, or other groups who have persistently experienced social disadvantage or discrimination. As a result, members of vulnerable populations that experience health inequities systematically experience worse health status or greater health risks than more advantaged social groups.[11]

Over the course of our lives, each of us has the potential to experience vulnerability. This could come as a normal and inevitable part of our lives such as when we age, lose a job, or suffer a significant loss, or it can be created and continued by social factors within our society such as the stigmatization of people with AIDS. Certain groups have traditionally been identified as being at greater risk, or more vulnerable, experiencing disparities in health. Members of these vulnerable populations often lack resources such as having limited educational backgrounds, decreased physical capabilities, poor communicative skills, and/or inadequate financial assets, exposing them to increased risk and making it difficult to adequately safeguard their own health.[12]

Examples of groups typically viewed as vulnerable include people living in poverty, people of color, the uninsured, those experiencing homelessness, older adults, those with disabilities, those with increased frailty, those suffering from noncommunicable diseases, those who do not speak English, immigrants, refugees, people marginalized by sexual preference, and those who are incarcerated. Each of these diverse groups has in common an enhanced level of risk as well as an overlap of other risk factors that predispose them to vulnerability. It is important to note that the groups listed as examples of vulnerable populations are found usually to be at higher risk for vulnerability from the

perspective of health and health-care outcomes. However, these groups are composed of diverse individuals, and each individual has his or her own unique set of risk factors, making him or her more or less vulnerable.

There are many reasons it is important for nurses to understand the health needs of vulnerable populations. Shi and Stevens[13] identified four reasons health-care providers and the country as a whole should focus attention on vulnerable populations:

- Because of their increased risk for poor physical and mental health, vulnerable populations have greater rates of morbidity and mortality than the general population, exacting an enormous toll on their health and well-being.
- The number of vulnerable groups is increasing.
- It is a social issue and is best solved not at the individual but at the community/population level.
- The health-care needs of vulnerable populations place an increased demand on the limited capacity and resources of our health-care system.

There is greater emphasis today on reducing health disparity and increasing equity as reflected in the *Healthy People 2020 (HP 2020)* goals and in multiple new interventions (see Chapter 7). All nurses, including public health nurses (PHNs), are uniquely positioned to provide care that encompasses the societal mandate to deliver quality individual- and population-based care to everyone. This approach to care utilizes the personal, social, and health resources available to reduce the impact of vulnerability on health. The American Nurses Association has issued a Nursing Social Policy Statement that describes the duties of our profession to meet the health needs of all human beings through delivery of care that is grounded in comprehensive knowledge of the determinants of human health.[14] Therefore, an understanding of vulnerability and vulnerable populations, from a public health perspective, is crucial to providing this holistic care. In addition, this understanding allows nurses to advocate on behalf of vulnerable populations to reduce their vulnerability.

● APPLYING PUBLIC HEALTH SCIENCE
The Case of the Sheltered Mom
Public Health Science Topics Covered:

- Community assessment
- Health planning
- Policy development

Twenty-two-year old pregnant Rosa Gonzalez and her 2-year-old son Henry arrived at a homeless shelter that was currently housing an overcapacity population. She managed to secure a cot for herself and Henry in the crowded dorm of the shelter. One of the student nurses, Mary, doing her public health clinical rotation at the shelter that day, approached Rosa to see whether she could be of any help. Rosa sighed, placing her son on her lap, but didn't respond. Mary tried again to speak to Rosa, this time in Spanish, asking her whether she was okay. Rosa just sighed and said, "De nada."

The next day, Mary saw Rosa sitting, watching her son play at her feet. Mary went over and asked Rosa whether she could sit with her for a while. Rosa agreed. At first, Rosa didn't say much, so Mary sat quietly next to her. After some time passed, Rosa slowly began to talk. In Spanish, she shared how she and her husband James had moved 3 years ago from California to Anytown (a hypothetical town), a community located in southwest Detroit. James had gotten a temporary job in a local car plant. Rosa had not wanted to move because it meant leaving her extended family behind, but the money was good. At first, all went well and they were even able to save a little money toward a house. Then last year James was laid off. As a temporary worker, he didn't qualify for unemployment benefits. Despite walking the streets all day, he couldn't find another job. Rosa herself tried looking for work without luck. With English as a second language, she had trouble with job interviews. She said that she had her immigration papers, but had come to the United States in her late teens, had not gone to schools in the United States, and did not have a high school diploma. Prior to meeting James, she lived in a Mexican-American community in California and hadn't needed to learn English. Right before James lost his job in Detroit, she had enrolled in a general educational development (GED) program for persons with English as a second language, but without regular childcare and James coming home very late most nights, she had dropped out.

Without jobs, Rosa and her husband quickly used up their savings and couldn't pay the rent or the utility bills. Back in California, they would have been able to move in with their relatives, but here there was no one, and now no money to use to return to California. Though the Hispanic community in Anytown was large, Rosa had kept to herself and had not made any friends. James became depressed and started drinking. Rosa said everything fell apart the night James, obviously drunk, came in late from the bar. She had been sitting up worrying about him and their lack of money. As soon as he walked in the door, she complained that he had no right to spend money on liquor when there was no money to pay for heat and the landlord was threatening them with eviction. James flew into a rage and hit her.

Tears rolled down Rosa's cheeks as she told her story to Mary. She talked of being afraid of her husband, being hungry and cold, and being evicted. A few nights ago, James failed to come home at all, so she came to the shelter with the few belongings she could carry. Just today, Rosa discovered that James had been arrested for assault and drug distribution. Rosa asserted that James was trying hard to find the money to pay the rent. She had heard one of the men he had met at the bar telling him about a way to make big money. She hadn't realized it involved selling drugs. Now that James was in jail, Rosa felt trapped and didn't know what to do.

Rosa is one of the many faces of vulnerability. Pregnancy increases a woman's vulnerability. When that is coupled with other risk factors such as homelessness, lack of job skills, experiences of domestic violence, English as a second language, and no family social network, a woman's vulnerability increases dramatically. She is faced with what appears to be insurmountable challenges and few resources to meet these challenges.

Mary had a complex set of tasks in front of her if she wished to help Rosa. Rosa needed a place to stay, food, and a job. Rosa also needed legal support related to her husband's arrest and incarceration, and psychological support related to her history of being a victim of domestic violence (see Chapter 12). In addition, Rosa was in need of prenatal and well childcare. Mary began to provide beginning support for Rosa's health needs, but to tackle all the other issues required an interdisciplinary team.

When Mary discussed Rosa with her instructor, the instructor asked her to look at Rosa's story from a broader viewpoint. A population perspective can lead nurses to the creation of interventions aimed at helping whole population groups and preventing those who are more vulnerable from experiencing adverse health consequences. This requires applying public health science, especially community assessment, program planning, and creating new health policies. If Mary continues to focus only on Rosa as an individual, she may miss opportunities to improve outcomes for many others who are vulnerable and suffer inequities in their health.

Based on numerous population-level studies, as mentioned above, we know that multiple factors contribute to vulnerability such as age, female gender, income, education status, lack of regular health care, and lack of health insurance.[12,15] As in Rosa's case, many of the factors that contribute to increased vulnerability are external to the individual. For example, the economic downturn experienced by the automakers in 2008 directly affected the city of Detroit, resulting in the city declaring bankruptcy in 2013. In Detroit, the unemployment rate of 10.5 in 2013 was one of the highest in the nation for a major metropolitan statistical area. The loss of James's job began the cascade of events that ended with Rosa living at a crowded shelter. Vulnerability does not occur in isolation. Prior to James's loss of his job, the family had the resources they needed to care for themselves. However, when the economy had an impact on their ability to earn an income, those risk factors increased their vulnerability and resulted in an inability to meet the needs of their family.

Mary began with a focused community assessment (see Chapter 4). She first examined demographic information on Anytown and found a thorough report released in 2013 on child health in Detroit with specific information on Anytown.[16] The report supported targeted community-level interventions, but in the hard economic times little action by the city had begun. With the encouragement of the instructor, Mary began a search to see whether there were any other successful evidence-based public health interventions that had occurred in Detroit with nongovernmental organizations or elsewhere in the United States with similar populations.

Based on the findings from her community assessment, Mary recognized that policy initiatives were needed that would address the wider issues of free or affordable prenatal care, increased shelters, GED programs for women with English as a second language that included daycare, and counseling and legal support for women who had suffered domestic violence. When Mary included in her clinical experience a population perspective, she had a better understanding of the risk factors that contributed to Rosa's vulnerability and how external events shaped Rosa's experience. Moving the plan of care to one that included the continuum of care across individuals, families, groups, and populations allowed Mary to identify policy opportunities that could provide possible solutions for the vulnerable homeless women that were not possible on the individual level. Just as understanding the natural history of the disease helps in the development of primary, secondary, and tertiary prevention for that disease (see Chapter 2), understanding vulnerability risk factors is essential to the development of interventions that help to minimize vulnerability and improve health and social outcomes.

Mary was able to provide direct support for Rosa because of population-level interventions that had been developed in Detroit. These included services for women who have experienced domestic violence, access to subsidized housing, and other support services available for women and children living in the Detroit metropolitan area. She worked to link Rosa with members of the Hispanic community in Detroit and encouraged her to build social support networks. She also located a support group for families of prisoners and went with Rosa to her first meeting with this support group. Finally, she located a family health clinic that accepted Medicaid and could provide prenatal and well childcare for Rosa. Mary discovered that many resources were available. In Rosa's case, the key was to begin by building a trusting relationship with Rosa that provided that initial support needed to link her with the other people and programs available to her.

Ethics: Concepts Related to Vulnerability

The majority of the literature on ethics and health care with vulnerable populations revolves around their inclusion in research. Health-care research focused on vulnerable populations includes participants who are at greatest risk for coercion and may not be able to give informed consent. These groups include prisoners, pregnant women, children, those who are mentally incapacitated, refugees, the poor, older adults, sexual minorities, and persons with a substance use disorder.[17,18]

However, the issue of ethics and vulnerability is much larger. Though the term *vulnerability* is useful when conceptualizing the risks and barriers to optimal health and health care, labeling a group as vulnerable must be done with care to avoid paternalism and stereotyping, which further stigmatizes individuals, families, and populations. Conceptualizing those who are vulnerable as "less than" can lead to blaming the victim, when in reality the forces creating vulnerability may be beyond a person's or a population's control. To address this issue, it is important to consider frameworks of vulnerability that extend beyond traditional discussions of individual-level risk factors that contribute to vulnerability. This broader approach incorporates the social forces that shape the lives, and therefore contributes to the vulnerability of, certain segments of our society.

Nursing care of vulnerable populations uses a framework of cultural competence, social justice, and human rights. The ethical code of nursing has the expectation that all individuals, families, groups, and communities will receive equal nursing care.[19] Nurses who demonstrate competence with advocacy for social justice and protection of human rights are better able to address the social inequities of vulnerable populations. There is always a tension between availability of scarce resources and the perceived worthiness of the individual receiving these resources. Christine Ferguson, a long-term public servant who has sought out these scarce resources, feels that the vulnerable population has been divided into three groups by the community:

- A deserving group who has become vulnerable as the equivalent of an "act of God," such as cancer or prematurity
- An undeserving group that is viewed as suffering as a result of their own actions, such as those who use alcohol and other drugs at harmful levels, prisoners, those experiencing homelessness, single mothers, and persons with sexually transmitted infections (STIs)
- Children of people who have made "bad choices," such as illegal immigrants and women using the federal program Temporary Assistance to Needy Families (TANF).[20] TANF is a block grant federal program that replaced prior welfare programs such as the Aid to Families With Dependent Children program.[21]

Marginalization

Marginalization is a social process through which a person or group is on the periphery of society based on identity, associations, experiences, or environment.[22] To marginalize someone is to treat the person as though she is of little or no consequence, or is unimportant. The marginalization of certain groups conveys the idea that individuals in those groups do not matter or are of little concern to the rest of society. Often, group differences, such as gender, ethnicity, or race, education or income, geographical location, or sexual preference, contribute to marginalization. Women, racial and ethnic minorities, and persons living in poverty are examples of groups that have a long history of marginalization within our society.

Marginalization is exclusionary and isolating. As a result, this process can lead to negative health outcomes and therefore contribute to vulnerability. It can limit an individual's or a group's opportunities for establishing beneficial relationships necessary for accessing health-care services. In addition, those who are marginalized can experience heightened levels of stress and despair related to their sense of powerlessness.[23] Historically, many if not all of the groups designated as vulnerable populations have been marginalized within the larger society. Because marginalization is a force outside of the control of the person being marginalized, some public health experts suggest that marginalization is a more accurate terminology to use when discussing health and health-care disparities than the concept of vulnerability, because the latter can be used to imply a degree of personal control and "victim blaming."[24]

Stigma and Discrimination

Stigma can be thought of as a characteristic of a person or a group of persons that is contrary to those characteristics of the larger group. Stigmatized individuals either possess, or are believed to possess, some attribute that is not valued in a particular social context.[25] For example, in many societies, mental illness is seen as a stigmatizing characteristic, as it sets those individuals who have a mental illness apart in a demeaning way from those who are perceived as being "normal."

Stigma can also be seen as a relationship between an attribute of a certain group and a **stereotype.** A stereotype is an exaggerated, usually negative, belief or image applied to an entire category of people. Members of vulnerable populations who are stigmatized experience loss of status within society, which can then result in **discrimination.** Discrimination is the differential and negative treatment of an individual based on his or her race, ethnicity, gender, socioeconomic status, or other group membership. This discriminatory treatment leads to further stigma and further loss of status, thus perpetuating a cycle that enhances vulnerability and marginalization that is, once again, beyond the control of the individual.

Stigma and discrimination are social processes that can affect the health and health care of vulnerable populations. A great deal of stress is associated with the constant threat of being stigmatized.[26] As a result of these forces, individuals and groups are also placed at a distinct social disadvantage with regard to resources such as knowledge, money, power, prestige, and social connections, thus adding to their risks and level of vulnerability to negative health and health-care outcomes.[27] In addition, when people are seen as responsible for their life circumstances, such as in the case of a person who engages in harmful substance use, unwed mothers, or prisoners, there is less public compassion and the perception that these individuals contributed to their own vulnerability can result in further stigmatization for other members of these groups.[20] From a public health perspective, vulnerability is perceived as a temporary situation that can be addressed at the individual, family, and community levels.

Risk Factors Related to Vulnerability

Risk factors associated with vulnerability and the social determinants of health have been discussed in detail in Chapter 7. Various risk factors such as lower socioeconomic status, lifestyle behaviors, poverty, genetics, race, ethnicity, and gender increase individual or group vulnerability and the associated ill health. Vulnerability is influenced by the interrelationship of these multiple factors that act in an additive or even multiplicative way to increase risk for poor health outcomes. For example, middle-aged women diagnosed with diabetes would be considered at risk for negative health outcomes because of their diabetes and would then be considered a vulnerable population. If those same women were recent immigrants to this country, did not speak English, and lacked a regular source of medical care, they would have even greater risks for poor health status because of increased vulnerability.

Social Determinants of Health and Vulnerability

As explained in Chapter 7, another approach to understanding vulnerability is that of the community- or societal-level determinants of health. Social determinants associated with vulnerable populations include economic determinants, environmental determinants, social capital, and health system determinants.[9] From this perspective, the concept of vulnerability moves beyond individual risk factors to community and population factors that contribute to the vulnerability of at-risk groups within our society.

Poverty

Economic factors are, perhaps, the most important in influencing the health status of an individual or group. When household income falls below the threshold considered to be adequate to support the number of persons in the household, the members of that household are considered to be living in **poverty**.[27] There are multiple aspects to defining this poverty threshold and the applications of this threshold to determine poverty rates.

In the United States, the **poverty threshold** is the measurement used by the U.S. Bureau of the Census to calculate all official poverty population statistics.[28] The poverty threshold is a yearly determination of a standard of living below which a family has the lack of goods and

services commonly taken for granted by mainstream society. Table 24-1 provides the income figures used in 2013 to determine whether a family was living in poverty. As shown in the table, there are adjustments made for family size. The poverty threshold income numbers were initially created based on poverty measurement work done by the economist Mollie Orshansky in the mid-1960s.[28] With very few adaptations, the U.S. government's measurement of poverty has remained unchanged for 40 years, although the basis on which the initial calculations were made has shifted significantly. For example, the percentage of income spent on food has decreased and the percentage spent on such categories as transportation, health care, and childcare have significantly increased.

There are also considerable variances between costs in different parts of the United States and in urban and rural areas, and these variances are not considered in the current poverty threshold. In 1995, the National Academy of Science asked to reexamine the measurements and made several suggestions to make the threshold currently more meaningful. None of these have been officially implemented and the poverty threshold continues to be based on the original structure.

The poverty threshold is primarily used for statistical purposes, so a consistent method of measurement is used at the national level. The other federal measure used is the **poverty guidelines**. These guidelines simplify the poverty thresholds and are used for administrative

TABLE 24–1	2013 Poverty Guidelines for the 48 Contiguous States and the District of Columbia
Persons in Family/ Household	Poverty Guideline
1	$11,490
2	$15,510
3	$19,530
4	$23,550
5	$27,570
6	$31,590
7	$35,610
8	$39,630
	For families/households with more than 8 persons, add $4,020 for each additional person

Source: See reference 28.

purposes such as determining who is eligible for federal programs aimed at providing assistance to those living in poverty.[29] Both poverty guidelines and poverty thresholds are established on a yearly basis, and are issued by the U.S. Department of Health and Human Services.[30]

In 2012, the median household income had not recovered from the economic recession that occurred in 2007.[31] More people were living in poverty. There was a significant increase in the U.S. poverty rate from 2000 (11.1%) to 2012 (15.0%). This translated into 46.5 million people living in poverty in 2012, the largest actual number in 51 years.[31] This is not the highest percentage, as more than 20% lived in poverty in the early 1960s. The War on Poverty under the Johnson administration decreased the poverty rate to 11.1% in 1973. Unfortunately, the number rose again in the 1980s and has since fluctuated based on economic growth and recession, even with multiple programs directed at decreasing poverty in the United States (Fig. 24-1).

Poverty has a significant impact on a person's health. Persons living in poverty are unable to meet their most basic needs of food, clothing, and shelter, and health care becomes a luxury that they simply cannot afford. They have higher rates of infant mortality, complex health problems, and complications owing to poor management of noncommmunicable disease. Certain diseases are more common among people living in poverty than in middle- or high-income groups, including anemia, asthma, diabetes, pneumonia, and hypertension. Individuals living in poverty also experience increased rates of mental illness resulting from chronic stress and a disproportionate exposure to trauma and violence. Poor neighborhoods have higher rates of crime and substance abuse when compared with more affluent communities.

Socioeconomic status (SES) is a composite measure of the interrelated concepts of income, education, and occupation. With higher levels of education, a person is more likely to secure a better job, which in turn provides a higher rate of pay. In contrast, a person who doesn't earn a high school diploma has more difficulty finding a job that pays a living wage (a wage that provides access to the means of a healthy living, e.g., housing, food, and health care) Therefore, individuals at a lower SES level have increased vulnerability to poor health because of lack of economic resources. The link of SES to health outcomes was illustrated through the work of Sir Michael Marmot, who studied the health of British civil servants.[32] What Marmot discovered in his studies was that there was a striking inverse social gradient in morbidity and mortality. That is, as a person's social status increased (higher SES), the risk for morbidity and mortality decreased. When considering the influence of SES on health, it becomes clear that health-care providers must focus their efforts on improving not just health outcomes, but also social determinants of health such as educational and employment opportunities (see Chapter 7).

Social Capital and Vulnerability

Social capital is a term that has numerous definitions in the literature. The central point of social capital is the benefits that occur through social networks. One example is that persons often secure a job based on who they know rather than what they know. Thus, social capital usually refers to a person's or a community's capacity to obtain support from the social connections available to the person. Social capital resides in the quantity and quality of interpersonal ties among people and communities.[33] These relationships represent a resource (capital) that can be drawn upon during challenging times. Social capital is reflected in the institutions, organizations, and informal practices of giving that people create to share resources and build attachments with others. The values and norms of a community influence the health and well-being, and vulnerability, of individuals and populations. Community-level attributes such as social stability, recognition and valuing of diversity, safety, good working relationships, and a cohesive community provide a supportive environment in which to live, thereby reducing a person's potential risk for poor health. These ties may be with family, friends, or colleagues, as well as with

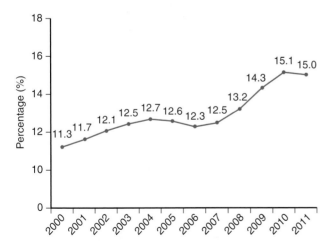

Figure 24-1 Poverty rates between 2000 and 2011. *(From the Office of the Assistant Secretary for Planning and Evaluation of the U.S. Department of Health and Human Services. Retrieved from http://aspe.hhs.gov/hsp/12/povertyandincomeest/ib.shtml.)*

various community institutions and agencies. When a person or group has reduced social capital, he or she is at greater risk for vulnerability at all times, but especially when faced with a challenge.

A good example of community-level social capital is the case of the community referred to as Little Italy in Baltimore, Maryland. In the summer of 2013, the neighborhood located east of downtown Baltimore experienced a number of assaults and robberies. The community already had a long-standing community committee. The committee called a community meeting and invited the Baltimore police and their state representative to attend. Because of the relationships this community had built over time with the city of Baltimore and their state representative, they were able to obtain heightened police presence in the community. The members of the community also banded together and began to pool their resources so that they could obtain further security for the community. As a result, the number of assaults and robberies fell. The community had developed strong social capital over time within the community through the building of a sense of pride in the community felt by the residents, the support between community businesses, and the ability to gain the attention of lawmakers and the city police department. In addition, the community came together for one assault victim who had sustained serious injuries, and raised funds to help cover his hospital expenses.

A person's culture is another important social resource (see Chapter 23). Feeling a sense of connection to a supportive community of individuals who share one's culture can enhance health. In contrast, the level of vulnerability may increase for those who are separated, either physically or emotionally, from their cultural group. It is important to note that an individual may have social attachments with other individuals, yet remain vulnerable because of a lack of social capital. For example, during Hurricane Katrina, many of the individuals who were most vulnerable lacked connections with individuals or agencies that could assist them with evacuation during the disaster. While these individuals and families no doubt had social connections with supportive family and friends, many of those same individuals lacked the capacity to provide needed support for evacuation in the form of money, transportation, and shelter.

Multiple Determinants of Vulnerability

In order to reduce vulnerability, it is necessary to examine the root causes in a comprehensive manner. Although it is important to consider both individual and

social determinants of health and vulnerability, we must also acknowledge the synergistic effect that multiple levels of risk have on the health of certain populations. Approaches to understanding vulnerability from the lens of individual-level determinants of health fail to reveal the impact that larger social influences have on the individual or population.[34] Conversely, approaches to vulnerability that focus entirely on the social determinants of health fail to recognize the manifestation of these influences as they are filtered through our unique biological characteristics and personal strengths, capacities, and weaknesses.

From a *multiple determinants of vulnerability* approach, overlap of risk across many of the determinants of health results in increased vulnerability. That is, the more risk factors for poor health that a person or group has, distributed across the individual and societal levels, the more likely it is that the person or group will be vulnerable. Therefore, in order to adequately assess vulnerability and design interventions to reduce its incidence, it is necessary to examine vulnerability using this comprehensive multiple determinants framework.

As an illustration of the concept of overlap of risk, let's examine the public health threat of infant mortality. Overall, infant mortality has an impact on the health of every American citizen, either directly or indirectly, through personal and health-care system costs. Based on infant mortality rates, African American infants are twice as likely to die in the first year of life compared with non-Hispanic white infants (see Chapter 18). At first glance, it might appear that race by itself is the determinant. However, using the overlap of risk approach, African American infants born to mothers living in poverty would be considered to be more vulnerable than African American infants born to mothers with middle- or high-level SES.

Strategies for Reducing Vulnerability

In order to reduce vulnerability, all nurses must move beyond traditional conceptualizations of health as they work to address not only individual but also social determinants of health. Guidelines from *HP 2020* demonstrate a unified effort to improve the health of all of our citizens (see Chapter 2). Strategies for reducing vulnerability must also be grounded in knowledge of the core principles guiding health promotion and reduction of risk for vulnerable populations. Foundational knowledge related to health equity, health inequality, social justice and injustice, human rights, cultural competence, and health literacy is crucial for guiding nurses in the planning, delivery, and evaluation of meaningful, competent health promotion and risk reduction interventions that target vulnerable populations.

Finally, nurses must ground care delivery in an understanding of those resources that are readily available and are known to reduce vulnerability. These resources include not just societal-level resources, but the strengths and assets inherent in all groups and individuals, including those considered most vulnerable. Indeed, recognition and valuing of these resources for resilience must provide the foundation for the development of any strategy aimed at reducing vulnerability.

Healthy People 2020

The vision of *HP 2020* is to create "a society in which all people live long, healthy lives." Two of the overarching goals of this agenda that directly relate to the care of vulnerable individuals, families, and populations are to:[35]

- Achieve health equity, eliminate disparities, and improve the health of all groups
- Create social and physical environments that promote good health for all

The *Healthy People* vision provides useful guiding principles for improving the health of all Americans, especially those who are vulnerable to poor health outcomes. A topic specific to vulnerability in *HP 2020* is social determinants of health. The goal is to create social and physical environments that promote health. This topic is a new addition to *HP 2010* and was included in recognition of the complexity of health. As stated:

> A range of personal, social, economic, and environmental factors contribute to individual and population health. For example, people with a quality education, stable employment, safe homes and neighborhoods, and access to preventive services tend to be healthier throughout their lives. Conversely, poor health outcomes are often made worse by the interaction between individuals and their social and physical environment.[36]

HP 2020 includes a model that illustrates this reality (Fig. 24-2).[35] Many of the leading health indicators for *HP 2020* focus on improving the health of vulnerable populations through several initiatives, including a focus on reduction of gender- and age-based health disparities, enhanced educational opportunities as a means to improving overall health, and strategies targeting the built environment.[36]

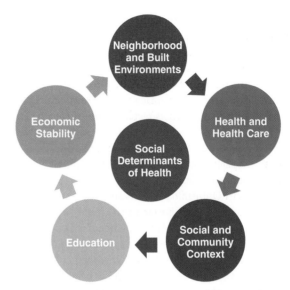

Figure 24-2 *Healthy People 2020* social determinants of health. *(From United States Department of Health and Human Services. [2013]. Healthy People 2020 topic: Social determinants. Retrieved from http://healthypeople.gov/2020/topicsobjectives2020/overview.aspx?topicid=39.)*

■ HEALTHY PEOPLE 2020
Vulnerable Populations

Targeted Topic: Social Determinants of Health

Goal

Create social and physical environments that promote good health for all.

Overview

Health starts in our homes, schools, workplaces, neighborhoods, and communities. We know that taking care of ourselves by eating well and staying active, not smoking, getting the recommended immunizations and screening tests, and seeing a doctor when we are sick all influence our health. Our health is also determined in part by access to social and economic opportunities; the resources and supports available in our homes, neighborhoods, and communities; the quality of our education; the safety of our workplaces; the cleanliness of our water, food, and air; and the nature of our social interactions and relationships. The conditions in which we live explain in part why some Americans are healthier than others and why Americans more generally are not as healthy as they could be.

Healthy People 2020 highlights the importance of addressing the social determinants of health by including

"Create social and physical environments that promote good health for all" as one of the four overarching goals for the decade.[36] This emphasis is shared by the World Health Organization, whose Commission on Social Determinants of Health in 2008 published the report *Closing the Gap in a Generation: Health Equity Through Action on the Social Determinants of Health*. The emphasis is also shared by other U.S. health initiatives such as the National Partnership for Action to End Health Disparities and the National Prevention and Health Promotion Strategy.

The Social Determinants of Health topic area within *Healthy People 2020* is designed to identify ways to create social and physical environments that promote good health for all. All Americans deserve an equal opportunity to make the choices that lead to good health. But to ensure that all Americans have that opportunity, advances are needed not only in health care but also in fields such as education, childcare, housing, business, law, media, community planning, transportation, and agriculture. Making these advances involves working together to:

- Explore how programs, practices, and policies in these areas affect the health of individuals, families, and communities
- Establish common goals, complementary roles, and ongoing constructive relationships between the health sector and these areas
- Maximize opportunities for collaboration among federal-, state-, and local-level partners related to social determinants of health

Source: See reference 35.

Nursing Care of Vulnerable Populations—Roles of the Nurse

Nurses in all settings fulfill a variety of roles when providing care or coordinating services and developing interventions for at-risk and vulnerable populations. Following the guidelines set forth in the nursing process, nurses caring for vulnerable populations assess and identify needs, plan and deliver interventions, and evaluate outcomes as a result of those interventions. Each of these steps takes place in partnership with clients. As part of the process, nurses function to identify resources available to meet identified needs (resources that are both internal and external to the client). PHNs are asked to fill the many roles identified in the Minnesota Model: Public Health Intervention Wheel including those of advocate, case manager, educator and counselor, collaborator, researcher, and

partner (see Chapter 2). As PHNs function in these multiple roles, they meet the societal mandate to ensure delivery of quality nursing care to all people in a spirit of respect that is unaltered by differences in gender, race, class, or culture. These roles are also central to the delivery of quality care for nurses working in settings outside of public health.

■ EVIDENCE-BASED PRACTICE
Transdisciplinary Collaboration

Practice Statement: Transdisciplinary collaboration is designed to build partnerships and combine resources to help improve health outcomes for vulnerable populations.

Targeted Outcome: Improved health outcomes for vulnerable populations

Evidence to Support: There has been increased attention on the need for transdisciplinary practice as a means to decrease health inequities. Transdisciplinary health-care delivery requires that knowledge be integrated from multiple disciplines so that all of the team members use this knowledge and provide a consistent approach within an intervention. Much of the current evidence is related to the effectiveness of interprofessional education programs, but evidence is beginning to emerge that transdisciplinary practice in the field is also effective. An example is a service learning project implemented by PHN students in a community setting. The students sought out agency partners outside of the nursing discipline as collaborators on their projects. The students found that with collaboration across disciplines, they experienced more cultural awareness, increased competency in planning interventions, and better met community needs. Additional student benefits included expertise in caring for vulnerable populations, evidence of effective interventions, role models, and increased knowledge of community resources. In another study, researchers reported that the use of a transdisciplinary model improved the effectiveness of a tobacco-use intervention. The intervention delivered to smokers was enhanced through the assurance that each member of the team provided patients with the same information. In addition, through sharing of knowledge, the team members reinforced the interventions through pooled evidence across disciplines as well as tying together the different aspects of the health issue from the perspective of each discipline.

Recommended Approaches

The use of a transdisciplinary approach to education, practice, and research has the potential to strengthen the use of evidence-based practices across disciplines in public health practice. This requires the development of multidisciplinary teams across a health-care issue who share knowledge and work to tie together the different aspects of the health issue.

Sources

1. Gargano, L.M., Gallagher, P.F., Barrett, M., Howell, K., Wolfe. C., Woods C., et al. (2013). Issues in the development of a research and education framework for One Health [Conference summary]. *Emerging Infectious Disease.* Retrieved from http://dx.doi.org/10.3201/eid1903.121103.

2. Jacobs, J.A., Jones, E., Gabella, B.A., Spring, B., & Brownson, R.C. (2012). Tools for implementing an evidence-based approach in public health practice. *Prevention of Chronic Disease, 9.* doi:http://dx.doi.org/10.5888/pcd9.110324.

3. Sternas, K.A., & Scharf, M.A. (2007). *Advancing evidenced-based practice with vulnerable populations through transdisciplinary collaboration on service learning projects.* Paper presented at the 18th International Nursing Research Congress Focusing on Evidence-Based Practice, Vienna, Austria. Retrieved from http://stti.confex.com/stti/congrs07/techprogram/paper_34952.htm.

4. Hoffman, M.A., & Little, V. (2011). Trans-disciplinary care: A new approach to improving effectiveness of tobacco use interventions. *Journal of the Health Care for the Poor and Underserved, 22*(2), 409-414.

5. Picard, M., Sabiston, C.M., & McNamara, J.K. (2011). The need for a trans disciplinary global health framework. *Journal of Alternative Care Medicine, 17*(2), 179-184.

Homelessness and Vulnerability

Although not a disease, homelessness kills.[37] This is partly the result of limited access to health-care insurance, leaving the hospital emergency department (ED) as the primary accessible source of health care for homeless adults.[38] When lack of access is coupled with the high prevalence of noncommunicable diseases, both life expectancy and quality of life are negatively affected.[39,40] Forty to over fifty percent of homeless adults have at least one noncommunicable disease.[40] They are four to nine times more likely to die than their housed counterparts,[41,42] and have a reduced life expectancy of 45 years compared with the U.S. life expectancy of 77.9 years, a 33-year difference.[43, 44]

Who exactly experiences homelessness? Is it someone who lives on the street or someone who lives in a shelter? What about someone sleeping on the couch of a friend or family member? To answer these questions, the U.S. government has a two-part definition of **homelessness.** According to the U.S. Department of Housing and Urban Development, someone who is homeless meets one or both of the following criteria:[45]

- One who lacks a fixed, regular, and adequate nighttime residence
- One who lives in a supervised shelter or institution designed for temporary residence, or one who lives in a place that is not normally used as accommodation for people

Using this definition of homelessness, a person who lives on the street, in a shelter, or is couch-surfing is experiencing homelessness. If a person moves from home to home constantly, then that person is lacking a fixed and/or regular nighttime residence, and therefore is homeless.

There are then clearly different types or levels of homelessness. Just as we separate prevention into three levels—primary, secondary, and tertiary—the standard for defining the degree of homelessness is to place those experiencing homelessness into three groups:[46]

- **Primary homelessness** includes everyone who is living without adequate shelter—those living in vehicles, surviving on the streets, staying in parks, or squatting in abandoned buildings.
- **Secondary homelessness** includes those who are staying in a temporary form of housing because they have nowhere else to go—those living with friends or family, or in shelters.
- **Tertiary homelessness** includes those who rent single rooms on a long-term basis without security of a fixed or permanent residence.[46]

Prevalence of Homelessness

Obtaining estimates of the numbers of persons who experience homelessness is a challenge because of the difficulty in collecting the data.[47] The overall numbers of persons experiencing homelessness was 610,042 in January of 2013.[48] Of these, 17% were experiencing chronic homelessness and 38% were experiencing primary homelessness. In some areas, such as New York City, there was a rise in the number of persons experiencing homelessness and seeking shelter.[49] Thus, although there was an overall decline at the national level, there was variability across states with 7 states experiencing an increase.[48] In addition, depending on weather and other issues, the number of persons experiencing homelessness on any given night can range from 450,000 to more than 900,000.[41] Obtaining data related to how many are experiencing homelessness on a given night is called a **point in time estimate** of homelessness, because a single night, or one point in time, was used to determine prevalence. Table 24-2 shows some the change in point in time estimates for select U.S. cities from 2005 to 2011, demonstrating the variability based on geography.[50]

There are other ways to look at the epidemiology of homelessness. Estimating the prevalence can be done by the type of homelessness (primary, secondary, or tertiary) or the different populations experiencing homelessness, for example, families, single youths, and single adults do not experience the same rates of homelessness. Further, minorities are largely overrepresented in the U.S. homeless population, so it affects minorities disproportionately.[50] Locale can play a role in homelessness; warmer climates make it easier to deal with issues related to weather. Certain segments of the population are at greater risk for experiencing homelessness. In the general population, the odds of experiencing homelessness are one in 194. For those who are doubling up with friends and neighbors, the odds are one in 12, for those who have been in prison the odds are one in 13, and for those who grew up in foster care the odds are one in 11.[50]

Single or solitary adults, mostly males, are more likely to experience primary homelessness than those who are either solitary youths or in families. Homeless families are more likely to experience secondary homelessness than primary homelessness, as are solitary youths. Most cities responded that this was likely the result of the policies in place to protect families with children from experiencing homelessness, including policies that made it more difficult to evict families who had fallen behind on their rent. Between 2009 and 2011, there was a 2.4% decline in homelessness experienced by persons in families.[50]

The prevalence of homelessness in the United States also varies based on racial background. African Americans are largely overrepresented in the sheltered homeless population (Table 24-3). Whereas African Americans comprised 12.6% of the U.S. population in 2010, nearly 40% of the sheltered homeless during that same period were African Americans. White non-Hispanics are underrepresented. Whereas whites made up 56.1% of the U.S. population, there were only a little more white persons in shelters than there were African Americans (41.6% vs. 37%).[51,52]

Homelessness is not just a big city problem; rural homelessness does exist. Those who experience homelessness in a rural setting are much more difficult to locate and, thus, their homelessness is more difficult to address.[50,53-55] In comparison with urban homeless populations, the rural homeless are more likely to have jobs, but are less likely to be educated. About two-thirds of the rural homeless population fall into the age range of 35 to 44, and nearly eight out of 10 are men. Further, those experiencing homelessness in a rural setting are much more likely to stay with friends or family than are those experiencing homelessness in an urban setting. Lastly, according to clinicians, rural homeless populations tend to have more advanced health-care problems than do their urban counterparts.[55,56]

TABLE 24–2	Point in Time Estimates of Homelessness in Selected U.S. Cities	
U.S. City	Point in Time Estimate 2005	Point in Time Estimate 2011
Phoenix, AZ	1,906	5,831
San Francisco, CA	6,248	5,669
Washington, DC	5,518	6,546
Boston, MA	5,819	5,476
Baltimore, MD	2,904	4,094
Detroit, MI	14,827	3,138
New York, NY	48,155	51,123
Philadelphia, PA	6,653	6,180

Source: See reference 50.

TABLE 24–3	Racial and Ethnic Statistics of Sheltered Individuals in the United States, 2009–2010	
Ethnic Background	Percentage of Secondary Homeless Population (2009–2010)	Percentage of U.S. Population (2009)
Black or African American	37.0%	12.6%
White, non-Hispanic	41.1%	56.1%
White, Hispanic	9.7%	16.3%
Multiple races	7.2%	2.9%
Other single race	4.5%	12.1%

Sources: See references 51 and 52.

Impact on Health

The impact of homelessness on health is a major public health issue that affects one out of every 15 adults during their lifetime.[57,58] The homeless adult is faced with an excess disease burden, a shorter life expectancy, limited access to care, and consumption of significantly more health-care resources when she or he does finally receive care.[58-60] The homeless experience higher rates of non-communicable diseases compared with the general U.S. population, including asthma (18% vs. 10%), hypertension (up to 29% vs. 16.5%), and chronic back pain (up to 18% compared with 4.6%).[59,60]

Between 25% to 33% of homeless persons have mental health issues, including schizophrenia, depression, and bipolar disorder.[61] In the general U.S. population, only about 6% experience the same severe mental health issues.[61] In relation to behavioral health, up to 37% report depression compared with 5% to 10% in the general adult population, and 22% to 43% report drug use compared with 14.4% in the general population. Alcohol use disorders are as high as 84% in homeless men and 58% of homeless women compared with only 8% in the general population (Table 24-4).[59,62-64]

About one-half of persons experiencing homelessness who have mental health issues also have a concurrent substance abuse disorder, some of which is a result of attempts to self-medicate with drugs and/or alcohol.[65,66] Persons who are experiencing homelessness experience an abundance of health issues, including cardiovascular disease, respiratory disorders, ulcers, and skin diseases, and have an higher risk than the greater population to contract communicable diseases or suffer from cardiovascular disease.[39,67] A person experiencing homelessness is much more likely to arrive at the hospital in an ambulance, be uninsured, be admitted, and is also more likely to have a longer stay.[58]

Risk Factors for Poor Health

First, the living conditions of those experiencing primary homelessness are not optimal. If a homeless patient is admitted to the hospital for surgery, it will be much more difficult for that patient to keep an incision infection free postdischarge than it will be for someone who is living in a place that is suitable for human shelter. Second, transportation costs make it difficult for a patient experiencing homelessness to receive follow-up care and testing. Third, the nutritional intake of a homeless patient is irregular and less healthy than that of the general population, making diet instructions hard to follow. Another problem concerns the unmet dental and vision needs of the homeless population. Two-thirds of those experiencing homelessness have clinically significant dental problems, while 40% have vision problems that interfere with their function.[68] If two out of every five of the homeless population have trouble reading due to unmet vision needs, it seems to follow that it would be much more difficult for them to adhere to written medical directions, such as discharge instructions. As previously mentioned, the high rate of mental health disorders in the homeless population could further complicate care. There are other complicating factors that are easily overlooked. For example, where can a diabetic homeless patient store insulin? How does such a patient keep a medication from being stolen?

In addition to considering the challenges from a health-care provider's point of view, we should also consider the barriers to access for those experiencing homelessness. Other than cost, there are also barriers such as language and culture and the availability of health care in a given community, among others.

TABLE 24-4	Characteristics of Persons Experiencing Homelessness Versus That of the U.S. General Population	
Characteristic	Percentage of Homeless Population (2009)	Percentage of U.S. Population (2008)
Mental Health Disorder	26.0%	6.0%
Disability	37.8%	15.5%
Drug Use Disorder*	38.0%	15.0%
Veteran	14.0%	11.2%

Source: See reference 62.

* This row compares the percentage of persons experiencing homelessness who reported that they had a drug dependence (excluding alcohol) and the percentage of the general population, over the age of 12, who reported using drugs (excluding alcohol) at least once in the past 12 months.

● APPLYING PUBLIC HEALTH SCIENCE

The Case of the Rubbermaid Storage Box

Public Health Science Topics Covered:

- Community assessment
- Community diagnosis
- Organization and management
  - Community partnerships

While in graduate school pursuing a degree as an advanced public health nurse (APHN), Adele was asked to supervise a group of undergraduate nursing students who were assigned to take weekly blood pressure readings at a local homeless shelter, the City Gospel Mission. This faith-based nondenominational mission was located in downtown Cincinnati and provided multiple services including meals and shelter beds but did not offer health care. From her first trip to the City Gospel Mission, Adele felt compelled to reach out to this vulnerable population.

Adele recognized that these men had very few options for health care, and she wanted to offer more than blood pressure screenings. As part of her practicum experience, she went to the mission on a weekly basis to provide nursing assessments, health education, and nursing care. She began to interact more with the men when they came to the clinic and worked with them to help identify their health needs and, in some cases, offer referrals. All of her supplies, including her blood pressure cuff and a glucometer, fit into a Rubbermaid storage box, which she left at the shelter. Although she was providing some assistance, she knew these men needed more. When she approached her faculty preceptor, she was encouraged to apply the health planning process, do a focused assessment that would help her to understand whether there was a need for expanding the care, and consider developing the model of a nurse-managed clinic if there was a need. The faculty member explained that the assessment could provide the data she needed to develop a plan to address the health needs of the men she was seeing.

In conducting part of their assessment, Adele and a fellow APHN student asked key informants, homeless men at the mission, where they sought health care. They all mentioned the ED at a nearby major urban medical center. The students' assessment at the medical center focused on identifying the costs associated with nonurgent emergency department (ED) care for patients experiencing homelessness. The students presented the findings to the hospital performance improvement committee. The committee agreed that an intervention aimed at providing nonurgent care to homeless men outside the ED would result in a cost benefit to the hospital, and that a nurse-managed clinic model had the potential to meet that need.

After Adele graduated, she no longer had time to continue to provide even the small amount of nursing care she had offered at the mission. Having established

a need, Adele together with her faculty preceptor sought sources of possible funding for expanding Adele's practicum experience to establish a permanent nurse-managed clinic at the City Gospel Mission.

The success of this project depended on the application of public health science and the public health competencies that Adele had acquired. First, a team was formed that included Adele, two faculty members from the University of Cincinnati College of Nursing, the chief nursing officer from the hospital, and the director of the City Gospel Mission. The next step was to flesh out the initial needs assessment. Adele's assessment of ED use by the homeless was crucial information for the potential cost benefit of the clinic. However, to help understand the breadth of the problem, further assessment was done using aggregate data from the City Gospel Mission on the number of potential clients for the clinic as well as secondary analysis of available data on the prevalence of primary homelessness in the city of Cincinnati. These data provided a clear picture of the need for the clinic. The final step was to develop the program expanding on Adele's Rubbermaid container of supplies to include a more comprehensive nurse-managed clinic model.

The team chose a nurse-managed clinic model that would link with other resources in the city. Thus, patients of the clinic would receive nursing assessments, health education, and nursing care under the direction of Adele and be referred to other clinics for more complex medical problems. To do this, the project needed start-up funds to provide supplies, equipment, and a method to keep clinic medical records and to conduct an evaluation.

The first grant application was not funded. The team took the grant reviews, refined the application, and submitted it to another funding agency. They were successful this time in obtaining a 2-year start-up grant. The grant application succeeded based on three key elements: (1) a clear delineation of the need for the clinic; (2) evidence of sustainability of the clinic once the funding was exhausted; and (3) a clear plan to evaluate the effectiveness of the clinic. **Sustainability** refers to the ability of a program to be maintained once the funding period has been completed. In this case, the three organizations that supported the grant—the college, the hospital, and the shelter—all committed to maintaining the clinic if the evaluation demonstrated that it was effective. The college committed to sending students to the clinic for clinical experiences, the hospital agreed to be the "owner" of the clinic, that is, staff would maintain the medical records and provide salary support for Adele to continue her work at the clinic. City Gospel Mission agreed to continue to provide the space and utilities for the clinic. The homeless men also became partners, offering suggestions about time, location, and some of the health needs they would like to see met. They also saw a role in helping with the running of the clinic.

After 2 years of clinic implementation, the evaluation team was able to demonstrate that the clinic had indeed improved the health outcomes. One of the faculty members from the college conducted the evaluation. Attendees at the clinic were asked to complete a survey the first day they used the clinic and at least 2 months after they had begun to use the clinic. Forty-five homeless adults completed both a baseline survey and a survey after starting care at the clinic. There was a significant increase in the percentage of participants who were very satisfied in relation to perceived quality and availability of health care. In addition, there was a significant improvement in health-related quality of life in relation to mental health, physical problems, and vitality.[39]

Adele's story is true. The grant ended in 2006; 8 years later the clinic was still functioning, seeing 20 to 30 men a night. The clinic is staffed by volunteer nurses, nursing students, and, of course, Adele, who provides information and conversation to her patients in this vulnerable population. The important issue here is that Adele alone with her Rubbermaid container was not enough. Adele took her enthusiasm and concern for a vulnerable population and built a team. The use of solid public health approaches resulted in organizational commitment. Addressing the health-care challenges for those who are vulnerable requires this approach and can be successfully initiated, implemented, and sustained by nurses.

Interventions and Services for Persons Experiencing Homelessness

Even in the best of circumstances, health-care providers experience problems in an acute care setting in helping any patient manage personal health for the long term. For example, sometimes it is difficult to ensure that after discharge patients will follow up on time with their health-care providers. Other times, patients may not take their medicines as prescribed, which makes it even more problematic to ensure that conditions are treated in the best way possible. In primary care, patients might not get recommended testing because of embarrassment (e.g., colonoscopy) or because of costs associated with that testing. Each of these problems is magnified for patients who are also experiencing homelessness.

Shelter

Housing is the biggest need of the homeless. Simply providing housing can improve the health of the homeless and reduce the number of hospital visits and hospital admissions.[68] Homeless shelters provide an immediate and temporary solution, usually for a stipulated and limited amount of time (e.g., 3 months) for an individual or a family. It is a safe and warm place to sleep and in areas of the United States when the winter weather is more severe, an essential service. Shelters are frequently sponsored by nonprofit organizations that have religious and/or government sponsorship. Most shelters limit their service to certain groups of people, frequently not allowing any alcohol or illegal drugs, and have in place strict rules about there being no violence in the shelter. Many provide separate space or facilities for adolescents and families with children. Most shelters open late in the afternoon and close early in the morning, leaving the person staying at the shelter on the street for the daylight hours. Usually, shelters offer their service free of charge and some will provide an evening meal for those staying at the shelter. Some communities supplement their night shelters with day shelters where people can go during the time the night shelters are closed. These facilities usually have an array of social services to help with permanent housing, job placements, mental health care and services for those with addictions, and job training. There may also be showers, laundry facilities, used clothing available as well as other amenities to help individuals and families secure more permanent housing.

A step above the shelters is the more permanent *transitional housing,* which is affordable owing to significant subsidies, but again there is usually a time limit (6 months to 2 years). People who agree to live in transitional housing usually must participate in programs that provide counseling, job searches, and job and educational training. People are taught skills on how to maintain more permanent housing and manage their money.

Permanent affordable housing is the long-term solution. If the rent is subsidized based on the resident's income, the person is usually allowed to stay as long as he or she remains in the low-income bracket. Permanent supportive housing combines this housing assistance with services for homeless persons with disabilities. Usually, they serve individuals and members of that household who have serious mental illnesses, chronic substance abuse problems, physical disabilities, or AIDS and related diseases. People may receive these services either at the housing site or through partnering agencies.

Preventing homelessness is a cost-effective intervention. Funds can be used to pay expenses and resolve situations in certain circumstances so that individuals and households can avoid homelessness, receive support services to help them pay for the cost of their housing, and develop skills and employment to avoid a recurrence of the problem. Moving people rapidly into permanent housing has also been shown to be cost effective and is the goal now of several nongovernmental organizations.

Food

When families and individuals live in poverty, they frequently have to make impossible choices between paying the rent, buying food, or buying essential medications. This can lead to homelessness and decreased ability to provide adequate food. Homelessness and hunger are inseparably linked. The United Nations World Food Summit in 1996 defined **food security** as existing "when all people at all times have access to sufficient, safe, nutritious food to maintain a healthy and active life."[69] This definition of food security usually is considered to include both physical and economic access to food that meets people's dietary needs as well as their food preferences. In 2012, in the United States one in six (18%) households experienced food insecurity at some time during the year.[70] This was up from a little over 10% of households in 2007 just before the economic recession. In 2011, 5.7% of households experienced very low food security. Also 10% of households with children experienced food insecurity and 1% experienced very low food security.[71]

Homeless individuals and homeless families often experience food insecurity. During the recession that began in 2008, there was a growing request by poor Americans for food assistance. The available assistance was through food stamps, referred to as the Supplemental Nutrition Assistance Program, the Women, Infants, and Children supplemental nutrition program, and the National School Lunch Programs and School Breakfast Programs. In 2011, 57% of food-insecure households utilized federal assistance programs to obtain food.[71] Nonprofit organizations frequently help to provide food security through private donations to food pantries, food banks, and soup kitchens.[66]

Health Care

Steps are being taken to help address some of the barriers faced by the homeless in trying to attain health care,

especially access to health care. In many cities, health-care services are provided at places frequented by those experiencing homelessness, for example, soup kitchens and shelters. Outreach workers often go to the locations where the homeless are and tell them about the availability of different health-care resources. Finally, many communities are implementing mobile medical units that can travel to the patients' locations. Some of these mobile medical units are very specialized (such as only providing dental care) and others provide primary care and referral services.[72,73] Patients who are experiencing homelessness are resourceful when it comes to health care, and some may even have underground networks of health resources.[73]

As previously mentioned, other barriers faced by the homeless might stem from their providers. If providers speak at a health literacy level that is above the understanding of a homeless patient, the patient will be much less likely to understand such things as follow-up instructions. Furthermore, one recent study showed that 55% of patients felt they had been discriminated against because they had no permanent residence.[39] Thus, training on how to provide care for their patients who are experiencing homelessness will be beneficial to health-care providers.

Policy

Providing immediate housing with supportive services seems to be the most effective policy both related to cost and to improving the health of the homeless.[74] Supportive housing is very effective for those who have had a long history of homelessness, for homeless veterans, and for those who are homeless with mental health and addiction problems. Preventing families from becoming homeless, along with very rapid rehousing if the family does become homeless, is also effective policy. Preventing individuals with disabilities from becoming homeless is also effective and requires the collaboration of health-care providers, social workers, and individuals who monitor subsidized supportive housing. Providing more and better mental health services, effective services to individuals who have suffered domestic violence, and creation of additional addiction treatment centers also will have an impact on preventing homelessness and, for the homeless, will provide the additional support service necessary for individuals to keep their housing.

Migrant Workers, Immigrants, Refugees, and Asylees

In the United States, three populations that are often grouped together are migrants, immigrants, and refugees.

They each actually comprise distinct, though sometimes overlapping, populations with different risk factors for vulnerability and different barriers to achieving optimal health.

Immigrants are defined as persons who have legally emigrated from one country to another to become permanent residents of the new country.[75] In the United States, those who enter a country to become permanent residents without formal permission are illegally residing in the country and are usually referred to as illegal aliens, but more recent terms that carry fewer stigmas are *undocumented workers* and *undocumented immigrants*.

The 1980 Refugee Act in the United States defines a **refugee** as "a person outside of his or her country of nationality who is unable or unwilling to return because of persecution or a well-founded fear of persecution."[76] This current definition is based on a United Nations 1951 Convention that states, "any person who, owing to a well-founded fear of being persecuted for reasons of race, religion, nationality, membership in a particular social group or political opinion, is outside the country of his nationality and is unable or, owing to such fear, is unwilling to avail himself of the protection of that country; or who not having a nationality and being outside the country of his former habitual residence as a result of such events, is unable or, owing such fear, is unwilling to return to it."[77]

Migrant Workers

The term **migrant worker** is used to describe those who move from place to place to get work.[78] Globally there are approximately 175 million migrant workers.[79] In the US most of the migrant workers are employed in agricultural jobs.[78] Under Title 29 of the U.S. Code, "A **migrant agricultural worker** is a person employed in agricultural work of a seasonal or other temporary nature who is required to be absent overnight from his or her permanent place of residence. Exceptions are immediate family members of an agricultural employer or a farm labor contractor, and temporary H-2A foreign workers. (H-2A temporary foreign workers are nonimmigrant aliens authorized to work in agricultural employment in the United States for a specified time period, normally less than 1 year.)"[80] Migrant workers can be composed of groups from other countries, as well as U.S. citizens such as the migrant workers during the Great Depression.

Most of the 3.1 million migrant workers in the United States are employed in agriculture and support the $28 billion fruit and vegetable industry.[81] Because migrant workers move around or are frequently away from their permanent place of residence, establishing residency for benefits (e.g., federal assistance through food stamps) is often difficult for this group. Most of these workers have no access to workers' compensation or disability compensation. Many migrant farmworkers employed in planting and harvesting follow the crops for jobs. For example, major agricultural work starts in California, Texas, and Florida. These starting points result in three streams of workers: the western stream from California to Washington State, the midwestern stream from Texas to all the midwestern states, and the eastern stream from Florida through Ohio to Maine (Fig. 24-3). These streams represent how migrant workers follow the jobs, especially in agriculture, where the time to harvest crops changes with the seasons. In the past few years, these streams have been less distinct.[82]

This group is particularly vulnerable for multiple reasons. Only small portions (30%) of migrant agricultural workers reported that they could speak English well, so language is an obvious barrier.[82,83] Further, it is difficult to establish what the health needs are, as migrant workers are often isolated in rural areas, living miles away from major roads.[82] Another obvious barrier is financial. Twenty-three percent of farmworker families have incomes below the poverty guidelines and most do not qualify for workers' compensation.[84] This, in turn, can affect their access to care.

Prevalence of Seasonal Farmworkers

Based on the most recent National Agricultural Workers Survey, there were approximately 3 million migrant and seasonal agricultural workers in the United States in 2001, with 72% of them being foreign born.[84] Of these, 79% were men, the mean age was 32 with a sixth grade education, 93% were foreign born, 78% were foreign citizens, and 53% were not authorized to work in the United States.[84] According to the U.S. Bureau of Labor, in 2010 agricultural workers had a median annual income of $18,970.[83]

Impact on Health

Poor, substandard housing is frequently a part of the life of a migrant or seasonal farmworker. If a person has to continually move to find work, it is more likely that the person moving will not have long-term or stable housing, putting him or her into one of the groups of tertiary, secondary, or possibly even primary homelessness. More than just being connected by the lack of stable shelter, migrant workers may also experience negative psychosocial outcomes.[85] One group of researchers conducted a study in the 1990s with migrant workers and found that

Major Migratroy Streams for Farmworkers in the United States

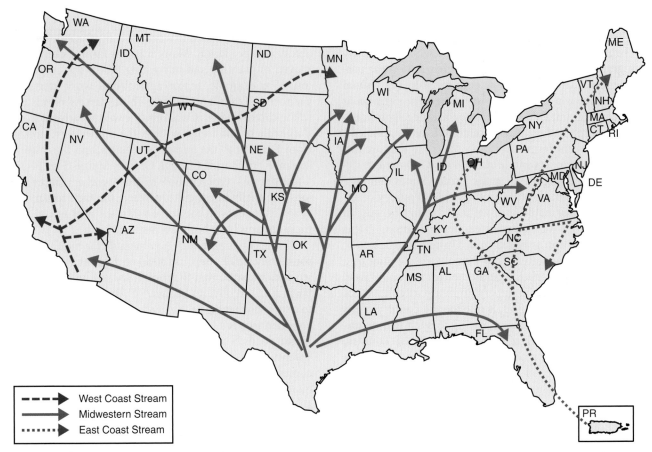

Figure 24-3 Migratory patterns of migrant farmworkers. *(Copyright © 1985–2002 National Center for Farmworker Health, Inc. Used with permission. Retrieved from http://www.ncfh.org/?pid=4&page=3.)*

the psychological stressors exhibited by migrant workers and depressive tendencies were similar to those seen in the homeless.[86]

The health of migrant workers reflects their poverty and poor living situations, making them vulnerable to conditions no longer thought of as being prevalent in the United States. Most foreign workers are from Mexico[81] and have a higher incidence of tuberculosis, other communicable diseases, and poor nutrition in addition to having the daily exposure to the dangerous occupation of farming and to pesticides. The workers live in crowded housing and working conditions, making them at higher risk for increased chances of developing tuberculosis during their lifetime and six times more likely to develop tuberculosis when compared with other workers.[81,87]

● APPLYING PUBLIC HEALTH SCIENCE
The Case of the Wandering Diabetic
Public Health Science Topics Covered:

- Focused community assessment
- Partnership building
- Advocacy

Sara, a nurse at the local nurse-managed clinic run by the hospital, met Steven and listened to his story. Steven told Sara he had lived in 12 states, following the jobs. He had dropped out of high school to help raise his siblings, and with the tough economy and his lack of education he couldn't find anything except seasonal and or other temporary work. He knew about the scenery of New Mexico, the Smokies in the fall, the hustle and bustle of New York, and the Seattle rain. His friends and family let him know of odd jobs, and he hitchhiked across the country multiple times to take those jobs. He had been a ranch hand, done construction work, and had plenty of factory jobs. He then got a job in California, working at a forge. He slept on friends' couches the first few months he was in town, but wore out his welcome. Steven liked the job and hoped for promotion, so he was able to pay rent at a trailer in a park that he heard was cheap.

Little did Steven know that low rent also meant power blackouts, sewage overflowing into the streets, and constant fires from poor electrical wiring. Steven said that this was the only place he could afford and did not have anyone else to stay with. He was reluctant to talk with his landlord about the conditions at the trailer park because his neighbor once called the city for an inspection, and that neighbor's rent was increased in retaliation from the landlord.

Steven came to the clinic because he was a type I diabetic, and with the inconsistent electricity, he was no longer able to store his insulin and hoped that Sara had some ideas about where he could store it. He also had sores on his feet that worried him. He told Sara that many people in his trailer park were living in these conditions, some of which were illegal, such as the water spigot that served as the main source of water for the park (Fig. 24-4).

Sara has other patients from the same trailer park, and while she suspected less-than-optimal living conditions, she never imagined anything to this extent. After assessing her patient, Sara decided that something needed to be done immediately. She started by gathering data about the trailer park and its residents. She investigated the unmet health needs of this group of people and examined the impact of the squalid living conditions using a qualitative survey of the residents (see Chapter 4). She also examined available data using the census track data for the locality of the trailer park. Many of the respondents to the survey stated that they had recently experienced infections. Others had noncommunicable diseases that they were unable to manage properly.

Based on this preliminary assessment Sara collaborated with other health partners to come up with solutions. She contacted her colleagues at the hospital, including the diabetes management experts and

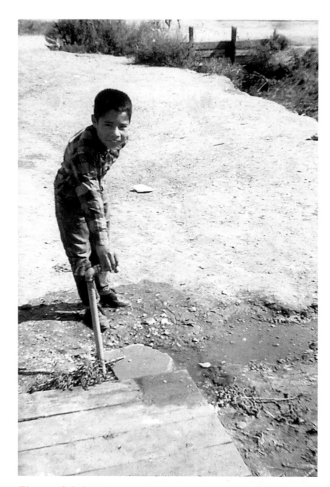

Figure 24-4 Water sanitation in migrant worker camps. *(From the Centers for Disease Control and Prevention, 1975.)*

communicable disease experts. She also contacted the local health department to assist in examining legal options for this group. Next, she formed a coalition with her colleagues and other agencies, and used this coalition to inform policymakers about the situation at the trailer park. By doing so, she advocated for the health of her patients. Sara also applied for a grant to extend the clinic services to include a weekly outreach clinic at the trailer park, and found a local company to donate a generator so that Steven and other residents would have electricity for refrigeration to safely store their medications.

Sara used a public health approach to the problem. She gathered data to examine the problem, and applied her problem-solving skills in helping a population. Sara also found that Steven's story was not unique.[85]

Because of this, she worked with the public health department and the hospital to evaluate the outreach program so that they would have evidence to share that would help other free clinics and public health departments trying to solve the same problem.

Intervention and Services for Migrant Workers

There has always been limited and inadequate housing for migrant farmworkers. There has been some improvement through the Federal Farmworker Housing Program, but housing continues to be an issue.[82] There is the option of housing located on the farm, but that generally means lower wages because housing rent is removed from the base salary, and there's no guarantee that the housing will be adequate. The off-the-farm option usually consists of very makeshift shelters, not close to any basic infrastructure, and with no or limited water access and sanitation. A 2007 study of migrant and seasonal farmworkers found that 82% of households experienced food insecurity and 49% of them reported hunger.[88]

Farmworkers as a vulnerable population (low literacy levels, different culture and language, poverty) have difficulty accessing health care, paying for health care, and participating in prevention activities. Migrant farmers usually work for an hourly wage or per item harvested or planted, and do not have the luxury of sick time or paid time to visit the health-care provider. According to the National Center for Farmworker Health, migrant workers are faced with numerous barriers related to accessing adequate health care. These include the cost of coverage, lack of health-care providers in the area, and lack of transportation to health-care services.[81] Another issue is the cultural and language barrier that prevents workers from knowing about accessible services.[86] Also, 80% of Mexican farmworkers interviewed in one study rarely sought dental care, and those who did sought it out in Mexico.[88]

Migrant workers often come from cultures different from the surrounding community. Specific strategies for this population can help with the cultural assessment (see Chapter 23) and serve as guidelines for school personnel in cross-cultural interactions around health or other issues (Box 24-1).[88,89]

Children of migrant workers are especially susceptible to unmet health needs. In one study, more than half the children (53%) had unmet health needs, which is 24 times higher than U.S. children in general and still significantly higher than housed Hispanic and African American children in the United States.[89] The migrant lifestyle that includes separation from family, constantly moving,

---

BOX 24-1 — A Multicultural Approach to Health Care With Immigrants and Refugees

The following strategies for cultural assessment serve as guidelines for school personnel in cross-cultural interactions concerning health or other issues:

- Remember that your cultural beliefs may be as foreign to the student as the student's beliefs may be to you.
- Practice "cultural competence"—a continuous process of learning characterized by respect for differences and appreciation of how your culture interacts with that of students and their families.
- Consider students and their families as individuals before considering them as members of a specific cultural group.
- Never presume that an individual's ethnic identity is any indication of his cultural values or patterns of behavior.
- Treat all presumptions about cultural values and traits as hypotheses to be tested anew with each individual. Turn "facts" into questions. Learn what expectations the student and/or family have of you and your role, as well as how they view themselves and their role in the interaction.
- Keep in mind that newcomers are bicultural and that they face the task of integrating at least two different cultures that may conflict.
- Some aspects of an individual's cultural history, values, and lifestyle may prove relevant to a school health situation, but others may not. Do not prejudge which aspects are relevant to an individual's understanding of any health issue.

Source: See reference 89.

---

having sex with prostitutes, needle sharing, and use of injection drugs make the migrant farmworker more at risk for HIV.[90]

The Primary Health Care Center program under the Health Resources and Services Administration provided health services to more than 900,000 agricultural workers in 2012, about one-third of that population. The service provides accessible primary and preventive health care for farmworkers, and all charges are provided on a sliding scale regardless of immigration status.[91]

Policy

The Affordable Care Act (ACA) does not directly benefit migrant workers, especially those who are undocumented. Employers with 50 or more employees are mandated to provide health-care insurance. Because farms use seasonal workers, the ACA uses a different formula. If the farm employs on average more than 50 full-time seasonal workers for fewer than 121 days, then the farm is not required to provide health-care coverage. In addition, workers who are undocumented are not required to purchase individual health-care insurance. This may leave a segment of the workforce uninsured. In some cases, large farms are establishing clinics. Many migrant workers currently pay for health care out of pocket. Thus, further policy may be needed to cover the cost of health care to this population.

As in working with all vulnerable populations, the effort is to have policies that decrease health disparity and increase social justice. Nurses can encourage the use of government monies to build new or utilize local low-income housing for the migrants. They can encourage experimentation with alternative building materials and other creative solutions for cost-cutting purposes to provide safer and healthier living conditions. Nurses can also raise awareness among public officials and the general public about the situation of farmworkers, especially the migrant workers and the need for even more consistent primary care.[92]

Immigrants

The United States is a country founded on immigrants. Until the early 1900s, immigration into the United States was encouraged and over time the influx of immigrants from all over the world brought a rich diversity to the country. In the United States, immigrants may or may not have legal status. Those with legal status are referred to as **legal permanent residents (LPRs)** by the Department of Homeland Security. These are immigrants who have been granted legal permanent residence in the United States and are holders of green cards but who have not yet become U.S. citizens.[93] Another population of immigrants is referred to under a number of lay terms including illegal aliens, undocumented workers, and illegals. The Department of Homeland Security uses the term **unauthorized immigrant,** which defines this population as persons born outside of the United States who are residing in the United States without obtaining legal status.[94]

Prevalence

Immigration, regulated within the federal government, was first limited in the 1920s with quotas for different ethnic groups, but these quotas have since been removed. In the 1980s and 1990s, legal immigration increased significantly, peaking in 1991 with over 1,800,000 people.[93] Of the LPRs entering the country, the majority (85%) were from developing countries, 50% from the Caribbean and Latin America, and about 33% from Asia.[93,94] The number of LPRs held steady at around 1,000,000 from 2004 to 2012.[93]

The United States has accepted more LPRs than all other countries in the world combined.[95] Since the removal of ethnic quotas in immigration in 1965, the number of first generation immigrants living in the United States has increased from 9.6 million in 1970 to about 13.3 million in 2012.[93] Between a little more than 600,000 to more than 700,000 were naturalized each year from 2009 to 2011.[96] The leading emigrating countries to the United States were Mexico, India, the Philippines, and China.[93,97,98]

Contemporary immigrants tend to be younger than the population of the United States, with a substantially higher percentage of immigrants aged between 15 and 34 years. Immigrants are also more likely to be married and less likely to be divorced than native-born Americans of the same age.[93,96,98]

The unauthorized immigrant population estimates stayed steady from 2005 to 2010 at between 10 million to 11 million a year.[94] The majority are from Mexico, and the states with the highest numbers are California followed by Texas and Florida. The age distribution was similar to LPRs. In 2010, 63% of unauthorized immigrants were between 25 and 44 years of age and only 4% were aged 55 years or older.[94]

Impact on Health for Both Legal and Unauthorized Immigrants

Although immigrants have increased risk factors for poor health such as poverty and less access to care, they experience what is known as the healthy immigrant effect. They are less likely to experience poor health and lower mortality. This phenomenon appears to be associated with less acculturation into the U.S. culture and unfortunately disappears the longer the immigrant lives in the United States.[99]

There is some concern that all immigrants who come from areas with a high incidence of certain communicable diseases could provide a resurgence of these diseases in the United States where incidence is now low, specifically tuberculosis, Chagas' disease, and hepatitis. To reduce this risk, all immigrants are currently screened before they enter the United States to prevent unnecessary transmission.

Immigrants face multiple health challenges that can include a lack of health insurance, limited access to care, culture and language barriers, and a cultural adjustment to the U.S. health-care system. Acculturation can be partially responsible for the diminished health of the immigrants as they remain in the United States and can include a less healthy diet of fewer grains and vegetables and more foods high in fat, increased smoking, loss of family support, and increased drug and alcohol abuse.[100] Recent immigrants have significantly lower rates of substance abuse than U.S. citizens, but those immigrants residing in the United States for more than 15 years use illicit drugs at rates similar to the native-born population.[101]

Recent and low-income immigrants, although working full-time, frequently work in low-wage jobs, are self-employed, or work in agriculture and are less likely to have health insurance sponsored by their employers. In 2003, only one-third of noncitizens had such insurance coverage.[102] Under the ACA there is now limited federal coverage for legal immigrants.[103]

Policy

The ebb and flow of immigration reflects the economic and political conditions in the United States and the presence or absence of immigration restrictions. After September 11, 2001, there was a backlash against immigrants that has continued, with numerous attempts at the federal level to institute immigration reform. An obvious need is for immigrants to have access to health insurance. With the ACA, health insurance is more available and the increased funding for federal health insurance programs such as Medicaid provides more opportunities for immigrant children to receive better health care. However, the ACA does not apply to everyone equally. Factors that will affect immigrants include income, immigration status, and how long they've lived in this country. Other areas to address from a policy perspective include increased opportunities for immigrants to learn English, clear implementation and enforcement of interpreter services when receiving health care, and culturally focused health care (see Chapter 23). The Centers for Disease Control and Prevention (CDC) works to help immigrants and refugees achieve optimal health (Box 24-2). For example, the CDC has developed flu vaccination information written in the native language of immigrant and refugee groups.[104]

Refugees and Asylees

Refugees and **asylees** for resettlement in the United States constitute a special type of immigrant. A refugee or asylee is a person "who is unable or unwilling to return to his or her country of nationality because of persecution or a well-founded fear of persecution on account of race, religion nationality, membership in a particular social group of political opinion."[105] A person asking to receive refugee status is outside the United States while an asylee is residing in the United States when applying for asylum.[105] As part of the Migration and Refugee Assistance program and in collaboration with the United

---

BOX 24–2	**Centers for Disease Control and Prevention Immigrant Health**

As a world leader in health promotion and disease prevention, the CDC works with immigrant, refugee, and migrant groups to improve their health by:

- Providing guidelines for disease screening and treatment in the United States and overseas
- Tracking and reporting disease in these populations
- Responding to disease outbreaks in the United States and overseas
- Advising U.S. partners on health care for refugee groups
- Educating and communicating with immigrant and refugee groups and partners.

Source: See reference 104.

Nations High Commission on Refugees, the U.S. State Department works with multiple nongovernmental organizations (NGOs) to provide resources and to assist in the resettlement of a number of these refugees. Some of the major NGOs that work on resettlement in the United States include the United States Conference of Catholic Bishops, Lutheran Immigrant Aid Society, International Rescue Committee, World Relief Corporation, Immigrant and Refugee Services of America, Hebrew Immigrant Aid Society, and Church World Service.[106]

Prevalence

In 2010, there were 43.3 million people worldwide forced from their homes by disasters, conflict, and persecution. This included 15.2 million refugees who were compelled to cross an international border to a host country, usually traveling to the closest safe area, and 27.1 million were displaced within their own countries. The largest numbers of refugees in 2010 were from Afghanistan, Iraq, Somalia, D.R. Congo, Myanmar, Colombia, Sudan, Eritrea, and Serbia. Worldwide, Pakistan (1.7 million), Iran (1 million), and Syria (1 million) hosted the largest number of refugees. Refugees are usually seen as temporary visitors to the host country, which frequently is also struggling and would have difficulty assimilating them into its own political, economic, and cultural structure.[106]

Refugees are often in a position of insecurity and unknown outcomes, many remaining in refugee camps for several years as the problems resolve in their own country. There currently are three suggestions for a permanent solution to the temporary refugee settlements. The preferred solution is for the refugees and asylees to be repatriated, returning to their home country when it is once more safe. However, this must be voluntary, and currently is occurring less frequently. If they can't go home, there are two other options—they can stay in the host country which most host countries do not want, or request resettlement to a third country.[107]

For many years, the United States has had the humanitarian commitment to resettle refugees from overseas. The most refugees worldwide are resettled from the host country to the United States (three times more than the rest of the industrialized world). This included 58,179 refugees and 29,484 asylees in 2012.[108] The United States is one of only 19 countries in the world that has agreed to resettles refugee, with these countries each year taking considerably fewer than does the United States.[109]

Impact on Health

The refugees victimized by war and/or political repression, famine, or natural disasters frequently experience food insecurity, poor sanitation, exposure to multiple communicable diseases, violence, and mental health issues with limited medical care both while fleeing their country of origin and while in refugee settlement camps in the host country. Their life in the refugee camp, which persists for several years, makes a major impact on their health. Post-traumatic stress disorder and depression are common diagnoses among those in the resettlement programs who have had severe exposure to violence.[110–113] Mental health risk factors are influenced by the premigration exposure, the stresses during migration, and what happens during resettlement.[114] Many of the refugees come from poor countries and have experienced limited resources all of their lives. Others come from more developed countries and have been educated and accustomed to adequate resources until they were forced to flee. Each of these groups has its own unique set of health issues.

In general, in the refugee camps the individuals experience higher rates of tuberculosis and hepatitis B, and have fewer immunizations, making them more exposed to the communicable diseases. Because of the nature of war and persecution and the violence and rape that occur both outside and inside the camps, there is increased exposure to STIs, including HIV. Refugees have also shown, depending on the location, higher rates of lead poisoning, malaria, and parasitic disease. Torture and major mental health issues are also very common. All of these health problems, many not common in the industrialized countries, should be considered when caring for a refugee in the United States. Current emphasis in the United States has been to encourage not only evaluation for these communicable diseases and mental health issues, but also a thorough evaluation of the refugees for noncommunicable diseases (e.g., cardiovascular disease and diabetes) that have demonstrated increased prevalence worldwide.[115]

Intervention and Services

The U.S. Public Health Service requires a health screening for all immigrants and refugees prior to departure from their country of origin or their host countries. Refugees can be kept from immigrating if they have untreated communicable disease, untreated substance abuse, or a mental illness that causes them to respond violently. If the refugee agrees to treatment, then he or she can be reconsidered for immigration.

The refugee families are provided broad health screening upon arrival in the United States. They can receive short-term health insurance, Refugee Medical Assistance, for the first eight months.[115] This 8-month period is the time for the family to get initial health screening, begin to understand the health-care system, begin to learn English, and to seek out and secure paid employment. After the 8-month period is over, many are then eligible for expanded health insurance options under the ACA.[103, 117] They are also encouraged to apply if eligible for other subsidy programs, such as Supplemental Security Income, for which they are entitled in their status as a refugee.

There are several barriers for the refugee to receive health care in the United States. Morris and colleagues found that language and poor communication skills, lack of acculturation that increased stress and isolation, and cultural beliefs about health delayed health seeking and health care.[118] There has been an effort in some of the states that receive large numbers of refugees for resettlement to educate health-care providers about diseases that they may never have seen, to provide training in cultural sensitivity, and to teach the health workers how to use translators and translating systems. Other care providers have noted the importance of inquiring about torture and recognizing its effects in women as well as men. One study of African refugees identified a prevalence of having been tortured in the range of 25% to 69% based on ethnicity and gender, a percentage much higher than expected.[119]

Incarceration and Vulnerability

In 2012, the U.S. imprisonment rate was 480 persons per 100,000 residents in the United States.[120] The United States has 5% of the world's population and 25% of its prisoners.[121] This is an alarming statistic for the sheer numbers, but equally important because once individuals have a history of incarceration, they have limited opportunities for employment, education, housing, and a stable family life. This in turn has significant impact on health.[122] In addition, it destroys community cohesiveness, especially in areas where there are high incarceration rates, another factor that contributes to poor health.[123]

Prevalence

In 2012, about 1.6 million people in the United States were in a state or federal correctional institution.[120] The breakdown for adults under correctional control in the United States was as follows: 910 per 100,000 male residents and 63 per 100,000 female residents. African Americans are overrepresented in the prison population. In 2012, 38% of prisoners were African American compared with 35% non-Hispanic whites and 21% who were Hispanic. A little over 60% were under 40 years of age.[120] Although the prison population quadrupled between 1980 and 2009, there was a decline from 2010 to 2012.[120]

Impact on Health

Under the 1976 U.S. Supreme Court ruling *Estelle v. Gamble*, states are compelled to provide a constitutionally adequate level of medical care for those who are incarcerated, or care that generally meets a "community standard."[124] As the cost of health care continues to increase, the cost to the state prison system has been increasing dramatically. The prison population is made up of vulnerable subpopulations, which puts them at much higher need for health care, and there are specifically larger numbers infected with hepatitis C and HIV, an increasing prevalence of noncommunicable diseases, and a high prevalence of mental health and substance use disorders.[122] Another emerging health issue is the increased number of older adults who are incarcerated, up by 62% from 2009 to 2012.[124] This population has a higher prevalence of noncommunicable diseases as well as cognitive disorders such as Alzheimer's disease.[125]

The health needs of the incarcerated population reflect the health needs of the population they represent—in general, a vulnerable population of poverty with limited access to health care, low education levels, addictions to alcohol and drugs, mental health issues, and communicable disease such as hepatitis and HIV. Women offenders display rates of HIV that are three to five times higher than rates in the general population. It is not clear why this occurs but some suggestions include higher levels of drug use, mental illness, history of sexual victimization, relational violence, high-risk sexual partners, and homelessness.[126,127] All of these problems are amplified

in prison. The stresses of prison life, poor diet, and frequently less than adequate medical care often exacerbate noncommunicable conditions such as diabetes and hypertension.

Incarcerated men and women experience higher rates of comorbidities of substance use and psychiatric disorders. These psychiatric diagnoses include major depressive disorder, antisocial personality disorder, anxiety, post-traumatic stress disorder (PTSD), borderline personality disorders, and eating disorders. In one study, incarcerated substance abusing women were nearly twice as likely to have affective disorder, a major depressive disorder, PTSD, or borderline personality disorder as were women in the community.[128] With 2.5 million schoolchildren having an incarcerated parent, there is also a collateral impact on families, both a significant economic effect and major mental health effects on the children.

Policy

There might be less damage to the individual, to the family, and to the community if we as a country could discover how to reduce incarceration, especially that of nonviolent offenders. Implementing primary prevention, especially by working with high-risk youth in the communities to prevent the crime that would result in incarceration, could affect the largest group, young males, by keeping them out of prison. Offering better education opportunities, providing better community-level health care to diagnosis and treat mental health issues, and providing more addiction services and other interventions to prevent or diminish noncommunicable diseases would help to prevent some of the issues that lead to incarceration. Assistance should widen to provide more help to the families of those who are incarcerated, whereas the family member and the incarcerated individual need additional help when the individual is released. Limiting the disenfranchisement of released offenders can also assist in better integration back into the community.

Lesbian, Gay, Bisexual, and Transgender Population

Based on current research findings, being gay, lesbian, bisexual, or transgender (LGBT) is a normal variation of human sexuality. These individuals have normal mental health and social adjustment. Researchers have consistently shown that gay and lesbian parents are as good at parenting as are heterosexual parents and their children are as healthy and as well-adjusted as children raised by heterosexual parents.[129,130] In addition, LGBT persons are becoming accepted into the mainstream of American society as evidenced by the increasing numbers of states that have passed legislation recognizing lesbian and gay marriages. Historically, however, those who identify themselves as LGBTs have experienced discrimination from friends, family, and others. This in turn has sometimes also led to violence and a negative effect on physical and mental health.[131]

The Williams Institute at the University of California, Los Angeles School of Law estimated that in 2011 approximately 9 million (about 3.8%) Americans identified themselves as gay, lesbian, bisexual, or transgender. The institute found that bisexuals make up 1.8% of the population, whereas 1.7% are gay or lesbian. Transgender adults make up 0.3% of the population.[132]

Impact on Health

LGBTs have special health concerns in addition to the usual ones experienced by both men and women.[131] As a vulnerable population, they frequently experience social inequality, which is associated with poorer health status. The leading cause of death for all men, including gay men, is heart disease and cancer. However, gay men also have higher rates of HIV, other STIs, tobacco and drug use, and depression. The CDC encourages specific screening tests for this population (Box 24-3).[133]

For lesbians, there are similar concerns. Although much more research is needed, LGBT people appear to be slightly more prone to developing breast, ovarian, and endometrial cancers, and experiencing stress-related conditions such as obesity, smoking-related illnesses, and mental health conditions (such as anxiety disorders, depression, and substance use disorders). Health care should also place emphasis on avoiding STIs (Box 24-4).[134,135]

Mental health for LGBTs can be affected by marginalization and discrimination, internalization of negative stereotypes, and limited social support. Violence is a concern, especially bullying that occurs in the school or workplace. In October 2009, the Matthew Shepard and James Byrd, Jr., Hate Crimes Prevention Act was signed into law and makes hate crime based on sexual orientation, among other offenses, a federal crime in the United States.[136] A recent survey of 37 European countries found that more than half of LGBT young people had experienced bullying in school. The bullying was also directed at young people who appeared different from their gender type, even though they were not LGBT.[137] Many gay and lesbian adults reported receiving little to no information about LGBT when in school.[138]

Interventions and Policy

Community-based organizations can be supportive of LGBT people and can influence the general community to provide a more inclusive environment. Public campaigns are a way to reach a large number of people with messages challenging homophobia. Schools also can educate young people, confronting widely accepted prejudices. This might include specific curriculums and action against bullying, creating a school environment wherein all students feel comfortable.[139,140] Political leaders, police forces, health services, broadcasters, and

BOX 24–3	Centers for Disease Control and Prevention Recommended Screenings for Gay Men

- HIV (at least annually)
- Syphilis
- Chronic hepatitis B infection
- Hepatitis C for men who engage in risky behaviors, such as rough sex or sex with multiple partners
- Genital herpes if directed by health-care provider
- Chlamydia and gonorrhea testing of the throat if they have had receptive oral sex in the past year
- Chlamydia and gonorrhea testing of the penis (urethra) is needed if they have had insertive anal or oral sex in the past year
- Chlamydia and gonorrhea testing of the rectum is needed if they have had receptive anal sex in the past year

Source: See reference 133.

BOX 24–4	Recommended Health Behaviors of Gay Men, Lesbians, and Bisexuals

- Avoid contact with a woman's menstrual blood and with any visible genital lesions.
- Cover sex toys that penetrate more than one person's vagina or anus with a new condom for each person; consider using different toys for each person.
- Use a barrier (e.g., latex sheet, dental dam, condom, plastic wrap) during oral sex.
- Use latex or vinyl gloves and lubricant for any manual sex that might cause bleeding.

Source: See references 134 and 135.

employers can all positively influence the way that the LGBT populations is treated.[141] Nurses can also take action to help provide culturally and clinically appropriate care (Box 24-5).[142]

■ Summary Points

- Many factors at both the individual and community levels combine to increase the vulnerability of certain populations, thus having an impact on their physical and mental health.
- Social forces such as discrimination and stigma can lead to the marginalization of certain segments of our society, resulting in increased levels of marginalization overall.
- Health disparities disproportionately affect members of racial, ethnic, minority, underserved, and vulnerable groups and affect the overall health of the United States.
- Social determinants of health including poverty, access to care, cultural barriers, and education play a role in increasing the vulnerability of certain populations.
- Nurses are uniquely positioned to provide care for vulnerable populations, functioning in a variety of roles through which they enhance health and reduce vulnerability.
- Certain populations like the homeless, migrant workers, immigrants, refugees, the incarcerated, and LGBT people are more likely to be vulnerable and benefit from specific interventions and changes in policy.

| BOX 24–5 | Nursing Care for the LGBT Community |

- Become well educated about the LGBT community and help educate others so that they can provide culturally and clinically appropriate health care. Emphasize the importance of health screening with an established primary care provider who is sensitive to LGBT issues.
- Keep up to date on the new research and understand the *Healthy People 2020* objectives and outcomes.
- Work to prevent violence against the LGBT community and implement antibullying program in the schools.
- Utilize social service collaboration in working with LGBT community, especially the youths, to reduce the risk of suicide and homelessness.
- Support policies that expand domestic partner health insurance.
- Be aware that older LGBT people are frequently more isolated, have fewer family to provide supportive care, and may need increased social service benefits.

Sources: See references 141 and 142.

▲ CASE STUDY
Poverty

Objectives: At the end of this case study, the student will be able to:

1. Discuss the role poverty plays in health, especially maternal-child health.
2. Examine the resources available to provide care to women and children living in poverty.
3. Identify resources available to women and children living in poverty.
4. Explore the contextual factors that affect the health of women and children living in poverty.

You are working with a group of five young unmarried women in a prenatal clinic run by the metropolitan public health department that is located close to a large area of subsidized housing. All of the women qualify for the Children's Health Insurance Program. They have expressed interest in knowing more about their pregnancies and the care of their newborns. However, their biggest concern is figuring out how they will support themselves and their newborns. Two are in post–high school education programs, but all five of them need to find work and childcare. None of them has any real economic resources, but currently they all have places to live with family.

1. Identify and list any associations or thoughts you have about poverty.
2. Review the government definitions of poverty, then the types of health insurance available under the ACA and other income-assistance programs available to people living in poverty and for women who are pregnant.
3. What additional programs are available to pregnant women that can encourage economic self-sufficiency?
4. What are some of the prime issues related to poverty and women caring for their children? Whom do these issues affect and how? Do these issues vary by race, ethnicity, age, and/or physical ability?
5. Who are some of the key players who can assist these women?
6. What are solutions for these women in their desire to be financially independent and what connected issues need to be discussed to help them reach their goals?

REFERENCES

1. Centers for Disease Control and Prevention. (2013). *Minority health.* Retrieved from http://www.cdc.gov/minorityhealth/populations.html#Other.
2. Urban Institute Health Policy Center. (2010). *Vulnerable populations.* Retrieved from http://www.urban.org/health_policy/vulnerable_populations/.
3. Aday, L.A. (2001). *At risk in America: The health and health care needs of vulnerable populations in the United States* (2nd ed.). San Francisco, CA: Jossey-Bass.
4. Vulnus. (2004). *Oxford Latin dictionary.* Oxford, England: Oxford University Press.
5. Vulnerability. (2010). *Merriam-Webster online dictionary.* Retrieved from http://www.merriam-webster.com/dictionary/vulnerability.
6. Smedley, B.D. Stith, A.Y, & Nelson, A.R. (Eds.). (2002). *Institute of Medicine: Unequal treatment; Confronting racial and ethnic disparities in health care.* Washington, DC: National Academies Press.
7. The Organization for Economic Co-operation and Development. (2013). *OECD Health Data 2013: How does the United States compare?* Retrieved from http://www.oecd.org/unitedstates/Briefing-Note-USA-2013.pdf.
8. Office of Minority Health and Health Equity, Centers for Disease Control and Prevention. (2013). *Minority health.* Retrieved from http://www.cdc.gov/minorityhealth/omhhe.html.
9. Brulle, R.J., & Pellow, D.N. (2006). Environmental justice: Human health and environmental inequalities. *Annual Reviews of Public Health, 27,* 103-124.
10. Giger, J., Davidhizar, R.E., Purnell, L., Harden, J.T., & Strickland, O. (2007). American Academy of Nursing Expert Panel report: Developing cultural competence to eliminate health disparities in ethnic minorities and other vulnerable populations. *Journal of Transcultural Nursing, 18*(2), 95-102.
11. National Center on Minority Health and Health Disparities. (2002). *Review of minority aging research at the NIA: Recommendations.* Bethesda, MD: National Institute on Aging.
12. World Health Organization. (2013). *Vulnerable groups.* Retrieved from http://www.who.int/environmental_health_emergencies/vulnerable_groups/en/.
13. Shi, L., & Stevens, G.D. (2005). Vulnerability and unmet health care needs: The influence of multiple risk factors. *Journal of General Internal Medicine, 20,* 148-154.
14. American Nurses Association. (2010). *Nursing's social policy statement: The essence of the profession.* Silver Spring, MD: Nursesbooks.org.
15. Shi, L., Stevens, G.D., Lebrun, L.A., Faed, P., & Tsai, J. (2008, November). Enhancing the measurement of health disparities for vulnerable populations. *Journal of Public Health Management Practice,* (Supp.), S45-S52.
16. Data Driven Detroit. (2013). *State of the Detroit child.* Retrieved from http://datadrivendetroit.org/projects/2012-state-of-detroits-child/.
17. United States Department of Health and Human Services. (2005). *Research involving vulnerable populations.* Retrieved from http://grants.nih.gov/grants/policy/hs/populations.htm.
18. Miracle, V.A. (2010). Vulnerable populations in research. *Dimensions of Critical Care Nursing, 29*(5), 242-245.
19. American Nurses Association. (2001). *American Nurses Association Code of Ethics for Nurses.* Retrieved from http://www.nursingworld.org/MainMenuCategories/EthicsStandards/CodeofEthicsforNurses.aspx.
20. Ferguson, C. (2007). Barriers to serving the vulnerable: Thoughts of a former public official. *Health Affairs, 26*(5), 1358-1365.
21. U.S. Department of Health and Human Services. (2013). *Temporary Assistance for Needy Families (TANF).* Retrieved from http://www.hhs.gov/recovery/programs/tanf/.
22. Hall, J.M., Stevens, P.E., & Meleis, A.I. (1994). Marginalization: A guiding concept for valuing diversity in nursing knowledge development. *Advances in Nursing Science, 16*(4), 23-41.
23. Lynam, M., & Cowley, S. (2007). Understanding marginalization as a social determinant of health. *Critical Public Health, 17*(2), 137-149.
24. Anderson, E.T., & McFarlane, J. (2008). *Community as partner: Theory and practice in nursing* (5th ed.). Philadelphia, PA: Lippincott, Williams & Wilkins.
25. Link, B.G., & Phelan, J.C. (2001). Conceptualizing stigma. *Annual Review of Sociology, 27,* 363-385.
26. Link, B.G., & Phelan, J.C. (2006). Stigma and its public health implications. *The Lancet, 367,* 528-529.
27. Mechanic, D., & Tanner, J. (2007). Vulnerable people, groups, and populations: Societal view. *Health Affairs, 26*(5), 1220-1230.
28. U.S. Census Bureau. (2013). *2013 poverty guidelines.* Retrieved from http://aspe.hhs.gov/poverty/13poverty.cfm.
29. U.S. Department of Health and Human Services. (2013). *2013 poverty guidelines.* Retrieved from http://aspe.hhs.gov/poverty/13poverty.cfm#thresholds.
30. U.S. Department of Health and Human Services. (2013). *Further resources on poverty measurement, poverty lines and their history.* Retrieved from http://aspe.hhs.gov/poverty/contacts.cfm.
31. DeNavas-Walt, C., Proctor, B.D., & Smith, J.C. (2012). *U.S. Census Bureau, income, poverty, and health insurance coverage in the United States: 2012* (Current Population Reports, P60-243). Washington, DC: U.S. Government Printing Office.
32. Marmot, M., & Wilkinson, R.G. (Eds.). (2006). *Social determinants of health* (2nd ed.). Oxford, England: Oxford University Press.
33. World Bank. (2011). *What is Social Capital?* Retrieved from http://web.worldbank.org/WBSITE/EXTERNAL/TOPICS/EXTSOCIALDEVELOPMENT/EXTTSOCIALCAPITAL/0,,contentMDK:20185164~menuPK:418217~pagePK:148956~piPK:216618~theSitePK:401015,00.html.

34. Shi, L., & Stevens, G.D. (2005). *Vulnerable populations in the United States.* San Francisco, CA: Jossey-Bass.

35. U.S. Department of Health and Human Services. (2013). *Healthy People 2020 Topic: Social determinants.* Retrieved from http://healthypeople.gov/2020/topicsobjectives2020/overview.aspx?topicid=39.

36. U.S Department of Health and Human Services. (2013). *Healthy People 2020. Leading health indicators: Social determinants.* Retrieved from http://www.healthypeople.gov/2020/leading-health-indicators/2020-lhi-topics/Social-Determinants.

37. Peate, I. (2013). The other silent killer: Homelessness. *British Journal of Nursing, 22*(11), 607.

38. Nwakeze, P.C., Magura, S., Rosenblum, A., & Joseph, H. (2003). Homeless substance misuse and access to public entitlements in a soup kitchen population. *Substance Use & Misuse, 38,* 645-668.

39. Savage, C.L., Gillespie, G.L., Lee, R.J., & Lindsell, C. (2008). The effectiveness of a United States nurse managed clinic for the homeless in improving health status. *Health and Social Care in the Community, 16,* 469-475.

40. Substance Abuse and Mental Health Services Administration. (2011). *Current statistics on the prevalence and characteristics of people experiencing homelessness in the United States.* Retrieved from http://homeless.samhsa.gov/ResourceFiles/hrc_factsheet.pdf.

41. U.S. Interagency Council on Homelessness. (2013). *People experiencing chronic homelessness.* Retrieved from http://www.usich.gov/population/chronic.

42. Baggett, T.P., Hwang, S.W., O'Connell, J.J., Porneala, B.C., Stringfello, E.J., & Rigottie, N.A. (2013). Mortality among homeless adults in Boston: Shifts in cause of death over a 15-year period. *JAMA Internal Medicine, 173*(3), 189-195.

43. Centers for Disease Control and Prevention. (2012). *National Homeless Persons' Memorial Day.* Retrieved from http://www.cdc.gov/features/homelessness/.

44. National Coalition for the Homeless. (2011). *Dying without dignity.* Retrieved from http://www.nationalhomeless.org/publications/dyingwithdignity/summary.html.

45. U.S. Department of Health and Human Services. (2009). *The McKinney-Vento Homeless Assistance Act As amended by S. 896 The Homeless Emergency Assistance and Rapid Transition to Housing (HEARTH) Act of 2009.* Retrieved from http://portal.hud.gov/hudportal/documents/huddoc?id=HAAA_HEARTH.pdf.

46. Government of Western Australia, Department for Child Protection. (n.d.). *What is homelessness?* Retrieved from http://www.childprotection.wa.gov.au/Resources/Documents/StatisticsForMedia/WAHomelessness.pdf.

47. National Coalition for the Homeless. (2009). *How many people experience homelessness?* Retrieved from http://www.nationalhomeless.org/factsheets/How_Many.html.

48. National Alliance to End Homelessness. (2014). *The state of homelessness in America 2014.* Retrieved from http://www.ncsha.org/resource/state-homelessness-america-2014.

49. Coalition for the Homeless. (2012). *State of homelessness 2012: If not now when?* Retrieved from http://www.coalitionforthehomeless.org/pages/state-of-the-homeless-2012.

50. U.S. Department of Housing and Urban Development. (2012). *The 2011 point-in-time estimates of homelessness: Supplement to the Annual Homeless Assessment Report.* Retrieved from https://www.onecpd.info/resources/documents/pit-hic_supplementalaharreport.pdf.

51. Substance Abuse and Mental Health Services Agency, Homeless Resource Center. (2011). *Current statistics on the prevalence and characteristics of people experiencing homelessness in the United States.* Retrieved from http://homeless.samhsa.gov/Resource/Current-Statistics-on-the-Prevalence-and-Characteristics-of-People-Experiencing-Homelessness-in-the-United-States-48841.aspx .

52. U.S. Census Bureau. (n.d.). 2010 *Census data.* Retrieved from http://www.census.gov/2010census/data/.

53. US Department of Housing and Urban Development, Office of Planning and Development. (2013). *The 2013 annual homeless assessment report (AHAR) to Congress: point in time estimates.* Retrieved from https://www.hudexchange.info/resources/documents/AHAR-2013-Part1.pdf.

54. Rollinson, P. (2007). A rural problem, too: Homelessness beyond the big cities. *Planning, 73*(6), 20-23.

55 National Coalition for the Homeless. (2009). *Rural homelessness.* Retrieved from http://www.nationalhomeless.org/factsheets/rural.html .

56. Post, P.A. (2002). *Hard to reach: Rural homelessness & health care* (pp. 1-32). Nashville, TN: National Health Care for the Homeless Council.

57. Frankish, C.J., Hwang, S.W., & Quantz, D. (2005). Homelessness and health in Canada. *Canadian Journal of Public Health, 96*(Suppl.), S23-S29.

58. Oates, G., Tadros, A., & Davis, S.M. (2009). A comparison of national emergency department use by homeless versus non-homeless people in the United States. *Journal of Health Care for the Poor and Underserved, 20,* 840-845.

59. National Coalition for the Homeless. (2009). *Health care and homelessness.* Retrieved from http://www.nationalhomeless.org/publications/facts/Health.pdf.

60. Jones, C.A., Perera, A., Chow, M., Ho, I., Nguyen, J., & Davachi, S. (2009). Cardiovascular disease risk among the poor and homeless—what we know so far. *Current Cardiology Reviews, 5*(1), 69-77.

61. National Coalition for the Homeless. (2009). *Mental illness and homelessness.* Retrieved from http://www.nationalhomeless.org/factsheets/Mental_Illness.html.

62. National Coalition for the Homeless. (2009). *Substance abuse and homelessness.* Retrieved from http://www.nationalhomeless.org/factsheets/addiction.html.

63. Savage, C.L., Gillespie, G., & Lindsell, C. (2008). Substance use and health care needs in a homeless

population attending a free nurse managed clinic. *Journal of Addictions Nursing, 19*, 27-33.

64. Baggett, T.P., O'Connell, J.J., Singer, D.E., & Rigotti, N.A. (2010). The unmet health care needs of homeless adults: A national study. *American Journal of Public Health, 100*(7), 1326-1333.

65. Douglass, J.M. (2005). Mobile dental vans: Planning considerations and productivity. *Journal of Public Health Dentistry*, 65(1), 110-113.

66. Matins, D.C. (2008). Experiences of homeless people in the health care delivery system: A descriptive phenomenological study. *Public Health Nursing, 25*(5), 420-430.

67. Larimer, M., Malone, D., Garner, M., Atkins, D., Burlingham, B., Lonczak, H., et al. (2011). Health care and public service use and costs before and after provision of housing for chronically homeless persons with severe alcohol problems. *JAMA, 301*(13), 1349-3157.

68. Sadowski, L.S. (2009). Case management and housing among homeless adults. *JAMA, 301*(17), 1771–1778.

69. World Food Summit. (1996). *Rome declaration on world food security.* Retrieved from http://www.fao.org/docrep/003/w3613e/w3613e00.htm.

70. Food Research and Action Center. (2013). *Food hardship in America 2012.* Retrieved from http://org2.democracyinaction.org/o/5118/p/salsa/web/common/public/content?content_item_KEY=10884.

71. Nord, M., Andrews, M., & Carlson, S. (2008). *USDA: Household food security in the United States.* Retrieved from http://www.ers.usda.gov/publications/err66/err66.pdf.

72. Coleman-Jensen, A., Nord, M., Andrews, M., & Carlson, S. (2012). *Household food security in the United States, 2011* (Economic Research Reports No. ERR-141). Retrieved from http://www.ers.usda.gov/publications/err-economic-research-report/err141.aspx.

73. Douglass, J.M. (2005). Mobile dental vans: Planning considerations and productivity. *Journal of Public Health Dentistry*, 65(1), 110-113.

74. Matins, D.C. (2008). Experiences of homeless people in the health care delivery system: A descriptive phenomenological study. *Public Health Nursing, 25*(5), 420-430.

75. Immigrant. (n.d.). *Dictionary.com.* Retrieved from http://dictionary.reference.com/browse/immigrant.

76. *Refugee Act of 1980, Pub. L. No. 96-212.* (1980). Retrieved from http://www.answers.com/topic/refugee-act-of-1980.

77. UNHCR. (1992). *Handbook on procedures and criteria for determining refugee status.* Geneva, Switzerland: UNHCR.

78. Migrant. (n.d.). *Dictionary.com.* Retrieved from http://dictionary.reference.com/browse/migrant.

79. International Labor Organization. (2014). *International Labour Standards on Migrant workers.* Retrieved from http://www.ilo.org/global/standards/subjects-covered-by-international-labour-standards/migrant-workers/lang—en/index.htm.

80. US. Department of Agriculture, Office of the Chief Economist. (2002). *Migrant and seasonal agricultural worker protection act.* Retrieved from http://www.thecre.com/fedlaw/legal19/mspasumm.htm.

81. National Center for Farmworker Health. (2012.) *Facts about farmworkers.* Retrieved from http://www.ncfh.org/docs/fs-Facts%20about%20Farmworkers.pdf.

82. National Center for Farmworker Health. (n.d.). *About American farmworkers: Population demographics.* Retrieved from http://www.ncfh.org/?pid=4&page=3.

83. U.S. Department of Labor. (2005). *Findings from the national agricultural workers survey (2001–2002): A demographic and employment profile of United States farmworkers.* Retrieved from www.doleta.gov/agworker/report9/naws_rpt9.pdf.

84. U.S. Department of Labor, Bureau of Labor Statistics (2012). *Agricultural workers.* Retrieved from http://www.bls.gov/ooh/farming-fishing-and-forestry/agricultural-workers.htm.

85. Arcury, T.A., & Quandt, S.A. (2007). Delivery of health services to migrant and seasonal farmworkers. *Annual Review of Public Health, 28,* 345-363.

86. Lindquist, C.H., Lagory, M., & Ritchey, F.J. (1999). The myth of the migrant homeless: An exploration of the psychosocial consequences of migration. *Sociological Perspectives, 42*(4), 691-709.

87. National Center for Farmworker Health. (2013). *Tuberculosis.* Retrieved from http://www.ncfh.org/docs/fs-What%20is%20TB.pdf.

88. Quandt, S., Hiott, A., Davis, S.W., Arcury, T.A. (2007). Oral health and quality of life of migrant and seasonal farmworkers in North Carolina. *Journal of Agricultural Safety and Health, 13*(1), 45-55.

89. Commonwealth of Massachusetts Department of Public Health, School Health Manual. (2007). *Refugee and immigrant health.* Retrieved from http://www.mass.gov/eohhs/gov/departments/dph/programs/community-health/primarycare-healthaccess/school-health/publications/comprehensive-school-health-manual.html.

90. Weathers, A., Minkovitz, C., O'Camp, P., & Diener-West, M. (2003). Health service use by children of migratory agricultural workers: Exploring the role of need for care. *Pediatrics*, *111*(5), 39.

91. Health Research and Services Administration. (n.d.). *Primary care: The health center program.* Retrieved from http://bphc.hrsa.gov/about/specialpopulations/index.html.

92. Farmworker Justice. (2010). *Migrant health centers.* Retrieved from http://www.farmworkerjustice.org/migrant-health-centers.

93. Rytina, L., & U.S. Homeland Security Office of Immigration Statistics. (2013). *Estimates of the legal permanent resident population in 2012.* Retrieved from http://www.dhs.gov/publication/estimates-legal-permanent-resident-population-2012.

94. Hoefer, M., Rytina, N., Baker, B.C., & U.S. Homeland Security. (2013). *Estimates of the unauthorized immigrant population residing in the United States: January 2010.* Retrieved from http://www.dhs.gov/publication/refugees-and-asylees-2012.

95. Segal, U.A., Elliott, D., & Mayadas, N.S. (2010). *Immigration worldwide: Policies, practices and trends.* New York, NY: Oxford University Press.

96. Lee, J., & U.S. Homeland Security Office of Immigration Statistics. (2012). *U.S. naturalization, 2011.* Retrieved from http://www.dhs.gov/xlibrary/assets/statistics/publications/natz_fr_2011.pdf.

97. Homeland Security. (2013). *Yearbook of immigration statistics. Data table 8.* Retrieved from http://www.dhs.gov/yearbook-immigration-statistics.

98. United States Immigration Support. (2012). *Immigration to the United States.* Retrieved from http://www.usimmigrationsupport.org/immigration-us.html.

99. Flores, G., & Brotanek, J. (2005). The healthy immigrant effect: A greater understanding might help us improve the health of all children. *Archives of Pediatrics and Adolescent Medicine, 159*(3), 295-297.

100. Derose, K., Escarce, J., & Lurie, N. (2007). Immigrants and health care: Sources of vulnerability. *Health Affairs, 26*(5), 1258-1268.

101. Brown, J.M., Council, C.C., Penne, M.A., Gfroer, J.C. (2005). *Immigrants and Substance Use: Findings from the 1999–2001 National Surveys on Drug Use and Health.* Retrieved from http://www.samhsa.gov/data/immigrants/immigrants.htm#1.5.1.

102. Ku, L., & Waidmann, T. (2003). *How race/ethnicity, immigration status, and language affect health insurance coverage, access to and quality of care among the low income population.* Washington, DC: Kaiser Commission on Medicaid and the Uninsured.

103. National Immigration Law Center. (2014). *Affordable Care Act.* Retrieved from http://www.nilc.org/immigrantshcr.html.

104. Centers for Disease Control and Prevention. (2013). *Immigrant and refugee health.* Retrieved from http://www.cdc.gov/immigrantrefugeehealth/.

105. U.S. Homeland Security. (2013). *Refugees and asylees: 2012.* Retrieved from http://www.dhs.gov/publication/refugees-and-asylees-2012.

106. Migration Policy Institute. (2011). *The U.S. refugee resettlement program.* Retrieved from http://www.migrationinformation.org/USFocus/display.cfm?ID=229.

107. United Nations High Commission for Refugees. (2009). *World Refugee Day: 42 million uprooted people waiting to go home.* Retrieved from http://www.unhcr.org/4a3b98706.html.

108. Martin, D.C., & Yankey, J.E. (2012). *U.S. Homeland Security Office of Immigration Statistics. Annual flow report.* Retrieved from http://www.dhs.gov/sites/default/files/publications/ois_rfa_fr_2012.pdf.

109. Refugee Resettlement Watch. (2010). *Refugee resettlement fact sheet.* Retrieved from http://refugeeresettlementwatch.wordpress.com/refugee-resettlement-fact-sheets/.

110. Khamis, V. (2005). Post-traumatic stress disorder among school age Palestinian children. *Child Abuse & Neglect, 29*(1), 81-95.

111. Sundquist, K., Johansson, L.M., DeMarinis, V., Johansson S.E., & Sundquist J. (2005). Posttraumatic stress disorder and psychiatric co-morbidity: Symptoms in a random sample of female Bosnian refugees. *European Psychiatry, 20*(2), 158-164.

112. Geltman, P.L., Grant-Knight, W., Mehta, S.D., Lloyd-Travaglini, C., Lustig, S., Landgraf, J.M., & Wise, P.H. (2005). The "lost boys of Sudan": Functional and behavioral health of unaccompanied refugee minors re-settled in the United States. *Archives of Pediatrics and Adolescent Medicine, 159*(6), 585-591.

113. Fazel, M., Wheeler, J., & Danesh, J. (2005). Prevalence of serious mental disorder in 7,000 refugees resettled in western countries: A systematic review. *Lancet, 365*(9467), 1309.

114. Kirmayer, L., Narasiah, L., Munoz, M., Rashid, M., & Pottie, K. (2010). Common mental health problems in immigrants and refugees: General approach in primary care. *Canadian Medical Association Journal. 183*(12), E959-E967. doi:10.1503/cmaj.090292.

115. Dookeran, N.M., Battaglia, T., Cochran, J., & Geltman, P.L. (2010). Chronic disease and its risk factors among refugees and asylees in Massachusetts, 2001–2005. *Preventing Chronic Disease, 7*(3). Retrieved from http://www.cdc.gov/ped/issues/2010/may/09_0046.htm.

116. U.S. Department of Health and Human Services, Office of Refugee Resettlement. (2014). Retrieved from http://www.acf.hhs.gov/programs/orr/health.

117. Refugee Health Technical Assistance. (2011). *Access to care.* Retrieved from http://refugeehealthta.org/access-to-care/.

118. Morris, M., Popper, W., Rodwell, T., Brodine, S., & Brouwer, K. (2009). *Journal of Community Health, 34,* 529-538.

119. Jaranson, J., Butcher, J., Halcon, L., Johnson, D., Robertson, C., David, K., & Westermeyer, J. (2004). Somali and Oromo refugees: Correlates of torture and trauma history. *American Journal of Public Health, 94*(4), 591-598.

120. Carson, A.E., Golinelli, D., & U.S. Department of Justice, Bureau of Justice Statistics (2012). *Prisoners in 2012—advanced counts.* Retrieved from http://www.bjs.gov/content/pub/press/p12acpr.cfm.

121. Leary, B., & Sidel, V. (Eds.). (2006). *Social injustice and public health.* New York, NY: Oxford University Press.

122. Centers for Disease Control and Prevention. (2013). *Correctional health.* Retrieved from http://www.cdc.gov/correctionalhealth/.

123. Young, A.M.W. (2006). Incarceration as a public health crisis. *American Journal of Public Health, 129*(6), 249.

124. *Estelle v. Gambelle, 429 U.S. 97 (1976).* Retrieved from http://caselaw.lp.findlaw.com/cgi-bin/getcase.pl?court=US&vol=429&invol=97.

125. Fellener, J. (2013, August 19). Graying prisons. *The New York Times.* Retrieved from http://www.nytimes.com/2013/08/19/opinion/graying-prisoners.html?_r=0.

126. Epperson, M., Khan, M., Miller, D., Perron, B., El-Bassel, N., & Gilbert, L. (2010). Assessing criminal justice involvement as an indicator of Human Immunodeficiency Virus risk among women in

methadone treatment. *Journal of Substance Abuse Treatment, 38*, 375-383.

127. Leenerts, M. (2003). From neglect to care: A theory to guide HIV-positive incarcerated women in self-care. *Journal of the Association of Nurses in AIDS Care, 14*(5), 25–38.

128. Zlotnick, C., Clarke, J., Friedmann, P., Roberts, M., & Melnick, G. (2008). Gender differences in comorbid disorders among offenders in prison substance abuse treatment programs. *Behavioral Sciences and the Law, 26*, 403-412.

129. Short, E., Riggs, D., Perlesz, A., Brown, R., & Kane, G. (2007). *Lesbian, gay, bisexual and transgender (LGBT) parented families—a literature review prepared for the Australian Psychological Society.* Retrieved from http://www.psychology.org.au/Assets/Files/LGBT-Families-Lit-Review.pdf.

130. American Academy of Pediatrics Committee on Psychosocial Aspects of Child and Family Health. (2013). Promoting the wellbeing of children whose parents are gay or lesbian. *Pediatrics, 131*(4), 827-830.

131. Centers for Disease Control and Prevention. (2011). *Gay and bisexual men's health: Stigma and discrimination.* Retrieved from http://www.cdc.gov/msmhealth/stigma-and-discrimination.htm.

132. Gate, G. (2011). *How many people are gay, lesbian, bisexual and transgender?* Los Angeles, CA: William Institute at ULCA. Retrieved from http://www3.law.ucla.edu/williamsinstitute/pdf/How-many-people-are-LGBT-Final.pdf.

133. Centers for Disease Control and Prevention. (2011). *Gay and bisexual men's health.* Retrieved from http://www.cdc.gov/msmhealth/for-your-health.htm.

134. Catalyst, K., Sr., & Mravack, S. (2006). Primary care for lesbians and bisexual women. *American Family Physician, 74*(2) 279-286.

135. Centers for Disease Control and Prevention. (2013). *Lesbian and gay women.* Retrieved from http://www.cdc.gov/lgbthealth/women.htm.

136. Human Rights Campaign. (2009). *President Barack Obama signs hate crimes legislation into law.* Retrieved from http://www.hrc.org/13699.htm.

137. Do something.org. (n.d.). *11 facts about gay rights.* Retrieved from http://www.dosomething.org/tipsandtools/11-facts-about-gay-rights?gclid=CPiNq-_x-6gCFaR95QodlWQXUA.

138. IGLYO & ILGA-Europe. (2006). *Social exclusion of young lesbian, gay, bisexual and transgender (LGBT) people in Europe.* Retrieved from http://www.coe.in/t/dg4/youth/Source/Coe...ESG.../2007_NCC_Report_4.pdf.

139. Stonewall. (2007). *The school report: Experiences of young gay people in Britain's schools.* Retrieved from http://www.stonewall.org.uk/at_school/education_resources/4121.asp.

140. Educational Action Challenging Homophobia. (2008). *Ten things you can do to challenge homophobia.* Retrieved from http://www.avert.org/homophobia.htm.

141. Department for Children, Schools, and Families. (2007). *Safe to learn: Embedding anti-bullying work in schools—preventing and responding to homophobic bullying in schools.* Retrieved from http://www.devon.gov.uk/cyps-prejudicerelatedbullying2010-web.pdf.

142. National Academy of Sciences. (2011). *The health of lesbian, gay, bisexual, and transgender people: Building a foundation for better understanding* (IOM Report). Washington, DC: Author.

Chapter 25

Emergency Preparedness and Disaster Management

LEARNING OUTCOMES

After reading this chapter, the student will be able to:

1. Describe the impact of natural and man-made disasters on population health.
2. Appreciate the unique role of nurses during disasters and public health emergencies.
3. Discuss the five areas of focus in emergency and disaster planning: (1) preparedness, (2) mitigation, (3) response, (4) recovery, and (5) evaluation.
4. Apply the emergency preparedness theoretical framework to a public health disaster scenario.
5. Describe the structure and organization of local and national disaster mitigation efforts.
6. Describe the process of epidemiological surveillance during community disaster mitigation and recovery.
7. Recognize the role of functional needs support services to optimize the health outcomes of vulnerable populations affected by a disaster event.

KEY TERMS

Bioterrorism
Blast events
Crown fire
Disaster
Disaster epidemiology
Disaster management
Disaster planning
Emergency information systems (EISs)
Emergency preparedness
Emergency preparedness and disaster management (EPDM)
Evacuation
Extreme heat
Ground fire
Hazardous materials
Man-made disaster
Mass casualty event
Mitigation
Natural disaster
Preparedness
Point of dispensing
Quarantine
Recovery
Response
Response evaluation
Risk communication
Surface fire
Surge
Triage

■ Introduction

The necessity of a strategic emergency preparedness and disaster management for man-made disasters was made all too clear in 2001 during the attacks on the World Trade Center and the Pentagon. The lesson was reinforced for natural disasters with Hurricane Katrina and the Haitian earthquake of 2010 (Fig. 25-1). The world watched in dismay at the impact these disasters had on the communities involved. Despite the horror of the September 11 attack on New York, the city had learned from the 1993 World Trade Center bombing and had an emergency preparedness and disaster management plan in place. For Katrina and the Haiti earthquake, in con-trast, the lack of clear plans resulted in increased mortality and exacerbated the effect of the disasters on the communities affected in both the short and long terms. These and other events resulted in an increase in concentrated training by health-care providers and first responders. The benefits of this relentless training resulted in minimal loss of life during the 2013 Boston Marathon bombings.

Because weather-related events are ubiquitous and can occur without warning, humans have had little recourse but to prepare to respond to the wrath of the environment in which they live. Environmental devastation caused by natural hazards of terrestrial origin (earthquakes, tsunamis, blizzards, tornadoes, hurricanes,

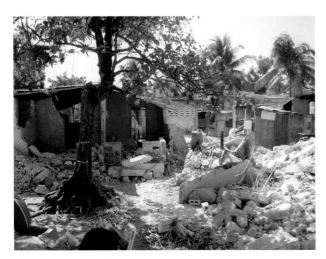

Figure 25-1 Devastation from the Haiti earthquake. *(From the CDC, photograph by Lt. Cmdr. Gary Brunette, 2010.)*

floods, wildfires, and extreme heat) is inevitable. Events such as the tornado that hit Joplin, Missouri (2011), the tsunami in Japan and the subsequent Fukushima nuclear disaster (2011), and Superstorm Sandy in the eastern United States (2012) reveal an increasing intensity in disaster impact and destruction. The number of people affected and the human and economic losses associated with these events have placed an imperative on disaster planning for emergency preparedness. Global warming, climate shift, sea-level rise, and societal factors may coalesce to create future calamities. Population shifts to urban coastal settings and the growth of megacities contribute to increased risk.[1,2]

Concurrent to these events is the ever-present risk of a man-made disaster such as an accidental or deliberate release of a biological, chemical, or radiological agent or the use of an explosive device. Forced migration and people forcibly displaced by war (complex human emergencies),[3] acts of aggression, political upheaval, populist uprisings such as the Arab Spring, and the increasing incidence of global terrorist attacks are reminders of the potentially deadly consequences of our inhumanity toward one another. The enormous human costs of forced migration—destroyed homes and livelihoods, increased vulnerability, disempowered communities, and collapsed social networks and common bonds—demand urgent and decisive action by disaster relief agencies.[3,4]

Natural disasters result not only in increased morbidity and mortality but also in destruction of property and natural resources. They can result in a reduction in

economic productivity and harm to both the natural and man-made environments. The mental health impact on a community may be extensive, debilitating, and long lasting. The negative impact of natural and man-made disasters can, at a minimum, be mitigated or perhaps prevented entirely. In expecting the unexpected,[5,6] much can be done in advance to anticipate and mitigate the devastating effects of natural and man-made disasters. Ongoing research in disaster science is paving the way to a world prepared to prevent and manage disaster (Box 25-1).

Disaster Nursing

Adequate disaster preparedness and response is essential for the delivery of lifesaving interventions and the optimization of population health outcomes.[7-9] Nursing is the single largest profession in the health-care system, so many of the first responders and most of the "first-receivers" during a disaster event are nurses. In the wake of any catastrophic event, communities will need nurses who will respond quickly and who are clinically competent to

---

BOX 25-1   Current Disaster Science Sources

Disaster science, accompanied by major advances in technology and meteorology, has provided a better understanding of the hallmark characteristics of natural/environmental hazards and the disasters that they cause.

- Eric Noji notes in his sentinel disaster book that "understanding the way that people are injured or die as a result of a natural or man-made disaster is a prerequisite to preventing or reducing deaths and injuries during future disasters."[6]
- Better scientific evidence enables nurses, health-care planners, and public health officials to prepare for these types of events and to develop advance-warning systems to minimize injuries and the loss of life. Advance preparation for a major disaster can later result in significant reductions in mortality.[7]
- Postdisaster research has demonstrated that both access to care and health-seeking behaviors are affected by natural disasters[8–10] and advance planning can anticipate and accommodate these changes.
- The mere availability of response and recovery services will not limit the burden of disasters if the victims of these events are unwilling or unable to use the services.[11] Rapid assessment of disaster-related injuries and outreach efforts to meet the identified physical, mental health, and behavioral needs are critical.

provide safe, appropriate, individual and population-based care.[10-12]

During a disaster, priorities change and the need to establish crisis standards of care may occur.[13,14] The objective quickly shifts from providing high-quality, individualized care to population-based care with the goal of saving as many lives as possible. Valuable lessons were learned from recent disasters such as the Indian Ocean Southeast Asian tsunami (2004), Hurricane Katrina (2005), and the powerful 9.0-magnitude earthquake that hit Japan (2011). Prior to such epic disasters, many nurses had only imagined what such events would be like. A heightened awareness now exists concerning what these disasters will demand of both responders and hospital-based first receivers. Nurses are clearly needed across the disaster continuum during all phases.[10] Nurses as victim advocates and as health educators adopt a population focus during the emergency preparedness and disaster planning process by engaging community participation in the process and disseminating vital health and safety information throughout a disaster event. Nurses help to shape disaster policy in their role as planners, evaluators, and leaders in health care.[10,12]

Imagine that you wake up in the middle of the night to find that an earthquake has occurred, devastating your community. Your first response is to think about your family, friends, and pets. Children, parents, and other loved ones immediately enter your mind. Where are they? Are they safe? Your next thought may be to see whom you can help, where should you go and what can you do? Your desire to help is compelling and you want to respond. But, are you ready?

Disaster experts encourage taking time *in advance of an event* to evaluate your personal and professional readiness to respond (Fig. 25-2). All nurses should be able to answer basic questions related to disaster preparedness (Box 25-2). Much work remains to be done to ensure that *all* members of the nursing profession possess the knowledge and skills necessary to respond appropriately to any type of disaster. The responsibility lies within our profession to engender a broad-based professional culture of excellence, both in disaster nursing care and in our health systems' management of catastrophic events.[11]

Emergency Preparedness and Disaster Management

Emergency preparedness is the planning process focused on avoiding or ameliorating the risks and hazards resulting from the impact of a disaster in order to optimize population health and safety. In contrast, **disaster management** is the integration of emergency response plans engaged throughout the life cycle of a disaster event. Disaster management efforts are stimulated by the population perception of risk related to the hazards associated with the disaster.[15]

Disasters pose a unique threat to the health of the populations affected and require strategic planning prior to an event occurrence and efficient management during the emergency.[16-18] Public health emergency preparedness and disaster management form a shared responsibility that extends far beyond local and state health departments and government organizations. A collaboration among private health organizations, social organizations, community health providers, community agencies, and the population at large is crucial for success.

A **disaster** is defined as an emergency of such severity and magnitude that the resultant combination of death, injury, illness, and property damage cannot be effectively managed with routine resources or procedures.[18] Disasters can result from a variety of specific hazards including natural disasters such as communicable disease epidemics and severe weather, as well as man-made disasters such as terrorism and chemical spills.[19] Disasters have the ability to cause catastrophic morbidity and mortality in a population. The impact on public health may be immediate or insidious, developing slowly in the days and weeks following the event. The issue of widespread morbidity and mortality associated with a disaster was evidenced following a major earthquake in Haiti (2010). The disaster caused massive acute injury to the population as a result of the collapse of buildings and flying debris, but also an additional long-term health impact because of the total destruction of the existing health-care system. Superstorm Sandy (2012) demonstrated the devastating impact of a massively large, slow-moving event on multiple states on the East Coast. Homes were washed away and thousands of individuals and families sought refuge in shelters. Many were stranded in high-rise apartment buildings in New York City and New Jersey. Community outreach efforts by nurses to provide needed supplies and health care to victims in their homes helped mitigate the long-term health impact of the event. The 2013 Boston Marathon bombing resulted in injury and death in a small area with no collateral damage to buildings, but this terror event affected an entire city. Because of the risk posed by the suspects while they were still at large, a citywide order to shelter in place was enforced until shortly before the suspect was apprehended.

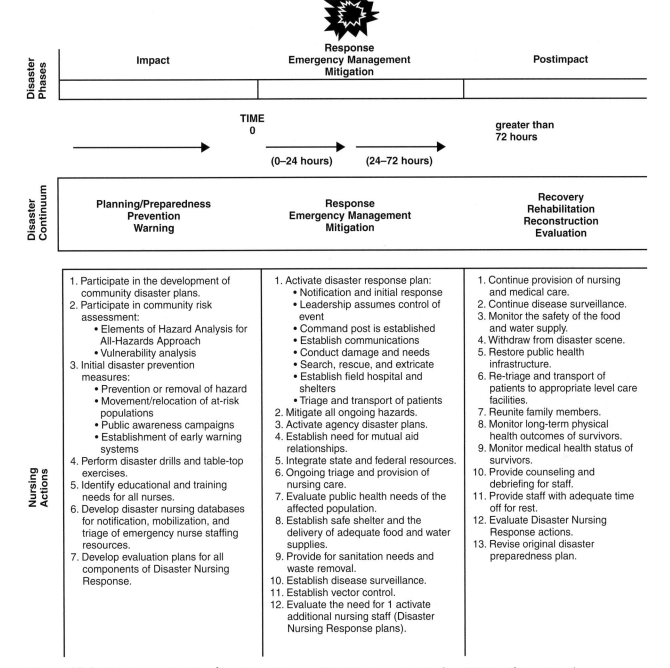

Figure 25-2 Disaster nursing time line. *(From Veenema, T.G. Disaster nursing timeline. 2000©, with permission.)*

Emergency Preparedness Theoretical Framework

Emergency preparedness and disaster management (EPDM) is a continuous cycle lacking a true beginning or end. The overarching concept of the emergency preparedness framework is prevention as it relates to public health. Public health practitioners are constantly learning from the events of the past and present and trying to foresee issues of the future. To effectively prepare for emergencies and manage disasters when they occur, EPDM plans are needed at the community, state, national, and global levels. Disaster plans must be developed

Do you possess the disaster specific knowledge and skill set needed to respond in a timely and appropriate way? Below are essential questions that all nurses, regardless of the setting in which they are working, level of educational preparation, or previous work experience, must know the answers to in order to contribute to an effective response:
- Do you understand the incident command system and your role in it?
- Do you have the knowledge to keep yourself and others safe if the event involves the release of a biological, chemical, or radiological hazard?
- Do you know whether your community has a plan to deal with natural disasters?
- Do you know what that plan is and what your role is within that plan?
- Do you understand the nature of the disaster?
- Do you have a plan in place to keep your family safe?

Sources: See references 10 and 12.

so that timely interventions can be rapidly disseminated when a threat surfaces.

The four key concepts of the preparedness framework include preparedness, response, recovery, and mitigation (Fig. 25-3) and a fifth component, evaluation.[16,17,19,20] The life cycle of a disaster is generally referred to as the disaster continuum and is characterized by three major phases: preimpact (before), impact (during), and postimpact (after), which provides the foundation for the disaster

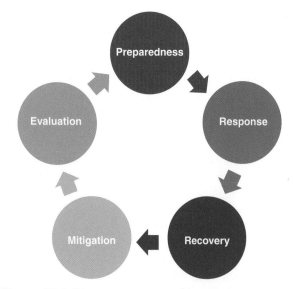

Figure 25-3 Disaster continuum framework.

time line. Specific actions taken during these three phases, along with the nature and scope of the planning, will affect the extent of the illness, injury, and death that occur. There is a degree of overlap across phases, but each phase has distinct activities associated with it. Each phase incorporates vital components necessary for the overall success of the response and occurs over the time line.

Disaster Planning

Disaster planning addresses the problems posed by various potential events, ranging in scale from mass casualty incidents, such as blast explosions with multiple victims, to extensive flooding or earthquake damage, to armed conflicts and acts of terrorism.[20] Disaster planning is broad in scope and should always address collaboration and mutual aid agreements across agencies and organizations. It should define all advance preparations as well as describe needs assessments, event management, and recovery efforts. The ability of a community and outside support systems to rapidly respond and provide needed medical treatment and supplies, shelter, food, and clean water are essential in the prevention of morbidity and mortality associated with the aftereffects of the disaster. This is more apt to occur when there is a plan in place that specifies the three critical "Cs" of disaster response: communication, coordination, and collaboration. In addition to immediate needs, a plan must also include a method to address the long-term effects of the disaster that exist in a population after the dust has settled. Thus, emergency preparedness can avert or reduce both the short-term and long-term effects of a disaster.

In addition, during the disaster, a well-developed infrastructure is needed to manage the disaster. For example, on January 12, 2010, a massive earthquake struck the nation of Haiti, causing catastrophic damage inside and around the capital city of Port-au-Prince. Disaster management of the Haiti earthquake was hampered by the lack of emergency preparedness; the outpouring of aid from multiple countries and agencies was backlogged because there was no plan in place to coordinate the distribution of aid or to deal with the damage to the transportation infrastructure.

● APPLYING PUBLIC HEALTH SCIENCE
The Case of the Impending Storm
Public Health Science Topics Covered:

- Development of an EPDM plan
- Environmental assessment
- Advocacy

Susan Doe, RN, MPH, worked as the vice president of community outreach at a regional hospital located near Atlantic Ocean coastal areas. After Hurricane Katrina, a team was convened to revamp the EPDM plan for the region to help avoid the problems encountered in New Orleans. The team began by evaluating the risk for severe weather events, identifying the populations at greatest risk, examining the role of various responders, and evaluating potential problems posed by a hurricane.

Of particular concern to the team was that the recent building of vacation homes by nonresidents of the state and the building of sophisticated beach barricades by owners of multimillion-dollar homes to protect those properties might also increase damage to the shoreline following storms. Although the recent construction had been beneficial to the economy and had been able to take place because of a lack of updated ordinances, the building had resulted in changes to the coastline that potentially reduced the natural ecological defenses to hurricane damage that protected the community in the past. In addition, construction had increased the number of residences at risk for hurricane-related damage as well as the number of persons at risk should a hurricane hit while the summer people were in town. Another concern was that the summer residents might not be as knowledgeable about evacuation and emergency shelters that permanent residents knew about through word of mouth. To help develop an EPDM plan that addressed these concerns, the team members realized they needed to educate themselves on the concepts of preparedness, response, mitigation, and recovery in order to organize an emergency preparedness and disaster management plan for their community.

The team began by looking at prevention. Prevention during emergency preparedness and disaster planning includes efforts at multiple levels with the aim of preventing not only injury and mortality directly related to the disaster, but also reducing damage to the infrastructure of the community, thus preventing long-term negative health consequences. Sue and her team realized that during a hurricane, injury and death directly related to the storm surge are the most immediate health concerns and often result in the greatest loss of life. A storm surge is an abnormal rise of water generated by a storm, over and above predicted astronomical tides, which can cause extreme flooding in coastal areas, particularly when it coincides with normal high tide, resulting in storm tides reaching up to 20 feet or more. However, after the event has passed,

damage to the infrastructure of the community could result in serious health consequences owing to lack of access to the essentials of food, water, shelter, and medical care. If the community is seriously damaged, a large segment may be unable to return to their homes, resulting in long-term negative economic and mental health issues. They concluded that their EPDM plan needed to include mechanisms for prevention of both the direct and indirect negative consequences potentially related to a disaster event.

Sue invited a consultant from the International Federation of Red Cross and Red Crescent Societies to help educate the team. The consultant suggested that the team begin with primary prevention. This part of the planning process focuses on the development of strategies that include both what to do when the event occurs and what prevention efforts can be done to decrease the threat to persons and infrastructure. The consultant explained that the prevention efforts of an EPDM plan related to a hurricane event would address their concern about evacuation, since they would now have a clear evacuation plan prior to the storm reaching coastal lands. This would help prevent injury, death, or exposure to communicable disease. The team began to develop a plan that included how to mobilize members of the community to follow the plan. Based on the lessons learned from Katrina, the team included instructions in the plan that would help direct members of the community in gathering life-sustaining items. They also began to work on the evacuation plan with particular attention to communicating the plan to those who were visiting the coastal area as tourists and renters as well as the year-round population. They realized that efficiently evacuating the community at risk prior to a hurricane reaching land was more complex than originally thought. Based on the events during Superstorm Sandy in 2012, they realized that the area affected by a hurricane could be quite large and require moving a large population well inland. To effectively design their plan, they brought in the state police and transit authorities.

The team began to see that prevention efforts also include building an infrastructure to prevent damage. Thus, their hurricane EPDM plan was expanded to include the development of hurricane-specific building codes and the construction of seawalls. They began to examine the impact of private barriers being built around the wealthier beach communities. Based on the success of communities in other states that had instituted these policies to reduce risk, the team began to draw up recommendations to their community for requiring that construction of new buildings near the coastal area be resistant to the effect of high winds, storm surge, and floodwaters.

Sue's team put their EPDM plan in place. The following fall, a hurricane hit their area. It was listed as a Category 2 hurricane and did not require mandatory evacuations. Luckily, the team had put in place an evacuation system that included a plan for both voluntary and mandatory evacuations. The community was well informed about evacuation routes and a system was in place to inform seasonal renters. The majority of the population, especially the seasonal renters, chose to evacuate. The evacuations began a good 24 hours prior to the storm, and there was little difficulty in handling the traffic headed out of the area. Because of the smooth evacuation process, there was minimal need to rescue people in harm's way after the storm made landfall.

The team also included secondary prevention components in the plan. The secondary prevention components of their plan began with a focus on preventing injury and disease by designating safe places for residents to shelter. They realized that not everyone would be able to evacuate and that this population would include those most vulnerable, especially the elderly or those with disabilities. Thus, they designated shelters that included a mechanism for providing for health needs during the storm. The goal of this part of their plan was to prevent initial or secondary injury. Residents who were unable to evacuate were directed to these safe locations throughout the area. These were shelters that could withstand the hurricane storm forces.

The team also incorporated tertiary prevention strategies into the plan, that is, strategies designed to minimize the disease effects among those previously ill in the community. They discussed the need to provide short-term pharmaceutical supplies to members of the population with noncommunicable illness, such as insulin, oxygen, and heart medications.

After the hurricane, Sue and her team reviewed the event to see how the plan had worked. They found that once people were safely in a temporary shelter, the strategies used to prevent the spread of disease and to maintain health among the victims of the storm seemed to work. During the planning, Sue had informed her team that without careful planning, respiratory and gastrointestinal disease could spread quickly in an area of mass population relocation.[18] The plan had

helped ensure that uncontaminated food and water, as well as proper personal hygiene supplies, were available at each of the designated shelters. In addition, key medical supplies were available, not only to treat injury, but also to provide care, for example, adequate supplies of medications including antibiotics and insulin for diabetic residents. Each shelter had designated nurses to help care for the relocated population as a vital asset in the community's effort to maintain health during a hurricane.

Sue and her team concluded that their EDMP had helped to reduce mortality and morbidity. However, following the hurricane an inspection of the beachfront property most hard hit by the storm confirmed their suspicion that private barriers erected by home owners may have protected those homes, but resulted in further beach erosion in other areas. The team concluded that a Category 4 or 5 hurricane could result in higher threats to morbidity and mortality owing to the instability of the beaches and that further action was needed for primary prevention that would require possible legislation as well as allocation of funds to further protect the coastline.

Preparedness

Preparedness refers to the proactive planning efforts designed to structure the disaster response prior to its occurrence. Disaster planning encompasses evaluating potential vulnerabilities (assessment of risk) and the propensity for a disaster to occur. *Warning* (also known as *forecasting*) refers to monitoring events to look for indicators that predict the location, timing, and magnitude of future disasters. Preparedness begins with defining the precise role of public health providers during the various disaster events. Multiple agencies join forces during a disaster to form an organized web of responders. Each agency must be aware of its role in the plan and the chain of command appropriate for the situation.[20-23] For example, in preparing for a major hurricane, the EPDM plan would include a clear delineation of the role of the state and local officials in the chain of command and agencies would be identified to serve as support staff. National agencies are included as appropriate, such as the Federal Emergency Management Agency (FEMA), the U.S. Coast Guard, Centers for Disease Control and Prevention (CDC), Environmental Protection Agency, National Guard, and the Department of Homeland Security (DHS). Nongovernmental stakeholders are included in the plan as needed for a hurricane event such as local hospitals, the American Red Cross, and the utility companies.

Once the final EPDM plan developed for the impending storm is established, each state and local agency included in the plan must develop an individualized response plan and disseminate the information to the organizational and public stakeholders. A key component to emergency preparedness is that each responding organization can independently and collectively demonstrate their role during a disaster. Drills must be conducted that involve both the community and the organizations identified in the plan prior to an event to help identify and improve on the areas of weakness and improve the efficiency of the response across multiple levels to a disaster event.[21–24] Establishing interorganizational communication becomes a priority during a disaster drill, as well as communication with the members of the community.

Mitigation

Mitigation includes measures taken to reduce the harmful effects of a disaster by attempting to limit its impact on human health, community function, and economic infrastructure. These are all steps that are taken to lessen the impact of a disaster should one occur and can be considered as prevention measures. Mitigation usually requires a significant amount of forethought, planning, and implementation of measures *before* the incident occurs. The mitigation phase focuses on long-term measures, taken prior to a disaster, that can reduce or eliminate risk. Previously established response plans guide the endeavor. The first priority is to identify the affected population and environment and adjust the plan as needed to specifically target the community of interest. Each disaster is a unique event that affects populations with varying severity. Flexibility and creative problem-solving techniques are vital for an effective public health response. Continuous evaluation of the mitigation plan must continue throughout the response to ensure maximum effectiveness. For example, relief shelters should be identified in coastal regions prior to a hurricane event. However, the storm forces could compromise the integrity of a relief shelter. Mitigation includes establishing immediate changes to the response plan and identifying a safe structure to which to relocate the population.

Mitigation also involves the prevention actions referred to above that improve the infrastructure of the community, thus mitigating the risk posed by the impending storm. Examples of hurricane-related mitigation strategies that are put in place prior to an event include building flood levees, developing flood zones, establishing clearly marked evacuation routes, and enforcing building codes.

Response

The **response** phase is the actual implementation of the disaster plan. Disaster *response,* or *emergency management,* is the organization of activities used to address the event. Traditionally, the emergency management field has organized its activities in sectors, such as fire, police, hazardous materials management *(HAZMAT),* and emergency medical services. The response phase focuses primarily on emergency *relief:* saving lives, providing first aid, minimizing and restoring damaged systems such as communications and transportation, and providing care and basic life requirements to victims (food, water, and shelter). Disaster response plans are most successful if they are clear and specific, simple to understand, use an incident command system, are routinely practiced, and are updated as needed. Response activities need to be continually evaluated and adjusted to the changing situation.[10–12]

Recovery

Recovery actions focus on stabilizing and returning the community (or an organization) to normal (its preimpact status). This can range from rebuilding damaged buildings and repairing infrastructure to relocating populations and instituting mental health interventions. *Rehabilitation* and *reconstruction* involve numerous activities to counter the long-term effects of the disaster on the community and future development. In the case of the major hurricane, recovery begins when hurricane storm forces end and floodwaters recede. The length of recovery varies depending on the type and intensity of the disaster. Short-term and long-term population impacts are identified after the initial event is mitigated. Evidence-based science should be applied to ensure continuous population protection. The structural stability of buildings and homes becomes a concern as well as the availability of the resources necessary for survival. Power outages can continue for an extensive amount of time. Contamination from the floodwaters and displaced sewage can pose long-term population affects. Epidemiological surveillance is needed to identify a possible increase of communicable diseases in the region, especially waterborne and foodborne diseases.

Response Evaluation

Response evaluation is the phase of disaster planning and response that often receives the least attention. FEMA only recognizes the four previously mentioned phases of the disaster life cycle. However, the importance of response evaluation cannot be underestimated. After a disaster, it is essential that evaluations be conducted immediately to determine what worked; what did not work; and what specific problems, issues, and challenges can be identified. This quality assurance process should involve all responding agencies and participants including volunteers. Revisions to the disaster plan then become incorporated into future drills, exercises, and mitigation efforts. The quality assurance process does not cease until all gaps have been addressed and alternative planning is in place. Future disaster planning should always be based on empirical evidence derived from previous disasters.[25]

Disaster Epidemiological Surveillance

Principles of epidemiology are utilized during a disaster to determine the immediate and long-term effects to public health. The key focus of **disaster epidemiology** is to prevent or decrease morbidity and mortality associated with acute or noncommunicable illness associated with a disaster event.[18]

A community rapid needs assessment identifies the priority health issues in the population and assesses the availability of accessibility of health services (see Chapter 4). As noted above, primary, secondary, and tertiary methods of prevention play a critical role during disaster mitigation. Other strategies include education of the population to address possible hazards such as safe handling of exposed electrical lines, avoiding contaminants that have the potential to cause illness, and safe stabilizing practices on unstable structures.

Emergency Information Systems

The collection and dissemination of disaster-related disease and injury data form a core component of epidemiological surveillance. **Emergency information systems (EISs)** are designed to collect population data during the impact, mitigation, and recovery phases. Rapid data collection and analysis during a disaster ensure a timely flow of information to the appropriate responders.[26] Ongoing population data collection and surveillance allow public health providers to identify the needs of the population and design interventions to decrease morbidity and mortality. Disaster surveillance concentrates on the incidence, prevalence, and severity of illness and injury related to the event. An increase in endemic or communicable disease can follow the disaster impact owing to population displacement, overcrowded shelters, disruption in normal sanitation, and loss of health services. Data focused on communicable disease or exacerbation of noncommunicable illness help guide population treatment.

All health-care facilities, including hospitals and clinics, must participate in the collection of emergency information. Minimal data collection includes the surge capacity of an organization that specifies the number of available beds, staffing needs, and supply shortages. Tracking the name and number of patients who have been treated and are awaiting treatment assists public health officials with the overall population surveillance. Community health-care providers and private laboratories are important sources of patient-related disease and injury data. Community providers are also a frontline tool to educate individuals about communicable diseases and injury treatment. An integrated EIS should be developed during the planning phase and made accessible to all emergency responding agencies.

The National Notifiable Diseases Surveillance System (NNDSS) is an example of an electronic reporting database.[27] The NNDSS facilitates electronically transferring public health surveillance data from the health-care system to public health departments. It is a conduit for exchanging information that supports NNDSS. Today, when states and territories voluntarily submit notifiable disease surveillance data electronically to the CDC, they use data standards and electronic disease information systems and resources supported in part by the NNDSS. This ensures that state data shared with CDC are submitted quickly, securely, and in an understandable form. The NNDSS helps connect the health-care system to public health departments and those health departments to the CDC by providing leadership and resources to state and local health departments to adopt standards-based systems needed to support national disease surveillance strategy. This enables health agencies to use information technology more effectively by developing patient-centered systems that help health departments identify issues such as comorbidities (multiple diseases or conditions) that occur in the same individual over time. The NNDSS also defines and implements content (i.e., disease diagnosis, risk factor information, lab confirmation results) standards for the health-care industry to use.[27]

Postimpact Epidemiological Surveillance

Population disease and injury outcomes can be anticipated based on the specific type of disaster affecting the population. For example, an increase in diarrheal disease is common after a flood because of the disruption in sanitation practices and the integrity of the public health infrastructure. Respiratory illness increases after a wildfire as a result of the atmosphere contaminants released into the air.[28] Epidemiologists determine the association between the exposure, the disaster event, and the outcome. A standard case definition is established to identify and monitor the affected persons. Detection thresholds must be flexible to capture the changing levels of risks and priorities related to population illness and injury. For example, respiratory illnesses and long-term burn treatment will be anticipated following a wildfire. Postimpact surveillance monitors the increase in respiratory disease from baseline and tracks burn cases caused by the environmental exposures. Epidemiologists anticipate a spike in respiratory disease and bodily injury postimpact. Surveillance continues until levels stabilize back to the regional baseline. Data collected and dissemination during a disaster assist in future planning efforts by helping to predict expected health issues and prioritize health education needs of a population affected by a similar disaster.

Natural Disasters

In 2005, the world watched in awe as the forces of Hurricane Katrina assaulted the Gulf Coast of the United States and devastated the population of New Orleans. Floodwaters destroyed buildings, power sources, potable water supplies, and transportation systems. The community suffered injuries from hurricane debris and unstable structures. Contaminated water and food supplies left the people without adequate nutritional support. Medical infrastructures lay in ruins, leaving victims without access to treatment and medication supplies. The images of an event such as this guide the efforts for future preparedness efforts.

Natural disasters are events that occur from forces in nature that are not the result of human activity. These events lack controllability and may vary in their predictability. Their onset can be acute and rapid or slow and progressive. Natural disasters vary in the type and degree of population impact. The probability of an event occurring will vary depending on geographical region and season. In understanding the various types of natural disasters and determining the likelihood of these events occurring in a specific region, nurses can be active participants in the planning process, the management of a disaster, and the evaluation of the plan.

Cyclones, Hurricanes, and Typhoons

Cyclones are large-scale storms characterized by low pressure in the center surrounded by circular wind motion. The U.S. National Weather Service's (NWS) technical definition of a tropical cyclone is "non-frontal, warm-core, low pressure system of synoptic scale, developing over tropical or subtropical waters and having a definite organized circulation."[29]

In practice, that circulation is a closed airflow at the earth's surface, going counterclockwise in the Northern Hemisphere and clockwise in the Southern Hemisphere. Severe storms arising in the Atlantic waters are known as hurricanes, whereas those developing in the Pacific Ocean and the China seas are called typhoons. The precise classification (e.g., tropical depression, tropical storm, hurricane) depends on the wind force (measured on the Beaufort scale, introduced in 1805), wind speed, and manner of creation (Box 25-3).

A hurricane is a tropical storm with winds that have reached a constant speed of 74 miles per hour or more.[29] Hurricane winds blow in a large spiral around a relatively calm center known as the *eye*. The eye is generally 20 to 30 miles wide, and the storm may extend outward 400 miles. As a hurricane approaches, the skies will begin to darken and winds will grow in strength. As a hurricane nears land, it can bring torrential rains, high winds, and storm surge. A single hurricane can last for more than 2 weeks over open waters and can run a path along the entire length of the Eastern Seaboard. August and September are peak months during the hurricane season, which lasts from June 1 through November 30. Satellites track hurricanes from the moment they begin to form, so warnings can be issued many days before a storm strikes. The greatest damage to life and property is not from the wind, however, but from tidal surges and flash flooding. Hurricanes are typically rated on a scale of 1 to 5, known as the Saffir-Simpson Hurricane Wind Scale. Category 3, 4 and 5 hurricanes are considered to be major storms.[30] Owing to its violent nature, its potentially prolonged duration, and the extensive area that could be affected, the hurricane or cyclone is potentially the most devastating of all storms.

BOX 25–3 Cyclone Terminology

A tropical cyclone is a rotating, organized system of clouds and thunderstorms that originates over tropical or subtropical waters and has a closed low-level circulation. Tropical cyclones rotate counterclockwise in the Northern Hemisphere. They are classified as:
- **Tropical Depression:** A tropical cyclone with maximum sustained winds of 38 mph (33 knots) or less
- **Tropical Storm:** A tropical cyclone with maximum sustained winds of 39 to 73 mph (34 to 63 knots).
- **Hurricane:** A tropical cyclone with maximum sustained winds of 74 mph (64 knots) or higher; also called typhoons in the western North Pacific or cyclones in the Indian Ocean or and South Pacific Ocean.

Source: See reference 29.

A distinctive characteristic of hurricanes is the increase in sea level, often referred to as *storm surge* (referred to earlier in The Case of the Impending Storm). This increase in sea level is the result of the low-pressure central area of the storm creating suction, the storm winds piling up water, and the tremendous speed of the storm. Rare storm surges have risen as much as 14 meters above normal sea level. This phenomenon can be experienced as a large mass of seawater pushed along by the storm with great force. When it reaches land, the impact of the storm surge can be exacerbated by high tide, a low-lying coastal area with a gently sloping seabed, or a semi-enclosed bay facing the ocean.[30]

The severity of a storm's impact on humans is exacerbated by deforestation, which often occurs as a result of population pressure. When trees disappear along coastlines, winds and storm surges can enter land with greater force. Deforestation on the slopes of hills and mountains increases the risk of violent flash floods and landslides caused by the heavy rain associated with tropical cyclones. At the same time, the beneficial effects of the rainfall, replenishment of the water resources, may be negated because of the inability of a deforested ecosystem to absorb and retain water.

In anticipation of a hurricane making landfall, disaster planners and health-care providers should note that the Saffir-Simpson Hurricane Wind Scale does not address the potential for other hurricane-related impacts such as storm surge, rainfall-induced floods, and tornadoes. It should also be noted that these wind-caused damages are to some degree dependent on the local building codes in effect and how well and how long they have been enforced. For example, building codes enacted during the 2000s in Florida, North Carolina, and South Carolina are likely to reduce the damage to newer structures from that described below. However, for a long time to come, the majority of the building stock in existence on the coast will not have been built to a higher code. Hurricane wind damage is also very dependent on other factors, such as duration of high winds, change of wind direction, and age of structures.[30, 31]

Deaths and injuries from hurricanes occur because victims fail to evacuate the affected area or take shelter, do not take precautions in securing their property, and do not follow guidelines on food and water safety or injury prevention during recovery. Nurses need to be familiar with the commonly used definitions for severe weather watches and storm warnings in order to assist with timely evacuation or finding shelter for affected populations. Morbidity during and after the storm itself results from drowning, electrocution, lacerations, or punctures from flying debris, and blunt trauma or bone fractures from falling trees or other objects. Heart attacks and stress-related disorders can arise during the storm or its aftermath. Gastrointestinal, respiratory, vector-borne disease, and skin disease as well as accidental pediatric poisoning can all occur during the period immediately following a storm.[28] Injuries from improper use of chain saws or other power equipment, disrupted wildlife (e.g., bites from mammals, snakes, or insects), and fires are common. Fortunately, the ability to detect, track, and warn communities about cyclones, hurricanes, and tropical storms has helped reduce morbidity and mortality in many countries.

The Anatomy of a Natural Disaster: Lessons Learned From Hurricane Katrina

The National Hurricane Center in Miami, Florida, noted the increasing force of a tropical storm over the Bahamas on August 23, 2005, and issued the first advisory, stating that the weather system would become Hurricane Katrina. The storm continued to strengthen over the next 2 days and came ashore late Thursday evening on the coast of Miami. The hurricane caused significant damage to the coast as well as two fatalities. During Thursday night into early Friday morning, the storm weakened in intensity and was reclassified as a tropical storm. Hurricane Katrina emerged from the Florida peninsula around 5 a.m. Friday morning and immediately intensified after encountering the warm Gulf of Mexico waters. The strength of the hurricane grew over the next several hours. By 5 a.m. on Sunday, August 28, 2005, the storm had been declared a Category 4 hurricane and continuous public warnings were being aired to the potentially affected population.

The National Hurricane Center stated that Hurricane Katrina was a potentially catastrophic storm at this time. Rough storm waters began placing stress on the levees of New Orleans as the storm continued to increase in severity throughout Sunday. Fears were expressed that flooding could occur around the levees and along the Gulf of Mexico coastline. Hurricane Katrina entered the Gulf at Category 5. Late Sunday night, thousands of people who were unable or chose not to evacuate Louisiana took shelter in the Louisiana Superdome. At approximately 5 a.m. Monday, August 29, 2005, hurricane forces moved within 100 miles from the Louisiana shore, creating strong winds, waves greater than 40 feet in height, and heavy rainfall. The storm came ashore again around 11 a.m. Monday at the Louisiana and Mississippi border, causing devastation to the cities of Biloxi and Gulfport. Around this same time, a major levee in New Orleans failed, sending floodwaters throughout the city. Floodwater continued to pour into the city of New Orleans during the day on Tuesday.

All remaining residents were ordered to evacuate the city on Wednesday, August 31, 2005. However, floodwater and hurricane debris prevented trucks or buses from traveling through the area. Cries for help poured from New Orleans throughout Wednesday and Thursday as residents were stranded without food, water, or other essential life-sustaining supplies. The 3 days following the failure of the New Orleans levee presented unbearable challenges to those staying in the overcrowded Superdome and Convention Center. The U.S. National Guard arrived in New Orleans on Friday, September 2, 2005, with food, water, and medical supplies and the U.S. Congress approved a bill containing $10.5 billion in relief aid.

Thousands of residents evacuated New Orleans and the Gulf Coast following the initial warnings from the National Hurricane Center. Thousands more lacked resources and modes of transportation to evacuate the target area. These residents were directed to the Louisiana Superdome and were warned of the treacherous conditions that would become reality during the weeks following the storm. People were left without clean water, food, or medical supplies. In the days following the levee break, responding agencies encountered confusion and disorganization. Responders faced challenges associated with jurisdictional authority and lacked a clear disaster management structure necessary to provide prompt and effective disaster relief. Vulnerable populations including the poor, older adults, and the disabled faced the greatest impact following the hurricane devastation. Physical and financial resources and personal handicaps prevented effective evacuation.

Thousands of residents from the Gulf Coast were displaced following Hurricane Katrina. The Category 5 hurricane destroyed cities along the coast and displaced residents for long periods of time to various areas around the country. Many residents suffered extreme economic loss with the destruction of their homes and businesses. The process of rebuilding the lost cities was a feat that continued for years following the tragic event.

The lessons learned from Hurricane Katrina stimulated new emphasis on disaster management and emergency preparedness efforts. States organized legislative actions as well as policies and procedures regarding evacuation following the declaration of severe weather events. Emergency response efforts were organized into a standard structure to distinguish the role and authority of each responding agency and organization. Evidence of the successful reorganization and planning was made evident in 2008 during the Hurricane Gustav resident evacuation along the Gulf Coast. The efficient emergency preparedness structure put in place was directly responsible for reducing injury and death as well as mitigating any long-term effects.

Earthquakes

An earthquake, generally considered to be the most destructive and frightening of all forces of nature, is a sudden, rapid shaking of the earth caused by the breaking and shifting of rock beneath the earth's surface. This shaking can cause buildings and bridges to collapse; disrupt gas, electric, and phone service; and sometimes trigger landslides, avalanches, flash floods, fires, and huge, destructive ocean waves (tsunamis). Aftershocks of similar or lesser intensity can follow the main quake. Buildings with foundations resting on unconsolidated landfill, old waterways, or other unstable soil are most at risk. Buildings or trailers and manufactured homes not tied to a reinforced foundation anchored to the ground are also at risk because they can be shaken off their mountings during an earthquake.

Worldwide, earthquakes were four of the top eight deadliest disasters in 2010.[32] Earthquakes can occur at any time of the year. Earthquake losses, like those of other disasters, tend to cause more financial losses in industrialized countries and more injuries and deaths in undeveloped countries.[33]

The Richter scale, used as an indication of the force of an earthquake, measures the magnitude and intensity or energy released by the quake. This value is calculated based on data recordings from a single observation point for events anywhere on earth, but it does not address the possible damaging effects of the earthquake. According to global observations, an average of two earthquakes of a Richter magnitude 8 or slightly more occur every year. A one-digit drop in magnitude equates with a 10-fold increase in frequency. In other words, earthquakes of magnitude 7 or more generally occur 20 times in a year, whereas those with a magnitude of 6 or more occur approximately 200 times a year.[33]

Earthquakes can result in a secondary disaster, a catastrophic tsunami, discussed in a following section of this chapter. Geologists have identified regions where earthquakes are likely to occur. With the increasing population worldwide and urban migration trends, higher death tolls and greater property losses are more likely in many areas prone to earthquakes. At least 70 million Americans face significant risk of death or injury from earthquakes because they live in the 39 states that are seismically active. In addition to the significant risks in

California, the Pacific Northwest, Utah, and Idaho, six major cities with populations greater than 100,000 are located within the seismic area of the New Madrid fault (Missouri).[33] Cities in low- and middle-income countries where large numbers of people live on earthquake-prone land in structures unable to withstand damage include Lima, Peru; Santiago, Chile; Quito, Ecuador; and Caracas, Venezuela.

Deaths and injuries from earthquakes vary according to the type of housing available, time of day of occurrence, and population density. Common injuries include cuts, broken bones, crush injuries, and dehydration from being trapped in rubble. Stress reactions are also common. Morbidity and mortality can occur during the actual quake, the delayed collapse of unsound structures, or cleanup activity. Disruption of the earth may release pathogens that, when inhaled, can lead to increased reports of communicable disease. Mitigation involves developing and implementing strategies for reducing losses from earthquakes by incorporating principles of seismic safety into public and private decisions regarding the setting, design, and construction of structures (i.e., updating building and zoning codes and ordinances to enhance seismic safety), and regarding buildings' nonstructural elements, contents, and furnishings.

Extreme Heat

Extreme heat from a population perspective is a weather phenomenon characterized by substantially elevated outdoor temperatures or humidity conditions.[34] Extreme heat can result in an elevated body temperature, which then leads to hyperthermia, dehydration, heat exhaustion, or heat stroke. These conditions can cause internal organ damage when the body loses the ability to regulate temperature. Humid or muggy conditions, which add to the discomfort of high temperatures, occur when a dome of high atmospheric pressure traps hazy, damp air near the ground.

Over time, populations can acclimate to hot weather. However, mortality and morbidity rise when daytime temperatures remain unusually high several days in a row and nighttime temperatures do not drop significantly. Because populations acclimate to summer temperatures over the course of the summer, heat waves in June and July have more of an impact than those in August and September. There is often a delay between the onset of a heat wave and adverse health effects. Deaths occur more commonly during heat waves when there is little cooling at night and taper off to baseline levels if a heat wave is sustained.[35]

Heat is the number one weather-related killer in the United States, resulting in hundreds of fatalities each year. In fact, on average, excessive heat claims more lives each year than do floods, lightning, tornadoes, and hurricanes combined. In the disastrous heat wave of 1980, more than 1,250 people died. In the heat wave of 1995, more than 700 deaths in the Chicago area were attributed to heat; and in August 2003, a record heat wave in Europe claimed an estimated 50,000 lives.[36] Heat kills by pushing the human body beyond its limits. On average, about 175 Americans succumb to the taxing demands of heat every year. Our bodies dissipate heat by varying the rate and depth of blood circulation, by losing water through the skin and sweat glands, and, as a last resort by panting, when blood is heated above 98.6°F. Sweating cools the body through evaporation. However, high relative humidity retards evaporation, robbing the body of its ability to cool itself.[36] When heat gain exceeds the level the body can remove, body temperature begins to rise, and heat-related illnesses and disorders may develop. Most heat disorders occur because the victim has been overexposed to heat or has overexercised for his or her age and physical condition. Other conditions that can induce heat-related illnesses include stagnant atmospheric conditions and poor air quality.[35]

Heat waves result in adverse health effects in cities more than in rural areas. During periods of sustained environmental heat—particularly during the summer—the numbers of deaths classified as heat related (e.g., heatstroke) and attributed to other causes (e.g., cardiovascular, cerebrovascular, and respiratory diseases) increase substantially. Those at an increased risk for heat-related mortality are older adults, infants, persons with noncommunicable conditions (including obesity), patients taking medications that predispose them to heatstroke (e.g., neuroleptics or anticholinergics), and persons confined to bed or who otherwise are unable to care for themselves.

Adverse health outcomes associated with high environmental temperatures include heatstroke, heat exhaustion, heat syncope (fainting), and heat cramps. Heatstroke (i.e., core body temperature greater than or equal to 105°F (40.4°C) is the most serious of these conditions and is characterized by rapid progression of lethargy, confusion, and unconsciousness; it is often fatal despite medical care directed at lowering body temperature. Heat exhaustion is a milder syndrome that occurs following sustained exposure to hot temperatures and results from dehydration and electrolyte imbalance. Manifestations of heat exhaustion include dizziness, weakness, or fatigue; treatment is supportive. Heat syncope and heat cramps are usually related to physical exertion during hot weather.

Basic behavioral and environmental measures are essential for preventing heat-related illness and death. Personal prevention strategies should include increasing time spent in air-conditioned environments, increasing the intake of nonalcoholic beverages, and incorporating cool baths into a daily routine. When possible, activity requiring physical exertion should be conducted during cooler parts of the day. Sun exposure should be minimized and light, loose cotton clothing should be worn. The risk for heat-induced illness is greatest before persons become acclimated to warm environments. Athletes and workers in occupations requiring exposure to either indoor or outdoor high temperatures should take special precautions, including allowing 10 to 14 days to acclimate to an environment of predictably high ambient temperature.[35] Nurses and other health-care providers can assist in preventing heat-related illnesses and deaths by disseminating community prevention messages to persons at high risk (e.g., older people and persons with preexisting medical conditions) using a variety of communication techniques. They may also establish emergency plans that include provision of access to artificially cooled environments.

Floods and Mudslides

Prolonged rainfall over several days can cause a river or stream to overflow and flood surrounding areas. A flash flood from a broken dam or levee or after intense rainfall of 1 inch (or more) per hour often catches people unprepared. Global statistics show that floods are the most frequently recorded destructive events, accounting for almost 40% of the world's disasters in 2012. Worldwide, flooding incidents were five of the top ten deadliest disasters in 2012.[32] Floods are the most common type of disaster in the United States. The frequency of floods is increasing faster than any type of disaster. Much of this rise in incidence can be attributed to uncontrolled urbanization, deforestation, and the effects of climate change. Moreover, the risk of flooding is expected to increase.[36] Floods may also accompany other natural disasters, such as sea surges during hurricanes and tsunamis following earthquakes.[36,37]

Except for flash floods, flooding directly causes few deaths. Instead, widespread and long-lasting detrimental effects include damage to homes and mass homelessness, disruption of communications and health-care systems, and heavy loss of business, livestock, crops, and grain, particularly in densely populated, low-lying areas. The frequent, cyclic nature of flooding can mean a constant and ever-increasing drain on the economy of rural populations. Flood-related morbidity and mortality vary

from country to country. Flash flooding, such as from excessive rainfall or sudden release of water from a dam, is the cause of most flood-related deaths. Many victims become trapped in their cars and drown when attempting to drive through rising or swiftly moving water. Wading, bicycling, or other recreational activities in flooded areas have caused other deaths. The health impacts of flooding include communicable disease morbidity exacerbated by crowded living conditions and compromised personal hygiene, contamination of water sources, disruption of sewage service and solid waste collection, and increased vector populations. Water-borne diseases (e.g., enterotoxigenic *Escherichia coli, Shigella,* hepatitis A, leptospirosis, and giardiasis) become a significant hazard, as do other vector-borne diseases and skin disorders. Injured and frightened animals, hazardous waste contamination, molds and mildew, and dislodging of graves pose additional risks in the period following a flood.[38] Food shortages that are due to water-damaged stocks may occur because of flooding and sea surges. The stress and exertion required for cleanup following a flood also cause significant morbidity (mental and physical) and mortality (e.g., myocardial infarction). Fires, explosions from gas leaks, downed live electrical wires, and debris can all cause significant injury.

Mudslides are another disaster that is weather related. They usually occur after heavy rains. A mudslide involves the rapid movement of rocks, earth, and other debris down a slope. They can be associated with floods, earthquakes, and volcanoic eruptions. The risk of a mudslide is increased when the natural vegetation on a slope has been modified following a wildfire or human activities.[19] Mudslides occur in all 50 states, with many mudslides occurring in California as a result of drought and wildfires. In 2013, mudslides were responsible for deaths in Colorado Springs, Ecuador, and Mexico. The deadliest mudslide occurred in 1999, killing 30,000 to 50,000 people in Vargas, Venezuela.

Tornadoes

Tornadoes are rapidly whirling, funnel-shaped air spirals that emerge from a violent thunderstorm and reach the ground. Tornadoes can have a wind velocity of up to 200 miles per hour and generate sufficient force to destroy even massive buildings. The average circumference of a tornado is a few hundred meters, and it is usually exhausted before it has traveled as far as 20 kilometers. Knowing some facts about tornados is useful when putting together an EPDM plan for communities living in a tornado prone area of the country (Box 25-4).[39]

BOX 25–4 **Tornado Facts**

- They may strike quickly, with little or no warning.
- They may appear nearly transparent until dust and debris are picked up or a cloud forms in the funnel.
- The average tornado moves southwest to northeast, but tornadoes have been known to move in any direction.
- The average forward speed of a tornado is 30 mph, but may vary from stationary to 70 mph.
- Tornadoes can accompany tropical storms and hurricanes as they move on to land.
- Waterspouts are tornadoes that form over water.
- Tornadoes are most frequently reported east of the Rocky Mountains during spring and summer months.
- Peak tornado season in the southern states is March through May; in the northern states, it is late spring through early summer.
- Tornadoes are most likely to occur between 3 p.m. and 9 p.m., but can occur at any time.

Source: See reference 39.

Approximately 1,000 tornadoes occur annually in the United States, and none of the lower 48 states is immune. Certain geographical areas are at greater risk because of recurrent weather patterns; tornadoes most frequently occur in the midwestern and southeastern states. Although tornadoes often develop in the late afternoon and more often from March through May, they can arise at any hour of the day and during any month of the year. Injuries from tornadoes occur from flying debris or people being thrown by the high winds (e.g., head injuries, soft tissue injury, secondary wound infection). Stress-related disorders are more common, as is disease related to loss of utilities, potable water, or shelter.

Because tornadoes can occur so quickly, communities should develop redundant warning systems (e.g., media alerts and automated telephone warnings), establish protective shelters to reduce tornado-related injuries, and practice tornado shelter drills. In the event of a tornado, the residents should take shelter in a basement if possible, away from windows, while protecting their heads. Special outreach should be made to people with special needs, who should make a list of their limitations, capabilities, and medications and have ready an emergency box of needed supplies. People with special needs should have a buddy who has a copy of the list and who knows of the emergency box.

Tsunamis

A tsunami is a single or multiple tidal wave(s) created from an earthquake on the ocean floor.[29] On December 26, 2004, a 9.0 magnitude earthquake struck at approximately 7 a.m. about 100 miles from the coast of Sumatra, Indonesia. The quake caused a massive tsunami that killed more than 225,000 people and displaced another 1.2 million. This disaster quickly elevated to a crisis situation, affecting 11 countries and requiring global relief aid and disaster responders. Seven years later, on March 11, 2011, 31,000 people lost their lives from a tsunami that struck Japan.

Initial tsunami-related morbidity and mortality occur from the force of the water, impact with moving debris, or crush injuries from falling structures. Long-term effects are similar to those of a severe flood event, with an increase in water- and foodborne communicable disease, an increase in respiratory disease related to large numbers of displaced individuals in crowded relief shelters, and a lack of necessary medical and fiscal resources. In the case of the 2011 Japanese tsunami, damage to a nuclear reaction power plant added the hazard for release of radioactivity into the environment. In addition, the Japanese tsunami has had a global impact. We now know that the Fukushima nuclear power plant affected by the tsunami has been leaking radioactive water into surrounding groundwater, which then makes its way into the Pacific Ocean. Also, debris that was swept into the ocean has already made its way to the Pacific shores of the United States, creating a long-term environmental problem.[40]

Submarine landslides and volcanic eruptions beneath the sea or on small islands can also be responsible for tsunamis, but their effects are usually limited to smaller areas. Tsunamis are often mistakenly referred to as tidal waves because they can resemble a violent tide rushing to shore. Tsunamis are powerful enough to move through any obstacle; therefore, damage from tsunamis results from both the destructive force of the initial wave and the rapid flooding that occurs as the water dissipates. Depending on the strength of the initiating event, underwater topology, and the distance from its epicenter to the shore, the effects of a tsunami can vary greatly, ranging from being barely noticeable to total destruction.

Tsunami waves can be described by their wavelength (measured in feet or miles), period (minutes or hours it takes one wavelength to pass a fixed point), speed (miles per hour), and height. Tsunamis may travel long distances, increasing in height abruptly when they reach shallow water, causing great devastation far away from the source. In deep water, a person on the surface may not realize that a tsunami is forming while the wave increases to great heights as it approaches the coastline. The Pacific Tsunami Warning Center maintained by the

National Oceanic and Atmospheric Administration (NOAA) monitors the Pacific Ocean for possible tsunamis and issues warnings.[41] Though this type of warning system is not yet available in other parts of the world, they are being developed to provide alerts about impending tsunamis across the globe. Tsunamis are not preventable, nor predictable, but there are warning signs. A number of events or signs are indicative of a possible tsunami (Box 25-5).

In the immediate aftermath of a tsunami, the first health interventions are to rescue survivors and provide medical care for any injuries. For people caught in the waves, the force of the water pushes people into debris, resulting in the broadest range of injuries, such as broken limbs and head injuries. Drowning is the most common cause of death associated with a tsunami. Tsunami waves and the receding water are very destructive to structures in the run-up zone. Other hazards include flooding and fires from ruptured gas lines or tanks.

The floods that accompany a tsunami result in potential health risks from contaminated water and food supplies. Loss of shelter leaves people vulnerable to exposure to insects, heat, and other environmental hazards. Further, the lack of medical care may result in exacerbations of noncommunicable disease. Tsunamis have long-lasting effects and recovery necessitates long-term surveillance of infectious and water- or insect-transmitted diseases, an infusion of medical supplies and medical personnel, and the provision of mental health and social support services.

Potential waterborne diseases that follow tsunamis include cholera; diarrheal or fecal-oral diseases, such as amebiasis, cryptosporidiosis, cyclosporiasis, giardiasis, hepatitis A and E, leptospirosis, parasitic infections, rotavirus, shigellosis, and typhoid fever; animal- or mosquito-borne illness, such as plague, rabies, malaria, Japanese encephalitis, and dengue fever (and the potentially fatal complication dengue hemorrhagic shock syndrome); and wound-associated infections and diseases, such as tetanus. Mental health concerns are another serious consequence of tsunami events.

Volcanic Eruptions

A volcano is a mountain that opens downward to a reservoir of molten rock below the surface of the earth. Unlike most mountains, which are pushed up from below, volcanoes are built up by an accumulation of their own eruptive products. When pressure from gases within the molten rock becomes too great, an eruption occurs. Extremely high temperature and pressure cause mantle, located deep inside the earth between the molten iron core and the thin crust at the surface, to melt and become liquid rock or magma. When a large amount of magma is formed, it rises through the denser rock layers toward the earth's surface. Eruptions can be quiet or explosive. There may be lava flows, flattened landscapes, poisonous gases, and flying rock and ash.

Because of their intense heat, lava flows are great fire hazards. Lava flows destroy everything in their path, but most move slowly enough that people can move out of the way. Fresh volcanic ash, made of pulverized rock, can be abrasive, acidic, gritty, gassy, and odorous. Although not immediately dangerous to most adults, the acidic gas and ash can cause lung damage to small infants, to older adults, and to those suffering from severe respiratory illnesses. Volcanic ash can affect people hundreds of miles away from the cone of a volcano.[42]

Sideways-directed volcanic explosions, known as lateral blasts, can shoot large pieces of rock at very high speeds for several miles. These explosions can kill by impact, burial, or heat. They have been known to knock down entire forests. Volcanic eruptions can be accompanied by other natural hazards, including earthquakes, mudflows and flash floods, rock falls and landslides, acid rain, fire, and (under special conditions) tsunamis. Active volcanoes in the United States are found mainly in Hawaii, Alaska, and the Pacific Northwest. The danger area around a volcano covers approximately a 20-mile radius. Some danger may exist 100 miles or more from a volcano.

Volcanic eruptions can endanger the lives of people and property located both near to and far from a volcano. The range of adverse health effects on the population resulting from volcanic activity is quite broad and extensive. Immediate, acute, and nonspecific irritant effects have been reported in the eyes, nasal passages, and upper airways of persons exposed to volcanic ash. Victims can experience exacerbations of their asthma and chronic obstructive pulmonary disease and can asphyxiate due

---

BOX 25–5 **Signs of a Possible Tsunami**

- There has been a recent submarine earthquake.
- The sea appears to be boiling, as large quantities of gas rise to the surface of the water.
- The water is hot, smells of rotten eggs, or stings the skin.
- There is an audible thunder or booming sound followed by a roaring or whistling sound.
- The water may recede a great distance from the coast.
- Red light might be visible near the horizon and, as the wave approaches, the top of the wave may glow red.

to inhalation of ash or gases. Eruptions can result in blast injuries and lacerations from projectile rock fragments. Volcanic flow can cause fires and the destruction of buildings, with victims experiencing trauma and thermal burns.[43]

Prior to an eruption, communities living near a volcano that may become active need to develop an EPDM plan. During an eruption the first steps are to evacuate, avoiding river beds and low lying areas. Another concern is the potential for mudslides and exposure to falling ash.[42] Following the Mount St. Helens eruption, the falling ash was so thick that motorists could not see more than a few feet in front of their cars. After an eruption, it is important to have shelters for the population, especially for those whose homes may not be safe to return to.[42]

Winter Weather

Winter weather brings ice, snow, cold temperatures, and often dangerous driving conditions, and a major winter storm can be lethal. Even small amounts of snow and ice can cause severe problems for southern states where such storms are infrequent. Nurses need to be familiar with winter storm warning messages, such as wind chill, winter storm watch, winter storm warning, and blizzard warning. The NOAA defines a blizzard as an event lasting greater than 3 hours with winds over 35 miles per hour, heavy snowfall, and decreased visibility. An avalanche results when a mass of snow, rock, or ice rapidly slides down a mountain or incline; it is also referred to as a snow slide.[29] Other issues with winter weather include ice storms and extreme cold.

These extreme conditions can prevent people from using established routes of transportation and obtaining life sustaining supplies and sources of power. The severity of the event can prevent emergency personnel from gaining access to the affected population. Blizzards, ice storms, and avalanches can strand individuals in places without heat or electricity, preventing the use of medical devices and exposing a population to the previously discussed conditions. Prolonged exposure to cold weather conditions can result in conditions such as hypothermia and frostbite (Table 25-1).

Transportation accidents are the leading cause of death during winter storms. Preparing vehicles for the winter season and knowing how to react if stranded or lost on the road are the keys to safe winter driving. Morbidity and mortality associated with winter storms include frostbite and hypothermia, carbon monoxide poisoning, blunt trauma from falling objects, penetrating trauma from the use of mechanical snow blowers, and cardiovascular events usually associated with snow removal. Frostbite is a severe reaction to cold exposure that can permanently damage its victims. A loss of feeling and a light or pale appearance in fingers, toes, nose, or earlobes are symptoms of frostbite. Hypothermia is a condition brought on when the body temperature drops to less than 90°F. Symptoms of hypothermia include uncontrollable shivering, slow speech, memory lapses, frequent stumbling, drowsiness, and exhaustion.

TABLE 25–1	Centers for Disease Control and Prevention Recommendations for Cold Weather Injuries	
Health Effect	Symptoms	Treatment
Frostbite	• Numbness usually located on cheeks, toes, nose, chin, ears, and fingers • White or grayish-yellow discoloration • Waxy or firm skin	• Submerse affected area in warm, not hot, water. • Remain in a warm area. • Do not walk on or use effected parts. • Do not rub or massage. • Do not use a heating pad.
Hypothermia	• Decreased consciousness • Altered mental status • Shallow respirations • Pallor of the skin • Shivering • Confusion or disorientation	• Remove wet clothing. • Keep victim in a warm room. • Make skin-to-skin contact under cover of blanket. • Warm the center of body first (i.e., chest, head, and groin). • Use electric blanket if available. • Provide warm beverage to increase core body temperature.

Source: See reference 19.

Communities include in their disaster plans preparation for cold weather events. Individuals can invest in preventive mitigation steps such as home winterization activities (insulating pipes, installing storm windows) to help reduce the impact of winter weather. At the population level, communities must have plans to handle interruption to transportation, loss of power, injury, and access to needed medical care. Of particular concern are vulnerable populations such as older adults or the homeless. Again, shelters may be needed to provide care in the event of a power outage. Many urban communities will increase capacity to provide shelter to the homeless during extreme cold.

Wildfires

Wildfires are raging and rapidly spreading fires that can sweep quickly across large areas of land. They lack predictability and often require great resources to contain and extinguish. The Santa Barbara, California, wildfire of 2009 forced thousands of people from their homes and consumed a great number of structures. In 2011, multiple wildfires burned thousands of acres in Texas, resulting in the dealths two firefighters. Three deaths occurred in a wildfire in Colorado in 2012, and a wildfire in 2013 in Pigeon Forge, Tennessee, burned 230 acres and required 20 fire departments to respond before being controlled. As residential areas expand into relatively untouched forests, wild lands, and remote mountain sites, forest fires increasingly threaten people living in these communities.[43] Protecting structures from fire poses special problems, often stretching firefighting resources to the limit.

Morbidity and mortality associated with wildfires include burns, inhalation injuries, respiratory complications, and stress-related cardiovascular events (exhaustion and myocardial infarction experienced while fighting or fleeing the fire).[29,44] Compromised respiratory conditions can result from the air pollution caused by the vast amount of smoke generated by the fires. Another concern is taking precautions to protect those who respond to fires. Responders are at increased risk for morbidity and mortality. Volunteer firefighters are at greatest risk; for example, 19 firefighters lost their lives combating a wildfire in Arizona in July 2013. The CDC provides specific guides for protecting firefighters during cleanup to reduce their risk of adverse consequences following the fire (Box 25-6).[45]

FEMA identified three areas of concern for public health preparedness—before a fire, during a fire, and after a fire.[43] Prefire population considerations focus on community education regarding actions that will enhance personal and public safety. Families are encouraged to

BOX 25–6	**CDC Fact Sheet: Worker Safety During Fire Cleanup**

Have available:
- First aid
- Protective equipment
  Workers face hazards even after fires are extinguished.
In addition to a smoldering or new fire, dangers include:
- Carbon monoxide poisoning
- Musculoskeletal hazards
- Heavy equipment
- Extreme heat and cold
- Unstable structures
- Hazardous materials
- Fire
- Confined spaces
- Worker fatigue
- Respiratory hazards

Source: See reference 45.

have an evacuation plan, especially for vulnerable members of the family children, older people, and persons with handicaps, at the first warning of fire outbreak. People are the encouraged to wear protective clothing, shut off gas at the source, and gather all essential valuables and place them a safe place for easy access. During the fire, homeowners are asked to leave all lights on inside the home, place a ladder outside in a highly visible area, leave all doors unlocked, and evacuate immediately. These measures are vital for responders to effectively manage structure fires and protect the population. Families should remain together in a central area of the home if they become trapped by the wildfire. After the wildfire is controlled, active embers and sparks can settle on roofs and in attics, creating the potential for further structure fires. It is important for people to watch for these sources that can cause a home to reignite, and safely alleviate the threat.[46]

Wildfires often begin unnoticed and spread quickly by igniting brush, trees, and homes. There are three different classes of wildfires. A **surface fire,** the most common type, burns along the floor of a forest, moving slowly and killing or damaging trees. A **ground fire** is usually started by lightning and burns on or below the forest floor in the humus layer down to the mineral soil. **Crown fires** spread rapidly by wind and move quickly by jumping along the tops of trees. Depending on prevailing winds and the amount of water in the environment, wildfires can quickly spread out of control, causing extensive damage to personal property and human life. If heavy rains follow a fire, other natural disasters can occur, including landslides, mudflows, and floods. Once ground cover has been burned away, little is left to hold soil in place on steep slopes and hillsides, increasing the risk for mudslides. A major wildfire can leave a large amount of scorched and barren land. These areas may not return to prefire conditions for decades. Danger zones include all wooded, brushy, and grassy areas, especially those in Kansas, Mississippi, Louisiana, Georgia, Florida, the Carolinas, Tennessee, California, Massachusetts, and the national forests of the western United States.[43]

Epidemics

An epidemic occurs when there is an increase in cases significantly higher than the usual number of cases. A pandemic describes epidemics that are occurring across the globe (see Chapter 8). In the case of communicable diseases, EPDM plans are needed to handle the emergence of a communicable disease at epidemic proportions that puts a population or populations at risk. Quick response is essential because epidemics develop rapidly, resulting in human and economic losses and political difficulties. An epidemic or threatened epidemic can become an emergency when certain characteristics are present (Box 25-7). The categorization of an emergency differs from country to country, depending on two local factors: whether the disease is endemic and whether a means of transmitting the agent exists. Frequently, the introduction of a pathogen and the start of an epidemic may occur through an animal vector; thus, veterinarians may be the first to identify a disease new to a community.

BOX 25-7   Epidemic Disaster Planning: Emergency Signs

Note: Not every characteristic need be present and each must be assessed with regard to its relative importance locally:

• There is a risk of the introduction to and spread of the disease in the population.
• A large number of cases may reasonably be expected to occur.
• The disease involved is of such severity that it may lead to serious disability or death.
• There is a risk of social or economic disruption resulting from the presence of the disease.
• There is an inability of authorities to cope adequately with the situation because of insufficient technical or professional personnel, organizational experience, and necessary supplies or equipment (e.g., drugs, vaccines, laboratory diagnostic materials, vector-control materials).
• There is a risk of international transmission.

Man-Made Disasters

The events of September 11, 2001, in the United States stimulated the worldwide emergence of preparedness planning for terrorism. **Man-made disasters** differ from natural disasters based on the human element associated with high levels of morbidity and mortality in a population. These events can be accidental exposures or intentional terrorist events. An expansive consortium of responders is vital for an effective reaction to a man-made event.

Blast Events

Explosions have the potential to affect a population by causing immediate physical injuries and destruction of property and well as long-term emotional distress, disability, and damage to the community's perception of safety. **Blast events** are the result of a device explosion. Immediate considerations following an explosion include identifying the causative agent, the affected geographical area, and extent of injury and damage. Responders must be aware of the appropriate personal protective equipment necessary for the situation and be proficient in the proper techniques in using the equipment. Only trained personnel should be involved in explosion mitigation until the safety of the blast scene is established. An explosion generates a blast wave that moves outward from the point of origin. In confined spaces, irregular, high-pressure blast waves will cause unpredictable injury patterns.[47,48]

The four stages of blast injuries include primary, secondary, tertiary, and quaternary (Table 25-2). Primary reflects injuries due to the blast wave, which is the overpressurization impulse created by the blast. The injuries from a blast result in the changes to the body brought about by the overpressurization force that impacts the surface of the human body. Most common blast injuries associated with the primary stage of impact include rupture of the tympanic membrane, causing temporary or permanent hearing loss and injury to the air-filled organs in the body.[47]

Secondary injuries are the result of flying debris from the blast. In the Boston Marathon bombing, the majority of the injuries that required care were secondary injuries that resulted in damage to lower extremities, which, in some cases, required amputation. In this same event, there was also tertiary damage, with images of runners falling to the ground shortly after the bomb went off played over and over again by the media. Quaternary injuries include exacerbations of existing noncommunicable diseases as well as the threat of infection at the site of the wounds inflicted by the flying debris.

TABLE 25–2	Blast Injuries		
Category	Characteristics	Body Part Affected	Types of Injuries
Primary	Unique to high-order explosives (HE), results from the impact of the overpressurization wave with body surfaces	Gas-filled structures are most susceptible—lungs, gastrointestinal tract, and middle ear.	Blast lung (pulmonary barotrauma) Tympanic membrane rupture and middle ear damage Abdominal hemorrhage and perforation Globe (eye) rupture Concussion (traumatic brain injury without physical signs of head injury)
Secondary	Results from flying debris and bomb fragments	Any body part may be affected.	Penetrating ballistic (fragmentation) or blunt injuries Eye penetration (can be occult)
Tertiary	Results from individuals being thrown by the blast wind	Any body part may be affected.	Fracture and traumatic amputation Closed and open brain injury
Quaternary	All explosion-related injuries, illnesses, or diseases not due to primary, secondary, or tertiary mechanisms. Includes exacerbation or complications of existing conditions	Any body part may be affected.	Burns (flash, partial, and full thickness) Crush injuries Closed and open brain injury Asthma, chronic obstructive pulmonary disease or other breathing problems from dust, smoke, or toxic fumes Angina Hyperglycemia, hypertension

Source: See reference 47.

The response to Boston Marathon bombings in the spring of 2013 is an excellent example of effective EPDM planning on the part of a city to deal with a blast-related disaster. The health-care providers and first responders followed the plan, hospitals were ready to receive the influx of wounded, and emergency care was provided that saved lives. When interviewed by the media, the physicians and nurses stated that they did what they had been trained to do.

Chemical Exposure

Chemicals are found everywhere from industrial workplaces to home cleaning products. Releases can range from a small-scale, contained spill to a large release that causes widespread environmental contamination. Immediate priorities associated with a chemical exposure are to evacuate the contaminated area and identify the chemical. For example, visualize an auto accident involving a tanker vehicle transporting gasoline. Damage to the vehicle could result in a chemical spill on the roadway. Urgent actions involve restoring safety to the scene of the accident, the surrounding environment, and the exposed population. Chemical explosions can cause widespread destruction and contaminate the air,

soil, and water. The explosive, flammable, poisonous, radioactive, and combustible properties of a substance must be identified immediately following a potential or active release.[49,50]

Hazardous materials are substances found in multiple forms that have the potential to cause death, morbid health effects, and property damage. These materials pose dangers to population health during production, storage, use, and disposal. A placard, a card or plaque containing a numerical code that identifies the type of chemical or hazardous material being transported by railway, vehicle, or waterway, is required by the U.S. Department of Transportation and allows emergency responders to immediately identify the substance in question.[49] Preparedness actions to ensure patient and employee safety from potential chemical exposures in a health-care organization are also important. It is important to know the commonly used chemicals in a hospital or health-care setting and educate those handling the substance on proper use and how to respond to a spill or human exposure.[51] Material safety data sheets contain information that is pertinent to planning, such as safe handling techniques, toxic effects of the material, and first aid considerations following human exposure.

Radiation Exposure

Ionizing radiation exposure has the potential to cause immediate and long-term negative health effects in a community. The explosion at the Chernobyl nuclear power plant on April 26, 1986, is the largest nuclear disaster in world history and continues to plague parts of Europe. The accident created a release of nuclear material, causing the evacuation of approximately 116,000 people from the highly contaminated area surrounding the reactor. Serious contamination resulted in Ukraine, Belarus, and the Russian Federation, all of which were part of the former Soviet Union. Trace contamination spread by wind and water throughout eastern and western Europe.[52] More than 600,000 people have been involved with the mitigation of this radiation exposure during the subsequent three decades.

The health effects associated with various types of alternative energy sources have become a priority public health planning component during the 21st century. Considering the Chernobyl case, the World Health Organization (WHO) conducted a longitudinal study following the nuclear disaster and found an increase in thyroid disease, leukemia, solid cancers, and mental disease among the population in the three severely contaminated countries.[53] The lessons learned following the Chernobyl disaster have guided the development of regulations associated with general radiation use. A proficient knowledge of the regional contamination potential will focus emergency preparedness and disaster planning priorities specific to the population of interest.

Bioterrorism

Bioterrorism is a deliberate release of a pathogen that is either naturally occurring or man-made and can create a public health emergency. The agent is bacterial or viral in origin. An event would typically present with a single definitively diagnosed case of an illness to be known as a bioterrorism agent, a cluster of patients presenting with a similar clinical syndrome lacking clear etiology or explanation, or an unexplained increase of a common syndrome above seasonal expectations.[19] The CDC prioritizes infectious agents into three categories based on the impact and speed of transmission arranged from highest priority to emerging agents (Table 25-3).[19] Disaster mitigation would mimic that of an infection epidemic; however, the rapid spread of disease and origin identification present unique challenges. Primary care providers and community hospitals will be the first to

TABLE 25–3	Bioterrorism Agents by Category	
Category A Agents (Highest Priority Agents)	**Category B Agents**	**Category C Agents (Emerging Infections)**
Anthrax	Q Fever	Nipah virus
Bacillus anthracis	*Coxiella burnetii*	(1)
Botulism	Brucellosis	Hantaviruses
Clostridium botulinum	*Brucella* species	(2)
Smallpox	Glanders	Tick-borne hemorrhagic fever
Variola major	*Burkholderia mallei*	(3)
Pneumonic plague	Castor beans	Tick-borne encephalitis
Yersinia pestis	*Ricinus communis*	(4)
Tularemia	Clostridium perfringens	Yellow fever
Francisella tularensis	Epsilon toxin	(5)
	Water or foodborne agents	Multidrug-resistant tuberculosis
	Salmonella	
	Shigella dysenteriae	
	Escherichia coli	
	Vibrio cholerae	
	Cryptosporidium	

Source: See reference 19.

experience the influx of patients following the use of a biological weapon; therefore, detection and diagnosis would be made at the local level.

Disaster Response Structure and Organization

All disasters are local yet have the potential to affect health on regional, national, and international levels. Local health departments and government officials engage disaster response plans specific to the event and call on the resources necessary to effectively manage and mitigate the situation. Disaster events present challenges associated with the increased need for emergency personnel and resources.

Consider the possibility of a major crash of a passenger jet airplane. The potential for a large number of victims with life-threatening injuries increases the importance of a solid response structure for this event. Increased numbers of medical responders and medical supplies are needed to manage the number of potential victims. Responders from local governmental and volunteer agencies will be required to increase the power of the workforce. The initial priority of the emergency medical personnel is to identify the extent of illness and injury, communicate the gravity of the situation to local stakeholders and medical facilities, and begin victim medical treatment.

Disaster Triage and Patient Tracking

Emergency responders (usually paramedics and other emergency medical team members) begin victim treatment with a field triage. **Triage** is derived from a French term meaning *to sort*.[12,18] Disaster triage determines the severity of illness or injury suffered by the victim and assists responders with systematically distributing patients evenly among the local hospitals. The system is a color-coded, four-level process ranging from minor injuries to those expired at the scene. A large-scale disaster can produce greater numbers of victims stretching beyond the capabilities of the emergency medical system in a community. These scenarios are known as **mass casualty events (MCEs)** and require special considerations during the disaster planning process.[20] A chain of medical care is established between emergency responders and medical facilities. Though the plan of response varies between communities, most share standardized similarities.

During a disaster, patient and population tracking is a core function of state and local public health officials. Tracking becomes complicated when people evacuate to areas other than public shelters. Population tracking becomes an even greater challenge when considering the homeless, incarcerated victims, shelters that do not register the injured, and the deceased. Established communication networks between hospitals, mass treatment facilities, and health departments help to identify the location of the injured victims seeking treatment.

Federal Response and Organization

The U.S. DHS is authorized by law to activate federal resources and assistance under certain circumstances. Federal agencies can act on their own authority when appropriate. For example, the Federal Bureau of Investigation has established authority when an act of bioterrorism is suspected, and the Federal Aviation Administration maintains authority following an airplane crash. State and local officials can also request federal assistance when the disaster expands beyond the resources and capabilities of local responders. Resource assistance includes financial support, personnel assistance, and physical supplies. The U.S. president has the authority to direct the secretary of the DHS to assume responsibility for managing a disaster when the event merits such an action.

Federal Emergency Management Agency

FEMA is the lead agency for and assumes coordination of disaster response following a presidential declaration of authority under the Stafford Act. FEMA has direct access to federal resources and funding. Federal financial resources can be allotted for various functions including preparedness, response, and recovery efforts for large-scale disasters. FEMA is one of more than 27 agencies, along with the American Red Cross, that provide technical support and personnel for the purpose of disaster planning and mitigation.

National Response Framework

The National Response Framework (NRF), enacted in January 2008, supersedes the previous National Response Plan and serves as a guide to how the nation conducts comprehensive incident response using an all-hazards approach to respond to natural and man-made disasters. Built on its predecessor, it includes guiding principles that detail how federal, state, local, tribal, and private-sector partners, including the health-care sector, prepare for and provide a unified domestic response through improved coordination and integration. The plan provides national direction for all responders during a domestic disaster.

National Incident Management System

The National Incident Management System (NIMS) enhances the ability to oversee a national response to an event through a single, comprehensive management model. Several key elements are incorporated into the NIMS system, which functions to increase the effectiveness of a national disaster response. An established Incident Command System organizes areas such as command, operation, planning, logic, and finances during event mitigation and recovery. A unified command is established to assist with clearly defining objectives and joint decision making. Preparedness is another key element of the system and enhances the readiness of responders regarding the performance of vital disaster functions. The NIMS also provides organizational design for an interoperable communication infrastructure and information systems. The Joint Information System ensures that all levels of government are releasing the same information and coordinate to deliver a unified message to the public.[17] Each key element of the NIMS involves an intricate process and directly affects the overall effectiveness of the systems.

Strategic National Stockpile

A large-scale disaster response will require access to large amounts of pharmaceutical and medical supplies. The Strategic National Stockpile (SNS) is a national repository of antibiotics, chemical antidotes, antitoxins, life-support medications, IV administration, airway maintenance supplies, and medical-surgical items. Federal agencies such as the Department of Health and Human Services, and primarily the CDC, are responsible for maintenance and delivery of SNS assets, but state and local authorities must plan to receive, store, stage, distribute, and dispense the assets. During a disaster, the SNS program is designed to deliver pharmaceuticals, vaccines, medical supplies, and equipment to states and local jurisdictions affected by the event. Each state is responsible for management of the stockpile under which it resides. Relationships with public and private agencies are established within each state to ensure the maintenance and delivery of supplies. Upon request, push packs filled with medical and pharmaceutical supplies can be delivered to any area in the United States in less than 12 hours and readied for distribution by local health departments.

For example, a disease outbreak infecting large numbers of people in a rapid time frame will demand resources outweighing the capabilities of the local health departments. Local public health officials would request the deployment of supplies from the SNS. Bulk push packs will then be delivered to the predetermined destination for distribution to the local care sites and medical facilities. Local public health providers are then responsible for maintenance and distribution of the allotted

supplies. Mass care facilities are ideal for the treatment of large numbers of patients in a timely manner. An example of a mass care facility is a disaster treatment center opened in a local venue large enough to house high volumes of community members. These care facilities provide disaster triage and basic medical care. Patients with critical or life-threatening injuries are stabilized at these facilities and transported to the appropriate health-care institution.

Point of Dispensing

A **point of dispensing (POD)** site is set up when the population requires rapid medical treatment, prophylaxis, or vaccination. PODs are designed to provide treatment to the population in a rapid and organized fashion. Multiple stations work in assembly-line fashion, providing services from screening to treating.[18] Patients begin with registration, at which a log is maintained of all persons receiving care in the POD. Patients are then screened for eligibility of treatment and epidemiological background related to the event. Once screened, patients move through to a triage area staffed by licensed health-care providers, such as nurses or physicians, where patients are assessed to determine whether dispensing treatment is appropriate or whether further evaluation is needed from a health-care facility. The acutely ill are transferred immediately to a hospital for evaluation. Individuals who are receiving prophylaxis or medical treatment for minor symptoms then move to the dispensing station. Licensed health-care providers (including pharmacists), where medication or treatment is provided, also staff dispensing stations. Counseling services, POD security, and medical record-keeping are also vital components of the services provided. Patients can receive medical and psychological treatment while at the distribution center.

Multiple-Agency Consortiums

One concept that becomes obvious during emergency preparedness and disaster planning is the need for multiple agencies employing collective expertise to decrease disaster-related morbidity and mortality. The collaboration of public health personnel, law enforcement agencies, emergency responders, fire officials, and trained volunteers is essential for effective population medical treatment and physical protection. Organizational models such as NRF and NIMS provide guidance for local and state health departments to develop a consortium of disaster responders. The Medical Reserve Corps (MRC) is a federally sponsored program that provides an organized structure for community public health and medical volunteers. The program supports adequate training and exercises to ensure safety and competence of responding personnel.[18] The local MRC is activated during both emergency situations and nonemergent events, such as blood and immunization drives.

Health-Care Facility Disaster Response

Health-care facility preparedness is the cornerstone of effective mass casualty management.[8] Disasters present the unique challenge of large numbers of patients seeking medical attention in amounts that reach beyond the typical capacity. A sudden increase of patients is referred to as a **surge.** Large volumes of patients are associated with disaster-related surge events, creating a demand for health services in which additional capacity and capabilities are required.[53] Routinely practiced disaster drills and exercises in an organization are the most effective strategies to increase the effectiveness of health-care facility disaster response. Each member of the institution must have proficient knowledge of her or his role in the mitigation efforts as well as proper internal and external communication procedures. It is important that surge plans are developed, documented, communicated, and exercised prior to a mass casualty event.

Health-Care Facility Surge Planning

Surge plans developed by a health-care facility should be compatible with the previously discussed national norms. Allocation of roles and responsibilities are established through the developed chain of command and planning structure. The health-care organization must have a command group or an emergency management group. These individuals are the leaders in the chain of command and will hold the ultimate authority of the event mitigation. Protocols should be developed in the institution pertaining to internal events and communication with state or local coordination centers. The organizational response varies depending on the size of the incident. The predetermined command staff is responsible for initiating and deactivating a facility surge plan. A plan to scale up or scale down the surge response is determined during the disaster mitigation to meet the medical needs of the affected population. An emerging issue regarding health-care facility disaster response is the need for a community-based network of local health-care providers. This network ensures the continuation of health-care operations if the infrastructure is damaged during the disaster.

Specific key components are essential for the development of a facility surge plan. Efforts begin with discharging the less acutely ill persons. Those who can be managed as an outpatient are released to create space for disaster victims. Elective procedures are canceled until the surge plan is deactivated. The events may call for additional beds being placed in predetermined locations and conversion of inpatients to hold multiple individuals. Supplemental staff is essential to carry out mass casualty care. Each facility should develop a plan to call back staff for additional shifts to meet the needs of the community. During a surge, hospitals and clinics work with the same amount of supplies as they would under normal daily function. Equipment and pharmaceutical resource management requires conserving and rationing until additional supplies are delivered to the health-care organization from local, state, or federal stockpiles.

The network of health-care providers must derive a unified plan for greater levels of surge. The need to share equipment and resources may arise during event mitigation. Documented agreements on the procedure used to distribute medical resources need to be established at a local level during the planning phase. Established procedures to call up facility volunteers should also be arranged during the planning phase and authority granted to a member of the chain of command to activate the volunteers. The need to provide rapid care to large numbers of patients often requires relaxed documentation, an increased staff-to-patient ratio, and reduced testing procedures. Documentation protocols would be developed and exercised during the planning phase by all staff and volunteers. Documentation should coincide with local, state, and national norms to increase the ease in transfer of patient-related information.

Training and Exercises

Training exercises should be established with local and internal personnel. Each facility must plan to the capacity of the organization, and then provide disaster continuing education to all staff members and volunteers. Disaster plans and training are most effective when internal personnel and organizational stakeholders participate in the design process. The materials used for training must be specific to the surge plan established by the organization and easily accessible by all involved persons. A key factor involved in training exercises is the development of a structure that maintains organizational function and prevents confusion or poor communication among the responders. Training exercises scheduled at regular intervals provide continuing education for new and senior staff and allow for staff evaluation of surge mitigation effectiveness (Fig. 25-4). Problems that arise during a disaster drill must be addressed and incorporated into a new plan appropriate for the institution.

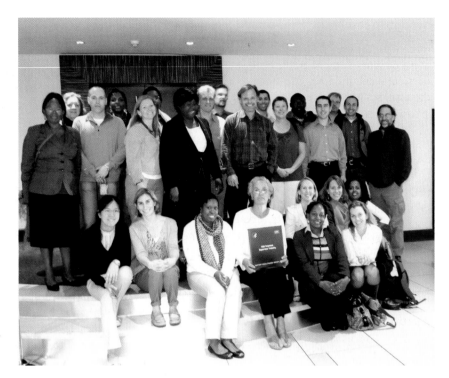

Figure 25-4 This was a group photograph captured at the Center for Global Health's (CGH) Overseas Supervisor Training seminar. The gathering took place during the 2012 South African Regional Training meeting. *(From the CDC, Nasheka Powell, photograph by Yvonne Green, RN, CNM, MSN.)*

● APPLYING PUBLIC HEALTH SCIENCE

The Case of the Chemical Ka Boom

Public Health Science Topics Covered:

- Health planning
  - Instituting a EPDM plan
- Managing a surge

During the EPDM planning process for his community John, a nurse working at the emergency department (ED) at the larger (urban) hospital in the community, volunteered to be a member of the command staff at the hospital in the event of a disaster affecting his community. While working in the ED, John received a call that there had just been an explosion at a local chemical plant located 15 miles from his hospital. It was midday and all of the plant employees were in the building during the time of the event. The buildings and surrounding structures had suffered great damage. Unknown chemicals had been released into the atmosphere. Emergency responders were on the scene to evacuate the uninjured and transport the injured to local health-care facilities, taking the most severely injured to John's ED.

John's hospital received a call that there were mass casualties, with many of the injured in need of medical care. The command team activated the surge plan. Additional personnel and volunteers were activated to respond to the institution. Each of the trained staff in the ED responded by performing his or her specific role in the process. These roles varied from triaging, determining which patients were safe to treat and discharge and which needed immediate medical treatment, to actually delivery of care. John was assigned to organizing the mass treatment areas inside the facility.

In this case, John also established a decontamination zone as a priority given the chemical nature of the event. As patients arrived at the ED, triage personnel directed the individuals through a rapid registration and triage process before moving patients to the appropriate area for treatment and/or decontamination. Internal and communitywide communication flowed through the command team. External coordinators of the disaster's aftermath determined the status of the various health-care facilities and the extent of patient casualties still requiring medical treatment. Of particular concern was the possibility that community members not directly affected by the explosion may have had complications from the release of chemicals into the air and would also need treatment. John prepared the staff for a possible influx of walk-in patients and made sure the staff followed the same process for these patients as those transported via medical responders. John and his team continued to work, following the plan, scaling up or down based on the volume of influx, until all was clear for the surge to be deactivated.

Finally, John noted that the surge of patients had slowed, all victims were accounted for, and those who needed it were receiving medical treatment. Decreasing the surge response began as soon as John was notified that the rapid influx of patients had ceased. One responsibility of being a team leader is to continuously communicate the needs of the surge to staff and patients. Also, ongoing communication to victim family members is crucial during a disaster scenario.

Once the disaster was over and the hospital had returned to normal daily functions, John led a quality improvement meeting. The purpose of the quality improvement effort was to collaboratively decide the functions that worked effectively and those in need of enhancement. The effectiveness of population disaster care for a health-care facility in an event such as this would be directly related to the level of preparedness and the amount of training received by the staff and volunteers.

Disaster Communication

Communication is central to disaster planning and mitigation. Natural and man-made events are frequently accompanied by power outages, damage to telephone towers, and interference in cell phone communication, which present challenges to responders and victims. It is critical that multiple agencies have the ability to exchange information rapidly during and after the impact regardless of the technological limitations. Furthermore, communication with the affected population must clearly emphasize the potential for disaster-related illness and injury as an event approaches without creating panic. Population communication educates individuals and families as to the appropriate actions necessary to prevent disaster-related morbidity and mortality.

Risk Communications

Risk communication is an interactive process involving individuals, groups, and institutions through the exchange of information regarding the nature, magnitude, significance, control, and management of the an associated public health risk.[54] The use of risk communication

principles assists the communicator in identifying the strengths and weaknesses of various communication outlets and maximizing the outreach potential of each. Disasters are associated with fear, confusion, anger, and worry. These emotions prevent individuals from comprehending complex messages. Thus, the use of clear, concise, and easy-to-understand messages is essential in the communication of information to a population confronted with a disaster.

The two main goals of risk communication are to decrease the mental noise associated with a disaster event and establish trust among the affected population. When a person is in a state of high concern, the ability to process information is severely impaired. During a disaster, individuals experience a wide range of emotions ranging from fear to anger. The mental agitation generated from strong feelings and emotions is known as *mental noise* and can interfere with the ability to engage in rational communication. Further complicating an individual's ability to comprehend information during a disaster is the level of trust people in an affected community have in the person or persons communicating the information. The establishment of trust is essential in all risk communication strategies. It helps to decrease the mental noise experienced by the affected population. Only after trust has been established can other goals, such as disaster event education and mitigation principles, be accomplished.

Four main factors must be engaged to develop and maintain trust among the population. Risk communication must be caring and empathetic, portray dedication and commitment to the population, demonstrate competence and expertise, and be honest and open.[54] Community leaders should identify individuals or groups that have a high level of trust with the population prior to an event and seek their expert opinion during a crisis situation. Such groups typically include citizen groups, health-care providers, safety professionals, scientists, and educators. For example, building on The Case of the Impending Storm, one of the stakeholders included in the team was the local fire chief. He was well respected by the community. He was chosen as the spokesperson for promotion of the plan to the community as well as the point person for all media communication during and immediately following a disaster. It is essential that those who are communicating the information are all in agreement on the information being communicated. Trust decreases when there is a disagreement between experts and communication can break down. For example, if there is a lack of organization coordination, then multiple messages are released that can contain conflicting information. The best choice for a spokesperson is one with the ability to engage in sensitive and effective listening. In addition, leaders must be willing to acknowledge the risks and disclose information. During the severe acute respiratory syndrome outbreak, China withheld information related to the severity of the outbreak, thus delaying global efforts needed to prevent a pandemic.

Emotions and fear surge when communities are faced with crisis situations and disaster events and effective communication can reduce panic responses that occur related to fear and misinformation. Population risk communication is often viewed as the most important component of disaster mitigation and receives the greatest attention during the preparedness process. The seven rules of population risk communication are used by public officials to guide their communication strategies (Box 25-8).[54] A well-prepared leader has arranged what he or she will communicate and has practiced communication techniques prior to the occurrence of an event by anticipating the information that will be pertinent to the population. An excellent example is Mayor Rudy Giuliani during the September 11 attack on the World Trade Center. After the 1993 bombing of the World Trade Center, Mayor Giuliani, who took office in 1994, sought training in risk communication and prepared for the possibility of another disaster event. His preparation paid off, providing the citizens of New York with clear communications that helped to reduce panic.

Social and Mass Media Systems

The technological advancements of the 21st century that have made the rapid exchange of information possible have revolutionized disaster communications.[55,56] Social and mass media systems such as the Internet, Twitter, Facebook, and other social networking sites increase the communication outreach potential of public health providers. Using both traditional (television and radio) and newer social media sources is an important component of disaster communication.

BOX 25–8	**Seven Rules of Risk Communication**

1. Accept and involve the public as a legitimate partner.
2. Plan carefully and evaluate your efforts.
3. Listen to the public's specific concerns.
4. Be honest, frank, and open.
5. Coordinate and collaborate with other credible sources.
6. Meet the needs of the media.
7. Speak clearly and with compassion.

Source: See reference 54.

Disaster events occur in rapid progression and population communication must follow quickly. Media messages must be consistent across the various communication sources and answer the most frequently asked questions. Media messages must include information regarding what has happened, what is being done to resolve the issues, when and why it happened, if it will happen again, and actions that should be taken by community members. For example, the Japan tsunami (March 2011) provided an example of the application of social and mass media systems to disaster communications. Japan's highly advanced early warning system proved key in saving lives, but greatly underestimated the likely height of the tsunami and people perished by failing to evacuate to higher ground. Many failed to receive updated warnings about the tsunami height when local relays such as community wireless speakers were damaged by the earthquake or disabled by power cuts. A major social media and technical emergency response provided a vital information lifeline to survivors, but was blunted by the large-scale power blackouts, the disruption of mobile telecommunications networks, and the demographics of the disaster that affected coastal areas where 30% of the population is over 60 years old and less accustomed to accessing information online.

Emergency Alert System

The Emergency Alert System (EAS) is a national public warning system in the United States managed by the Federal Communication Commission in conjunction with FEMA, and the NWS. The EAS requires all radio and television broadcasters to provide population-level communication during an emergency. Emergency alerts can be activated by state and local authorities for use during serve weather conditions. The U.S. president has sole discretion over use at a national level. An audible siren is accompanied by broadcasted instructions during an emergency. The NWS develops the weather-related information and disseminates pertinent instructions about dangerous conditions to the affected community. System effectiveness is established and maintained through routine drills and exercises conducted on state, local, and national levels.

Population Communication With Limited Technology

Interruption to landline telephones and electronic communication devices such as cell phones is likely to occur during a disaster. Planning for this disruption in standard communication is an essential communication concept for emergency responders. Emergency telecommunication systems must be established prior to the loss of function or a call volume overload. Cellular telephones are the telecommunication network of choice during a disaster. These wireless systems can also experience an overload, limiting the capabilities available for emergency responders. Organizations must create an emergency backup communication system designed for activation following technological failure. An illustration of communication devices that support disaster mitigation includes handheld radios, wireless Internet devices, satellite phones, and beeper paging systems.

Public Health Law

Public health laws grant the authority for federal organizations to provide resources and expertise to state, local, and private institutions during planning, direction, and delivery of health-care services. The Pandemic and All-Hazards Preparedness Act, passed in 2006, and reauthorized in March 2013, amended the Public Health Service Act to require the Secretary of Health and Human Services (HHS) to lead all federal public health and medical responses to public health emergencies.[57] Included in this legislation are many requirements to improve the ability of the nation to respond to a public health or medical disaster or emergency, such as the creation of the office of the Assistant Secretary for Preparedness and Response (ASPR) and the requirement to establish a near real-time, electronic, nationwide public health situational awareness capability to enhance early detection of, rapid response to, and management of potentially catastrophic infectious disease outbreaks and other public health emergencies. This legislation also tasked HHS/ASPR to disseminate novel and best practices of outreach to, and care of, at-risk individuals before, during, and following public health emergencies.[57]

Proposed Model State Acts

Following the events of September 11, the National Governors Association, the National Conference of State Legislatures, the Association of State and Territorial Health Officials, and the National Association of County and City Health Officials recognized the need to revamp state public health laws to increase the ability of states to deal with a public health crisis. A few states, either through their statutes or administrative regulations, adopted legal frameworks to deal with a bioterrorist attack. Most, however, lacked a legal response framework, or had only outdated or inadequate measures in place.[58] The Center for Law and the Public's Health at Georgetown and Johns Hopkins Universities drafted a model law, the Model State Emergency Health Powers Act (MSEHPA or Model Act), to give state governments a clear legal framework for dealing with a public health crisis, particularly one caused by an act of bioterrorism. The Model Act is one that states are free to adopt or not, and to amend in any way they wish.

The Model Act grants to the governor of the state the power to declare a public health emergency in the event of a bioterrorist attack (and some other types of events such as a chemical attack or a nuclear accident). The declaration of the public health emergency would give the state health department (or other designated state agency) certain powers during the duration of the public health emergency. The Model Act is structured to reflect five basic public health functions to be facilitated by law: (1) *preparedness,* comprehensive planning for a public health emergency; (2) *surveillance,* measures to detect and track public health emergencies; (3) *management of property,* ensuring adequate availability of vaccines, pharmaceuticals, and hospitals as well as providing power to abate hazards to the public's health; (4) *protection of persons,* powers to compel vaccination, testing, treatment, isolation, and quarantine when clearly necessary; and (5) *communication,* providing clear and authoritative information to the public. The Model Act also contains a modernized, extensive set of principles and requirements to safeguard personal rights. An analysis shows that 41 states have adopted at least some portion of the Model Act, as of August 1, 2011. (For a list of states adopting all or part of the Model Act, visit http://www.networkforphl.org/_asset/80p3y7/MSEHPA-States-TableFINAL.pdf.)

Following hurricanes Katrina and Rita (in 2005), the Uniform Laws Commission proposed the Uniform Emergency Volunteer Health Practitioners Act (UEVHPA).[59] Its scope is more limited than MSEHPA. Generally, the UEVHPA would provide some protection from civil liability for volunteer emergency health-care providers and allow volunteer emergency health-care providers to work in states other than where they are licensed.

Legal Considerations: Quarantine and Evacuation

The process of disaster management can interfere with the civil liberties of an individual. State and local legislation supports disaster planning and grants legal authority to responding agencies and organizations to interfere with normal social functions and force individuals to take action they may not want to do, such as mandatory evacuations or quarantine. Legislation is specific to the function of the responding agency. For example, disaster laws define law enforcement procedures and actions during a bioterrorism event and specific public health functions when considering a quarantine order. Although voluntary actions are encouraged during a disaster, such as individual isolation or prophylactic medication administration, there are times when individuals are required to take the action whether they wish to or not. Thus, the principle of public health, that the public's good overrides individual rights, is very much in play during a disaster. However, quarantine must be addressed legally to prepare for events that lack community voluntary compliance. The need for mandated actions arises during planning for disaster mitigation that requires comprehensive legislative support. National public health laws serve as a guide to state and local officials that can be altered to meet the needs of the community.

Health-care providers have an ethical obligation to prevent the spread of communicable disease within a community. Isolation of infectious individuals is a voluntary process that offers the least restrictive form of transmission prevention. Physicians and public health officials have the authority to institute a legal quarantine if individuals refuse voluntary isolation. **Quarantine** is a compulsory act that mandates infected persons to remain confined to a home or health-care institution. Legal issues associated with involuntary confinement arise during a mandated quarantine, which require judicial review, typically within 48 hours of initiation. Quarantine preparedness actions involve the development of legislation at the local and state levels, granting the authority to institute short-term quarantine when warranted.[18] Health officials must consider the best interest of the community, while respecting individual autonomy, when considering isolation or quarantine.

Evacuation, as with quarantine, begins as a voluntary action following a recommendation from public health officials. Levels of evacuation can vary from single buildings to a large-scale population event. Buildings with known contamination from communicable disease warrant the need for a small-scale evacuation. However, an infectious outbreak of a highly virulent agent could require a large-scale population evacuation. Severe weather warning systems provide evacuation recommendations through the EAS, prompting individuals and families to leave prior to impact. Mandatory evacuation becomes an important action when community members refuse voluntary evacuation.[18] These situations require strategic legal planning prior to a disaster event.

The case of anthrax used as a bioterrorism agent provides a clear illustration of the importance of public health isolation and quarantine. One confirmed case of anthrax exposure is considered an outbreak. Isolation can begin as a voluntary action by the source patient. A physician or public health official can mandate quarantine if the infected individual refuses voluntary isolation. Community-based isolation could be necessary if a greater percentage of the population becomes infected. Voluntary evacuation of a contaminated house or building is a primary prevention action taken to protect uninfected community members from contracting disease. As with quarantine, legally mandated evacuation can be ordered if individuals refuse to voluntarily evacuate a contaminated building or geographical location. Protecting a population from harm is a core function of the public health service and must remain the central focus when considering quarantine or evacuation. Proactive disaster planning, with emphasis on legal preparation, can decrease the overall burden created when individual civil liberties are disrupted.

Vulnerable Populations and Disaster

Some groups in society are more prone than others to damage, loss, and suffering in the context of differing disaster events. The poor, racial and ethnic minorities, immigrants and nonnative speakers, women, children, older adults, and persons with disabilities have all been identified as among those most at risk for the adverse impacts of disaster.[60] Although these groups differ in many ways, they demonstrate similarities in that they often lack access to vital economic and social resources, have limited autonomy and power, and have low levels of social capital. These groups of individuals often live and work in the most hazardous regions and in the lowest-quality buildings, thus further exposing them to risks associated with natural hazards.[61]

Demographic characteristics not limited to socioeconomic status, race, gender, age, and disability frequently intersect in complex ways that may increase the vulnerability of any given member of a social group. During the past decade, there has been some movement away from simple taxonomies or checklists of vulnerable groups to vulnerable *situations*. This approach adds a vital temporal and geographical dimension to examining vulnerability and the social contexts and circumstances in which people live.[60] Cutter and colleagues did extensive work to help determine how much of the variability in risk was accounted for by certain social and environmental factors. They found that such things as age, stage of development, and economic status increased risk (Box 25-9).[62]

BOX 25–9	**Factors Associated With Social Vulnerability**

The eleven factors at the county level associated with social vulnerability to environmental hazards that accounts for more than 75% of the variance in risk include the following:

- Age
- Racial and ethnic disparities
- Occupation
- Personal wealth
- Housing stock and tenancy
- Density of the built environment
- Single-sector economic dependence
- Infrastructure dependence
- Persons with disabilities

Source: See reference 62.

When trying to understand why disasters happen and who is affected most, it is crucial to recognize that natural events are not the only cause. As discussed earlier, disasters are the product of social, political, and economic environments that structure the lives and life chances of different groups of people. The capacity for resiliency following a disaster varies based on the population and the environment.[60,61] Certain populations are more vulnerable to disease and injury and less apt to recover physically, socially, and economically from the impact of a large-scale disaster. Persons that are poor and living in poverty are among those at greatest risk for adversity following a large-scale disaster. The poor are at greater risk for decreased health, homelessness, long-term displacement, and death.[63]

Children

Children are at special risk for increased morbidity and mortality from disaster events because of their size, anatomy and physiology, and their developmental status. Owing to the increased potential for injury and disease, public and emergency health-care providers need to be trained in how to communicate at an age-appropriate level for children, the normal child assessment, and pediatric emergency care. Many hospitals are ill prepared to receive and care for severely injured children, and their capacity to accommodate a sudden demand for pediatric care may be limited.[63] Pediatric-specific equipment, supplies, and medications should be available to provide emergent care during the aftermath of a disaster.[63] Children may be separated from their parents as a result of the disaster itself or during the intervention phase when, in an effort to expedite and provide appropriate treatment, parents are separated from their

children. Efforts should be made to keep siblings together as well as ensure the children's security until an adult family member is able to assume custody.

■ EVIDENCE-BASED PRACTICE
Pediatric Triage Tool

Practice Statement: Children affected by a disaster require a specialized triage approach.

Targeted Outcome: Optimize the triage of injured children based on pediatric physiology during a multicasualty incident.

Evidence to Support: The JumpSTART tool was designed to provide an objective framework for identifying the severity of injury in children. The tool acknowledges key differences that exist between pediatric and adult injury victims. It was specifically designed for multicasualty settings and not for ED triage. It is recognized as the gold standard for pediatric triage during disasters. It was designed to take into account the physiological differences between pediatric victims and adult victims. The materials are available online and include a clear algorithm that can be copied and distributed.

Recommended Approaches and Resources:

1. Romig, L. (2013). *The JumpSTART pediatric MCI triage tool*. Retrieved from http://www.jumpstarttriage.com/.
2. Romig, L. (2008). Pediatric triage on-scene in disasters. In G. Foltin, A. Cooper, & M. Trieber (Eds.), *Pediatric disaster preparedness: A resource for planning, management and provision of out-of-hospital emergency care*. New York, NY: Center for Pediatric Emergency Medicine.
3. Kelly, F. (2010). Keeping PEDIATRICS in pediatric disaster management: Before, during and in the aftermath of complex emergencies. *Critical Care Nursing Clinics of North America, 22*, 465-480.

Maternal-Infant

Pregnant and perinatal women and infants are at increased risk during a disaster event. Disasters limit the availability and access to prenatal care, birthing centers, and neonatal care. Following Hurricane Katrina, there were no organized services for pregnant women and neonates. Hospitals with maternity patients and low-birth-weight newborns were evacuated, and many births took place during the disaster in the Louie B. Armstrong New Orleans International Airport without benefit of clean water or electricity.[64]

Older Adults

Older adults are more likely to have one or more non-communicable illnesses such as hypertension, cardiovascular disease, arthritis, and diabetes as well as limitations to mobility. Even with proper disaster planning, older adults may experience complications. They are not as easily able or willing to evacuate as their younger counterparts and they may struggle to adapt to a new environment. Nursing home patients are also at increased risk for poor health and safety outcomes. During the Hurricane Katrina disaster aftermath, nursing home staff worked in understaffed conditions, without air-conditioning during the hot, humid summer month, and with reduced supplies. The older adults were not able to contact their family members who had already evacuated to seek their assistance.[63]

Special Needs Populations

Persons with a mobility or sensory disability may require special assistance during and after a disaster. Persons with a sensory disability have a limitation in the ability to hear (e.g., hard of hearing, deaf) or see (e.g., blind, tunnel vision).[65,66] Persons with a mobility disability include persons with little to no use of their arms or legs.[67] Assistive devices such as walkers, wheelchairs, or scooters may be required for ambulation or movement by persons with a mobility disability.

The person with a mobility or sensory disability may have difficulty evacuating a building structure that is determined to be unsafe (e.g., fire, earthquake). If the person is deaf, the person may need to be notified that a disaster situation has been declared and have instructions provided in writing or sign language. If the disaster is communicated by a strobe light, as with a building fire, or on the bottom ("crawl") of a television screen, as with a tornado warning, the blind will not be aware of the disaster.[18] Communications need to be oral or through the use of sirens or bells along with the strobes and television screens.

Disaster plans should be developed with comprehensive planning efforts to accommodate the needs of these populations. Representatives from vulnerable population groups should be included on disaster planning committees to inform and gain the population's input. Plans should address how individuals can prepare for, evacuate to safety if necessary, and protect themselves on site during the disaster until rescue help arrives when evacuation is not a possibility.[64-66] Disaster drills conducted in advance can test and ensure the plan's feasibility. Plans and drills should take into account both the use of and absence of service animals and assistive devices.

FEMA released *Guidance on Planning for Integration of Functional Needs Support Services in General Population Shelters*, commonly known as the FNSS, in November 2010.[68,69] This guidance is intended to ensure that individuals who have access and functional needs receive lawful and equal assistance before, during, and after public health emergencies and disasters. This guidance can be incorporated into existing shelter plans. It does not establish a new tier of sheltering or alter existing legal obligations. For example, the Americans With Disabilities Act, Fair Housing, and civil rights requirements are not waived in disaster situations, and emergency managers and shelter planners have the responsibility to ensure that sheltering services and facilities are accessible.

Functional Needs Support Services (FNSS) are services that enable individuals with access and functional needs to maintain their independence in a general population shelter. Individuals requiring FNSS may have physical, sensory, mental health, and cognitive and/or intellectual disabilities affecting their ability to function independently without assistance. Others who may benefit from FNSS include women in the late stages of pregnancy, seniors, and people whose body mass requires special equipment.[69]

Advanced planning is essential in order to ensure equal access and services. Making general population shelters accessible to persons with access and functional needs may require additional items and services, including durable medical equipment such as walkers and wheelchairs; consumable medical supplies such as medications and diapers; and personal assistance services.

Plans must also be made for how medical support will be implemented in general population shelters and how to assess when individuals are not appropriate for these settings because of medical needs. It is important for emergency planners and public health officials to know and understand the community's demographic profile in order to ascertain what services and equipment will be needed in an emergency. Meeting with community partners, stakeholders, providers, constituents, and service recipients, including individuals with access and functional needs, will enhance emergency planners' and public health officials' abilities to develop plans that successfully integrate individuals with access and functional needs into general population shelters. In addition, these collaboration efforts will help educate community members with access and functional needs about the importance of personal preparedness plans.[61,68,69]

Incarcerated Populations

U.S. Marshals became a box office hit when it was released by Warner Brothers Entertainment in 1998.

Near the movie's opening sequence, an airplane transporting incarcerated prisoners crash-landed along a small country road, then came to a stop as it rolled upside down into a river. The prisoners who survived the disaster were secured along the river's bank until emergency medical assistance arrived. In a real disaster, such as the Hurricane Katrina disaster, concern was raised about the incarcerated population in New Orleans. Disaster plans need to include both protection of the inmates from the disaster and plans to address possible release of prisoners into the general public. Disasters involving incarcerated prison populations outside the prison pose unique issues for disaster mitigation because the safety of the general public must be considered as well as the safety of the prisoners. Disasters within a prison facility require careful consideration of the safety of first responders.

Mental Health and Disaster

Stress and anxiety occur normally in populations in the aftermath of a disaster. Most often, the symptoms usually resolve within a short time frame depending on the ability of each individual and family to cope with stressful situations. A small percentage of the population will experience severe symptomatology or have symptoms that persist for months or years following the disaster event.

Mental Health Disorders Following Disaster

Acute stress disorder (ASD) and post-traumatic stress disorder (PTSD) are mental health disorders that are experienced following a stressful event such a disaster.[70,71] Criteria for ASD and PTSD include exposure to a specific event that causes a sense of fear, helplessness, or horror. Persons experiencing the stress disorders may also have flashbacks or recurrent images of the trauma; actively avoid reminders of the trauma; and/or are in a hyperarousal state that affects their startle response, sleep, and concentration. Because the symptomatology of stress disorders may initially be a normal stress response, ASD cannot be diagnosed until the symptoms have persisted for at least 2 days. After 1 month of persistent symptoms, affected persons will be diagnosed with PTSD. Many victims of complex human emergencies experience PTSD.[3]

Somatization occurs to persons experiencing psychological stress and the absence of a physical problem to explain their symptoms.[63] Survivors of disasters may develop a variety of somatic symptoms affecting their neurological, digestive, and immune systems. Symptoms may include abdominal pain, back pain, chest pain, diarrhea, headaches, impotence, and vomiting.[72]

The mental health consequences of stress and somatization primarily affect survivors of a disaster in varying degrees. Other groups affected by a disaster are the friends and relatives of disaster victims, the first responders, health-care providers who participate in disaster-related activities, and community members who either believe they are at risk for a similar disaster or empathize with the disaster victims.[73–78] Other persons reported as being at higher risk for the development of PTSD are those who knew someone who worked, was injured, or died at the site of a disaster. Factors that contribute to risk for PTSD are seeing dead bodies or body bags and being disturbed by the smells emanating from the disaster site.[79,80] The negative mental health effects may last only a few days or may persist for years.

The occurrence of negative psychological reactions varies across affected populations. Negative reactions are most common for children and adolescents; persons living in a developing country; those who experience a violence-related disaster (e.g., terrorism); females; ethnic minorities; people living in poverty or at a low socioeconomic status; those who have a preexisting mental disease or disorder; and those individuals lacking a support system. Although these population groups have a greater risk, anyone who directly or indirectly experiences a disaster (e.g., family members of disaster victims) may be at psychological risk.

Stress Among Health-Care Workers

Health-care workers, including community/public health nurses (PHNs), are at risk for experiencing negative stress related to rendering postdisaster care. Nurses may experience secondary traumatic stress as a result of their caring, compassion, and empathy with disaster victims. Secondary traumatic stress is a psychological stress disorder that mimics ASD and PTSD, except the symptoms are a direct result of the caregiving experience and not a result of being the disaster victim.[76,77] Nurses identified as experiencing secondary traumatic stress need to be referred to employee assistance programs or other professional or community services to receive interventions that can help the nurses to protect their mental health.

Mental Health Interventions

Psychological and psychosocial interventions need to be initiated with persons experiencing negative mental health consequences of a disaster. Interventions have been identified at the level of the individual, family, neighborhood, community, and society that may protect their mental health.[81,82] Individual-level interventions include religious affiliation, maintenance of a normal routine, traditional healing, clinical treatment, play therapy, and cognitive behavioral therapy. Family-level interventions include family self-help networks and family education. Community-level interventions include capacity building, public education, service coordination, and religion-related social interactions such as a mass gathering for prayer or worship.[83-85]

Nurses can apply specific strategies for identifying persons at risk for and exhibiting ASD/PTSD following a disaster.[86,87] Referrals should be made to primary care providers, mental health specialists, and community resources that are able to provide diagnostic testing and mental health care for affected persons. There are a number of community mental health resources that can be used to assist with potential mental health issues following a disaster. Debriefing and counseling are additional interventions that can be offered to the survivors and responders in individual or group sessions following a disaster as soon as feasible. Although it is prudent to offer debriefing and counseling, offering the interventions immediately following the disaster event may worsen future symptomatology. It may be more beneficial to offer the interventions 2 to 3 days after the disaster.[87] In addition, not everyone will be able to participate in these interactive interventions because of the risk for further trauma by having to relive the disaster experience.

Interventions for the mental health consequences associated with disaster start as soon as the awareness of an impending disaster is known. Even though advance warning may occur prior to some natural disasters such as hurricanes and blizzards, the public may not be adequately prepared for the devastation, lack of resources, and isolation that occur during the immediate aftermath of a natural, technological, or man-made disaster.

Disaster Management, Ethics, and Culture

During a disaster, ethics often comes to the forefront. Decisions have to be made that may result in choosing whom to rescue and how to prioritize the response. In addition, there are a multitude of nongovernmental organizations that respond to disasters, some of which are well known, such as the International Red Cross and Oxfam America and Oxfam International. Often during a disaster, it is assumed that anything done under the umbrella of charitable work is acceptable. However, the ethics decisions made by these responders must be looked at from the broader ethical perspective.

In 2010, a group of church members from the United States were arrested for attempting to transport children

from Haiti into the Dominican Republic following the Haiti earthquake. They initially stated that the children were orphans, but it soon became apparent that some of the children still had living parents. Had the church workers attempted to kidnap the children? Had they coerced the parents into giving up the children with the promise of a better life for the children? The church members were eventually let out of prison and returned to the United States. Their case demonstrates that persons who are attempting to provide assistance during a disaster can end up making decisions without thinking through the ethics of their actions or understanding the culture of the people they are trying to help.

When a disaster occurs, the immediacy of the situation can result in nongovernmental agencies putting pressure on themselves, which results in short-sighted efforts that ignore the culture of the people in distress. In 1994, six of the world's largest nongovernmental relief agencies established a code of ethics (Box 25-10). It is not a binding code, but rather one that is voluntary and helps guide charities providing disaster relief. The code is made up of 10 principal commitments,

BOX 25–10 **Principles of Conduct for the International Red Cross and Red Crescent Movement and NGOs in Disaster Response Programs**

1. The humanitarian imperative comes first.
2. Aid is given regardless of the race, creed or nationality of the recipients and without adverse distinction of any kind. Aid priorities are calculated on the basis of need alone.
3. Aid will not be used to further a particular political or religious standpoint.
4. We shall endeavor not to act as instruments of government foreign policy.
5. We shall respect culture and custom.
6. We shall attempt to build disaster response on local capacities.
7. Ways shall be found to involve program beneficiaries in the management of relief aid
8. Relief aid must strive to reduce future vulnerabilities to disaster as well as meeting basic needs.
9. We hold ourselves accountable to both those we seek to assist and those from whom we accept resources.
10. In our information, publicity and advertising activities, we shall recognize disaster victims as dignified human beings, not hopeless objects.

Source: See reference 88.

beginning with the commitment that "the humanitarian imperative comes first."[88] The principles include respect for culture and the commitment to build on local capacities.

During a disaster, difficult choices are made when resources are scarce. As demonstrated in the 2010 Haiti earthquake disaster, in the first week there was a scarcity of water and food. When water and food arrived, choices were made to provide women and children with water first. A good EPDM plan includes a process for priority setting. Who will get medical assistance, those who are the most ill or those who are healthier and apt to have a longer life span? Answering these questions require a systems approach that includes organizations and policy makers and should occur during the planning phase.[61] According to Stone, a moral framework that begins at the community level is needed to address the needs of vulnerable and marginalized populations. This framework should be built on the concepts of social justice.[89]

Not only is EPDM a key component to health care today, but ethics plays a big role in the development and execution of EPDM plans. Natural and man-made disasters have taken untold lives over the history of mankind. In our modern world we have increased our capacity to respond quickly to disasters and through prevention, preparedness, mitigation, and recovery we can reduce the short- and long-term adverse affects of disasters more effectively than ever before. However, increasing our capacity has also increased the ethical issues confronting responders.[89] EPDM requires a culturally grounded plan that addresses the hard choices that have to be made in a way that provides the greatest help to the greatest number and includes all those affected.

Healthy People 2020

Because of the increased awareness of the need for preparedness in the event of a disaster, *Healthy People 2020* added a new objective, Preparedness. It is built on the National Health Security Strategy released in 2009. This strategy was developed to help pull together the various approaches to EPDM so that the nation as a whole can prepare for and respond in the event of a disaster. The goal is to reduce the impact on health. The inclusion of preparedness reflects the commitment the nation has made in the years since September 11, 2001, and Hurricane Katrina to improve our ability to prepare for and respond to disasters both natural and man-made.

■ HEALTHY PEOPLE 2020

Targeted Topic: Preparedness
Goal: Improve the nation's ability to prevent, prepare for, respond to, and recover from a major health incident
Overview: Preparedness involves government agencies, nongovernmental organizations, the private sector, communities, and individuals working together to improve the nation's ability to prevent, prepare for, respond to, and recover from a major health incident. The *Healthy People 2020* objectives for preparedness are based on a set of national priorities articulated in the *National Health Security Strategy of the United States of America (NHSS)*. The overarching goals of NHSS are to build community resilience and to strengthen and sustain health and emergency response systems.
Source: See references 90 and 91.

■ Summary Points

- Preparedness and sound disaster planning can provide a community with the ability to respond effectively to both man-made and natural disasters.
- Disaster epidemiological surveillance provides early recognition and identification of infectious disease outbreaks.
- Nurses should play a key role in the planning phase, contribute to prevention efforts related to disasters, and provide needed services that help mitigate the effects of a disaster. They are essential to the response and recovery phases of a disaster.
- Effective communication throughout the disaster continuum will help to mitigate the adverse effects of the disaster.
- Vulnerable populations require special consideration in emergency preparedness and disaster management planning.
- There are acute and long-term mental health issues following a disaster.

▲ CASE STUDY
Flooding and the Older Adult
Learning Outcomes:

By the end of this case, the student will be able to:

- Gain understanding of how to participate in the emergency and disaster management process

- Describe the challenges encountered when planning for a major natural disaster
- Identify functional needs support services needed related to a specific subset of the population

A local 200-bed nursing home has been ordered to evacuate because of its location in a flood plain. Many of the residents require oxygen and have a mobility disability. More than half of the patients suffer from Alzheimer's disease. You are the nursing director in the public health department and part of the communitywide team responsible for the community's EPDM plan. The community is located along a major river. It has never flooded before but a hundred-year flood has been predicted. When you review the community's plan, you find that the nursing home was not included in it. You call the team together and point out that they must be ready to include the nursing home in their plan before the water starts rising.

1. Design a disaster plan in the event that the nursing home experiences a flood and needs to be evacuated. Questions to address include:
   a. What members are essential for the planning committee?
   b. How will residents be notified of the need for evacuation?
   c. Where will residents be relocated?
   d. How will residents be relocated?
   e. How will the relocation of residents be tracked?
   f. What items need to be relocated with the residents?
2. How will you address the following issues?
   a. A resident with a sensory disability
   b. A resident with a mobility disability
   c. A resident requiring continuous oxygen
   d. A resident with no limitations or special needs
   e. How will residents be notified of the need for evacuation?
   f. Where will the residents be relocated?
   g. How will residents be relocated?
   h. How will the relocation of residents be tracked?
   i. What items need to be relocated with the residents? .

Finally, identify how the plan will differ based on time from notification for facility evacuation and the time that evacuation needs to be completed (e.g., 1 day's warning vs. 1 hour's warning).

REFERENCES

1. International Federation of Red Cross and Red Crescent Societies. (2010). *World disasters report 2010: Focus on urban risk.* Geneva, Switzerland: Author.
2. Khan, O., & Pappas, G. (2011). *Megacities and global health.* Washington, DC: American Public Health Association.
3. Burkle, F. (2007). Complex humanitarian emergencies. In D.E. Hogan & J.L. Burstein (Eds.), *Disaster medicine* (pp. 86-94). Philadelphia, PA: Lippincott Williams & Wilkins.
4. International Federation of Red Cross and Red Crescent Societies. (2012). *World disasters report 2010: Focus on forced migration and displacement urban risk.* Geneva, Switzerland: Author.
5. Jennex, M.E. (Ed.). (2011). *Crisis response and management and emerging information systems: Critical applications.* Hershey, PA: IGI Global.
6. Noji, E.K. (Ed.). (1996). *The public health consequences of disasters.* New York, NY: Oxford University Press.
7. Bissell, R.A., Pinet, L., Nelson, M., & Levy, M. (2004). Evidence of the effectiveness of health sector preparedness in disaster response: The example of four earthquakes. *Family & Community Health, 27*(3), 193-203.
8. Noji, E.K. (2005). Disasters: Introduction and state of the art. *Epidemiologic Reviews, 27*(1), 3-8.
9. Noji, E.K. (2005). Public health in the aftermath of disasters. *BMJ, 330*(7504), 1379-1381.
10. Veenema, T.G. (2011). Disaster preparedness 10 years after 9/11. *American Journal of Nursing, 111*(9), 7.
11. Veenema, T.G., & Toke, J. (2007). When standards of care change in mass-casualty events. *American Journal of Nursing, 107*(9), 72A-72F.
12. Veenema, T.G. (Ed.). (2012). *Disaster nursing and emergency preparedness for chemical, biological, and radiological terrorism and other hazards* (3rd ed.). New York, NY: Springer.
13. Rodriguez, H., & Aguirre, B.E. (2006). Hurricane Katrina and the healthcare infrastructure: A focus on disaster preparedness, response, and resiliency. *Frontiers of Health Services Management, 23*(1), 13.
14. Stimpson, J.P., Wilson, F.A., & Jeffries, S.K. (2008). Seeking help for disaster services after a flood. *Disaster Medicine and Public Health Preparedness, 2*(3), 139-141.
15. Institute of Medicine. (2009). *Guidance for establishing crisis standards of care for use in disaster situations: A letter report.* Retrieved from http://www.iom.edu.
16. Koenig, K.L., Cone, D.C., Burstein, J.L., & Camargo, C.A, Jr. (2006). Surging to the right standard of care. *Academic Emergency Medicine, 13*(2), 195-198.
17. Landesman, L., & Morrow, C. (2008). Roles and responsibilities of public health in disaster preparedness and response. In F. Novick, C. Morrow, & G. Mays (Eds.), *Public health administration: Principles for population-based management* (pp. 657-714). Sudbury, MA: Jones & Bartlett.

18. Landesman, L.Y. (2011). *Public health management of disasters: The practice guide* (3rd ed.). Washington, DC: American Public Health Association.

19. Centers for Disease Control and Prevention. (2013). *Emergency preparedness and response.* Retrieved from http://www.bt.cdc.gov/.

20. Rowitz, L. (2005). *Public health for the 21st century: The prepared leader.* Sudbury, MA: Jones & Bartlett.

21. Koh, H.K., Shei, A.C., Bataringaya, J., Burstein, J., Biddinger, P.D., Crowther, M.S., et al. (2006). Building community-based surge capacity through a public health and academic collaboration: The role of community health centers. *Public Health Reports, 121*(2), 211.

22. Kaji, A.H., Langford, V., & Lewis, R.J. (2008). Assessing hospital disaster preparedness: A comparison of an on-site survey, directly observed drill performance, and video analysis of teamwork. *Annals of Emergency Medicine, 52*(3), 195-201.

23. Hsu, E.B., Jenckes, M.W., Catlett, C.L., Robinson, K.A., Feuerstein, C., Cosgrove, S.E., & Bass, E.B. (2004). Effectiveness of hospital staff mass-casualty incident training methods: A systematic literature review. *Prehospital and Disaster Medicine, 19*(03), 191-200.

24. Thomas, T.L., Hsu, E.B., Kim, H.K., Colli, S., Arana, G., & Green, G.B. (2005). The incident command system in disasters: evaluation methods for a hospital-based exercise. *Prehospital and Disaster Medicine, 20*(01), 14-23.

25. Auf der Heide, E. (2006). The importance of evidence-based disaster planning. *Annals of Emergency Medicine, 47*(1), 34.

26. Rains, A.B. (2012). Information technology in disaster management. In T. Veenema (Ed.), *Disaster nursing and emergency preparedness for chemical, biological, and radiological terrorism and other hazards* (3rd ed.). New York, NY: Springer.

27. Centers for Disease Control and Prevention. (2013). *National notifiable diseases surveillance system.* Retrieved from http://wwwn.cdc.gov/nndss/script/nedss.aspx.

28. Waring, S., & Brown, B. (2005). The threat of communicable disease following natural disasters: A public health response. *Disaster Management and Response,* 3(2), 41–47. DOI: 10.1016/j.dmr.2005.02.003.

29. National Weather Service. (2013). *Glossary.* Retrieved from http://w1.weather.gov/glossary/.

30. National Weather Service. (2013). *Tropical cyclones.* Retrieved from http://www.nws.noaa.gov/os/hurricane/resources/TropicalCyclones11.pdf.

31. National Weather Service. (2013). *National Hurricane Center.* Retrieved from http://www.nhc.noaa.gov.

32. United Nations Office for Disaster Reduction (n.d.). *2012 Disaster in numbers.* Retrieved from http://www.preventionweb.net/files/31685_factsheet2012.pdf.

33. Federal Emergency Management Agency. (2013). *Earthquakes.* Retrieved from http://www.fema.gov/earthquake.

34. Centers for Disease Control and Prevention. (2012). *Emergency preparedness and response: Extreme heat.* Retrieved from http://emergency.cdc.gov/disasters/extremeheat/heat_guide.asp.

35. Federal Emergency Management Agency. (2013). *Dealing with extreme heat.* Retrieved March 20, 2013, from http://www.fema.gov/news-release/2012/08/15/dealing-extreme-heat.

36. National Weather Service. (2013). *Beat The Heat Weather Ready Nation Campaign.* Retrieved from http://www.nws.noaa.gov/os/heat/index.shtml.

37. Woodruff, R.E., McMichael, T., Butler, C., & Hales, S. (2007). Action on climate change: The health risks of procrastinating. *Australian and New Zealand Journal of Public Health, 30*(6), 567-571.

38. Federal Emergency Management Agency. (2013). *Floods.* Retrieved from http://www.ready.gov/floods.

39. National Weather Service. (2010). *Tornados: Nature's Most Violent Storms.* Retrieved from http://www.nws.noaa.gov/om/brochures/tornado.shtml.

40. Slodkowski, A., & Saito, M. (2013, August 6). *Japan nuclear body says radioactive water at Fukushima an emergency. Reuters.* Retrieved from http://in.reuters.com/article/2013/08/06/us-japan-fukushima-panel-idINBRE97408V20130806.

41. National Oceanic and Atmospheric Administration. (2013). *The Pacific Tsunami Warning Center.* Retrieved from http://ptwc.weather.gov/.

42. Federal Emergency Management Agency. (2103). *Volcanoes.* Retrieved from http://www.ready.gov/volcanoes.

43. Federal Emergency Management Agency. (2013). *Wildfires.* Retrieved from http://www.ready.gov/wildfires.

44. Centers for Disease Control and Prevention. (2012). *Emergency preparedness and response: Wildfires.* Retrieved from http://www.bt.cdc.gov/disasters/wildfires/index.asp.

45. Centers for Disease Control and Prevention. (2012). *Emergency preparedness and response: Worker safety during fire cleanup.* Retrieved from http://www.bt.cdc.gov/disasters/wildfires/cleanupworkers.asp.

46. Centers for Disease Control and Prevention. (2012). *Emergency preparedness and response: Wildfires cleanup.* Retrieved from http://www.bt.cdc.gov/disasters/wildfires/cleanupworkers.asp.

47. Centers for Disease Control and Prevention. (2012). *Explosions and blast injuries: A primer for clinicians.* Retrieved from http://www.bt.cdc.gov/masscasualties/explosions.asp#blast.

48. DePalma, R.G., Burris, D.G., Champion, H.R., & Hodgson, M.J. (2005). Blast injuries. *New England Journal of Medicine, 352*(13), 1335-1342.

49. Federal Emergency Management Agency. (2009). *Hazardous materials.* Retrieved from http://www.fema.gov/hazard/hazmat/index.shtm.

50. Environmental Protection Agency. (2014). *Risk Management Plan (RMP) rule.* Retrieved from http://www2.epa.gov/rmp.

51. Veenema, T.G. (2003). Chemical and biological terrorism preparedness for staff development specialists. *Journal for Nurses in Staff Development, 19*(5), 215.

52. World Health Organization. (2006). *Health effects of the Chernobyl accident and special health care programmes.* Retrieved from http://www.who.int/ionizing_radiation/chernobyl/WHO%20Report%20on%20Chernobyl%20Health%20Effects%20July%2006.pdf.

53. World Health Organization. (2007). *Mass casualty management systems.* Retrieved from http://whqlibdoc.who.int/publications/2007/9789241596053_eng.pdf.

54. Covello, V., Peters, R., Wojtecki, J., & Hyde, R. (2001). Risk communication, the West Nile virus epidemic, and bioterrorism. *Journal of Urban Health, 78*(2), 382-391.

55. Epstein, R., Ekbatani, A., Kaplan, J., Schechter, R., & Grunwald, Z. (2010). Development of a staff recall system for mass casualty using cell phone text messaging. *Anesthesia-Analgesia, 110*(3), 871.

56. Haddow, G., & Haddow, K. (2009). *Disaster communications in a changing media world.* Oxford, England: Butterworth-Heineman.

57. *Pandemic and All Hazards Preparedness Act, Pub. L. No. 109-417 (2006).* Retrieved from http://www.phe.gov/preparedness/legal/pahpa/.

58. Hodge, J.G. (2005). The legal framework for meeting surge capacity through the use of volunteer health professionals during public health emergencies and other disasters. *The Journal of Contemporary Health Law and Policy, 22*(11), 5-71.

59. Department of Health and Human Services. (2013). *The emergency system for advance registration of volunteer health professionals.* Retrieved from http://www.phe.gov/esarvhp/.

60. Warren, R.C., Walker, B., Maclin, S.D., Miles-Richardson, S., Tarver, W., & James, C. (2011). Respecting and protecting the beloved community, especially susceptible and vulnerable populations. *Journal of Health Care for the Poor and Underserved, 22*(3), 3-13. Retrieved from http://search.proquest.com/docview/906064956?accountid=11752.

61. Johns Hopkins Bloomberg School of Public Health (2014). *Human vulnerability to natural disasters.* Retrieved from http://www.jhsph.edu/research/centers-and-institutes/center-for-refugee-and-disaster-response/natural_disasters/.

62. Cutter, S.L., Boruff, B.J., & Shirley, W.L. 2003. Social vulnerability to environmental hazards. *Social Science Quarterly, 84*(2), 242-261.

63. Health Systems Research. (2005). *Altered standards of care in mass casualty events* (AHRQ Publication No. 05-0043). Rockville, MD: Agency for Healthcare Research and Quality. Retrieved from http://www.ahrq.gov/research/altstrand/altstrand.pdf

64. Harville, E.W., Xiong, X., & Buekens, P. (2009). Hurricane Katrina and perinatal health. *Birth, 36*(4), 325-331.

65. Federal Emergency Management Agency, American Red Cross . (2004). *Preparing for disaster for people with disabilities and other special needs* (FEMA Publication No. 476). Washington, DC: Federal Emergency Management Agency. Retrieved from http://www.fema.gov/media-library-data/20130726-1445-20490-6732/fema_476.pdf.

66. National Organization on Disability. (2010). *Disaster readiness tips for people with sensory disabilities* [Pamphlet]. Retrieved from http://www.nod.org/resources/PDFs/epips2sensory.pdf.

67. National Organization on Disability. (2010). *Disaster readiness tips for people with mobility disabilities* [Pamphlet]. Retrieved from http://www.nod.org/resources/PDFs/epips4mobility.pdf.

68. Federal Emergency Management Agency. (2013). *Guidelines for functional needs support services.* Retrieved from http://www.fema.gov/pdf/about/odic/fnss_guidance.pdf.

69. Federal Emergency Management Agency. (2013). *Public Health Emergency. Functional Needs Support Services.* Retrieved from http://www.phe.gov/Preparedness/planning/abc/Pages/funcitonal-needs.aspx.

70. Galea, S., Nandi, A., & Vlahov, D. (2005). The epidemiology of post-traumatic stress disorder after diseases. *Epidemiologic Reviews, 27,* 78-91.

71. Bryant, R.A., & Harvey, A.G. (2000). *Acute stress disorder: A handbook of theory, assessment, and treatment.* Washington, DC: American Psychological Association.

72. Vorvick, L., & Rogge, T.A. (2008). *Somatization disorder.* Retrieved from http://www.nlm.nih.gov/medlineplus/ency/article/000955.htm.

73. Herman, D., Felton, C., & Susser, E. (2002). Mental health needs in New York state following the September 11th attacks. *Journal of Urban Health, 79*(3), 322-331.

74. Giosan, C., Malta, L., Jayasinghe, N., Spielman, L., & Difede, J. (2009). Relationships between memory inconsistency for traumatic events following 9/11 and PTSD in disaster restoration workers. *Journal of Anxiety Disorders, 23,* 557-561.

75. Ketumarn, P., Sitdhiraksa, N., Pithayaratsathien, N., Piyasilpa, V., Plubrukan, R., Dumrongphol, H., et al. (2009). Prevalence of post-traumatic stress disorder in students 23 months after tsunami. *Asian Journal of Psychiatry, 2,* 144-148.

76. Stellman, J.M., Smith, R.P., Katz, C.L., Sharma, V., Charney, D.S., Herbert, R., et al. (2008). Enduring mental health morbidity and social function impairment in World Trade Center rescue, recovery, and cleanup workers: The psychological dimension of an environmental health disaster. *Environmental Health Perspectives, 116*(9), 1248-1253.

77. Gates, D.M., & Gillespie, G.L. (2008). Secondary traumatic stress in nurses who care for women. *Journal of Obstetric, Gynecologic, and Neonatal Nursing, 37*(2), 243-249.

78. Morrissette, P.J. (2004). *The pain of helping: Psychological injury of helping professionals.* New York, NY: Brunner-Routledge.

79. Marshall, R.D., & Suh, E.J. (2003). Contextualizing trauma: Using evidence-based treatments in a multicultural community after 9/11. *Psychiatric Quarterly, 7*(4), 401-420.

80. Mijanovich, T., & Weitzman, B.C. (2009). Disaster in context: The effects of 9/11 on youth distant from the attacks. *Community Mental Health Journal* [Online journal], 1-11. doi:10.1007/s10597-009-9240-5.

81. Brake, H.T., Duckers, M., de Vries, M., van Duin, D., Rooze, M., & Spreeuwenberg, C. (2009). Early psychosocial interventions after disasters, terrorism, and other shocking events: Guideline development. *Nursing and Health Sciences, 11*, 336-343.

82. Norris, F.H., Friedman, M.J., & Watson, P.J. (2002). 60,000 disaster victims speak: Part II. Summary and implications of the disaster mental health research. *Psychiatry, 65*(3), 240-260.

83. Norris, F.H., Friedman, M.J., Watson, P.J., Byrne, C.M., Diaz, E., & Kaniastry, K. (2002). 60,000 disaster victims speak: Part I. An empirical review of the empirical literature, 1981–2001. *Psychiatry, 65*(3), 207-239.

84. Bisson, J.I., Tavakoly, B., Witteveen, A.B., Ajdukovic, D., Jehel, L., Johansen, V.J., & Olff, M. (2010). TENTS guidelines: Development of post-disaster psychosocial care guidelines through a Delphi process. *British Journal of Psychiatry, 196*(1), 69-74.

85. Dugan, E.M., Snow, M.S., & Crowe, S.R. (2010). Working with children affected by Hurricane Katrina: Two case studies in play therapy. *Child and Adolescent Mental Health, 15*(1), 52-55.

86. Meisenhelder, J.B., & Cassem, E.H. (2009). Terrorism, posttraumatic stress, spiritual coping, and mental health. *Journal of Spirituality in Mental Health, 11*(3), 218-230.

87. Demaria, T., Barrett, M., & Ryan, D. (2006). Medical screenings as a trigger for PTSD in public safety workers. *Annals of the New York Academy of Sciences, 1071*, 478-480.

88. International Federation of Red Cross and Red Crescent Societies. (n.d.). *Code of conduct.* Retrieved from http://www.ifrc.org/publicat/conduct/index.asp?navid=09_08.

89. Stone, J.R. (2007). Importance of community input: A moral framework for disaster planning. *Clinical and Organizational Ethics, 2*(4), 9-11.

90. U.S. Department of Health and Human Services. (2013). *Healthy People 2020: Preparedness.* Retrieved from http://www.healthypeople.gov/2020/topicsobjectives2020/overview.aspx?topicid=34.

91. U.S. Department of Health and Human Services. (2011). *National health security strategy.* Retrieved from http://www.phe.gov/Preparedness/planning/authority/nhss/Pages/default.aspx.

Appendix A

Quality and Safety Education for Nurses Crosswalk

Overview: According to the Quality and Safety Education for Nurses (QSEN) Institute, the QSEN project focuses on providing nursing students with the knowledge and skills needed to actively participate in continuous quality improvement within the health-care systems that they work. The six domains within the QSEN framework include patient-centered care, teamwork and collaboration, evidence-based practice, quality improvement, safety, and informatics. This book builds on other QSEN content from other courses. The domains are presented through the lens of population level care. For example, domain one,

patient-centered care in this book includes community-centered care. Improving quality and safety for populations requires application of the public health sciences to help understand the underlying causes of adverse health outcomes, best practices for nursing interventions at the population level, building interdisciplinary teams to solve the problem, and the use of population level data bases to guide the health planning process for populations. The problem-based learning approach throughout the book helps the student meet the full complement of competencies required in pre-licensure programs.

Categories	Knowledge	Skills	Attitudes
Patient-Centered Care			
Chapter 2: Optimizing Population Health	X	X	
Chapter 17: Health Planning With Rural and Urban Communities	X	X	X
Chapter 16: Health Planning in Primary Care Settings	X	X	
Chapter 23: Culture and Public Health Nursing	X	X	X
Chapter 24: Vulnerable Populations	X	X	
Chapter 25: Disaster Management and Public Health Emergency Preparedness	X	X	
Teamwork and Collaboration			
Chapter 1: Public Health and Nursing Practice	X	X	
Chapter 2: Optimizing Population Health	X	X	
Chapter 15: Health Planning for Acute Care Settings	X	X	X
Chapter 16: Health Planning for Primary Care Settings	X	X	
Chapter 17: Health Planning with Rural and Urban Communities	X	X	X
Chapter 25: Disaster Management and Public Health Emergency Preparedness	X	X	
Evidence-based Practice			
Evidence-based boxes in Chapters 2–25	X	X	X
Quality Improvement			
Strategies for improving outcomes across clinical settings covered in Chapters 14–21	X	X	
Chapter 15: Health Planning for Acute Care Settings	X	X	X

Categories	Knowledge	Skills	Attitudes
Safety			
Chapter 12: Injury and Violence	X	X	
Chapter 20: Health Planning for Older Adults	X	X	
Chapter 21: Health Planning for Occupational Health	X	X	
Informatics			
Chapter 3: Epidemiology and Nursing Practice	X	X	
Chapter 4: Introduction to Community Assessment	X	X	

Index

Note: *b* indicates box; *f*, figure; *t*, table; CDC, Centers for Disease Control and Prevention; IOM, Institute of Medicine; and WHO, World Health Organization.